Primer on the Metabolic Bone Diseases and Disorders of Mineral Metabolism

Third Edition

An Official Publication of the American Society for Bone and Mineral Research

Primer on the Metabolic Bone Diseases and Disorders of Mineral Metabolism

Third Edition

EDITOR

Murray J. Favus, M.D.
Department of Medicine
The University of Chicago Medical Center
Chicago, Illinois

ASSOCIATE EDITORS

Sylvia Christakos, Ph.D.
University of Medicine and Dentistry of
New Jersey
New Jersey Medical School
Newark, New Jersey

Steven R. Goldring, M.D.
Harvard Medical School
Deaconess and New England Baptist
Hospitals
Boston, Massachusetts

Geoffrey N. Hendy, B.Sc., Ph.D.
McGill University
Royal Victoria Hospital
Montreal, Quebec, Canada

Michael F. Holick, M.D., Ph.D.
Boston University School of Medicine and
Medical Center
Boston City Hospital
Boston, Massachusetts

Frederick Kaplan, M.D.
University of Pennsylvania School of
Medicine
Philadelphia, Pennsylvania

Sundeep Khosla, M.D.
Mayo Clinic and Medical School
Rochester, Minnesota

Michael Kleerekoper, M.D.,
F.A.C.E.
Wayne State University School of Medicine
Harper Hospital
Detroit, Michigan

Craig B. Langman, M.D.
Northwestern University Medical School
Children's Memorial Hospital
Chicago, Illinois

Jane B. Lian, Ph.D.
University of Massachusetts Medical School
Worcester, Massachusetts

Elizabeth Shane, M.D.
Columbia University
College of Physicians and Surgeons
New York, New York

Dolores M. Shoback, M.D.
University of California, San Francisco
San Francisco Veterans Affairs Medical
Center
San Francisco, California

Andrew F. Stewart, M.D.
Yale University School of Medicine
Connecticut Veterans Affairs Medical Center
West Haven, Connecticut

Michael P. Whyte, M.D.
Washington University School of Medicine
Shriners Hospital for Crippled Children
St. Louis, Missouri

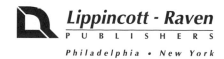

Lippincott - Raven
PUBLISHERS

Philadelphia • New York

Printed in the United States of America

9 8 7 6 5 4 3 2 1

Library of Congress Cataloging-in-Publication Data

Primer on the metabolic bone diseases and disorders of mineral metabolism / editor, Murray J. Favus : associate editors, Sylvia Christakos … [et al.]. — 3rd ed/

    p. cm.

    "An official publication of the American Society for Bone and Mineral Research"—Cover.

    Includes bibliographical references and index.

    ISBN 0-397-51763-7

    1. Bones—Metabolism—Disorders.   2. Mineral metabolism—Disorders. I. Favus, Murray J. II. Christakos, Sylvia. III. American Society for Bone and Mineral Research.

    [DNLM: 1. Bone Diseases, Metabolic. 2. Bone and Bones—metabolism. 3. Minerals—metabolism. WE 250 P953 1996]

RC930.P75   1996

616.7′16—dc20

DNLM/DLC

for Library of Congress   96-16184

Contents

Section I. Anatomy and Biology of Bone Matrix and Cellular Elements

Section II. Calcium, Magnesium, Phosphorus Homeostasis and Physiology, and Biochemistry of Calcium Regulating Hormones

Section III. Clinical Evaluation of Bone and Mineral Disorders

Section IV. Disorders of Serum Minerals

Section V. Metabolic Bone Diseases

Section VI. Genetic, Developmental, and Dysplastic Skeletal Disorders

Section VII. Acquired Disorders of Cartilage and Bone

Section VIII. Paget's Disease

Section IX. Extraskeletal (Ectopic) Calcification and Ossification

Section X. Nephrolithiasis

Section XI. Appendix

Contributing Authors

John S. Adams, M.D.
*Professor of Medicine, Department of Medicine,
University of California, Los Angeles, and Cedars Sinai
Research Institute, 8700 Beverly Boulevard, B131,
Los Angeles, California 90048*

Dennis L. Andress, M.D.
*Associate Professor of Medicine, Department of
Medicine, Veterans Affairs Medical Center (111A),
1660 South Columbian Way, Seattle, Washington 98108*

Louis V. Avioli, M.D., F.A.C.E.
*Shoenberg Professor of Medicine, and Professor of
Orthopedic Surgery, Departments of Medicine and
Orthopedic Surgery, Washington University Medical
Center, Barnes-Jewish North Campus, 216 South
Kingshighway, St. Louis, Missouri 63110*

Jane Aubin, Ph.D.
*Department of Anatomy and Cell Biology, Faculty of
Medicine, University of Toronto, 6th Floor Medical
Science Building, 1 King's College Circle, Toronto,
Ontario, Canada, M5S 1A8*

Daniel T. Baran, M.D.
*Professor of Medicine, Orthopedics, and Cell Biology,
Departments of Medicine, Orthopedics, and Cell Biology,
University of Massachusetts Medical Center, 55 Lake
Avenue, North, Worcester, Massachusetts 01655*

Roland Baron, D.D.S., Ph.D.
*Professor of Orthopedics and Cell Biology,
Department of Orthopedics and Cell Biology,
Yale University School of Medicine, 333 Cedar Street,
New Haven, Connecticut 06510*

Daniel D. Bikle, M.D., Ph.D.
*Professor of Medicine, Department of Medicine,
University of California, San Francisco, Veterans
Affairs Medical Center, 4150 Clement Street,
San Francisco, California 94121*

John P. Bilezikian, M.D.
*Department of Medicine, Columbia University, College
of Physicians and Surgeons, 630 West 168th Street,
New York, New York 10032*

Neil A. Breslau, M.D.
*Professor of Medicine, Center for Mineral Metabolism
and Clinical Research, Department of Medicine, and
Program Director, General Clinical Research Center,
University of Texas, Southwestern Medical Center, 5323
Harry Hines Boulevard, Dallas, Texas 75235*

Arthur E. Broadus, M.D., Ph.D.
*Professor of Medicine and Physiology, Department of
Internal Medicine, Yale University, 333 Cedar Street,
New Haven, Connecticut 06510-8020*

Edward M. Brown, M.D.
*Professor of Medicine, Department of Medicine,
Harvard Medical School; and Endocrine-Hypotension
Unit, Brigham and Women's Hospital, 221 Longwood
Avenue, Boston, Massachusetts 02115*

William J. Burtis, M.D., Ph.D.
*Emerson Practice Associates, John Cuming
Building # 210
131 ORNAC, Concord, Massachusetts 01719*

Ernesto Canalis, M.D.
*Professor of Medicine and Orthopedic Surgery, and
Director, Department of Research, The University of
Connecticut, St. Francis Hospital and Medical Center,
114 Woodland Street, Hartford,
Connecticut 06105-1299*

Thomas O. Carpenter, M.D.
*Associate Professor, Department of Pediatrics,
Yale University School of Medicine, P.O. Box 208064,
33 Cedar Street, New Haven, Connecticut 06520-8064*

Russell W. Chesney, M.D.
*Professor and Chairman, Department of Pediatrics,
University of Tennessee, Le Bonheur Children's
Medical Center, 50 North Dunlap Street, Memphis,
Tennessee 38103*

Sylvia Christakos, Ph.D.
*Professor of Biochemisty and Molecular Biology,
Department of Biochemistry and Molecular Biology,
University of Medicine and Dentistry of New Jersey,
New Jersey Medical School, 185 South Orange Avenue,
Newark, New Jersey 07103*

Thomas L. Clemens, B.A., M.S., Ph.D.
*Professor of Medicine and Molecular and Cellular
Physiology, Department of Endocrinology and
Metabolism, University of Cincinnati, 231 Bethesda
Avenue, Cincinnati, Ohio 45267-0547*

Jack W. Coburn, M.D., F.A.C.P.
*Professor of Medicine, Department of Medicine
University of California, Los Angeles, School of
Medicine; and West Los Angeles Veterans Affairs
Medical Center, 11301 Wilshire Boulevard, Los
Angeles, California 90073*

Fredric L. Coe, M.D.
Kidney Stone Program, Nephrology Section, Department of Medicine, University of Chicago Hospital, 5841 South Maryland Avenue, Chicago, Illinois 60637

David E. C. Cole, M.D., Ph.D., F.C.C.M.G., F.R.C.P.C.
Associate Professor of Clinical Biochemistry, Medicine and Genetics, Departments of Clinical Biochemisrty, Medicine, and Genetics, University of Toronto, Banting Institute, Room 415, 100 College Street, Toronto, Ontario, Canada M5G 1L5

John Connolly, M.B., B.Ch., M.R.C.P.
Renal Division, Barnes-Jewish Hospital, 216 South Kingshighway, St. Louis, Missouri 63110

Gilbert J. Cote, Ph.D.
Assistant Professor of Medicine, Section of Endocrine Neoplasia and Hormonal Disorders, University of Texas, M.D. Anderson Cancer Center, 1515 Holcombe Boulevard, Box 15, Houston, Texas 77030

Leonard J. Deftos, M.D., J.D.
Professor of Medicine, Department of Medicine, University of California, San Diego; and Veterans Affairs Medical Center, 3350 La Jolla Village Drive, San Diego, California 92161

Marc K. Drezner, M.D.
Professor of Medicine, Departments of Medicine and Cell Biology, and Sarah W. Stedman Center for Nutritional Studies, Duke University Medical Center, Box 3285, Durham, North Carolina 27710

Howard Duncan, M.D.
Division of Rheumatology, Henry Ford Hospital, 2799 West Grand Boulevard, Detroit, Michigan 48202

Thomas A. Einhorn, M.D.
Professor of Orthopedics, Department of Orthopedics, Mount Sinai School of Medicine, Fifth Avenue and 100th Street, New York, New York 10029-6574

David R. Eyre, Ph.D.
Professor, and Burgess Chairman of Orthopedic Research, Department of Orthopedics, University of Washington, 1959 Northeast Pacific, Box 356500, Seattle, Washington 98195

Murray J. Favus, M.D.
Director, Bone Program, Director, General Clinical Research Center, and Professor of Medicine, Department of Medicine, The University of Chicago Medical Center, 5841 South Maryland Avenue, MC5100, Chicago, Ilinois 60637

Robert F. Gagel, M.D.
Professor of Medicine, Section of Endocrine Neoplasia and Hormonal Disorders, University of Texas, M.D. Anderson Cancer Center, 1515 Holcombe Boulevard, Box 15, Houston, Texas 77030

Susan C. Galbraith, M.D.
Department of Medicine, Division of Endocrinology, Yale University School of Medicine, New Haven, Connecticut 06520

Harry K. Genant, M.D.
Skeletal Section, Department of Radiology, University of California, San Francisco, Box 0628, San Francisco, California 94143-0628

Francis H. Glorieux, M.D., Ph.D.
Departments of Surgery, Pediatrics, and Human Genetics, McGill University, and Genetics Unit, Shriners Hospital, 1529 Cedar Street, Montreal, Quebec, Canada, H3G 1A6

Steven R. Goldring, M.D.
Associate Professor of Medicine, Harvard Medical School; and Chief of Rheumatology, Deaconess and New England Baptist Hospitals, 110 Francis Street, Boston, Massachusetts 02215

David Goltzman, M.D.
Professor of Medicine, Department of Medicine, McGill University; and Royal Victoria Hospital, 687 Pine Avenue West, Montreal, Quebec, Canada H3A 1A1

William G. Goodman, M.D.
Department of Radiological Sciences, B3-227M CHS, University of California, Los Angeles School of Medicine, 10833 Le Conte Avenue, Los Angeles, California 90095

Robert P. Heaney, M.D.
John A. Creighton University Professor, Creighton University, 2500 California Plaza, Omaha, Nebraska 68178

Hunter Heath III, M.D.
Group Leader, Endocrinology, Medical Division, Lilly USA, Eli Lilly and Company, Lilly Corporate Center, Indianapolis, Indiana 46285

Geoffrey N. Hendy, B.Sc., Ph.D.
Professor of Medicine, Departments of Medicine and Physiology, McGill University; and Calcium Research Laboratory, Royal Victoria Hospital, 687 Pine Avenue West, Montreal, Quebec, Canada, H3A 1A1

Maurine Hobbs, Ph.D.
Research Associate, Department of Human Genetics, University of Utah School of Medicine, 2100 Eccles Institute of Human Genetics, Salt Lake City, Utah 84112

Michael F. Holick, M.D., Ph.D.
Professor of Medicine, Physiology, and Dermatology, Department of Medicine, Section of Endocrinology, Diabetes, and Metabolism, Boston University School of Medicine and Medical Center; and Boston City Hospital, 80 East Concord Street, M-1013, Boston, Massachusetts 02118

Mahalakshmi Honasonge, M.B.B.S., F.A.C.P.
Staff Physician, Bone and Mineral Division, Henry Ford Health System, 2799 West Grand Boulevard, Detroit, Michigan 48202

Keith A. Hruska, M.D.
Renal Division, Barnes-Jewish Hospital, 216 South Kingshighway, St. Louis, Missouri 63110

Karl L. Insogna, M.D.
Associate Professor of Medicine, Section of Endocrinology, Yale University School of Medicine, FMP 106, P.O. Box Z08020, New Haven, Connecticut 06520-8020

Jeffrey A. Jackson, M.D.
Associate Professor of Medicine, Division of Endocrinology, Scott & White Clinic, Texas A & M University Health Science Center, 2401 South 31st Street, Temple, Texas 76508

C. Conrad Johnston, Jr., M.D.
Professor of Medicine, Department of Medicine, Indiana University School of Medicine, 545 North Barnhill Drive, Emerson Hall 421, Indianapolis, Indiana 46202-5124

Frederick Kaplan, M.D.
Chief, Division of Metabolic Bone Diseases, Departments of Orthopaedic Surgery and Medicine , University of Pennsylvania School of Medicine, Silverstein Pavilion, 3400 Spruce Street, Philadelphia, Pennsylvania 19104

Arnold Kahn, Ph.D.
Department of Growth and Development, School of Dentistry, University of California, San Francisco, 521 Parnassus Avenue, San Francisco, California 94143-0640

Kastytis C. Karvelis, M.D.
Director, Division of Nuclear Medicine, Department of Diagnostic Radiology, Henry Ford Hospital, 2799 West Grand Boulevard, Detroit, Michigan 48202

Sundeep Khosla, M.D.
Associate Professor of Medicine, Department of Endocrinology, Mayo Clinic and Medical School, 200 First Street, Southwest, Rochester, Minnesota 55905

Michael Kleerekoper, M.D., F.A.C.E.
Professor of Medicine, Department of Internal Medicine, Wayne State University School of Medicine, Harper Hospital, 1 Webber South, 3990 John R, Detroit, Michigan 48201

Gordon L. Klein, M.D., M.P.H.
Professor of Pediatrics, Department of Pediatrics, University of Texas Medical Branch, Galveston, Texas 77555-0352

Sambasiva R. Kottamasu, M.D.
Associate Professor of Radiology, Wayne State University School of Medicine; and Vice-Chief, Department of Imaging, Children's Hospital of Michigan, 3901 Beaubien, Detroit, Michigan 48201-9985

Henry M. Kronenberg, M.D.
Professor of Medicine, Harvard Medical School; and Chief, Endocrine Unit, Department of Medicine, Massachusetts General Hospital, 50 Blossom Street, WEL 501, Boston, Massachusetts 02114

Craig B. Langman, M.D.
Professor of Pediatrics, Head, Nephrology and Mineral Metabolism, Department of Pediatrics, Northwestern University Medical School; and Children's Memorial Hospital, 2300 Children's Plaza, Box 37, Chicago, Illinois 60614

Michael A. Levine, M.D.
Professor of Medicine and Pathology, Division of Endocrinology and Metabolism, The Johns Hopkins University School of Medicine, Ross Research Building Room 1029, 720 Rutland Avenue, Baltimore, Maryland 21205

Jane B. Lian, Ph.D.
Professor of Cell Biology, Department of Cell Biology, University of Massachusetts Medical School, 55 Lake Avenue North, Worcester, Massachusetts 01655-0106

Uri A. Liberman, M.D., Ph.D.
Professor of Physiology and Medicine and Head, Division of Endocrinology and Metabolic Diseases, Rabin Medical Center-Beilinson Campus; and Sackler School of Medicine, Tel Aviv University, 49100 Petah-Tikva, Israel

Robert Lindsay, Ph.D., M.B., Ch.B., F.R.C.P.
Professor of Clinical Medicine, Columbia University New York, New York; and, Department of Medicine, Helen Hayes Hospital, Route 9 West, West Haverstraw, New York 10993

James E. Lingeman, M.D.
Director of Research, Methodist Hospital Institute for Kidney Stone Disease, 1801 North Senate Boulevard, Suite 655, Indianapolis, Indiana 46202

Barbara P. Lukert, M.D.
Professor of Medicine, Department of Medicine, University of Kansas Medical Center, 3901 Cambridge, Kansas City, Kansas 66160

Lawrence E. Mallette, M.D., Ph.D.
Associate Professor of Medicine, Division of Endocrinology and Metabolism, Baylor College of Medicine, One Baylor Plaza, Houston, Texas 77030

Robert Marcus, M.D.
*Professor of Medicine, Department of Medicine,
Stanford University, Veterans Affairs Medical Center,
3801 Miranda Avenue, Palo Alto,
California 94304*

Stephen J. Marx, M.D.
*Chief, Genetics and Endocrinology Section, National
Institute of Diabetes and Digestive and Kidney
Diseases, National Institutes of Health, Building 10,
Room 9C-101, Bethesda, Maryland 20892*

L. Joseph Melton III, M.D.
*Eisenberg Professor of Epidemiology, Department of
Health Sciences Research, Mayo Clinic and
Foundation, 200 First Street, Southwest, Rochester,
Minnesota 55905*

Gregory R. Mundy, M.D.
*Department of Medicine, Endocrinology and
Metabolism, University of Texas Health Science Center,
7703 Floyd Curl Drive, San Antonio, Texas 78284-7877*

Robert A. Nissenson, Ph.D.
*Professor of Medicine and Physiology, University of
California; and Veterans Affairs Medical Center, 4150
Clement Street, San Francisco, California 94121*

Michael E. Norman, M.D.
*Clinical Professor of Pediatrics, Department of
Pediatrics, University of North Carolina School of
Medicine, Chapel Hill, North Carolina 27599*

Eric S. Orwoll, M.D.
*Chief, Department of Endocrinology and Metabolism,
Portland Veterans Affairs Medical Center; and
Associate Professor of Medicine, Oregon Health
Sciences University, 3181 Southwest Sam Jackson Park,
Portland, Oregon 97201*

Socrates E. Papapoulos, M.D., Ph.D.
*Associate Professor of Medicine, Department of
Endocrinology and Metabolic Diseases, University
Hospital Leiden, Rijnsburgerweg 10, 2333 AA Leiden,
The Netherlands*

Joan H. Parks, M.S.
*Research Associate and Assistant Professor,
Administrator, Kidney Stone Program, Department of
Medicine, Section of Nephrology, University of
Chicago, 5841 South Maryland Avenue, Box 28,
Chicago, Illinois 60637*

Anthony A. Portale, M.D.
*Departments of Pediatrics and Medicine, University of
California, San Francisco, Room U-585, 533 Parnassus
Avenue, San Francisco, California 94143-0126*

Andrew K. Poznanski, M.D.
*Earl J. Frederick Professor of Radiology, Department
of Radiology, Northwestern University Medical School;
and Children's Memorial Hospital, 2300 North
Children's Plaza, Chicago, Illinois 60614-3394*

J. Edward Puzas, Ph.D.
*Donald and Mary Clark Professor of Orthopedics,
Department of Orthopedics, University of Rochester
School of Medicine, 575 Elmwood Avenue, Rochester,
New York 14642*

L. Darryl Quarles, M.D.
*Department of Medicine, Division of Nephrology,
Duke University Medical Center, 00570 Blue Zone,
Box 3036, Durham, North Carolina 27710*

D. Sudhaker Rao, M.B.B.S., F.A.C.P.
*Clinical Assistant Professor of Medicine, University of
Michigan, Head, Bone and Mineral Division, K-2,
Henry Ford Health System, 2799 West Grand
Boulevard, Detroit, Michigan 48202*

Robert R. Recker, M.D.
*Professor of Medicine, Department of Internal
Medicine, Creighton University, St. Joseph's
Hospital, 601 North 30th Street, Suite 5766,
Omaha, Nebraska 68131*

Pamela Gehron Robey, Ph.D.
*Chief, Bone Research Branch, National Insititutes of
Health, 9000 Rockville Pike MSC 4320, Bethesda,
Maryland 20892*

Robert K. Rude, M.D.
*Professor of Medicine, Department of Medicine,
University of Southern California, 2025 Zonal Avenue,
Los Angeles, California 90033*

Isidro B. Salusky, M.D.
*Professor of Pediatrics, Departments of Pediatrics and
Nephrology, University of California, Los Angeles
School of Medicine, 10833 Le Conte Avenue, A2-383,
Los Angeles, California 90095-1752*

Gino V. Segre, M.D.
*Associate Professor of Medicine, Department of
Medicine, Harvard Medical School, and Endocrine
Unit, Massachusetts General Hospital, Fruit Street,
Boston, Massachusetts 02114*

Elizabeth Shane, M.D.
*Associate Professor of Clinical Medicine, Department
of Medicine, Columbia University, College of
Physicians and Surgeons, 630 West 168th Street,
New York, New York 10032*

Dolores M. Shoback, M.D.
*Associate Professor of Medicine, Department of
Medicine, University of California, San Francisco, and
San Francisco Veterans Affairs Medical Center, 4150
Clement Street, San Francisco, California 94121*

Eileen Shore, Ph.D.
*Research Assistant Professor of Orthopaedic Surgery
and Genetics, Department of Orthopaedic Surgery,
University of Pennsylvania, 424 Stemmler Hall, Thirty-
Sixth and Hamilton Walk, Philadelphia,
Pennsylvania 19104-6081*

Richard M. Shore, M.D.
Assistant Professor of Radiology, Department of Radiology, Northwestern University Medical School; and Children s Memorial Hospital, 2300 Children's Plaza, Chicago, Illinois 60614-3394

Ethel S. Siris, M.D.
Professor of Clinical Medicine, Department of Medicine, Columbia University, College of Physicians and Surgeons, 630 West 168th Street, New York, New York 10032

Peter M. Sklarin, M.D.
Endocrine Fellow, Department of Endocrinology and Metabolism, Metabolic Research Unit HSW 1141, University of California, San Francisco, San Francisco, California 94143

Eduardo Slatopolsky, M.D.
Department of Medicine, Barnes-Jewish Hospital, 216 South Kingshighway, St. Louis, Missouri 63110

Charles W. Slemenda, M.P.H., Dr. P.H.
Associate Professor of Medicine, Department of Medicine, Indiana University School of Medicine, Riley Hospital, 702 Barnhill Drive, Indianapolis, Indiana 46202

Andrew F. Stewart, M.D.
Professor of Medicine, Department of Endocrinology, Yale University School of Medicine; and, Chief, Department of Endocrinology, Connecticut Veterans Affairs Medical Center, 950 Campbell Avenue, 151C, West Haven, Connecticut 06516

Gordon J. Strewler, M.D.
Professor of Medicine, University of California, San Francisco; and Chief of Endocrinology, Veterans Affairs Medical Center, 4150 Clement Street, San Francisco, California 94114

John D. Termine, Ph.D.
Executive Director, Lilly Research Laboratories, Eli Lilly and Company, Lilly Corporate Center, Indianapolis, Indiana 46285

David C. Wang, M.D.
Senior Staff, Division of Nuclear Medicine, Department of Diagnostic Radiology, Henry Ford Hospital, 2799 West Grand Boulevard, Detroit, Michigan 48202

Richard D. Wasnich, M.D., F.A.C.P.
Hawaii Osteoporosis Center, 401 Kamakee Street, Second Floor, Honolulu, Hawaii 96814

Michael P. Whyte, M.D.
Professor of Medicine and Pediatrics, Division of Bone and Mineral Diseases, Washington University School of Medicine; and Medical Director, Metabolic Research Unit, Shriners Hospital for Crippled Children, 2001 South Lindbergh Boulevard, St. Louis, Missouri 63131-3597

Kai H. Yang, M.D.
Associate Research Scientist, Department of Endocrinology, Yale University School of Medicine; and Staff Physician, Department of Endocrinology, Connecticut Veterans Affairs Medical Center, 950 Campbell Avenue, 151C, West Haven, Connecticut 06516

The American Society for Bone and Mineral Research

The American Society for Bone and Mineral Research (ASBMR) was founded in 1977 to bring together the increasing number of clinical and experimental scientists involved in the investigation of bone and mineral metabolism. Since then, the Society has experienced remarkable growth in its membership, and its annual meetings have become the premier event for exchange of new knowledge in this developing field. From its inception the Society has emphasized support and encouragement of its young members, whose contributions are recognized at the meeting. More than three years ago the Society started publishing the Journal of Bone and Mineral Research, which provides on a continuing basis an additional focus for the burgeoning interest in this field of inquiry and application.

Our areas of interest cross many disciplines—both basic and clinical—and, as is frequently the case with newly evolving disciplines, it has received relatively sparse coverage in the formal curricula of many of our schools. The Society has therefore taken the initiative to provide an up-to-date presentation of the principles and the tools applied to the diagnosis, investigation, and therapy of metabolic bone disorders. We wish to thank our members, who have generously devoted their time to put together this excellent edition of the *Primer*, which we hope will help students and practitioners in the health sciences and will attract new devotees to this field.

John G. Haddad, Jr., M.D.
Gideon A. Rodan, M.D., Ph.D.
Past Presidents, ASBMR
June 1990

Preface to the First Edition

Our understanding of the scientific basis for clinical bone and mineral disorders has grown rapidly since the founding of the American Society for Bone and Mineral Research (ASBMR) in 1977. The number of basic scientists and clinicians involved in either research or patient care in bone and mineral metabolism has grown dramatically, attracting the interest of medical students, house officers, and practitioners. While textbooks of Medicine, Pediatrics, Endocrinology, Nephrology, Radiology, and Orthopedic Surgery devote chapters or sections to metabolic bone disease, none provide a comprehensive description of the clinical manifestations of the diseases and the basic science necessary to understand pathophysiology. Three years ago the Education Committee of the ASBMR undertook the task of creating a comprehensive educational source, and this *Primer* is the result of our efforts.

The primary purpose of the *Primer* is to provide a comprehensive, yet concise description of the clinical manifestations, pathophysiology, diagnostic approaches, and therapeutics of diseases that come under the rubric of 'bone and mineral disorders'.

The organization of the *Primer* into twelve sections reflects the several basic science and clinical disciplines that contribute to the field. The first three sections contain the basic science core material that provides the underpinning of our understanding of normal bone and mineral structure and biology. Section I contains a thorough description of the gross anatomy and ultrastructure of bone, the physiology of skeletal growth, development and remodeling, the biochemistry of the bone matrix, and the unique structural features and functions of the cellular elements of bone. Section II provides a dynamic view of the biologic importance of the major elements of bone (usually referred to as the minerals) and their body distribution and balance, including the processes of accumulation and elimination across epithelial barriers in the intestine and kidney. Section III focuses on the details of the synthesis, secretion, metabolism, and biologic actions of the key hormones (parathyroid hormone, vitamin D, and calcitonin) that regulate skeletal growth and remodeling, calcium homeostasis, and the assimilation of minerals to support these processes.

The clinical portion of the *Primer* begins with the eleven chapters in Section IV. Laboratory assays, radiographic and imaging techniques, and bone histomorphometry used to evaluate patients suspected of having bone or mineral disorders are described. Section V contains 26 chapters that describe the many clinical entities that may present to the clinician with disordered levels of serum minerals including hyper- and hypo- calcemia, -phosphatemia, and -magnesemia. Chapters in Section VI describe the several genetic and acquired causes of the classic metabolic bone diseases of rickets, osteomalacia, osteoporosis and the many presentations of renal osteodystrophy.

Section VII contains the genetic and developmental disorders that primarily affect bone. These conditions may present in infancy, childhood, or adulthood as abnormal radiographs, fractures, growth retardation, or skeletal pain. Section VIII includes vascular, tumoral and degenerative processes that may cause bone pain, skeletal deformity, and fracture. Section IX is devoted solely to Paget's disease of bone, a common and important entiry with many presentations.

Diseases characterized by pathologic calcification of soft tissue are presented in Section X, and Section XI contains the metabolic disorders in which pathologic crystalization is selective for the urinary tract.

Section XII is the Appendix, composed of seven subsections containing information useful to the practitioner, including growth charts, ossification center tables, normal values for commonly used biochemical analyses, instructions on how to conduct and interpret dynamic tests of calciotropic hormone secretion, recommended daily mineral and vitamin D intake for all ages, and a drug formulary.

The full credit for any educational benefit that the *Primer* may offer goes to the many scientists and clinicians who have captured their knowledge and experience on the pages of their chapters. The high quality of their contributions and their cooperation are deeply appreciated. I am also deeply indebted to the seven Associate Editors of the *Primer*: Sylvia Christakos, Robert F. Gagel, Michael Kleerekoper, Craig B. Langman, Elizabeth Shane, Andrew F. Stewart, and Michael P. Whyte for their hard work and devotion to the project. Their ability to enlist the participation of over seventy authors, continued enthusiasm and critical editing served to forge the *Primer* into its final form. I also express my deepest appreciation to the presidents of ASBMR who held office during the development of the *Primer*—Norman Bell, Gideon Rodan, John Haddad, and Armen Tashjian. They were most generous in devoting time and effort to find the resources necessary to bring the *Primer* to publication.

I would also express my sincere appreciation to the people at Byrd Press for their guidance and assistance in the preparation and publication of the *Primer*. Finally, I would like to gratefully acknowledge Shirley Hohl, ASBMR Executive Secretary, and John Hohl for their much valued assistance in preparing the *Primer* for publication and distribution.

Murray J. Favus, M.D.
The University of Chicago
Pritzker School of Medicine

Preface to the Third Edition

As with the first two editions of the *Primer*, the *Third Edition* is written for those clinicians, basic scientists, students, residents, and fellows who seek a concise yet thorough description of basic bone biology, mineral metabolism, and the diseases that affect these systems. While the basic organization of the *Primer* has been retained the large volume of important new information in both the basic sciences and clinical realms has resulted in the extensive revision of nine chapters and the addition of 30 new chapters.

Over the past several years, the scientific contributions of a relatively small group of investigators have attracted increasing numbers of basic scientists and clinical investigators into the field of bone and mineral metabolism. The broad array of scientists entering the bone field also reflects the movement away from the traditional separation of disciplines, as research turns from descriptive science to the understanding of molecular processes. This general evolution of science is reflected in the basic science chapters, whose authors have backgrounds in cellular and molecular biology, physiology, biochemistry, embryology, and molecular genetics. The clinical chapters also show the breadth of interest in the field, with contributions from authors with backgrounds in internal medicine, endocrinology, genetics, nephrology, pediatrics, rheumatology, radiology, nuclear medicine, nutrition, and orthopedic surgery. The breadth and depth of the current expanding research effort has created an anticipation for further advances, making this an exciting time to be in this field.

Murray J. Favus. M.D.
Bone Program
University of Chicago Medical Center
June 1996

Acknowledgments

Credit for any success the *Primer* may enjoy is due to the contributing authors' devotion to their areas of interest, and their commitment to present their material in the most comprehensible manner. The high standards set by the authors of the first two editions are greatly appreciated and are responsible for the excellent chapters prepared for the Third Edition. Yet, the greatest asset continues to be the Associate Editors and members of the ASBMR Task Force for *Primer, Third Edition,* including Sylvia Christakos, Steven R. Goldring, Geoffrey N. Hendy, Michael F. Holick, Sundeep Khosla, Frederick Kaplan, Michael Kleerekoper, Craig B. Langman, Jane B. Lian, Elizabeth Shane, Dolores M. Shoback, Andrew F. Stewart, and Michael P. Whyte. I am deeply grateful for their hard work, creativity, dedication, and thoughtful criticism. I also wish to acknowledge the strong support we have received from our publisher, Lippincott-Raven. My deep appreciation is extended to Judy Hummel for her diligence and good spirit in coordinating the day-to-day communications between the authors, Associate Editors, and Lippincott–Raven Publishers.

Murray J. Favus, M.D.
June 1996

Primer on the Metabolic Bone Diseases and Disorders of Mineral Metabolism

Third Edition

An Official Publication of the American Society for Bone and Mineral Research

SECTION I

Anatomy and Biology of Bone Matrix and Cellular Elements

1. Anatomy and Ultrastructure of Bone

Roland E. Baron, D.D.S., Ph.D.

Departments of Orthopedics and Cell Biology, Yale University, School of Medicine, New Haven, Connecticut

Bone is a specialized connective tissue that makes up, together with cartilage, the skeletal system. These tissues serve three functions: (i) mechanical: support and site of muscle attachment for locomotion; (ii) protective: for vital organs and bone marrow; and (iii) metabolic: as a reserve of ions, especially calcium and phosphate, for the maintenance of serum homeostasis, which is essential to life.

In bone, as in all connective tissues, the fundamental constituents are the cells and the extracellular matrix. The latter is particularly abundant in this tissue and is composed of collagen fibers and noncollagenous proteins. In bone, cartilage, and the tissues forming the teeth, however, unlike in other connective tissues, the matrices have the unique ability to become calcified.

BONE AS AN ORGAN: MACROSCOPIC ORGANIZATION

Anatomically, two types of bones can be distinguished in the skeleton: flat bones (skull bones, scapula, mandible, and ileum) and long bones (tibia, femur, and humerus). These two types are derived by two distinct types of histogenesis, intramembranous and endochondral, respectively (see later section, Bone Histogenesis and Growth), although the development and growth of long bones actually involve both types of histogenesis.

External examination of a long bone (Fig. 1) shows two wider extremities (the epiphyses), a more or less cylindrical tube in the middle (the midshaft or diaphysis), and a developmental zone between them (the metaphysis). In a growing long bone, the epiphysis and the metaphysis, which originate from two independent ossification centers, are separated by a layer of cartilage, the *epiphyseal cartilage* (also called growth plate). This layer of proliferative cells and expanding cartilage matrix is responsible for the longitudinal growth of bones; it becomes entirely calcified and remodeled by the end of the growth period (see later section, Bone Histogenesis and Growth). The external part of the bones is formed by a thick and dense layer of calcified tissue, the *cortex* (compact bone) which, in the diaphysis, encloses the medullary cavity where the hematopoietic bone marrow is housed. Toward the metaphysis and the epiphysis, the cortex becomes progressively thinner and the internal space is filled with a network of thin, calcified trabeculae; this is the *cancellous bone,* also named spongy or *trabecular bone.* The spaces enclosed by these thin trabeculae are also filled with hematopoietic bone marrow and are in continuity with the medullary cavity of the diaphysis. The bone surfaces at the epiphyses that take part in the joint are covered with a layer of articular cartilage that does not calcify.

There are consequently two bone surfaces at which the bone is in contact with the soft tissues (Fig. 1): an external surface (the periosteal surface) and an internal surface (the endosteal surface). These surfaces, the *periosteum* and the *endosteum,* are lined with osteogenic cells organized in layers. Cortical and trabecular bone are constituted of the same cells and the same matrix elements, but there are structural and functional differences. The primary structural difference is quantitative: 80% to 90% of the volume of compact bone is calcified, whereas 15% to 25% of the trabecular bone is calcified (the remainder being occupied by bone marrow, blood vessels, and connective tissue). The result is that 70% to 85% of the interface with soft tissues is at the

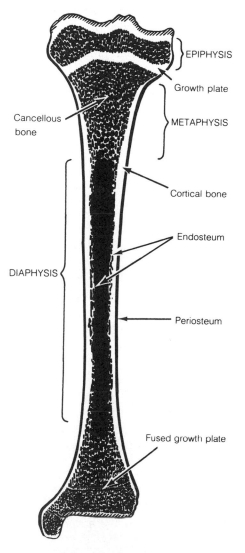

FIG. 1. Schematic view of a longitudinal section through a growing long bone. (From: Jee WSS. The skeletal tissues. In: Weiss L (ed) *Histology, Cell and Tissue Biology.* Elsevier Biomedical, New York, pp 200–255, 1983.)

endosteal bone surface, which leads to the functional difference: the cortical bone fulfills mainly a mechanical and protective function and the trabecular bone a metabolic function.

BONE AS A TISSUE

Microscopic Organization

Bone Matrix and Mineral

Bone is formed by *collagen fibers* (type I, 90% of the total protein), usually oriented in a preferential direction, and noncollagenous proteins. Spindle- or plate-shaped crystals of hydroxyapatite [$3Ca_3(PO_4)_2 \cdot (OH)_2$] are found on the collagen fibers, within them, and in the ground substance. They tend to be oriented in the same direction as the collagen fibers. The ground substance is primarily composed of glycoproteins and proteoglycans. These highly anionic complexes have a high ion-binding capacity and are thought to play an important part in the calcification process and the fixation of hydroxyapatite crystals to the collagen fibers.

Numerous noncollagenous proteins present in bone matrix have recently been purified and sequenced (see Chapter 4), but their role has been only partially characterized. Most of these proteins are synthesized by bone-forming cells, but not all: a number of plasma proteins are preferentially absorbed by the bone matrix, such as α_2-HS-glycoprotein, which is synthesized in the liver.

The preferential orientation of the collagen fibers alternates in adult bone from layer to layer, giving to this bone a typical *lamellar* structure, best seen under polarized light or by electron microscopy. This fiber organization allows the highest density of collagen per unit volume of tissue. The lamellae can be parallel to each other if deposited along a flat surface (trabecular bone and periosteum), or concentric if deposited on a surface surrounding a channel centered on a blood vessel (haversian system, Fig. 2). However, when

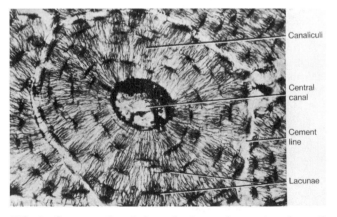

FIG. 2. Cross-sectional view of a haversian system in cortical bone, showing the lamellar organization of collagen in mature bone matrix, and the morphology and canalicular organization of osteocytes. (From: Jee WSS. The skeletal tissues. In: Weiss L (ed) *Histology, Cell and Tissue Biology.* Elsevier Biomedical, New York, pp 200–255, 1983.)

bone is being formed very rapidly (during histogenesis and fracture healing, or in tumors and some metabolic bone diseases), there is no preferential organization of the collagen fibers. They are then found in somewhat randomly oriented bundles: this type of bone is called *woven bone* (see later section, Bone Histogenesis and Growth), as opposed to lamellar bone.

Cellular Organizations Within the Bone Matrix: Osteocytes

The calcified bone matrix is not metabolically inert, and cells (osteocytes) are found embedded deep within the bone in small osteocytic lacunae ($25,000/mm^3$ of bone) (Figs. 2,3). They were originally bone-forming cells (osteoblasts), and they were trapped in the bone matrix that they produced and which later became calcified. These cells have numerous and long cell processes rich in microfilaments, which are in contact with cell processes from other osteocytes (i.e., there are frequent *gap junctions*), or with processes from the cells lining the bone surface (osteoblasts or flat lining cells in the endosteum or periosteum). These processes are organized during the formation of the matrix and before its calcification; they form a network of thin canaliculi permeating the entire bone matrix (Fig. 2).

Between the osteocyte's plasma membrane and the bone matrix itself is the *periosteocytic space*. This space exists both in the lacunae and in the canaliculi, and it is filled with extracellular fluid (ECF).

The physiological significance of this system is readily demonstrated by some numbers. The total bone surface area of the canaliculae and lacunae is 1000 to 5000 m^2 in an adult (compared to a surface area of 140 m^2 for lung capillaries); the volume of bone ECF is 1.0 to 1.5 L; and the surface calcium contained on bone mineral crystals is approximately 5 to 20 g, which accounts for a significant percentage of the total exchangeable bone calcium. The fact that the calcium concentration in the bone ECF (0.5 mmol/L) is lower than in plasma (1.5 mmol/L) suggests that there is a constant flow of calcium ions out of the bone.

The morphology of the osteocytes varies according to their age and functional activity. A young osteocyte has most of the ultrastructural characteristics of the osteoblast from which it was derived, except that there has been a decrease in cell volume and in the importance of the organelles involved in protein synthesis (rough endoplasmic reticulum, Golgi). An older osteocyte, located deeper within the calcified bone, shows these decreases further accentuated, and, in addition, there is an accumulation of glycogen in the cytoplasm. These cells have been shown to be able to synthesize new bone matrix at the surface of the osteocytic lacunae, which can subsequently calcify. Although historically they have been considered able to resorb calcified bone from the same surface, this point has recently been disputed. The fate of the osteocytes is to be phagocytized and digested, together with the other components of bone, during osteoclastic bone resorption. These cells may also play a role in local activation of bone turnover.

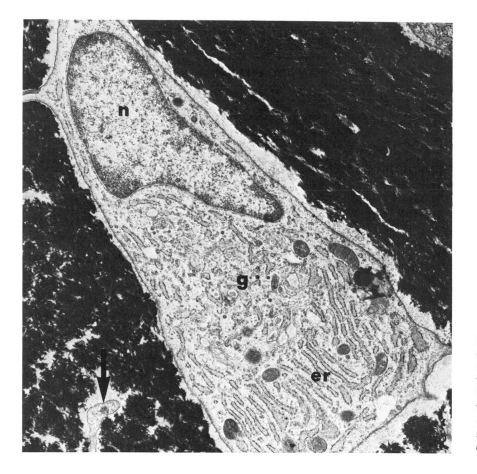

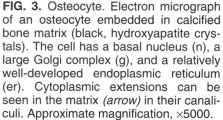

FIG. 3. Osteocyte. Electron micrograph of an osteocyte embedded in calcified bone matrix (black, hydroxyapatite crystals). The cell has a basal nucleus (n), a large Golgi complex (g), and a relatively well-developed endoplasmic reticulum (er). Cytoplasmic extensions can be seen in the matrix *(arrow)* in their canaliculi. Approximate magnification, ×5000.

The Bone Surface

Most of the bone tissue turnover occurs at the bone surfaces, mainly at the endosteal surface where it interfaces with bone marrow. This surface is morphologically heterogeneous, reflecting the various specific cellular activities involved in remodeling and turnover.

The Osteoblast and Bone Formation

The osteoblast is the bone lining cell responsible for the production of the matrix constituents (collagen and ground substance) (Fig. 4). It originates from a local mesenchymal stem cell (bone marrow stromal stem cell or connective tissue mesenchymal stem cell). These precursors, with the right stimulation, undergo proliferation and differentiate into preosteoblasts and then into mature osteoblasts. Osteoblasts never appear or function individually but are always found in clusters of cuboidal cells along the bone surface (~100–400 cells per bone-forming site). At the light microscope level, the osteoblast is characterized by a round nucleus at the base of the cell (opposite to the bone surface), a strongly basophilic cytoplasm, and a prominent Golgi complex located between the nucleus and the apex of the cell. Osteoblasts are always found lining the layer of bone matrix that they are producing, before it is calcified (called, at this point, *osteoid tissue*). Osteoid tissue exists because of a time lag between matrix formation and its subsequent calcification (the osteoid maturation period), which is approximately 10 days. Behind the osteoblast can usually be found one or two layers of cells: activated mesenchymal cells and preosteoblasts. At the ultrastructural level, the osteoblast is characterized by (i) the presence of an extremely well-developed rough endoplasmic reticulum with dilated cisternae and a dense granular content, and (ii) the presence of a large circular Golgi complex comprising multiple Golgi stacks. Cytoplasmic processes on the secreting side of the cell extend deep into the osteoid matrix and are in contact with the osteocyte processes in their canaliculi. Junctional complexes (gap junctions) are often found between the osteoblasts. The plasma membrane of the osteoblast is characteristically rich in alkaline phosphatase (whose concentration in the serum is used as an index of bone formation) and has been shown to have receptors for parathyroid hormone, but not for calcitonin. Osteoblasts also express receptors for estrogens and vitamin D_3 in their nuclei. Toward the end of the secreting period, the osteoblast becomes either a flat lining cell or an osteocyte.

The Osteoclast and Bone Resorption

The osteoclast is the bone lining cell responsible for bone resorption (Fig. 5).

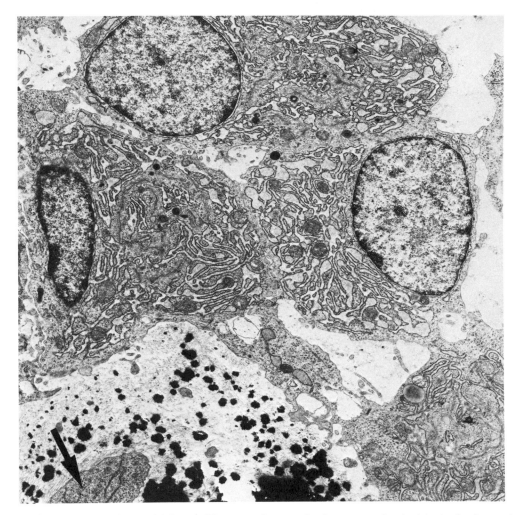

FIG. 4. Osteoblasts and osteoid tissue. Electron micrograph of a group of osteoblasts *(top)* covering a layer of mineralizing osteoid tissue *(bottom)* with a newly embedded osteocyte *(arrow)*. Basal nuclei, prominent Golgi, and endoplasmic reticulum, and characteristics of active osteoblasts. Approximate magnification, ×3000.

Morphology. The osteoclast is a giant multinucleated cell, containing four to 20 nuclei. It is usually found in contact with a calcified bone surface and within a lacuna (Howship's lacunae) that is the result of its own resorptive activity. It is possible to find up to four or five osteoclasts in the same resorptive site, but there usually are only one or two. Under the light microscope, the nuclei appear to vary within the same cell: some are round and euchromatic, and some are irregular in contour and heterochromatic, possibly reflecting the asynchronous fusion of mononuclear precursors. The cytoplasm is "foamy" with many vacuoles. The zone of contact with the bone (the sealing zone) is characterized by the presence of a ruffled border with dense patches on each side.

Characteristic ultrastructural features of this cell are the abundant Golgi complexes characteristically disposed around each nucleus, the mitochondria, and the transport vesicles loaded with lysosomal enzymes. The most prominent features of the osteoclast are, however, the deep foldings of the plasma membrane in the area facing the bone matrix, which form the sealing zone: the ruffled border surrounded by a ring of contractile proteins that serve to attach the cell to the bone surface, thus sealing off the subosteoclastic bone-resorbing compartment. The attachment of the cell to the matrix is performed via integrin receptors, which bind to specific sequences in matrix proteins. The plasma membrane in the ruffled border area contains proteins that are also found at the limiting membrane of lysosomes and related organelles, and a specific type of electrogenic proton ATPase involved in acidification. The basolateral plasma membrane of the osteoclast is highly and specifically enriched in (Na^+,K^+) ATPase (sodium-potassium pumps), HCO_3^-/Cl^- exchangers, and Na^+/H^+ exchangers.

A

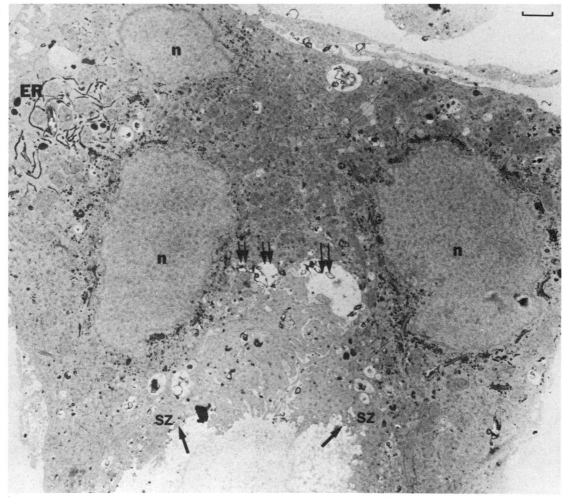

OSTEOCLAST

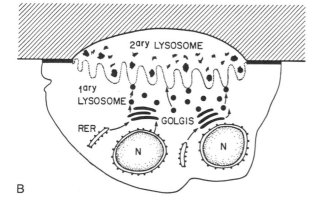

B

FIG. 5. Osteoclast. **A:** Section of an osteoclast stained for the lysosomal enzyme arylsulfatase. The osteoclast contains multiple nuclei (n), an endoplasmic reticulum where lysosomal enzymes are synthesized (ER), and prominent Golgi stacks around each nucleus. The cell is attached to bone matrix *(bottom)* and forms a separate compartment underneath itself, limited by the sealing zone (SZ) *(single arrows)*. The plasma membrane of the cell facing this compartment is extensively folded and forms the ruffled border, with pockets of extracellular space between the folds *(double arrows)*. Multiple small vesicles for transporting enzymes toward the bone matrix can be seen in the cytoplasm. Approximate magnification, ×9000. **B:** Schematic representation of enzyme secretion polarity in osteoclasts. (From: Baron R, Neff L, Louvard D, Courtoy PJ. *J Cell Biol* 101:2210–2222, 1985.)

Mechanisms of Bone Resorption. Lysosomal enzymes are actively synthesized by the osteoclast and are found in the endoplasmic reticulum, Golgi, and many transport vesicles. The enzymes are secreted, via the ruffled border, into the extracellular bone-resorbing compartment; they reach a sufficiently high extracellular concentration because this compartment is sealed off. The transport and targeting of these enzymes for secretion at the apical pole of the osteoclast involves mannose-6-phosphate receptors. Furthermore, the cell secretes nonlysosomal enzymes such as collagenase.

The acidifies the extracellular compartment by secreting protons across the ruffled-border membrane (by proton pumps). Recent evidence suggests the presence of an electrogenic proton-pump ATPase, related to but different from that of the kidney-tubule-acidifying cells. The protons are provided to the pumps by the enzyme carbonic anhydrase, and they are highly concentrated in the cytosol of the osteoclast; ATP and CO_2 are provided by the mitochondria. The basolateral membrane activity exchanges bicarbonate for chloride, thereby avoiding an alkalinization of the cytosol. The basolateral sodium pumps might be involved in secondary active transport of calcium and/or protons in association with a Na^+/Ca^{2+} exchanger and/or a Na^+/H^+ antiport. This cell could therefore function in a manner similar to that of kidney tubule or gastric parietal cells, which also acidify lumens.

The extracellular bone-resorbing compartment is therefore the functional equivalent of a secondary lysosome, with (i) a low pH, (ii) lysosomal enzymes, and (iii) the substrate. The low pH dissolves the crystals, exposing the matrix. The enzymes, now at optimal pH, degrade the matrix components; the residues from this extracellular digestion are either internalized, or they are transported across the cell (by transcytosis) and released at the basolateral domain, or they are released during periods of relapse of the sealing zone, possibly induced by a calcium sensor responding to the rise of extracellular calcium in the bone-resorbing compartment.

First, the hydroxyapatite crystals are mobilized by digestion of their link to collagen (the noncollagenous proteins) and dissolved by the acid environment. Then, the residual collagen fibers are digested either by the activation of latent collagenase or by the action of cathepsins at low pH.

Clinically, this explains why (i) bone resorption helps to maintain calcium and inorganic phosphate levels in the plasma, and (ii) the concentrations of hydroxyproline and N-terminal collagen peptides in the urine are used as indirect measurements of bone resorption in humans (collagen type I is highly enriched in hydroxyproline and pyridoxiline links).

Origin and Fate of the Osteoclast. It is the work of Walker on osteopetrotic mice that established the hematogenous origin of the osteoclast. Cells of the mononuclear/phagocytic lineage are the most likely candidates for differentiation into osteoclasts. Although this differentiation may occur at the promonocyte stage, monocytes and macrophages, already committed to their own lineage, might still be able to form osteoclasts under the right circumstances.

Recent work has suggested that, despite its mononuclear/phagocytic origin, the osteoclast membrane is devoid of Fc and C_3 receptors, as well as of several other macrophage markers; it is, however, rich in nonspecific esterases, it synthesizes lysozyme, and it expresses colony-stimulating factor 1 (CSF-1) receptors, as do mononuclear phagocytes. Monoclonal antibodies have been produced that recognize osteoclasts but not macrophages. Receptors for calcitonin, but not for parathyroid hormone, are present on the osteoclast membrane, and estrogen, but not vitamin D receptors, have been found in these cells.

BONE REMODELING

The previously described activity of bone cells is performed along the surfaces of bone, mainly the endosteal surface, and it results in bone remodeling, which is the process of bone growth and turnover. Bone formation and bone resorption do not, however, occur along the bone surface at random: they are part of the turnover mechanism by which old bone is replaced by new bone. In the normal adult skeleton, bone formation occurs only where bone resorption has

previously occurred. The sequence of events at the remodeling site (Figs. 6,7) is the activation-resorption-formation (ARF) sequence. During the intermediate phase between resorption and formation (the reversal phase), some macrophage-like, uncharacterized mononuclear cells are observed at the site of the remodeling, and a cement line is formed, which marks the limit of resorption and acts to cement together the old and the new bone. The duration of these various phases has been measured (Fig. 8): the complete remodeling cycle takes about 3 to 6 months.

Although cortical bone is anatomically different, its remodeling follows the same biological principles (Fig. 9). Lamellar bone being formed within such a system gives the characteristic structure of an haversian system when seen in cross section (see Fig. 2).

BONE HISTOGENESIS AND GROWTH

There are two types of histogenesis of bone: intramembranous ossification (flat bones) and endochondral ossification (long bones). The main difference between them is the presence of a cartilaginous phase in the latter.

Intramembranous Ossification

In intramembranous ossification, a group of mesenchymal cells within a highly vascularized area of the embryonic connective tissue undergoes division and differentiates directly into preosteoblasts and then into osteoblasts. These cells synthesize a bone matrix with the following characteristics: (i) the collagen fibers are not preferentially oriented but appear as irregular bundles, (ii) the osteocytes are large

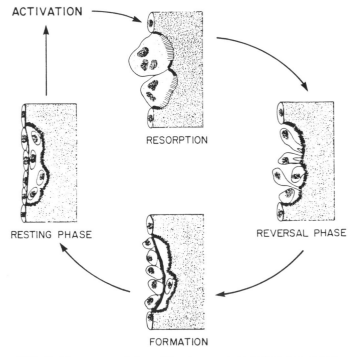

FIG. 6. Bone remodeling. The bone remodeling sequence as it occurs in trabecular bone. (The same principles apply to haversian remodeling; see text.)

Remodeling Sequence

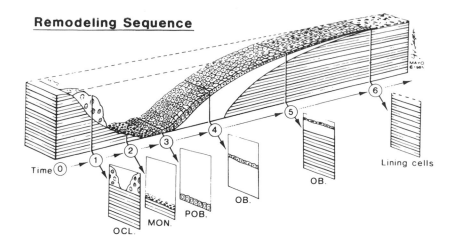

FIG. 7. Bone remodeling in cancellous bone as seen in longitudinal sequence and cross sections. Five different phases can be distinguished over time: (1) osteoclastic resorption, (2) reversal, (3) preosteoblastic migration and differentiation into osteoblasts, (4) osteoblastic matrix (osteoid) formation, and (5) mineralization. The end-product of remodeling in cancellous bone is the completed cancellous bone structural unit (BSU) covered by lining cells (6). (From: Eriksen EF, Axelrod DW, Melsen F. *Bone Histomorphometry*. Raven Press, New York, pp 3–12, 1994.)

and extremely numerous, and (iii) calcification is delayed and does not proceed in an orderly fashion but in irregularly distributed patches. This type of bone is called woven bone. At the periphery, mesenchymal cells continue to differentiate, following the same steps. Blood vessels incorporated between the woven bone trabeculae will form the hematopoietic bone marrow. Later, this woven bone is remodeled following the ARF sequence, and it is progressively replaced by mature lamellar bone.

Endochondral Ossification

Formation of a Cartilage Model

Mesenchymal cells undergo division and differentiate into prechondroblasts and then into chondroblasts. These cells secrete the cartilaginous matrix. Like the osteoblasts, the chondroblasts become progressively embedded within their own matrix, where they lie within lacunae, and they are then called chondrocytes. But, unlike the osteocytes, they continue to proliferate for some time, this being allowed in part by the gel-like consistency of cartilage. At the periphery of this cartilage (the perichondrium), the mesenchymal cells continue to proliferate and differentiate. This is called appositional growth. Another type of growth is observed in the cartilage by synthesis of new matrix between the chondrocytes (interstitial growth). In the growth plate, the cells appear in regular columns called

isogenous groups. Later on, the chondrocytes enlarge progressively, become hypertrophic, and die.

Vascular Invasion and Longitudinal Growth (Remodeling)

The embryonic cartilage is avascular. During its early development, a ring of woven bone is formed by intramembranous ossification in the future midshaft area under the perichondrium (which is then a periosteum). Just after the calcification of this woven bone, blood vessels (preceded by osteoclasts) penetrate it and the cartilage, bringing the blood supply that will form the hematopoietic bone marrow.

The growth plate in a growing long bone shows, from the epiphyseal area to the diaphyseal area, the following cellular events (Fig. 10). In a proliferative zone, chondroblasts divide actively, forming isogenous groups and actively synthesizing the matrix. These cells become progressively larger, enlarging their lacunae in the hypertrophic zone, and then they undergo programmed cell death (apoptosis). At this level of the epiphyseal plate, the matrix of the longitudinal cartilage septa selectively calcifies (zone of provisional calcification). Once calcified, the cartilage matrix is resorbed, but only partially, by osteoclasts, and then blood vessels appear in the zone of invasion. After resorption, osteoblasts differentiate and form a layer of woven bone on top of the cartilaginous remnants of the longitudinal septa.

Thus, the first ARF sequence is complete: the cartilage has been remodeled and replaced by woven bone. The

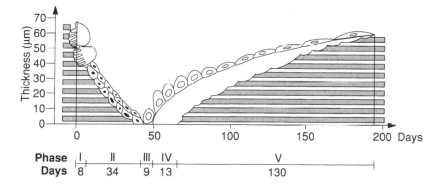

FIG. 8. Duration and depth of the various phases of the normal cancellous-bone-remodeling sequence, calculated from histomorphometric analysis of bone biopsy samples obtained from young individuals. Note the balance between the erosion depth and the mean wall thickness. (From: Eriksen EF, Axelrod DW, Melsen F. *Bone Histomorphometry*. Raven Press, New York, pp 13–20, 1994.)

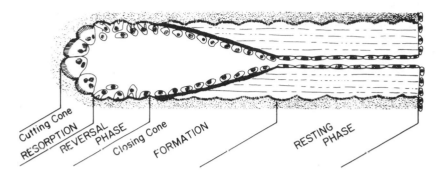

FIG. 9. The bone-remodeling activity in cortical bone as seen in longitudinal sequence. Osteoclasts dig out a tunnel, creating a "cutting cone." Subsequently, new bone is formed in the area of the "closing cone," leading to the creation of a new BSU (i.e., the haversian system).

resulting trabeculae are called the primary spongiosum. Still lower in the growth plate, this woven bone is subjected to further remodeling (a second ARF sequence), in which the woven bone and the cartilaginous remnants are replaced with lamellar bone, resulting in the mature state of trabecular bone called secondary spongiosum (Fig. 11).

Growth in Diameter, and Shape Modification (Modeling)

Growth in the diameter of the shaft is the result of a deposition of new membranous bone beneath the periosteum that will continue throughout life. In this case, resorption does not immediately precede formation. The midshaft is narrower than the metaphysis, and the growth of a long bone progressively destroys the lower part of the metaphysis and transforms it into a diaphysis, accomplished by continuous resorption by osteoclasts beneath the periosteum (Fig. 10).

SUGGESTED READINGS

1. Baron R, Chakraborty M, Chatterjee D, Horne W, Lomri A, Ravesloot J-H: Biology of the osteoclast. In: Mundy GR, Martin TJ (eds) *Physiology and Pharmacology of Bone.* Springer-Verlag, New York, 111–147; 1993
2. Eriksen EF, Axelrod DW, Melsen F: *Bone Histomorphometry.* Raven Press, New York, 1994
3. Jee WSS: The skeletal tissues. In: Weiss L (ed) *Histology, Cell and Tissue Biology.* Elsevier Biomedical, New York, pp 200–255, 1983
4. Nijweide P, Burger EH, Feyen JHM: Cells of bone: Proliferation, differentiation and hormonal regulation. *Physiol Rev* 66:855–886, 1986
5. Suda T, Takahashi N, Martin TJ: Modulation of osteoclast differentiation. *Endocr Rev* 13:66–80, 1992

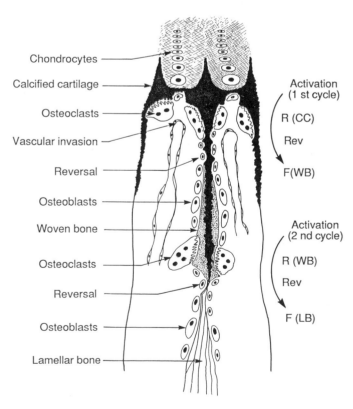

FIG. 10. Bone growth and remodeling at the epiphyseal plate. Schematic representation of the cellular events occurring at the growth plate in long bones. R, resorption; Rev, reversal; F, formation; CC, calcified cartilage; WB, woven bone; LB, lamellar bone.

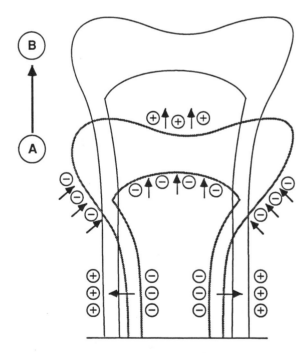

FIG. 11. Resorption (–) and formation (+) activities during the longitudinal growth of bones. During growth from A to B, the cortex in the diaphysis must be resorbed inside and reformed outside *(bottom).* The growth plate moves upward (see Fig. 10), and the wider parts of the bone must be reshaped into a diaphysis. (From: Jee WSS. The skeletal tissues. In: Weiss L (ed) *Histology, Cell and Tissue Biology.* Elsevier Biomedical, New York, pp 200–255, 1983.)

2. Osteoblast Cell Biology—Lineage and Functions

J. Edward Puzas, Ph.D.

Department of Orthopedics, University of Rochester School of Medicine, Rochester, New York

Bone-forming cells are, by definition, the cells responsible for the production of authentic bone. For the purposes of this discussion, bone is defined as the tissue that is formed by the deposition of mineral ions within a collagenous framework. The mineral must be in the form of carbonated hydroxyapatite and the collagen must be predominantly type I collagen. Although this definition seems self-evident, it does exclude a number of mineralized tissues that, through the years, have been grouped with authentic bone. Some examples of such mineralizing nonbone tissues are dentin and enamel in teeth, calcifying cartilage in the developing growth plate of long bones, virtually any organ undergoing pathologic calcification (e.g., arterial and aortic walls), and renal stones. There are, however, some forms of ectopic or heterotopic bone which do fit the criteria of authentic bone. These forms of bone frequently occur after orthopedic surgery or in rare metabolic disease states. A discussion of this type of pathologic bone or related calcification syndromes is found in Section IX. The reader is also referred to review articles on the topic (1,2).

The term *bone-forming cell* can be equated with the term *osteoblast*. That is, wherever there is authentic bone being formed, there must be present a population of osteoblasts. This dissertation is organized into four categories: (i) the ultrastructural and functional properties of osteoblasts, including specific characteristics and biochemical markers of the cells, (ii) the osteoblast lineage, (iii) key processes involved in bone formation, and (iv) unique regulatory mechanisms related to these cells.

ULTRASTRUCTURE AND PROPERTIES OF BONE-FORMING CELLS

The ultrastructural and histologic features of osteoblasts underscore the fact that these are very metabolically active cells. They have an extensive rough endoplasmic reticulum composed of polysomal structures that stain intensely basophilic. The predominant genes that are transcribed and translated in these cells are those dealing with the synthesis of an extracellular matrix, i.e., collagenous and noncollagen matrix proteins. Fully 20% of the total protein produced by osteoblasts is type I collagen. When one considers the number of genes that need to be expressed to maintain function, for a cell to devote one fifth of its activity to a single gene product is extraordinary. The predominant noncollagen protein secreted by osteoblasts is osteocalcin [bone gla-protein (BGP)], making up approximately 1% of extracellular matrix protein. Moreover, a host of regulatory factors are produced and deposited in bone by osteoblasts. These include the family of bone morphogenetic proteins (BMPs), the beta transforming growth factors (TGF-βs), the insulin-like growth factors (IGFs), platelet-derived growth factors (PDGFs), and basic fibroblast growth factor (bFGF), among others. Though these proteins represent a minor component of the extracellular matrix, they play a critical role in bone remodeling (see later).

A well-developed Golgi apparatus is also present in osteoblasts. This cellular structure is responsible for the secretion of collagen and noncollagen proteins. It is usually found near the center of the cell as a negatively stained organelle. The negative staining results from the high lipid composition of the Golgi lamellae.

All osteoblasts are mononuclear. The nucleus is usually positioned eccentrically in the cell opposite the rough endoplasmic reticulum. The nuclear material is similar to that of other eukaryotic cells and remains in a diffuse, uncondensed state during interphase. There are usually present one to three nucleoli. A mature, functioning osteoblast does not divide. That is, the mitotic forms of prophase, metaphase, anaphase, and telophase do not appear in osteoblasts. If ever such structures are observed, the cell must be considered, by convention, a progenitor form of an osteoblast or a pre-osteoblast.

Figure 1, an electron micrograph of five osteoblasts and one osteoprogenitor cell, shows examples of osteoblasts with well-developed rough endoplasmic reticulum, Golgi apparatus, and nuclei with nucleoli.

A characteristic of osteoblasts that can be demonstrated histochemically is the presence of a substantial amount of the enzyme alkaline phosphatase. Bone-specific alkaline phosphatase has been localized to the plasma membrane of osteoblasts, and, although it is known to be present in large amounts, its true function has not yet been determined. Speculations as to its role in mineralization have been published since 1923 (3); it is clear that alkaline phosphatase activity correlates with bone formation, but its exact mechanism of action is not yet known. Elevated levels of bone-specific alkaline phosphatase in the blood indicate excessive osteoblast activity, or bone formation. Normal levels in an adult would be 20 to 70 international units (IU); in a growing child, 100 to 150 IU; and, in pathologic high-bone-turnover states such as Paget's disease, 350 to 700 IU.

The osteoblast also plays a key role in bone resorption. Recent evidence has shown that osteoblasts possess receptors for a number of bone-resorbing stimulatory factors, such as parathyroid hormone, vitamin D, prostaglandins, interleukins, and TGF-β, and that the primary target for these agents in the modulation of osteoclast activity is the osteoblast (or stromal lining cells) (4–7). The hypothesis under which most investigators are working is that the systemic signal to resorb bone is received and processed by osteoblasts, which then elaborate a molecule (or molecules) that recruits and stimulates the activity of osteoclasts. Also, because osteoclasts do not resorb bone that is lined by intact osteoblasts or stromal cells (8), the presence or absence of these cells can determine what bony sites are to be resorbed. Thus, it is clear that the osteoblast plays a pivotal role in directing both when and where bone resorption will occur.

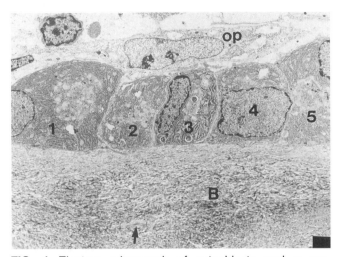

FIG. 1. Electron micrograph of osteoblasts and a pre-osteoblast; five osteoblasts line the bone surface. A well-developed rough endoplasmic reticulum and Golgi apparatus can be seen in most of the cells. The elongated cell with an elongated nucleus immediately above the osteoblasts is an osteoprogenitor cell, or pre-osteoblast. This cell still has the capacity for division, and it will take the place of one of the osteoblasts when the latter becomes encased in the bone matrix as an osteocyte. The *arrow* indicates the presence of a canaliculus from an osteocyte deeper within the bone. (From: Marks SC, Popoff SN. *Am J Anat* 183:1–44, 1988.)

THE OSTEOBLAST LINEAGE

Three forms of the osteoblast cell lineage are recognized. They are progenitor osteoblasts (pre-osteoblasts), mature osteoblasts, and osteocytes. From a phylogenetic point of view, it is known that osteoblasts arise from cells in the condensing mesenchyme, and as such they are one form of connective tissue. Because mesenchymal cells can give rise to a number of tissue types, it is not until a cell is committed to the osteoblast lineage that it can be classified as a bone-forming cell.

Figure 2 summarizes the osteoblast lineage pathways.

The Pre-osteoblast

A committed progenitor cell destined to become an osteoblast has a number of distinguishing features. First, these cells are physically near bone-forming surfaces. That is, they are usually present where active mature osteoblasts are synthesizing bone. They are elongated cells, each with an elongated nucleus (Fig. 1). Most often, they are found in a stratum type of configuration, a few cell layers distant from the active osteoblasts. Second, they have the capacity to divide. Frequently, mitotic characters can be found in these cells. Third, these cells usually stain less intensely for alkaline phosphatase and there is no evidence of a developed rough endoplasmic reticulum. That is, they have not yet acquired many of the protein-synthesizing characteristics of mature osteoblasts.

Pre-osteoblasts give rise to osteoblasts at two distinctly different sites: the endosteum and the periosteum. Endosteal pre-osteoblasts are those bone-forming cells that are active on trabecular and endocortical bone surfaces. They are derived from the stromal group of cells that, along with the hemopoietic group, populate marrow spaces. These stromal cells are self-renewing (9), and with each cell division they have the capacity to create a determined osteoprogenitor cell (DOPC) that will ultimately become a mature osteoblast, and an inducible osteoprogenitor stem cell (IOPC) that will retain stem cell potentiality. The nomenclature of DOPC and IOPC was coined by Friedenstein et al. (10).

The periosteal pre-osteoblast is one of the cells that form the fibrous periosteum surrounding all bones. These cells give rise to osteoblasts on the bone surfaces and may also provide progenitor cells for the fibroblasts in the fibrous layers. They are derived from a pool of cells that more closely resemble DOPCs than IOPCs. That is, there is no evidence for the presence of a stromal stem cell such as those in the marrow space. Nevertheless, the periosteal cell layers are also a self-renewing population (11).

Differentiation of an osteoprogenitor cell into an osteoblast is not a quantal process. Osteoblasts express all of the genes necessary for bone formation, but they are not all expressed

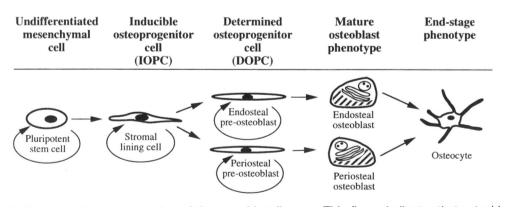

FIG. 2. Diagrammatic representation of the osteoblast lineage. This figure indicates that osteoblasts have their origin from undifferentiated mesenchymal stem cells that have the potential for differentiation into many connective tissue cell types. The first stage of differentiation is into a noncommitted osteoprogenitor cell (IOPC) and then to a committed osteoprogenitor cell (DOPC). All three of these cell phenotypes have the capacity for proliferation and self-renewal. Mature osteoblasts are found on both endosteal and periosteal surfaces. Eventually, osteoblasts may encase themselves in a bony matrix, at which point they become osteocytes.

simultaneously. A number of cell models (both *in vivo* and *in vitro*) have been used to investigate this, but perhaps the most information has come from the molecular models of Stein et al. (12). Although their model is an *in vitro* one, it does provide a framework for studying the differentiation process. It is clear that in the early stages of bone development there is extensive proliferation of progenitor cells with expression of growth-related genes (such as c-*myc* and c-*fos*). Also during the proliferative phase, a number of matrix genes begin to be expressed (i.e., type I collagen, fibronectin, and some growth factors such as TGF-β). These genes remain active for a number of days and are joined by gene products that are associated with a mature matrix, such as alkaline phosphatase and matrix gla-protein. As the matrix and matrix-maturing proteins are suppressed, new gene products associated with the mineralization phase begin to be expressed (i.e., osteocalcin and osteopontin), thus leading to hydroxyapatite accumulation and complete mineralization.

When viewed as a continuum, the maturation of a pre-osteoblast into a mature osteoblast is quite a complex process. Gene products are expressed and repressed at specified stages, and unless all of the actions are in concert, a normal bone matrix will not be formed.

Osteoblast

A mature osteoblast is derived from a pre-osteoblast and expresses all of the differentiated functions required to synthesize bone. As discussed above, there is a gradient of differentiation which becomes fully expressed when the mature form of the cell reaches the bone surface. Once the osteoblast has reached the surface, its function is to synthesize and secrete collagen, noncollagen matrix proteins, and regulatory factors into a structured array, and to ultimately mineralize it. Usually, active osteoblasts are found within a matrix that they themselves have synthesized. It is within this matrix at the mineralization front that the process of hydroxyapatite crystal growth occurs. The mineralization front is the advancing edge of calcification and is usually 5 to 50 microns away from the osteoblast surface. The area between the osteoblast and the mineralizing front is often referred to as an osteoid seam. The depth and character of the osteoid seam can be diagnostic for some forms of bone disease, such as osteomalacia and rickets. (See Chapters 25, 58, 65).

Osteocyte

An osteocyte is an osteoblast which has become encased in calcified bone. During the process of bone formation, the osteoblast determines its own fate by calcifying itself into a lacunae. Approximately 15% of osteoblasts eventually become osteocytes, and, although it can be said that not all osteoblasts survive as osteocytes, it is true that all osteocytes had their origin from osteoblasts. At the point of total encasement, the metabolic activity of the cell dramatically decreases as a result of the lack of nutrient diffusion. The only source of nutrients and gas exchange to which the osteocyte has access is that which can occur through small canals known as canaliculi. These channels are actually the remnants of cellular processes which extended from the osteoblast during bone mineralization. The canaliculi form an extensive array of connecting tubules, and it has been speculated that these tubules form a communication as well as a nutrient network. Figure 3 is a photomicrograph of

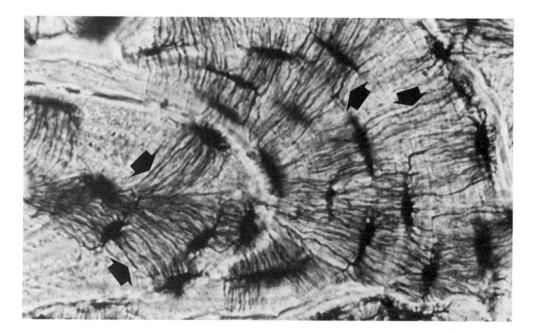

FIG. 3. Photomicrograph of mature bone. This unstained section of bone was prepared by hand grinding a fragment of adult bone until it became translucent. The osteocytes form concentric layers around a central nutrient vessel. The canaliculi of the osteocytes *(arrows)* form a fine network of tubules through which diffusion of solutes and gases can occur. The canaliculi may also form a communication network between the cells.

mature bone in which a number of osteocytes and the numerous canaliculi between them are visible.

Progression Through the Osteoblast Lineage

Many very enlightening studies demonstrating the origin and fate of pre-osteoblasts, osteoblasts, and osteocytes were performed a number of years ago (13,14). These works utilized timed radiolabeled-thymidine exposure to monitor the progression of a cell through the osteoblast lineage. Because thymidine is incorporated only into newly forming DNA, the bone cells that were labeled immediately after the injection were pre-osteoblasts in the process of cell division. There was no label in osteoblasts or osteocytes. A few days after the injection, the cells that contained the radioactive label were the osteoblasts, and after a few weeks the cells with the label were the osteocytes. Because it is known that osteoblasts and osteocytes do not divide, it was evident that the label that appeared in these cells originated in the pre-osteoblasts. In fact, the lifetime and differentiation time for osteoblasts could be calculated with these and other techniques, and it was shown that mature osteoblast appearance required not more than a few days and that they were active for up to 12 weeks before progressing into osteocytes (15,16).

KEY PROCESSES IN BONE FORMATION

Matrix Maturation

One of the major and yet poorly understood areas of collagen metabolism in bone formation is the so-called maturation of the osteoid matrix. This alteration of collagen fibers must occur before the matrix is competent to support mineralization. The best way to illustrate this is to describe the process of bone formation at a remodeling site, which involves three distinct stages of collagen synthesis and its mineralization. In the first stage, collagen is deposited at a rapid rate, and an ever-thickening osteoid seam is produced. In the second stage, the rate of mineralization increases to match the rate of collagen synthesis, and the osteoid seam width remains constant. In the third stage, the rate of collagen synthesis decreases and mineralization continues until the osteoid seam disappears. The maturation of the collagen matrix is expressed as the ratio of the mineralization rate (in microns per day) to the osteoid seam width (in microns). Thus, the maturation of the collagen has a unit of time (days). This ratio has become known as the mineralization lag time: the length of time it takes for the osteoid matrix to acquire the characteristics necessary to support mineralization. The mineralization lag time is roughly 5 to 15 days in adults, and its

magnitude can sometimes be diagnostic for metabolic bone diseases. Biochemically, the mineralization lag time remains undefined. Some theories support a role for crosslinking of collagen in the osteoid, others support the removal of a mineralization inhibitor (see later). Whatever the actual mechanism of osteoid maturation, it is apparent that newly deposited collagen cannot provide a substrate for normal mineralization until it has matured.

Mineralization

Mineralization of the collagen substructure is another unique function of the osteoblast. Although not all the details of this process are known, many important pieces of data have been collected. For example, the mineral in mature, fully calcified bone is mostly in the form of carbonated hydroxyapatite crystals. These crystals are needle-shaped and rodlike, with a diameter of 30 to 50Å and a length of up to 600Å. They lie linearly along the collagen fibrils and in some instances may penetrate some of the larger fibers. The actual process of mineral precipitation, however, remains obscure. In fact, a number of paradoxical observations have been made in trying to experimentally examine the process of calcification. For example, it appears that once the hydroxyapatite has been formed, further growth of the crystal can occur in the absence of cell activity. In other words, under physiologic conditions, the extracellular fluid is supersaturated with calcium and phosphate in the presence of hydroxyapatite. If crystal growth were not somehow mediated, the extracellular fluid would be depleted of calcium and phosphate at the expense of hydroxyapatite formation. This finding was one of the major pieces of evidence for proposing an ionic barrier between bone and blood, and it is the reason that devitalized bone will support mineralization if implanted in tissue fluids or bathed in physiologic solutions of calcium and phosphate. Therefore, the continuing processes of mineralization appear to be controlled at both the initiation stages and the deposition stages of hydroxyapatite formation.

Measurements of Bone Formation

Although we may not understand all the physical and chemical processes of osteoid maturation and mineralization, it has been possible to define and measure many parameters of bone formation. An entire histologic discipline has grown up around the methods needed to make these accurate measurements of skeletal activity. Variables such as sampling sites, embedding and sectioning techniques, and staining and quantification techniques must be considered when measuring formation (and resorption) rates. Table 1 is

Table 1. *Parameters of bone formation under the control of osteoblasts*

Bone volume (microscopic area that is cancellous bone)	22.8%
Osteoid volume (volume of uncalcified osteoid, compared to bone)	4.4 mm^3/cm^3 bone
Osteoid surface (bone surface covered by osteoid)	7.5%
Osteoid seam width	10.0 μ
Mineral apposition rate	0.65 μ/day
Trabecular diameter (mean diameter of trabeculae in cancellous bone)	283.0 μ
Bone–osteoblast interface (bone surface in direct contact with osteoblasts)	3.8%

Table 2. *Endocrine, paracrine, and autocrine factors affecting osteoblasts*

Endocrine hormones	Paracrine factors	Autocrine factors
Parathyroid hormone	Parathyroid-hormone-related protein	
Vitamin D	TGF-β1, -β2, and -β3	TGF-β1, -β2, and -β3
Glucocorticoid hormones	Fibroblast growth factors (1 and 2)	Fibroblast growth factors (1 and 2)
Calcitonin	Insulin-like growth factors	Insulin-like growth factors
Gonadal steroids (estrogen and testosterone)	Platelet-derived growth factors	Platelet-derived growth factors
Insulin	BMPs 2–7	BMPs 2–7
	Interleukin-6	

a brief list of some of the normal values that have been obtained from human bone. Typically, over 50 different measurements (or calculations from measurements) can be made from a bone section, and with these measurements an accurate picture of the metabolic activity of osteoblasts can be obtained. A detailed discussion of bone histomorphometry with excellent histologic and morphometric examples has recently been published (17), and the reader is referred also to Chapter 25.

UNIQUE REGULATORY MECHANISMS RELATED TO OSTEOBLASTS

This area is one of the most active and important topics being investigated in bone research today. It is in this arena that molecular biologic, immunologic, and biochemical techniques have been merged in an attempt to understand not only the disease processes but the normal processes of bone metabolism. It is probably from these lines of research that new therapies will emerge for diseases such as osteoporosis.

Control of osteoblast function occurs at three levels: endocrine, paracrine, and autocrine (Table 2). Endocrine control is exerted through the action of hormones such as parathyroid hormone (PTH), 1,25-dihydroxyvitamin D_3, growth hormone, glucocorticoid hormones, and gonadal steroids. These agents are secreted into the circulation by endocrine glands, and they ultimately affect all bone, no matter how distant from the site of hormone synthesis. Of these agents, PTH and 1,25-dihydroxyvitamin D_3 have been the most widely studied with regard to bone formation. Although both of these hormones are known to be responsible for increasing the level of calcium in the blood, PTH by stimulating bone resorption and 1,25-dihydroxyvitamin D_3 by stimulating intestinal calcium transport, they have also been shown to have important effects on bone formation. For example, in osteoblasts, PTH mediates ion and amino acid transport, stimulates cyclic adenosine monophosphate, regulates collagen synthesis, and binds to a specific receptor (18–22). 1,25-dihydroxyvitamin D_3 also stimulates matrix and alkaline phosphatase synthesis, production of bone-specific proteins, and binds to a receptor. In fact, we now have direct evidence that under certain conditions both PTH and 1,25-dihydroxyvitamin D_3 are direct anabolic agents for skeletal mass (23–26).

Paracrine control of osteoblast activity occurs when cells adjacent to the osteoblasts produce and release locally acting factors that influence bone formation. There are many examples of this in the skeleton, ranging from (i) the initial developmental stages in the embryo, (ii) long-bone growth and fracture healing, and (iii) the basal remodeling that occurs throughout life. Specific examples include the role of bFGF (or FGF-2) in development and expression of the limb rudiments, the production of the TGF-βs and BMP-2 by chondrogenic cells in the growth plate and fracture callus, and the production of interleukins by osteoclasts at sites of bone remodeling. These examples demonstrate the synthesis of a key factor by a nonosteoblast cell type that influences the activity of a nearby osteoblast.

Last, autocrine regulation of osteoblasts also occurs: factors produced by osteoblasts are eventually used to regulate their own activity. In the bone remodeling process, this pathway is best represented by the growth factors embedded in bone by osteoblasts, which are released to influence these cells at a later time. Some of the best studied of these factors are the insulin-like growth factors, IGF-I and IGF-II. These molecules can be extracted from bone and have been shown to have proliferation- and differentiation-stimulating activity for osteoblasts.

SUMMARY

Osteoblasts are complex and pivotal cells that participate in all aspects of bone metabolism. They serve two main functions: they form the structural components of bone (i.e., matrix and mineral) and they produce regulatory factors that influence both bone formation and bone resorption. Osteoblasts are derived from a progenitor mesenchymal cell through the expression of a series of genes that are coordinately regulated. These cells ultimately develop receptors that recognize endocrine hormones, and they translate these hormonal signals to control both bone formation and bone resorption at locally specific sites. The end-stage phenotype of an osteoblast is an osteocyte. Although viable, osteocytes are completely encased in bone and have a very much reduced metabolic activity. A clear-cut regulatory action for osteocytes has not been identified.

REFERENCES

1. Sawyer JR, Myers MA, Rosier RN, Puzas JE: Heterotopic ossification: Clinical and cellular aspects. *Calcif Tissue Int* 49:208–215, 1991
2. O'Conner JM: *Soft Tissue Ossification*. Springer-Verlag, New York, 1983
3. Robison R: The possible significance of hexosephosphoric esters in ossification. *Biochem J* 17:286–293, 1923
4. Rodan GA, Martin TJ: Role of osteoclasts in hormonal control of bone resorption—a hypothesis. *Calcif Tissue Int* 33:349 351, 1981

5. Burger EH, Van der Meer JWM, Nijweide PJ: Osteoclast formation from mononuclear phagocytes: Role of bone forming cells. *J Cell Biol* 99:1901–1905, 1984
6. Chambers TJ, McSheehy PMJ, Thomson BM, Fuller K: The effect of calcium–regulating hormones and prostaglandins on bone resorption by osteoclasts disaggregated from neonatal rabbit bones. *Endocrinology* 116:234–239, 1985
7. Martin TJ, Ng KW: Mechanism by which cells of the osteoblast lineage control osteoclast formation and activity. *J Cell Biochem* 56:357–366, 1994
8. Zambonin-Zallone A, Teti A, Primavera MV: Resorption of vital or devitalized bone by isolated osteoclasts in vitro: The role of lining cells. *Cell Tissue Res* 235:561–564, 1984
9. Owen ME: Bone growth at the cellular level: A perspective. In: Dixon AD, Sarnat BG (eds) *Factors and Mechanisms Influencing Bone Growth.* Alan R Liss, New York, 1982, pp 19–28
10. Friedenstein AY, Chailakhyan RK, Latsinik NY, Panasyuk AF, Keiliss-Borok IV: Stromal cells responsible for transferring the microenvironment of the hemopoietic tissues. *Transplantation* 17:331–340, 1974
11. Nijweide PJ, van der Plas A: Embryonic chick periosteum in tissue culture: osteoid formation and calcium uptake. *Proc K Ned Akad Wet C* 78:410–417, 1975
12. Stein GS, Lian JB, Own TA: Relationship of cell growth to the regulation of tissue-specific gene expression during osteoblast differentiation. *FASEB J* 4:3111–3123, 1990
13. Tonna EA, Cronkite EP: The periosteum: Autoradiographic studies on cellular proliferation and transformation utilizing tritiated thymidine. *Clin Orthop* 30:218–232, 1963
14. Tonna EA, Cronkite EP: An autoradiographic study of periosteal cell proliferation with tritiated thymidine. *Lab Invest* 11:455–461, 1962
15. Kimmel DB, Jee WSS: Bone cell kinetics during longitudinal bone growth in the rat. *Calcif Tissue Int* 32: 123–133, 1980
16. Tran VPT, Vignery A, Baron R: Cellular kinetics of the bone remodeling sequence in the rat. *Anat Rec* 202:445–451, 1982
17. Malluche HH, Faugere M-C: *Atlas of Mineralized Bone Histology.* Karger, New York, 1986
18. Donahue HJ, Fryer MJ, Eriksen EF, Heath H: Differential effects of parathyroid hormone and its analogs on cytosolic calcium ion and cAMP levels in cultured rat osteoblast-like cells. *J Biol Chem* 263:13522–13527, 1988
19. Rosenbusch JP, Nichols G Jr: Parathyroid hormone effects on amino acid transport into bone cells. *Endocrinology* 81:553–557, 1967
20. Lomri A, Marie PJ: Effect of parathyroid hormone and forskolin on cytoskeletal protein synthesis in cultured mouse osteoblastic cells. *Biochim Biophys Acta* 970:333–42, 1988
21. Kream BE, Rowe D, Smith MD, Maher V, Majeska R: Hormonal regulation of collagen synthesis in a clonal rat osteosarcoma cell line. *Endocrinology* 119:1922–1928, 1986
22. Hesch RD, Brabant G, Rittinghaus EF, Atkinson MJ, Harms H: Pulsatile secretion of parathyroid hormone and its action on a type I and type II PTH receptor: A hypothesis for understanding osteoporosis. *Calcif Tissue Int* 42:341–344, 1988
23. Harrison JR, Clark NB: Avian medullary bone in organ culture: Effects of vitamin D metabolites on collagen synthesis. *Calcif Tissue Int* 39:35–43, 1986
24. Fritsch J, Grosse B, Lieberherr M, Balsan S: 1,25-dihydroxyvitamin D is required for growth-independent expression of alkaline phosphatase in cultured rat osteoblasts. *Calcif Tissue Int* 37: 639–645, 1985
25. Price PA, Baukol SA: 1,25-dihydroxyvitamin D increases synthesis of the vitamin K dependent bone protein by osteosarcoma cells. *J Biol Chem* 255:11660–11663, 1980
26. McDonnell DP, Pike JW, O'Malley BW: The vitamin D receptor: A primitive steroid receptor related to thyroid hormone receptor. *J Steroid Biochem* 30:41–46, 1988

3. Bone-Resorbing Cells

Gregory R. Mundy, M.D.

Department of Medicine, Endocrinology and Metabolism, University of Texas Health Science Center, San Antonio, Texas

The major and possibly sole bone-resorbing cell is the osteoclast, and this cell will be the focus of attention in this chapter. Other cells, however, have been linked to bone resorption. These include osteocytes, monocytes, tumor cells, and osteoblasts. Osteocytic bone resorption, also called osteocytic osteolysis, was first described over 30 years ago by histologists examining light microscopy sections. It was thought that osteocytic osteolysis resulted from expansion of the osteocyte lacunae, in which osteocytes are embedded in bone. However, more recent observations with scanning electron microscopy make it unlikely that osteolysis by osteocytes occurs (1). Using this technique, it is apparent that bone resorption is characterized by easily discernible degradative changes in the bone matrix, which are not observed around osteocytes. Jones and coworkers (1) consider apparent osteolysis by osteocytes an artifact of observations made in bone that is rapidly turning over (fetal or woven bone). From time to time, other cells have also been linked to bone resorption. Monocytes and macrophages have been shown to degrade devitalized bone (2,3). These observations strengthen the notion that monocytes

and osteoclasts have a common precursor, a concept that, in light of subsequent data, appears likely to be true. However, there are no resorption pits associated with monocytes or macrophages when they lie against bone surfaces, and it is unlikely that they have a major role in bone degradation. Similarly, tumor cells have also been shown to resorb devitalized bone by causing release of previously incorporated calcium (4), but resorption pits are not found around tumor cells, even *in vivo* (5). It has been suggested that osteoblasts may act as helper cells in the process of osteoclastic resorption by preparing the bone surface for later attack by osteoclastic enzymes, although there is still little direct evidence to support this interesting concept.

Although osteoclasts are clearly the major bone-resorbing cells, osteoclast activity may be modulated by other cells such as osteoblasts and immune cells.

OSTEOCLAST MORPHOLOGY

Osteoclasts have been studied extensively using light microscopy, transmission electron microscopy, and scanning electron microscopy. They are unique and highly specialized cells. They are localized on endosteal bone surfaces, in haversian systems, and also occasionally on periosteal surfaces. They are not commonly seen on normal bone surfaces but are found frequently at sites of actively remodeling bones, such as the metaphyses of growing bones or in pathologic circumstances, such as adjacent to collections of tumor cells. They are large, multinucleated cells, varying in size up to 100 μ in diameter in pathologic states and containing, on average, 10 to 20 nuclei. The number of nuclei in osteoclasts is related to the species, more being seen in the cat and fewer in the mouse. The nuclei are centrally placed and usually contain 1 to 2 nucleoli. Osteoclasts have primary lysosomes, numerous and pleomorphic mitochondria, and a specific area of the cell membrane, known as the ruffled border, which abuts against the bone surface. This area of the cell membrane is composed of folds and invaginations that allow intimate contact with the bone surface. This is the site at which resorption of bone occurs and the resorption bay (also known as the Howship's lacuna) is formed. Some workers have considered the confined and circumscribed space between the ruffled border and the bone surface to be equivalent to a secondary lysosome (6). The ruffled border is surrounded by a clear zone which appears free of organelles but in fact contains actin filaments and appears to anchor the ruffled border area to the bone surface undergoing resorption.

CRITERIA FOR DEFINITION OF THE OSTEOCLAST

Some of the morphologic features of the osteoclast have been used as criteria for identification. These include multinuclearity, pleomorphic mitochondria, and presence of the ruffled border adjacent to areas of resorbed bone. These criteria have received much attention in recent years as investigators have attempted to isolate osteoclasts *in vitro* and distinguish them from other cells. Osteoclasts are difficult to distinguish from macrophage polykaryons, which are related cells with a similar lineage. Some of the features of the osteoclast that aid in the distinction from macrophage polykaryons include the capacity to resorb bone, capacity to form a ruffled border, contraction of the cytoplasm on exposure to calcitonin, presence of calcitonin receptors, crossreactivity with osteoclast-specific monoclonal antibodies (although it has not been convincingly shown that any antibody is absolutely specific for the osteoclast), appropriate responses to calciotropic hormones, and absence of the Fc receptor. The presence of tartrate-resistant acid phosphatase is a helpful marker, but it is not useful for distinguishing human osteoclasts from macrophage polykaryons. Responsivity to osteotropic hormones also has been used as a criterion for identification of osteoclasts. Osteoclast-stimulating agents, including parathyroid hormone, interleukin-1, tumor necrosis factor, transforming growth factor α, and 1,25-dihydroxyvitamin D, activate osteoclasts. Inhibitors of osteoclast activity include calcitonin, gamma interferon, and transforming growth factor. However, the effects of some of these factors are not specific for osteoclasts. For example, 1,25-dihydroxyvitamin D promotes not only the fusion of osteoclasts but also enhances the fusion of macro-

phages to form polykaryons (7). Moreover, some of these factors are species specific. For example, calcitonin may not cause contraction of avian osteoclast cytoplasmic membranes. The evidence suggests that macrophages can be induced to form multinucleated cells, form resorption pits, and respond to calcitonin. A reasonable compromise is to denote cells as functional osteoclasts if they form resorption pits, are multinucleated, and respond to calcitonin, while recognizing that some authentic osteoclasts are not multinucleated, do not form resorption pits, and do not respond to calcitonin.

MOLECULAR MECHANISMS OF BONE RESORPTION

Osteoclasts resorb bone by the production of proteolytic enzymes and hydrogen ions in the localized environment under the ruffled border of the cell. Hydrogen ions are generated in the cell by the enzyme carbonic anhydrase type II. They are then pumped across the ruffled border by a proton pump, apparently similar, but not identical, to the complex vacuolar ATPase in the intercalated cells of the kidney (8). Lysosomal enzymes are also released by the osteoclast, and the hydrogen ions produced by the proton pump ATPase provide an optimal environment for these proteolytic enzymes to degrade the bone matrix.

The extrusion of protons across the ruffled border of the cell (apical surface) requires the presence of a number of ion exchanges, pumps, and channels in the basolateral membrane of the cell to maintain electrochemical balance of the osteoclast. These include an Na^+/H^+ antiporter, an Na^+/K^+ ATPase, an HCO_3^-/Cl^- exchanger, a Ca^{2+} ATPase, and a K^+ channel.

The osteoclast is a motile cell. It resorbs bone to form a lacuna and then moves across the bone surface to resorb a separate area of bone. The tracks of its path can often be followed (1). Periods of locomotion are not associated with resorption. When the cell stops moving, it usually starts resorbing bone.

Some diseases are caused by disturbances in the molecular mechanisms responsible for bone resorption. For example, it has been shown that there is an unusual form of inherited osteopetrosis in children, in which there is a deficiency of the carbonic anhydrase type II isoenzyme (9). The osteoclasts in this disease are incompetent, bone is not resorbed, and the bone marrow cavity is not formed. Children with this disease also have renal tubular acidosis, caused by a similar enzyme defect in renal tubular cells, leading to impairment of hydrogen ion secretion.

Several other processes may be involved in the complex process of osteoclastic bone resorption. Some workers have suggested that the surface of the bone is prepared for the osteoclast by the actions of collagenase released by bone lining cells or osteoblasts. The osteoclasts then produce acid and lysosomal enzymes that complete the process. Because osteoblasts have the capacity to produce enzymes that could activate latent collagenase, such as plasminogen activator, such a mechanism is possible. However, it has already been shown that osteoclasts also secrete cysteine proteinases that are capable of degrading collagen in the acid environment under the ruffled border.

Recent data have suggested that oxygen-derived free radicals are involved in the resorption of bone by osteoclasts (10). Many degradative processes of phagocytic cells are associated with free radical production, and bone resorption seems another. The use of radical-generating systems *in vivo* and *in vitro* shows that enzymes that deplete tissues of radicals, such as superoxide dismutase, block osteoclastic bone resorption stimulated by parathyroid hormone or interleukin-1. Staining reactions with nitroblue tetrazolium show that radical generation occurs within osteoclasts. Radicals could be involved in the degradation of bone under the ruffled border. However, the demonstration that radical generation is associated with new osteoclast formation suggests that radicals also have a cellular effect on the formation of osteoclasts.

The active resorbing osteoclast is a highly polarized cell. The ruffled border is the highly specialized area of the osteoclast cell membrane that lies adjacent to the bone surface. The attachment of the osteoclast to the bone surface has been shown to be an essential requirement for resorption to occur. This attachment process involves, at least in part, cell-membrane-bound proteins called integrins. Integrins attach to specific proteins in the bone matrix. One of the integrins important for osteoclast function is the vitronectin receptor (11), also known as the α_{v3} integrin. Antibodies to this receptor preferentially recognize osteoclasts. Attachment to bone matrix proteins involves specific Arg-Gly-Asp (RGD) amino acid sequences in the bone matrix proteins, and synthetic peptides are being developed that compete with osteoclast integrins for binding to these proteins, preventing osteoclast attachment to the bone surface and thereby inhibiting bone resorption. The snake venom *Echistatin* binds to this integrin and inhibits bone resorption *in vitro* and *in vivo* (12).

Recent observations have shown that the 60-kilodalton non receptor tyrosine kinase that is the product of the c-*src* proto-oncogene is required for osteoclasts to form resorption pits. This proto-oncogene is a ubiquitous intracellular tyrosine kinase which is membrane bound and has been linked to function of the cytoskeleton. In experiments in which the c-*src* gene was deleted from mice by targeted disruption in embryonic stem cells, it has been possible to breed mice that do not have the capacity to express *src*. In these mice, it was found unexpectedly that the mice have osteopetrosis, the bone disease characterized by nonfunctioning osteoclasts (13). More detailed examination of these mice has shown that multinucleated cells form on bone surfaces in *src*-deficient animals, but these multinucleated cells cannot form ruffled borders and resorb bone (14). These results indicate that this intracellular tyrosine kinase is essential for normal bone resorption, and they suggest a potential therapeutic target for the development of new inhibitors of bone resorption. Even more recently, gene knockout of the proto-oncogene c-*fos* has also been shown to cause osteopetrosis (15).

FORMATION AND ACTIVATION OF OSTEOCLASTS

Osteoclasts arise from hematopoietic mononuclear cells in the bone marrow (7). Mononuclear osteoclast precursors can circulate in the blood. At endosteal bone surfaces, the precursors proliferate, fuse to form multinucleated cells, form ruffled borders, and resorb bone. The cell of origin for the osteoclast in the bone marrow is still debated. The weight of evidence suggests it is a pluripotent stem cell that has the capacity, in response to appropriate stimuli, to differentiate into a granulocyte, monocyte, or osteoclast. The most likely stem cell is a CFU-GM (colony-forming unit for the granulocyte-macrophage series).

It was shown over 20 years ago that osteoclasts formed by fusion of precursors at the bone surface. These precursors circulated in the blood as mononuclear cells (16,17).

OSTEOCLAST APOPTOSIS

The disappearance of osteoclasts from bone remodeling sites may be as important as their formation for the control of bone resorption. Recent observations have suggested that osteoclasts undergo apoptosis at the conclusion of the resorbing phase of the bone remodeling process (18). Osteoclast apoptosis can be recognized by characteristic morphologic appearances of the osteoclast, including condensation of the nuclear chromatin. Another characteristic feature is loss of the ruffled border and detachment of the osteoclast from the surfaces of mineralized bone matrix. Apoptosis is modulated by drugs which regulate osteoclast function (but in an inverse manner). Drugs that inhibit bone resorption, such as bisphosphonates and estrogen, induce osteoclast apoptosis both *in vitro* and *in vivo* (18).

LESSONS FROM OSTEOPETROSIS

Osteopetrosis is the bone disorder characterized by impaired osteoclast function. It is clearly a heterogeneous disorder. There are a number of different variants in rodents that have now been well described, as well as a number of different forms that occur in humans. Although a rare disease, this is a very informative condition for osteoclast biologists. Because specific molecular and genetic defects have been found in some types of osteopetrosis, studies of variants of this disorder have characterized some of the molecular mechanisms responsible for osteoclastic bone resorption. For example, in one rare variant seen in humans, there is deficient expression of the osteoclast enzyme carbonic anhydrase type II, which is responsible for proton production in osteoclasts (9). Because proton production is necessary for normal bone resorption, patients with abnormalities in expression of this enzyme have impaired bone resorption and subsequent osteopetrosis. In several of the murine models of osteopetrosis, it has been possible to identify genes that are essential for osteoclast function. For example, in one naturally occurring animal model of osteopetrosis, the op/op murine variant, there is impaired production of colony-stimulating factor 1 (CSF-1) by stromal cells in the osteoclast microenvironment (19). As a consequence, osteoclasts fail to form and bone is not resorbed. This model shows that during the neonatal period in mice, production of normal CSF-1 is required for normal osteoclast formation. In another murine variant, tumor biologists experimenting with specific disruption of the *src* proto-oncogene have shown that this proto-oncogene, which encodes an intracellular tyrosine kinase, is required for normal osteoclastic bone resorption (13). However, the defect is different from that seen in the op/op variant of osteopetrosis. In *src*-deficient mice, osteoclasts form, but they do not become polarized and are incapable of forming ruffled borders and resorbing bone. Unlike the op/op variant, the defect in *src* deficiency is not in the microenvironment of the osteoclast, but rather in the mature osteoclast itself. More recently, similar gene knockout experiments in mice with the c-*fos* proto-oncogene have also led unexpectedly to osteopetrosis (15). The precise mechanism is not known.

TECHNIQUES FOR STUDYING OSTEOCLASTS

Osteoclasts are very inaccessible cells, and so direct studies on these cells have been difficult to perform. Detailed information on their behavior was therefore not available until isolation techniques were developed for studying them *in vitro*. Techniques are now available for studying isolated preformed osteoclasts obtained from chicks, rodents, and baboons, as well as from human giant-cell tumors, and for studying the formation of osteoclasts from marrow precursors (7,20). These techniques are providing a tremendous boon to advances in this area of bone cell biology, for they allow the determination of the modes of actions of factors that stimulate and inhibit bone resorption.

REGULATION OF OSTEOCLAST ACTIVITY

Osteoclasts lie on bone surfaces in a bed of elliptical or fusiform, spindle-shaped cells called lining cells, which are probably members of the osteoblast lineage. When exposed to a bone-resorbing agent, the first response is that these lining cells retract and the osteoclasts insinuate an arm into the retracted area; then a ruffled border forms, and bone is resorbed at the exposed surface (1). The molecular mechanisms by which these complicated processes are controlled are unknown. Why lining cells retract at specific sites and how the osteoclast is activated is still not clear. It appears most likely that the osteoclast is activated by a soluble signal released from the lining cell (21,22).

Many hormones and factors have now been shown to stimulate osteoclast activity. Their mechanisms of action differ. Osteoclastic resorption may be stimulated by factors that enhance proliferation of osteoclast progenitors, which cause differentiation of committed precursors into mature cells or activation of the mature multinucleated cell to resorb bone (23). Similarly, osteoclasts could be inhibited by agents that block proliferation of precursors, that inhibit differentiation or fusion, or that inactivate the mature multinucleated resorbing cell. Current evidence indicates that most factors that stimulate or inhibit osteoclasts act on at least two of these steps (Fig. 1).

Systemic Hormones

The systemic hormones parathyroid hormone (PTH), 1,25-dihydroxyvitamin D, and calcitonin all influence osteoclast activity.

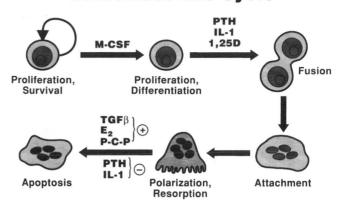

FIG. 1. Events involved in osteoclastic bone resorption. Osteoclasts develop from pluripotent mononuclear precursors (CFU-GM) present in the bone marrow. Early cells in the osteoclast lineage can differentiate along the granulocyte-macrophage lineage or the osteoclast lineage and have high proliferative capacity. As these cells become further committed to the osteoclast lineage, they gradually lose proliferative potential. Monocyte–macrophage colony-stimulating factor (M-CSF) is an important cytokine required for survival of these precursors. As the mononuclear cells proceed down the osteoclast lineage, they become further differentiated and eventually fuse to form immature osteoclasts. This process may involve cell attachment molecules such as E-cadherin. It is enhanced by systemic factors such as parathyroid hormone, 1,25-dihydroxyvitamin D, and cytokines such as interleukin-1. In the presence of bone, the mature osteoclast becomes polarized, forms a ruffled border, and, with appropriate stimulation, begins to resorb bone. A number of the molecular mechanisms that are required in the osteoclast for polarization include the expression of the *src* proto-oncogene, a nonreceptor tyrosine kinase. The osteoclast also utilizes other specialized molecules to resorb bone, including a vacuolar ATPase which is responsible for pumping protons across the ruffled border. The osteoclast undergoes apoptosis (programmed cell death) during bone remodeling and in response to agents such as transforming growth factor-β (TGF-β), estrogens, and bisphosphonates.

Parathyroid Hormone

PTH stimulates differentiation of committed progenitors to fuse, forming mature multinucleated osteoclasts. It also activates preformed osteoclasts to resorb bone. However, it does not increase CFU-GM, the earliest detectable cells in the osteoclast lineage. The activation of osteoclasts is probably indirect, probably mediated through cells in the osteoblast lineage such as the lining cells (22). The mechanisms by which osteoblasts send the second signal to the multinucleated osteoclasts in response to PTH is not known.

Parathyroid-hormone-related protein (PTH-rP) has effects on osteoclasts identical to those of PTH.

1,25-Dihydroxyvitamin D

1,25-Dihydroxyvitamin D is a potent stimulator of osteoclastic bone resorption. Like PTH, it stimulates osteoclast progenitors to differentiate and fuse (7). It has a similar effect on macrophage polykaryons, which are not osteoclasts. It also activates mature preformed osteoclasts, possibly by a similar mechanism to that of PTH. 1,25-Dihydroxyvitamin D also has other effects on bone resorption, which are indirect. It is a potent immunoregulatory molecule (24). It inhibits T cell proliferation and the production of the cytokine interleukin-2. Under some circumstances, it can enhance interleukin-1 production in cells with monocyte characteristics. Thus, the overall effects of 1,25-dihydroxyvitamin D on bone resorption are multiple and complex.

Calcitonin

Calcitonin is a polypeptide hormone that is a potent inhibitor of osteoclastic bone resorption, but its effects are only transient. Osteoclasts escape from the inhibitory effects of calcitonin following continued exposure (25). Thus, patients treated for hypercalcemia with calcitonin will respond for only a limited period of time (usually 48 to 72 hours) before hypercalcemia recurs. Even in patients with Paget's disease, the beneficial effects of calcitonin may eventually be lost with continued treatment. The "escape" phenomenon is likely a result of down-regulation of mRNA for the receptor (26). Calcitonin causes cytoplasmic contraction of the osteoclast cell membrane, which has been correlated with its capacity to inhibit bone resorption (27). It also causes the dissolution of mature osteoclasts into mononuclear cells. However, it also inhibits osteoclast formation, both inhibiting proliferation of the progenitors and inhibiting differentiation of the committed precursors. The effects of calcitonin on osteoclasts are mediated by cyclic adenosine monophosphate.

Local Hormones

Local hormones may be more important than systemic hormones for the initiation of physiologic bone resorption and for the normal bone remodeling sequence. Because bone remodeling occurs in discrete and distinct packets throughout the skeleton, it seems probable that the cellular events are controlled by factors generated in the microenvironment of bone. A number of potent local stimulators and inhibitors of osteoclast activity have been identified.

Interleukin-1

There are two interleukin-1 molecules, interleukin-1α and β. Their effects on bone appear to be the same and are mediated through the same receptor. Interleukin-1 is released by activated monocytes, but also by other types of cells including osteoblasts and tumor cells. It is a potent stimulator of osteoclasts. It works at all phases in the formation and activation of osteoclasts. It stimulates proliferation of the progenitors and differentiation of committed precursors into mature cells (28). It also activates the mature multinucleated osteoclast indirectly through another cell (possibly a bone lining cell) (29).

Interleukin-1 also stimulates osteoclastic bone resorption when infused *in vivo,* and it causes a substantial increase in the plasma calcium (30,31). At least part of its effects may be mediated via prostaglandin generation. It has been implicated as a potential mediator of bone resorption and increased bone turnover in osteoporosis (32). It may be responsible for the increase in bone resorption seen in some malignancies, as well as the localized bone resorption associated with collections of chronic inflammatory cells in diseases such as rheumatoid arthritis.

Lymphotoxin and Tumor Necrosis Factor

Lymphotoxin and tumor necrosis factor (TNF) are molecules that are related functionally to interleukin-1. Many of their biologic properties overlap with those of interleukin-1. They share the same receptor with each other, which is distinct from that of interleukin-1. They are synergistic with interleukin-1 in their effects on bone. Lymphotoxin is released by activated T-lymphocytes, and TNF by activated macrophages. TNF is one of the mediators of the systemic effects of endotoxic shock. It also causes wasting (cachexia) and suppresses erythropoiesis (red blood cell formation). Lymphotoxin and TNF stimulate proliferation of osteoclast progenitors, cause fusion of committed precursors to form multinucleated cells, and activate multinucleated cells (through cells in the osteoblast lineage) to resorb bone (33–35). Lymphotoxin may be an important mediator of bone resorption in myeloma (36). Lymphotoxin and TNF cause osteoclastic bone resorption and hypercalcemia when infused or injected *in vivo* (34,36,37).

Colony-Stimulating Factor-1

The growth regulatory factor CSF-1, which was once thought to be specific for the monocyte-macrophage lineage, has been shown to be required for normal osteoclast formation in rodents during the neonatal period. In the op/op variant of osteopetrosis, there is impaired production of CSF-1, and the consequence is osteopetrosis because of decreased normal osteoclast formation (see earlier). The disease can be cured by treatment with CSF-1 (38). CSF-1 is produced by stromal cells in the osteoclast microenvironment. Presumably, cells in the osteoclast lineage contain the CSF-1 receptor (a receptor tyrosine kinase), and this is the mechanism by which CSF-1 mediates osteoclast formation.

Osteoclastpoietic Factor

Since the osteoclast shares a common precursor with the formed elements of the blood, and CFU-GM are precursors for the osteoclast, it has long been wondered if there is a lineage-specific growth-regulatory factor for osteoclast formation. Two reports have suggested that such a factor may exist (39,40). Tumors that are associated with hypercalcemia often also cause leukocytosis due to production of various colony-stimulating factors. In human and murine tumors associated with the hypercalcemia–leukocytosis syndrome, in addition to colony-stimulating factors, these tumors have been shown to produce a 17-kDa peptide that stimulates osteoclast formation. Complete purification and cloning of this factor are awaited with interest.

Interleukin-6

Interleukin-6 is a pleiotropic cytokine that has important effects on bone. It is expressed and secreted by normal bone cells in response to osteotropic hormones such as PTH, 1,25-dihydroxyvitamin D, and interleukin-1 (41). The osteoclast is the most prodigious cell source of interleukin-6 so far described. Interleukin-6 is a fairly weak stimulator of osteoclast formation, and less powerful than other cytokines such as interleukin-1, TNF, and lymphotoxin (42,43). It has recently been implicated in the bone loss associated with estrogen withdrawal (ovariectomy) in the mouse (44).

Gamma Interferon

Gamma interferon is a multifunctional lymphokine produced by activated T-lymphocytes. In contrast to the other immune cell products, it inhibits osteoclastic bone resorption (45,46). Its major effect appears to be to inhibit differentiation of committed precursors to mature cells (47). It also has less potent effects on osteoclast precursor proliferation. Unlike calcitonin, it does not cause cytoplasmic contraction of isolated osteoclasts.

Transforming Growth Factor-β

TGF-β is a multifunctional polypeptide that is produced by immune cells but is also released from the bone matrix during resorption. TGF-β has unique effects on osteoclasts. In most systems, it inhibits osteoclast formation by inhibiting both proliferation and differentiation of osteoclast precursors (28,48). In addition, it directly inhibits the activity of mature osteoclasts by decreasing superoxide production, and it inhibits accumulation of tartrate-resistant acid phosphatase in osteoclasts. Because TGF-β has a powerful effect on osteoblasts (it stimulates proliferation and synthesis of differentiated proteins and increases mineralized bone formation) (49), it may be a pivotal factor in the bone-remodeling process. For example, it could be released during this resorption process and then be available as a natural endogenous inhibitor of continued osteoclast activity. At the same time, working in conjunction with other bone factors, it may lead to osteoblast stimulation and the eventual formation of new bone. However, the effects of TGF-β are complex and may differ in different species. In one system, neonatal mouse calvariae, it stimulates prostaglandin generation, which in turn leads to bone resorption, which is the opposite effect to that seen in the rat or human systems (50).

Other Factors

A number of other factors whose precise role in physiologic and pathologic bone resorption are still to be delineated.

Retinoids

Vitamin A is the only fully characterized factor that has a direct stimulatory effect on osteoclasts (51). Vitamin A excess eventually leads to increased bone resorption in vivo and hypercalcemia. It is unknown if the effects of vitamin A on osteoclasts have physiologic significance.

Transforming Growth Factor-α

TGF-α, like the related compound epidermal growth factor (EGF), is a powerful stimulator of osteoclastic bone resorption (50,52–54). TGF-α is produced by many tumors and is likely involved in increased bone resorption associated with cancer. It is probably produced normally during embryonic life. It stimulates the proliferation of osteoclast progenitors and probably also acts on immature multinucleated cells. Its actions on osteoclasts are comparable to those of the CSFs on other hematopoietic cells (55). The effects of TGF-α on bone cells are mediated through the EGF receptor, although it is more potent than EGF for bone resorption. Injections or infusions of TGF-α increase the plasma calcium levels in vivo (37).

Neutral Phosphate and Calcium

Neutral phosphate inhibits osteoclast activity in organ cultures (56). The precise mode of action is not clear. Phosphate is a useful form of therapy in patients with increased bone resorption, diseases such as cancer, or primary hyperparathyroidism, although it may have other effects in addition to those of inhibiting bone resorption, such as impairment of calcium absorption from the gut.

High extracellular calcium concentrations also lead to decreased osteoclast activity, associated with an increase in intracellular calcium concentrations. This suggests that increased local calcium concentrations may be another mechanism by which osteoclast activity to resorb bone may be regulated.

Prostaglandins

Prostaglandins have complex and multiple effects on osteoclasts, depending on the species. Prostaglandins have been linked to the hypercalcemia and increased bone resorption associated with malignancy and chronic inflammation (57). However, the effects of prostaglandins are confusing. Prostaglandins of the E series stimulate osteoclastic bone resorption in organ culture. Moreover, some bone-resorbing factors, and particularly growth factors, appear to mediate their effects through the production of prostaglandins in mouse bones. Prostaglandins inhibit the formation of human osteoclasts and cause cytoplasmic contraction of isolated osteoclasts in much the same way as calcitonin. However, prostaglandins stimulate the formation of mouse multinucleated osteoclasts from marrow progenitors. The overall significance of prostaglandins depends on the species studied. Their overall effects on bone resorption in humans are still a mystery.

Leukotrienes

Leukotrienes, like prostaglandins, are arachidonic acid metabolites that have been linked to osteoclastic bone resorption (58). They are produced by the metabolism of arachidonic acid by a 5-lipoxygenase enzyme. Several of these leukotrienes have been shown to activate osteoclasts *in vitro,* and they may be related to the bone resorption seen in giant cell tumors of bone. These arachidonic acid metabolites have effects on osteoclasts that are different from those of the E series prostaglandins, which stimulate osteoclastic bone resorption in organ culture and cause transient inhibition of the activity of isolated osteoclasts. In contrast, the leukotrienes stimulate osteoclastic bone resorption in organ culture, but they also enhance the capacity of isolated osteoclasts to form resorption pits.

Thyroid Hormones

The thyroid hormones thyroxine and triiodothyronine stimulate osteoclastic bone resorption in organ cultures (59). Some patients with hyperthyroidism have increased bone loss, increased osteoclast activity, and hypercalcemia. Thyroid hormones act directly on osteoclastic bone resorption, but their precise mode of action is unknown.

Glucocorticoids

Glucocorticoids inhibit osteoclast formation *in vitro* and inhibit osteoclastic bone resorption in organ cultures. Their efficacy depends on the stimulus to bone resorption. They are less effective in inhibiting bone resorption stimulated by parathyroid hormone than they are in inhibiting bone resorption stimulated by cytokines such as interleukin-1 (60).

In vivo, glucocorticoid administration is associated with increased bone resorption. This is an indirect effect that results from the effects of glucocorticoids to inhibit calcium absorption from the gut. As a consequence, parathyroid gland activity is stimulated and secondary hyperparathyroidism leads to a generalized increase in osteoclastic bone resorption.

Estrogens and Androgens

Estrogen lack is associated with increased osteoclastic bone resorption in the 10 years following the menopause (61). The mechanisms are not clear. It has been suggested that estrogens may affect osteoclasts directly (62) but, in addition, estrogens may mediate their effects on osteoclasts indirectly by suppressing the production of bone-resorbing cytokines such as interleukin-1 and interleukin-6 (32,44,63). These notions suggested that estrogen withdrawal, for example at the menopause, leads to enhanced bone resorption.

Pharmacologic Agents

A number of pharmacologic agents have been used as inhibitors of bone resorption and are useful therapies in patients with diseases such as malignancy associated with hypercalcemia. These include plicamycin (mithramycin), gallium nitrate, and the bisphosphonates (23). All of these agents inhibit osteoclastic activity, although their mechanism of action is unknown. In the case of the cytotoxic drugs plicamycin and gallium nitrate, it is possible that their actions are mediated through cytotoxic effects on osteoclasts or inhibition of proliferation of the osteoclast progenitors.

Bisphosphonates are very important inhibitors of osteoclastic bone resorption *in vivo;* they are achieving increased use in diseases associated with increased bone resorption, and particularly in osteoporosis, hypercalcemia of malignancy, Paget's disease of bone, and osteolytic bone disease. Their molecular mechanism of action is still debated. Some investigators suggest they work primarily by coating bone surfaces and rendering mineralized bone surfaces toxic to resorbing osteoclasts (64), while others postulate a cellular effect, in bone cells in the osteoclast lineage during their formation (65), or in osteoblastic cells that control osteoclastic bone resorption (66). Whatever their target, it has recently been shown that the end result is osteoclast apoptosis (18).

Sex hormone deficiency increases osteoclastic bone resorption. The mechanism is still unclear. Thus, estrogens or androgens may be used as therapy in postmenopausal women or hypogonadal men, respectively. Estrogens and androgens cause increases in all cells at all stages in the osteoclast lineage. Although relatively small numbers of estrogen receptors are present in osteoclasts (62), it is likely that the main primary cellular target is not the osteoclast, and that inhibitory effects on osteoclasts are mediated through accessory cells for bone resorption. Several cytokines have been implicated in the increased bone resorption associated with estrogen withdrawal, including interleukin-1, interleukin-6, TGF-β, and prostaglandins of the E series. As indicated earlier, evidence from *in vivo studies* suggest that both interleukin-1 and interleukin-6 may be involved (32,44). Because the majority of patients will not take estrogens, attempts are now being made to develop drugs that have estrogen-like effects on bone and the cardiovascular system, but not the deleterious effects of estrogens on the breast and endometrium of the uterus. One member of this group of estrogen agonists/antagonists is raloxifene (67).

REFERENCES

1. Jones SJ, Boyde A, Ali NN, Maconnachie E: A review of bone cell substratum interactions. *Scanning* 7:5–24, 1985
2. Mundy GR, Altman AJ, Gondek M, Bandelin JG: Direct resorption of bone by human monocytes. *Science* 196:1109–1111, 1977
3. Kahn AJ, Stewart CC, Teitelbaum SL: Contact-mediated bone resorption by human monocytes in vitro. *Science* 199:988–990, 1978
4. Eilon G, Mundy GR: Direct resorption of bone by human breast cancer cells in vitro. *Nature* 276:726–728, 1978
5. Boyde A, Maconnachie E, Reid SA, Delling G, Mundy GR: Scanning electron microscopy in bone pathology: Review of methods. Potential and application. *Scanning Electron Microsc* IV:1537–1554, 1986
6. Baron R, Vignery A, Horowitz M: Lymphocytes, macrophages and the regulation of bone remodeling. In: Peck WA (ed) *Bone and Mineral Research*, vol II. Elsevier, New York, pp 175–242, 1983
7. Roodman GD, Ibbotson KJ, MacDonald BR, Kuehl TJ, Mundy GR: 1,25(OH)$_2$ vitamin D3 causes formation of multinucleated

cells with osteoclast characteristics in cultures of primate marrow. *Proc Natl Acad Sci* 82:8213–8217, 1985

8. Blair HC, Teitelbaum SL, Ghiselli R, Gluck S: Osteoclastic bone resorption by a polarized vacuolar proton pump. *Science* 245: 855–857, 1989

9. Sly WS, Whyte MP, Sundaram V, et al.: Carbonic anhydrase II deficiency in 12 families with the autosomal recessive syndrome of osteopetrosis with renal tubular acidosis and cerebral calcification. *N Engl J Med* 313:139–145, 1985

10. Garrett IR, Boyce BF, Oreffo ROC, Bonewald L, Poser P, Mundy GR: Oxygen-derived free radicals stimulate osteoclastic bone resorption in rodent bone in vitro and in vivo. *J Clin Invest* 85: 632–639, 1990

11. Davies J, Warwick J, Totty N, Philip R, Helfrich M, Horton M. The osteoclast functional antigen, implicated in the regulation of bone resorption, is biochemically related to the vitronectin receptor. *J Cell Biol* 109:1817–1826, 1989

12. Fisher JE, Caulfield MP, Sato M, Quartuccio HA, Gould RJ, Garsky VM, Rodan GA, Rosenblatt M: Inhibition of osteoclastic bone resorption in vivo by echistatin, an arginyl-glycyl-aspartyl (RGD)-containing protein. *Endocrinology* 132:1411–1413, 1993

13. Soriano P, Montgomery C, Geske R, Bradley A: Targeted disruption of the c-src proto-oncogene leads to osteopetrosis in mice. *Cell* 64:693–702, 1991

14. Boyce BF, Byars J, McWilliams S, et al.: Histological and electron microprobe studies of mineralization in aluminum-related osteomalacia. *J Clin Pathol* 45:502–508, 1992

15. Grigoriadis AE, Wang ZQ, Cecchini MG, Hofstetter W, et al.: c-fos: a key regulator of osteoclast-macrophage lineage determination and bone remodeling. *Science* 266:443–4438, 1994

16. Kahn AJ, Simmons DJ: Investigation of the cell lineage in bone using a chimera of chick and quail embryonic tissue. *Nature* 258:325–327, 1975

17. Walker DG: Control of bone resorption by hematopoietic tissue. The induction and reversal of congenital osteopetrosis in mice through the use of bone marrow mononuclear phagocytes. *J Exp Med* 156:1604–1614, 1975

18. Hughes DE, Wright KR, Uy HL, Sasaki A, Yoneda T, Roodman GD, Mundy GR, Boyce BF: Bisphosphonates promote apoptosis in murine osteoclasts in vitro and in vivo. *J Bone Miner Res* 10:1478–1487, 1995

19. Wiktor-Jedrzejczak W, Urbanowska E, Aukerman SL, et al.: Correction by CSF-1 of defects in the osteopetrotic op/op mouse suggests local, developmental, and humoral requirements for this growth factor. *Exp Hematol* 19:1049–1054, 1991

20. Zambonin Zallone A, Teti A, Primavera MV: Isolated osteoclasts in primary culture: First observations on structure and survival in cultured media. *Anat Embryol* 165:405–413, 1982

21. Rodan GA, Martin TJ: Role of osteoblasts in hormonal control of bone resorption—a hypothesis. *Calcif Tissue Int* 33:349–351, 1981

22. McSheehy PMJ, Chambers TJ. Osteoblastic cells mediate osteoclastic responsiveness to parathyroid hormone. *Endocrinology* 118:824–828, 1986

23. Mundy GR, Roodman GD: Osteoclast ontogeny and function. In: Peck W (ed) *Bone and Mineral Research*, vol V. Elsevier, New York, pp 209–280, 1987

24. Tsoukas CD, Provvedini DM, Manolagas SC: 1,25 dihydroxyvitamin D3: a novel immunoregulatory hormone. *Science* 224: 1438–1440, 1984

25. Wener JA, Gorton SJ, Raisz LG: Escape from inhibition of resorption in cultures of fetal bone treated with calcitonin and parathyroid hormone. *Endocrinology* 90:752–759, 1972

26. Takahashi S, Goldring S, Katz M, Hilsenbeck S, Williams R, Roodman GD: Down regulation of calcitonin receptor mRNA expression by calcitonin during human osteoclast-like cell differentiation. *J Clin Invest* 95:167–171, 1995

27. Chambers TJ, Magnus CJ: Calcitonin alters the behavior of isolated osteoclasts. *J Pathol* 136:27–40, 1982

28. Pfeilschifter JP, Seyedin S, Mundy GR: Transformed growth factor inhibits bone resorption in fetal rat long bone cultures. *J Clin Invest* 82:680–685, 1988

29. Thomson BM, Saklatvala J, Chambers TJ: Osteoblasts mediate interleukin-1 stimulation of bone resorption by rat osteoclasts. *J Exp Med* 164:104–112, 1986

30. Sabatini M, Boyce B, Aufdemorte T, Bonewald L, Mundy GR: Infusions of recombinant human interleukin-1α and β cause hypercalcemia in normal mice. *Proc Natl Acad Sci* 85: 5235–5239, 1988

31. Boyce BF, Aufdemorte TB, Garrett IR, Yates AJP, Mundy GR: Effects of interleukin-1 on bone turnover in normal mice. *Endocrinology* 123:1142–1150, 1989

32. Pacifici R, Rifas L, McCracken R, et al.: Ovarian steroid treatment blocks a postmenopausal increase in blood monocyte interleukin-1 release. *Proc Natl Acad Sci* 86:2398–2402, 1989

33. Bertolini DR, Nedwin GE, Bringman TS, Mundy GR: Stimulation of bone resorption and inhibition of bone formation in vitro by human tumour necrosis factors. *Nature* 319:516–518, 1986

34. Johnson RA, Boyce BF, Mundy GR, Roodman GD: Tumors producing human TNF induce hypercalcemia and osteoclastic bone resorption in nude mice. *Endocrinology* 124:1424–1427, 1989

35. Thomson BM, Mundy GR, Chambers TJ: Tumor necrosis factors alpha and beta induce osteoblastic cells to stimulate osteoclastic bone resorption. *J Immunol* 138:775–779, 1987

36. Garrett IR, Durie BGM, Nedwin GE, et al.: Production of the bone resorbing cytokine lymphotoxin by cultured human myeloma cells. *N Engl J Med* 317:526–532, 1987

37. Tashjian AH Jr, Voelkel EF, Lazzaro M, et al.: Tumor necrosis factor-alpha (cachectin) stimulates bone resorption in mouse calvaria via a prostaglandin-mediated mechanism. *Endocrinology* 120:2029–2036, 1987

38. Felix R, Cecchini MG, Fleisch H: Macrophage colony stimulating factor restores in vivo bone resorption in the op/op osteopetrotic mouse. *Endocrinology* 127:2592–2594, 1990

39. Lee MY, Eyre DR, Osborne WRA: Isolation of a murine osteoclast colony-stimulating factor. *Proc Natl Acad Sci USA* 88:8500–8504, 1991

40. Yoneda T, Kato I, Bonewald LF, Chisoku H, Burgess WH, Mundy GR: A novel osteoclastpoietic peptide: Purification and characterization. *J Bone Miner Res* 6(suppl):454, 1991

41. Feyen JHM, Elford P, Dipadova FE, Trechsel U: Interleukin-6 is produced by bone and modulated by parathyroid hormone. *J Bone Miner Res* 4:633–638, 1989

42. Black K, Garrett IR, Mundy GR: Chinese hamster ovarian cells transfected with the murine interleukin-6 gene cause hypercalcemia as well as cachexia, leukocytosis and thrombocytosis in tumor-bearing nude mice. *Endocrinology* 128:2657–2659, 1991

43. Ishimi Y, Miyaura C, Jin CH, Akatsu T, Abe T, Nakamura Y, Yamaguchi M, Yoshiki S, Matsuda T, Hirano T, Kishimoto T, Suda T: IL-6 is produced by osteoblasts and induces bone resorption. *J Immunol* 145:3297–3303, 1990

44. Jilka RL, Hangoc G, Girasole G, Passeri G, Williams DC, Abrams JS, Boyce B, Broxmeyer H, Manolagas SC: Increased osteoclast development after estrogen loss—mediation by interleukin-6. *Science* 257:88–91, 1992

45. Gowen M, Mundy GR: Actions of recombinant interleukin-1, interleukin-2 and interferon gamma on bone resorption in vitro. *J Immunol* 136:2478–2482, 1986

46. Gowen M, Nedwin G, Mundy GR: Preferential inhibition of cytokine stimulated bone resorption by recombinant interferon gamma. *J Bone Miner Res* 1:469–474, 1986

47. Takahashi N, Mundy GR, Kuehl TJ, Roodman GD: Osteoclast like formation in fetal and newborn long term baboon marrow cultures is more sensitive to 1,25-dihydroxyvitamin D3 than adult long term marrow cultures. *J Bone Miner Res* 2:311–317, 1987

48. Chenu C, Pfeilschifter J, Mundy GR, Roodman GD: Transforming growth factor inhibits formation of osteoclast-like cells in long-term human marrow cultures. *Proc Natl Acad Sci* 85: 5683–5687, 1988

49. Noda M, Camilliere JJ: In vivo stimulation of bone formation by transforming growth factor-beta. *Endocrinology* 124:2991–2994, 1989

50. Tashjian AH Jr, Voelkel EF, Lloyd W, et al.: Actions of growth factors on plasma calcium. Epidermal growth factor and human transforming growth factor-alpha cause elevation of plasma calcium in mice. *J Clin Invest* 78:1405–1409, 1986

51. Fell HB, Mellanby E: The effect of hypervitaminosis A on embryonic limb bones cultured in vitro. *J Physiol* 116:320–349, 1952

52. Ibbotson KJ, D'Souza SM, Smith DD, Carpenter G, Mundy GR: EGF receptor antiserum inhibits bone resorbing activity produced by a rat Leydig cell tumor associated with the humoral hypercalcemia of malignancy. *Endocrinology* 116:469–471, 1985

53. Ibbotson KJ, Harrod J, Gowen M: Human recombinant transforming growth factor alpha stimulates bone resorption and inhibits formation in vitro. *Proc Natl Acad Sci* 83:2228–2232, 1986

54. Stern PH, Krieger NS, Nissenson RA, et al.: Human transforming growth factor alpha stimulates bone resorption in vitro. *J Clin Invest* 76:2016–2020, 1985

55. Takahashi N, MacDonald BR, Hon J, Winkler ME, Derynck R, Mundy GR, Roodman GD: Recombinant human transforming growth factor alpha stimulates the formation of osteoclast-like cells in long term human marrow cultures. *J Clin Invest* 78:894–898, 1986

56. Raisz LG, Niemann I: Effect of phosphate, calcium and magnesium on bone resorption and hormonal responses in tissue culture. *Endocrinology* 85:446–452, 1969

57. Tashjian AH, Voelkel EF, Levine L, et al.: Evidence that the bone resorption-stimulating factor produced by mouse fibrosarcoma cells is prostaglandin E2: A new model for the hypercalcemia of cancer. *J Exp Med* 136:1329–1343, 1972

58. Gallwitz WE, Mundy GR, Oreffo ROC, Gaskell SJ, Bonewald LF: Purification of osteoclastotropic factors produced by stromal cells: Identification of 5-lipoxygenase metabolites. *J Bone Miner Res* 6(suppl):457, 1991

59. Mundy GR, Shapiro JL, Bandelin JG, Canalis EM, Raisz LG: Direct stimulation of bone resorption by thyroid hormones. *J Clin Invest* 58:529–534, 1976

60. Mundy GR, Rick ME, Turcotte R, Kowalski MA: Pathogenesis of hypercalcemia in lymphosarcoma cell leukemia. Role of an osteoclast activating factor-like substance and mechanism of action for glucocorticoid therapy. *Am J Med* 65:600–606, 1978

61. Lindsay R, Hart DM, Forrest C, et al.: Prevention of spinal osteoporosis in oophorectomised women. *Lancet* 2:1151–1153, 1980

62. Oursler MJ, Osdoby P, Pyfferoen J, Riggs BL, Spelsberg TC: Avian osteoclasts as estrogen target cells. *Proc Natl Acad Sci USA* 88:6613–6617, 1991

63. Girasole G, Jilka RL, Passeri G, et al.: 17 beta-estradiol inhibits interleukin-6 production by bone marrow-derived stromal cells and osteoblasts in vitro—a potential mechanism for the antiosteoporotic effect of estrogens. *J Clin Invest* 89:883–891, 1992

64. Sato M, Grasser W, Endo N, Akins R, Simmons H, Thompson DD, Golub E, Rodan GA: Bisphosphonate action—Alendronate localization in rat bone and effects on osteoclast ultrastructure. *J Clin Invest* 88:2095–2105, 1991

65. Hughes DE, MacDonald BR, Russell RGG, Gowen M: Inhibition of osteoclast-like cell formation by bisphosphonates in long-term cultures of human bone marrow. *J Clin Invest* 83:1930–1935, 1989

66. Sahni M, Guenther HL, Fleisch H, Collin P, Martin TJ: Bisphosphonates act on rat bone resorption through the mediation of osteoblasts. *J Clin Invest* 91:2004–2011, 1993

67. Black LJ, Sato M, Rowley ER, Magee DE, Bekele A, Williams DC, Cullinan GJ, Bendele R, Kauffman RF, Bensch WR, Frolik CA, Termine JD, Bryant HU: Raloxifene (LY139481 HCl) prevents bone loss and reduces serum cholesterol without causing uterine hypertrophy in ovariectomized rats. *J Clin Invest* 93:63–69, 1994

4. Bone Matrix Proteins and the Mineralization Process

John D. Termine, Ph.D., and *Pamela Gehron Robey, Ph.D.

Lilly Research Laboratories, Eli Lilly and Company, Indianapolis, Indiana
Bone Research Branch, National Institutes of Health, Bethesda, Maryland

The largest proportion of the body's connective tissue mass is bone. It consists of extracellular matrix proteins and the cells that first make, then mineralize, and finally maintain them (1,2). Unlike other connective tissues, bone matrix is physiologically mineralized with small crystallites of a basic, carbonate-containing calcium phosphate called hydroxyapatite. In this regard, bone mineral most closely resembles a geological mineral crystalline form called dahlite. Further, the bone matrix is unique among connective tissues in that it is constantly regenerated throughout life as a consequence of bone turnover.

COLLAGEN

Some 85% to 90% of the total bone protein consists of collagen fibers made almost exclusively of type I collagen (unlike other tissues that contain fibers of mixed collagen types). Type I collagen is the most abundant form of collagen in the body and is widely distributed in connective tissue. Bone collagen fibers are highly insoluble as a result of many covalent intra- and intermolecular cross-links, the type and pattern of which differ from those in soft connective tissues (3). The basic building block of the bone matrix

fiber network is the type I collagen molecule, which is a triple-helical, coiled coil (a supercoil), containing two identical α1(I) chains and a structurally similar, but genetically different, α2(I) chain. The collagen coil can form because every third residue in each chain's helical domain (~1000 amino acids, or 300 nm in length) is glycine. This amino acid has no bulky side chain and conveys the ability to coil. Collagen chains also contain a high proportion of proline, a cyclic amino acid, most of which immediately follow glycine. The gly-X-Y repeating triplet (where X is often proline, and Y is often a modified form of proline) makes the collagen structure unique in biology (4).

All of the information necessary to fold into native molecules (see below) and then pack into fibrous protein resides in the primary sequence of the individual collagen chain. In the matrix, individual collagen molecules pack end to end with a short space (or gap) between them, and then pack laterally in a one-quarter-stagger array, so that each molecule is offset from its neighbor by approximately one fourth of its length. This three-dimensional arrangement constitutes the fiber structure found in the bone extracellular space.

The genes for the α1(I) and α2(I) chains of collagen are found on chromosomes 17 and 7, respectively (5). As in most genes, each consists of multiple small regions (called exons) that code for protein, interspersed by larger, noncoding DNA regions (introns). The messenger RNA for each collagen chain encodes a biosynthesized precursor procollagen chain, ~160,000 Da in size. Following removal of a short (~20-amino-acid residue) signal sequence, the procollagen chains consist of propeptide extensions at the amino and carboxy termini of ~25,000 and 35,000 Da, respectively, attached to a central region (a chain of ~100,000 Da). The carboxy-terminal propeptide facilitates molecular folding of the trimeric procollagen molecule, which is secreted in an unprocessed form. Either concomitant with, or subsequent to, secretion from the cell, the procollagen peptide extensions are removed as fiber formation occurs (6). These propeptide extensions seem to assist in fibril formation and eventually become entrapped, at least in part, in the final matrix of bone (7). The propeptide extensions of type I collagen can also escape to serum, where they have proved to be useful markers of bone formation (8). The preponderance of propeptide type I collagen extensions found in serum come from bone turnover. The propeptide extensions of type III collagen are often measured (along with those of type I) to correct for nonbone collagen synthesis (8). Such propeptide extension measurements have correlated significantly with direct histomorphometric measurements of bone formation (9).

Several posttranslational modifications of collagen occur during its biosynthesis and secretion. Intracellular modifications include hydroxylation of some proline and lysine residues, addition of galactose to certain hydroxylysines, and serine phosphorylation. Extracellular modifications include cleavage of the peptide extensions from the procollagen molecule by specific peptidases, and, after fibril formation, complexation with noncollagen proteins (see below) and cross-link formation. Intra- and intermolecular covalent cross-links are formed by lysyl oxidase action on collagen lysine and/or hydroxylysine residues (10,11). In bone, multiple cross-linking sites combine extracellularly to form pyridinium ring structures (the pyridinolines), tying several collagen monomer molecules together within the fiber, thereby rendering it completely insoluble (3). These pyridinium cross-links are released only on degradation of the mineralized collagen fibrils during bone resorption. Measurement of these ringed cross-link structures in urine have proved to be good measures of bone resorption (12).

NONCOLLAGENOUS PROTEINS

Noncollagenous proteins (NCPs) account for 10% to 15% of the total bone protein content. Approximately one fourth of the bone NCP is exogenously derived, being adsorbed or entrapped in the bone matrix space (13). This fraction is largely composed of serum-derived proteins that are acidic in character and become bound to the hydroxyapatite mineral of bone. Some of these proteins may be advantageous to the tissue. For example, trapped growth factors [e.g., platelet-derived growth factor (PDGF)] could easily contribute to the regeneration of bone upon injury (13). Other proteins, such as serum albumin, may be present merely adventitiously.

On a mole-to-mole basis, however, it can be calculated that the bone cell synthesizes and secretes as many molecules of NCP as it does of collagen. Remember, triple helical collagen has a molecular weight of over 300,000, whereas most bone NCPs are approximately one-tenth that size. Thus, a considerable portion (~50%) of the osteoblast's matrix-directed biosynthetic activities are devoted to NCP molecules. These can be broken down into four general groups of protein products: (i) proteoglycans, (ii) growth-related proteins, (iii) cell attachment proteins, and (iv) γ-carboxylated (gla) proteins. These classifications are often overlapping, and most of the physiologic roles for individual bone protein constituents remain undefined at present (Table 1).

Proteoglycans are macromolecules that contain acidic polysaccharide side chains (glycosaminoglycans) attached to a central core protein. In bone, two types of glycosaminoglycan are predominately found: chondroitin sulfate, a polymer of sulfated N-acetylgalactosamine and glucuronic acid, and heparan sulfate, a polymer of sulfated N-acetylglucosamine and glucuronic acid. The bone cell heparan sulfate proteoglycan product is membrane associated and, as for all connective tissues, probably facilitates interaction of the osteoblast with extracellular macromolecules (some of which are cell attachment proteins) and heparin-binding growth factors (14,15). During development, high levels of hyaluronan, an unsulfated glycosaminoglycan that is not attached to a protein core, are also found.

Chondroitin sulfate in bone is attached to three separate core proteins (15). One of these is approximately 300,000 Da in size (resultant proteoglycan, ~600 to 800 kDa) |and resembles a proteoglycan product synthesized by fibroblasts called *versican* (16). Its role is not yet understood, but it may be important in delineating areas that will become bone (17). The vast bulk of the glycosaminoglycans of bone are attached to two small (~40 kDa) core proteins that are composed of a leucine-rich repeat sequence. While they are very similar, they are separate gene products (18). *Decorin* has one attached 50,000-Da chondroitin sulfate chain and *biglycan* has two attached chains, based on their relative electrophoretic migration on sodium dodecyl sulfate gels (18). Decorin is found in all stages of bone development and biglycan is more abundant in developing (i.e., fetal or young) than in adult bone. Decorin is distributed predominantly in the extracellular matrix space of connective tissues, whereas biglycan tends to be found in pericellular locales (19). A similar developmental distribution for these two proteoglycans is found in other connective tissues (19). Decorin, so called because it binds to collagen fibrils, has been implicated in the regulation of collagen fibrillogenesis (reviewed in ref. 20). Although the exact physiologic functions of the small proteoglycans have not been definitively elucidated, they are generally assumed to be important for the integrity of most connective tissue matrices. One function might arise from their ability to bind and modulate the activity of transforming growth factor-β (TGF-β) family in the extracellular space (21,22). By this property, decorin and biglycan can influence cell proliferation and differentiation in a variety of connective tissues, including bone.

TABLE 1. *Stages of osteoblast maturation and their principal noncollagenous products*

Stage of maturation	Protein (M$_r$ kDa)	Chemical features	Potential function
Osteoprogenitors	Type I collagen (300,000)	[α1(I)$_2$α2(I)], RGD	Matrix organization
	Type III collagen (300 kDa)	[α1(III)]$_3$, disulfide bonds	Matrix organization
	Versican (~1 × 10^6)	360-kDa core with EGF-like sequences, 45-kDa CS chains	"Capture space" destined to become bone
Pre-osteoblasts	Collagen I, III, versican		
	Alkaline phosphatase (200–160 kDa)	Bone/liver/kidney isoforms, tissue-specific glycosylation, disulfide-bonded dimer	Hydrolyze phosphates, ion carrier protein
	Thrombospondin (~450 kDa)	Three identical disulfide-bonded subunits of ~150 kDa, RGD	Cell attachment, growth factor binding
	Matrix gla protein (19 kDa)	Gla residues	Unknown
	Decorin (~160 kDa)	~40-kDa core with leucine repeats, 50-kDa CS chains	Collagen fibril diameter, binds to TGF-β
Osteoblasts	Alkaline phosphatase, thrombospondin, decorin		
	Fibronectin (~400 kDa)	Two non-identical disulfide-bonded subunits of ~200 KD, RGD	Major protein in serum, cell attachment
	Osteonectin (~45 kDa)	Glycosylated, phosphorylated, EF hand structure	High and low affinity Ca^{2+}-binding, apatite binding, matrix protein binding
	Biglycan (~280 kDa)	~40-kDa core with leucine repeats, 50-kDa CS chains	Pericellular environment, growth factor binding
	Osteopontin (~90–45 kDa)	Glycosylated, phosphorylated, RGD	Cell proliferation, cell attachment
	Bone sialoprotein (~85 kDa)	Heavily glycosylated (50%), sulfated, RGD	Cell attachment, marker of mineralization
	Type I collagen (only)	Different posttranslational modifications (gal-hyl cross-links, phosphorylation of N-propeptide), RGD	May orient nucleators of matrix mineralization
Osteocytes	Fibronectin, biglycan		
	Osteocalcin (5800)	Gla-residues, one disulfide bridge	Binds Ca^{2+}, marker of bone turnover

The proteins listed for each stage of maturation do not exist only in that stage, but they are maximally detected at that point in maturation (see Chapter 6). M$_r$, molecular weight; RGD, Arg-Gly-Asn cell attachment consensus sequence; CS, chondroitin sulfate.

Other bone cell products (primarily glycoproteins that are differentially, posttranslationally modified) may be associated with the growth and/or differentiation of the osteoblast in an indirect or as yet undefined fashion. One of the hallmarks of the osteoblast phenotype is the synthesis of high levels of *alkaline phosphatase* (23). This enzyme is first found on the osteoblast plasmalemma, and some may be cleaved from the cell surface and adsorbed within the mineralized bone matrix space. The function of alkaline phosphatase in bone cell biology has been the subject of much speculation, but it remains undefined to the present day.

The most abundant NCP produced by bone cells is *osteonectin,* a phosphorylated glycoprotein accounting for approximately 2% of the total protein of developing bone in most animal species. The protein has high affinity for binding ionic calcium and physiologic hydroxyapatite (24). It also binds to collagen (24) and thrombospondin (25). Osteonectin protein is found in platelets (26) and in nonbone tissues that are rapidly proliferating, remodeling, or undergoing profound changes in tissue architecture (27,28). Thus, the protein is associated with growing tissue, and in nonbone systems, its transcription and synthesis are down-regu-

lated under steady-state conditions. Osteonectin biosynthesis is up-regulated, again in nonbone systems, during wound repair, and in some conditions of cell culture. Its function(s) in bone may be multiple, with potential association with osteoblast growth and/or proliferation, as well as with matrix mineralization (see below). Using synthetic peptides specific for parts of the osteonectin molecule, a number of different activities have been identified (primarily in endothelial cells), such as binding to PDGF-AB, cell cycle regulation, and modulation of shape change (reviewed in ref. 29). However, it is not known if the effects of these synthetic peptides (taken out of the context of the entire molecule) also pertain to cells in the osteoblastic lineage.

All connective tissue cells interact with their extracellular environment in response to chemical stimuli that direct or coordinate specific cell functions, such as proliferation, migration, and differentiation. These particular interactions involve cell attachment and spreading, via transient, focal adhesions to extracellular macromolecules. This is done via the integrin family of cell surface receptors that transduce signals to the cytoskeleton (30). Bone cells synthesize at least six proteins that affect cell attachment: type I collagen;

fibronectin; thrombospondin; and low levels of vitronectin (Dunlay, Grzesik, and Gehron Robey, *unpublished results*), osteopontin, bone sialoprotein (31–33), and most likely BAG-75 (34). Three of these *(thrombospondin, osteopontin, and bone sialoprotein)* are strong binders of ionic calcium and are found in the mineralized bone extracellular space (1,2). Osteopontin is a phosphoprotein that, like fibronectin and thrombospondin, is found also in nonbone tissue systems (35). Bone sialoprotein is almost exclusively found in the skeleton (36), and its appearance is tightly correlated with the appearance of mineral (37). Both osteopontin and bone sialoprotein bind Ca^{2+} via polyacidic amino acid sequences, and both are known to anchor osteoclasts to the bone extracellular space in cell regions called clear zones (36,38). Specific extracellular matrix receptors called integrins bind to these molecules allowing the osteoclasts to first form ruffled borders and then resorb bone (39).

Vitamin K–dependent γ-carboxylation occurs on three bone NCPs: *osteocalcin* (bone gla-protein) and *matrix gla-protein* (MGP), which are both made by bone cells (40), and protein S, which is made primarily in the liver (41). Dicarboxylic glutamyl (gla) residues also occur in blood-clotting proteins, where enhanced calcium binding to gla side chains is important to the bioactivity of these molecules. Osteocalcin (~6 kDa) is somewhat bone specific, although the related mRNA has been found in platelets and megakaryocytes (42), whereas MGP (~9 kDa) is found also in cartilage (40). In human bone, osteocalcin is concentrated in osteocytes (43) and its release may provide a signal in the bone turnover cascade (44). Osteocalcin and MGP are partially homologous structurally (40), but it is as yet unclear how they function physiologically, either together or separately in bone tissue. Nevertheless, determination of osteocalcin in serum has proved valuable as a marker of bone turnover in metabolic disease states (45).

A number of proteins in bone appear to be associated with the life cycle and function of the osteoblast. These proteins may be *morphogens* (46), growth factors such as TGF-β1 through -β5 and insulin-like growth factors, osteoblast secretion products that can stimulate osteoblast cell growth in an autocrine or paracrine fashion (47,48). Thus, the growth potential of a bone cell may result from its own genetic activity and may involve transcription of both factors and their receptors in the same cell population.

MINERALIZATION

Two mechanisms for bone mineralization have been described, one that predominates in both calcified cartilage and primitive woven bone, the other in lamellar bone (49–52). In some instances, calcified cartilage and woven bone seem to mineralize via matrix vesicles (49), membrane-bound bodies that exocytose from the plasma membrane and migrate to the loose extracellular matrix space. The lipid-rich inner membrane of these vesicles becomes the nidus for hydroxyapatite crystal formation, and eventually crystallization proceeds to the point of obliteration of the vesicle membrane, producing a spherulite of clustered, small (50Å × 200Å × 400Å) crystals. In this context, the matrix vesicle is on a suicide mission, and its "death" leads to mineral encrustation. Recent studies indicate that osteoblasts secrete matrix

components that have been preorganized within the cell, and, upon secretion, these packets of matrix proteins (including bone sialoprotein) become mineralized immediately (37). These spherulites conglomerate until a continuous mineralized mass is achieved throughout the matrix space. The driving force for this mineral cascade, once initiated, seems to be the mineral crystals themselves that are first associated with the matrix vesicle membrane. The rate of mineralization in both woven and (see below) lamellar bone seems to depend on the presence of inhibitor molecules (e.g., pyrophosphate and acidic NCPs), which in solution seem to regulate the kinetics of the mineralization process (50). Thus, in this type of calcification, the cell buds off organelles capable of mineral accumulation and then synthesizes proteins that can control the rate at which crystallization proceeds.

The extracellular matrix in nonfetal and more abundant lamellar bone is tightly packed with well-aligned collagen fibrils that are "decorated" with complexed NCPs (e.g., proteoglycan and osteonectin). Either because there is simply insufficient space for them or for developmental reasons, matrix vesicles are rarely (if ever) seen in lamellar bone. Instead, mineralization proceeds in association with the heteropolymeric (collagen–NCP complex) matrix fibrils themselves. Somewhat more mineral appears associated with aligned gap regions (or "hole" zones) of the fibers (three-dimensional channels resulting from the spaces between longitudinally associated collagen monomers), which have more room for inorganic ions that the rest of the fibril structure. Other loci for the bone mineral appear to be between the collagen fibrils in a brick-and-mortar fashion (51). It is unlikely that the driving force for mineralization is bone collagen, because purified collagen appears to be a poor initiator of crystal deposition. Consequently, it is probable that the NCPs are responsible for this process. The extent of mineralization in the bone matrix space appears limited by the volume of bone occupied by its insoluble organic fibrous protein content alone. Decreased mineralization seems to occur under conditions of mineral ion deprivation, such as osteomalacia, and is fully reversible by increasing the pool of ions available for this purpose.

REFERENCES

1. Gehron Robey P, Bianco P, Termine JD: The cellular biology and molecular biochemistry of bone formation. In: Coe FL, Favus MJ (eds) *Disorders of Mineral Metabolism*. Raven Press, New York, pp 241–263, 1992
2. Gehron Robey P, Boskey AL: The biochemistry of bone. In: Marcus RA, Feldman D, Kelsey J (eds) *Osteoporosis*. Academic Press, New York, 95–183, 1996
3. Eyre DR, Dickson IR, Van Ness K: Collagen cross-linking in human bone and articular cartilage. Age-related changes in the content of mature hydroxypyridinium residues. *Biochem J* 252: 495–500, 1988
4. Hulmes DJ: The collagen superfamily—diverse structures and assemblies. *Essays Biochem* 27:49–67, 1992
5. Vuorio E, de Crombrugghe B: The family of collagen genes. *Annu Rev Biochem* 59:837–872, 1990
6. Fleischmajer R, Perlish JS, Olsen BR: Amino and carboxyl propeptides in bone collagen fibrils during embryogenesis. *Cell Tissue Res* 247:105–109, 1987
7. Fisher LW, Gehron Robey P, Tuross N, Otsuka A, Tepen DA, Esch FS, Shimasaki S, Termine JD: The M_r 24,000 phosphoprotein from developing bone is the NH_2-terminal propeptide of the α1 chain of type I collagen. *J Biol Chem* 262:13457–13463, 1987

8. Krane SM, Munoz AJ, Harris ED: Urinary polypeptides related to collagen synthesis. *J Clin Invest* 49:716–720, 1970

9. Parfitt AM, Simon LS, Villanueva AR, Krane SM: Procollagen type I carboxy-terminal extension peptide in serum as a marker of collagen biosynthesis in bone. Correlation with iliac bone formation rates and comparison with total alkaline phosphatase. *J Bone Miner Res* 2:427–436, 1987

10. Yamauchi M, Katz EP, Mechanic GL: Intermolecular cross-linking and stereospecific molecular packing in type I collagen fibrils of the periodontal ligament. *Biochemistry* 25:4907–4913, 1986

11. Robins SP, Duncan A: Pyridinium cross-links of bone collagen and location in peptides isolated from rat femur. *Biochim Biophys Acta* 914:233–239, 1987

12. Uebelhart D, Gineyts E, Chapuy M-C, Delmas PD: Urinary excretion of pyridinium cross-links; a new marker of bone resorption in metabolic bone disease. *Bone Miner* 8:87–96, 1990

13. Termine JD: Non-collagen proteins in bone. In: Evered D, Harnett S (eds) *Cell and Molecular Biology of Vertebrate Hard Tissues.* Ciba Foundation Synposium 136. John Wiley and Sons, Chichester, pp 178–190, 1988

14. Hook M, Woods A, Johansson S, Kjellen L, Couchman Jr: Functions of proteoglycans at the cell surface. In: Evered E, Whelan J (eds) *Functions of the Proteoglycans.* Ciba Foundation Symposium 124. John Wiley and Sons, Chichester, pp 143–156, 1986

15. Beresford JN, Fedarko NS, Fisher LW, Midura RJ, Yanagishita M, Termine JD, Gehron Robey P: Analysis of the proteoglycans synthesized by human bone cells in vitro. *J Biol Chem* 262: 17164–17172, 1987

16. Krusius T, Gehlsen KR, Ruoslahti E: A fibroblast chondroitin sulfate proteoglycan core protein contains lectin-like and growth factor-like sequences. *J Biol Chem* 262:13120–13125, 1987

17. Fisher LW: The nature of the proteoglycans of bone, In: Butler WT (ed) *The Chemistry and Biology of Mineralized Tissues.* EBSCO Media, Birmingham, AL, pp 188–196, 1985.

18. Fisher LW, Hawkins GR, Tuross N, Termine JD: Purification and partial characterization of small proteoglycans I and II, bone sialoproteins I and II and osteonectin from the mineral compartment of developing human bone. *J Biol Chem* 262:9702–9708, 1987

19. Bianco P, Fisher LW, Young MF, Termine JD, Gehron Robey P: Expression and localization of the two small proteoglycans biglycan and decorin in developing human skeletal and nonskeletal tissues. *J Histochem Cytochem* 38:1549–1563, 1990

20. Ruoslahti E: Structure and biology of proteoglycans. *Annu Rev Cell Biol* 4:229–255, 1988

21. Yamaguchi Y, Mann DM, Rouslahti E: Negative regulation of transforming growth factor-β by the proteoglycan decorin. *Nature* 346:281–284, 1990.

22. Takeuchi Y, Kodama Y, Matsumoto T: Bone matrix decorin binds transforming growth factor-β and enhances its bioactivity. *J Biol Chem* 51:32634–32638, 1994.

23. Rodan GA, Heath JK, Yoon K, Noda M, Rodan SB: Diversity of the osteoblast phenotype. In: Evered D, Harnett S (eds) *Cell and Molecular Biology of Vertebrate Hard Tissues.* Ciba Foundation Symposium 136. John Wiley and Sons, Chichester, pp 78–85, 1988

24. Termine JD, Kleinman HK, Whitson SW, Conn KM, McGarvey ML, Martin GR: Osteonectin, a bone-specific protein linking mineral to collagen. *Cell* 26:99–105, 1981

25. Clezardin P, Malaval L, Ehrensperger AS, Delmas P, Dechavanne M, McGregor JL: Complex formation of human thrombospondin with osteonectin. *Eur J Biochem* 175:275–284, 1988

26. Stenner DD, Tracy RP, Riggs BL, Mann KG: Human platelets contain and secrete osteonectin, a major protein of mineralized bone. *Proc Natl Acad Sci USA* 83:6892–6896, 1986

27. Holland PWH, Harper SJ, McVey JH, Hogan BLM: In vivo expression of mRNA for the Ca^{+2}-binding protein SPARC (osteonectin) revealed by in situ hybridization. *J Cell Biol* 105:473–482, 1987

28. Wewer UM, Albrechtsen R, Fisher LW, Young MF, Termine JD: Osteonectin/SPARC/BM-40 in human decidua and carcinoma, tissues characterized by de novo formation of basement membrane. *Am J Pathol* 132:345–355, 1988

29. Lane TF, Sage EH: The biology of SPARC, a protein that modulates cell–matrix interactions. *FASEB J* 8:163–73, 1994.

30. Ruoslahti E, Pierschbacher MD: New perspectives in cell adhesion: RGD and integrins. *Science* 238:491–497, 1987

31. Gehron Robey P, Young MF, Fisher LW, McClain TD: Thrombospondin is an osteoblast-derived component of mineralized extracellular matrix. *J Cell Biol* 108:719–727, 1988

32. Somerman MJ, Fisher LW, Foster RA, Sauk JJ: Human bone sialoprotein I and II enhance fibroblast attachment in vitro. *Calcif Tissue Int* 43:50–53, 1988

33. Grzesik WJ, Gehron Robey P: Bone matrix RGD glycoproteins: immunolocalization and interaction with human primary osteoblastic bone cells in vitro. *J Bone Miner Res* 9:487–496, 1994

34. Gorski JP: Acidic phosphoproteins from bone matrix: a structural rationalization of their role in biomineralization. *Calcif Tissue Int* 50:391–396, 1992

35. Mark MP, Prince CW, Gay S, Austin RL, Butler WT: 44kDal bone phosphoprotein (osteopontin) antigenicity at ectopic sites in newborn rats: kidney and nervous tissues. *Cell Tissue Res* 251:23–30, 1988

36. Bianco P, Fisher LW, Young MF, Termine JD, Gehron Robey P: Expression of bone sialoprotein (BSP) in developing human tissues. *Calcif Tissue Int* 49:421–426, 1991

37. Bianco P, Riminucci M, Silvestrini G, Bonucci E, Termine JD, Fisher LW, Gehron Robey P: Localization of bone sialoprotein (BSP) to golgi and post-golgi secretory structures in osteoblasts and to discrete sites in early bone matrix. *J Histochem Cytochem* 41:193–203, 1993

38. Reinholt FP, Hultenby K, Oldberg A, Heinegard D: Osteopontin—A possible anchor osteoclasts to bone. *Proc Natl Acad Sci USA* 87:4473–4475, 1990

39. Zambonin-Zallone A, Teti A, Grano M, Rubinacci A, Abbadini M, Gaboli M, Marchisio: Immunocytochemical distribution of extracellular matrix receptors in human osteoclasts; a β$_3$ integrin is co-localized with vinculin and talin in the podosomes of osteoclastoma giant cells. *Exp Cell Res* 182:645–652, 1989

40. Price PA: Vitamin K-dependent bone proteins. In: Cohn DV, Martin TJ, Meunier PJ (eds) *Calcium Regulation and Bone Metabolism: Basic and Clinical Aspects,* vol 9. Elsevier Science, Amsterdam, pp 419–425, 1987

41. Maillard C, Berruyer M, Serre CM, Dechavane M, Delmas PD: Protein S, a vitamin K-dependent protein, is a bone matrix component synthesized and secreted by osteoblasts. *Endocrinology* 130:1599–1604, 1992

42. Thiede MA, Smock SL, Petersen DN, Grasser WA, Thompson DD, Nishimoto SK: Presence of messenger ribonucleic acid encoding osteocalcin, a marker of bone turnover, in bone marrow megakaryocytes and peripheral blood platelets. *Endocrinology* 135:929–937, 1994

43. Kasai R, Bianco, P, Gehron Robey P, Kahn AJ: Production and characterization of an antibody against the human bone GLA protein (BGP/osteocalcin) propeptide and its use in immunocytochemistry of bone cells. *Bone Miner* 25:167–182, 1994

44. Glowacki J, Lian JB: Impaired recruitment of osteoclast progenitors by osteocalcin-deficient bone implants. In: Butler WT (ed) *The Chemistry and Biology of Mineralized Tissues.* EBSCO Media, Birmingham, AL, pp 164–169, 1985

45. Price PA, Parthemore JG, Deftos LJ: New biochemical marker for bone metabolism. *J Clin Invest* 66:878–883, 1980

46. Wozney JP: Bone morphogenetic proteins and their gene expression. In: *Cellular Molecular Biology of Bone*, Academic Press, New York, pp 131–168, 1993

47. Gehron Robey P, Young MF, Flanders KC, Roche NS, Kondaiah P, Reddi AH, Termine JD, Sporn MB, Roberts AB: Osteoblasts synthesize and respond to TGF-beta in vitro. *J Cell Biol* 105:457–463, 1987

48. Canalis E, McCarthy T, Centrella M: Isolation and characterization of insulin-like growth factor I (somatomedin C) from cultures of fetal rat calvariae. *Endocrinology* 122:22–27, 1988

49. Bonucci E: The locus of initial calcification in cartilage and bone. *Clin Orthop* 78:108–139, 1971

50. Glimcher MJ: The nature of the mineral component of bone and the mechanism of calcification. In: Coe FL, Favus MJ (eds) *Disorders of Bone and Mineral Metabolism.* Raven Press, New York, pp 265–286, 1992

51. Termine JD, Eanes ED, Conn KM: Phosphoprotein modulation of apatite crystallization. *Calcif Tissue Int* 31:247–251, 1980

52. Weiner S, Traub W: Organization of hydroxyapatite crystals within collagen fibrils. *FEBS Lett* 206:262–266, 1986

5. Regulation of Bone Remodeling

Ernesto Canalis, M.D.

Department of Research, The University of Connecticut and St. Francis Hospital and Medical Center,
Hartford, Connecticut

Bone remodeling is a complex process involving a number of cellular functions directed toward the coordinated resorption and formation of new bone. Bone remodeling is regulated by systemic hormones and by local factors, which affect cells of the osteoclast or osteoblast lineage and exert their effects on (i) the replication of undifferentiated cells, (ii) the recruitment of cells, and (iii) the differentiated function of cells. The endproduct of remodeling is the maintenance of a mineralized bone matrix, and the major organic component of this matrix is collagen. Bone metabolism is regulated by polypeptide, steroid, and thyroid hormones, as well as by local factors, which play a direct and important role in bone remodeling (see Tables 1,2) (1,2). The local factors are synthesized by skeletal cells and include growth factors, cytokines, and prostaglandins. Growth factors are polypeptides that regulate the replication and differentiated function of cells. Growth factors have effects on cells of the same class (autocrine factors) or on cells of another class within the tissue (paracrine factors). Prostaglandins are currently the only known local regulators of bone remodeling that do not have a polypeptide structure. The presence of local factors is not unique to the skeletal system, because nonskeletal tissues also synthesize and respond to autocrine and paracrine growth factors. Growth factors also are present in the circulation and may act as systemic regulators of skeletal and nonskeletal metabolism, but the locally produced factor has a more direct and possibly important function in cell growth. Circulating hormones may act on skeletal cells either directly or indirectly, modulating the synthesis, activation, receptor binding, and binding proteins of a local growth factor, which in turn stimulates or inhibits bone formation or bone resorption. It is likely that hormones are important in the targeting of growth factors to tissues expressing specific hormonal receptors. Growth factors may play a critical role in the coupling of bone formation to bone resorption, and possibly in the pathophysiology of bone disorders.

Bone remodeling occurs in small packets of cells called basic multicellular units (BMUs), which turn bone over in multiple bone surfaces (3). This bone remodeling is likely modulated by local cytokines, it is more active near the marrow cavity, and it occurs in cycles. A change in a single remodeling cycle does not result in a change in bone mass. A bone remodeling transient is a series of cellular events that occurs when there is a change in the remodeling rate, and that persists for only one remodeling cycle (4). Consequently, it does not involve changes in the ultimate balance between bone formation and bone resorption at a site. This concept has clinical relevance, because drugs affecting bone remodeling in the first cycle of the process do not necessarily cause a permanent change in bone mass.

HORMONAL REGULATION OF BONE REMODELING

Bone metabolism is regulated by a variety of systemic hormones that act on bone-forming and bone-resorbing cells (Table 1) (Fig. 1).

Polypeptide Hormones

Parathyroid Hormone and Calcitonin

Parathyroid hormone (PTH) is a polypeptide with a molecular weight (MW) of 9500. It stimulates bone resorption, although the effect is not direct because the osteoclast does not respond to PTH, and the presence of osteoblasts or osteoblast-derived factors is necessary to observe its resorptive action. PTH has complex effects on bone formation, and it can stimulate and inhibit bone collagen and matrix synthesis (5,6). Continuous treatment with PTH results in an inhibition of bone formation *in vitro*. This effect results from a direct inhibition of bone collagen synthesis by PTH occurring at the transcriptional level. In contrast, intermittent treatment with PTH results in a stimulation of bone collagen synthesis and bone formation. The anabolic effect of PTH appears to be mediated at least in part by an increased synthesis or release of local factors such as insulin-like growth factor (IGF)-I and possibly transforming growth factor-β (TGF-β) (5,6). The stimulation of skeletal IGF-I synthesis results from an increase in cyclic adenosine monophosphate (cAMP), and other inducers of cAMP mimic the effect of PTH on IGF-I production (7). PTH also has a mitogenic effect on bone, although the exact cells affected have not been defined, and the response is not mediated by IGF-I. The dual role of PTH, stimulating bone resorption and bone formation, should not be a surprise, because these processes are coupled, and it is possible that specific growth factors, such as IGF-I, are important in the coupling of bone formation and bone resorption. The effect of PTH *in vivo* also is complex, and when the hormone is administered intermittently, an anabolic effect is observed. Patients with hyperparathyroidism display osteopenia primarily in cortical and not in trabecular bone.

Calcitonin (CT), a 32-amino-acid polypeptide with an MW of 3000, is known to inhibit bone resorption, but it does not modify bone formation. Most of the actions of CT have been observed at a relatively high dose, and this peptide may be more important as a pharmacologic than physiologic hormone.

Insulin

Insulin is a polypeptide with an MW of 6000 synthesized by the beta cells of the pancreas. Insulin does not regulate

TABLE 1. *Hormones that regulate bone remodeling*

Polypeptide hormones
  Parathyroid hormone (PTH)
  Calcitonin (CT)
  Insulin
  Growth hormone (GH)
Steroid hormones
  1,25-Dihydroxyvitamin D_3 [1,25(OH)$_2$D$_3$]
  Glucocorticoids
  Sex steroids
Thyroid hormones

bone resorption, but it causes a marked stimulation of bone matrix synthesis and cartilage formation, making it among the most important systemic hormones modulating normal skeletal growth (8). In addition, insulin is necessary for normal bone mineralization, and individuals and experimental animals with untreated diabetes mellitus have impaired skeletal growth and mineralization. Insulin has direct stimulatory effects on the skeletal tissue, but it also increases IGF-I production by the liver; therefore, some of its *in vivo* effects could be mediated by IGF-I. Insulin stimulates bone matrix synthesis, but at physiologic concentrations it does not alter bone cell replication. The stimulatory effect of insulin on matrix synthesis is a result of its actions on the differentiated function of the osteoblast, rather than a result of an increase in the number of collagen-producing cells (8). Proinsulin is 100-fold less potent than insulin in stimulating bone collagen synthesis, and C-peptide does not modify this process. The actions of insulin and IGF-I are somewhat different, because, in addition to its effects on osteoblast differentiated function, IGF increases the number of bone-matrix-synthesizing cells.

Growth Hormone

Growth hormone (GH), a pituitary polypeptide with an MW of 21,000, does not have direct effects on bone resorption, and its direct stimulatory actions on bone formation are of a modest magnitude. Growth hormone causes a small stimulation of IGF-I production by skeletal cells and through this local factor GH may regulate bone formation (9). The direct effect of GH on bone formation is limited. Less controversial is the stimulatory effect of GH on bone formation *in vivo*, and GH is necessary for the maintenance of normal bone mass (10). This is substantiated by clinical studies demonstrating that patients with GH deficiency have decreased bone mass, which is restored by treatment with GH. The effect of GH *in vivo* is secondary to an increase in IGF-I production by the liver, and IGF-I is likely responsible for the anabolic actions of GH on the musculoskeletal system. In addition, GH increases calcium absorption in the gastrointestinal tract; this action is mediated by an increase in 1,25-dihydroxyvitamin D_3 [1,25(OH)$_2$D$_3$] production and may be important for normal bone mineralization.

Steroids

Vitamin D

1,25-Dihydroxyvitamin D_3, a hormone synthesized primarily but not exclusively by the kidney, has functions similar to those of PTH. The most critical action of vitamin D is the stimulation of calcium absorption in the gastrointestinal tract, and it is necessary for normal bone mineralization. 1,25(OH)$_2$D$_3$ stimulates bone resorption and has complex effects on bone formation (11). Whereas 1,25(OH)$_2$D$_3$ is essential for normal growth and bone mineralization, it does not stimulate bone formation directly: it enhances the synthesis of osteocalcin (bone gla protein), a peptide known to be exclusively synthesized by the osteoblast, indicating that 1,25(OH)$_2$D$_3$ has direct stimulatory effects on this cell (12). Although osteocalcin is expressed by the osteoblast, its exact role in bone remodeling is not known. The complex effects of 1,25(OH)$_2$D$_3$ on bone formation may be related to a variety of actions of this steroid. It directly inhibits bone collagen synthesis, but it increases the binding of IGF-I to its receptor in cells of the osteoblastic lineage. 1,25(OH)$_2$D$_3$ also stimulates the synthesis of selected IGF binding proteins, which may modify IGF actions and concentrations (13). In addition to 1,25(OH)$_2$D$_3$, other metabolites of vitamin D_3 may play a more important role in bone formation.

Glucocorticoids

Glucocorticoids are steroid hormones that have marked effects on bone and mineral metabolism (14). Glucocorticoids stimulate bone resorption *in vivo*, possibly because they decrease calcium absorption, with a subsequent increase in PTH secretion. This may result in continuous exposure of bone tissue to high levels of PTH. However, when bone tissue is exposed directly to glucocorticoids, these steroids have direct inhibitory effects on bone resorption (15). The actions of glucocorticoids on bone formation are complex. Although glucocorticoids induce the differentiation of cells of the osteoblastic lineage, their long-term effects on bone remodeling are the result of an inhibition of bone resorption and formation. This seems to be secondary to multiple and diverse effects. Glucocorticoids decrease the replication of bone cells, reducing the number of bone-forming and bone-resorbing cells (16). Glucocorticoids also affect genes that are central to the function of the osteoblast. They decrease type I collagen expression by transcriptional and posttranscriptional mechanisms, and they increase the expression of matrix metalloproteinase (MMP)-13 or interstitial collagenase 3 by posttranscriptional mechanisms (17).

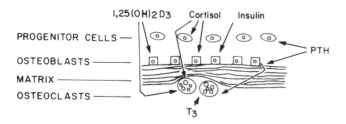

FIG. 1. Regulation of bone formation and bone resorption by hormones.

Because type I collagen is the major component of the bone matrix and MMP-13 is a protease essential for collagen degradation, these two actions of glucocorticoids result in decreased bone collagen and matrix.

Glucocorticoids have additional indirect effects on bone formation and alter the synthesis and activity of skeletal growth factors (14). Glucocorticoids have profound effects on the IGF axis in osteoblasts (18). They inhibit IGF-I synthesis, IGF-II receptor number, and the expression of IGF binding proteins (IGFBP)-2 through -5, and they enhance IGFBP-1 and -6 expression. Glucocorticoids activate TGF-β and shift its binding from signal-transducing to non-signal-transducing receptors (19). As a result of this effect, they inhibit the actions of TGF-β on bone cell replication and collagen synthesis. The effects of glucocorticoids on cell replication, collagen, and skeletal growth factors probably play a role in their inhibitory actions on bone mass and the pathogenesis of osteoporosis.

Sex Steroids

Estrogens and androgens are important in the skeletal maturation of growing individuals and in the prevention of bone loss. Estrogen receptors are expressed at a low level by bone cells; consequently, it is difficult to demonstrate direct effects of estrogens on bone formation or bone resorption. *In vivo,* estrogens decrease bone resorption and by doing so they prevent bone loss, but their actions may be indirect. Recently, estrogens have been shown to decrease the synthesis of cytokines, such as interleukin-1 and -6, which are present in the bone microenvironment and play a role in the stimulation of bone resorption (20,21). The inhibition of their synthesis may be important in the mechanism of action of estrogens decreasing bone resorption. Less compelling is the evidence for a stimulatory effect of estrogens on bone formation, and patients on estrogens stabilize, but do not increase their bone mass.

Thyroid Hormones

Thyroid hormones are necessary for normal growth and development, acting primarily on cartilage formation, possibly in conjunction with IGF-I. In contrast to their important role on cartilage and linear growth, thyroid hormones do not stimulate bone matrix synthesis or cell replication; they do, however, stimulate bone resorption. This effect has clinical consequences: hyperthyroid patients may have hypercalcemia and postmenopausal patients on chronic thyroid suppression may be prone to develop osteoporosis (22,23).

LOCAL REGULATION OF BONE REMODELING

Bone is a rich source of growth factors with important actions in the regulation of bone formation and bone resorption (Table 2) (Fig. 2). Frequently, these local factors are synthesized by skeletal cells, although some cytokines are secreted by stromal cells and by cells of the immune or hematological system, and as such they are present in the bone microenvironment (24).

TABLE 2. *Skeletal growth factors*

Insulin-like growth factors (IGF)

Transforming growth factor-β (TGF-β) family of peptides, including selected bone morphogenetic proteins (BMPs)

Fibroblast growth factors (FGF), or heparin-binding growth factors

Platelet-derived growth factors (PDGF)

Selected cytokines of the interleukin (IL), tumor necrosis factor (TNF), and colony-stimulating factor (CSF) families

Polypeptide Growth Factors

Insulin-like Growth Factors

IGFs are polypeptides with an MW of 7600 (25). Two IGFs have been characterized, IGF-I and IGF-II. These peptides are present in the systemic circulation and are synthesized by multiple tissues, including bone, where they act as local regulators of cell metabolism. Systemic IGF-I is secreted by the liver, and its synthesis is growth-hormone dependent, whereas the synthesis of IGF-I in peripheral tissues is regulated by diverse hormones (13,25). In the circulation, IGFs are bound to IGFBPs and to an acid-labile subunit (25). The most abundant IGFBP in serum is IGFBP-3, which also is growth-hormone dependent. Cells that secrete IGF also synthesize IGFBPs, and the expression of IGFBPs varies with the cell type.

IGF-I and -II have similar biologic activities, although in bone IGF-I is 4 to 7 times more potent than IGF-II (26). However, IGF-II is present in bone at higher concentrations than IGF-I. IGFs may act on the skeleton as systemic agents, but local IGFs have a direct and probably more significant effect on this tissue. *In vitro,* IGF enhances bone collagen and matrix synthesis and stimulates the replication of cells of the osteoblast lineage (27). The effect of IGF-I on matrix synthesis is in part dependent on an increased number of cells, but IGF-I directly modulates the differentiated function of the osteoblast. IGF-I increases type I collagen transcription and it decreases the transcription of MMP-13, a collagen-degrading protease (28). As a consequence of a decrease in MMP-13 levels, IGF-I inhibits bone collagen degradation. This dual effect, an increase in collagen syn-

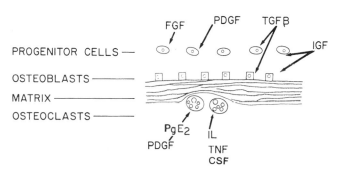

FIG. 2. Regulation of bone formation and bone resorption by growth factors and cytokines.

thesis and a decrease in its degradation, is central to the maintenance of bone matrix and bone mass. Short-term infusions of IGF-I to humans cause a generalized anabolic effect and an increase in bone remodeling (29). In view of the significant effects of IGF-I on bone cell function, it is likely that it plays a fundamental role in the process of bone formation and in the maintenance of bone mass.

IGFs can be modified by changes in their synthesis, receptor binding, and binding proteins (Table 3). The synthesis of skeletal IGF-I is regulated by hormones and growth factors, whereas the synthesis of IGF-II is regulated by growth factors and not by hormones (30,31). PTH and other agents that stimulate cAMP in bone cells, such as prostaglandin E_2, are the major stimulators of IGF-I synthesis (7). In contrast, GH plays a modest role in enhancing IGF-I production in bone. Glucocorticoids inhibit skeletal IGF-I synthesis, and this may be important in the mechanism of glucocorticoid action in bone (18). Skeletal growth factors with mitogenic properties, such as TGF-β, fibroblast growth factor (FGF), and platelet-derived growth factor (PDGF), inhibit the synthesis of IGF-I and -II by the osteoblast (30,31). This effect correlates with a decrease in the differentiated function of the osteoblast. Glucocorticoids inhibit IGF-II receptor synthesis, but the function of the IGF-II receptor is not completely understood: it may behave more as a binding protein, and store IGF-II, than as a signal-transducing receptor. Bone cells also secrete the six known IGFBPs, termed IGFBP-1 through -6. The precise role of the IGFBPs is not understood; they may prolong the half-life of IGF, neutralize or enhance its biologic activity, or be involved in the transport of IGF to its target cells. Some binding proteins, like IGFBP-4, have inhibitory activity. In contrast, IGFBP-5 stimulates bone cell growth and enhances the effects of IGF-I (13). The regulation of IGFBP synthesis in bone cells is complex. Selected IGFBPs, such as IGFBP-3, -4, and -5, are under cAMP control, and others are under IGF-I and -II control. The expression of IGFBP-5 is to an extent coordinated with that of IGF-I, and it is stimulated by retinoids and inhibited by glucocorticoids and mitogenic growth factors (32). IGFBPs are degraded by specific and nonspecific proteases, secreted by skeletal cells, and under hormonal control. Some of these proteases include serine proteases and MMPs.

Transforming Growth Factor-β Family

Transforming growth factors are polypeptides that were initially defined by their ability to induce nonneoplastic indicator cells (surface-adherent, density-dependent, growth-regulated fibroblasts) to form anchorage-independent colonies in soft agar suspension cultures. This process was considered linked to neoplastic transformation, because

tumor-derived cells can form colonies spontaneously. However, it is now known that TGF-β plays multiple functions in the regulation of normal cell metabolism. TGF-β is a polypeptide with an MW of 25,000 and is synthesized by many tissues, including bone. Three forms of TGF-β, which seem to have similar biologic activities, are present in various mammalian tissues including bone. They are TGF-β1, -β2, and -β3 (2). TGF-β stimulates the replication of precursor cells of the osteoblast lineage, and it has a direct stimulatory effect on bone collagen synthesis (33). Therefore, TGF-β modulates bone matrix synthesis by various mechanisms, including an increase in the number of cells capable of expressing the osteoblast phenotype, as well as direct actions on the differentiated function of the osteoblast. TGF-β also decreases bone resorption, possibly by inducing apoptosis of osteoclasts (34). The levels of TGF-β can be modified by changes in its synthesis and activity. The gene elements responsible for the control of TGF-β1, -β2, and -β3 expression are different (2). Consequently, different hormones and factors regulate the synthesis of the three forms of TGF-β. This factor is released in an inactive form bound to a precursor and to a binding protein (35). Hormones capable of inducing bone resorption, such as PTH, activate and increase the release of TGF-β from bone. The available TGF-β could be instrumental in suppressing bone resorption and initiating the bone-forming phase of remodeling (34). TGF-β binds to two signal-transducing receptors, termed TGF-β receptors I and II, and to a non-signal-transducing receptor termed TGF-β receptor III, or betaglycan. Changes in the expression of betaglycan can regulate the amount of TGF-β available for biologic effects (19).

There are a number of additional polypeptides that share amino acid sequence homology with TGF-β. These include a large family of bone morphogenetic proteins (BMP), or osteogenic proteins (36). BMPs are osteoinductive factors that induce normal endochondral bone formation, and they share some activities with TGF-β. However, they have specific receptors and induce the differentiation of cells of the osteoblast lineage. Because of their ability to increase the formation of new bone, BMPs may be important in the treatment of fractures.

Fibroblast Growth Factors

Acidic and basic FGFs, or heparin-binding growth factors 1 and 2, are polypeptides with an approximate MW of 17,000 (37). Initially these two factors were obtained from the central nervous system, but subsequently they were shown to be synthesized by a variety of normal and malignant tissues including bone (38). FGFs are members of a family of at least nine related genes. FGFs have angiogenic properties and are considered important for neovascularization and wound healing. Acidic and basic FGFs stimulate bone cell replication, which results in an increased bone cell population capable of synthesizing bone collagen (39). Basic FGF is more potent than acidic FGF. Bones treated with FGF synthesize a higher amount of collagenous matrix because they contain a greater number of collagen-synthesizing cells, but not because of a direct effect of FGF on the differentiated function of the osteoblast. In fact, basic FGF

TABLE 3. Levels of regulation of skeletal growth factors by systemic and local factors

Synthesis
Activation
Receptor binding
Binding proteins
    Synthesis
    Distribution
    Degradation by proteases

inhibits type I collagen transcription in osteoblasts (40). The stimulatory effects of FGFs on neovascularization, in association with those on bone cell replication, suggest that they are important in the process of healing and bone repair; particularly, because their release from cells may occur after cell injury or death. Neither acidic nor basic FGF modifies bone resorption, but basic FGF increases the expression of MMP-13, indicating a possible function in bone collagen degradation and remodeling. The systemic administration of basic FGF causes an early increase in the number of preosteoblasts, followed by a recruitment of osteoblasts and an increase in bone formation (41).

Studies on the synthesis of FGF in osteoblasts have been limited, but TGF-β and basic FGF increase FGF expression in osteoblast cell lines (42). There are four related FGF receptor (FGFR) genes, termed FGFR-1 to -4 (43). Their expression in bone cells has not been studied, but in other cells, FGFR-1, -2, and -3 mediate the mitogenic response to FGF. Recent studies have demonstrated diverse skeletal abnormalities in patients with mutations of FGFR-1, -2, and -3. These abnormalities vary with the mutated receptor and include achondroplasia, a common cause of dwarfism, and early closure of cranial sutures (44). FGFs bind to proteoglycans in the extracellular matrix and these molecules can modulate the biologic activity of FGFs.

Platelet-Derived Growth Factor

PDGF, a polypeptide with an MW of 30,000, was initially isolated from blood platelets and was considered important in the early phases of wound repair (45). Normal and neoplastic tissues also synthesize PDGF, indicating that it may act as a systemic or local regulator of tissue growth. PDGF is a dimer of the products of two genes, PDGF-A and -B, so that mature peptides can exist as a PDGF-AA or -BB homodimer or as a PDGF-AB heterodimer. PDGF-AB and -BB are the predominant isoforms present in the systemic circulation. Normal osteoblasts and osteosarcoma cells express both the PDGF-A and -B genes and have the potential to synthesize all the PDGF isoforms (46). PDGF has activities similar to those described for FGF. It stimulates bone cell replication and, as a consequence of an increased number of cells, PDGF stimulates bone collagen synthesis. However, PDGF does not stimulate the differentiated function of the osteoblast and it inhibits bone matrix apposition rates (47). PDGF-BB also stimulates bone resorption by increasing the number of osteoclasts, and it induces the expression of MMP-13 by the osteoblast.

The synthesis of the locally produced PDGF is regulated by growth factors (46). PDGF-A expression is enhanced by TGF-β and PDGF itself, but not by systemic hormones. PDGF-B expression is stimulated by TGF-β. There are two PDGF receptors, α and β, and the activity of PDGF can be regulated by changes in receptor binding (48). There are no specific binding proteins for PDGF, but PDGF-B chains bind to osteonectin (SPARC), which modifies the activity of PDGF by decreasing its binding to specific receptors (49). PDGF may act primarily as a systemic agent and, when released by the aggregating platelet, it may increase cells critical for the process of fracture and wound repair.

Other Cytokines

A number of cytokines with important effects on the immune and hematological system also act on skeletal cells. It is believed they act directly on bone cells, either because they are derived from marrow cells and are present in the bone microenvironment, or because they are synthesized by stromal cells and osteoblasts (24). These cytokines include interleukin (IL)-1, -4, -6, and -11, macrophage and granulocyte/macrophage (GM) colony-stimulating factors (CSFs), and tumor necrosis factors (TNFs). These cytokines have important effects in bone remodeling, and they stimulate bone resorption most likely by enhancing the recruitment of osteoclasts, the bone-resorbing cells.

IL-1 exists in two forms: IL-1α and IL-1β. They have partial amino acid homology and similar biologic activities. IL-1 has complex effects on bone remodeling and it stimulates bone resorption. IL-1 seems relevant in the mechanism of hypercalcemia in certain hematological malignancies, and increased IL-1 levels are found in selected cases of osteoporosis (21). IL-1 increases the synthesis of IL-6 by stromal cells, and IL-6 stimulates bone resorption by increasing the recruitment of cells of the osteoclast lineage. The synthesis of IL-1 and IL-6 is diminished by estrogens (21,24). It is postulated that the two cytokines are responsible for the increased bone resorption observed after estrogen withdrawal, such as in postmenopausal osteoporosis. IL-1 and IL-6 do not have a prominent effect on bone formation.

TNFα, or cachectin, is a cytokine known for its cytostatic, cytolytic, and antiviral actions. However, TNFα is also important in a variety of normal cellular responses, and, in contrast to its growth inhibitory effects on tumor cells, it stimulates the growth of nontransformed cells. TNFα stimulates bone resorption and bone cell replication (50). CSFs play a role in the maturation of osteoclasts and GM-CSF-1 deficiency causes osteopetrosis.

In summary, bone remodeling is a complex process regulated by systemic hormones and by local factors. Hormones regulate the synthesis, activation, effects, and binding proteins of the local factors that have a direct action on cellular metabolism, and they modify the replication or differentiated function of cells of the osteoblast or osteoclast lineage. It is possible that the role of the hormones is to provide tissue specificity for a given growth factor, because most of these factors are synthesized by a variety of skeletal and nonskeletal cells. Bone-associated factors may play a role in the maintenance of normal bone remodeling, have a function in wound and fracture healing, or play a role in the pathogenesis of specific bone diseases and hypercalcemia.

REFERENCES

1. Canalis E: The hormonal and local regulation of bone formation. *Endocr Rev* 4:62–77, 1983
2. Canalis E, Pash J, Varghese S: Skeletal growth factors. *Crit Rev Eukaryot Gene Expr* 3:155–166, 1993
3. Frost H: A new direction for osteoporosis research: A review and proposal. *Bone* 12:429–437, 1991
4. Heaney R: The bone-remodeling transient: Implications for the interpretation of clinical studies of bone mass change. *J Bone Miner Res* 9:1515–1523, 1994
5. Canalis E, Hock JM, Raisz LG: Parathyroid hormone: Anabolic

and catabolic effects on bone and interactions with growth factors. In: Bilezikian JP, Marcus R, Levine MA (eds) *The Parathyroids.* Raven Press, New York, pp 65–82, 1994

6. Canalis E, Centrella M, Burch W, McCarthy, TL: Insulin-like growth factor I mediates selective anabolic effects of parathyroid hormone in bone cultures. *J Clin Invest* 83:60–65, 1989

7. McCarthy TL, Centrella M, Canalis E: Cyclic AMP induces insulin-like growth factor I synthesis in osteoblast-enriched cultures. *J Biol Chem* 265:15353–15356, 1990

8. Canalis E: Effect of insulin-like growth factor I on DNA and protein synthesis in cultured rat calvaria. *J Clin Invest* 66:709–719, 1980

9. McCarthy TL, Centrella M, Canalis E: Parathyroid hormone enchances the transcript and polypeptide levels of insulin-like growth factor I in osteoblast-enriched cultures from fetal rat bone. *Endocrinology* 124:1247–1253, 1989

10. Canalis E: Growth hormone, skeletal growth factors and osteoporosis. *Endocr Pract* 1:39–43, 1995

11. DeLuca HF: Vitamin D revisited. *Clin Endocrinol Metab* 9:1–26, 1980

12. Lian JB, Coutts M, Canalis E: Studies of hormonal regulation of osteocalcin synthesis in cultured fetal rat calvariae. *J Biol Chem* 260:8706–8710, 1985

13. Delany AM, Pash JM, Canalis E: Cellular and clinical perspectives on skeletal insulin-like growth factor I. *J Cell Biochem* 55:1–6, 1994

14. Delany AM, Dong Y, Canalis E: Mechanisms of glucocorticoid action in bone cells. *J Cell Biochem* 56:295–302, 1994

15. Raisz LG, Trummel CL, Wener JA, Simmons H: Effect of glucocorticoids on bone resorption in tissue cultures. *Endocrinology* 90:961–967, 1972

16. Canalis E: Effects of glucocorticoids on type I collagen synthesis, alkaline phosphatase activity, and deoxyribonucleic acid content in cultured rat calvariae. *Endocrinology* 112:931–939, 1983

17. Delany A, Gabbitas B, Canalis E: Cortisol down-regulates osteoblast 1α (I) procollagen mRNA by transcriptional and post-transcriptional mechanisms. *J Cell Biochem* 57:488–494, 1995

18. McCarthy TL, Centrella M, Canalis E: Cortisol inhibits the synthesis of insulin-like growth factor I in skeletal cells. *Endocrinology* 126:1569–1575, 1990

19. Centrella M, McCarthy TL, Canalis E: Glucocorticoid regulation of transforming growth factor β_1 (TGF β_1) activity and binding in osteoblast-enriched cultures from fetal rat bone. *Mol Cell Biol* 11:4490–4496, 1991

20. Jilka RL, Hangoc G, Girasole G, Passeri G, Williams DC, Abrams JS, Boyce B, Broxmeyer H, Manolagas SC: Increased osteoclast development after estrogen loss: mediation by interleukin 6. *Science* 257:88–91, 1992

21. Horowitz MC: Cytokines and estrogen in bone: Anti-osteoporotic effects. *Science* 260:626–627, 1993

22. Mundy GR, Shapiro JL, Bandelin JG, Canalis EM, Raisz LG: Direct stimulation of bone resorption by thyroid hormones. *J Clin Invest* 58:529–534, 1976

23. Baran DT, Braverman LE: Thyroid hormones and bone mass (editorial). *J Clin Endocrinol Metab* 72:1182–1183, 1991

24. Manolagas SC, Jilka R: Bone marrow, cytokines, and bone remodeling. Emerging insights into the pathophysiology of osteoporosis. *N Engl J Med* 232:305–311, 1995

25. Jones JI, Clemmons DR: Insulin-like growth factors and their binding proteins: Biological actions. *Endocr Rev* 16:3–34, 1995

26. McCarthy TL, Centrella M, Canalis E: Regulatory effects of insulin-like growth factor I and II on bone collagen synthesis in rat calvarial cultures. *Endocrinology* 124:301–309, 1989

27. Hock JM, Centrella M, Canalis E: Insulin-like growth factor I (IGF-I) has independent effects on bone matrix formation and cell replication. *Endocrinology* 122:254–260, 1988

28. Canalis E, Rydziel S, Delany A, Varghese S, Jeffrey J: Insulin-like growth factors inhibit interstitial collagenase synthesis in bone cell cultures. *Endocrinology* 136:1348–1354, 1995

29. Ebeling PR, Jones JD, O'Fallon WM, Janes CH, Riggs BL: Short-term effects of recombinant human insulin-like growth factor I on bone turnover in normal women. *J Clin Endocrinol Metab* 77:1384–1387, 1993

30. Gabbitas B, Pash J, Canalis E: Regulation of insulin-like growth factor II synthesis in bone cell cultures by skeletal growth factors. *Endocrinology* 135:284–289, 1994

31. Canalis E, Pash J, Gabbitas B, Rydziel S, Varghese S: Growth factors regulate the synthesis of insulin-like growth factor I in bone cell cultures. *Endocrinology* 133:33–38, 1993

32. Canalis E, Gabbitas B: Skeletal growth factors regulate the synthesis of insulin-like growth factor binding protein-5 in bone cell cultures. *J Biol Chem* 270:10771–10776, 1995

33. Centrella M, McCarthy T, Canalis E: Transforming growth factor beta is a bifunctional regulator of replication and collagen synthesis in osteoblast-enriched cell cultures from fetal rat bone. *J Biol Chem* 262:2869–2874, 1987

34. Pfeilschifter J, Seyedin SM, Mundy GR: Transforming growth factor beta inhibits bone resorption in fetal rat long bone cultures. *J Clin Invest* 82:680–685, 1988

35. Centrella M, McCarthy TL, Canalis E: Transforming growth factor-beta and remodeling of bone. *J Bone Joint Surg* 73(A):1418–1428, 1991

36. Wozney JM, Rosen V, Celeste AJ, Mitsock LM, Whitters MJ, Kriz RW, Hewick RM, Wang EA: Novel regulators of bone formation: Molecular clones and activities. *Science* 242:1528–1534, 1988

37. Burgess WH, Maciag T: The heparin-binding (fibroblast) growth factor family of proteins. *Annu Rev Biochem* 58:575–606, 1989

38. Globus RK, Plouet J, Gospodarowicz D: Cultured bovine bone cells synthesize basic fibroblast growth factor and store it in their extracellular matrix. *Endocrinology* 124:1539–1547, 1989

39. Canalis E, Centrella M, McCarthy T: Effects of basic fibroblast growth factor on bone formation in vitro. *J Clin Invest* 81:1572–1577, 1988

40. Hurley MM, Abreu C, Harrison JR, Lichtler AC, Raisz LG, Kream BE: Basic fibroblast growth factor inhibits type I collagen gene expression in osteoblastic MC3T3-E1 cells. *J Biol Chem* 268:5588–5593, 1993

41. Nakamura T, Hanada K, Tamura M, Sibanushi T, Nigi H, Tagawa M, Fukumoto S, Matsumoto T: Stimulation of endosteal bone formation by systemic injections of recombinant basic fibroblast growth factor in rats. *Endocrinology* 136:1276–1284, 1995

42. Hurley MM, Abreu C, Gronowicz G, Kawaguchi H, Lorenzo J: Expression and regulation of basic fibroblast growth factor mRNA levels in mouse osteoblastic MC3T3-E1 cells. *J Biol Chem* 269:9392–9396, 1994

43. Wang J, Gao G, Goldfarb M: Fibroblast growth factor receptors have different signaling and mitogenic potentials. *Mol Cell Biol* 14:181–188, 1994

44. Shiang R, Thompson LM, Zhu YZ, Church DM, Fielder TJ, Bocian M, Winokur ST, Wasmuth JJ: Mutations in the transmembrane domain of FGFR3 cause the most common genetic form of dwarfism, achondroplasia. *Cell* 78:335–342, 1994

45. Heldin CH, Westermark B: PDGF-like growth factors in autocrine stimulation of growth. *J Cell Physiol* 5:31–34, 1987

46. Rydziel S, Shaikh S, Canalis E: Platelet-derived growth factors AA and BB enhance the synthesis of platelet-derived growth factor AA in bone cell cultures. *Endocrinology* 134:2541–2546, 1994

47. Hock JM, Canalis E: Platelet-derived growth factor enhances bone cell replication but not differentiated function of osteoblasts. *Endocrinology* 134:1423–1428, 1994

48. Centrella M, McCarthy TL, Kusmik WF, Canalis E: Isoform specific regulation of platelet-derived growth factor activity and binding in osteoblast-enriched cultures from fetal rat bone. *J Clin Invest* 89:1076–1084, 1992

49. Raines EW, Lane TF, Iruela-Arispe ML, Ross R, Sage EH: The extracellular glycoprotein SPARC interacts with platelet-derived growth factor (PDGF)-AB and -BB and inhibits the binding of PDGF to its receptors. *Proc Natl Acad Sci USA* 89:1281–1285, 1992

50. Bertolini DR, Nedwin GE, Bringman TS, Smith DD, Mundy GR: Stimulation of bone resorption and inhibition of bone formation in vitro by human tumor necrosis factors. *Nature* 319:516–518, 1986

6. The Osteoblast Lineage—Embryologic Origins and the Differentiation Sequence

Jane E. Aubin, Ph.D., and *Arnold Kahn, Ph.D.

Department of Anatomy and Cell Biology, Faculty of Medicine, University of Toronto, Toronto, Ontario, Canada
*Department of Growth and Development, School of Dentistry, University of California, San Francisco, San Francisco, California

Osteoblasts are the skeletal cells responsible for bone formation: they synthesize and regulate the deposition and mineralization of the extracellular matrix (type I collagen and a spectrum of noncollagenous proteins) of bone. This chapter presents an overview of osteoblast ontogeny and the transitions from immature precursor to mature, fully functional, bone-forming osteoblast, with reference to some of the experimental approaches used to characterize these stages.

WHERE DO OSTEOBLASTS AND BONE COME FROM?

The pre-osteoblast, osteoblast, osteocyte, and bone-lining cells are the most differentiated and easily recognizable cell types in the osteoblast family. Distinct morphologic features and histochemical markers define these populations in the tissue (and have been discussed in Chapter 2). However, the precursors of these cells, the osteoprogenitor cell and the osteogenic stem cell (Fig. 1), are not readily identifiable. In general, it is believed that the farther away from the bone surface an osteogenic cell is, the less differentiated it will be. Thus, osteoprogenitors are thought to reside within the zone of proliferating cells, behind the pre-osteoblast/osteoblast layer in periosteal tissues, and in bone marrow stroma; such cells are morphologically fibroblast-like cells with an elongated nucleus. It has been proposed that osteoprogenitor cells arise from mesenchymal stem cells that are multipotential (pluripotential) in nature and capable of giving rise to a number of committed and restricted cell lineages, including the osteogenic line (1–3). Early evidence for this point of view was provided by Freidenstein and his colleagues (4). In brief, these investigators argued that there is apparently not one but two types of osteoprogenitor cells, the determined osteogenic precursor cell (DOPC) and the inducible osteogenic precursor cell (IOPC). The DOPC is found in bone marrow as a member of the stromal cell family. It is clonogenic in nature, fibroblastic in morphology, highly proliferative, and capable of giving rise to bone, cartilage fibrous connective tissue, and fat when implanted *in vivo*. The IOPC, on the other hand, is found in lymphoid tissues, among peritoneal macrophages, and in blood; it is clonogenic, proliferative, and capable of undergoing osteogenesis, but only if placed in contact with an osteoinductive agent (e.g., transitional epithelium, decalcified bone matrix). It is likely that the IOPC (or its equivalent) is present in many soft tissues (e.g., skeletal muscle, dermal connective tissue) and is responsible for the ectopic bone formation that can occur at these sites.

Additional evidence for the existence of multipotential, mesenchymal progenitors has been provided by *in vitro* studies on several clonal cell populations isolated from different starting tissues by different investigators (4). These lines are multipotential in that they are able to differentiate into one or several phenotypes, including bone and cartilage, depending on experimental conditions. Many researchers are actively pursuing the identity of the regulatory molecules responsible for controlling the differentiation of these multipotential cells. Among the most intensively studied of the possible regulatory molecules are the members of the TGF-β superfamily, including the bone morphogenetic proteins (BMPs).

It is also important to recognize that not all bones of the body arise in the same way or from the same embryonic tissues. First, two types of bone formation processes are evident: intramembranous and endochondral. Intramembranous ossification occurs when mesenchymal progenitors aggregate (condense) and then differentiate *directly* into osteoblasts capable of forming bone. Intramembranous ossification is responsible for the development of the flat bones of the skull and the addition of bone on the periosteal or outer surfaces of long bones. Endochondral bone formation, on the other hand, occurs through a process in which mesenchymal cells condense to form first a cartilage model (template), which is later *replaced* by bone. This process involves the mineralization of the cartilage matrix, neovascularization, and the recruitment of osteoblasts and osteoclasts (bone- and cartilage-resorbing cells). Endochondral bone formation is responsible for forming most of the bones of the body, including the long bones of the appendicular skeleton and the vertebrae of the axial skeleton.

In addition to these different processes of bone formation, there are also separate embryonic lineages involved in forming different parts of the skeleton, whether by the endochondral or the intramembranous route. Both neural crest (from ectoderm) and mesoderm contribute to the skeleton (Fig. 2). Craniofacial skeletal tissues arise from neural crest, whereas rib and appendicular skeletons and the skull base originate from mesoderm. Some of the cranial skeleton forms from mesoderm, but classical embryological studies (including extirpation of particular regions of neural crest before migration, and transplantation experiments in which particular neural crest cells are grafted into recipient embryos) showed that all of the facial skeletal elements (maxillary, mandibular, and hyoid bones) come from neural crest. Cranial neural crest has the capacity to form the cartilage, bone, connective tissue, and tooth odontoblasts of the facial skeleton. Dorsal paraxial mesoderm gives rise to somites, the sclerotome, and eventually the axial skeleton. Lateral plate mesoderm gives rise to appendicular skeleton, while cephalic mesoderm gives rise to the cranial bones. By the time these lineages appear, the number and identity of the

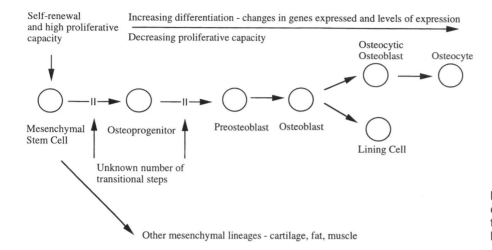

FIG. 1. Schematic of the osteoblast lineage from mesenchymal stem cell through transitional stages, to osteoblast, osteocyte, and lining cell.

derived skeletal elements have already been programmed. Recent molecular genetic approaches involving the *in vivo* manipulation of specific transcriptional regulators, or growth and differentiation factors (or their receptors), coupled to analyses of genes responsible for known mutations affecting human and mouse skeletal growth, show that skeletal patterning and bone growth and development are under tight genetic control. This control is manifest not only from mutational and gene manipulation analyses, but also from the pattern of expression of putative regulatory genes, a pattern that shows that such genes are active in particular places and particular times during development. Some genes (e.g., homeobox genes) specify early mesenchymal lineages, skeletal primordial shape, and the identity of individual skeletal elements. Other genes (e.g., growth and differentiation factors and hormones) further refine bone shape and size. Examples of both these levels of regulation are given in Table 1.

POTENTIAL NEW MARKERS OF THE OSTEOBLAST PHENOTYPE

It is clear that osteoblastic cells synthesize collagenous and noncollagenous proteins, and cytokine receptors and ligands. This has facilitated identification of subpopulations of osteoblasts based on the relative abundance of either mRNA transcripts or protein (Table 2). However, the molecular mechanisms responsible for the coordinate expression and regulation of these genes during osteoblast differentiation and development are only beginning to be deciphered. Transcription factors are DNA-binding proteins that play central roles in regulating cell growth, development, and differentiation by interacting with DNA cites that regulate gene transcription. New studies suggest that certain classes of transcription factors may play roles in gene regulation during specific stages of osteoblast development and differentiation. For example, hXBP-1 (a member of the basic region leucine zipper family) is expressed in osteoblasts and pre-osteoblasts in areas of ossification (5), whereas a novel transcription coactivator termed 1.9.2 is present in osteoblasts (6). Msx-2 protein, a homeodomain gene family member, is expressed in undifferentiated, but not in differentiated, mouse calvarial osteoblasts (7), it seems to be a transcriptional suppressor of the rat osteocalcin promoter (8,9), and it is mutated in some forms of human craniofacial synostosis that are characterized by premature suture closure in the calvaria (10) (Table 1). The roles of these and other transcription factors recently found in osteoblast lineage cells are not fully known, but their

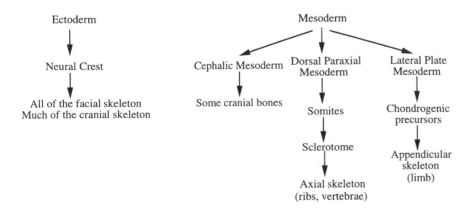

FIG. 2. Embryonic origins of different bones of the body.

TABLE 1. *Results of mutations of a few genes that affect skeletal patterning and growth*

Gene absent or altered	Phenotype
Hox genes	
hoxa-2	2nd branchial arch replaced by 1st branchial arch
hoxd-13	4th sacral vertebra replaced by 3rd, and deletions and additions in distal limb elements
msx-1	cleft palate
msx-2	craniosynostosis
Growth and differentiation factors	
BMP-5 (se)	altered shape in sternum and external ear cartilage
GDF-5 (bp)	reduced size of appendicular long bones
IGF-I	overall reduced size of skeleton
TGF-β2 (overexpression)	osteoporosis-like phenotype
Growth factor receptors	
FGFR-1, FGFR-2	craniosynostosis and/or limb defects, depending on the mutation
FGFR-3	achondroplasia
Hormones	
PTHrP	reduced proliferation and premature differentiation of chondrocytes, and increased endochondral ossification
Matrix proteins	
type I collagen	osteogenesis imperfecta
type XI collagen	chondrodysplasia (wider and shorter bones)

From: refs. 10, 16.

presence suggests a potential involvement in the regulation of certain osteoblast-associated genes. In addition, their pattern of expression may provide landmarks in the establishment of the osteoblast cell phenotype.

Other tools for tracking the stages of osteogenesis include monoclonal antibodies directed not only against matrix-derived antigens such as type I collagen (COLL-I), alkaline phosphatase, and osteopontin (OPN), but also against differentiation-stage-specific cellular epitopes (11,12). For example, Nijweide and colleagues (12) prepared a monoclonal antibody (OB 7.3) that reacts with only chick osteocytes. Although the epitope recognized by OB 7.3 is still unknown, this antibody has already proved a useful tool for isolation and characterization of chick osteocytes (12). Several other investigators have likewise described antibodies against different subpopulations of chick, human, or rat osteoblastic and osteosarcoma cells, many of which should prove invaluable in further studies of osteoblast development and maturation (11).

PROGRESSION FROM AN IMMATURE PROGENITOR CELL TO A MATURE OSTEOBLAST AND OSTEOCYTE

How do cells progress from early progenitors to fully functional matrix-synthesizing osteoblasts—through quantum leaps or gradual transitions? The majority of evidence, based on a combination of cell morphology, immunocytochemistry, and *in situ* hybridization, suggests that the transition is gradual (Fig. 1). However, the present panel of stage-specific markers is clearly incomplete and is heavily weighted in favor of the more differentiated osteoblast and osteocyte; many fewer markers are available for the pre-osteoblast and even fewer for less mature cells (Table 2). Although in general there is good agreement between the expression of a marker and cell morphology and function,

there are exceptions in which unexpected variation in marker expression is observed. Some of these discrepancies may be for technical reasons (e.g., species and methodological differences), but still to be rigorously investigated are variations that result from developmental or postnatal age, anatomic site (e.g., calvaria, vertebra, mandible), bone origin (intramembranous or endochondral), and the part of the bone studied (trabecular or cortical). Despite these caveats, it is generally accepted that alkaline phosphatase is expressed at least as early as the pre-osteoblast stage and is an earlier differentiation marker than osteopontin. These are followed by bone sialoprotein (BSP) and osteocalcin (OCN) as indicators of the more mature osteoblast phenotype (Table 2).

A variety of studies on cell culture models have augmented observations on bone tissue *in situ*. Important *in vitro* models include clonal cell lines derived either from bone tumors (e.g., rat ROS 17/2.8 or UMR 106; human MG-63 or SaOS-2) or from primary bone cell cultures (e.g., MC3T3-E1, UMR 201, and RCJ cell lines). Based on the profile of expression of osteoblastic characteristics and morphologic features reminiscent of osteoblasts *in vivo*, MC3T3-E1 cells have been described as relatively immature, UMR 106 as pre-osteoblastic cells, and ROS 17/2.8 as more differentiated osteoblasts (13). However, various features of the lines suggest that most are not normal in regulation or expression of at least some osteoblast properties (2). Given this less than normal behavior and the inherent instability of some clonal cell lines, primary cultures of bone-derived cells (e.g., rat, mouse, calf, or chick calvaria; rat, mouse, bovine, or human trabecular bone) are also being used. Of course, primary cultures also have limitations, including the important fact that they contain a heterogeneous mixture of osteoblastic cells at different stages of differentiation and cells of other lineages (2). Nonetheless, freshly isolated bone marrow stromal populations derived from bones such as fetal rat calvaria are being extensively

TABLE 2. *Expression of markers of the osteoblast (OB) phenotype at different stages of differentiation*

Species	Marker	Immunocytochemistry				*In situ* hybridization			
		Pre-OB	OB	Lining cell	Osteocyte	Pre-OB	OB	Lining cell	Osteocyte
Rat	COLL-I	—	+	—	—	—/+	+	—	—
	ALP	+	+	—	—	+	+	—	—
	OPN	+	+	—	+	—	+	+	+
	BSP	—	+	—	—	—	+	±	±
	OCN	—/+	+	—	+	—	+	—	+
	PTH/PTHrP-R	+	±	—	—	±	+	—	—
Human	COLL-I	+	+	—	±	+	+	—	—
	OPN	—	+	+	—	—	—	—	—
	BSP	—	+	—	+	—	+	—	+
	OCN	—	—	—	+	—	—	—	—

+, positive expression; —, negative expression; ±, weak expression; —/+, negative or positive expression, depending on study. From: refs 2,3,14.

studied. These isolated osteoblastic cells express alkaline phosphatase activity, synthesize COLL-I and all the noncollagenous bone proteins discussed above, and respond to various hormones and cytokines. Of particular note for the present discussion is that when these cells are maintained under suitable culture conditions, they will form bonelike nodules with the histologic, ultrastructural, and immunohistochemical appearance of embryonic/woven bone. The process of nodule formation has been most extensively studied in rat calvaria populations, in which it has been subdivided into three developmental stages: (i) proliferation, (ii) extracellular matrix development and maturation, and (iii) mineralization, with characteristic changes in genes associated with proliferative and cell cycling activity (e.g., c-*fos*, c-*myc*, cyclins) and those associated with specific osteoblast activities (2,3,14). Cells virtually identical to the same morphologic stages described *in vivo* can be identified, and the nodular matrix contains the major bone matrix proteins; it also mineralizes with crystals of hydroxyapatite. Also, like bone *in vivo,* these nodules appear to represent the endproduct of the proliferation and differentiation of relatively rare osteoprogenitor cells present in the starting cell population. In this process, the osteoprogenitor cells undergo a series of transitional stages in which new genes are turned in and others alter their expression levels in a manner replicating what is observed *in vivo* (Table 2) (Fig. 1) (2,3,14). In addition, the *in vitro* analyses are providing evidence for considerable flexibility in the repertoire of osteoblast-associated genes expressed at multiple differentiation stages as osteoprogenitors mature and form functional osteoblasts (3,15). Much remains to be done to assess the biologic meaning of this plasticity and to capture similar transitional events in different bones at different sites in the body throughout the entire developmental lifetime of vertebrate organisms.

REFERENCES

1. Caplan AI, Boyan BD. Endochondral bone formation: the lineage cascade. In: Hall BK, ed. *Bone. Volume 8: Mechanisms of Bone Development and Growth.* Boca Raton: CRC Press, 1–46, 1991

2. Aubin JE, Turksen K, Heersche JNM. Osteoblastic cell lineage. In: Noda M, ed. *Cellular and Molecular Biology of Bone.* San Diego: Academic Press, 1–45, 1993
3. Aubin JE, Liu F, Malaval L, Gupta AK. Osteoblast and chondroblast differentiation. *Bone* 17:77S–83S, 1995
4. Friedenstein AJ, Chailakhyan RK, Gerasimov UV. Bone marrow osteogenic stem cells: in vitro cultivation and transplantation in diffusion chambers. *Cell Tissue Kinet* 20:263–272, 1987
5. Clauss IM, Gravallese EM, Darling JM, Shapiro F, Glimcher MJ, Glimcher LH. In situ hybridization studies suggest a role for the basic region-leucine zipper protein hXBP-1 in exocrine gland and skeletal development during mouse embryogenesis. *Dev Dyn* 197:146–156, 1993
6. Yotov WV, Glorieux FH, St. Arnaud R. A novel transcriptional coactivator linking the basal transcriptional machinery to activating transcription factors is expressed specifically in bone during embryogenesis. *J Bone Miner Res* 10(suppl.1):S171, 1995
7. Dodig M, Keonenberg MS, Kream B, Pan Z, Upholt WB, Lichtler AC. Msx-2 inhibits COL1A1 promoter-CAT construct expression in osteoblastic cells. *J Bone Miner Res* 10(suppl.1):S421, 1995
8. Hoffman HM, Catron KM, van Wijnen AJ, McCabe LR, Lian JB, Stein GS, Stein JL: Transcriptional control of the tissue-specific developmentally regulated osteocalcin gene requires a binding motif for the MSX-family of homeodomain proteins. *Proc. Natl. Acad. Sci. USA*, 91:12887–12891, 1994
9. Towler DA, Rutledge SJ, Rodan GA: Msx-2/Hox 8.1: a transcriptional regulator of the rat osteaocalcin promoter. *Mol Endocrinol*; 8:1484–1493, 1994
10. Jabs EW, Muller U, Li X, et al. A mutation in the homeodomain of the human MSX2 gene in a family affected with autosomal dominant craniosynostosis. *Cell* 75:443– 450, 1993
11. Aubin JE, Turksen K. Monoclonal antibodies as tools for studying the osteoblast lineage. *Microscopy Research and Technique* 33:128–140, 1996
12. van der Plas A, Aarden EM, Feijen JHM, et al. Characteristics and properties of osteocytes in culture. *J Bone Miner Res* 9:1697–1704, 1994
13. Rodan GA, Noda M. Gene expression in osteoblastic cells. *Critical Reviews in Eukaryotic Gene Expression* 1:85–98, 1991
14. Stein GS, and Lian JB. (1993) Molecular mechanisms mediating proliferation / differentiation interrelationships during progressive development of the osteoblast phenotype. *Endocrine Reviews*, Vol. 14:424–442, 1993
15. Liu F, Malaval L, Gupta AK, Aubin JE. Simultaneous detection of multiple bone-related mRNAs and protein expression during osteoblast differentiation: polymeraise chain reaction and immunocytochemical studies at the single cell level. *Dev Biol* 166:220–234, 1994
16. Erlebacher A, Filvaroff EH, Gitelman ST, Dernyck R: Toward a molecular understanding of skeletal development. *Cell* 80:371–378, 1995

SECTION II

Calcium, Magnesium, Phosphorus Homeostasis and Physiology, and Biochemistry of Calcium Regulating Hormones

7. Calcium, Magnesium, and Phosphorus: Intestinal Absorption

Neil A. Breslau, M.D.

Center for Mineral Metabolism and Clinical Research, Department of Medicine, and General Clinical Research Center, University of Texas, Southwestern Medical Center, Dallas, Texas

The intestinal absorptions of calcium (Ca), magnesium (Mg), and phosphorus (P) are considered together because adequate absorption of all three elements is necessary for normal mineral homeostasis, including control of the blood ionized calcium level, skeletal growth in childhood, and maintenance of skeletal mass in adulthood. The quantities of Ca, Mg, and P that are absorbed by the intestine are determined by the availability of these minerals in the diet and by the capacity of the intestine to absorb them. Vitamin D, through its active metabolite 1,25-dihydroxyvitamin D [1,25(OH)$_2$D], plays a role in the transport processes of each of these elements. In general, intestinal mineral absorption represents the sum of two transport processes: saturable transcellular absorption that is physiologically regulated, and nonsaturable paracellular absorption that is dependent on mineral concentration within the lumen of the gut.

CALCIUM ABSORPTION

About 200 to 300 mg of calcium is absorbed each day in the adult, from a total luminal content of 1000 mg, assuming an average daily intake of 800 mg plus about 200 mg entering the intestinal tract via pancreatic, biliary, and intestinal secretions. Thus, overall efficiency of calcium absorption is only about 30% (1). There are three major influences on calcium absorption: cellular and paracellular transport, systemic modulators of cell function, and intraluminal factors.

Cellular and Paracellular Events

Absorption across the intestinal mucosa is achieved by two parallel processes: an active, transcellular transport process and a passive, paracellular diffusional process (2). Under normal dietary conditions, the duodenum is the major site for active transport, whereas passive, paracellular transfer occurs throughout the small intestine. Despite this localization of the active transport site, quantitatively more calcium may be absorbed in the jejunum and ileum than in the duodenum because of the relative amounts of time luminal contents spend in these regions of the intestine. The human jejunum absorbs calcium at a greater rate than the ileum, and absorption rates in all intestinal segments are increased by treatment with vitamin D.

Cellular Transport

The transcellular route involves transport across the apical membrane, transfer across the cytoplasm, and exit across the basolateral membrane (Fig. 1) (3). Entry probably occurs by way of specific calcium channels in the apical membrane and down the prevailing electrochemical gradient. Within the cytoplasm, binding to a calcium-binding protein, calbindin, is a key step. Maximum transport rates correlate closely with calbindin concentrations. This protein must rapidly take up the calcium entering the cell because intracellular free calcium concentrations are carefully maintained at very low values (about 10^{-7}M). Transient rises in intracellular calcium act as key second messenger signals for secretory responses in the enterocyte. Absorbed calcium is thus presumably segregated from that concerned with cell signaling, and calbindin plays a vital part in this.

The calbindins also act as a "ferry" to bring calcium to the transporter at the basolateral membrane. Initially, calcium enters into intestinal epithelial cells across the luminal brush-border plasma membrane. The calcium associates transiently with components of the brush border inside the cell. Calbindin has about a fourfold greater affinity for calcium than do components of the brush border. By acting as a calcium carrier, the vitamin-D-dependent increased concentration of calbindin, facilitates more rapid diffusion of calcium across the cell. The ATP-dependent Ca^{2+} pump in the basolateral membrane has still greater affinity (approximately 2.5-fold) for calcium than does calbindin. This progressively increasing gradient of Ca-binding affinity from the brush border to the basolateral membrane facilitates rapid calcium transcellular absorption (4).

The movement of calcium from the cell, where the calcium concentration is low (10^{-7}M) into the extracellular fluid, where the calcium concentration is high (10^{-3}M), is mediated mainly by the plasma membrane Ca^{2+} pump and to a much lesser extent by the Na$^+$-Ca^{2+} exchanger. The plasma membrane Ca^{2+} pump is a Ca^{2+}-Mg^{2+}-dependent ATPase that uses ATP to pump Ca^{2+} out of the cell against a concentration gradient and an electrical gradient. It has been localized by immunohistochemical methods to the basolateral membrane of the intestine (4). Expression of the plasma membrane Ca^{2+} pump has been shown to be vitamin D dependent (3). Both calmodulin and calbindins increase the affinity of the plasma membrane Ca^{2+} pump for calcium, and they increase the maximum rate of calcium transport (3).

Paracellular Transport

The vitamin-D-dependent active component of intestinal calcium absorption described above becomes saturated at rather low levels of calcium intake (<400 mg/day) (5).

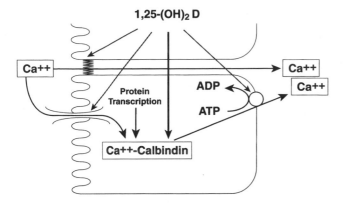

1,25-(OH)₂D

FIG. 1. Mechanisms of transport of calcium across the intestinal epithelium. A paracellular route allows a bidirectional flux. Transport into the epithelial cell occurs by way of specific channels down an electrochemical gradient. A critical step is the binding to calbindin, which then presents calcium for export by way of a calcium-dependent ATPase on the basolateral membrane. Each of these processes appears to be influenced by 1,25(OH)₂D, although the maximal effect is felt to be on the synthesis of fresh calbindin. (From: Turnberg LA, Riley SA. Digestion and absorption of nutrients and vitamins. In: Sleisenger MH, Fordtran JS, et al. (eds) *Gastrointestinal Disease: Pathophysiology, Diagnosis, Management*, 5th ed. WB Saunders, Philadelphia, pp 977–1008, 1993.)

When calcium concentrations in the intestinal lumen are high, paracellular passive transfer occurs. Paracellular calcium transport may occur independently of vitamin D, it is passively mediated, and it is nonsaturable. Hence, it is linearly correlated with luminal calcium concentration, which in turn is dependent on calcium intake. It has been estimated that such passive absorption could account for 31 mg for each 100-mg increment in meal calcium intake (5). Paracellular absorption occurs by way of the tight junctions. Recent evidence suggests that tight junctional permeability may be increased by 1,25(OH)₂D treatment and during sugar transport (2,6).

Role of Vitamin D in Intestinal Calcium Transport

The active metabolite of vitamin D is 1,25(OH)₂D, which acts in a manner similar to other steroid hormones. It exerts its biologic effects primarily through intracellular 1,25(OH)₂D receptors (VDRs). The VDRs are part of the steroid–thyroid receptor gene superfamily of nuclear transcription factors. In the cell, VDRs exist predominantly in the nucleus. The receptor protein contains a hormone-binding domain near the carboxy-terminus, and a DNA-binding domain near the amino-terminus. 1,25(OH)₂D regulates transcription of more than 60 genes, including those for the VDR itself, for calbindins, and for the plasma membrane Ca^{2+} pump. When 1,25(OH)₂D is administered exogenously, there are increases in intestinal VDR, calbindins, and Ca^{2+} pumps, which are associated with a corresponding increase in intestinal calcium absorption (Fig. 1) (3).

A rapid nongenomic effect of vitamin D on intestinal calcium transport also has been proposed (7). This mode of action involves a pathway that is independent of the regulation of gene transcription. The hormone interacts with the cell membrane, resulting in the opening of calcium channels in a response that is too rapid to be a result of gene transcription. This very rapid stimulation of intestinal calcium transport (transcaltachia) appears within seconds to minutes after treatment with 1,25(OH)₂D compared with 1 or more hours required for genomic responses. Transcaltachia is observed only in vitamin-D-replete animals, indicating that the calcium absorption system must somehow be "preprimed" with vitamin D.

Krejs et al., using the triple-lumen tube perfusion technique, investigated the effects of 1,25(OH)₂D administration on calcium absorption in normal humans (8). In the basal state, net calcium absorption in the jejunum was 3 times that in the ileum. Administration of 1,25(OH)₂D for 1 week resulted in significant increases in calcium absorption in both jejunum and ileum, with the ileal absorption rate reaching that of the jejunum. There is evidence, too, that colonic absorption of calcium occurs and can be enhanced in response to 1,25(OH)₂D (9). The presence of the colon has advantages for calcium absorption in patients with the short bowel syndrome (10,11).

Role of 1,25(OH)₂D in Intestinal Adaptation

Normal intestinal adaptation is a process that allows the body to avoid extremes of calcium deficiency or excess, by augmenting fractional calcium absorption during periods of low calcium intake and reducing it during high calcium intake. It is now known that parathyroid hormone (PTH)-dependent synthesis of 1,25(OH)₂D is responsible for this regulation. Thus, during low calcium intake, the stimulated 1,25(OH)₂D synthesis (from increased PTH secretion) enhances fractional calcium absorption (12). In contrast, during high calcium intake, the fraction of calcium absorbed is reduced from the suppression of 1,25(OH)₂D synthesis. This type of adaptation may partly explain the limited risk of kidney stone formation in women receiving chronic calcium supplements (Fig. 2) (13).

Loss of intestinal adaptation may play a role in the development of senile osteoporosis. In the elderly, the fractional intestinal calcium absorption is low, and its stimulation by the institution of a low calcium diet is blunted (14). Most (14–16), but not all (17), studies have shown that with advancing age and declining renal function, there is an impairment of 1,25(OH)₂D synthesis. One study also implicated an age-related decrease in intestinal VDR as contributing to blunted 1,25(OH)₂D action (18). It is likely that reduced 1,25(OH)₂D production in the elderly contributes to diminished intestinal calcium absorption, which may lead to negative calcium balance, especially at low calcium intakes.

A high salt intake also may impair calcium balance in those who have diminished intestinal adaptation. Excessive intake of sodium causes renal hypercalciuria by impairing renal calcium reabsorption, resulting in a compensatory increase of PTH secretion. In young individuals and premenopausal women in whom the capacity for 1,25(OH)₂D production is intact, stimulation of intestinal calcium

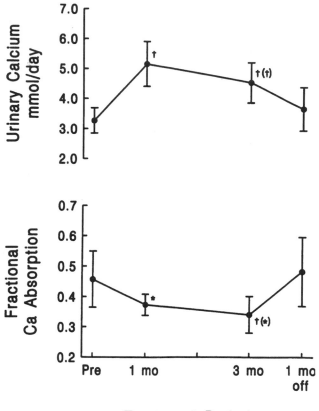

FIG. 2. Effect of long-term calcium citrate treatment on urinary calcium and fractional intestinal calcium absorption. Vertical bars, mean ± SD; * and † indicate significant differences between control and other phases. (*) and (†) indicate significant differences between 1-month and 3-month calcium citrate treatments, respectively. (From: Sakhaee K, Baker S, Zerwekh J, Poindexter J, Garcia-Hernandez PA, Pak CYC. Limited risk of kidney stone formation during long-term calcium citrate supplementation in nonstone forming subjects. *J Urol* 152:324–327, 1994.)

absorption ensues from the sodium load consequent to PTH-dependent augmentation of 1,25(OH)₂D synthesis (19). Thus, calcium balance is maintained. However, in elderly women, the compensatory rise in intestinal calcium absorption does not develop following sodium-induced calciuria because of impaired 1,25(OH)₂D synthesis (relating to aging kidney or estrogen deficiency) (20). Elderly women are therefore theoretically at risk for bone loss from habitual high sodium intake. The influence of urinary sodium excretion was examined in a 2-year, longitudinal study of bone density in 124 postmenopausal women (21). Urinary sodium excretion was negatively correlated with changes in bone density at the hip.

Other Systemic Modulators of Intestinal Calcium Absorption

As noted above, 1,25(OH)₂D is the most potent modifier of calcium absorption. In vitamin D deficiency, active cal-

cium transport is absent. 25-hydroxyvitamin D [25(OH)D] also stimulates calcium absorption, but is only about 1% as potent as 1,25(OH)₂D. In addition, intestinal calcium absorption may be increased or decreased by a variety of hormones or agents, which act either directly on the enterocyte or indirectly through alterations in the circulating level of 1,25(OH)₂D (Table 1).

Systemic Agents That Increase Calcium Absorption

Parathyroid Hormone. PTH increases intestinal calcium absorption indirectly through stimulation of the renal biosynthesis of 1,25(OH)₂D. PTH-generated renal cyclic adenosine monophosphate (cAMP) and phosphate excretion are involved in the stimulation of the renal 1α-hydroxylase. Infusion of cAMP or induction of phosphate depletion with phosphate-binding antacids can stimulate renal production of 1,25(OH)₂D independently of PTH, and hence raise intestinal calcium absorption (22).

Calcitonin. Initially, it was believed that the stimulation of 1,25(OH)₂D synthesis following calcitonin injection into rats depended on stimulation of the parathyroid glands by calcitonin-induced hypocalcemia. More recently, calcitonin has been shown to stimulate 1,25(OH)₂D synthesis (and intestinal calcium absorption) in thyroparathyroidectomized rats (23). However, available data in humans are contradictory. If there is an effect of calcitonin on net calcium transport, it is probably small.

Growth Hormone. Administration of growth hormone to healthy humans and pituitary dwarfs increases net intestinal calcium absorption. There is controversy as to whether this action is mediated by stimulation of 1,25(OH)₂D synthesis or by some other mechanism (24).

Estrogen. Postmenopausal women may have a defective synthesis of 1,25(OH)2D and reduced intestinal calcium absorption (14). Estrogen therapy restores normal 1,25(OH)₂D synthesis, raises intestinal calcium absorption, and converts calcium balance from negative to positive (25). Enhanced 1,25(OH)₂D production also is the likely cause of the enhanced calcium absorption seen during pregnancy and lactation. During pregnancy, the placenta produces 1,25(OH)₂D in addition to that produced by the kidneys.

Furosemide. Furosemide increases urinary calcium excretion, and intestinal calcium absorption increases to

TABLE 1. *Systemic modulators of intestinal calcium absorption*

Increase	Decrease
Vitamin D	Aging
Low calcium diet	High calcium diet
High sodium diet	Low sodium diet
PTH	Glucocorticoids
Phosphate depletion	Phosphate loading
Growth hormone	Thyroid hormone
Estrogen	Metabolic acidosis
Pregnancy	Thiazides
Lactation	
Furosemide	

match urinary calcium losses (26). One would anticipate a compensatory increase in PTH, stimulating $1,25(OH)_2D$ synthesis, but this is not always found (26).

Systemic Agents That Reduce Calcium Absorption

Glucocorticoids. Spontaneous Cushing syndrome and chronic treatment with pharmacologic doses of glucocorticoids suppress intestinal calcium absorption, without altering vitamin D levels (27). Expression of vitamin-D-dependent genes may be altered by glucocorticoids. For example, dexamethasone treatment results in a 75% decrease in rat intestinal calbindin-D_{9K} mRNA (28). Pharmacologic doses of vitamin D metabolites can increase calcium absorption during glucocorticoid therapy and thus overcome the inhibitory actions on calcium transport (29).

Thyroid Hormone. In hyperthyroidism, there is a net calcium efflux from the skeleton. This calcium and phosphate load may in turn suppress $1,25(OH)_2D$ formation and decrease calcium absorption (30).

Metabolic Acidosis. In rats, chronic metabolic acidosis induced by ingestion of ammonium chloride reduces intestinal calcium absorption by decreasing serum $1,25(OH)_2D$ (31). $1,25(OH)_2D$ is reduced because production rates decline with elevation in the blood ionized calcium level (31). A diet high in animal protein results in an acid load because of the sulfur-containing amino acids. An animal-protein-rich diet may provoke bone calcium release, hypercalciuria, and suppression of the PTH– $1,25(OH)_2D$ axis (32).

Thiazide Diuretics. Thiazide diuretics reduce intestinal calcium absorption in patients with renal hypercalciuria and kidney stones (33). In these patients, administration of thiazide corrects the renal calcium leak, reverses secondary hyperparathyroidism, and consequently restores normal serum $1,25(OH)_2D$ concentration (33). In rats, chlorthalidone decreases intestinal calcium absorption without altering serum $1,25(OH)_2D$ levels (34). It is not yet clear whether thiazide diuretics reduce intestinal calcium absorption in normal humans.

Intraluminal Factors

Food Sources. About 60% to 75% of daily calcium intake in adults is derived from milk and other dairy products. In animal products, calcium is present largely bound to protein, from which it is liberated by proteases and then absorbed. Many dark-green leafy vegetables are known to have relatively high calcium contents. However, the calcium of spinach is very poorly absorbed, presumably because of the high oxalate content of spinach (35). In contrast, kale, a low-oxalate vegetable, exhibits excellent absorbability of its calcium (36). Other low-oxalate, high-calcium vegetable greens that are believed to be good sources of dietary calcium include broccoli and turnip, collard, and mustard greens (36).

Calcium Supplements. Calcium supplements are available in many forms, including calcium gluconate, calcium lactate, calcium citrate, calcium carbonate, and calcium phosphate. It is expected that calcium bioavailability, or the amount of calcium available for intestinal absorption, may vary among these calcium preparations because of low aqueous solubility of some salts (calcium carbonate and calcium phosphate) and the ability of some anionic components (e.g., citrate) to form soluble complexes with calcium (37). In the normally acid environment of the gastric juice, most calcium salts will probably dissolve and become bioavailable, except at high dosages. However, when gastric acidity is reduced (as in the elderly, in patients with achlorhydria, and after treatment with antacids or H_2-blockers), calcium bioavailability from calcium carbonate and calcium phosphate may be low because of their incomplete dissolution. When calcium salts of lactate, citrate, and carbonate are given, the anions released may neutralize some of the gastric acid and further impair solubility of calcium salts.

The bioavailability of calcium carbonate, the most widely used calcium supplement, may be particularly dependent on pH because of low aqueous solubility. Calcium absorption from calcium carbonate given alone has been reported to be impaired in patients with achlorhydria (38), although another study, conducted under nonphysiologic conditions, reported that calcium absorption was independent of gastrointestinal acid secretion (39).

Because of its relatively high aqueous solubility and evidence that the calcium citrate complex itself may be absorbed (37), this salt may provide optimum calcium bioavailability. One study compared the calcium bioavailability from calcium citrate with that of calcium carbonate (40). Fourteen normal subjects (22 to 37 years old) took 1000 mg of calcium orally as calcium citrate or calcium carbonate. The amount of calcium absorbed was estimated from the rise in urinary calcium, which was significantly higher after oral administration of calcium citrate than calcium carbonate, whether it was expressed as the total amount or as an increase from basal (fasting) excretion. The mean difference between the two calcium salts ranged from 20% for total calcium excreted after the dose, to 52% for the increase in urinary calcium over the 4-hr post-load period, to 66% for the increase in calcium excretion during the second half of the post-load period. The higher calcium absorbability of calcium citrate compared to calcium carbonate was also demonstrated by radiolabeling the calcium in each salt and measuring fecal recovery of the radioisotope (37).

Other Intraluminal Factors. Many compounds decrease calcium absorption when they are present in the lumen, because of the formation of insoluble complexes (41) (Table 2). These include long-chain fatty acids (steatorrhea), phosphate, oxalate, phytate, and dietary fiber. Because calcium is thought to be absorbed primarily in the ionic form, less than complete absorption of dietary calcium occurs when there is complexation of calcium in the intestinal lumen. As much as 500 mg of calcium can be found in fatty acid soaps during steatorrhea (1). Owing to the large amount of phosphate in the diet (often 1.0 g or more, compared to less than 1.0 g of calcium), calcium phosphate is a major complex in the intestinal lumen. Because calcium phosphate formation is pH dependent, with a pKa of about 6.1, increases in luminal pH above 6.1 favor complexation and reduction of the amount of ionic Ca^{2+} available for absorption.

Table 2. *Intraluminal factors that affect intestinal calcium absorption*

Decrease	Increase
Long-chain fatty acids	Lysine
Phosphate	Arginine
Oxalate	Penicillin
Phytate	Chloramphenicol
Fiber	Lactose
Sodium cellulose phosphate (Calcibind)	
Tetracycline	
Small bowel resection	

Calcium complexation with oxalate and phytate is not as sensitive to pH and is not readily reversible. Ingestion of food rich in oxalate (nuts, rhubarb, spinach, brewed tea) or phytate (whole wheat products) may result in reduced calcium absorption. Dietary fiber, including cellulose and noncellulose types, decreases calcium absorption by binding dietary calcium in proportion to the uronic acid content of the fiber.

Additional factors that may reduce absorption of calcium from the intestinal lumen include drugs such as sodium cellulose phosphate (Calcibind) and tetracycline, which bind calcium. Intestinal resection reduces absorptive surface and quickens transit time. For example, in one study, calcium absorption decreased in direct proportion to the amount of small bowel resected, in the absence of the colon (10).

Other luminal compounds can enhance calcium absorption, possibly by forming more soluble complexes and preventing formation of less soluble calcium phosphate. These compounds include certain amino acids (lysine, arginine), certain antibiotics (penicillin, chloramphenicol), and monosaccharides or disaccharides, especially lactose. Lactose, the major disaccharide in milk and other dairy products, increases net calcium absorption in humans by a direct action on the intestinal cell that is independent of vitamin D (41). The breakdown of lactose to glucose and galactose may be important, because lactose fails to stimulate calcium absorption in lactose-intolerant people. This action of lactose may explain the finding by some investigators that milk calcium is better absorbed than equal amounts of calcium from other foods (1).

MAGNESIUM

Food Sources

In contrast to calcium, magnesium is highly concentrated in cells and thus is widely distributed in foods, largely bound by protein and phosphate. In vegetables and green plants, magnesium is complexed with porphyrins in chlorophyll. Like calcium, it must be solubilized by proteases, acid pH, or the presence of anions capable of forming soluble magnesium salts, before it is absorbed.

Intestinal Absorption

The average daily intake of magnesium in a Western diet is 300 mg, of which about 30% to 35% is absorbed. Over the range of normal magnesium intake, there is a linear relationship between intake and absorption. However, at very high magnesium intake, absorption is lower than predicted, suggesting that the magnesium absorptive mechanism in humans may be saturable. Net magnesium absorption was measured in normal subjects after they ingested a standard meal, plus magnesium supplements in a range from 36 mg to 960 mg (42). Although absorption increased with each increment in intake, the percent of magnesium absorbed fell progressively, from 65% at the lowest to 11% at the highest magnesium intake. It is believed that magnesium absorption is mediated by both a saturable carrier and by passive diffusion, with the carrier primarily responsible for mediating absorption when magnesium intake is normal or only slightly elevated, and with passive absorption accounting for the continual rise in absorption when intake is elevated further.

At very low levels of intake, there is net secretion rather than net absorption of calcium (5). By contrast, there is no suggestion that net secretion of magnesium would occur if magnesium intake was extremely low. On the other hand, at higher levels of intake, calcium absorption is much higher than magnesium absorption. It thus appears that the normal intestine is somewhat protective against net loss of magnesium when magnesium intake is low, and against hyperabsorption of magnesium when intake is high (42). A relatively restricted passive diffusion across the mucosa of magnesium in comparison with calcium would explain such behavior.

Relatively little is known about the sites of intestinal magnesium absorption in humans. Based on the appearance of radioactive isotope in blood after oral ingestion, magnesium is thought to be absorbed throughout the small intestine, with maximal absorption in the proximal small bowel (41). Magnesium absorption has been studied in human jejunum and ileum using the triple-lumen perfusion technique (8). In contrast to calcium, magnesium absorption in the basal state is greater in the ileum than in the jejunum. Little information is available on magnesium absorption by the large bowel; however, hypermagnesemia following rectal enemas indicates that magnesium may also be absorbed by the colon.

Role of Vitamin D

There is considerable evidence that vitamin D increases net magnesium absorption in humans. For example, patients with low $1,25(OH)_2D$, as in chronic renal failure, have lower net magnesium absorption which is restored to normal with $1,25(OH)_2D$ (43). Additional convincing evidence for a stimulatory effect of $1,25(OH)_2D$ on magnesium net absorption has been obtained using the triple-lumen perfusion technique in healthy humans (8). Treatment with $1,25(OH)_2D$ for 7 days increases jejunal, but not ileal, net magnesium absorption. As noted previously, fractional calcium absorption is increased by a low, and reduced by a high, calcium diet. This adaptation process is mediated by $1,25(OH)_2D$. Calcium intake influences intestinal magnesium absorption in a similar fashion (12). There is no evidence that the PTH–vitamin D axis adapts to a chronic high or low magnesium intake, as it does with calcium.

PHOSPHORUS

Food Sources

Most foods contain phosphorus, but the most important dietary sources are dairy products, grains, and meats. In the American diet, food additives present in baked goods, cheeses, and carbonated beverages can contribute as much as 30% of the dietary phosphorus intake. Organic phosphorus is released during the digestive process. Phosphorus absorption can be reduced by a high intake of calcium or by aluminum-hydroxide-containing compounds, because both calcium and aluminum bind phosphorus to form relatively insoluble salts in the intestinal lumen.

Intestinal Absorption

The normal diet contains 800 to 2000 mg of phosphorus per day. Throughout this range, approximately 65% of dietary phosphorus is absorbed. This percentage absorption is relatively independent of the intake of phosphorus, because absorption occurs primarily by a diffusional process, although there is a small saturable component. Passive absorption of phosphorus by the paracellular route occurs when the luminal concentration exceeds 1.5 mmol, or 47 mg/L, as probably occurs postprandially. This is quantitatively the most significant process. A separate cellular pathway for phosphorus uptake involves sodium-coupled phosphorus entry by a carrier (Na-P cotransporter) in the brush-border membrane (Fig. 3) (41). Energy for this elec-

trochemically uphill process is provided by the sodium gradient, which is maintained by sodium-potassium ATPase. The exit of phosphorus across the basolateral membrane into the blood is believed to be passive, down electrical and perhaps concentration gradients. Overall, the evidence favors (i) Na-dependent active cotransport at low luminal phosphorus concentrations, and (ii) passive diffusional forces driving phosphorus transport at luminal phosphorus concentrations above the concentration that saturates the cotransporter (41). The highest basal and 1,25(OH)$_2$D-stimulated phosphorus absorption occurs in the jejunum.

Role of Vitamin D

Metabolic balance studies have shown that administration of vitamin D or 1,25(OH)$_2$D to animals or humans enhances net intestinal phosphorus absorption (41). The site of action of 1,25(OH)$_2$D to increase cellular phosphorus transport appears to be the brush border (Fig. 3). The Na-dependent phosphorus uptake process is saturable, with a dissociation constant (Kd) of less than 1 mM (44). Pretreatment with 1,25(OH)$_2$D increases Na-dependent phosphorus influx into brush-border membrane vesicles through an increase in V$_{max}$ without a significant change in Kd (44). No vitamin-D-dependent proteins have been identified that are specific for phosphorus transport.

In response to dietary phosphorus-deprivation or to hypophosphatemia, the kidney increases 1,25(OH)$_2$D production. This results in an influx of calcium and phosphorus from bone and intestine, with suppression of PTH secretion, thereby reducing renal phosphorus excretion. This entire sequence represents an adaptation to phosphorus depletion. In response to an excessive phosphorus load, the reverse sequence would ensue, although the overall effect of reduced 1,25(OH)$_2$D concentration on net phosphorus absorption would be limited. Even in the presence of very low serum 1,25(OH)$_2$D levels, patients with chronic renal failure exhibit significant concentration-dependent jejunal phosphorus absorption (45). Thus, the availability of phosphorus in the diet appears to be the major determinant of net phosphorus input to the body from the intestine.

TECHNIQUES FOR MEASUREMENT OF CA, MG, AND P ABSORPTION IN MAN

Serum and urinary concentrations of Ca, Mg, and P are easily and routinely measured in the evaluation and care of patients with disorders of mineral metabolism and bone. However, quantitation of their intestinal absorption is difficult and has generally been assessed only in a research setting. Several available techniques are listed in Table 3, with comments on their specific drawbacks and with appropriate references provided for those seeking more detailed information (8,39,46–52).

Fast and Oral Ca Load Test

This test, although indirect, provides a readily available assessment of intestinal calcium absorption (50–52). After

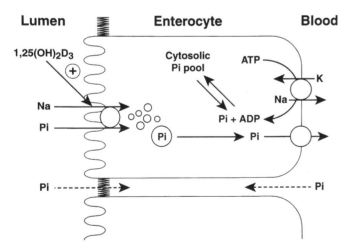

FIG. 3. Schematic of inorganic phosphorus (Pi) absorption (from lumen to blood) and secretion (from blood to lumen) across intestinal epithelium. *Solid arrows* indicate transcellular pathway and *broken arrows* indicate paracellular pathway. 1,25(OH)$_2$D stimulates Na-coupled Pi influx into membrane vesicles. Transcellular movement of Pi may be sequestered in structures that are presently unidentified. Exit is down electrical and perhaps concentration gradients. (From: Favus MJ. Intestinal absorption of calcium, magnesium, and phosphorus. In: Coe FL, Favus MJ (eds) *Disorders of Bone and Mineral Metabolism.* Raven Press, New York, pp 57–81, 1992.)

TABLE 3. *Techniques for measurement of Ca, Mg, and P absorption in humans*

Technique	Major drawbacks	Reference
Metabolic balance	Requires metabolic kitchen; prolonged time period for equilibration and sample collection (weeks); errors caused by inaccuracies of fecal collection.	46
Absorption from a single meal, following intestinal washout	Requires intestinal lavage; not physiologic.	39
Absorption of isotopic minerals	May require fecal collections; radioisotopes involve safety and hazardous waste issues; high cost of radiocalcium; instrumentation required for measurement of ^{47}Ca; no suitable radioisotope for Mg or P measurement; stable isotopes require mass spectrometer.	47–49
Segmental intestinal perfusion	Requires passage of triple-lumen tube; measures absorption only in isolated intestinal segment.	8
Fast and oral Ca load test	Requires restricted calcium and sodium diet 1 week prior to testing; an indirect test: both renal function and bone status can influence results.	50–52

overnight fasting, a 2-hr urine is collected and urinary calcium excretion expressed in terms of urinary creatinine, or glomerular filtration rate (GFR). The fasting urinary calcium level is normally less than 0.11 mg/dl GFR, and elevated values suggest either a renal calcium leak or increased bone resorption. The 2-hr fasting urinary calcium excretion is critical to the test calculations and hence to the assessment of calcium absorption. To obtain an optimum fasting urinary calcium level that is not exaggerated by excess sodium intake or by an incomplete clearance of absorbed calcium, the subject should be on a daily diet of 400 mg calcium and 100 meq sodium for a week prior to the testing.

In the test, subjects are given a 1000-mg oral calcium load in either milk or a liquid synthetic diet. Urine is collected for 4 hours after the oral calcium load. Either the absolute amount of urinary calcium excretion (expressed per mg creatinine), or the increment in urinary calcium excretion, is utilized as a measure of intestinal calcium absorption. Normal urinary calcium following an oral calcium load is .06 to .20 mg/mg creatinine. Patients with malabsorption may fail to increase urinary calcium levels appropriately. Conversely, greater increases in urinary calcium after an oral calcium load provide evidence for increased intestinal calcium absorption (e.g., nephrolithiasis due to absorptive hypercalciuria). The major advantage of this technique is its simplicity in performance and analysis, without requiring the use of radioisotopes. It can be repeated frequently and correlates very well with isotopic methods of calcium absorption (Fig. 4) (52).

For the proper use and interpretation of this test, its limitations should be understood. Both renal function and bone status can influence the results. Situations in which renal handling of calcium is altered, such as impaired renal function or use of thiazide diuretics, would invalidate test results. An avid calcium uptake by bone can also lead to erroneous results using this technique.

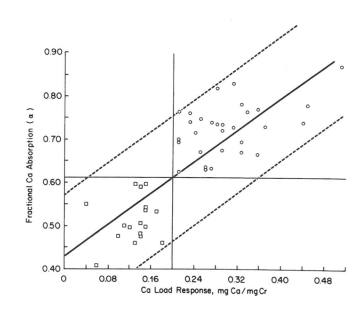

FIG. 4. Correlation of fractional intestinal calcium absorption (α) with urinary calcium excretion after a 1-g oral calcium load. Data are presented for normal subjects (□) and patients with absorptive hypercalciuria (o). The *solid diagonal line* represents the regression line correlating α with calcium load response, and the *dashed diagonal lines* represent ± 2 SD of the regression line. The correlation coefficient was 0.81 ($p <$ 0.001). Calcium load response was expressed as total urinary calcium per mg creatinine over a 4-hr period after ingestion of 1 g calcium. The *solid horizontal and vertical lines* indicate the upper limit of normal for α (0.61) and calcium load response (0.20), respectively. Values for α and calcium load response in absorptive hypercalciuria were significantly higher than those of the control group. (From: Zerwekh JE, Sakhaee K, Pak CYC. Utility and limitation of calciuric response to oral calcium load as a measure of intestinal calcium absorption: Comparison with isotopic fractional calcium absorption. *Invest Urol* 19:161—164, 1981.)

REFERENCES

1. Alpers DH: Absorption of vitamins and divalent minerals. In: Sleisenger MH, Fordtran JS (eds) *Gastrointestinal Disease*, 4th ed. WB Saunders, Philadelphia, pp 1045–1062, 1989
2. Turnberg LA, Riley SA: Digestion and absorption of nutrients and vitamins. In: Sleisenger MH, Fordtran JS, et al. (eds) *Gastrointestinal Disease: Pathophysiology, Diagnosis, Management*, 5th ed. WB Saunders, Philadelphia, pp 977–1008, 1993
3. Johnson JA, Kumar R: Renal and intestinal calcium transport: Roles of vitamin D and vitamin D-dependent calcium binding proteins. *Semin Nephrol* 14:119–128, 1994
4. Wasserman RH, Chandler JS, Meyer SA, et al.: Intestinal calcium transport and calcium extrusion processes at the basolateral membrane. *J Nutr* 122:662–671, 1992
5. Sheikh MS, Ramirez A, Emmett M, Santa Ana C, Schiller LR, Fordtran JS: Role of vitamin D-dependent and vitamin D-independent mechanisms in absorption of food calcium. *J Clin Invest* 81:126–132, 1988
6. Karbach U: Paracellular calcium transport across the small intestine. *J Nutr* 122:672–677, 1992
7. Norman AW, Nemere I, Zhou L-X, et al.: 1,25-(OH)$_2$-vitamin D$_3$: A steroid hormone that produces biologic effects via both genomic and nongenomic pathways. *J Steroid Biochem Mol Biol* 41:231–240, 1992
8. Krejs GJ, Nicar MJ, Zerwekh JE, Norman DA, Kane MG, Pak CYC: Effect of 1,25-dihydroxyvitamin D$_3$ on calcium and magnesium absorption in the healthy human jejunum and ileum. *Am J Med* 75:973–976, 1983
9. Grinstead WC, Pak CYC, Krejs GJ: Effect of 1,25-dihydroxyvitamin D$_3$ on calcium absorption in the colon of healthy humans. *Am J Physiol* 247:G189–G192, 1984
10. Hylander E, Ladefoged K, Jarnum S: The importance of colon in calcium absorption following small-intestinal resection. *Am J Physiol* 15:55–60, 1980
11. Hylander E, Ladefoged K, Jarnum S: Calcium absorption after intestinal resection. The importance of a preserved colon. *Scand J Gastroenterol* 25:705–710, 1990
12. Norman DA, Fordtran JS, Brinkley LJ, Zerwekh JE, Nicar MJ, Strowig SM, Pak CYC: Jejunal and ileal adaptation to alterations in dietary calcium. Changes in calcium and magnesium absorption and pathogenetic role of parathyroid hormone and 1,25-dihydroxyvitamin D. *J Clin Invest* 67:1599–1603, 1981
13. Sakhaee K, Baker S, Zerwekh J, Poindexter J, Garcia-Hernandez PA, Pak CYC: Limited risk of kidney stone formation during long-term calcium citrate supplementation in nonstone forming subjects. *J Urol* 152:324–327, 1994
14. Gallagher JC, Riggs BL, Eisman J, Hamstra A, Arnaud SB, DeLuca HF: Intestinal calcium absorption and serum vitamin D metabolites in normal subjects and osteoporotic patients. *J Clin Invest* 64:729–736, 1979
15. Slovik DM, Adams JS, Neer RM, Holick MF, Potts Jr JT: Deficient production of 1,25-dihydroxyvitamin D in elderly osteoporotic patients. *N Engl J Med* 305:372–374, 1981
16. Tsai KS, Heath H, Lumar R, Riggs BL: Impaired vitamin D metabolism with aging in women. Possible role of pathogenesis of senile osteoporosis. *J Clin Invest* 73:1668–1672, 1984
17. Christiansen C, Rodbro P: Serum vitamin D metabolites in younger and elderly postmenopausal women. *Calcif Tissue Int* 36:19–24, 1984
18. Ebeling PR, Sandgren ME, DiMagno EP, Lane AW, DeLuca HF, Riggs BL: Evidence of an age-related decrease in intestinal responsiveness to vitamin D: Relationship between serum 1,25-(OH)$_2$D and intestinal vitamin D receptor concentrations in normal women. *J Clin Endocrinol Metab* 75:176–182, 1992
19. Breslau NA, McGuire JL, Zerwekh JE, Pak CYC. The role of dietary sodium on renal excretion and intestinal absorption of calcium and on vitamin D metabolism. *J Clin Endocrinol Metab* 55:369–373, 1982
20. Breslau NA, Sakhaee K, Pak CYC: Impaired adaptation to salt-induced urinary calcium losses in postmenopausal osteoporosis. *Trans Assoc Am Physicians* 98:107–115, 1985
21. Devine A, Criddle RA, Dick IM, Kerr DA, Prince RL: A longitudinal study of the effect of sodium and calcium intakes on regional bone density in postmenopausal women. *Am J Clin Nutr* 62:740–745, 1995
22. Breslau NA, Weinstock R. Regulation of 1,25-(OH)$_2$D synthesis in hypoparathyroidism and pseudohypoparathyroidism. *Am J Physiol* 255:E730–E736, 1988
23. Jaeger P, Jones W, Clemens TL, Hayslett JP: Evidence that calcitonin stimulates 1,25-(OH)$_2$D production and intestinal absorption of calcium in vivo. *J Clin Invest* 78:456–461, 1986
24. Chipman JJ, Zerwekh J, Nicar M, Marks J, Pak CYC: Effect of growth hormone administration: Reciprocal changes in serum 1,25-(OH)$_2$D and intestinal calcium absorption. *J Clin Endocrinol Metab* 51:321–324, 1980
25. Gallagher JC, Riggs BL, DeLuca HF: Effect of estrogen on calcium absorption and serum vitamin D metabolites in postmenopausal osteoporosis. *J Clin Endocrinol Metab* 51:1359–1364, 1980
26. Bushinsky DA, Favus MJ, Langman CB, Coe FL: Mechanism of chronic hypercalciuria with furosemide: Increased calcium absorption. *Am J Physiol* 251:F17–24, 1986
27. Seeman E, Kumar R, Hunder GG, Scott M, Heath H III, Riggs BL: Production, degradation, and circulating levels of 1,25-dihydroxyvitamin D in health and in chronic glucocorticoid excess. *J Clin Invest* 66:664–669, 1980
28. Christakos S, Gill R, Lee S, Li H: Molecular aspects of the calbindins. *J Nutr* 122:678–682, 1992
29. Hahn TJ, Halstead LR, Teitelbaum SL: Altered mineral metabolism in glucocorticoid-induced osteopenia. Effect of 25-hydroxyvitamin D administration. *J Clin Invest* 64:655–665, 1979
30. Haldimann B, Kaptein EM, Singer FR, Nicoloff JT, Massry SG: Intestinal calcium absorption in patients with hyperthyroidism. *J Clin Endocrinol Metab* 51:995–997, 1980
31. Bushinsky DA, Riera GS, Favus MJ, Coe FL: Response of serum 1,25-(OH)$_2$D$_3$ to variation of ionized calcium during chronic metabolic acidosis. *Am J Physiol* 249:F361–365, 1985
32. Breslau NA, Brinkley L, Hill KD, Pak CYC: Relationship of animal protein-rich diet to kidney stone formation and calcium metabolism. *J Clin Endocrinol Metab* 66:140–146, 1988
33. Zerwekh JE, Pak CYC: Selective effects of thiazide therapy on serum 1,25-dihydroxyvitamin D and intestinal calcium absorption in renal and absorptive hypercalciuria. *Metabolism* 29:13–17, 1980
34. Bushinsky DA, Favus MJ, Coe FL: Mechanism of chronic hypocalciuria with chlorthalidone: Reduced calcium absorption. *Am J Physiol* 247:F746–752, 1984
35. Heaney RP, Weaver CM, Recker RR: Calcium absorbability from spinach. *Am J Clin Nutr* 47:707–709, 1988
36. Heaney RP: Calcium absorption from kale. *Am J Clin Nutr* 51:656–657, 1990
37. Pak CYC, Breslau NA, Harvey JA: Nutrition and metabolic bone disease. In: Scarpelli DG, Migaki G (eds) *Nutritional Diseases: Research Directions in Comparative Pathobiology*. Alan R. Liss, New York, pp 215–240, 1986
38. Recker RR: Calcium absorption and achlorhydria. *N Engl J Med* 313:70–73, 1985
39. Bo-Linn GW, Davis GR, Buddru DJ, Morawski SG, Santa Ana C, Fordtran JS: An evaluation of the importance of gastric acid secretion in the absorption of dietary calcium. *J Clin Invest* 73:640–647, 1984
40. Nicar MJ, Pak CYC: Calcium bioavailability from calcium carbonate and calcium citrate. *J Clin Endocrinol Metab* 61:391–393, 1985
41. Favus MJ: Intestinal absorption of calcium, magnesium, and phosphorus. In: Coe FL, Favus MJ (eds) *Disorders of Bone and Mineral Metabolism*. Raven Press, New York, pp 57–81, 1992
42. Fine KD, Santa Ana CA, Porter JL, Fordtran JS: Intestinal absorption of magnesium from food and supplements. *J Clin Invest* 88:396–402, 1991
43. Schmulen AC, Lerman M, Pak CYC, Zerwekh J, Morawski S, Fordtran JS, Vergne-Marini P: Effect of 1,25-(OH)$_2$D$_3$ on jejunal absorption of magnesium in patients with chronic renal disease. *Am J Physiol* 238:G349–352, 1980
44. Matsumoto T, Fontaine O, Rasmussen H: Effect of 1,25-dihydroxyvitamin D$_3$ on phosphate uptake into chick intestinal brush border membrane vesicles. *Biochem Biophys Acta* 599:13–23, 1980
45. Lemann Jr J: Intestinal absorption of calcium, magnesium and

phosphorus. In: Favus MJ (ed) *Primer on the Metabolic Bone Diseases and Disorders of Mineral Metabolism*, 2nd ed. Raven Press, New York, pp 46–50, 1993

46. Pak CYC, Stewart A, Raskin P, Galosy RA: A simple and reliable method for calcium balance using combined period and continuous fecal markers. *Metabolism* 29:793–796, 1980
47. Pak CYC, Ohata M, Lawrence EC, et al.: The hypercalciurias: Causes, parathyroid functions and diagnostic criteria. *J Clin Invest* 54:387–400, 1974
48. Birge SJ, Peck WA, Berman M, Whendon GD: Study of calcium absorption in man: A kinetic analysis and physiologic model. *J Clin Invest* 48:1705–1713, 1969
49. Mautalen CA, Cabrejas ML, Soto RJ: Isotopic determination of intestinal calcium absorption in normal subjects. *Metab Clin Exp* 18:395–405, 1969
50. Pak CYC, Kaplan RA, Bone H, Townsend J, Waters O: A simple test for the diagnosis of absorptive, resorptive and renal hypercalciurias. *N Engl J Med* 292:497–500, 1975
51. Broadus AE, Dominguez M, Bartter FC: Pathophysiologic studies in idiopathic hypercalciuria: Use of an oral calcium tolerance test to characterize distinctive hypercalciuric subgroups. *J Clin Endocrinol Metab* 47:751–760, 1978
52. Zerwekh JE, Sakhaee K, Pak CYC: Utility and limitation of calciuric response to oral calcium load as a measure of intestinal calcium absorption: Comparison with isotopic fractional calcium absorption. *Invest Urol* 19:161–164, 1981

8. Calcium, Magnesium, and Phosphorus: Renal Handling and Urinary Excretion

Neil A. Breslau, M.D.

Center for Mineral Metabolism and Clinical Research, Department of Medicine, and General Clinical Research Center, University of Texas, Southwestern Medical Center, Dallas, Texas

In the normal steady state, there is zero net external mineral exchange. During this zero mineral balance, bone acquisition equals bone resorption, and the calcium (Ca), magnesium (Mg), and phosphorus (P) contents in urine approximate those of net intestinal absorption. Large amounts of calcium, magnesium, and phosphorus continually enter and leave plasma via bone, kidney, and intestine, and these ion movements must be carefully regulated. In some respects, the renal tubule resembles the intestine. Each contains ion-transporting cells that are polarized, with a redundant plasma membrane on the side not exposed to plasma (i.e., renal tubular and intestinal mucosal cells possess a brush border). Moreover, each is responsive to one or more of the three major calcitropic hormones. In this chapter, we shall focus on the renal handling of calcium, magnesium, and phosphorus.

CALCIUM

General Features of Filtration, Reabsorption, and Clearance

Based on a daily calcium intake of 1000 mg, the net calcium absorbed each day by the intestine is about 200 mg. In a mature, calcium-replete individual, the kidney would excrete this amount of calcium to maintain calcium balance. Renal excretion of calcium begins with the filtration of about 8000 mg calcium at the glomerulus (1). A normal total plasma calcium of 10.0 mg/dl is made up of 4.5 mg/dl of nonfilterable, protein-bound calcium and 5.5 mg/dl of filterable calcium, which is in turn made up of 5.0 mg/dl of free calcium ions (Ca^{2+}) and 0.5 mg/dl of calcium complexed with a variety of anions such as citrate, bicarbonate, and phosphate. Assuming a GFR of 100 ml/min (i.e., 144 L/day), the filtered load of calcium will amount to about 8000 mg/day (5.5 mg/dl or 55 mg/L × 144 L/day). Of this 8000 mg of filtered calcium, 7800 mg is reabsorbed (97.5%) to yield a net urinary excretion of 200 mg.

Thus, the kidney has to reabsorb a large quantity of the filtered calcium, while at the same time excreting, with relative precision, the small amount of calcium absorbed by the gut. Compared with the intestine, which is known for its calcium absorptive potential, the renal tubule absorbs 40-fold (8000 mg vs. 200 mg) more calcium each day. As derived from micropuncture data, approximately 70% of the filtered calcium is reabsorbed in the proximal tubule, 20% in the thick ascending limb of the loop of Henle (TALH), 5% to 10% in the distal tubule, and a small fraction, less than 5%, in the collecting duct system (2). Bulk calcium reabsorption is accomplished in the proximal nephron and in the TALH, in association with sodium reabsorption, and with no additional energy requirements. Regulation of calcium excreted in the urine is mainly accomplished in the distal nephron, a locus where the active calcium reabsorptive mechanism and the action of important calcitropic hormones congregate. The specific characteristics of calcium handling by individual nephron segments have been reviewed (1,2).

Mechanisms of Tubular Calcium Reabsorption

In calcium-absorbing epithelia, such as those lining the renal tubule and the intestine, calcium fluxes across the epithelium can occur between the cells and through the cells (Fig. 1). The flow of sodium and water across the intercellular pathway can carry calcium with it in solution (solvent drag). A large fraction of calcium reabsorption in the proximal tubule is mediated by this mechanism. A second mechanism that moves calcium across the intercellular pathway is passive diffusion, down electrical or chemical gradients (3). For example, higher luminal calcium con-

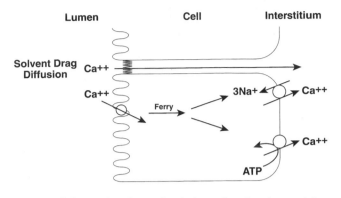

FIG. 1. Schematic of renal tubule cells showing calcium reabsorption through the intercellular and transcellular pathways.

centration [Ca] drives calcium in the absorptive direction toward lower [Ca] in the interstitium across most parts of the proximal convoluted tubule (PCT).

Transcellular transport of calcium across a renal tubular cell resembles that across an intestinal cell and would involve at least three steps: entry across the luminal membrane, ferry through the cytoplasm, and exit across the basolateral membrane (Fig. 1). A majority of the calcium reabsorbed in the PCT is reabsorbed via the paracellular pathway, but a small amount is reabsorbed via a transcellular pathway. The precise mechanisms of transcellular calcium reabsorption in the PCT are not clear. Presumably, calcium enters the cells via channels and is then extruded from the cell by the Na^+-Ca^{2+} exchanger or by a Ca^{2+} pump (4).

In the distal tubule, reabsorption of calcium can be dissociated from sodium reabsorption, and, unlike in the proximal tubule, calcium reabsorption occurs against steep concentration and electrical gradients. Parathyroid hormone (PTH) may activate channels permitting calcium to enter distal tubule cells (5). Following entry at the apical pole, calcium needs to be buffered so that the low intracellular Ca^{2+} environment is protected. It then has to traverse the cytoplasm to the basolateral pole for extrusion. Much interest has been focused on the vitamin-D-dependent Ca^{2+}-binding protein, calbindin-D (CaBP-D), an intracellular system both for buffering and for ferrying Ca^{2+} (1). A model of distal tubule renal calcium transport has been proposed, emphasizing similarities to calcium transport in the enterocyte (4,6) (see Chapter 7). At the basolateral membrane, calcium is actively transported out of the cell against electrochemical gradients. At least two mechanisms may participate in the cellular expulsion of calcium: (i) a calcium-sensitive, magnesium-dependent ATPase (Ca^{2+} pump), and (ii) a Ca^{2+}-Na^+ exchange system.

Factors Influencing Renal Handling of Calcium

The major factors influencing urinary calcium excretion are depicted in Fig. 2 (7). The maximum range of daily uri-

nary calcium excretion in healthy adults is from 40 mg/day to 300 mg/day, whereas in disease states, urinary calcium excretion may be <40 mg/d and can range upward to as much as 800 mg/day. Factors affecting renal handling of calcium may be divided into dietary factors, hormonal factors, metabolic perturbations, diuretics, and other factors.

Dietary Factors

Sodium

It has long been known that the clearance of calcium parallels that of sodium (8,9). One explanation is that salt loading, and the consequent volume expansion, cause reduction in sodium and calcium reabsorption in the proximal tubule, but inhibition of calcium reabsorption in the distal nephron may also contribute. Increases of urinary calcium excretion of 25 to 50 mg occur with each 100-mEq increment of urinary sodium excretion (7,9,10). The rise in urinary calcium following increases in dietary sodium intake may also be mediated through extrarenal causes (10). Increasing sodium intake is associated with increases in circulating levels of immunoreactive PTH, which in turn stimulates $1,25(OH)_2D$ production and intestinal calcium absorption.

Calcium

In a normal individual who is in calcium balance, the kidney excretes the amount of calcium absorbed by the intestine. When the relationship between urinary calcium excretion and dietary calcium intake was examined in normal individuals, Lemann and associates (7,11) found that only 6% to 8% of an oral calcium load appeared in the urine. Thus, a calcium supplement of 1000 mg/day would be expected to increase daily urinary calcium excretion by 60 to 80 mg. Urinary calcium excretion falls within 2 to 4 days

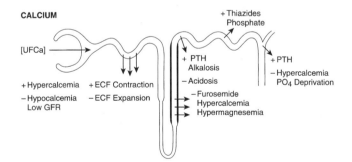

FIG. 2. Regulation of urinary calcium excretion. Reduction (-) in GFR of calcium reduces urinary calcium excretion, whereas inhibition (-) of renal tubular calcium reabsorption increases urinary calcium excretion. (From: Lemann J Jr. Urinary excretion of calcium, magnesium, and phosphorus. In: Favus MJ (ed) *Primer on the Metabolic Bone Diseases and Disorders of Mineral Metabolism*, 2nd ed. Raven Press, New York, 50–54, 1993.)

when subjects are fed diets providing 200 mg calcium/day or less (7). Even after subjects have been adapted to such diets for long periods, individual minimum urinary calcium excretion rates vary widely, from 20 to 200 mg/day, presumably because of individual differences in net bone resorption and the regulation of renal tubular calcium reabsorption.

Inorganic Phosphate

It is a long-established observation that oral and parenteral phosphate administration is associated with a fall in urinary calcium (12). The mechanism for this hypocalciuric effect is still not well understood. Micropuncture studies suggest increases in calcium reabsorption in the distal or terminal portion of the nephron (13). Phosphate administration or excess can also reduce urine calcium through extrarenal mechanisms (1). Thus, phosphate loading is associated with increased calcium sequestration in bone and/or soft tissues, which in turn, could reduce the calcium load for urinary excretion. Phosphate can also stimulate PTH secretion (possibly through reducing plasma ionized calcium concentration) and thereby augment distal calcium reabsorption. Increased phosphate ingestion can also reduce intestinal calcium absorption through complexing and rendering calcium less absorbable.

Other Dietary Factors

Increasing dietary protein intake is accompanied by increased urinary calcium excretion related to the increased production of fixed acid as amino acid sulfur is oxidized to sulfate, thereby inducing a mild acidosis (11,14,15). An animal protein diet with its higher sulfur-containing amino acid content (cysteine, methionine) produces greater hypercalciuria than a vegetarian protein diet (15). The ability of sulfate to complex calcium within renal tubular fluid, thus limiting calcium reabsorption, may also play a role in the hypercalciuric action of protein (7). Acute ingestion of rapidly metabolizable carbohydrates such as glucose and sucrose may be accompanied by increased urinary calcium excretion, as a consequence of inhibition of tubular calcium reabsorption (16). This effect may be magnified in stone-formers (16). However, chronic ingestion of a diet with increased simple or complex carbohydrates does not appear to augment urinary calcium excretion in normal subjects (17).

Hormonal Factors

Parathyroid Hormone

Patients with primary hyperparathyroidism generally have increased urinary calcium excretion secondary to the hypercalcemia (and thus a high filtered load of calcium) produced by the hormone. The direct action of PTH on the kidney is to enhance fractional reabsorption of calcium from the glomerular filtrate (18). This renal effect is readily apparent when calcium clearance is measured at various serum calcium concentrations, with or without the influence

of PTH (Fig. 3). At any given calcium load, calcium clearance is decreased under the influence of PTH, and is increased in the absence of PTH secretion.

In the proximal tubule, PTH actually decreases sodium and calcium absorption (18,19). However, the major physiologic effect of PTH (i.e., enhancement of calcium reabsorption) occurs in the TALH and the distal tubule (20). PTH action can be duplicated by cyclic adenosine monophosphate (cAMP) analogs (20,21).

1,25-Dihydroxyvitamin D

One of the many actions of PTH on the PCT is the stimulation of 1,25-dihydroxyvitamin D [1,25(OH)$_2$D] production (21). The effects of vitamin D and its metabolites on renal calcium transport are controversial. In a study in which serum calcium and PTH levels were independently controlled, vitamin D deficiency was clearly shown to reduce tubular calcium reabsorption (22). The precise locus of action of 1,25(OH)$_2$D on renal tubular calcium transport is still uncertain. Autoradiographic evidence localized nuclear transfer of 1,25(OH)$_2$D-receptor complex to the TALH and distal tubule (23), coinciding with sites for immunocytochemical localization of CaBP-D.

Calcitonin

The effects of calcitonin on the renal handling of calcium are also confusing. The principal physiologic action of this hormone is to lower serum calcium concentration. Doses of

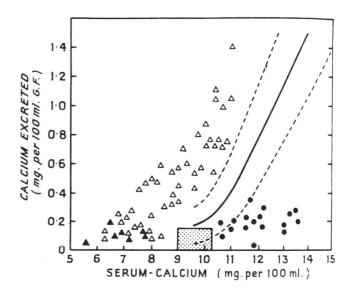

FIG. 3. Urinary excretion of calcium as a function of serum calcium concentration in normal subjects *(solid line)* and in patients with hypoparathyroidism (△▲) and hyperparathyroidism •. *Dashed lines,* ±2 SD; *shaded area,* the normal physiologic situation. (From: Nordin BEC, Peacock M. Role of kidney in regulation of plasma calcium. *Lancet* 2:1280–1283, 1969.)

calcitonin above physiologic levels have a hypercalciuric effect in dogs and humans (2).

Other Hormones

In the humoral hypercalcemia of malignancy, tumors secrete a factor known as PTH-related peptide (PTHrP) (24). This substance mimics most of the actions of PTH, including increased urinary cAMP excretion and renal calcium reabsorption, although it is immunochemically distinct from PTH. The cDNA encoding PTHrP has been cloned, and the sequence of the primary gene product has been defined (25). Since 8 of the first 13 amino acids at the amino-terminal end of these proteins are identical to those found in PTH, it is assumed that PTHrP interacts with the PTH receptor.

Chronic glucocorticoid excess can cause calciuria, partly through a net catabolic effect on the skeleton, but also by impairing renal tubular calcium reabsorption (26). Chronic mineralocorticoid excess can also augment urinary calcium excretion, possibly mediated through the mechanism of volume expansion (27). Insulin infusion and hyperinsulinemia are also associated with hypercalciuria (28).

Metabolic Perturbations

Acid-Base

Acute and chronic metabolic acidoses are associated with an increase in calcium excretion that is not attributable to changes in filtered load of calcium or in parathyroid activity (29,30). Micropuncture studies suggest that although acute acidosis reduced proximal calcium (and sodium) reabsorption, the hypercalciuria is attributable to an impairment in calcium reabsorption relative to sodium reabsorption in the distal nephron (29). Reduction in urinary calcium associated with alkali administration also appeared to be mediated by a distal effect (29). Decreased calcium excretion is more consistently demonstrated with potassium bicarbonate (31) or citrate (32) administration than with the administration of sodium salts. This is because sodium administration may cause natriuresis with parallel calciuresis, thus masking the alkali-induced hypocalciuria.

Hypercalcemia

There are numerous causes of resorptive hypercalcemia, including immobilization, osteolytic malignancy, and granulomatous disease with excess $1,25(OH)_2D$ production. Generally, PTH is suppressed, thereby reducing distal tubule calcium reabsorption and facilitating urinary calcium excretion. Renal calcium excretion forms a "safety valve" in the prevention and amelioration of hypercalcemia in these conditions.

Hypercalcemia may have direct effects on the tubule to decrease tubular calcium reabsorption (33,34). Recently, an extracellular Ca^{2+}-sensing receptor has been cloned and characterized by Brown and colleagues (35). This Ca^{2+}-sensing receptor has been found in the membrane of cells that need to respond to changes in extracellular ionized Ca^{2+}, such as the renal tubule (TALH), as well as the parathyroid and C-cells of the thyroid. Patients with familial hypocalciuric hypercalcemia (FHH) have a defective gene for the Ca^{2+}-sensitive receptor on chromosome 3 (36). Their renal tubules, unable to sense the hypercalcemia, continue to avidly reabsorb calcium. PTH secretion is also inappropriately elevated.

Idiopathic Hypercalciuria

Hypercalciuria (urinary calcium excretion >250 mg/day in women or >300 mg/day in men, or >4 mg/kg/day in either sex), in the absence of hypercalcemia, occurs in over 50% of patients having kidney stones composed of calcium oxalate and/or apatite, and it is one of the risk factors for the crystallization of these insoluble salts (7). The mechanism for the hypercalciuria generally involves a primary increase in intestinal calcium absorption, a renal calcium leak, enhanced bone resorption, or some combination of these derangements (37,38). Increased intestinal calcium absorption is the major source of the extra calcium appearing in the urine of these patients, either because of excessive $1,25(OH)_2D$ production or sensitivity, or because of a vitamin-D-independent mechanism.

Diuretics

The administration of furosemide, bumetanide, or other diuretics acting on the TALH is accompanied by inhibition of tubular calcium reabsorption at this site and increased urinary calcium excretion (1,7). This calciuretic effect of the diuretics that act on the loop of Henle (loop diuretics) may be used clinically for the treatment of hypercalcemia (39). In contrast, administration of thiazide diuretics is accompanied by increased tubular calcium reabsorption in the distal renal tubule and a fall in urinary calcium excretion (40,41). Because volume contraction is required for the hypocalciuric action of thiazides, it usually takes 2 to 4 days of drug treatment to observe the full hypocalciuric effect (42). The chronic hypocalciuric effect of thiazides has led to their use in the management of hypercalciuric calcium nephrolithiasis (43). The administration of chlorthalidone, amiloride, or indapamide also reduces urinary calcium excretion (7).

MAGNESIUM

Distribution and Regulation

Although the homeostatic control of magnesium is less well characterized than that of calcium and phosphorus, the same organ systems are involved: the intestine, bone, and kidneys. Thus far, no single hormone has been identified as a specific regulator of magnesium homeostasis. Total body magnesium for a 70-Kg person is about 26 g, of which 54% is in the skeleton, 45% in the soft tissues, and only 1% in the extracellular space. In the normal adult, neutral magnesium balance is maintained even with intakes as low as 25 mg/day, the average daily intake being 300 mg. Although the gastrointestinal absorption of magnesium is not regulated as closely as that of calcium, when intake is severely limited, fecal and urinary excretion fall profoundly.

General Features of Filtration, Reabsorption, and Clearance

In the normal adult, plasma magnesium ranges from 1.7 to 2.3 mg/dl. Approximately 30% of total plasma magnesium is protein bound and about 70% is filterable through artificial membranes (15% complexed, 55% free Mg^{2+} ions). With a glomerular filtration rate (GFR) of about 150 L/d and an ultrafilterable mg concentration of 14 mg/L, there is a filtered magnesium load of approximately 2100 mg/d. Normally, only 3% of the filtered magnesium appears in the urine; thus 97% is reabsorbed by the renal tubules. In contrast to sodium and calcium, only about 25% to 30% of filtered magnesium is reabsorbed in the proximal tubule. Approximately 60% to 65% of filtered magnesium is reabsorbed in the TALH, and 5% is reabsorbed in the distal nephron. Relatively little is known about cellular magnesium transport mechanisms.

Factors Influencing Renal Handling of Magnesium

Dietary Magnesium Intake and Absorption

Restriction of dietary magnesium leads by unknown mechanisms to rapid and selective renal conservation of magnesium without large decreases in serum concentration of magnesium (Fig. 4) (18). In patients with intestinal malabsorption, urinary magnesium declines before serum magnesium and is an earlier and more reliable indicator of evolving magnesium deficiency (44). The magnesium-loading test is the most widely accepted criterion with which to determine the magnitude of magnesium deficiency (45). Those with greater magnesium deficiency retain more of the infused magnesium. Because 24-hour urinary magnesium levels correlate inversely with magnesium retention in the magnesium-loading test (46), 24-hour urinary magnesium values are also helpful in detecting subclinical magnesium deficiency states.

Other Factors Influencing Urinary Magnesium Excretion

Figure 5 summarizes the major factors influencing urinary magnesium excretion (7). Hypermagnesemia induced by high dietary intake or magnesium infusion increases the filtered load of magnesium. This results in an increase in the load delivered to the loop of Henle. Reabsorption in the TALH is also depressed after elevation of the plasma magnesium. Urinary magnesium excretion increases with inhibition of proximal tubular reabsorption by extracellular fluid (ECF) volume expansion, or osmotic diuretics such as mannitol. Hypercalcemia causes a high peritubular concentration of calcium that directly inhibits the reabsorption of both calcium and magnesium at the TALH (2). Loop diuretics such as furosemide and bumetanide also inhibit tubular magnesium reabsorption at this site. It is worth noting that in contrast to the hypocalciuric

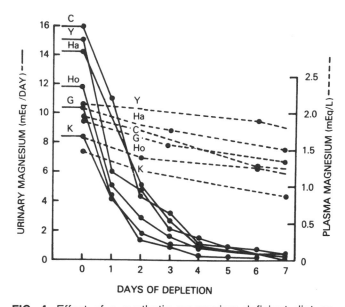

FIG. 4. Effect of a synthetic magnesium-deficient diet on plasma magnesium concentration and urinary magnesium excretion in six patients. (Modified from: Shils ME. Experimental human magnesium depletion. *Medicine (Baltimore)* 48:61–85, 1969.)

effect of thiazides, these diuretics may produce a mild but variable increase in magnesium excretion (43). Phosphate depletion causes defective magnesium reabsorption in the TALH and distal tubule. Several drugs that are associated with renal magnesium wasting (especially aminoglycoside antibiotics, the antineoplastic agent cisplatin, and the immunosuppressive agent cyclosporine) also inhibit magnesium reabsorption in Henle's loop (2).

Other factors enhance tubular magnesium absorption. Hypomagnesemia and hypocalcemia increase magnesium reabsorption at the TALH. PTH and metabolic alkalosis enhance magnesium reabsorption in the distal tubule (2,7).

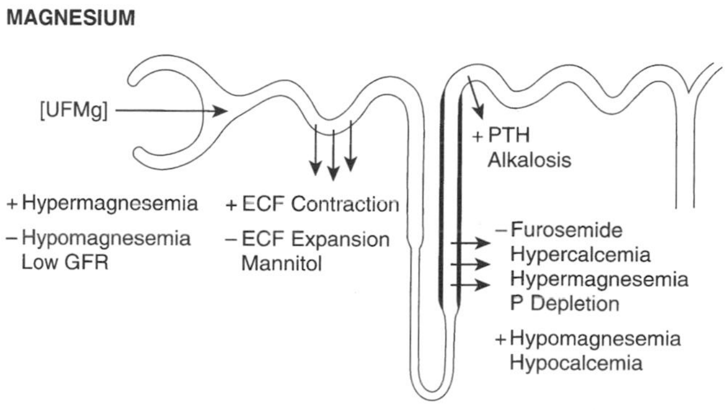

MAGNESIUM

FIG. 5. Regulation of urinary magnesium excretion. (Modified from: Lemann J Jr. Urinary excretion of calcium, magnesium, and phosphorus. In: Favus MJ (ed) *Primer on the Metabolic Bone Diseases and Disorders of Mineral Metabolism*, 2d ed. Raven Press, New York, 50–54, 1993.)

PHOSPHORUS

Distribution and Regulation

Plasma and intracellular phosphorus play an important role in many metabolic processes involving intermediary metabolism and energy-transfer mechanisms. Of the total body phosphorus content (500 to 800 g), 90% is in the skeleton and 10% is in soft tissue. Adults are normally in phosphorus balance, with intake equal to output. Approximately 60% of the dietary intake is absorbed by the intestine over a wide range of phosphorus intake (800 to 1500 mg/day), and an equivalent amount is excreted by the kidneys.

Phosphorus homeostasis is closely regulated in normal humans. Like serum calcium, serum phosphorus is maintained within a narrow range of values, and people with abnormal concentrations may have a predisposition to serious conditions such as hemolysis, myopathy, and osteomalacia. The principal organ that regulates phosphorus homeostasis is the kidney. This regulation is accomplished primarily through variation in proximal tubule reabsorption of phosphate.

General Features of Filtration, Reabsorption, and Clearance

Serum phosphorus is generally considered to be completely ultrafilterable across the glomeruli (7). Approximately 80% of the filtered load is reabsorbed by the renal tubules in a unidirectional reabsorptive process (1). Renal reabsorption of phosphorus is saturable. As plasma phosphorus concentration is increased, the amount of phosphorus reabsorbed also increases until the transport capacity is reached. This maximum rate is generally known as the maximum tubular reabsorptive rate for phosphorus, or TmP. The theoretical phosphorus threshold represents the plasma phosphorus level, below which most of the filtered phosphorus is reabsorbed and above which most of the filtered phosphorus is excreted. The theoretical phosphorus threshold (TmP/GFR) provides a useful index for assessing renal tubular phosphorus reabsorptive activity. A nomogram has been constructed so that TmP/GFR can be easily derived from the values of both fractional phosphorus reabsorption (TRP) and plasma phosphorus concentration (47).

The major portion of the filtered phosphorus is reabsorbed in the early PCT. Micropuncture studies show that 60% to 70% of the filtered phosphorus load is reabsorbed by the time the filtrate reaches the late PCT (1). Some phosphorus reabsorption also occurs along the distal and terminal part of the nephron, but this is of uncertain significance.

Cellular Mechanisms of Phosphorus Transport

The cellular events involved in phosphorus movement from the luminal fluid to the peritubular capillary blood have received much attention in recent years. Studies have

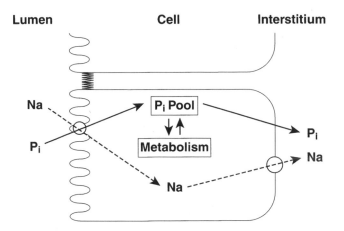

FIG. 6. Schematic of transcellular phosphorus transport across the proximal tubule cell.

focused on the proximal tubules where the principal portion of the filtered phosphorus is reabsorbed (Fig. 6) (1).

Phosphorus enters the cell from the lumen against its electrochemical gradient by an energy-requiring mechanism, and it leaves the cell on the contraluminal side, down the electrochemical gradient. Specific transport systems are located on the brush-border and the basolateral membranes. Brush-border membrane phosphorus transport is sodium-dependent [Na-Pi (inorganic phosphorus) cotransport] (48). The energy required to maintain the favorable electrochemical gradient for sodium is generated by Na^+, K^+-ATPase at the basolateral membrane. However, the exact mechanism coupling sodium to phosphorus transport remains unknown.

Physiological regulation of proximal tubular phosphorus reabsorption is most likely related to alterations in the function of the apical transporters (48–52). Important factors that regulate proximal tubular phosphorus reabsorption, such as PTH and dietary phosphorus, have been shown to alter brush-border membrane Na-P cotransporters (48).

Factors Influencing Renal Handling of Phosphorus

Figure 7 summarizes the major factors influencing urinary phosphorus excretion (1,7). Urinary phosphorus excretion appears to increase as serum phosphorus concentration increases, as a result of both increased filtration of phosphorus and inhibition of renal tubular phosphorus reabsorption. As the GFR falls progressively among patients with kidney disease, the early development of secondary hyperparathyroidism inhibits renal tubular phosphorus reabsorption and, despite the fall in the glomerular filtration of phosphorus, preserves normal rates of urinary phosphorus excretion, thereby preventing hyperphosphatemia until the GFR falls to about 25% of normal.

Urinary phosphorus excretion among healthy adults is directly related to dietary phosphorus intake. The renal tubule has an intrinsic ability to adjust the reabsorption rate

PHOSPHATE

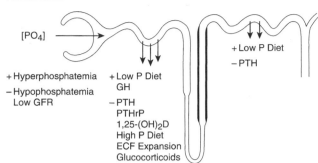

FIG. 7. Regulation of urinary phosphorus excretion. (Modified from: Lemann J Jr. Urinary excretion of calcium, magnesium, and phosphorus. In: Favus MJ (ed) *Primer on the Metabolic Bone Diseases and Disorders of Mineral Metabolism*, 2nd ed. Raven Press, New York, 50–54, 1993.)

of phosphorus according to its availability to the body. Urinary phosphorus excretion falls to <15 mg/day within 3 to 5 days when dietary phosphorus is reduced to 60 to 120 mg/day. Such avid renal phosphorus conservation can occur with minimal change in the serum phosphorus concentration. These adaptive responses occur primarily in the PCT (1), associated with changes in brush-border Na-P cotransporters (48).

Several hormones affect renal phosphorus handling. It is widely recognized that PTH is the major hormone regulator of renal phosphorus reabsorption. Parathyroidectomy decreases renal phosphorus excretion. Administration of PTH leads to phosphaturia by reducing the maximal transport rate of phosphorus reabsorption, TmP/GFR (21). The main site of action of PTH is in the PCT, but phosphorus transport in the distal tubule may also be sensitive to PTH. In the PCT, PTH action begins with receptor binding and activation of adenylate cyclase on the basolateral membrane. It has been postulated that PTH-stimulated cAMP may lead to phosphorylation of renal brush-border membranes and mediate the hormonal effect on phosphorus transport (53,54). PTHrP, the mediator of the humoral hypercalcemia of malignancy, is also a phosphaturic factor, presumably because it interacts with the PTH receptor (24).

Although there is controversy concerning the effects of vitamin D metabolites on renal phosphorus excretion, chronic administration of 1,25(OH)₂D enhances intestinal phosphorus absorption. The proximal tubule responds appropriately to the abundance of phosphorus and lowers phosphorus reabsorption (55). Glucocorticoids and calcitonin are also phosphaturic hormones believed to act at the proximal tubule (1).

Growth hormone (GH) has long been known to promote phosphorus reabsorption by the kidney (56). Because GH raises TmP/GFR, it is likely that GH affects the intrinsic tubular reabsorptive capacity for phosphorus. Such a notion was further supported by the finding that administration of GH increased phosphorus uptake by renal brush-border membrane (57). Growing children and patients with

acromegaly have increased serum phosphorus concentrations (with normal urinary phosphorus excretion) as a result of the action of GH.

An assortment of miscellaneous factors also influence phosphorus excretion. Expansion of the ECF volume causes phosphaturia (58). Many diuretics increase urinary phosphorus excretion. Of all the diuretics, the greatest phosphaturia is produced by the carbonic anhydrase inhibitor acetazolamide (59). Dipyridamole, a widely used platelet inhibitor, was reported to enhance renal tubular phosphorus reabsorption in humans (60).

Hypophosphatemia in patients with tumor-induced osteomalacia is a result of markedly diminished renal phosphorus reabsorption. Cai et al. (61) recently presented evidence that the syndrome, or at least the hypophosphatemia that characterizes it, may be caused by ectopic secretion of a heat-labile factor with a mass between 8000 and 25,000 daltons that inhibits renal tubular reabsorption of phosphorus. Unlike PTH or PTHrP, this substance did not stimulate cAMP production or increase bone resorption. Econs and Drezner (62) have speculated that a similar substance may be produced in patients with X-linked hypophosphatemic rickets, and they have termed this potential phosphate-regulating hormone phosphatonin.

REFERENCES

1. Yanagawa N, Lee DBN: Renal handling of calcium and phosphorus. In: Coe FL, Favus MJ (eds) *Disorders of Bone and Mineral Metabolism*. Raven Press, New York, pp 3–40, 1992
2. Suki WN, Rouse D: Renal transport of calcium, magnesium, and phosphate. In: Brenner BM (ed) *The Kidney*, 5th ed. WB Saunders, Philadelphia, 472–515, 1996
3. Wright E, Schulman G: Principles of epithelial transport. In: Maxwell MH, Kleeman CR, Narins RG (eds) *Clinical Disorders of Fluid and Electrolyte Metabolism*, 4th ed. McGraw-Hill, New York, 15–31, 1987
4. Johnson JA, Kumar R. Renal and intestinal calcium transport: Roles of vitamin D and vitamin D-dependent calcium binding proteins. *Semin Nephrol* 14:119–128, 1994
5. Bacskai BJ, Friedman PA. Activation of latent Ca²⁺ channels in renal epithelial cells by parathyroid hormone. *Nature* 347:388–391, 1990
6. Cai Q, Chandler JS, Wasserman RH, et al.: Vitamin D and adaptation to dietary calcium and phosphorus deficiencies increase intestinal plasma membrane calcium pump gene expression. *Proc Natl Acad Sci USA* 90:1345–1349, 1993
7. Lemann J Jr: Urinary excretion of calcium, magnesium, and phosphorus. In: Favus MJ (ed) *Primer on the Metabolic Bone Diseases and Disorders of Mineral Metabolism*, 2nd ed. Raven Press, New York, 50–54, 1993
8. Walser M: Calcium clearance as a function of sodium clearance in the dog. *Am J Physiol* 200:1009–1014, 1961
9. Kleeman CR, Bohannan J, Bernstein D, Ling S, Maxwell MH: Effect of variation in sodium intake on calcium excretion in normal humans. *Proc Soc Exp Biol Med* 115:29–32, 1964
10. Breslau NA, McGuire JL, Zerwekh JE, Pak CYC: The role of dietary sodium on renal excretion and intestinal absorption of calcium and on vitamin D metabolism. *J Clin Endocrinol Metab* 55:369–373, 1982
11. Lemann J Jr, Adams ND, Gray RW: Urinary calcium excretion in human beings. *N Engl J Med* 301:535–541, 1979
12. Albright F, Bauer W, Cockrill JR: Studies in parathyroid physiology. III. The effect of phosphate ingestion in clinical hyperparathyroidism. *J Clin Invest* 11:411–435, 1932
13. Wong NLM, Quamme GA, Sutton RAL, O'Callaghan T, Dirks

JH: Effect of phosphate infusion on renal phosphate and calcium transport. *Renal Physiol* 8:30–37, 1985

14. Lemann J Jr, Gray RW, Maierhofer WJ, Cheung HS: The importance of renal net acid excretion as a determinant of fasting urinary calcium excretion. *Kidney Int* 29:743–746, 1986

15. Breslau NA, Brinkley L, Hill KD, Pak CYC: Relationship of animal protein-rich diet to kidney stone formation and calcium metabolism. *J Clin Endocrinol Metab* 66:140–146, 1988

16. Lemann J Jr, Piering WF, Lennon EJ: Possible role of carbohydrate-induced calciuria in calcium oxalate kidney-stone formation. *N Engl J Med* 280:232–237, 1969

17. Garg A, Bonanome A, Grundy SM, Unger RH, Breslau NA, Pak CYC: Effects of dietary carbohydrates on metabolism of calcium and other minerals in normal subjects and patients with noninsulin-dependent diabetes mellitus. *J Clin Endocrinol Metab* 70:1007–1013, 1990

18. Aurbach GD, Marx SJ, Spiegel AM: Parathyroid hormone, calcitonin, and the calciferols. In: Wilson JD, Foster DW (eds) *Williams Textbook of Endocrinology*, 8th ed. WB Saunders, Philadelphia, pp 1397–1476, 1992

19. Agus ZS, Gardner LB, Beck LH, Goldberg M: Effects of parathyroid hormone on renal tubular reabsorption of calcium, sodium and phosphate. *Am J Physiol* 224:1143–1148, 1973

20. Suki WN, Rouse D: Hormonal regulation of calcium transport in thick ascending renal tubules. *Am J Physiol* 241:F171–174, 1981

21. Breslau NA, Weinstock RS: Regulation of 1,25(OH)₂D synthesis in hypoparathyroidism and pseudohypoparathyroidism. *Am J Physiol* 255 (*Endocrinol Metab* 18):E730–E736, 1988

22. Yamamoto M, Kawanobe Y, Takahashi H, Shimazawa E, Kimura S, Ogata E: Vitamin D deficiency and renal calcium transport in the rat. *J Clin Invest* 74:507–513, 1984

23. Stumpf WE, Sar M, Narbaitz R, Reid FA, DeLuca HF, Tanaka Y: Target cells for 1,25-dihydroxyvitamin D₃ in intestinal tract, stomach, kidney, skin, putuitary and parathyroid. *Proc Natl Acad Sci USA* 77:1149–53, 1980

24. Broadus AD, Mangin M, Ikeda K, et al.: Humoral hypercalcemia of cancer: Identification of a novel parathyroid hormone-like peptide. *N Engl J Med* 319:556–563, 1988

25. Mangin M, Webb AC, Dreyer BE, et al.: Identification of a cDNA encoding a parathyroid hormone-like peptide from a human tumor associated with humoral hypercalcemia of malignancy. *Proc Natl Acad Sci USA* 85:597–601, 1988

26. Laake H: The action of corticosteroids on the renal reabsorption of calcium. *Acta Endocrinol (Copenh)* 34:60–64, 1960

27. Suki WN, Schwettmann RS, Rector FC Jr, Seldin DW: Effect of chronic mineralocorticoid administration on calcium excretion in the rat. *Am J Physiol* 215:71–74, 1968

28. DeFronzo RA, Goldberg M, Agus ZS: The effects of glucose and insulin on renal electrolyte transport. *J Clin Invest* 58:83–90, 1976

29. Sutton RAL, Wong NLM, Dirks JH: Effects of metabolic acidosis and alkalosis on sodium and calcium transport in the dog kidney. *Kidney Int* 15:520–533, 1979

30. Lemann J Jr, Litzow JR, Lennon EJ: Studies of the mechanism by which chronic metabolic acidosis augments urinary calcium excretion in man. *J Clin Invest* 46:1318–1328, 1967

31. Lemann J, Gray RW, Pluess JA: Potassium bicarbonate, but not sodium bicarbonate, reduces urinary calcium excretion and improves calcium balance in healthy men. *Kidney Int* 35:688–695, 1989

32. Sakhaee K, Nicar M, Hill lK, Pak CYC: Contrasting effects of potassium citrate and sodium citrate therapies and crystallization of stone-forming salts. *Kidney Int* 24:348–352, 1983

33. Edwards BR, Sutton RAL, Dirks JH: Effect of calcium infusion on renal tubular reabsorption in the dog. *Am J Physiol* 227:13–18, 1974

34. Quamme GA: Effect of hypercalcemia on renal tubular handling of calcium and magnesium. *Can J Physiol Pharmacol* 60:1275–1280, 1982

35. Brown EM, Pollak M, Hebert SC: Sensing of extracellular Ca²⁺ by parathyroid and kidney cells: Cloning and characterization of an extracellular Ca²⁺-sensing receptor. *Am J Kidney Dis* 25:506–513, 1995

36. Pollak M, Brown EM, Chou Y-HC, et al.: Mutations in the human Ca²⁺-sensing receptor gene cause familial hypocalciuric hypercalcemia and neonatal severe hyperparathyroidism. *Cell* 75:1297–1303, 1993

37. Pak CYC, Ohata M, Lawrence EC, et al.: The hypercalciurias: Causes, parathyroid functions and diagnostic criteria. *J Clin Invest* 54:387–400, 1974

38. Breslau NA, Coe FL: Management of idiopathic hypercalciuria. In: Coe FL, Favus MJ, Pak CYC, Parks JH, Preminger GM (eds) *Kidney Stones: Medical and Surgical Management.* Lippincott-Raven, Philadelphia, pp 773–785, 1996

39. Suki WN, Yium JJ, Von Minden M, Saller-Herbert C, Eknoyan G, Martinez-Maldonado M: Acute treatment of hypercalcemia with furosemide. *N Engl J Med* 283:836–840, 1970

40. Costanzo LS, Weiner IM: On the hypocalciuric action of chlorothiazide. *J Clin Invest* 54:628–637, 1974

41. Costanzo LS, Windhager EE: Calcium and sodium transport by the distal convoluted tubule of the rat. *Am J Physiol* 235:F492–506, 1978

42. Breslau N, Moses AM, Weiner IM: The role of volume contraction in the hypocalciuric action of chlorothiazide. *Kidney Int* 10:164–170, 1976

43. Yendt ER, Cohanim M: Prevention of calcium stones with thiazides. *Kidney Int* 13:397–409, 1978

44. Fleming CR, George L, Stoner GL, Tarrosa B, Moyer TP: The importance of urinary magnesium values in patients with gut failure. *Mayo Clin Proc* 71:21–24, 1996

45. Ryzen E, Elbaum N, Singer FR, Rude RK: Parenteral magnesium tolerance testing in the evaluation of magnesium deficiency. *Magnesium* 4:137–147, 1985

46. Sjogren A, Floren CH, Nilsson A: Evaluation of magnesium status in Crohn's disease as assessed by intracellular analysis and intravenous magnesium infusion. *Scand J Gastroenterol* 23:555–561, 1988

47. Bijvoet OLM: Indices for the measurements of the renal handling of phosphate. In: Massry SG, Fleisch H (eds) *Renal Handling of Phosphate.* Plenum Press, New York, pp 1–37, 1980

48. Murer H, Biber J: Molecular mechanisms in renal phosphate reabsorption. *Nephrol Dial Transplant* 10:1501–1504, 1995

49. Magagnin S, Werner A, Markovich D, Sorribas V, Stange G, Biber J, Murer H: Expression cloning of human and rat renal cortex Na/Pi cotransport. *Proc Natl Acad Sci USA* 90:5979–5983, 1993

50. Werner A, Moore ML, Mantei N, Biber J, Semenza G, et al.: Cloning and expression of cDNA for a Na/Pi cotransport system of kidney cortex. *Proc Natl Acad Sci USA* 88:9608–9612, 1991

51. Tenenhouse HS, Werner A, Biber J, Ma S, Roy S, Murer H: Renal Na-phosphate cotransport in murine X-linked hypophosphatemic rickets. Molecular characterization. *J Clin Invest* 93:671–673, 1994

52. Kos CH, Tihy F, Econs MJ, Murer H, Lemieux N, Tenenhouse HS: Localization of a renal sodium-phosphate cotransporter gene to human chromosome 5q35. *Genomics* 19:176–177, 1994

53. Hammerman MR, Hruska KA: Cyclic AMP-dependent protein phosphorylation in canine renal brush border membrane vesicles is associated with decreased phosphate transport. *J Biol Chem* 257:992–999, 1982

54. Malmstroem K, Biber J, Gmaj P, Murer H: Possible mechanisms for the regulation of the Pi transport in brush border membrane vesicles. In: Bronner F, Peterlik M (eds) *Epithelial Calcium and Phosphate Transport: Molecular and Cellular Aspects.* Alan R. Liss, New York, pp 325–330, 1984

55. Bonjour JP, Preston C, Fleisch H: Effect of 1,25-dihydroxyvitamin D₃ on the renal handling of Pi: Effect of dietary Pi and diphosphates. *J Clin Invest* 60:1419–1428, 1977

56. Corvilain J, Abramow M: Effect of growth hormone on tubular transport of phosphate in normal and parathyroidectomized dogs. *J Clin Invest* 43:1608–1612, 1964

57. Hammerman MR, Karl IE, Hruska KA: Regulation of canine renal vesicle Pi transport by growth hormone and parathyroid hormone. *Biochim Biophys Acta* 603:322–335, 1980

58. Suki WN, Martinez-Maldonado M, Rouse D, Terry A: Effect of expansion of extracellular fluid volume on renal phosphate handling. *J Clin Invest* 48:1888–1894, 1969

59. Beck LH, Goldberg M: Effects of acetazolamide and parathyroidectomy on renal transport of sodium, calcium and phosphate. *Am J Physiol* 224:1136–1142, 1973

60. Michaut P, Prié D, Amiel C, Friedlander G: Dipyridamole for renal phosphate leak? *[letter]. New Engl J Med* 331:58–59, 1994

61. Cai Q, Hodgson SF, Kao PC, Lennon VA, Klee GG, Zinmeister AR, Kumar R: Brief report: Inhibition of renal phosphate transport by a tumor product in a patient with oncogenic osteomalacia. *N Engl J Med* 330:1645–1649, 1994

62. Econs MJ, Drezner MK: Tumor-induced osteomalacia—unveiling a new hormone. *N Engl J Med* 330:1679–1681, 1994

9. Mineral Balance and Homeostasis

Arthur E. Broadus, M.D., Ph.D.

Department of Internal Medicine, Yale University, New Haven, Connecticut

Life began in a primordial sea, rich in potassium and magnesium and poor in sodium and calcium, and it is felt that the present composition of the cytosol, also rich in potassium and magnesium and poor in sodium and calcium, reflects this ancient heritage. With time, geologic changes altered the composition of the seas to one rich in sodium and calcium, and primitive organisms adapted to this altered milieu by developing ion pumps in order to maintain the asymmetry of the concentrations of monovalent and divalent cations across their plasma membranes. The evolution of these pumps and channels may be viewed as one of the most fundamental developments in cell biology.

The progression to terrestrial life carried with it a complete dependence on minerals from the environment. With this came the evolution of the mineral exchange mechanisms in intestine, kidney, and bone (which subserve systemic mineral needs) as well as the key systemic hormones, parathyroid hormone (PTH) and 1,25-dihydroxyvitamin D [1,25(OH)$_2$D] (which regulate these exchange mechanisms). This integrated regulatory system has many checks and balances and is an elegant example of biologic control.

Calcium. An adult human contains approximately 1000 g of calcium (1,2). Some 99% of this calcium is in the skeleton in the form of hydroxyapatite, and 1% is contained in the extracellular fluids and soft tissues. About 1% of the skeletal content of calcium is freely exchangeable with the extracellular fluids. Although a small percentage of skeletal content, this exchangeable pool is approximately equal to the total content of calcium in the extracellular fluids and soft tissues, and it serves as an important buffer or storehouse of calcium. The extracellular concentration of calcium ions (Ca^{2+}) is in the range of 10^{-3} M, whereas the concentration of Ca^{2+} in the cytosol is about 10^{-6} M.

Calcium plays two predominant physiologic roles in the organism. In bone, calcium salts provide the structural integrity of the skeleton. In the extracellular fluids and in the cytosol, the concentration of Ca^{2+} is critically important in the maintenance and control of a number of biochemical processes, and the concentrations of Ca^{2+} in both compartments are maintained with great constancy.

Phosphorus. An adult human contains approximately 600 g of phosphorus. Some 85% of this phosphorus is present in crystalline form in the skeleton and plays a structural role. About 15% is present in the extracellular fluids, largely in the form of inorganic phosphate ions, and in soft tissues, almost totally in the form of phosphate esters. Intracellular phosphate esters and phosphorylated intermediates are involved in a number of important biochemical processes, including the generation and transfer of cellular energy. Intracellular and extracellular concentrations of phosphorus (as the phosphate divalent anion) are approximately 1×10^{-4} M and 2×10^{-4} M, respectively, and these concentrations are less rigidly maintained than are those of calcium and magnesium.

Magnesium. An adult human contains approximately 25 g or 2000 mEq of magnesium. About two thirds is present in the skeleton and one third in soft tissues. The magnesium in bone is not an integral part of the hydroxyapatite lattice structure but appears to be located on the crystal surface. Only a minor fraction of the magnesium in bone is freely exchangeable with extracellular magnesium. Magnesium is the most abundant intracellular divalent cation, and cellular magnesium is important as a cofactor for a number of enzymatic reactions and in the regulation of neuromuscular excitability. Approximately 1% of total body magnesium is contained in the extracellular compartment, and its concentration in plasma does not provide a reliable index of either total body or soft tissue magnesium content. The concentration of magnesium ions (Mg^{2+}) is about 5×10^{-4} M in the cytosol as well as in the extracellular fluids, and its concentration in both compartments is rigidly maintained.

EXTRACELLULAR MINERAL METABOLISM

Calcium. There are three definable fractions of calcium in serum: ionized calcium (about 50%), protein-bound calcium (about 40%), and calcium that is complexed, mostly to citrate and phosphate ions (about 10%) (3). Both the complexed and ionized fractions are ultrafilterable, so that about 60% of the total calcium in serum crosses semipermeable membranes. About 90% of the protein-bound calcium is bound to albumin and the remainder to globulins. Alterations in the serum albumin concentration have a major influence on the measured total serum calcium concentration. At pH 7.4, each gm/dl of albumin binds 0.8 mg/dl of calcium, and this simple relationship can be used to "correct" the total serum calcium concentration when circulating albumin is abnormal (e.g., given measured albumin and calcium concentrations of 2.0 gm/dl and 7.4 mg/dl, respectively, the corrected serum calcium concentration at an albumin concentration of 4.0 gm/dl is 9.0 mg/dl). Calcium is bound largely to the carboxyl groups in albumin, and this binding is highly pH-dependent. Acute acidosis decreases binding and increases ionized calcium, and acute alkalosis increases binding with a consequent decrease in ionized calcium. These changes are not reflected in the total serum calcium concentration and can only be appreciated by actual management of ionized serum calcium at the ambient pH. Calcium concentrations are typically recorded in mg/dl (mg%); these concentrations can be converted to molar units simply by dividing by 4 (e.g., 10 mg/dl converts to 2.5 mM).

It is the ionized fraction of calcium (Ca^{2+}) that is physiologically important and that is rigidly maintained by the combined effects of PTH and $1,25(OH)_2D$. Examples of the physiologic functions of extracellular Ca^{2+} include (i) serving as a cofactor in the coagulation cascade (e.g., for factors VII, IX, X, and prothrombin), (ii) maintenance of the normal mineral ion product required for skeletal mineralization, and (iii) contributing stability to plasma membranes by binding to phospholipids in the lipid bilayer and also regulating the permeability of plasma membranes to sodium ions. A reduction in ionized calcium increases sodium permeability and enhances the excitability of all excitable tissues; an increase in ionized calcium has the opposite effect. For example, the pH dependency of calcium binding to carboxyl groups noted above is the explanation for the reduction in ionized calcium that is responsible for the neuromuscular symptoms that characterize the hyperventilation syndrome.

Phosphorus. Serum inorganic phosphate also exists as three fractions: ionized, protein-bound, and complexed. Protein binding is relatively insignificant for phosphate, representing some 10% of the total, but about 35% is complexed to sodium, calcium, and magnesium. Thus, approximately 90% of the inorganic phosphate in serum is ultrafilterable. The major ionic species of phosphate in serum at pH 7.4 is the divalent anion (HPO_4^{2-}).

In contrast to the rigidly regulated concentration of calcium in serum, the serum phosphorus concentration varies quite widely throughout the day and is influenced by age, sex, diet, pH, and a variety of hormones. An adequate serum phosphate concentration is important in maintaining a sufficient ion product for normal mineralization.

Magnesium. About 55% of serum magnesium is ionized, with 30% being protein bound and 15% complexed. The protein-bound fraction interacts with the carboxyl groups of albumin and is influenced by pH in a fashion analogous to that of calcium. It is the ionized fraction of magnesium that is physiologically important (e.g., to plasma membrane excitability). The extracellular concentration of ionized magnesium is tightly controlled by the tubular maximum or threshold for magnesium in the nephron (4).

Only fasting measurements of serum calcium and phosphorus should be considered reliable.

CELLULAR MINERAL METABOLISM

A detailed summary of the numerous metabolic functions of calcium, magnesium, and phosphorus within cells is beyond the scope of this syllabus. This section attempts simply to highlight briefly some of the important roles of these ions in cellular physiology.

Calcium. The control of cellular calcium homeostasis is complex, and the regulation of the concentration of the calcium ion in the cytosol is as rigidly maintained as is its concentration in extracellular fluids (5). Cells are bathed in extracellular fluids containing approximately 10^{-3} M Ca^{2+}. The concentration of Ca^{2+} in the cytoplasm is approximately 10^{-6} M, or one-thousandth that in extracellular fluids. Cytosolic calcium is to some extent buffered by binding to other cytoplasmic constituents, and certain cells contain a specific calcium-binding protein that may serve as a buffer and/or a calcium transport protein within the cytosol. The mitochondria and microsomes contain 90% to 99% of the intracellular calcium, bound largely to organic and inorganic phosphates. The calcium content of these organelles is sufficient to replenish cytosolic calcium some 500 times.

The low Ca^{2+} concentration in the cytosol is maintained by three pump-leak transport systems: an external system located in the plasma membrane and two internal systems located in the microsomal membrane and the inner mitochondrial membrane, respectively. Calcium diffuses into the cytosol across these three membranes. Each of the three pumps is oriented in a direction of calcium egress from the cytosol; each requires energy, and each shares a high affinity for calcium (K_m approximately 10^{-6} M).

The importance of these three calcium transport systems in regulating cellular calcium metabolism varies considerably from cell to cell depending on the function of a particular cell type. Several examples serve to illustrate how the details of cellular calcium homeostasis have been adapted to subserve the specific physiologic function of a given cell type.

Calcium ion is the coupling factor linking excitation and contraction in all forms of skeletal and cardiac muscle (5). In striated muscle, the microsomes are extensively developed as the sarcoplasmic reticulum, which serves as the principal storehouse of intracellular calcium in muscle and which is the most highly developed calcium transport system known. Depolarization of the plasma membrane is accompanied by the entry of a small amount of extracellular calcium into the cell, and this acts as a trigger to release large quantities of calcium stored in the sarcoplasmic reticulum. The abrupt increase in cytosolic calcium interacts with troponin, a specific calcium-binding protein, leading to a conformational change and the actin–myosin interaction that constitutes muscle contraction. The reticulum vesicles are capable of reaccumulating the large quantity of cytosolic calcium with the extreme speed required by the relaxation process.

In most mammalian cells other than muscle, the principal internal calcium pump-leak system is that of the inner mitochondrial membrane. In a number of cells, calcium serves as a second messenger, mediating the effects of membrane signals on the release of secretory products (e.g., neurotransmitters, exocrine secretions such as amylase, and endocrine secretions such as insulin and aldosterone) (5). The calcium messenger system involves a flow of information along several pathways: (i) the calmodulin pathway and (ii) the phosphoinositide C-kinase pathway. It is now recognized that in many cells the several branches of the calcium messenger system and the cyclic adenosine monophosphate (cAMP) messenger system are intimately related, and that these systems are integrated in such a way that the net cellular response to a given stimulus is determined by a complex interplay ("cross-talk") between these systems (5).

Phosphorus. The transport of phosphate ions across the plasma membrane and the membranes of intracellular organelles proceeds passively but is determined by the movement of cations, mostly calcium. The phosphate content in mitochondria is high, where it is largely in the form of calcium salts. The cytoplasmic concentration of free phosphate ions is estimated to be quite low, and the remaining portion of intracellular phosphate is either bound or in the form of organic phosphate esters. These phosphate esters play a variety of critically important roles in cellular metabolism: purine nucleotides provide the cell with stored energy; phosphorylated intermediates are concerned with energy conservation and transfer; phospholipids are major constituents of cell membranes, and the phosphorylation of proteins is an important means of regulating their function.

Magnesium. Magnesium is the most abundant intracellular divalent cation and the second most abundant intracellular cation after potassium. Approximately 60% of cellular magnesium is contained in the mitochondria, and it is estimated that only 5% to 10% of intracellular magnesium exists as free ions in the cytoplasm. The transport mechanisms responsible for maintaining the asymmetric distribution of magnesium in intracellular compartments are less well studied than the corresponding calcium transport systems, but it is clear that the cellular metabolisms of calcium and magnesium are regulated independently. Magnesium is an essential cofactor in the functioning of a wide variety of key enzymes, including essentially all enzymes concerned with the transfer of phosphate groups, all reactions that require ATP, and each of the steps concerned with the replication, transcription, and translation of genetic information.

MINERAL ION BALANCE AND MECHANISMS FOR MAINTAINING SYSTEMIC MINERAL HOMEOSTASIS

Mineral ion influx and efflux in the intestine, bone, and kidney, and the regulation of these processes by PTH and $1,25(OH)_2D$ are described in detail in other chapters in this primer. The information in the sections that follow attempts to integrate these processes at the level of the intact organism, and it describes the fine set of checks and balances that regulate mineral homeostasis *in vivo*.

The term *mineral ion balance* refers to the state of mineral homeostasis in the organism vis-à-vis the environment. In zero balance, mineral intake and accretion exactly match mineral losses. In positive balance, mineral intake and accretion exceed mineral losses. In negative balance, mineral losses exceed mineral intake and accretion. A growing child is in positive mineral balance, whereas an immobilized patient is in negative mineral balance. Formal balance studies are a relic of the past and are no longer performed, but the concept of balance is central to even a cursory understanding of systemic mineral ion homeostasis. Figure 1 is a schematic representation of calcium, phosphorus, and magnesium metabolism in a normal adult on an average diet who is in zero mineral ion balance.

Calcium. The total extracellular pool of calcium is approximately 900 mg. This pool is in dynamic equilibrium with calcium entering and exiting via the intestine, bone, and renal tubule. In zero balance, bone resorption and formation are equivalent at about 500 mg/day, and the net quantity of calcium absorbed by the intestine, approximately 175 mg per day, is quantitatively excreted into the urine. Thus, under normal circumstances, net calcium absorption provides a surplus of calcium that considerably exceeds systemic requirements.

Several points illustrated in this schema merit some emphasis. The first is the quantitative importance of the kidney in the regulation of calcium homeostasis. The filtered load of calcium is a whopping 10,000 mg/day, and 10% of this, or 1000 mg/day, is under the control of PTH-regulated reabsorption in the distal nephron. The second is the elegance of biologic control that must underlie a system in which calcium absorption and excretion are matched on essentially a milligram-per-milligram basis.

Phosphorus. The extracellular pool of orthophosphate is approximately 550 mg (Fig. 1). This pool is in dynamic equilibrium with phosphate entry and exit via the intestine, bone, kidney, and soft tissues (not depicted in the figure). In zero balance, fractional net phosphorus absorption is about two thirds of phosphorus intake; this amount represents a vast excess over systemic requirements and is quantitatively excreted into the urine.

Again, several points merit emphasis. The first is that the absorption of phosphate in the intestine is far less rigidly regulated than is the absorption of calcium. The second is the dominant role of the kidney; in this case, the threshold for phosphate reabsorption in the proximal tubule [tubular maximum for phosphate/glomerular filtration rate (TmP/GFR)] is essentially the setpoint that defines the fasting serum phosphorus concentration, and it is the setpoint that is regulated by PTH.

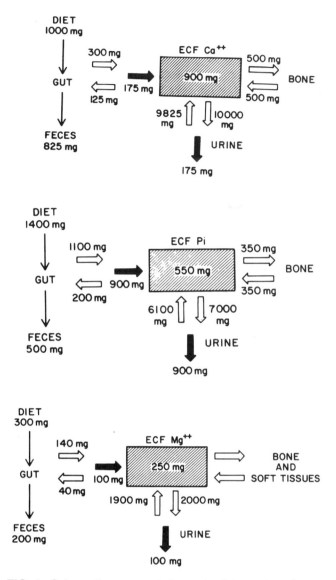

FIG. 1. Schematic representations of calcium, phosphorus, and magnesium fluxes in a normal adult in zero mineral ion balance. *Open arrows* denote unidirectional mineral fluxes, and *solid arrows* denote net fluxes; all values are given in mg/day. (From: Stewart AF, Broadus AE. Mineral metabolism. In: Felig P, Baxter JD, Broadus AE, Frohman LA (eds) *Endocrinology and Metabolism*, 2nd ed. McGraw-Hill, New York, 1987.)

Magnesium. The extracellular pool of magnesium is approximately 250 mg and is in bidirectional equilibrium with magnesium fluxes across the intestine, kidney, bone, and soft tissues (Fig. 1). In zero balance, the magnesium derived from net intestinal absorption, approximately 100 mg per day, represents a systemic surplus and is quantitatively excreted. The kidney is responsible for regulating the serum magnesium concentration by a setpoint or Tm-limited process that is reminiscent of the setpoint for phosphorus, except that the TmMg is not hormonally regulated.

Two key points are made in the preceding paragraphs : (i) normally, hormonal and/or intrinsic mechanisms of mineral ion absorption in the intestine provide the organism with a mineral supply that exceeds systemic mineral needs by a considerable measure, and (ii) the renal tubule plays the dominant quantitative role in maintaining normal mineral homeostasis. Within this framework, minor fluctuations in systemic requirements are easily met by the surfeit of normal mineral absorption and do not require hormonal adjustments.

SYSTEMIC CALCIUM HOMEOSTASIS AND MAINTENANCE OF A NORMAL SERUM CALCIUM CONCENTRATION

The parathyroid chief cell is exquisitely sensitive to the ionized serum calcium concentration and is capable of responding to changes in this concentration so small that they are unmeasurable by human hands (1,6). The recently identified calcium receptor is the sensing device that is at the core of the chief cell's sensitivity to the ambient calcium concentration.

The integrated actions of PTH on distal tubular calcium reabsorption, bone resorption, and 1,25(OH)$_2$D-mediated intestinal calcium absorption are responsible for the fine regulation of the serum ionized calcium concentration. The precision of this integrated control is such that, in a normal individual, serum ionized calcium probably fluctuates by no more than 0.1 mg/dl in either direction from its normal set-point value throughout the day.

Distal tubular calcium reabsorption and osteoclastic bone resorption are the major control points in minute-to-minute serum calcium homeostasis; of these two processes, the effect of PTH on the distal tubule is quantitatively the more important. Indeed, the 1000 mg/dl of calcium that is under PTH control as it passes through the distal nephron is clearly the centerpiece of the organism's ability to fine tune the serum calcium concentration on a minute-to-minute basis. The effects of PTH on the acute phase of bone resorption and calcium reclamation in the distal tubule together constitute a classic "short-loop" feedback system, in that the calcium so provided feeds back directly in the parathyroid chief cell.

The parathyroid–renal (PTH–1,25(OH)$_2$D) axis is reminiscent of the pituitary–adrenal (ACTH–cortisol) axis, and use of the axis concept and terminology is encouraged. Whereas 1,25(OH)$_2$D does influence PTH secretion directly as a short-loop feedback, the essence of the PTH–1,25(OH)$_2$D axis in practice is a long-loop feedback system in which 1,25(OH)$_2$D-mediated calcium absorption provides the ultimate feedback on the parathyroid chief cell. This long-loop system is the only means by which the organism can change its net capacity to obtain calcium from the environment, and it is therefore the centerpiece of the organism's response to either a prolonged or a major hypocalcemic challenge. Maximal adjustments to the rate of calcium absorption in the intestine via the PTH–1,25(OH)$_2$D axis require 24 to 48 hours to become fully operative, so that this system has little to do with minute-to-minute regulation.

A 12- to 15-hour fast in a normal individual represents a minor physiologic hypocalcemic challenge that requires only subtle hormonal readjustments for correction. The total quantity of calcium lost into the urine during this time is in the range of 50 to 75 mg. An unmeasurable fall in serum calcium occurs, leading to a slight increase in PTH secretion. The dip in serum calcium is corrected by an increased efficiency of calcium reclamation in the distal tubule and by the rapid resorptive response to PTH in bone; by 12 hours, only minor increases in 1,25(OH)$_2$D synthesis will have occurred.

An abrupt reduction in dietary calcium intake to less than 100 mg per day, or the administration of 80 mg of furosemide daily to a normal individual, represents a moderate hypocalcemic challenge; in each case, the initial deficit of calcium is in the range of 100 to 150 mg per day. A series of adjustments occurs, leading to a new steady state by 48 hours (Fig. 2). A moderate increase in the secretion rate of PTH results in: (i) increased calcium reabsorption from the distal tubule, (ii) increased mobilization of calcium and phosphorus from bone, and (iii) increased synthesis of 1,25(OH)$_2$D, which participates with PTH in bone resorption and increases the efficiency of calcium and phosphorus absorption in the intestine. The increased circulating concentration of PTH resets the renal tubular phosphate threshold (TmP/GFR) at a lower level so that the increased amount of phosphorus mobilized from bone and absorbed from the intestine is quantitatively excreted into the urine. In the new steady state, serum calcium has returned to normal, serum phosphorus is unchanged or slightly reduced, and a state of mild secondary hyperparathyroidism and efficient intestinal mineral absorption exists. At this point, the initial requirement for calcium mobilization from the skeleton is largely replaced by the enhanced absorption of calcium in the intestine.

The systemic mechanisms for the prevention of hypercalcemia consist largely of a reversal of the sequence just described, namely, an inhibition of PTH and 1,25(OH)$_2$D synthesis, with a reduction in calcium mobilization from bone, absorption from the intestine, and reclamation from the distal renal tubule. Whether the putative effects of calcitonin are of pathophysiologic importance in humans remains unclear. The bottleneck in the system's defense against hypercalcemia is the limited capacity of the kidneys to excrete calcium. In theory, normal kidneys can excrete a calcium load of 1000 mg or more per day. In practice, calcium excretion rates in this range are rarely seen. Limitations in the theoretical ability of the kidney to combat hypercalcemia include: (i) the fact that abnormalities in distal tubular reabsorption are actually involved in the genesis of hypercalcemia in a number of conditions (e.g., primary hyperparathyroidism), (ii) the fact that a degree of renal impairment frequently accompanies many hypercalcemic conditions, and (iii) the fact that an increased calcium concentration inhibits the ability of the renal tubule to conserve water, which may lead to a vicious cycle of dehydration, prerenal azotemia, and worsening hypercalcemia. One or more of these limitations can usually be demonstrated in any given patient with hypercalcemia.

A patient with advanced breast carcinoma metastatic to bone represents a severe hypercalcemic challenge. In such a patient, calcium is mobilized from bone by local osteolytic mechanisms, parathyroid function and 1,25(OH)$_2$D synthesis are appropriately suppressed, and the normal mechanisms of bone resorption, intestinal calcium absorption, and distal tubular calcium reabsorption are virtually eliminated. Initially, these adjustments may lead to a compensated steady state in which approximately 800 to 1000 mg per day of mobilized calcium is excreted, with a serum calcium that is high-normal or only slightly elevated. With advancing disease or, as often occurs, with immobilization resulting from the basic disease process or an intercurrent illness, the quantity of mobilized calcium overwhelms the renal capacity for calcium excretion, and the spiral of hypercalcemia, dehydration, azotemia, and worsening hypercalcemia begins. In this circumstance, the serum calcium may climb from 10.5 to 15 mg/dl within 48 hours.

SYSTEMIC PHOSPHORUS HOMEOSTASIS AND MAINTENANCE OF A NORMAL SERUM PHOSPHORUS CONCENTRATION

The kidney plays the dominant role in systemic phosphorus homeostasis and maintains the serum phosphorus concentration at a value very close to the tubular phosphorus threshold or TmP/GFR. Because of the normal efficiency and lack of fine regulation of phosphorus absorption in the intestine, only in unusual circumstances (e.g., prolonged use of phosphate-binding antacids) is the systemic supply of phosphorus a limiting factor in phosphorus homeostasis. Thus, most disorders associated with chronic hypophosphatemia and/or phosphorus depletion in humans result from either intrinsic (e.g., familial hypophosphatemic rickets) or extrinsic (e.g., primary hyperparathyroidism) alterations in TmP/GFR. Similarly, most conditions of chronic hyperphosphatemia result from either intrinsic (e.g., renal

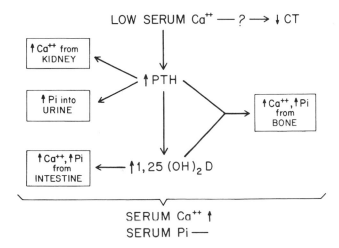

FIG. 2. The sequence of adjustments that are called into play in response to a moderate hypocalcemic challenge. (From: Stewart AF, Broadus AE. Mineral metabolism. In: Felig P, Baxter JD, Broadus AE, Frohman LA (eds) *Endocrinology and Metabolism*, 2nd ed. McGraw-Hill, New York, 1987.)

impairment) or extrinsic (e.g., hypoparathyroidism) abnormalities in the renal threshold for phosphorus. Acute hypophosphatemia most commonly results from the flux of extracellular phosphate ions into soft tissues.

The sequence of events initiated in the face of a hypophosphatemic challenge (Fig. 3) includes: (i) stimulation of 1,25(OH)$_2$D synthesis in the kidney, (ii) enhanced mobilization of phosphorus and calcium from bone, and (iii) a hypophosphatemia-induced increase in TmP/GFR (the exact mechanism of which is unknown). The increased circulating concentration of 1,25(OH)$_2$D leads to increases in phosphorus and calcium absorption in the intestine and provides an additional stimulus for phosphorus and calcium mobilization from bone. The increased flow of calcium from bone and the intestine results in an inhibition of PTH secretion, which diverts the systemic flow of calcium into the urine and further increases TmP/GFR. The net result of this sequence of adjustments is a return of the serum phosphorus concentration to normal without change in the serum calcium concentration.

The defense against hyperphosphatemia consists largely of a reversal of the sequence of adjustments just described. The principal humoral factor that combats hyperphosphatemia is PTH, but its action is indirect. The product of the concentrations of calcium and phosphorus in serum is referred to as the mineral ion (Ca × P) product. This product tends to be a biologic constant, in the sense that an increase in the concentration of one member leads to a reciprocal change in the concentration of the other. Thus, an acute rise in the serum phosphorus concentration produces a transient fall in the concentration of serum ionized calcium and a stimulation of PTH secretion, which reduces TmP/GFR and leads to a readjustment in serum phosphorus and calcium concentrations. A prolonged rise in the serum phosphorus concentration results in (i) an intrinsic downward adjustment in TmP/GFR that is independent of PTH and (ii) a persistent increase in PTH secretion that can ultimately lead to chief cell hyperplasia. If hyperphosphatemia is prolonged

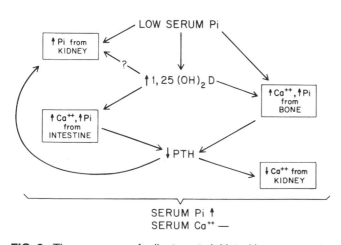

FIG. 3. The sequence of adjustments initiated in response to hypophosphatemia. (From: Stewart AF, Broadus AE. Mineral metabolism. In: Felig P, Baxter JD, Broadus AE, Frohman LA (eds) *Endocrinology and Metabolism*, 2nd ed. McGraw-Hill, New York, 1987.)

and severe (e.g., as occurs in chronic renal insufficiency), the degree of secondary hyperparathyroidism is sufficient to lead to the typical findings of parathyroid bone disease.

SYSTEMIC MAGNESIUM HOMEOSTASIS AND MAINTENANCE OF A NORMAL SERUM MAGNESIUM CONCENTRATION

The understanding of systemic magnesium homeostasis remains at a relatively primitive state. Unlike calcium and phosphorus, there appears to be no important systemic or hormonal regulation of the magnesium concentration in the extracellular fluids. Instead, maintenance of the serum magnesium concentration seems to result from the combined fluxes of magnesium at the levels of the intestine, kidney, intracellular fluids, and perhaps the skeleton. The kidney is primarily responsible for the regulation of the serum magnesium concentration.

The fractional absorption of magnesium is approximately 30%. In conditions of dietary magnesium excess, a smaller proportion may be absorbed, and in conditions of dietary magnesium deficiency, a higher proportion may be absorbed. The cellular mechanisms mediating magnesium absorption in the small intestine are poorly defined but would appear to consist of both passive and facilitated (but not active) elements. These elements do not seem to be sensitive to PTH, calcitonin, or 1,25(OH)$_2$D. Thus, the net quantity of magnesium absorbed appears to be primarily a function of magnesium intake.

Of the approximately 2000 mg of magnesium filtered per day, 96% is reabsorbed along the nephron and some 4% is excreted in the urine (fractional magnesium excretion). The mechanisms of magnesium reabsorption along the nephron at a cellular level are poorly understood, but, as is the case for calcium and phosphorus, it is possible to define a renal magnesium threshold or tubular maximum for magnesium (TmMg). The TmMg represents the net effects of magnesium reabsorption at different sites along the nephron. The TmMg is approximately 1.4 mg/dl when expressed as a function of the ultrafilterable serum magnesium concentration, or 2.0 mg/dl when expressed as a function of the total serum magnesium concentration (4). The tubular maximum functions essentially as a setpoint for reabsorption, such that magnesium filtered at a concentration above the TmMg is excreted and that filtered at a concentration beneath the TmMg is retained. As in the intestine, renal tubular magnesium handling does not appear to be regulated by systemic or hormonal mechanisms in any important way.

In summary, systemic magnesium homeostasis does not appear to be hormonally regulated and therefore reflects largely the quantitative interplay of net magnesium absorption in the intestine and the fractional excretion of magnesium by the kidney. The fractional excretion of magnesium functions as a Tm-limited process and is primarily responsible for maintaining the serum magnesium concentration within rather narrow limits. The fine regulation of the serum magnesium concentration in the absence of hormonal controls provides an excellent example of the biologic power of a Tm-limited transport process.

ACKNOWLEDGMENT

Supported in part by National Institutes of Health grant RR125.

REFERENCES

1. Bringhurst FR: Calcium and phosphate distribution, turnover and metabolic actions. In: DeGroot LJ (ed) *Endocrinology*, 3rd ed. Saunders, Philadelphia, 1015–1043, 1995
2. Krane SM: Calcium, phosphate and magnesium. In: Rasmussen H (ed) In: *International Encyclopedia of Pharmacology and Therapeutics*, vol 1. Pergamon Press, London, 19–59, 1970
3. Marshall RW: Plasma fractions. In: Nordin BEC (ed) In: *Calcium, Phosphate and Magnesium Metabolism*. Churchill Livingstone, London, 162–185, 1976
4. Rude RK, Singer FR: Magnesium deficiency and excess. *Ann Rev Med* 32:245–253, 1981
5. Rasmussen H, Rasmussen J: Calcium as intracellular messenger: From simplicity to complexity. *Curr Top Cell Regul* 31: 1–109, 1990
6. Stewart AF, Broadus AE: Mineral metabolism. In: Felig P, Baxter JD, Broadus AE, Frohman LA (eds) In: *Endocrinology and Metabolism*, 2nd ed. McGraw-Hill, New York: 1317–1453, 1987

10. Secretion, Circulating Heterogeneity, and Metabolism of Parathyroid Hormone

Gino V. Segre, M.D., and *Edward M. Brown, M.D.

Department of Medicine, Harvard Medical School; and Endocrine Unit, Massachusetts General Hospital, Boston, Massachusetts
*Department of Medicine, Harvard Medical School; and Endocrine-Hypertension Unit, Brigham and Women's Hospital, Boston, Massachusetts

It is important to distinguish parathyroid hormone (PTH) gene regulation and control of PTH synthesis from regulation of PTH secretion by parathyroid cells. The following discussion, which concerns factors that influence the plasma concentration of PTH, must be prefaced with a brief consideration of the regulation of the PTH gene and resultant effects on PTH secretion. Although the PTH gene is active under normal physiologic conditions, its expression is regulated; mRNA levels for prepro-PTH rise several-fold in rats made hypocalcemic *in vivo* (1), whereas the mRNA levels fall after exposure to high calcium concentrations or 1,25-dihydroxyvitamin D, both *in vivo* and *in vitro* (2–4). Additional factors have been shown to modulate expression of the PTH gene, such as estrogen (5) and retinoids (6), but their physiologic significance is unclear. An important, but poorly understood, level of control of parathyroid function is the regulation of cellular proliferation. Although it is likely that hypercalcemia inhibits, and, conversely, that hypocalcemia stimulates, parathyroid cellular proliferation, it is uncertain whether this is a direct action on the parathyroid cell (7). 1,25-Dihydroxyvitamin D appears to play an important role in tonically inhibiting parathyroid cell growth under normal circumstances (8,9). Conversely, 1,25-dihydroxyvitamin D deficiency, as occurs in renal insufficiency, probably contributes to parathyroid glandular enlargement.

SECRETION

Although the extracellular fluid (ECF) ionized calcium concentration $[Ca^{2+}]$ is the major determinant of PTH secretion, 1,25-dihydroxyvitamin D also appears to be an important regulator; this is presumably in large part a result of its control of PTH gene expression (3,4). Catecholamines and additional biogenic amines, other ions (such as magnesium, lithium, and aluminum), hormones (including glucagon, secretin, cortisol, and calcitonin), and other agents influence PTH secretion, but their relevance to normal physiology is uncertain (7,10). Several of these agents, however, modulate PTH secretion in pathophysiologic states. For example, both chronic magnesium depletion (7,10) and severe hypermagnesemia (11) inhibit PTH secretion. Lithium stimulates PTH secretion *in vivo* and *in vitro* (7,12), and the use of lithium in the therapy of bipolar affective disorder is associated with the development of PTH-dependent hypercalcemia in as many as 10% to 15% of cases. The latter is sometimes reversible following discontinuation of the drug, but it is more commonly associated with the presence of either a parathyroid adenoma or four-gland hyperplasia, possibly resulting from the pharmacologic actions of lithium on the parathyroid cell (13). Aluminum, which inhibits PTH secretion *in vitro* (14), may influence hormone secretion in patients with severe renal impairment who are dialyzed against solutions contaminated with aluminum, or who are treated with aluminum-containing phosphate binders for control of hyperphosphatemia.

PTH secretory dynamics have been studied *in vivo* in humans, calves, dogs, rats, and even mice during the infusion of calcium and of calcium chelators (10). These dose–response curves describe inverse sigmoidal relationships between blood PTH and serum $[Ca^{2+}]$, which can be defined by models incorporating four variables (14). The latter include maximally and minimally blood-immunoreactive (i) PTH, the midpoint or set-point of the curve, and the slope of the curve at its midpoint. The development of immunometric PTH assays that primarily detect intact PTH (1-84) (15) has greatly facilitated these studies. In normal subjects, iPTH levels, as measured with such assays, range from approximately 10 to 60 pg/ml, their maximally stimulated and maximally suppressed levels are about 100 to 150 pg/ml and 5 to 10 pg/ml, respectively, and the set-point is at a serum $[Ca^{2+}]$ of 1.2 to 1.25 mM (the normal range for serum $[Ca^{2+}]$ is about 1.15 to 1.35 mM).

In humans as well as in experimental animals, perturbations of the blood $[Ca^{2+}]$ by as little as 0.025 to 0.05 mM promptly change PTH secretion (16). The iPTH levels dramatically increase (by fivefold or more) when blood $[Ca^{2+}]$ is lowered to ~1 mM; further lowering of the calcium level, however, does not elicit any additional increase in iPTH. Upon raising the blood $[Ca^{2+}]$, iPTH secretion falls; however, it is not completely suppressed, even when blood $[Ca^{2+}]$ is strikingly elevated. iPTH secretion under normal, steady-state physiologic circumstances is only modestly higher than the maximally suppressed level (about 20 to 25 pg/ml, versus 5 to 10 pg/ml). Thus, the parathyroid glands are poised to best respond to a hypocalcemic challenge with a marked increase in PTH secretory rate.

Recent studies have shown certain deviations from the sigmoidal relationship between iPTH levels and blood $[Ca^{2+}]$ described above, which may be of physiologic relevance. When the serum $[Ca^{2+}]$ is reduced in normal humans by infusion of citrate, and the calcium level is then allowed to return to normal by discontinuing the infusion, there is hysteresis in the relationship between iPTH and blood $[Ca^{2+}]$ (17). That is, the iPTH level is higher at any given level of $[Ca^{2+}]$ when the calcium is rising than when it is falling, and there is an apparent shift of the sigmoidal curve between iPTH and $[Ca^{2+}]$ to the left. In addition, if citrate is infused at varying rates, with corresponding variations in the rate of fall of the serum $[Ca^{2+}]$, the more rapid reductions in $[Ca^{2+}]$ elicit substantially greater increases in iPTH levels (16). The physiologic relevance and the mechanisms underlying these hysteretic and rate-dependent relationships between PTH and $[Ca^{2+}]$ are uncertain.

PTH secretory dynamics in most patients with primary hyperparathyroidism show that the level of blood $[Ca^{2+}]$ at which PTH secretion is one half of its maximal level (the set-point) is higher than in normal subjects (18). Factors responsible for this set-point error are under intense study; they may relate to abnormalities in the ECF calcium-sensing mechanism(s) of the parathyroid cell, which are described in more detail later. Such abnormalities might be primary defects in the calcium-sensing mechanism, or they might represent secondary responses to defects in the regulation of parathyroid cell proliferation, because various forms of hyperparathyroidism appear to be the consequence of the proliferation of clones of abnormal cells with acquired or inherited [as in multiple endocrine neoplasia (MEN) syndromes] mutations in genes involved in control of growth, including oncogenes and tumor suppressor genes (19,20). Interestingly, recent studies show that the pathophysiologic disturbances in parathyroid gland function appear to differ between patients with primary and those with secondary hyperparathyroidism (at least secondary hyperparathyroidism associated with end-stage renal failure). Using similar techniques to test PTH secretory dynamics, Salusky, Goodman, and their associates (21,22) showed no change in the set-point for plasma intact iPTH in dialyzed patients, compared to normal subjects, either before or after treatment of their hyperparathyroidism with calcitriol.

In vitro, the PTH secretory response also shows an increase in set-point when there is concomitant exposure of parathyroid cells to high lithium concentrations (7,12) or when the cells are incubated under conditions favorable to cell division (23). Estrogen treatment of postmenopausal women also has been reported to lower the set-point slightly, perhaps contributing to estrogen-induced changes in calcium balance (24).

Recent studies have shed considerable light on the molecular mechanisms through which parathyroid cells and other cell types recognize and respond to or "sense" changes in the ambient $[Ca^{2+}]$. The technique of expression cloning in *Xenopus laevis* oocytes was used to isolate a cDNA clone encoding an extracellular calcium (Ca^{2+}_o)-sensing receptor from bovine parathyroid (25). Analysis of the nucleotide and predicted amino acid sequences of this clone indicate that it is a receptor belonging to the superfamily of G-protein-coupled receptors, which comprises multiple members, including the recently cloned receptors for PTH and calcitonin (CT) (Fig. 1). The calcium-sensing receptor couples to activation of phospholipase C and, perhaps, to inhibition of adenylyl cyclase.

The Ca^{2+}_o-sensing receptor is also present on the C-cells of the thyroid gland and probably mediates the stimulatory effects of ECF $[Ca^{2+}]$ on CT secretion. It is likewise expressed on a variety of other cells, including a number of those within the central nervous system, gastrointestinal tract, and kidney (25,26). In the last, it may mediate some of the poorly understood direct actions of ECF $[Ca^{2+}]$ on renal function (27). Although efforts to understand the signaling and physiologic properties of the Ca^{2+}_o-sensing receptor are in their infancy, the existence of such a receptor documents that ECF $[Ca^{2+}]$ acts, in effect, as a calciotropic hormone, analogous to other, more classical, hormones (i.e., PTH and CT) being used by cells involved in maintaining calcium homeostasis.

Direct evidence for the physiologic relevance of the Ca^{2+}_o-sensing receptor has come from studies of human diseases that result from either inactivating or activating mutations in the receptor gene. As discussed in more detail in Chapter 29, the hypercalcemic disorders, familial hypocalciuric (or benign) hypercalcemia (FHH or FBH) and neonatal severe hyperparathyroidism (NSHPT), represent, respectively, the clinical expression of inactivating mutations in the receptor when present in the heterozygous and homozygous states (27). In FHH, there is an increase in the set-point of the parathyroid gland (28), a PTH-independent increase in renal tubular calcium reabsorption at any given level of serum $[Ca^{2+}]$, and normal urinary concentrating ability despite hypercalcemia (29,30). These observations strongly support the role of the receptor in mediating the direct actions of calcium on PTH secretion as well as on the aspects of renal function noted above. While heterozygotes (i.e., those with FHH) have a mild and generally benign phenotype, the homozygous state (NSHPT) is often fatal unless parathyroidectomy is carried out in the newborn period to treat the severe hypercalcemia. Thus the Ca^{2+}_o-sensing receptor appears to play a central role in Ca^{2+}-regulated PTH

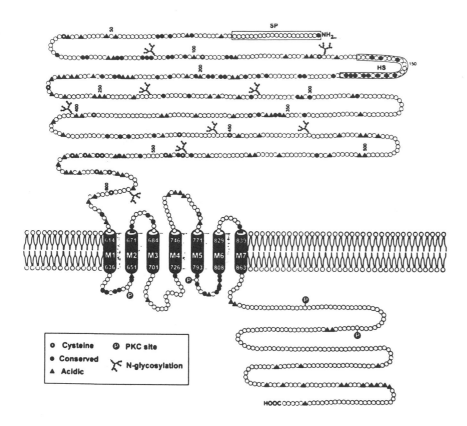

FIG. 1. Proposed model for the bovine parathyroid calcium-sensing receptor protein, which includes seven membrane-spanning helices. The large amino-terminal region is located extracellularly and contains nine potential glycosylation sites. Amino acids are indicated at intervals of 50 in this region. Potential intracellular protein kinase C phosphorylation sites are shown. Amino acids that are identical in the bovine parathyroid calcium-sensing receptor and in all metabotropic glutamate receptors are indicated. (From: Brown EM, Gamba G, Riccardi D, Lombardi M, Butters R, Kifor O, Sun A, Hediger MA, Lytton J, Hebert SC. Cloning and characterization of an extracellular Ca^{2+}-sensing receptor from bovine parathyroid. *Nature* 366:575–580, 1993.)

secretion. Individuals with FHH and NSHPT also show varying degrees of hypermagnesemia (29,30), suggesting that the receptor probably contributes to "setting" the ECF magnesium level as well, most likely by regulating renal tubular magnesium reabsorption in the thick ascending limb. Conversely, activating mutations in the receptor produce a form of autosomal dominant hypocalcemia (31). In this syndrome, the set-point of the parathyroid is reset downward, producing hypocalcemia, in contrast to the situation with FHH and NSHPT, where is it reset upward, resulting in hypercalcemia.

IMMUNOHETEROGENEITY OF PLASMA PARATHYROID HORMONE

In normal humans, intact PTH comprises only 5% to 30% of the circulating iPTH; inactive fragments that consist mostly of the two thirds of the intact hormone molecule at the carboxyl (C)-terminal end account for the remaining 70% to 95% (32). Although amino (N)-terminal fragments that circulate in certain pathologic conditions have been described, it is generally agreed that, if they circulate at all, they comprise only a very small fraction of the total iPTH. Fragments from the middle (M) portion of the hormone also have been reported. Both secretion of iPTH fragments by the parathyroid glands and peripheral metabolism of intact hormone into circulating fragments contribute to the immunoheterogeneity of circulating iPTH. Hormonal fragments from M and C-terminal portions of the hormonal

sequence have been detected in extracts of parathyroid glands, they are released by parathyroid tissue *in vitro,* and they are present in the parathyroid venous-effluent of both normal and hyperparathyroid glands. Interestingly, the relative circulating concentrations of intact iPTH and of its fragments appear to relate to control of their secretion by the blood $[Ca^{2+}]$. This was first demonstrated *in vivo* by directly sampling bovine parathyroid venous-effluent while the circulating blood $[Ca^{2+}]$ was exogenously perturbed; with hypercalcemia, the concentration of C-terminal fragments increased relative to that of intact hormone, whereas the converse was true when the animals were made hypocalcemic (10).

Subsequently, these observations have been confirmed and elegantly extended, mainly in studies by D'Amour and his associates in dogs (33,34) and humans (35,36). Whereas intact iPTH constituted no more than 25% of the total iPTH at normal $[Ca^{2+}]$ in dogs, it became the dominant immunoreactive form during induced hypocalcemia (33). In normal humans, C-terminal fragments were the predominant forms of circulating iPTH, even during induced hypocalcemia, and increased considerably during induced hypercalcemia (35). Patients with primary hyperparathyroidism had a higher set-point (as defined previously) than normal subjects. Interestingly, dynamic testing revealed that C-terminal fragments were not preferentially secreted in these patients, as they were both in normal subjects and in those with other hypercalcemic states (36). This suggests that intra-gland processing/degradation also is abnormal in patients with primary hyperparathyroidism.

METABOLISM OF CIRCULATING PARATHYROID HORMONE

Intact PTH is cleared very rapidly from the circulation, with a half-time of less than 4 minutes, mostly by high-capacity hepatic and renal mechanisms (10,37). Recently, the cloning of two PTH receptors has allowed a search for sites expressing their mRNAs. The first, a receptor that binds PTH and PTH-related protein with nearly equal affinities, is very widely distributed in nearly all tissues (38), whereas the second receptor appears to bind only PTH and is distributed mainly in the brain and the pancreas (39). Although no estimates have been made, it seems likely that biologically active PTH is also cleared from blood by high-affinity receptors encoded by these mRNAs.

Hepatic clearance exceeds renal clearance, at least under normal conditions. It is a complex process involving at least three different mechanisms: (i) hepatic macrophages, Kupffer cells, take up most of the hormone and degrade it to either free amino acids or very small fragments, (ii) Kupffer cells also cleave the hormone into discrete fragments and release some of them back into the circulation, and (iii) hepatocytes take up a relatively small amount of hormone, perhaps through receptor-mediated mechanisms. Kupffer cell clearance is of high capacity, and it discriminates poorly, if at all, between active and inactive PTH, whereas uptake by hepatocytes is of low capacity, but it specifically removes biologically active hormone. The C-terminal fragments generated and released by Kupffer cells *in vitro* reflect cleavage of the hormone mostly between residues 33-34 and 36-37 of the intact molecule. These are the same fragments that appear *in vivo* in the circulation of animals injected with intact hormone (10,37). Studies with isolated rat livers *ex vivo* indicate that uptake is modestly more efficient when the liver was perfused with a solution containing 4 mM of $[Ca^{2+}]$, than when perfused with one containing 1 mM of $[Ca^{2+}]$ (40). C-terminal fragments persist in blood for 5 to 10 times longer than does intact hormone, and they are cleared nearly exclusively by glomerular filtration; these fragments are minimally taken up by the liver, if at all (10,37,41). The fate of N-terminal fragments of PTH, presumably resulting from cleavage(s) by endopeptidase(s), is uncertain. The weight of evidence suggests that these fragments are not released back into the circulation, although, of course, they might have escaped detection because their blood levels were too low to be measured even by the high-resolution methods used. In sum, C-terminal fragments released by Kupffer cells, but not N-terminal fragments, substantially contribute to the heterogeneity of plasma PTH (10).

Renal clearance mechanisms for PTH also are complex. A small amount of biologically active hormone appears to be removed through mechanisms located on the basilateral surface of tubule cells, and this may represent receptor-mediated internalization. Large amounts of intact hormone and nearly all C-terminal fragments, however, are cleared efficiently by glomerular filtration (37). Filtered PTH is metabolized extensively by the kidney, and most studies show that neither intact hormone nor C-terminal fragments are excreted into the urine (10,37). In the isolated rat kidney, the clearance of PTH did differ when the perfusate calcium was changed from 1 mM to 4 mM, but there was release of M and C-terminal fragments back into the perfusate only when the solution $[Ca^{2+}]$ was 4 mM, but not when it was 1 mM in $[Ca^{2+}]$ (40).

The biologic consequences of these metabolic events has long been sought, in part because the sequence of PTH's C-terminal third is intensely homologous in the four mammalian species in which it has been defined, suggesting that this portion of the molecule serves an important biologic function. Very recently, reports have appeared that point to effects of C-terminal fragments on osteoclasts and/or their precursors (42), and putative receptors have been identified on a rat osteosarcoma cell line, ROS 17/2.8, and their properties partially characterized (43). Additionally, PTH metabolism potentially could generate biologically active N-terminal fragments with unique functions. Indeed, studies with isolated dog limbs showed that synthetic bovine PTH (1-34) has unique biologic properties in bone (10,37). Indeed, N-terminal fragments, some of which might be large enough to retain biologic activity, have been shown to accumulate in the liver and the kidney after bolus injection of intact hormone, although they have not been detected in blood (10,44,45). These fragments might play a yet unidentified local role in renal or hepatic physiology.

REFERENCES

1. Yamamoto M, Igarishi T, Muramatsu M, Fukagawa M, Ogata E: Hypocalcemia increases and hypercalcemia decreases the steady-state level of parathyroid hormone mRNA in the rat. *J Clin Invest* 83:1053–1056, 1989
2. Russell J, Lettieri D, Sherwood LM: Direct regulation by calcium of cytoplasmic messenger RNA coding for pre-pro-parathyroid hormone in isolated bovine parathyroid cells. *J Clin Invest* 72:1851–1855, 1983
3. Silver J, Russell J, Sherwood LM: Regulation by vitamin D metabolites of messenger RNA of parathyroid hormone in isolated parathyroid cells. *Proc Natl Acad Sci USA* 82:4270–4273, 1985
4. Silver J, Naveh-Many T, Mayer H, et al.: Regulation by vitamin D metabolites of parathyroid hormone gene transcription in vivo in the rat. *J Clin Invest* 78:1296–1301, 1986
5. Naneh-Many T, Almogi G, Livni N, et al.: Estrogen receptors and biological response in rat parathyroid tissue and C-cells. *J Clin Invest* 90:2434–2438, 1992
6. MacDonald PN, Ritter C, Brown AJ, Slatopolsky E: Retinoic acid suppresses parathyroid hormone (PTH) secretion and pre-proPTH levels in bovine parathyroid cell cultures. *J Clin Invest* 93:725–731, 1994
7. Brown EM: Extracellular Ca^{2+} sensing, regulation of parathyroid function, and role of Ca^{2+} and other ions as extracellular (first) messengers. *Physiol Rev* 71:391–411, 1991
8. Nygren P, Larsson R, Johansson H, Ljunghall S, Rastad J, Akerstrom G: $1,25(OH)_2D$ inhibits hormone secretion and proliferation but not functional differentiation in cultured bovine parathyroid cells. *Calcif Tissue Int* 42:213–218, 1988
9. Kremer R, Bolivar I, Goltzman D, Hendy GN: Influence of calcium and 1,25-dihydroxycholecalciferol on proliferation and proto-oncogene expression in primary cultures of bovine parathyroid cells. *Endocrinology* 125:935–941, 1989
10. Potts JT Jr, Bringhurst FR, Gardella T, Nussbaum SR, Segre GV, Kronenberg HM. Parathyroid hormone: physiology, chemistry, biosynthesis, secretion, metabolism, and mode of action. In: Degroot LJ (ed) *Endocrinology*, 3rd ed, vol 2. WB Saunders, Philadelphia, pp 920–960, 1995
11. Cholst IN, Sternberg SF, Tropper PJ, et al.: The influence of

hypermagnesemia on serum calcium and parathyroid hormone levels. *N Engl J Med* 301:1221–1225, 1984

12. Segre GV, Potts JT Jr. Differential diagnosis of hypercalcemia. In: DeGroot LJ (ed) *Endocrinology*, 3rd ed, vol 2. WB Saunders, Philadelphia, 1075–1063, 1995

13. Mallette LE, Eichhorn E: Effects of lithium carbonate on human calcium metabolism. *Arch Intern Med* 146:770–776, 1986

14. Brown EM: Four parameter model of the sigmoidal relationship between PTH release and the extracellular calcium concentration in normal and abnormal parathyroid tissue. *J Clin Endocrinol Metab* 56:572–581, 1983

15. Nussbaum SR, Zahradnik R, Lavigne J, et al.: Highly sensitive two-site immunoradiometric assay for parathyrin and its clinical utility in evaluating patients with hypercalcemia. *Clin Chem* 33:1364–1348, 1987

16. Grant FD, Conlin PR, Brown EM: Rate and concentration dependence of parathyroid hormone dynamics during stepwise changes in serum ionized calcium in normal humans. *J Clin Endocrinol Metab* 71:370–378, 1990

17. Conlin PR, Fajtova VT, Mortensen RM, LeBoff MS, Brown EM: Hysteresis in the relationship between serum ionized calcium and intact parathyroid hormone during recovery from induced hyper- and hypocalcemia in normal humans. *J Clin Endocrinol Metab* 69:593–599, 1989

18. Brown EM, Wilson RE, Thatcher JC, Marynich SP: Abnormal calcium-regulated PTH release in normal parathyroid glands from patients with an adenoma. *Am J Med* 71:565–570, 1981

19. Motokura T, Bloom T, Kim HG, et al.: A novel cyclin encoded by a bcl1-linked candidate oncogene. *Nature* 350:512–515, 1991

20. Friedman E, Sakaguchi K, Bale AE, et al.: Clonality of parathyroid tumors in familial multiple endocrine neoplasia type 1. *N Engl J Med* 321:213–218, 1989

21. Ramirez JA, Goodman WG, Gornbein J, Menezes C, Moulton L, Segre GV, Salusky IB: Direct in vivo comparison of calcium-regulated parathyroid hormone secretion in normal volunteers and patients with secondary hyperparathyroidism. *J Clin Endocrinol Metab* 76:1489–94, 1993

22. Ramirez JA, Goodman WG, Belin TR, Segre GV, Salusky IB: Calcitriol therapy and calcium-regulated PTH secretion in patients with secondary hyperparathyroidism. *Am J Physiol* 267:E961–967, 1994

23. LeBoff MS, Rennke HG, Brown EM: Abnormal reguilation of parathyroid cell secretion and proliferation in primary cultures of bovine parathyroid cells. *Endocrinology* 113:277–284, 1983

24. Boucher A, D'Amour P, Hamel L, Fugere P, Gascon-Barré M, et al.: Estrogen replacement decreases the setpoint of parathyroid hormone stimulation by calcium in normal postmenopausal women. *J Clin Endocrinol Metab* 68:831–836, 1989

25. Brown EM, Gamba G, Riccardi D, Lombardi M, Butters R, Kifor O, Sun A, Hediger MA, Lytton J, Hebert SC: Cloning and characterization of an extracellular Ca^{2+}-sensing receptor from bovine parathyroid. *Nature* 366:575–580, 1993

26. Riccardi D, Park J, Lee W-S, Gamba G, Brown EM, Hebert SC: Cloning and functional expression of a rat kidney extracellular calcium/polyvalent cation-sensing receptor. *Proc Natl Acad Sci USA* 92:131–135, 1995

27. Pollak M, Brown EM, Chou Y-HC, Hebert SC, Marx SJ, Steinman B, Levi T, Seidman CE, Seidman JG: Mutations in the human Ca^{2+}-sensing receptor gene cause familial hypocalciuric hypercalcemia and neonatal severe hyperparathyroidism. *Cell* 75:1297–1303, 1993

28. Khosla S, Ebeling PR, Firck AF, et al.: Calcium infusion suggests a "set-point" abnormality of parathyroid gland function in familial benign hypercalcemia and more complex disturbances

in primary hyperparathyroidism. *J Clin Endocrinol Metab* 76:715–720, 1993

29. Marx SJ, Attie MF, Levine MA, Spiegel AM, Downs RW Jr, Lasker RD: The hypocalciuric or benign variant of familial hypercalcemia: Clinical and biochemical features in fifteen kindreds. *Medicine (Baltimore)* 60:397–412, 1981

30. Law WM Jr, Heath III H: Familial benign (hypocalciuric) hypercalcemia. Clinical and pathogenic studies in 21 families. *Ann Intern Med* 102:511–519, 1985

31. Pollak MR, Brown EM, Estep HL, McLaine PN, Kifor O, Park J, Hebert SC, Seidman CE, Seidman JG: An autosomal dominant form of hypocalcemia caused by a mutation in the human Ca^{2+}-sensing receptor gene. *Nat Genet* 8:303–308, 1994

32. Segre GV, Habener JF, Dowell D, Tregear GW, Potts Jr JT: Parathyroid hormone in human plasma: Immunochemical characterization and biological implications. *J Clin Invest* 51:3163–3172, 1972

33. D'Amour P, Labelle F, Lecavalier L, Plourde V, Harvey D: Influence of serum calcium concentration on circulating forms of PTH in three species. *Am J Physiol* 251:E680–687, 1986

34. Cloutier M, Rousseau M, Gascon-Barré M, D'Amour P: Immunological evidence for post-translational control of parathyroid function ionized calcium in dogs. *Bone Miner* 22:197–207, 1993

35. D'Amour P, Palardy J, Bahsali G, Mallette LE, et al.: The modification of circulating parathyroid hormone immunoheterogeneity in man by ionized calcium concentration. *J Clin Endocrinol Metab* 74:525–532, 1992

36. Brossard JH, Whittom S, Lepage R, D'Amour P: Carboxyl-terminal fragments of parathyroid hormone are not secreted preferentially in primary hyperparathyroidism as they are in other hypercalcemic states. *J Clin Endocrinol Metab* 77:413–419, 1993

37. Martin KJ, Hruska KA, Freitage JJ, et al.: The peripheral metabolism of parathyroid hormone. *N Engl J Med* 301:1092–1098, 1979

38. Ureña P, Kong XF, Abou-Samra AB, Jüpper H, Kronenberg HM, Potts JT Jr, Sogre GV. Parathyroid hormone (PTH)/PTH-related peptide receptor mRNA is widely distributed in rat tissues. *Endocrinology* 133:617–623, 1993

39. Usdin TB, Gruber C, Bonner TI: Identification and functional expression of a receptor selectively recognizing parathyroid hormone, the PTH2 receptor. *J Biol Chem* 270:15455–15458, 1995

40. Daugaard H, Egfjord M, Olgaard K: Influence of calcium on the metabolism of intact parathyroid hormone by isolated perfused rat kidney and liver. *Endocrinology* 126:1813–1820, 1990

41. Segre GV, D'Amour P, Hultman A, Potts Jr JT: Effects of hepatectomy, nephrectomy and nephrectomy/uremia on the metabolism of parathyroid hormone in the rat. *J Clin Invest* 67:439–448, 1981

42. Kaji H, Sugimoto T, Kanatani M, et al.: Carboxyl-terminal PTH fragments stimulate osteoclast-like cells formation and osteoclastic activity. *Endocrinology* 134:1897–1904, 1994

43. Inomata N, Akiyama M, Kubota N, Jüppner H: Characterization of a novel parathyroid hormone receptor with specificty for the carboxyl-terminal region of PTH (1-84). *Endocrinology* 136:4732–4740, 1995

44. Bringhurst FR, Stern AM, Yotts M, et al.: Peripheral metabolism of parathyroid hormone: fate of the biologically active amino-terminus in vivo. *Am J Physiol* 255:E866–E893, 1988

45. Bringhurst FR, Stern AM, Yotts M, et al.: Peripheral metabolism of [^{35}S] parathyroid hormone in vivo: influence of alterations in calcium availability and parathyroid status. *J Endocrinol* 122:237–245, 1989

11. Parathyroid Hormone: Mechanism of Action

Henry M. Kronenberg, M.D.

Harvard Medical School; and Endocrine Unit, Department of Medicine, Massachusetts General Hospital, Boston, Massachusetts

Parathyroid hormone (PTH) regulates the levels of calcium and phosphate in blood by modulating the activity of specific cells in bone and kidney. These actions serve to (i) stimulate release of calcium and phosphate from bone, (ii) stimulate reabsorption of calcium and inhibit reabsorption of phosphate from glomerular filtrate, and (iii) stimulate the renal synthesis of 1,25-dihydroxyvitamin D [1,25(OH)$_2$D], thereby increasing intestinal absorption of calcium and phosphate. The net result of these actions is to raise the level of blood calcium and lower the level of blood phosphate. Blood calcium, in turn, is the major regulator of PTH secretion; a rise in blood calcium decreases PTH secretion. The mutual regulatory interactions of PTH and calcium serve to keep the blood level of calcium constant, despite moderate fluctuations in diet, bone metabolism, and renal function. In this chapter, I shall first detail the physiologic actions of PTH and then examine the cellular and subcellular mechanisms responsible for those actions.

Parathyroid hormone has complex and still poorly understood actions on bone. Administration of PTH leads to release of calcium from a rapidly turning-over pool of calcium near the surface of bone; after several hours, calcium is also released from an additional pool that turns over more slowly (1). Chronic administration of PTH (or increased secretion of PTH associated with primary hyperparathyroidism) leads to an increase in osteoclast cell number and activity (2). The release of calcium is accompanied by the release of phosphate and matrix components, such as collagen. Paradoxically, at low intermittent doses, PTH administration leads to the deposition of increased amounts of trabecular bone (3). The physiologic role of this anabolic action of PTH is uncertain.

Even though PTH causes a release of phosphate from bone, PTH administration leads to a fall in the blood level of phosphate because of the phosphaturia caused by PTH. This phosphaturia reinforces the effect of PTH on bone, because low levels of blood phosphate independently lead to resorption of bone (4). The normal dominance of the renal phosphaturic effect of PTH is well illustrated by the effect of PTH on blood phosphate in severe renal failure. In that setting, where PTH can effect little change in renal phosphate handling, the effects of PTH on bone dominate, and parathyroidectomy leads to a fall in blood phosphate (5,6).

Phosphate is normally reabsorbed from glomerular filtrate both in the proximal and distal tubules. Reabsorption at both these sites is inhibited by PTH (7). Parathyroid hormone administration leads to a decrease in calcium reabsorption in the proximal tubule as well, but the net effect of PTH on the kidney is to increase calcium reabsorption because of the effects of PTH on distal tubular sites (7). This increased reabsorption of calcium synergizes with PTH-induced bone resorption to increase the blood level of calcium.

Even though the PTH-stimulated kidney more efficiently reabsorbs calcium, the absolute amount of calcium in the urine usually increases when PTH blood levels are high. This increase in urine calcium is caused by the substantial increase in the filtered load of calcium resulting from increased bone resorption and increased intestinal absorption of calcium (see later).

Parathyroid hormone and vitamin D interact in a number of complex ways. In the kidney, PTH activates 25-hydroxyvitamin D 1-hydroxylase (8). This enzyme in the proximal tubule catalyzes the synthesis of the most active metabolite of vitamin D, 1,25(OH)$_2$D$_3$, which, in turn, is a potent inducer of intestinal calcium absorption. Calcium absorption can increase from 10% to 70% in response to 1,25(OH)$_2$D$_3$; this effect synergizes with the effect of PTH on bone and kidney to raise blood calcium. In the absence of vitamin D metabolites, bone is poorly mineralized. PTH cannot mobilize calcium efficiently from this poorly mineralized bone. At high levels, in contrast, 1,25(OH)$_2$D$_3$ causes bone resorption directly, without requiring PTH.

The important role of 1,25(OH)$_2$D$_3$ in partially mediating the effect of PTH on blood calcium has led to its widespread use, along with oral calcium, to treat hypoparathyroidism. Because 1,25(OH)$_2$D$_3$ cannot mimic the renal effects of PTH, however, urine calcium rises quickly when hypoparathyroid patients are treated with 1,25(OH)$_2$D$_3$. The blood calcium is best kept in the low normal range in such patients, in order to avoid the consequences of hypercalciuria.

CELLULAR ACTIONS OF PTH

Although the most obvious histologic consequence of PTH action on bone is an increase in osteoclast number and activity, osteoclasts paradoxically express no PTH receptors on their plasma membranes, and PTH has no direct effects on isolated osteoclasts (9). Instead, PTH receptors are found on bone-forming osteoblasts. When isolated osteoblasts are treated with PTH, they secrete a factor or factors that, in turn, stimulate osteoclasts to resorb bone. This functional linkage of osteoblasts and osteoclasts may partly explain the increase in osteoblast activity that accompanies the increased osteoclast activity in hyperparathyroidism. The increase in osteoclast cell number caused by PTH has been studied in a tissue culture system designed to analyze the development of differentiated osteoclasts from mononuclear progenitor cells that originate in the bone marrow (2). In this *in vitro* system, PTH stimulates the final steps in the differentiation of cells committed to the osteoclast pathway. Whether this effect of PTH is mediated indirectly by osteoblasts, or instead is a direct effect of PTH on pre-osteoclasts, has not been established.

The kidney responds to PTH without the dramatic changes in cellular composition found in bone. Instead, the activities of specific individual tubular cells are simulated. In the best-studied proximal tubule cell, phosphate is transported into the cell against an electrochemical gradient. The ATP used to accomplish this task does so indirectly: ATP fuels the sodium pump, which drives sodium from the cell. Sodium then travels back into the cell in response to the concentration gradient established by the sodium pump. Phosphate transport is coupled to the entry of sodium back into the cell through the action of a membrane co-transporter (10). Parathyroid hormone blocks this sodium-dependent phosphate co-transport. In the distal tubule, presumably PTH has a similar effect on phosphate transport. Also in the distal tubule, PTH stimulates calcium absorption against an electrochemical gradient. After PTH is administered *in vivo*, the Vmax of the sodium–calcium exchanger in subsequently isolated basolateral membrane vesicles is increased (11). The 1-hydroxylase responsible for hydroxylating 25-hydroxyvitamin D is located in mitochondria in proximal tubular cells and is activated both by PTH and low blood levels of phosphate.

INITIAL ACTIONS OF PTH

Intact PTH does not act directly in the cytoplasm of its target cells in kidney and bone. Instead, it binds to specific receptors on the surface of target cells; this binding triggers the release of cytoplasmic "second messengers" that then mediate the multiple distant effects of PTH. Binding of PTH to its receptors requires only the first 34 residues of the PTH molecule, which contains 84 amino acids. The function of the carboxyl portion of the molecule is unknown. The recently discovered factor, PTH-related protein (PTHrP), made by certain tumors that causes humorally mediated hypercalcemia resembles PTH in its first 13 residues (12). Peptide fragments of this protein bind to PTH receptors in bone and kidney (13); this action probably explains many of the activities of the protein and the similarities between hyperparathyroidism and the humoral hypercalcemia of malignancy (see Chapters 12, 32).

The number of PTH receptors on cells is regulated; this regulation probably modulates the effects of PTH on target cells. Prolonged exposure of cultured cells to PTH leads to a dramatic decrease in the number of receptors on the surface of such cells. This action may partly explain the decreased sensitivity to PTH of experimental animals after prolonged exposure to PTH (14).

The best-characterized mediator of PTH's action is cyclic adenosine monophosphate (cAMP). Exposure of bone or kidney cells to PTH results in a rapid intracellular accumulation of cAMP and an outpouring of cAMP into the urine (15). The rise in urinary cAMP occurs only in response to PTH and to the PTH-like factor associated with the humoral hypercalcemia of malignancy. Although an elevation in urinary cAMP cannot be used to distinguish hyperparathyroidism from malignant hypercalcemia, the measurement of renal cAMP generation has provided a useful bioassay of PTH action in clinical investigation.

Administration of analogs of cAMP can mimic many of the effects of PTH. The rapid elevation of cAMP in response to PTH and the actions of cAMP strongly suggest that cAMP mediates the effects of PTH. Binding of PTH to its receptor on the external surface of the cell triggers the release of guanosine diphosphate (GDP) from an intracellular protein called Gs and permits the binding of intracellular guanosine triphosphate (GTP) to Gs. GTP-Gs then stimulates membrane-bound adenylate cyclase. The cAMP produced by adenylate cyclase then binds to the regulatory subunit of cAMP-dependent protein kinase A. This binding causes the regulatory subunit to dissociate from the catalytic subunit of protein kinase. The free catalytic subunit then phosphorylates specific serines and threonines in target proteins. The relevant target proteins and their precise modes of action remain uncharacterized, although proteins that activate genes responsive to cAMP and ion channel proteins are strong candidates.

The human disease pseudohypoparathyroidism (Chapter 38) provides evidence for the physiologic relevance of the mechanism of PTH action outlined previously, and it also raises intriguing problems. Patients with pseudohypoparathyroidism are unresponsive to PTH: although PTH levels in their blood are high, they are hypocalcemic and hyperphosphatemic. Urinary cAMP does not rise in response to administration of exogenous PTH, a key diagnostic finding. Most of these patients have only 50% of the expected amount of Gs in membranes from a variety of accessible cells (16). This loss of Gs may well cause the unresponsiveness to PTH. Why loss of half of the normal amount of Gs leads to complete unresponsiveness to PTH is not understood. Further, the similar loss of half the normal amount of Gs in patients with pseudo-pseudohypoparathyroidism, who exhibit normal responsiveness to PTH, remains unexplained (17). Although the explanation of pseudohypoparathyroidism thus remains incomplete, what we already know strongly supports the role of cAMP in mediating PTH's effects. Further, bone cells engineered to contain a protein kinase unresponsive to cAMP have blunted responses to PTH (18). Thus, multiple types of evidence support the model that PTH action is mediated at least in part by cAMP.

Reality may be more complicated than this straightforward model, however. PTH stimulates phosphotidylinositol turnover in cultured cell lines (19), causes a rapid rise in levels of free cytosolic calcium (20), and causes a shift of protein kinase C to the cell membrane (21). These effects are different from the actions of cAMP analogs and suggest that multiple second messengers may mediate some actions of PTH. The physiologic importance of metabolites of phosphotidylinositol and intracellular calcium as PTH-induced second messengers has not yet been established.

This brief summary illustrates the recently delineated complexities associated with PTH action. Parathyroid hormone acts on several different tissues, sometimes with apparently paradoxical actions. For example, when administered continuously to animals, PTH causes net bone resorption; yet when it is administered by once-daily injection, PTH can cause net bone formation. Further, PTH acts through more than one second messenger system. Most intriguingly, both PTH and PTHrP, the mediator of the humoral hypercalcemia of malignancy, bind to the same receptor. How can the same receptor mediate the carefully regulated calcium homeostatic functions of PTH and, at the same time, mediate actions of PTHrP, a peptide that has no obvious involvement in feedback-regulated, normal calcium homeostasis?

The recent cloning of DNA encoding rat, opossum, and human PTH/PTHrP receptors has begun to clarify the mechanisms involved in the PTH signaling system (22,23). The DNA sequence encoding the receptor predicts that the receptor is a member of the large family of receptors that span the plasma membrane seven times and work by activating G proteins on the inner surface of the membrane. The PTH/PTHrP receptor belongs to a newly appreciated subfamily of that large family. Members of this new subfamily, which includes receptors for calcitonin and secretin, closely resemble each other in their primary sequences and in several functional properties, but they bear only a distant relationship to other members of the family. Precisely the same receptor is found in bone and kidney, both in rats and in humans. When the cloned receptor is expressed in cultured cells that do not normally bear PTH receptors, PTH binding stimulates both adenylate cyclase and phospholipase C. Thus, this one receptor is capable of stimulating both of the known second-messenger pathways used by PTH. The receptor binds and responds to PTH and to amino-terminal fragments of PTHrP equally well. Further, messenger RNA for the receptor is found not only in traditional PTH target tissues, but also in putative PTHrP target tissues, such as early embryonic cells. This one receptor is, therefore, apparently quite versatile: it mediates actions of both PTH and PTHrP in multiple tissues and signals through more than one second-messenger pathway. Data discussed in the next chapter suggest that PTHrP may well work through more than one receptor; the number of receptors for PTH is less certain.

The recent discovery of a disease caused by point mutations in the PTH/PTHrP receptor illustrates the importance of the receptor in mediating the actions of PTH and PTHrP (24). Patients with these mutations have receptors that are always active, even in the absence of PTH or PTHrP. As a consequence, these patients have high levels of calcium, low levels of phosphate, and high levels of $1,25(OH)_2D_3$ in their blood, but they have low levels of PTH. They also have short stature, probably a result of inappropriate PTHrP-like actions on the cartilaginous growth plate.

Further analysis of the properties of the cloned PTH/PTHrP receptor and the continuing search for more receptors should lead to a greater understanding of the biochemical underpinnings of this complicated physiologic signaling network.

REFERENCES

1. Talmage RV, Elliott JR: Removal of calcium from bone as influenced by the parathyroids. *Endocrinology* 62:717–722, 1958
2. Mundy GR, Roodman GD: Osteoclast ontogeny and function. In: Peck WA (ed) *Bone and Mineral Research,* vol 5. Elsevier, Amsterdam, pp 209–280, 1987
3. Slovik DM, Rosenthal DI, Doppelt SH: Restoration of spinal bone in osteoporotic men by treatment with human parathyroid hormone (1-34) and 1,25 dihydroxyvitamin D. *J Bone Miner Res* 1:377–381, 1q986
4. Raisz LG, Niemann I: Effect of phosphate, calcium and magnesium on bone resorption and humoral responses in tissue culture. *Endocrinology* 85:446–452, 1969
5. Gill G, Pallotta J, Kashgarian M, Kessner D, Epstein FH: Physiological studies in renal osteodystrophy treated by subtotal parathyroidectomy. *Am J Med* 46:930–940, 1969
6. Neer RM: Calcium and inorganic phosphate homeostasis. In: DeGroot LJ (ed) *Endocrinology,* vol II. Grune and Stratton, New York, pp 927–954, 1989
7. Bringhurst FR: Calcium and phosphate distribution, turnover, and metabolic actions. In: DeGroot LJ (ed) *Endocrinology,* vol II. Grune and Stratton, New York, pp 805–843, 1989
8. Garabedian M, Holick MF, DeLuca HF, et al.: Control of 25-dihydroxycalciferol metabolism by the parathyroid glands. *Proc Natl Acad Sci USA* 69:1673–1676, 1972
9. McSheehy PMJ, Chambers TJ: Osteoblastic cells mediate osteoclastic responsiveness to parathyroid hormone. *Endocrinology* 118:824–828, 1986
10. Cheng L, Sacktor B: Sodium gradient-dependent phosphate transport in renal brush border vesicles. *J Biol Chem* 256:1556–1564, 1981
11. Jayakumar A, Cheung L, Liang CT, Sacktor B: Sodium-gradient-dependent calcium uptake in renal basolateral membrane vesicles. *J Biol Chem* 259:10827–10833, 1984
12. Suva LJ, Winslow GA, Wettenhall REH: A parathyroid hormone-related protein implicated in malignant hypercalcemia: Cloning and expression. *Science* 237:893–896, 1987
13. Jüppner H, Abou-Samra AB, Uneno S, Gu WX, Potts JT Jr, Segre GV: The PTH-like peptide associated with humoral hypercalcemia of malignancy and PTH bind to the same receptor on the plasma membrane of ROS 17/2.8 cells. *J Biol Chem* 263:8557–8560, 1988
14. Mahoney CA, Nissenson RA: Canine renal receptors for parathyroid hormone—Down regulation in vivo by exogenous parathyroid hormone. *J Clin Invest* 72:411–421, 1983
15. Chase LR, Aurbach GD: Parathyroid function and the renal excretion of 3′,5′-adenylic acid. *Proc Natl Acad Sci USA* 58:518–525, 1967
16. Farfel Z, Brickman AS, Kaslow HR, Brothers VM, Bourne HR: Defect in receptor-cyclase coupling protein in pseudohypoparathyroidism. *N Engl J Med* 303:237–242, 1980
17. Levine MA, Downs RW, Moses AM, et al.: Resistance to multiple hormone in patients with pseudohypoparathyroidism. *Am J Med* 74:545–556, 1983
18. Bringhurst FR, Zajac JD, Daggett AS, Skurat RN, Kronenberg HM: Inhibition of parathyroid hormone responsiveness in clonal osteoblastic cells expressing a mutant form of 3′,5′-cyclic adenosine monophosphate-dependent protein kinase. *Mol Endocrinol* 3:60–67, 1989
19. Meltzer V, Weinreb S, Bellorin-Font E, Hruska KA: Parathyroid hormone stimulation of renal phosphoinositide metabolism is a cyclic nucleotide-independent effect. *Biochem Biophys Acta* 712:258–267, 1982
20. Yamaguchi DT, Hahn TJ, Iida-Klein A, Kleeman CR, Muallem S: Parathyroid hormone-activated calcium channels in an osteoblast-like clonal osteosarcoma cell line. *J Biol Chem* 262:7711–7718, 1987
21. Abou-Samra AB, Jüppner H, Westerberg D, Potts JT Jr, Segre GV: Parathyroid hormone causes translocation of protein kinase-C activity from cytosol to membranes in rat osteosarcoma cells. *Endocrinology* 124:1107–1113, 1989
22. Jüppner H, Abou-Samra AB, Freeman M, Kong XF, Schipani E, Richards J, Kolakowski LF, Kronenberg HM, Segre GV: A G protein-linked receptor for parathyroid hormone and parathyroid hormone-related peptide. *Science* 254:1024–1026, 1991
23. Abou-Samra AB, Jüppner H, Force T, Freeman MW, Kong XF, Schipani E, Urena P, Richards J, Bonventre JV, Potts JT Jr, Kronenberg HM, Segre GV: Expression cloning of a common receptor for parathyroid hormone and parathyroid hormone-related peptide from rat osteoblast-like cells: A single receptor stimulates intracellular accumulation of both cAMP and inositol triphosphates and increases intracellular free calcium. *Proc Natl Acad Sci USA* 89:2732–3736, 1992
24. Schipani E, Kruse K, Jüppner H: A constitutively active mutant PTH-PTHrP receptor in Jansen-type metaphyseal chondrodysplasia. *Science* 268:98–100, 1995

12. Parathyroid-Hormone-Related Protein

Gordon J. Strewler, M.D., and *Robert A. Nissenson, Ph.D.

*Departments of Medicine and Endocrinology, and *Department of Physiology, University of California, San Francisco; and Veterans Affairs Medical Center, San Francisco California*

A second member of the parathyroid hormone (PTH) family, the PTH-related protein (PTHrP) has recently been discovered. Over the past 8 years, the elucidation of the structure of PTHrP and our growing understanding of its unique biologic role have changed our view of hypercalcemia and have expanded our concept of the role of the PTH/PTHrP family beyond the horizons of calcium homeostasis, to include developmental and regulatory functions in a variety of tissues (1,2).

Parathyroid-hormone-related protein was first identified as the cause of hypercalcemia in malignancy (3). The characteristics of the clinical syndrome of humoral hypercalcemia are discussed in Chapter 32. As in primary hyperparathyroidism, hypercalcemia in malignancy is characterized by a decreased renal threshold for phosphate, leading to hypophosphatemia, and by increased urinary excretion of cyclic adenosine monophosphate (cAMP) (4). Yet PTH is suppressed in malignancy-associated hypercalcemia. The finding that PTH was suppressed in a syndrome that so resembled primary hyperparathyroidism biochemically, suggested that a distinct molecule secreted by tumors could mimic PTH, and this led to the development of bioassay techniques to search for a PTH-like factor in tumors that produced hypercalcemia. These assays guided the isolation and ultimate identification of what proved to be a PTHrP (also called PTH-like protein). As predicted, the tumor-derived protein proved to be an able mimic of PTH, for reasons that became clear when its structure could be determined.

As disclosed by molecular cloning, the amino acid sequence of PTHrP is homologous with the sequence of PTH only at the amino terminus, where 8 of the first 13 amino acids in PTH and PTHrP are identical (Fig. 1). This homologous domain, limited as it is, involves a crucial region of the molecule that is known to be required for activation of the PTH receptor. Beyond this region, the sequences of PTH and PTHrP have little in common. Even in the primary receptor-binding domain (amino acids 18–34), PTH and PTHrP do not have recognizable primary sequence similarities (however, the binding domain has a common α-helical secondary structure in both peptides). Compared with the 84-amino-acid peptide PTH, PTHrP is considerably longer, with three isoforms of 139, 141, and 173 amino acids, whose sequences are identical through amino acid 139. These isoforms arise from alternative RNA splicing. Their relative secretory rates and their relative importance in normal physiology and humoral hypercalcemia are unknown, but they may give rise to a large number of peptide fragments, as discussed below.

Human PTHrP is encoded by a single-copy gene located on chromosome 12 (2). The human PTHrP gene, with three promoters, nine exons, and complex patterns of alternative exon splicing, is much more complicated than the PTH gene. Yet it is clear from the protein structure and from similarities in gene organization that both arose from a common ancestral gene.

Parathyroid-hormone-related protein and PTH bind with equivalent affinities to a common receptor (5,6), and consequently they have very similar ranges of biologic activities. Both produce hypercalcemia, hypophosphatemia as a consequence of reduced renal reabsorption of phosphate, and accelerated production of 1,25-dihydroxyvitamin D [1,25(OH)$_2$D] by the kidney (1,5). Despite the latter action, patients with PTHrP-induced hypercalcemia have considerably lower serum levels of 1,25(OH)$_2$D than are seen in primary hyperparathyroidism (4) (see Chapter 32).

There is little doubt that PTHrP is the major cause of hypercalcemia in malignancy (3). Infusion of PTHrP can reproduce most aspects of the clinical syndrome of hypercalcemia, serum levels of PTHrP are increased in hypercalcemia (7) (see Chapter 32), and neutralizing antibodies to PTHrP can reverse hypercalcemia induced in animals by human tumor cells (8). This indicates that secretion of PTHrP is not merely associated with hypercalcemia but necessary for hypercalcemia.

The specific tumors that characteristically produce humoral hypercalcemia by secreting PTHrP include squamous, renal, and breast carcinoma. Parathyroid-hormone-related protein also plays a causative role in the hypercalcemia that is associated with islet cell tumors, pheochromocytoma, and the adult T-cell leukemia syndrome, where PTHrP is produced by malignant T-lymphocytes infected with the etiologic agent of this disorder, the human T-cell lymphotrophic virus (9).

The normal circulating level of PTHrP is considerably lower than the level of PTH, and it is doubtful that PTHrP has a major role in the day-to-day maintenance of calcium

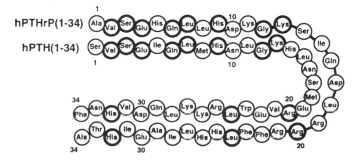

FIG. 1. Amino-terminal amino acid sequence of hPTHrP is compared with that of hPTH.

homeostasis. It is clear, however, that PTHrP has vital functions in development and in normal physiology, primarily local ones at the cell or tissue level. Parathyroid-hormone-related protein is widely present in fetal tissues, including cartilage, heart, distal renal tubules, hair follicles, placenta, and many epithelial surfaces (10,11). It has recently been possible to disrupt both copies of the PTHrP gene in the mouse by targeted mutations introduced by homologous recombination (12). Although mice heterozygous for the loss of PTHrP are phenotypically normal, in the homozygous state loss of the PTHrP gene is an embryonic lethal mutation. Homozygotes survive until near the time of parturition but have multiple anomalies in the development of cartilage and bone. From this phenotype it is apparent that PTHrP is crucial for the normal proliferation and differentiation of chondrocytes during endochondral bone formation.

Further studies of this and other models have begun to disclose other developmental effects of PTHrP as well. Parathyroid-hormone-related protein is present in the fetal placenta and parathyroid glands, and it regulates the placental calcium pump, which maintains a higher serum calcium in the fetus than in the mother (13–15). In humans, PTHrP is secreted by the amnion into the amniotic fluid, and it could thus play a role in parturition or in regulation of epithelia that are bathed in amniotic fluid (i.e, skin or gastrointestinal tract) (11).

The PTHrP gene is widely expressed in normal tissues of the adult, and it has been postulated to have a number of physiologic functions. Local production of PTHrP in developing breast tissue may regulate branching morphogenesis of mammary glands, because overexpression of the gene at this site leads to severe mammary hypoplasia (16). In lactating mammary tissue, expression of PTHrP is under the control of prolactin, and PTHrP is secreted into milk at concentrations 10,000-fold higher than its serum concentration (17). It is not clear whether these findings reflect a role for PTHrP in lactation itself, in the neonate who ingests large quantities of PTHrP in milk, or in both. PTHrP is expressed in epidermal keratinocytes (the parental cells for squamous carcinomas that characteristically secrete PTHrP as the cause of hypercalcemia), and it may be involved in differentiation of the skin and skin appendages. Forced overexpression of PTHrP in keratinocytes produces a failure of normal hair follicle development (18). The gene is also expressed in a variety of endocrine tissues, in the central nervous system (19), uterus (20), placenta (11), heart (21), and vascular smooth muscle (22) and other smooth muscle beds (22), where it is released in response to stretch (20) and serves as a muscle relaxant. Whether PTHrP serves in the short-loop feedback regulation of smooth muscle tone, as this suggests, is not yet known. However, the list of putative physiologic functions of PTHrP is already impressively long (Table 1).

The PTHrP molecule contains a number of potential processing sites, suggesting that PTHrP could function as a polyhormone precursor of a number of biologically active fragments (6). Both an amino-terminal fragment, PTHrP (1–36), and a midregion fragment beginning with amino acid 38 are generated in cells that secrete PTHrP (23), and a carboxyl-terminal fragment recognized by PTHrP (109–138) antibodies is also detectable in the circulation (7,24). (The latter could arise from peripheral, rather than cellular, processing of PTHrP.) It

TABLE 1. *Sites of expression and proposed actions of parathyroid-hormone-related protein*

Sites of expression	Proposed actions
Fetal tissues	
Cartilage	Regulation of chondrogenesis and mineralization
Parathyroid	Regulation of placental calcium transport
Placenta	Regulation of placental calcium transport
Heart, kidney, epithelia, hair follicles	Unknown
Amnion	Secreted into amniotic fluid; may regulate differentiation of epidermis/GI tract
Endocrine tissues	
Pituitary	Unknown
Pancreatic islets	Regulation of insulin secretion and somatic growth
Parathyroid	Unknown
Smooth muscle	Released in response to stretch, relaxes smooth muscle
Vascular	
Urinary bladder	
Myometrium	Regulation of parturition
Gastrointestinal	
Mammary gland	Regulation of branching morphogenesis of glands Regulation of lactation Regulation of neonatal metabolism
Skin	Regulation of hair follicle Regulation of epidermal differentiation
Central nervous system	Unknown

has been reported that the actions of PTHrP on placental calcium transport (13) and renal bicarbonate transport may be functions not of the PTH-like amino terminus, but of the midregion of the molecule. It is thus likely that PTHrP is a multifunctional molecule, like the neuropeptide pro-opiomelanocortin—the precursor not only of ACTH, but also of opiate peptides and melanocyte-stimulating hormones. To date, the only PTHrP receptor to be identified is the PTH/PTHrP receptor coupled to adenylyl cyclase, which recognizes the PTH-like amino-terminus of PTHrP. However, it is likely that some of the actions of PTHrP in "nonclassical" target tissues are initiated by binding to other PTHrP receptors that recognize determinants in the midregion or carboxyl-terminus of PTHrP (6). Our understanding of PTHrP and its distinct biologic actions is in its infancy.

REFERENCES

1. Halloran BP, Nissenson RA: *Parathyroid Hormone-Related Protein: Normal Physiology and Its Role in Cancer.* CRC Press, Boca Raton, FL, 1992

2. Broadus A, Stewart A: Parathyroid hormone-related protein: structure, processing, and physiological actions. In: Bilezikian J, Levine M, Marcus R (eds) *The Parathyroids.* Raven Press, New York, p. 259, 1994

3. Wysolmerski JJ, Broadus AE: Hypercalcemia of malignancy—the central role of parathyroid hormone-related protein. *Annu Rev Med* 45:189–200, 1994

4. Stewart AF, Horst R, Deftos LJ, Cadman EC, Lang R, Broadus AE: Biochemical evaluation of patients with cancer-associated hypercalcemia. *N Engl J Med* 303:1377–1383, 1980

5. Orloff JJ, Wu TL, Stewart AF: Parathyroid hormone-like proteins: Biochemical responses and receptor interactions. *Endocr Rev* 10:476–495, 1989

6. Orloff JJ, Reddy D, de Papp AE, Yang KH, Soifer NE, Stewart AF: Parathyroid hormone-related protein as a prohormone: Posttranslational processing and receptor interactions. *Endocr Rev* 15:40–60, 1994

7. Burtis WJ, Brady TG, Orloff JJ, Ersbak JB, Warrell RP Jr, Olson BR, Wu TL, Mitnick ME, Broadus AE, Stewart AF: Immunochemical characterization of circulating parathyroid hormone-related protein in patients with humoral hypercalcemia of cancer. *N Engl J Med* 322:1106–1112, 1990

8. Kukreja SC, Shevrin DH, Wimbiscus SA, Ebeling PR, Danks JA, Rodda CP, Wood WI, Martin TJ: Antibodies to parathyroid hormone-related protein lower serum calcium in athymic mouse models of malignancyassociated hypercalcemia due to human tumors. *J Clin Invest* 82:1798–1802, 1988

9. Ikeda K, Ohno H, Hane M, Yokoi H, Okada M, Honma T, Yamada A, Tatsumi Y, Tanaka T, Saitoh T, Hirose S, Mori S, Takeuchi Y, Fukumoto S, Terukina S, Iguchi H, Kiriyama T, Ogata E, Matsumoto T: Development of a sensitive two-site immunoradiometric assay for parathyroid hormone-related peptide: Evidence for elevated levels in plasma from patients with adult T-cell leukemia/lymphoma and B-cell lymphoma. *J Clin Endocrinol Metab* 79:1322–1327, 1994

10. Moseley JM, Hayman JA, Danks JA, Alcorn D, Grill V, Southby J, Horton MA: Immunohistochemical detection of parathyroid hormone-related protein in human fetal epithelia. *J Clin Endocrinol Metab* 73:478–484, 1991

11. Ferguson JE 2d, Gorman JV, Bruns DE, Weir EC, Burtis WJ, Martin TJ, Bruns ME: Abundant expression of parathyroid hormone-related protein in human amnion and its association with labor. *Proc Natl Acad Sci USA* 89:8384–8388, 1992

12. Karaplis AC, Luz A, Glowacki J, Bronson RT, Tybulewicz VLJ, Kronenberg HM, Mulligan RC: Lethal skeletal dysplasia from targeted disruption of the parathyroid hormone-related peptide gene. *Genes Dev* 8:277–289, 1994

13. Care AD, Abbas SK, Pickard DW, Barri M, Drinkhill M, Findlay JB, White IR, Caple IW: Stimulation of ovine placental transport of calcium and magnesium by mid-molecule fragments of human parathyroid hormone-related protein. *Exp Physiol* 75:605–608, 1990

14. Abbas SK, Pickard DW, Rodda CP, Heath JA, Hammonds RG, Wood WI, Caple IW, Martin TJ, Care AD: Stimulation of ovine placental calcium transport by purified natural and recombinant parathyroid hormone-related protein (PTHrP) preparations. *Q J Exp Physiol* 74:549–552, 1989

15. Kovacs CS, Lanske B, Karapllis A, Kronenberg HM: PTHrP-knockout mice have reduced ionized calcium, fetal-maternal calcium gradient and 45-calcium transport in utero (Abstr). *J Bone Miner Res* 10(suppl 1):S157, 1995

16. Wysolmerski JJ, McCaughern-Carucci JF, Daifotis AG, Broadus AE, Philbrick WM: Overexpression of parathyroid hormone-related protein or parathyroid hormone in transgenic mice impairs branching morphogenesis during mammary gland development. *Development* 121:3539–3547, 1995

17. Budayr AA, Halloran BP, King JC, Diep D, Nissenson RA, Strewler GJ: High levels of a parathyroid hormone-like protein in milk. *Proc Natl Acad Sci USA* 86:7183–7185, 1989

18. Wysolmerski JJ, Broadus AE, Zhou J, Fuchs E, Milstone LM, Philbrick WM: Overexpression of parathyroid hormone-related protein in the skin of transgenic mice interferes with hair follicle development. *Proc Natl Acad Sci USA* 91:1133–1137, 1994

19. Weir EC, Brines ML, Ikeda K, Burtis WJ, Broadus AE, Robbins RJ: Parathyroid hormone-related peptide gene is expressed in the mammalian central nervous system. *Proc Natl Acad Sci USA* 87:108–112, 1990

20. Thiede MA, Daifotis AG, Weir EC, Brines ML, Burtis WJ, Ikeda K, Dreyer BE, Garfield RE, Broadus AE: Intrauterine occupancy controls expression of the parathyroid hormone-related peptide gene in preterm rat myometrium. *Proc Natl Acad Sci USA* 87:108, 1990

21. Deftos LJ, Burton DW, Brandt DW: Parathyroid hormone-like protein is a secretory product of atrial myocytes. *J Clin Invest* 92:727–735, 1993

22. Hongo T, Kupfer J, Enomoto H, Sharifi B, Giannella-Neto D, Forrester JS, Singer FR, Goltzman D, Hendy GN, Pirola C, et al.: Abundant expression of parathyroid hormone-related protein in primary rat aortic smooth muscle cells accompanies serum-induced proliferation. *J Clin Invest* 88:1841–1847, 1991

23. Soifer NE, Dee KE, Insogna KL, Burtis WJ, Matovcik LM, Wu TL, Milstone LM, Broadus AE, Philbrick WM, Stewart AF: Parathyroid hormone-related protein. Evidence for secretion of a novel mid-region fragment by three different cell types. *J Biol Chem* 267:18236–18243, 1992

24. Orloff JJ, Soifer NE, Fodero JP, Dann P, Burtis WJ: Accumulation of carboxy-terminal fragments of parathyroid hormone-related protein in renal failure. *Kidney Int* 43:1371–1376, 1993

13. Vitamin D: Photobiology, Metabolism, Mechanism of Action, and Clinical Applications

Michael F. Holick, M.D., Ph.D.

Department of Medicine, Section of Endocrinology, Diabetes and Metabolism, Boston University School of Medicine and Medical Center, and Boston City Hospital, Boston, Massachusetts

Vitamin D is a secosteroid that is made in the skin by the action of sunlight (1). Vitamin D is biologically inert and must undergo two successive hydroxylations in the liver and kidney to become the biologically active 1,25-dihydroxyvitamin D (1,25(OH)$_2$D) (1–3). The main biologic effect of 1,25(OH)$_2$D is to maintain the serum calcium level within the normal range. This is accomplished by increasing the efficiency of intestinal absorption of dietary calcium and by recruiting stem cells in the bone to become mature osteoclasts which, in turn, mobilize calcium stores from the bone into the circulation. The renal production of 1,25(OH)$_2$D is tightly regulated by serum calcium levels through the action of parathyroid hormone (PTH) and phosphorus. There are a wide variety of inborn and acquired disorders in the metabolism of vitamin D that can lead to both hypo- and hypercalcemic conditions. Recently, it has been appreciated that 1,25(OH)$_2$D not only regulates calcium metabolism but also is capable of inhibiting the proliferation and inducing terminal differentiation of a variety of cells not associated with calcium metabolism (1). This unique property of 1,25(OH)$_2$D has been effectively used to develop a new generation of active vitamin D compounds for the treatment of the hyperproliferative skin disease psoriasis.

PHOTOBIOLOGY OF VITAMIN D$_3$

The skin is the organ responsible for the production of vitamin D$_3$. During exposure to sunlight, 7-dehydrocholesterol (7-DHC, provitamin D$_3$), the immediate precursor of cholesterol, absorbs solar radiation with energies between 290 and 315 nm [ultraviolet B (UVB)], which, in turn, causes the transformation of 7-DHC to previtamin D$_3$ (Fig. 1) (4). Once formed, previtamin D$_3$ undergoes a thermally induced isomerization over a period of a few hours and is transformed into vitamin D$_3$. Vitamin D$_3$ is translocated from the skin into the circulation, where it is bound to the vitamin-D-binding protein (4).

There are no documented cases of vitamin intoxication resulting from excessive exposure to sunlight. The likely reason for this is that once previtamin D$_3$ is formed, it absorbs solar UVB radiation and is transformed into biologically inert photoproducts, lumisterol and tachysterol. Furthermore, vitamin D$_3$ that is made in the skin is exquisitely sensitive to sunlight and is photoisomerized to suprasterol 1, suprasterol 2, and 5,6-trans-vitamin D$_3$ (Fig. 1) (4).

There are a variety of factors that can alter the cutaneous production of vitamin D$_3$. Melanin is an excellent natural sunscreen and competes with 7-DHC for UVB photons.

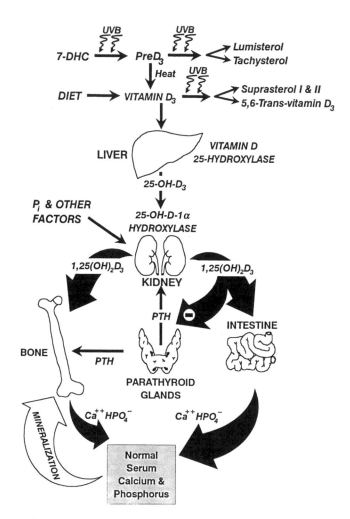

FIG. 1. Photosynthesis of vitamin D$_3$ and the metabolism of vitamin D$_3$ to 25(OH)D$_3$ and 1,25(OH)$_2$D$_3$. Once formed, 1,25(OH)$_2$D$_3$ carries out the biologic functions of vitamin D$_3$ on the intestine and bone. Parathyroid hormone (PTH) promotes the synthesis of 1,25(OH)$_2$D$_3$, which, in turn, stimulates intestinal calcium transport and bone calcium mobilization, and regulates the synthesis of PTH by negative feedback.

Therefore, increased skin melanin pigmentation decreases the photosynthesis of vitamin D$_3$ (1). People with darker skin color require longer exposure to sunlight to make the same amount of vitamin D$_3$ as those with lighter skin color (4). Aging significantly diminishes the concentration of unesterified 7-DHC in the epidermis. This results in a marked reduction in the production of vitamin D_3. Compared with a young adult, a person over the age of 70 years produces less than 30% of the amount of vitamin D_3 when exposed to the same amount of simulated sunlight (Fig. 2) (5). Latitude, time of day, and season of the year can dramatically affect the production of vitamin D_3 in the skin. At a latitude of 42°N (Boston), sunlight is incapable of producing vitamin D_3 in the skin between the months of November through February. At 52°N (Edmonton, Canada), this period is extended to include the months of October through March (4). Casual exposure to sunlight provides most of our vitamin D requirement. For children and young adults, the cutaneous production of vitamin D_3 during the spring, summer, and fall is adequate to produce enough that can be stored in the fat for use during the winter months. However, since the elderly may not make enough vitamin D_3 and therefore would have insufficient stores for winter use, the inability of the sun to produce vitamin D_3 in northern and southern latitudes during the winter may require them to take a vitamin D supplement to prevent vitamin D deficiency. Exposure to sunlight at lower latitudes, such as Los Angeles, (24°N), Puerto Rico (18°N), and Buenos Aires (34°S), results in the cutaneous production of vitamin D_3 during the entire year (4). During the summer months in Boston, exposure to sunlight from the hours of 700 to 1700 Eastern Daylight Savings Time (EDT) contains sufficient UVB radiation to produce vitamin D_3 in the skin. In the spring and fall months, vitamin D_3 production commences at ~900 and ceases after 1500 EDT. The topical use of a sunscreen with a sun protection factor of 8 will substantially reduce, by greater than 95%, the cutaneous production of vitamin D_3 (4). Chronic use of sunscreens can result in vitamin D insufficiency (4). Although sunscreen use is extremely valuable for the prevention of skin cancer and the damaging effects of excessive exposure to the sun, the elderly who depend on sunlight for their vitamin D_3 should consider exposure to suberythemal amounts of sunlight before topically applying a sunscreen.

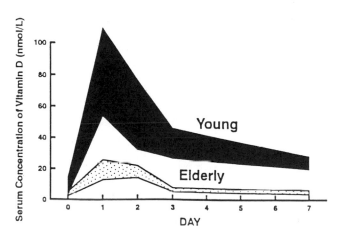

FIG. 2. Circulating concentrations of vitamin D in response to a whole-body exposure to one minimal erythemal dose in healthy young and elderly subjects. (Adapted from: Holick MF, Matsuoka LY, Wortsman J. Age, vitamin D, and solar ultraviolet radiation. *Lancet* 4:1104–1105, 1989.)

Thus, they can take advantage of the beneficial effect of sunlight while preventing the damaging effects of chronic excessive exposure to sunlight.

FOOD SOURCES OF VITAMIN D AND THE RDA

Vitamin D (either vitamin D_2 or vitamin D_3) is rare in foods. The major natural sources of vitamin D are fatty fish, such as salmon and mackerel, and fatty fish oils, including cod liver oil. Vitamin D can also be obtained from foods fortified with vitamin D, including some cereals, bread products, and milk. Other dairy products, including ice cream, yogurt, and cheese, are not fortified with vitamin D. A recent survey of the vitamin D content in milk throughout the United States and Canada, however, revealed that approximately 80% of the samples did not contain between 400 (10 mg) and 500 IU/qt (6). Almost 50% of the milk samples did not contain within 50% of the amount of vitamin D stated on the label, and approximately 15% of skim milk samples contained no detectable vitamin D. Multivitamin preparations containing vitamin D were found to contain between 400 and 600 IU of vitamin D, and pharmaceutical preparations labeled as 50,000 IU of vitamin D_2 contained the stated amount ±10%. The recommended daily allowances (RDA) for vitamin D for infants (birth to 6 months), children older than 6 months of age, and adults over 24 years of age are 300 IU, 400 IU, and 200 IU, respectively. For pregnant and lactating women of all ages, the RDA is 400 IU. There is mounting evidence that in the absence of sunlight, the RDA for vitamin D in adults is between 600 and 800 IU (4,7,8).

METABOLISM OF VITAMIN D

Vitamin D_2, which comes from yeasts and plants, and vitamin D_3, which is found in the fatty fish and cod liver oil and is made in the skin, have the same biologic potency in humans. The only difference between vitamin D_2 and vitamin D_3 is that vitamin D_2 contains a double bond between C_{22} and C_{23}, and a methyl group on C_{24} (Fig. 3) (1). Once either vitamin D_2 or vitamin D_3 enters the circulation, it is bound to the vitamin-D-binding protein and transported to the liver, where the cytochrome P_{450}-vitamin D-25-hydroxylase introduces an OH on carbon 25 to produce 25-hydroxyvitamin D [25(OH)D] (Fig. 3) (1–4). 25(OH)D enters the circulation and is the major circulating form of vitamin D. Because the hepatic vitamin D-25-hydroxylase is not tightly regulated, an increase in the cutaneous production of vitamin D_3 or ingestion of vitamin D will result in an increase in circulating levels of 25(OH)D (1,3). Therefore, its measurement is used to determine whether a patient is vitamin D deficient, vitamin D sufficient, or vitamin D intoxicated (1).

25(OH)D is biologically inert. It is transported to the kidney where the cytochrome P_{450}-mono-oxygenase, 25(OH)D-1α-hydroxylase, metabolizes 25(OH)D to 1,25-dihydroxyvitamin D [1,25(OH)$_2$D] (Fig. 3) (1–3). Although the kidney is the major source of the circulating 1,25(OH)$_2$D, there is strong evidence that a wide variety of cells, including

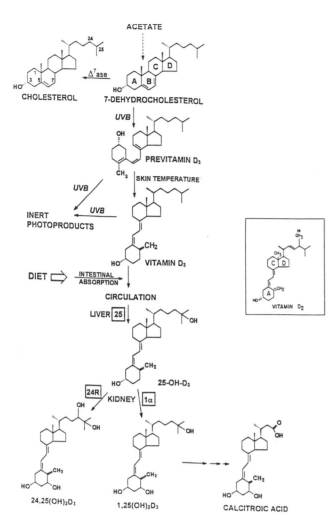

FIG. 3. The photochemical, thermal, and metabolic pathways for vitamin D$_3$. *Boxed letters* and *numbers* denote specific enzymes: Δ^7ase, 7-dehydrocholesterol reductase; 25, vitamin D-25-hydroxylase; 1α, 25(OH)D-1α-hydroxylase; 24R, 25(OH)D-24R-hydroxylase. **Inset:** the structure of vitamin D$_2$.

lating concentrations of 1,25(OH)$_2$D, respectively (12). A variety of other hormones associated with growth and development of the skeleton or calcium regulation including growth hormone and prolactin indirectly increase the renal production of 1,25(OH)$_2$D (1). Aged osteoporotic patients may lose their ability to up-regulate the renal production of 1,25(OH)$_2$D by PTH (Fig. 4) (13,14). This may help explain the age-related decrease in the efficiency of intestinal calcium absorption (13,14).

1,25(OH)$_2$D is metabolized in its target tissues (the intestine and bone) as well as in the liver and kidney (1–3). It undergoes several hydroxylations in the sidechain, resulting in the cleavage of the sidechain between carbons 23 and 24, resulting in the biologically inert, water-soluble acid, calcitroic acid (Fig. 3) (1,2). Both 25(OH)D and 1,25(OH)$_2$D undergo a 24-hydroxylation to form 24,25-dihydroxyvitamin D (24,25(OH)$_2$D) and 1,24,25-trihydroxyvitamin D, respectively. These metabolites are considered to be biologically inert and are the first step in the biodegradation. Although more than 40 different metabolites of vitamin D have been identified, only 1,25(OH)$_2$D is believed to be important for most if not all of the biologic actions of vitamin D on calcium and bone metabolism (1,3).

MOLECULAR BIOLOGY OF VITAMIN D

Once vitamin D is dihydroxylated, it becomes more hydrophilic. However, this hormone is still very lipid soluble, and therefore it acts like a steroid hormone. The mechanism of action of this hormone is similar to that of estrogen and other steroids. All target tissues for vitamin D contain a nuclear vitamin D receptor (VDR) for 1,25(OH)$_2$D. This vitamin D receptor has a 1000-fold higher affinity for 1,25(OH)$_2$D, compared to 25(OH)D and other dihydroxylated metabolites of vitamin D (1,3). Analogous to other steroid hormones, the free 1,25(OH)$_2$D in the circulation enters its target cell, where it is recognized by its nuclear receptor (Fig. 5). The exact sequence by which 1,25(OH)$_2$D interacts with its receptor and causes activation of transcription of specific genes whose products are involved in the stimulation of biologic responses to vitamin D has not been completely clarified (Fig. 5). However, it is known that the VDR must complex with a retinoic acid X receptor (RXR) to form a heterodimeric complex with 1,25(OH)$_2$D$_3$ (15). Once formed, this heterodimer complex interacts with a specific vitamin-D-responsive element within the DNA. The DNA binding motif for VDR, which is present in the N-terminus part of the molecule containing the zinc fingers (Fig. 6), interacts with the vitamin-D-responsive element (VDRE), which is composed of two tandemly repeated hexanucleotide sequences separated by three base pairs (Fig. 5). This interaction leads to the transcription of the gene and the synthesis of new mRNAs for a variety of proteins (1) (Fig. 5). The best-characterized proteins identified to date from osteoblasts are osteocalcin, osteopontin, and alkaline phosphatase, and, from the intestine, calcium-binding protein (CaBP) (1,3,16,17).

The VDR gene has nine exons that give rise to the VDR, which contains a DNA-binding domain in the N-terminal

bone and skin cells, have the ability to produce 1,25(OH)$_2$D (1,9). In addition, during pregnancy, the placenta produces 1,25(OH)$_2$D (1,10). However, because anephric patients have very low or undetectable levels of 1,25(OH)$_2$D in their blood, the extrarenal sites of 1,25(OH)$_2$D production do not appear to play a role in calcium homeostasis. The local production of 1,25(OH)$_2$D in tissues not associated with calcium homeostasis may be for the purpose of regulating cell growth (1,2,9,11).

When serum ionized calcium declines, there is an increase in the production and secretion of PTH, which has a variety of biologic functions on calcium metabolism (see Chapters 8,9,11). It also regulates calcium homeostasis by enhancing the renal conversion of 25-OH-D to 1,25(OH)$_2$D (Fig.1)(1-3). It does this indirectly through its renal wasting of phosphorus resulting in decreased intracellular and blood levels of phosphorus. Hypophosphatemia and hyperphosphatemia are associated with increased and decreased circu-

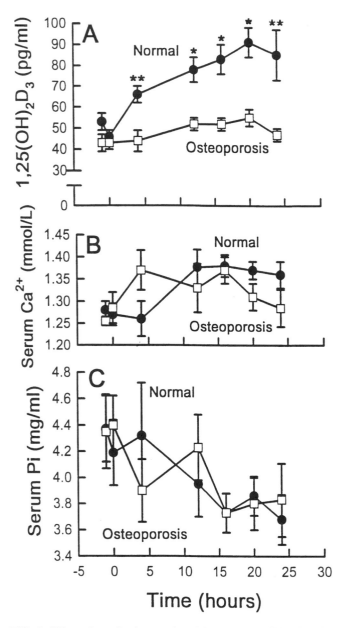

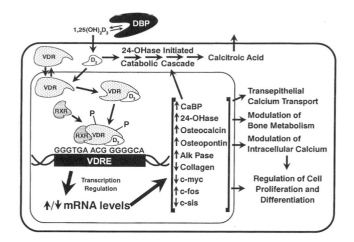

FIG. 5. Proposed mechanism of action of $1,25(OH)_2D_3$ in target cells resulting in a variety of biologic responses. The free form of $1,25(OH)_2D_3$ (D_3) enters the target cell and interacts with its nuclear vitamin D receptor (VDR), which is phosphorylated (P). The $1,25(OH)_2D_3$–VDR complex combines with the retinoic acid X receptor (RXR) to form a heterodimer, which, in turn, interacts with the vitamin-D-responsive element (VDRE) causing an enhancement or inhibition of transcription of vitamin D responsive genes such as the 25(OH)D-24-hydroxylase (24-OHase).

FIG. 4. Effect of synthetic parathyroid hormone [hPTH-(1-34)] on levels of $1,25(OH)_2D$ in normal subjects ● and patients with untreated osteoporosis (□)**(A)**. All values are expressed as the mean ±SEM. The *single asterisk* denotes significant differences at $p < 0.01$, and the *double asterisk* at $p < 0.05$, between the level in the patients and that in the controls at corresponding timepoints. *Asterisks* also refer to significant differences between the preinfusion baseline levels and the levels at particular timepoints. Effect of hPTH-(1-34) on serum levels of ionized calcium (Ca^{2+}) **(B)**, and of inorganic phosphate (P_i) **(C)** in normal subjects (●) and patients with osteoporosis (□). All values are expressed as mean ±SEM. There was no significant difference between the levels in the two groups. (Reproduced and modified with permission from: Slovik DM, Adams JS, Neer RM, Holick MF, Potts JT. Deficient production of 1,25-dihydroxyvitamin D in elderly osteoporotic patients. *N Engl J Med* 305:372–374, 1981.)

region and a hormone-binding domain in the C-terminal region (Fig. 6). Specific exon mutations have been identified that cause resistance to $1,25(OH)_2D$, causing vitamin-D-dependent rickets type II (18). There are also mutations in the exons and introns that can lead to polymorphisms of the VDR gene that do not cause any alteration in the amino acid composition of the VDR. These polymorphisms are thought to be important in the transcription of the VDR gene and/or stabilization of the resultant VDR mRNA (19). There is

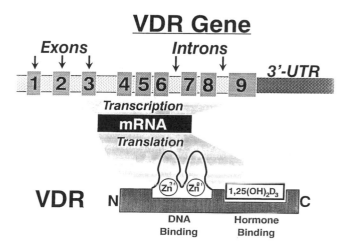

FIG. 6. Structure of the vitamin-D-receptor (VDR) gene showing the nine exons and intervening introns and the 3'-untranslated region (3'-UTR). The nine exons are transcribed into the VDR mRNA, which, in turn, is translated into the VDR that contains a DNA- and a hormone-binding domain.

some evidence that these polymorphisms may lead to a differential responsiveness to 1,25(OH)$_2$D$_3$ in the intestine and bone, thereby playing a role in peak bone mass and the development of osteoporosis (19). Although several studies have supported the concept that homozygotes for bb, TT VDR genotypes have a higher bone mineral density at various sites, other studies have not found the association (20).

BIOLOGIC FUNCTION OF VITAMIN D IN THE INTESTINE

The major biologic function of vitamin D is to maintain calcium homeostasis by increasing the efficiency of the small intestine to absorb dietary calcium (see Fig. 1). Specific nuclear receptors for 1,25(OH)$_2$D (VDR) are found in nuclei throughout the small intestine, with the highest concentration in the duodenum. 1,25(OH)$_2$D directly affects the entry of calcium through the plasma membrane into the intestinal absorptive cell, enhances the movement of calcium through the cytoplasm, and transfers the calcium across the basilateral membrane into the circulation (1–3,16,17). Although the exact mechanism by which 1,25(OH)$_2$D alters the flux of calcium across the intestinal absorptive cell is not known, 1,25(OH)$_2$D increases the production and activity of several proteins in the small intestine, including the CaBP, alkaline phosphatase, low-affinity Ca ATPase, brush-border actin, calmodulin, and brush-border proteins of 80 to 90 kDa (1–3,16,17). CaBP is specifically induced by 1,25(OH)$_2$D and is thought to be one of the major proteins responsible for the alteration in the flux of calcium across the gastrointestinal mucosa. When 1,25(OH)$_2$D is given as a single intravenous dose to vitamin-D-deficient animals, it causes a biphasic response. A rapid response occurs within 2 hours and peaks by 6 hours, and another begins after 12 hours and peaks at 24 hours, implying that several mechanisms may be involved in intestinal calcium absorption (1,2,16,17). 1,25(OH)$_2$D$_3$ also increases the efficiency of the small intestine to absorb dietary phosphorus. Although both calcium and phosphorus absorption occur along the entire length of the small intestine, most of the phosphorus transport activity is located in the jejunum and ileum, whereas calcium absorption occurs principally in the duodenum (1,2).

PHYSIOLOGIC ACTIONS OF 1,25(OH)$_2$D ON BONE

The major biologic function of vitamin D on bone is to enhance the mobilization of calcium stores at a time when dietary calcium is inadequate to maintain blood calcium in the normal range (see Fig. 1). 1,25(OH)$_2$D accomplishes this by inducing monocytic stem cells in the bone marrow to differentiate into osteoclasts (1). Once the osteoclasts have matured, they lose their ability to recognize 1,25(OH)$_2$D (21). Osteoclastic activity appears to be regulated indirectly by 1,25(OH)$_2$D$_3$ through its action on osteoblasts, which produce a variety of osteoclast-sensitive cytokines and hormones. Mature osteoblasts in the bone possess nuclear receptors for 1,25(OH)$_2$D. 1,25(OH)$_2$D increases the expression of alkaline phosphatase, osteopontin, and osteo-

calcin, as well as a variety of cytokines in these cells (1). Although vitamin D has long been recognized as important for bone mineralization, there is little direct evidence that 1,25(OH)$_2$D actively participates in this process (1,2). Instead, 1,25(OH)$_2$D promotes the mineralization of osteoid laid down by osteoblasts, by maintaining the extracellular calcium and phosphorus concentrations within the normal range, which results in the deposition of calcium hydroxyapatite into the bone matrix (1,2).

BIOLOGIC FUNCTION OF 1,25(OH)$_2$D$_3$ IN NONCALCEMIC TISSUES

A wide variety of tissues and cells possess nuclear receptors for 1,25(OH)$_2$D (Table 1) (1–3,9,11). Tumor cells that possess a VDR, when exposed to 1,25(OH)$_2$D, decrease their proliferative activity and may also terminally differentiate (22). For example, cells from the promyelocytic leukemic cell line HL-60, when exposed to physiologic amounts of 1,25(OH)$_2$D$_3$, are induced to become biochemically functioning macrophages (1,23). Of great interest is that, whereas resting T- and B-lymphocytes do not possess VDR, when the cells are activated, they express a VDR and become responsive to 1,25(OH)$_2$D (24). Activated T-lymphocytes respond to 1,25(OH)$_2$D$_3$ by decreasing the production of interleukin-2. 1,25(OH)$_2$D$_3$ has also been reported to inhibit DNA synthesis and immunoglobulin production in stimulated B-lymphocytes (1). Peripheral mononuclear cells have a VDR, and, when exposed to 1,25(OH)$_2$D *in vitro,* they are induced to become macrophages. Epidermal skin cells also possess a VDR (1,4,9,11). 1,25(OH)$_2$D$_3$ inhibits

TABLE 1. *Vitamin D activity in calcemic and noncalcemic tissues*

Vitamin D receptor activity in calcemic tissues
Small intestine
Bone
Kidney
Vitamin D receptor activity in noncalcemic tissues
Pituitary
Prostate
Gonads
Thymus
Parathyroids
Pancreas
Breast
Stomach
Placenta
Epidermis
Melanocytes
Hair follicles
Dermis
Monocytes
Lymphocytes
Myocytes
Cardiac muscle

Reproduced with permission from: Holick MF. Noncalcemic actions of 1,25-dihydroxyvitamin D$_3$ and clinical applications. *Bone* 17:107S–111S, 1995.

the proliferation of cultured human keratinocytes and induces them to terminally differentiate (1,4,9). The clinical use of 1,25(OH)$_2$D$_3$ for treating hyperproliferative diseases such as breast cancer and leukemia has not yet appeared to be promising because of recurrence of disease and complications resulting from hypercalcemic activity of the vitamin D compounds (11,25). However, the potent antiproliferative activity of 1,25(OH)$_2$D$_3$ and its analog calcipotriene (Dovonex), with its attendant prodifferentiating properties, has been effectively used for the treatment of the nonmalignant hyperproliferative skin disorder psoriasis (4,26,27).

REGULATION OF PARATHYROID HORMONE SECRETION BY 1,25(OH)$_2$D$_3$

Parathyroid hormone is the principal regulator for the renal production of 1,25(OH)$_2$D (1,2). 1,25(OH)$_2$D, in turn, increases serum calcium levels through its action on the intestine and bone, which results in the decrease in synthesis and production of PTH.

In addition to its action of increasing serum ionized-calcium concentrations, 1,25(OH)$_2$D$_3$ is also recognized by the VDR that is present in chief cells in the parathyroid glands. 1,25(OH)$_2$D$_3$ decreases the expression of the PTH gene, thereby decreasing the production and secretion of PTH (28). Patients with longstanding secondary and tertiary hyperparathyroidism can develop nests of PTH-secreting cells that have little or no VDR, and, therefore, they are probably not responsive to the PTH lowering effect of 1,25(OH)$_2$D (29). Therefore, the treatment of patients with moderate and severe renal failure with 1,25(OH)$_2$D$_3$ not only maintains calcium homeostasis but also helps decrease the risk of secondary hyperparathyroidism (30).

CLINICAL APPLICATIONS

Hypocalcemic Disorders

There are a variety of hypocalcemic disorders that are directly associated with acquired and inherited disorders in the acquisition of vitamin D and its metabolism to 1,25(OH)$_2$D (1,2,31). Vitamin D deficiency can be caused by a decreased synthesis of vitamin D$_3$ in the skin resulting from (i) excessive sunscreen use, (ii) clothing of all sun-exposed areas, (iii) aging, (iv) changes in season of the year, and (v) increased latitude. Intestinal malabsorption of vitamin D associated with fat malabsorption syndromes, including Crohn's disease, sprue, Whipple's disease, and hepatic dysfunction, is recognizable by low or undetectable concentrations of circulating 25(OH)D. Dilantin and phenobarbital can alter the kinetics for the metabolism of vitamin D to 25(OH)D, requiring that such patients receive 2 to 5 times the RDA for vitamin D in order to correct this abnormality (1,31). Because the liver has such a large capacity to produce 25(OH)D, usually more than 90% of the liver has to be dysfunctional before it is incapable of making an adequate quantity of 25(OH)D. Often, the fat malabsorption associated with the liver failure is the cause for vitamin D deficiency (1,31,32). Patients with nephrotic syndrome, who

excrete more than 4 gm of protein per 24 hours, can have lower 25(OH)D because of the coexcretion of the vitamin-D-binding protein with its 25(OH)D (1,31,33).

Acquired disorders in the metabolism of 25(OH)D to 1,25(OH)$_2$D can cause hypocalcemia. Patients with chronic renal failure with a glomerular filtration rate of less than 30% of normal have decreased reserve capacity to produce 1,25(OH)$_2$D (1,3,31). Hyperphosphatemia and hypoparathyroidism will result in the decreased production of 1,25(OH)$_2$D (1,31). Oncogenic osteomalacia, a rare acquired disorder, is associated with hypocalcemia, hypophosphatemia and low levels of 1,25(OH)$_2$D (31).

There are two rare inherited hypocalcemic disorders that are caused by either a deficiency in the renal production of 1,25(OH)$_2$D (vitamin-D-dependent rickets type I) or a defect in or deficiency of the VDR (vitamin-D-dependent rickets type II, or 1,25(OH)$_2$D-resistant syndrome) (3,31,34). Although patients with X-linked hypophosphatemic rickets have low normal or normal 1,25(OH)$_2$D levels, they are considered to have a defect in the renal production of 1,25(OH)$_2$D because these levels are inappropriately low for the degree of hyposphosphatemia (31).

Hypercalcemic Disorders

Excessive ingestion of vitamin D (usually greater than that 5000 to 10,000 IU/d) for many months can cause vitamin D intoxication that is recognized by markedly elevated levels of 25(OH)D (usually >125 ng/ml), hypercalcemia, and hyperphosphatemia (1,31). Ingestion of excessive quantities of 25(OH)D$_3$, 1α(OH)D$_3$, 1,25(OH)$_2$D$_3$, dihydrotachysterol, or exuberant use of topical calcipotriene (Dovonex) for psoriasis can cause vitamin D intoxication (4,31). Because activated macrophages convert in an unregulated fashion 25(OH)D to 1,25(OH)$_2$D, chronic granulomatous diseases such as sarcoidosis and tuberculosis are often associated with increased serum levels of 1,25(OH)$_2$D, which results in hypercalciuria and hypercalcemia (1,31,35). Rarely, lymphoma associated with hypercalcemia is caused by increased production of 1,25(OH)$_2$D by lymphomatous tissue (1). Primary hyperparathyroidism and hypophosphatemia are also associated with increased renal production of 1,25(OH)$_2$D (1,12,31).

Consequences and Treatment of Vitamin D Deficiency

Vitamin D plays a critically important role in the mineralization of the skeleton at all ages. As the body depletes its stores of vitamin D because of lack of exposure to sunlight or a deficiency of vitamin D in the diet, the efficiency of intestinal calcium absorption decreases from approximately 30% to 50%, to no more than 15%. This results in a decrease in the ionized calcium concentration in the blood, which signals the calcium sensor in the parathyroid glands, resulting in an increase in the synthesis and secretion of PTH. PTH not only tries to conserve calcium by increasing renal tubular reabsorption of calcium, but it also plays an active role in mobilizing stem cells to become active calcium-resorbing osteoclasts. PTH also increases tubular excretion of phosphorus, causing hypophosphatemia. The net effect of vitamin D insufficiency and vitamin D deficiency is a normal serum calcium, elevated PTH and alkaline phosphatase, and a low or low normal serum phosphorus. The hallmark of vitamin D insufficiency and deficiency is low normal (between 10 and 20 ng/ml) and low or undetectable (<10 ng/ml) 25(OH)D, respectively, in the blood. The secondary hyperparathyroidism and low plasma calcium × phosphorus product are thought to be responsible for the increase

in unmineralized osteoid, which is the hallmark of rickets/osteomalacia. In addition, the secondary hyperparathyroidism causes increased osteoclastic activity, resulting in calcium wasting from the bone, which in turn exacerbates osteoporosis in older adults.

Vitamin D insufficiency and vitamin D deficiency are now recognized as significant causes of metabolic bone disease in older adults. It has been estimated that upwards of 40% of patients with acute hip fracture are vitamin D deficient (4). In New England during the winter, when sunlight is incapable of producing sufficient quantities of vitamin D in the skin, a marked loss of bone mineral density of the hip and spine can be detected, which can be related to a decrease in circulating levels of 25(OH)D and secondary hyperparathyroidism. During the summer, serum 25(OH)D levels increase, PTH levels decrease, and the bone density partially or completely recovers (Fig. 7) (8,36).

A multivitamin that contains 400 IU of vitamin D is an excellent source of the vitamin and will help maintain circulating concentrations of 25(OH)D. However, in the absence of sunlight, a multivitamin may not be adequate to maintain a normal vitamin D status. For patients who are vitamin D deficient, treatment once a week with 50,000 IU of vitamin D_2 for 8 weeks increases serum 25(OH)D levels from less than 15 ng/ml, to 25 to 40 ng/ml. This treatment will maintain 25(OH)D levels in the normal range for 2 to 4 months.

Casual exposure to sunlight provides most of our vitamin D requirement. The skin has a large capacity to produce vitamin D_3. For a young adult, a whole body exposure to a minimal erythemal dose of simulated sunlight is equivalent to taking a single oral dose of between 10,000 and 75,000 IU of vitamin D (4). Therefore, adults over the age of 50 years will benefit from exposure of hands, face, and arms to suberythemal doses of sunlight. For example, in Boston, 5 to 15 minutes a day (depending on the skin's sensitivity to sunlight) in the spring, summer, and fall is usually adequate, as is sitting in sunlight on a verandah for 15 to 30 minutes in New Zealand (37).

CONCLUSIONS

When evaluating patients for hypo- and hypercalcemic conditions, it is appropriate to consider the patient's vitamin D status, as well as whether they suffer from either an acquired or inherited disorder in the acquisition and/or metabolism of vitamin D. Because the assay for vitamin D is not available to clinicians, the best compound to assay to determine vitamin D status is 25(OH)D. Only when there is a suspicion that there is an acquired or inherited disorder in the metabolism of 25(OH)D is it reasonable to measure circulating $1,25(OH)_2D$ concentrations. The measurement of other vitamin D metabolites, of which there are a variety in the circulation, has not proved to be of any significant value. It has been suggested that there may be a correlation of the development of metabolic bone disease with polymorphism for the vitamin D receptor gene (19,20). Although these data are intriguing, the information is, at this time, of limited clinical value; it may someday provide an insight as to a person's potential maximum bone den-

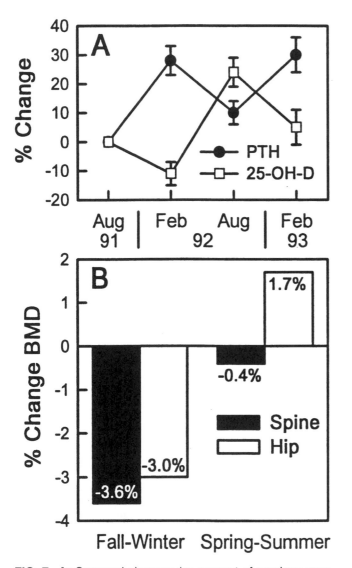

FIG. 7. A: Seasonal changes (as percent of previous measurement) in serum parathyroid hormone (PTH) and 25-hydroxyvitamin D [25(OH)D] over 18 months of the study period. Results are ±SEM. **B:** Percent change in the bone mineral density of the average L2-L4 spine and femoral neck of 15 older rural Maine women, from fall and winter, to spring and summer. (Reproduced with permission from: Rosen CJ, Morrison A, Zhou H, Storm D, Hunter SJ, Musgrave K, Chen T, Wen-Wei L, Holick MF. Elderly women in northern New England exhibit seasonal changes in bone mineral density and calciotropic hormones. *Bone Miner* 25:83–92, 1994.)

sity. The noncalcemic actions of $1,25(OH)_2D_3$ have great promise for clinical applications in the future. Already activated vitamin D compounds such as $1,25(OH)_2D_3$, $1,24(OH)_2D_3$, and calcipotriene herald a new pharmacologic approach for treating psoriasis. $1,25(OH)_2D_3$ and its analogs are actively being tested for treating autoimmune disorders such as diabetes type I and some cancers (11).

ACKNOWLEDGMENTS

This work was supported in part by National Institutes of Health grants AR 36963, DK 43690, M01RR 00533, and AG 04390.

REFERENCES

1. Holick MF: Vitamin D: Photobiology, metabolism, and clinical applications. In: DeGroot L, Besser H, Burger HG, et al. (eds) *Endocrinology*, 3rd ed. WB Saunders, Philadelphia, 990–1013, 1995
2. DeLuca H: The vitamin D story: A collaborative effort of basic science and clinical medicine. *Fed Proc Am Soc Exper Biol* 1988;2:224–236.
3. Reichel H, Koeffler HP, Norman AW: The role of the vitamin D endocrine system in health and disease. *N Engl J Med* 320:981–991, 1989
4. Holick MF: Vitamin D: New horizons for the 21st century. *Am J Clin Nutr* 60:619–630, 1994
5. Holick MF, Matsuoka LY, Wortsman J: Age, vitamin D, and solar ultraviolet radiation. *Lancet* 4:1104–1105, 1989
6. Holick MF, Shao Q, Liu WW, Chen TC: The vitamin D content of fortified milk and infant formula. *N Engl J Med* 326:1178–1181, 1992
7. Chapuy MC, Arlot M, Duboeuf F, et al.: Vitamin D_3 and calcium to prevent hip fracture in elderly women. *N Engl J Med* 327:1637–1642, 1992
8. Dawson-Hughes B, Dallal GE, Krall EA, Harris S, Sokoll LJ, Falconer G: Effect of vitamin D supplementation on wintertime and overall bone loss in healthy postmenopausal women. *Ann Int Med* 115:505–512, 1991
9. Pillai S, Bikle DD, Elias PM: 1,25-dihydroxyvitamin D production and receptor binding in human keratinocytes varies with differentiation. *J Biol Chem* 263:5390–5395, 1987
10. Gray TK, Lester GE, Lorenc RS: Evidence for extrarenal 1-hydroxylation of 25-hydroxyvitamin D_3 in pregnancy. *Science* 204:1311–1313, 1979
11. Holick MF: Noncalcemic actions of 1,25-dihydroxyvitamin D_3 and clinical applications. *Bone* 17:107S–111S, 1995
12. Portale AA, Booth BE, Halloran BP, Morris RC Jr: Effect of dietary phosphorus on circulating concentrations of 1,25-dihydroxyvitamin D and immunoreactive parathyroid hormone in children with moderate renal insufficiency. *J Clin Invest* 73:1580–1589, 1984
13. Slovik DM, Adams JS, Neer RM, Holick MF, Potts JT: Deficient production of 1,25-dihydroxyvitamin D in elderly osteoporotic patients. *N Engl J Med* 305:372–374, 1981
14. Riggs BL, Hamstra A, DeLuca HF: Assessment of 25-hydroxyvitamin D 1α-hydroxylase reserve in postmenopausal osteoporosis by administration of parathyroid extract. *J Clin Endocrinol Metab* 53:833–835, 1981
15. Ozono K, Sone T, Pike JW: Perspectives: The genomic mechanism of action of 1,25-dihydroxyvitamin D_3. *J Bone Miner Res* 6:1021–1027, 1991
16. Norman AW, Putkey JA, Nemere I: Intestinal calcium transport: Pleiotropic effects mediated by vitamin D. *Fed Proc* 41:78–83, 1982
17. Wasserman RH, Fullmer CS, Shimura F: Calcium absorption and the molecular effects of vitamin D_3. In: Kumar R (ed) *Vitamin D: Basic and Clinical Aspects*. Nijhoff, Boston, pp 233–257, 1984
18. Yagi H, Ozono K, Miyake H, Nagashima K, Kuroume T, Pike JW: A new point mutation in the deoxyribonucleic acid-binding domain of the vitamin D receptor in a kindred with hereditary 1,25-dihydroxyvitamin D-resistant rickets. *J Clin Endocrinol Metab* 76:509–512, 1992
19. Morrison NA, Qi JC, Tokita A, et al.: Prediction of bone density from vitamin D receptor alleles. *Nature* 367:284–287, 1994
20. Hustmyer FG, Peacock M, Hui S, Johnston CC, Christian J: Bone mineral density in relation to polymorphism at the vitamin D receptor gene locus. *J Clin Invest* 94:2130–2134, 1994
21. Merke J, Klaus G, Hugel U, et al.: No 1,25-dihydroxyvitamin D_3 receptors on osteoclasts of calcium-deficient chicken despite demonstrable receptors on circulating monocytes. *J Clin Invest* 77:312–314, 1986
22. Miyaura C, Abe E, Suda T, Kuroki T: Alternative differentiation of human promyelocytic leukemia cells (HL-60) induced selectively by retinoic acid and 1,25-dihydroxyvitamin D_3. *Cancer Res* 45:4244–4248, 1985
23. Tanaka H, Abe E, Miyaura C, et al.: 1,25-Dihydroxycholeciferol and human myeloid leukemia cell line (HL-60): The presence of cytosol receptor and induction of differentiation. *Biochem J* 204:713–719, 1982
24. Provvedine DM, Tsoukaas CD, Deftos LJ, Manolagas SC: 1,25-dihydroxyvitamin D_3 receptors in human leukocytes. *Science* 221:118, 1983
25. Koeffler HP, Hirjik J, Iti L, the Southern California Leukemia Group: 1,25-Dihydroxyvitamin D_3: In vivo and in vitro effects on human preleukemic and leukemic cells. *Cancer Treat Rep* 69:1399–1407, 1985
26. Smith EL, Pincus SH, Donovan L, Holick MF: A novel approach for the evaluation and treatment of psoriasis. *J Am Acad Dermatol* 19:516–528, 1988
27. Kragballe K: Treatment of psoriasis by the topical application of the novel vitamin D3 analogue MC 903. *Arch Dermatol* 125:1647–1652, 1989
28. Naveh-Many T, Silver J: Regulation of parathyroid hormone gene expression by hypocalcemia, hypercalcemia, and vitamin D in the rat. *J Clin Invest* 86:1313–1319, 1990
29. Fukuda N, Tanaka H, Tominaga R, Fukagawa M, Kurokawa K, Seino Y: Decreased 1,25-dihydroxyvitamin D_3 receptor density is associated with a more severe form of parathyroid hyperplasia in chronic uremic patients. *J Clin Invest* 92:1436–1443, 1993
30. Delmez JA, Tindira C, Grooms P, Dusso A, Windus DW, Slatopolsky E: Parathyroid hormone suppression by intravenous 1,25-dihydroxyvitamin D: A role for increased sensitivity to calcium. *J Clin Invest* 83:1349–1355, 1989
31. Holick MF, Krane S, Potts JR Jr: Calcium, phosphorus, and bone metabolism: Calcium-regulating hormones. In: Isselbacher KJ, Braunwald E, Wilson JD, et al. (eds) *Harrison's Principles of Internal Medicine*, 13th ed. McGraw-Hill, New York, pp 2137–2151, 1994
32. Bengoa JM, Sitrin MD, Meredith S, et al.: Intestinal calcium absorption and vitamin D status in chronic cholestatic liver disease. *Hepatology* 4:261–265, 1984
33. Pietrek J, Kokot F: Serum 25-hydroxyvitamin D in patients with chronic renal disease. *Eur J Clin Invest* 7:283–287, 1977
34. Demay MB: Hereditary defects in vitamin D metabolism and vitamin D receptor defects. In: Degroot LJ (ed), Cahil GF Jr, Martini L, Nelson DH (consulting eds) *Endocrinology*, vol. 2, 13th ed. Saunders, Philadelphia, pp 1173–1178, 1995
35. Adams JS, Gacad MA, Anders A, Endres DB, Sharma OP: Biochemical indicators of disordered vitamin D and calcium homeostasis in sarcoidosis. *Sarcoidosis* 3:1–6, 1986
36. Rosen CJ, Morrison A, Zhou H, Storm D, Hunter SJ, Musgrave K, Chen T, Wen-Wei L, Holick MF: Elderly women in northern New England exhibit seasonal changes in bone mineral density and calciotropic hormones. *Bone Miner* 25:83–92, 1994
37. Reid IR, Gallagher DJA, Bosworth J: Prophylaxis against vitamin D deficiency in the elderly by regular sunlight exposure. *Age Ageing* 15:35–40, 1985

14. Calcitonin

Leonard J. Deftos, M.D.,J.D.

Department of Medicine, University of California, San Diego; and San Diego Veterans Affairs Medical Center, San Diego California

Calcitonin (CT) is a 32-amino-acid peptide that is secreted primarily by thyroidal C-cells. Its main biologic effect is to inhibit osteoclastic bone resorption. This property has led to its use for disorders characterized by increased bone resorption. Calcitonin is an FDA-approved drug. Parenteral and nasal formulations of the peptide are used for the treatment of Paget's disease, osteoporosis, and the hypercalcemia of malignancy. The secretion of CT is regulated acutely by blood calcium and chronically by gender and perhaps age. Calcitonin is metabolized by the kidney and the liver. It is also a tumor marker for medullary thyroid carcinoma, and the signal tumor of multiple endocrine neoplasia (MEN) type II (1–3).

BIOCHEMISTRY

Structures have been determined for 12 species of CT, including that of humans (3) (Fig. 1). Common features include a 1–7 amino-terminal disulfide bridge, a glycine at residue 28, and a carboxy-terminal proline amide residue. Five of the 9 amino-terminal residues are identical in all CT species. The greatest divergence resides in the interior 27 amino acids. Basic amino acid substitutions enhance potency. Thus, the nonmammalian CTs have the most potency, even in mammalian systems. Unlike for parathyroid hormone (PTH), a biologically active fragment of CT has not been discovered. However, an amphipathic backbone seems to enhance potency.

MOLECULAR BIOLOGY

The CT gene consists of six exons separated by introns (3) (Fig. 2). Two distinct mature mRNAs are generated from differential splicing of the exon regions in the initial gene transcript. One translates as a 141-residue CT precursor, the other as a 128-residue precursor for calcitonin gene-related peptide (CGRP). Calcitonin is the major posttranslationally processed peptide in C-cells, whereas CGRP, a 37-amino-acid peptide, is the major processed peptide in neurons. The main biologic effect of CGRP is vasodilation, but it also functions as a neurotransmitter and does react with the CT receptor. The relevance of CGRP to skeletal metabolism is unknown, but it may be produced locally in skeletal tissue and exert a local regulatory effect. An alternative splicing pathway for the CT gene has been recently described. It produces a carboxy-terminal C-pro CT with eight different terminal amino acids (7). The CT gene predicts the presence of other processed peptides, and there is more than one copy of this gene (4–7).

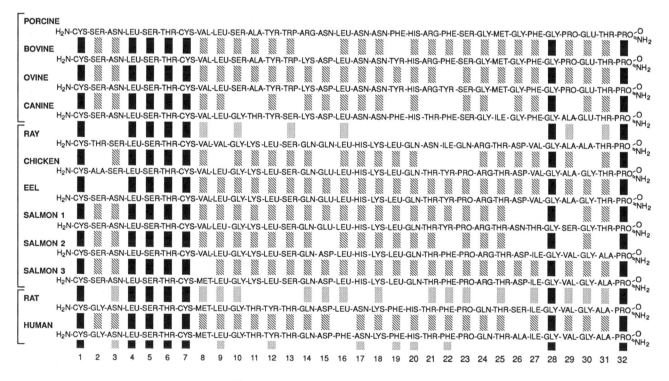

FIG. 1. Amino acid structure of the CTs.

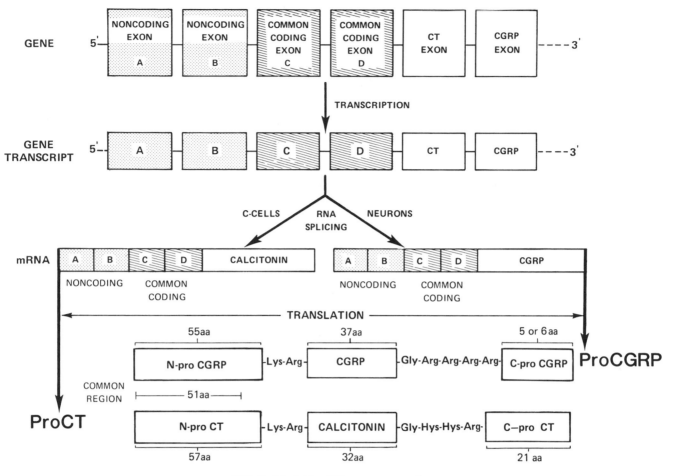

FIG. 2. Model for CT gene expression.

BIOSYNTHESIS

Thyroidal C-cells are the primary source of CT in mammals, and the ultimobranchial gland is the primary source in submammals (1–5). C-cells are neural crest derivatives and they also produce CGRP, the second CT gene product. Other tissue sources of CT have been described, notably the pituitary cells and widely distributed neuroendocrine cells (5,8,9). Although CT may have paracrine effects at these sites, the nonthyroidal sources of CT are not likely to contribute to its peripheral concentration. However, malignant transformation can occur in both ectopic and eutopic cells that produce CT, and the peptide then becomes a tumor marker. The best example of the latter is medullary thyroid carcinoma, and of the former, small-cell lung cancer. Many of the tumors associated with ectopic CT production probably derive this potential from their common neural crest origin with thyroidal C-cells (1).

BIOLOGIC EFFECTS

The main biologic effect of CT is to inhibit osteoclastic bone resorption (10). Within minutes of its administration, CT causes the osteoclast to shrink in size and to decrease its bone-resorbing activity (10,11). This dramatic and complex event is accompanied by the production of cyclic adenosine monophosphate (cAMP) and by increased cytosolic calcium in the osteoclast (1–3,11). In a situation where bone turnover is sufficiently high, CT will produce hypocalcemia and hypophosphatemia. Calcitonin has also been reported to inhibit osteocytes and stimulate osteoblasts, but these effects are controversial (10). Analgesia is a commonly reported effect of CT treatment (4). Calciuria, phosphaturia, and gastrointestinal effects on calcium flux have been reported for CT, but they occur at concentrations of the hormone that are supraphysiologic (1). It should be noted, however, that the concentration of the peptide at its several sites of biosynthesis may be sufficiently high to explain some extraskeletal effects of CT by a paracrine mechanism (12). Thus, CT may exert physiologic effects on the pituitary and central nervous system (5,8). Furthermore, the demonstration of CT and CT receptors at intracranial sites may qualify CT as a neurotransmitter (13). Other effects of CT have been reported. It has been observed to act as an anti-inflammatory agent, to promote fracture and wound healing, to be uricosuric, to be antihypertensive, and to impair glucose tolerance. Calcitonin may regulate and be regulated by other calcitropic hormones, and there is some evidence to suggest that it exerts an autoregulatory effect (12). The importance of these effects is yet to be determined (1–3).

CT as a Drug

The main biologic action of CT—its inhibition of osteoclastic bone resorption—has resulted in its successful use in disease states characterized by increased bone resorption and the consequent hypercalcemia. Calcitonin is widely used in Paget's disease, in which osteoclastic bone resorption is dramatically increased. Calcitonin is also used in osteoporosis, in which the increase of bone resorption may be more subtle, and in the treatment of hypercalcemia of malignancy (14). Newer pharmacologic preparations of CT may have improved therapeutic effects (17). A nasal preparation of CT is receiving increasing clinical application (18).

SECRETION

Calcium

Ambient calcium concentration is the most important regulator of CT secretion (1). When blood calcium rises acutely, there is a proportional increase in CT secretion, and an acute decrease in blood calcium produces a corresponding decrease in plasma CT. However, the effects of chronic hypercalcemia and chronic hypocalcemia are not fully defined, and conflicting results have been reported (19,20). It seems likely that the C-cells can respond to sustained hypercalcemia by increasing CT secretion, but, if the hypercalcemia is severe and/or prolonged, the C-cells probably exhaust their secretory reserve (1). The inhibitory effect on CT secretion by hypocalcemia is difficult to demonstrate. Chronic hypocalcemia seems to decrease the secretory challenge to C-cells and they increase their stores of CT; these stores can be released on appropriate stimulation (21).

Metabolism

The metabolism of CT is a complex process that involves many organ systems. Evidence has been reported for degradation of the hormone by kidney, liver, bone, and even the thyroid gland (3). Like many other peptide hormones, CT disappears from plasma in a multiexponential manner that includes an early half-life measured in minutes. In most studies, the kidney seems to be the most important organ of clearance for CT. Inactivation of the hormone seems more important than renal excretion, because relatively little CT can be detected in urine (1–4).

Gastrointestinal Factors

Gastrointestinal peptides, especially those of the gastrin-cholecystokinin family, are potent CT secretagogues when administered parenterally in supraphysiologic concentrations (1,2). This observation has led to the postulate that there is an entero-C-cell regulatory pathway for CT secretion. However, only meals that contain sufficient calcium to raise the blood calcium have been demonstrated to increase CT secretion in humans (19). Thus, the secretory relationship between the gastrointestinal tract and C-cells in human needs further exploration to determine its physiologic significance.

Other Factors

Although a variety of neuroendocrine and ionic factors have been demonstrated to regulate CT secretion under experimental conditions (1), it is unlikely that these agents participate in the physiologic regulation of CT secretion (1–5).

Provocative Testing for CT-Producing Tumors

The stimulatory effect of calcium and gastrin-related peptides, especially pentagastrin, on CT secretion has led to the use of these agents as provocative tests for the secretion of CT (2). These procedures are widely used in patients suspected of having medullary thyroid carcinoma (MTC), especially when the basal concentration of the hormone is not diagnostically elevated. Medullary thyroid carcinoma is a neoplastic disorder of thyroidal C-cells that can occur in a familial pattern as part of MEN type II, for which genetic tests are now available. Most tumors respond with increased CT secretion to the administration of either calcium or pentagastrin or their combination, but either agent can sometimes give misleading results. Therefore, in clinically compelling situations, both agents should be considered for diagnostic testing. Calcitonin measurements can also be used to evaluate the effectiveness of therapy in patients with CT-producing tumors.

Gender and Age

Most investigators find that women have lower CT levels than men (22,23). The mechanism of this difference is unclear but may be accounted for in part by a stimulating effect of gonadal steroids on CT secretion (24,25). The effect of age on CT secretion is more controversial (22,23,26): newborns seem to have a higher serum level of the hormone, and in adults, a progressive decline with age has been reported by several laboratories (1,22,26). However, stable adult levels have also been observed (23). It is likely that the different assay procedures used in different studies account for the conflicting results (Fig. 3). Thus, the serum concentration of some forms of CT may decline with age, whereas others do not (22,23). The physiologic significance of the various circulating forms of CT measured by different assay procedures has not been defined. Non-monomeric, as well as monomeric, forms of circulating CT species are biologically active (1,27), and some procedures may not accurately reflect biologically active CT in blood.

CLINICAL ABNORMALITIES OF CT SECRETION

Medullary Thyroid Carcinoma

Medullary thyroid carcinoma is a tumor of the CT-producing C-cells of the thyroid gland (2). Although a rare tumor, it can occur in a familial pattern as part of MEN type II (Table 1). Medullary thyroid carcinoma is generally regarded as intermediate between the aggressive behavior of anaplastic thyroid carcinoma and the more indolent behavior of papil-

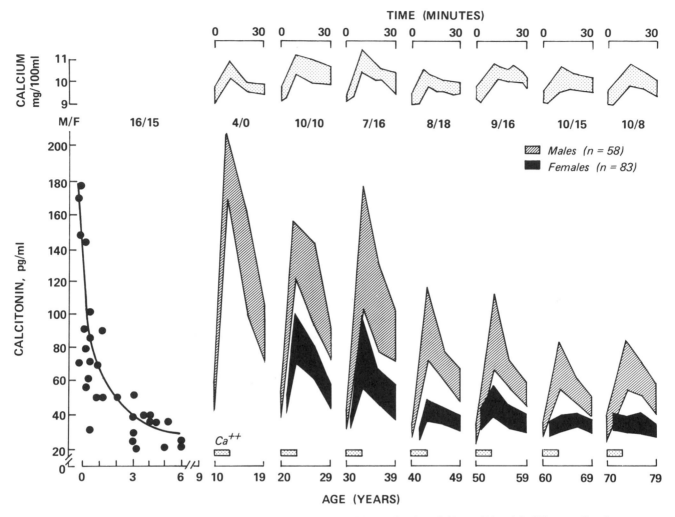

FIG. 3. Effects of age and gender on basal and calcium-stimulated (3 mg/10 min) CT secretion in humans. (Data from: Deftos LJ, Weisman MH, Williams GH, Karpf DB, Frumar AM, Davidson BH, Parthemore JG, Judd HL. Influence of age and sex on plasma calcitonin in human beings. *N Eng J Med* 302:1351–1353, 1980; and Klein GL, Wadlington EL, Colllins ED, Catherwood BD, Deftos LJ. Calcitonin levles in sera of infants and children: Relation to age and periods of bone growth. *Calcif Tissue Int* 36:635–638, 1984.)

lary and follicular thyroid carcinoma. The most common presentation is a thyroid nodule, and the most common symptom is diarrhea. These tumors usually produce diagnostically elevated serum concentrations of CT. Therefore, the radioimmunoassay for CT in serum can be used to diagnose the presence of MTC with an exceptional degree of accuracy

TABLE 1. *Components of multiple endocrine neoplasia (MEN) type II, and their frequency*

Component	MEN type IIA (%)	MEN type IIB (%)
Medullary thyroid carcinoma	97	90
Pheochromocytoma	30	45
Hyperparathyroidism	50	Rare
Mucosal neuroma syndrome	—	100

and specificity. In a small but increasing percentage of patients, however, basal hormone levels are indistinguishable from normal. Many of these subjects represent the early stages of C-cell neoplasia or hyperplasia most amenable to surgical cure. To identify these patients with early disease, provocative tests for CT secretion, previously discussed, have been developed that can identify MTC in a patient whose diagnosis could have been missed if basal CT determinations only had been performed (see Appendix iii). Abnormalities of the RET oncogene are the genetic basis for inherited MTC and provide the basis for genetic testing (1).

Other CT-Producing Neoplasms

Neoplastic disorders of other neuroendocrine cells can also produce abnormally elevated amounts of CT. The best known example is small-cell lung cancer. However, other tumors, such as carcinoids and islet cell tumors of the pancreas, can do the same (1,2).

Renal Disease

There are increases in immunoassayable CT with both acute and chronic renal failure, but considerable disagreement exists regarding the mechanism and significance of these increases (1–3). Because the secretion and/or metabolism of CT is abnormal in renal disease, and because renal osteodystrophy is characterized by increased bone resorption, CT, which acts to inhibit bone resorption, has been implicated in the pathogenesis of uremic osteodystrophy (3).

Hypercalciuria

Elevated levels of CT have been demonstrated in patients with hypercalciuria (28). The physiologic significance of enhanced CT secretion is unknown, but it may represent a compensatory response to intestinal hyperabsorption of calcium. Although CT in high concentrations has both phosphaturic and calciuric actions in humans, it is not likely that a primary alteration in CT secretion contributes to the development of hypercalciuria (1).

Bone Disease

No skeletal disease has been conclusively attributed to CT abnormalities (3,27). Although women have lower CT levels than men, there is conflicting evidence as to whether endogenous secretion of the hormone contributes to the pathogenesis of osteoporosis (25,29,30). Nevertheless, CT has been of therapeutic benefit in osteoporosis (17).

Reduced CT reserve in women may contribute to the greater severity of osteitis fibrosa cystica in women with primary hyperparathyroidism (20).

Hypercalcemia and Hypocalcemia

Calcium challenge is a well-documented stimulus for CT secretion. Although increased CT secretion has only inconsistently been associated with chronic hypercalcemia (19,20), an exaggerated response of CT to secretagogues has been convincingly observed in several hypocalcemic states (21).

Calcitonin Receptor

The CT receptor has been recently cloned (31). It has seven putative transmembrane domains, but it shows no homology to other classical receptor families. Rather it is structurally related to the secretin receptor and the PTH/PTH-related-protein receptor (Fig. 4). The CT receptor serves a dual signal transduction function in that it can activate effector pathways mediated by both cAMP and by the phosphoinositol/Ca^{2+} pathway (32).

Several isoforms of the human CT receptor have been cloned. They derive from alternate splicing of the mRNA from a single gene located on chromosome 7, and corresponding receptor isoforms have been identified in pig and rat (32). The CT receptor isoforms exhibit different CT affinities and signal transduction mechanisms, which may account for the pleiotropic effects of the hormone (32,33).

Role of Calcitonin in Mineral Metabolism

The exact physiologic role of CT in calcium homeostasis and skeletal metabolism has not been established in humans,

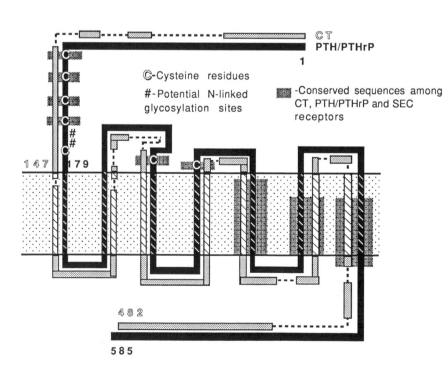

FIG. 4. Comparison of the deduced amino acid sequences of the receptors for CT, PTH/PTH-related protein, and secretin (SEC). Breaks in the sequences have been inserted to align the conserved amino acids. *Shaded areas* represent the regions of greatest identity and similarity. (From Lin HY, et al. Expression cloning of an adenylate cyclase-coupled calcitonin receptor. *Science* 254:1022–1024, 1991.)

and many questions remain unanswered about the significance of this hormone in humans. Does CT secretion decline with age? Do gonadal steroids regulate the secretion of CT? Do the lower levels of serum CT in women contribute to the pathogenesis of age-related loss of bone mass and osteoporosis? Do extrathyroidal sources of CT participate in the regulation of skeletal metabolism? Are there primary and secondary abnormalities of CT secretion in diseases of skeletal and calcium homeostasis? The conclusive answers to these questions await clinical studies with an assay procedure that directly measures the biologic activity of CT in blood. Furthermore, accurate local measurements of CT and its effects may be necessary to elucidate the emerging role of CT as a paracrine and autocrine agent.

ACKNOWLEDGMENTS

This work was supported by the National Institutes of Health, the National Cancer Institute, and the Department of Veterans Affairs.

REFERENCES

1. Deftos LJ: Calcitonin and medullary thyroid carcinoma. In: Bennett JC and Plum F (eds) *Cecil Textbook of Medicine,* 20th ed. WB Saunders, Philadelphia, pp 1372–1375, 1996
2. Deftos LJ: Calcitonin secretion in humans. In: Cooper CW (ed) *Current Research on Calcium Regulating Hormones.* University of Texas Press, Austin, pp 79–100, 1987
3. Deftos LJ: *Medullary Thyroid Carcinoma.* S Karger, New York, pp 1–114, 1983
4. Deftos LJ, Roos B: Medullary thyroid carcinoma and calcitonin gene expression. In: Peck WA (ed) *Bone and Mineral Research.* Excerpta Medica, Amsterdam, pp 267–316, 1989
5. Fischer JA, Born W: Calcitonin gene products: Evolution, expression and biological targets. *Bone Miner* 2:347–353, 1987
6. Cote GJ, Gould JA, Huang SC, Gagel RF: Studies of short-term secretion of peptides produced by alternative RNA processing. *Mol Cell Endocrinol* 53:211–219, 1987
7. Minvielle S, Giscard-Dartevelle S, Cohen R, Taboulet, Labye F, Jullienne A, Rivaille P, Milhaud G, Moukhtar MS, Lasmoles F: A novel calcitonin carboxyl-terminal peptide produced in medullary thyroid carcinoma by alternative RNA processing of the calcitonin/calcitonin gene-related peptide gene. *J Biol Chem* 266: 24627–24631, 1991
8. Deftos LJ: Pituitary cells secrete calcitonin in the reverse hemolytic plaque assay. *Biochem Biophys Res Commun* 146: 1350–1356, 1987
9. Becker KL, Monaghan KG, Silva OL: Immunocytochemical localization of calcitonin in Kulchitsky cells of human lung. *Arch Pathol Lab Med* 104:196–198, 1980
10. Deftos LJ, Glowacki J: Mechanisms of bone metabolism. In: Kem DC, Frohlich E (eds) *Pathophysiology.* JB Lippincott, Philadelphia, pp 445–468, 1984
11. Moonga BS, Alam AS, Bevis PJ, Avaldi F, Soncini R, Huang CL, Zaidi M: Regulation of cystosolic free calcium in isolated osteoclasts by calcitonin. *J Endocrinol* 132:241–249, 1992
12. Deftos LJ, Burton DW, Brown TF, Fieck A, Brandt DW: Calcitonin responsive elements are present in the calcitonin and PTH-like protein genes. *J Bone Miner Res* 7:5235, 1992
13. Goltzman D, Tannenbaum GS: Induction of hypocalcemia by intracerebroventricular injection of calcitonin: Evidence for control of blood calcium by the nervous system. *Brain Res* 416:1–6, 1987
14. Avioli LV: Calcitonin therapy for bone disease and hypercalcemia. *Arch Intern Med* 142:2076–2080, 1982
15. Singer FR, Schiller AL, Pyle EB, Krane SM: Paget's disease of bone. In: Avioli LV, Krane SM (eds) *Metabolic Bone Disease,* Academic Press, New York, pp 490–567, 1978
16. Gruber H, Ivey JL, Baylink DJ, Matthews M, Nelp WB, Sisom K, Chestnut CH III: Long-term calcitonin therapy in postmenopausal osteoporosis. *Metabolism* 33:295–298, 1984
17. Buclin T, Randin JP, Jacquet AF, Azria M, Attinger M, Gomez F, Burckhardt P: The effect of rectal and nasal administration of salmon calcitonin in normal subjects. *Calcif Tissue Int* 41:252–254, 1987
18. Carslens JH, Feinblatt JD: Future horizons for calcitonin. *J Bone Miner Res* 49:2–6, 1991
19. Austin LA, Heath H III: Calcitonin—Physiology and pathophysiology. *N Engl J Med* 304:269–278, 1981
20. Parthemore JG, Deftos LJ: Secretion of calcitonin in primary hyperparathyroidism. *J Clin Endocrinol Metab* 49:223–226, 1979
21. Deftos LJ, Powell D, Parthemore JG, Potts JT Jr: Secretion of calcitonin in hypocalcemic states in man. *J Clin Invest* 52:3109–3114, 1973
22. Deftos LJ, Weisman MH, Williams GH, Karpf DB, Frumar AM, Davidson BH, Parthemore JG, Judd HL: Influence of age and sex on plasma calcitonin in human beings. *N Engl J Med* 302:1351–1353, 1980
23. Tiegs RD, Body JJ, Barta JM, Health H III: Secretion and metabolism of monomeric human calcitonin: Effects of age, sex, and thyroid damage. *J Bone Miner Res* 1:339–343, 1986
24. Foresta C, Scanelli G, Zanatta GP, Busnardo B, Scandellari C: Reduced calcitonin reserve in young hypogonadic osteoporotic men. *Horm Metab Res* 19:275–277, 1987
25. Stevenson JC, White MC, Joplin GF, MacIntyre I: Osteoporosis and calcitonin deficiency. *Br Med J* 285:1010–1011, 1982
26. Klein GL, Wadlington EL, Collins ED, Catherwood BD, Deftos LJ: Calcitonin levels in sera of infants and children: Relations to age and periods of bone growth. *Calcif Tissue Int* 36:635–638, 1984
27. Tashjian AH Jr: Calcitonin 1976: A review of some recent advances. In: James VHT (ed) *International Congress Series Proceedings of the V International Congress of Endocrinology.* Excerpta Medica, Amsterdam, New York, pp 256–261, 1976
28. Ivey JJ, Roos BA, Shen FH, Baylink DJ: Increased immunoreactive calcitonin in idiopathic hypercalciuria. *Metab Bone Dis Relat Res* 3:29–32, 1981
29. Taggart HM, Ivey JJ, Sisom K, Chestnut CH III, Baylink DJ, Huber MB: Deficient calcitonin response to calcium stimulation in postmenopausal osteoporosis. *Lancet* 1:475–478, 1982
30. Tiegs RD, Body JJ, Wahner HW, Barta J, Riggs BL, Heath H III: Calcitonin secretion in postmenopausal osteoporosis. *N Engl J Med* 312:1097–2000, 1985
31. Lin HY, Harrus TL, Flannery MS, Aruffo A, Kaji EH, Gorn A, Kolakowski LF Jr., Lodish HF, Goldring SR: Expression cloning of an adenylate cyclase-coupled calcitonin receptor. *Science* 254: 1022–1024, 1991
32. Gorn AH, Rudolph SM, Flannery MR, Morton CC, Weremowicz S, Wang TZ, Krane SM, Goldring SR: Expression of two human skeletal calcitonin receptor isoforms cloned from a giant cell tumor of bone. *J Clin Invest* 95:2680–2691, 1995
33. Chabre O, Conklin BR, Lin HY, Wilson E, Ives HE, Catanzariti L, Hemmings BA, Bourne HR: A recombinant calcitonin receptor independently stimulates cAMP and Ca^{2+}/inositol phosphate signalling pathways. *Mol Endocrinol* 6:551–556, 1992

Clinical Evaluation of Bone and Mineral Disorders

15. History and Physical Examination

Peter M. Sklarin, M.D., and *Dolores M. Shoback, M.D.

*Department of Endocrinology and Metabolism, Metabolic Research Unit, and *Department of Medicine, University of California at San Francisco; and San Francisco Veterans Affairs Medical Center, San Francisco, California*

With the availability of treatments that can cure, prevent, or control most metabolic bone diseases, early recognition is essential. An experienced clinician can accurately diagnose many bone disorders by history and physical examination alone. Because many of these diseases have a subtle and insidious onset, they may not be recognized until they have reached a severe stage. The clinician's challenge, therefore, is not only early diagnosis of existing disease, but also the identification of patients at risk. A careful history and thorough physical examination are the physician's most powerful tools in choosing whom to screen with diagnostic tests and deciding which patients will benefit most from preventive intervention.

MEDICAL HISTORY

Initial assessment should include the patient's age, gender, race, menopausal status, and a complete medical, pharmacologic, nutritional, and family history.

In some situations, the chief complaint leads directly to the diagnosis: for example, a hip fracture from osteoporosis, bowing deformity of the legs from rickets, or numbness and tingling around the mouth and in the tips of the fingers in a patient with hypocalcemia. Other factors may provide strong evidence that an unspecified bone disease is present and prompt the physician to explore further. For example, severe back pain or bone pain, history of fracture with minimal trauma, prolonged immobilization, loss of height in elderly people, and sunlight deprivation, all raise the index of suspicion for the presence of skeletal disease. In children, growth retardation or short stature, bone pain, muscle weakness, skeletal deformities, extraskeletal calcifications, and waddling gait, all suggest metabolic bone disease.

The duration of symptoms is also important—are they lifelong or new? Does the diet contain adequate calcium, phosphorus, and vitamin D? If the diet is insufficient, is there adequate sunlight exposure? Does the patient engage in regular weight-bearing exercise? Does an adult or child with osteopenia engage in activities at play or work that involve a high risk of trauma?

A drug history is of vital importance, because many medicines, including over-the-counter preparations, can adversely affect the skeleton. Glucocorticoids, thyroid hormone, anticonvulsants, and heparin may cause osteoporosis. Current use of long-acting benzodiazepines and high caffeine intake may increase the risk of osteoporotic hip fracture. Excessive alcohol intake is associated with hypomagnesemia, nutritional deficiencies of calcium, vitamin D, and protein, reduced sunlight exposure, and tendency to fall. Alcohol ingestion also may directly impair osteoblast function. Antacids containing aluminum may lead to aluminum-induced bone disease, typically in the setting of renal insufficiency. Cancer chemotherapy also can affect bone. Long-term lithium therapy is associated with hypercalcemia and parathyroid hormone (PTH) hypersecretion. Chronic use of sodium fluoride or the bisphosphonate etidronate can result in osteomalacia. Hypervitaminosis A is associated with excessive bone resorption and bone pain, and vitamin D excess can result in hypercalcemia. Gonadotropin-releasing hormone agonists induce an estrogen-deficient state when given in a continuous manner and may result in reduced bone mass. Diuretics can confound test interpretation by increasing or decreasing urine calcium, or by increasing serum alkaline phosphatase activity.

The patient should be asked about any history of endocrine, renal, or gastrointestinal disease. Hyper- and hypoparathyroidism, hyperthyroidism, Cushing's syndrome, and sex hormone deficiency all may affect bone remodeling. Gastrectomy or gastric stapling, intestinal malabsorption syndromes, chronic obstructive biliary disease, and pancreatic insufficiency all can result in osteopenia.

Recent data from the Study of Osteoporotic Fractures (SOF), a multicenter cohort of 970 white women 65 years of age or older, identify historical factors that help to predict hip fracture in older women (3). This study suggests that the risk of hip fracture is higher among women who have had previous fractures of any type after the age of 50, women who rate their own health as fair or poor, and women who spend 4 hours a day or less on their feet. Among the SOF cohort, investigators found that the more weight a woman had gained since the age of 25, the lower her risk of hip fracture. However, if a woman weighed less than she had at age 25, this doubled her risk of hip fracture. Women who were tall at the age of 25 also had a greater risk.

Because many of the metabolic bone disorders are heritable, a careful family history is important for purposes of screening and educating those at risk, or for recommending genetic counseling. In the SOF cohort, women with a maternal history of hip fracture had a twofold increased risk of hip fracture, independent of bone mass, height, and weight (3). In certain conditions, the diagnosis is firmly established when other family members are tested. For example, in X-linked hypophosphatemic vitamin-D-resistant rickets, the presence of isolated hypophosphatemia in a heterozygous woman confirms the presence of the trait and its hereditary pattern.

PHYSICAL EXAMINATION

Height and weight should be measured in all patients. The clinician should look specifically for any bony deformities or masses, leg-length inequality, vertebral tenderness, a surgical scar on the neck (suggesting previous thyroid or parathyroid surgery), and abnormal gait. Often, a single physical finding leads to a specific diagnosis. Blue or gray sclerae suggest osteogenesis imperfecta. These patients also may have deafness, ligamentous laxity with joint hypermobility, diaphoresis, dental defects, and they may bruise easily. Cafe-au-lait spots are present in the McCune-Albright syndrome, soft-tissue or mesenchymal tumors in oncogenic rickets/osteomalacia, and premature loss of deciduous teeth in hypophosphatasia. Alopecia, ranging from sparse hair to total alopecia without eye lashes, occurs in two thirds of kindreds with vitamin-D-dependent rickets type II.

In rickets, a constellation of physical findings provides the diagnosis. The patient may have short stature, bony tenderness, softened skull (craniotabes), parietal flattening, and frontal bossing. There is often palpable enlargement of the costochondral junctions (the "rachitic rosary"), thickening of the wrists and ankles, flared wrists from metaphyseal widening, Harrison's groove (a horizontal depression along the lower border of the chest, corresponding to the costal insertions of the diaphragm), bowing deformity of the long bones from weight bearing, and waddling gait. The patient also may have reduced muscle strength and tone, lax ligaments, an indentation of the sternum in response to the force exerted by the diaphragm and intercostal muscles, delayed eruption of permanent teeth, and enamel defects. Rickets affects the most rapidly growing bone. Because the skull is growing rapidly at birth, craniotabes is found in congenital rickets. Rachitic rosary is prominent during the first year of life, when the rib cage grows rapidly. Late rickets, which occurs at the time of the adolescent growth spurt, results in the knock-knee deformity. In infants and young children, listlessness and irritability are common. In infants, floppiness and hypotonia are characteristic.

Hypocalcemia is characterized by neuromuscular irritability. This may include varying degrees of tetany, which usually begins with numbness and tingling around the mouth and in the tips of fingers, followed by muscle spasms in the extremities and face. There may be thumb adduction, metacarpophalangeal joint flexion, and interphalangeal joint extension. Latent tetany can be demonstrated by eliciting Chvostek's sign or Trousseau's sign. Chvostek's sign is spasm of facial muscles elicited by tapping the facial nerve in the region of the parotid gland, just anterior to the ear lobe, below the zygomatic arch or between the zygomatic arch and the corner of the mouth. The response ranges from a twitching of the lip at the corner of the mouth to a twitching of all of the facial muscles on the stimulated side. Slightly positive reactions may occur in up to 10% to 15% of normal adults. To elicit Trousseau's sign, a sphygmomanometer is inflated on the arm to 20 mm above the systolic blood pressure for 2 to 5 minutes. A positive response consists of carpal spasm with relaxation occurring 5 to 10 seconds after the cuff is deflated. Relaxation should not be immediate. Both Chvostek's and Trousseau's signs can be absent, however, even in severe hypocalcemia.

In patients with idiopathic hypoparathyroidism, the physician should look for signs of the polyglandular failure syndromes: chronic mucocutaneous candidiasis, Addison's disease, alopecia, vitiligo, premature ovarian failure, diabetes mellitus, autoimmune thyroid disease, and pernicious anemia. Most patients with primary hyperparathyroidism have no abnormal physical findings. Enlarged parathyroid glands are usually palpable only when parathyroid carcinoma is present, and band keratopathy (calcium-phosphate deposition in the medial and lateral limbic margins of the cornea) is seen rarely and usually only by slit-lamp exam.

Pseudohypoparathyroidism presents with a constellation of signs, including those of longstanding hypocalcemia and hyperphosphatemia. Symptoms of tetany are common and include carpopedal spasm, tetanic convulsions, paresthesias, muscle cramps, and stridor. There may be soft-tissue calcifications, and posterior subcapsular cataracts develop frequently. Albright's hereditary osteodystrophy refers to a constellation of findings seen in pseudohypoparathyroidism or pseudo-pseudohypoparathyroidism. It includes round facies, short stature, obesity, shortening of the digits (brachydactyly), subcutaneous ossification, and dental hypoplasia. Many patients are mentally retarded. A characteristic shortening of the fourth and fifth digits can be recognized as dimpling over the knuckles of a clenched fist (Archibald's sign).

Patients with renal osteodystrophy often have characteristic physical findings. Spontaneous tendon rupture may occur in patients with advanced renal failure, almost always in association with marked secondary hyperparathyroidism. Bone deformities are common, especially in patients with severe aluminum toxicity. A "funnel chest" abnormality may be produced by rib deformities and kyphoscoliosis. Pseudoclubbing may result from enlargement of the distal tufts of the fingers as a result of osteitis fibrosa. Bowing of long bones, genu valgum, and ulnar deviation of the wrist are common in children under 10 years of age, and slipped epiphyses may occur in the preadolescent period.

Patients with Paget's disease usually have no signs of the disease. Over many years, however, progressive cranial involvement can produce increased head size, while bowing and enlargement of the long bones may occur with disease of the femur and tibia. Slowly progressive hearing loss, vertigo, and/or tinnitus can occur in up to 25% of patients with skull involvement. Commonly, there is redness with increased skin temperature over an affected bone. Defects in Bruch's membrane of the retina, termed angioid streaks, may be observed in about 10% of patients. Deformity of the facial bones (leontiasis ossea) may be seen in Paget's disease but is more common in fibrous dysplasia.

Patients with established osteoporosis often exhibit dorsal kyphosis or a gibbus (Dowager's hump) and loss of height. They may have a protuberant abdomen (that the patient may confuse with obesity), ribs within the pelvic rim that may be bruised, paravertebral muscle spasm, and thin skin (McConkey's sign). The clinician should look for signs of secondary causes of osteoporosis (e.g., hypogonadism, Cushing's syndrome). In the SOF, four physical findings indicated an increased risk of hip fracture: the inability to rise from a chair without using one's arms, a resting pulse rate of more than 80 beats per minute, poor depth perception, and poorer low-frequency contrast sensitivity (3). By combining these clinical findings with a careful history and bone density measurement, it may be possible to make a good assessment of hip fracture risk.

With the availability of sophisticated diagnostic techniques to assess bone density and remodeling, the clinician is faced with new and difficult decisions about test interpretation and resource allocation. A complete history and physical examination continue to be the clinician's most important guides, often providing crucial clues to the etiology of skeletal disorders.

REFERENCES

1. Bilezikian JP, Silverberg SJ, Gartenberg F, Kim T, Jacobs TP, Siris ES, Shane E, Coburn JW, Salusky IB, Levine MA, Schwindinger WF, Downs RW, Moses AM. In: Bilezikian JP, Marcus R, Levine MA (eds) *The Parathyroids, Basic and Clinical Concepts.* Raven Press, New York:457–470; 721–746; 781–800, 1994

2. Levine MA, Spiegel AM, Goldring SR, Krane SM, Avioli LV, Singer FR. In: DeGroot LJ, Besser M, Burger HG, et al. (eds) *Endocrinology.* WB Saunders, Philadelphia:1136–1150; 1204–1227; 1259–1273, 1995

3. Cummings SR et al., and The Study of Osteoporotic Fractures Research Group: Risk factors for hip fracture in white women. *N Engl J Med* 322:767–773, 1995

16. Blood, Calcium, Phosphorus, and Magnesium

Anthony A. Portale, M.D.

Departments of Pediatrics and Medicine, University of California at San Francisco, San Francisco, California

SERUM CALCIUM CONCENTRATION

Calcium in serum exists in three separate fractions: protein-bound calcium (40%), which is not ultrafilterable by the kidney, and ionized (48%) and complexed (12%) calcium, which are ultrafilterable (1). Complexed calcium is that bound to various anions, such as phosphate, citrate, and bicarbonate. For clinical purposes, the total concentration of calcium in serum is the most commonly evaluated index of calcium status.

Total Calcium Concentration

Albumin accounts for 90% of the protein-bound calcium in serum; globulins account for the remainder. Calcium binds to anionic carboxylate groups on the albumin molecule, and in normal serum, fewer than 20% of the binding sites are occupied. Conditions that change the serum concentration of albumin, such as nephrotic syndrome or hepatic cirrhosis, will affect the measurement of total calcium concentrations. Under such circumstances, the total calcium concentration may not then accurately reflect the calcium status of the patient. Several algorithms or nomograms have been developed to correct the total calcium concentration for abnormal values of total protein or albumin or to estimate the "free" calcium concentration (2). For routine clinical interpretation of serum calcium levels, the simplest formula for correction of the total serum calcium concentration for changes in albumin concentration is the following (3):

Corrected total calcium concentration (mg/dL) =
measured total calcium concentration (mg/dL) –
albumin concentration (g/dL) + 4.

Such algorithms, however, do not provide precise estimates of the free calcium concentration, and they incorrectly predict the calcium status, as judged from actual measurement of ionized calcium concentration, in 20% to 30% of

subjects (2). Given that the measurement of blood ionized calcium concentration is now widely available in clinical laboratories, the use of estimated values for free calcium should be abandoned.

Calcium binding to albumin is strongly pH dependent between pH 7 and pH 8: an acute increase or decrease in pH of 0.1 pH units will increase or decrease, respectively, protein-bound calcium by about 0.12 mg/dL. In hypocalcemic patients with metabolic acidosis, rapid correction of acidemia with sodium bicarbonate can precipitate tetany, because the increased binding of calcium to albumin results in a decrease in ionized calcium concentration.

The total calcium concentration in serum exhibits a circadian rhythm characterized by a single nadir and peak, with amplitude (nadir to peak) of approximately 0.5 mg/dL (Table 1) (4,5). This rhythm is thought to reflect hemodynamic changes in serum albumin concentration that result from changes in body posture (6). Prolonged upright posture or venostasis can cause hemoconcentration and thus potentially misleading increases of 0.4 to 0.6 mg/dL in serum total calcium concentration. There is negligible difference between values taken in fasting and nonfasting states.

Normal values for serum total calcium concentration vary somewhat among clinical laboratories, in general ranging from 9.0 to 10.6 mg/dL. The concentration decreases with advancing age in men, from a mean of about 9.6 mg/dL at age 20 to about 9.2 mg/dL at age 80 years, and the decrease can be accounted for by decrease in serum albumin concentration (7). In women, no change is observed with age. In children, the serum calcium concentration is higher than in adults, being highest at 6 to 24 months of age, with a mean of 10.2 mg/dL, decreasing to a plateau of about 9.8 mg/dL at 6 to 8 years, and decreasing further to adult values at 16 to 20 years (8,9) (Table 2).

For routine determination of total serum calcium concentration, most clinical laboratories use automated spectrophotometric techniques, such as the *o*-cresolphthalein complexone method; the reference method is atomic absorption

TABLE 1. *Characteristics of the circadian rhythms in blood mineral concentration in humans*

	Concentration (mg/dL)		Amplitude (mg/dL)	Phase (hr)	
	Fasting	24-hr mean	(Nadir to peak)	Nadir	Peak
Total serum calcium	9.6	9.4	0.5	0300	1300
Blood ionized calcium	4.67	4.52	0.3	1900	1000
Serum phosphorus	3.6	4.0	1.2	1100	0200

From refs. 4,17.

spectrophotometry (10). Calcium concentrations expressed in mg/dL can be converted to mmol/L (mM) by dividing by 4, and to mEq/L by dividing by 2. (The atomic weight of calcium is 40.08 and its valence is 2.)

Ionized Calcium

Ionized calcium is the fraction of plasma calcium that is important for physiologic processes, such as muscle contraction, blood coagulation, nerve conduction, hormone secretion (parathyroid hormone and 1,25-dihydroxyvitamin D) and action, ion transport, bone mineralization, and integrity of plasma membranes. In the past, measurement of blood ionized calcium concentration was technically difficult and not widely available in clinical settings. With the advent of newer, semiautomated instruments using ion-selective electrodes, the concentration of ionized calcium can now be readily and accurately measured (11). This measurement is most useful in critically ill patients, particularly those in whom serum protein levels are decreased, acid–base disturbances are present, or to whom large amounts of citrated blood products are given, such as with cardiac surgery or liver transplantation.

The range of values of ionized calcium for normal individuals must be established for each laboratory, and it will vary depending on which technique is used and whether the measurement is made in serum, plasma, or heparinized whole blood. Measured with currently available, ion-selective electrodes, serum ionized calcium concentrations in healthy adult men and women range from approximately 4.5 to 5.2 mg/dL or 1.12 to 1.30 mmol/L, without significant sex differences (10,11). In healthy infants, ionized calcium levels decrease from about 5.8 mg/dL at birth to a nadir of 4.9 mg/dL at 24 hr of life (12), and they increase slightly

during the first week of life to 5.4 mg/dL (13). Values in young children are slightly higher (by about 0.1 mg/dL) than those in adults until after puberty (10,14).

Blood ionized calcium concentrations exhibit a low-amplitude circadian rhythm characterized by a peak at 1000 hr and a nadir at 1800 to 2000 hr, with amplitude (nadir to peak) of 0.3 mg/dL (4). Thus, specimens for analysis drawn after the morning give slightly lower values. Specimens must be obtained anaerobically to avoid spurious results from *ex vivo* changes in pH. Measurements made in heparinized whole blood tend to be slightly lower than those in serum, because of binding of calcium by heparin. Calcium binding to heparin can be minimized by using calcium-titrated heparin (Radiometer Corporation, Copenhagen, Denmark) at a concentration of 50 IU/ml or less, or sodium or lithium heparin at a concentration of 15 U/ml or less (15); under these circumstances, values from serum, plasma, and whole blood are similar. For hospitalized patients, it is recommended that specimens be obtained in the morning fasting state to avoid possible effects of posture, diurnal variation, and food ingestion.

SERUM PHOSPHORUS CONCENTRATION

Phosphorus exists in plasma in two forms: an organic form principally consisting of phospholipids, and an inorganic form (16). Of the total phosphorus in plasma (approximately 14 mg/dL), about 8 mg/dL is in the organic form and 4 mg/dL in the inorganic form. In clinical settings, only the inorganic orthophosphate form is routinely measured. About 15% of total inorganic phosphorus in plasma is protein bound. The remaining 85%, which is ultrafilterable by the kidneys, exists principally either as the undissociated or free ions, HPO_4^{2-} and $H_2PO_4^-$, which are present in serum in

TABLE 2. *Representative normal values for concentrations (in mg/dL) of blood ionized calcium, serum total calcium, phosphorus, and magnesium*

	Age (yr)	Blood ionized calcium	Serum total calcium	Phosphorus	Magnesium
Infants	0–0.25	4.9–5.6	8.8–11.3	4.8–7.4	1.6–2.5
	1–5	4.9–5.3	9.4–10.8	4.5–6.2	"
Children	6–12	4.6–5.3	9.4–10.3	3.6–5.8	1.7–2.3
Men	20	4.5–5.2	9.1–10.2	2.5–4.5	1.7–2.6
	50	"	8.9–10.0	2.3–4.1	"
	70	"	8.8–9.9	2.2–4.0	"
Women	20	4.5–5.2	8.8–10.0	2.5–4.5	1.7–2.6
	50	"	"	2.7–4.4	"
	70	"	"	2.9–4.8	"

Values are approximate, and normal ranges must be determined for each laboratory. From refs. 7–9,11–14,21–23.

a ratio of 4:1 at pH 7.4, or as phosphate complexed with sodium, calcium, or magnesium.

The terms *phosphorus concentration* and *phosphate concentration* are often used interchangeably, and for clinical purposes the choice matters little. It is phosphorus in the form of the phosphate ion that circulates in blood, is filtered by the glomerulus, and is transported across plasma membranes. However, the content of phosphate in plasma, urine, tissue, or foodstuffs is measured and expressed in terms of the amount of elemental phosphorus contained in the specimen, hence use of the term *phosphorus concentration.*

In healthy subjects ingesting typical diets, the serum phosphorus concentration exhibits a circadian rhythm, characterized by a decrease to a nadir just before noon, an increase to a plateau in late afternoon, and a small further increase to a peak shortly after midnight (Table 1) (4,17). The amplitude (nadir to peak) is approximately 1.2 mg/dL, or 30% of the 24-hr mean level. Increases or decreases in dietary intake of phosphorus induce substantial increases or decreases, respectively, in serum phosphorus levels during late morning, afternoon, and evening, but less or no change in morning fasting phosphorus levels (17). To minimize the effect of dietary phosphorus on the serum phosphorus concentration, specimens for analysis should be obtained in the morning in the fasting state. Specimens obtained in the afternoon are more likely to be affected by diet; they may be more useful in monitoring the effect of changes in dietary phosphorus on serum levels of phosphorus, as in patients with renal insufficiency receiving phosphorus binders to suppress secondary hyperparathyroidism. With administration of aluminum hydroxide, a phosphorus binding agent, a decrease in morning fasting phosphorus levels can underestimate the severity of hypophosphatemia that exists throughout much of the day (17,18).

Factors other than time of day and diet can affect the serum phosphorus concentration. Presumably by inducing movement of phosphorus into the cell, a decrease in phosphorus concentration can be acutely induced by intravenous infusion of glucose or insulin, ingestion of carbohydrate-rich meals, acute respiratory alkalosis, and infusion or endogenous release of epinephrine. The decrease in phosphorus concentration induced by acute respiratory alkalosis can be as great as 2.0 mg/dL (19). Serum phosphorus concentration can be acutely increased by metabolic acidosis and by intravenous infusion of calcium, the latter presumably because of the efflux of inorganic phosphate from red blood cells (20).

There are substantial effects of age on the fasting serum concentration of phosphorus. Phosphorus levels are high in infants, ranging from 4.8 to 7.4 mg/dL (mean 6.2 mg/dL) in the first 3 months of life, and decreasing to 4.5 to 5.8 mg/dL (mean 5.0 mg/dL) at age 1 to 2 years (21). In mid-childhood, values range from 3.5 to 5.5 mg/dL (mean 4.4 mg/dL) and decrease to adult values by late adolescence (8,9,22). In adult men, serum phosphorus levels decrease with age from about 3.5 mg/dL at age 20, to 3.0 mg/dL at age 70 (7,22). In women, the values are similar to those of men until after the menopause, when they increase slightly from about 3.4 mg/dL at age 50 to 3.7 mg/dL at age 70.

The normal range for serum phosphorus concentration is laboratory specific. Phosphorus concentration is most commonly determined using automated spectrophotometric techniques based on the reaction of phosphate ions with molybdate (10). In men, representative normal ranges are 2.5 to 4.5 mg/dL at age 20, 2.3 to 4.1 mg/dL at age 50, and 2.2 to 4.0 mg/dL at age 70. In women, representative normal ranges are 2.7 to 4.4 mg/dL at age 50 and 2.9 to 4.8 mg/dL at age 70 (Table 2).

Phosphorus concentrations should be determined in serum or plasma that has been separated promptly from red blood cells. Prolonged standing or hemolysis of the specimen can lead to a spurious increase in phosphorus concentration. Concentrations of phosphorus expressed as mg/dL can be converted to mmol/L by dividing by 3.1. (The atomic weight of phosphorus is 30.98.) Because plasma phosphate is a mixture of monovalent and divalent ions, the composite valence of phosphorus in serum (or intravenous solutions) at pH 7.4 is 1.8. At this pH, 1 mmol phosphorus is equal to 1.8 mEq.

SERUM MAGNESIUM CONCENTRATION

As is the case for calcium, magnesium exists in serum in three distinct forms, protein-bound magnesium (30%), which is not ultrafilterable, and ionized (55%) and complexed (15%) magnesium, which are ultrafilterable (15). Magnesium is bound principally to albumin in a pH-dependent manner similar to that of calcium. Ionized magnesium is the fraction that is important for physiologic processes, including neuromuscular transmission and cardiovascular tone. Measurement of ionized magnesium concentration is rarely available, and for most clinical purposes, the total concentration of magnesium in serum is determined. Most laboratories use automated spectrophotometric techniques; the reference method is atomic absorption spectrophotometry (10).

The serum concentration of magnesium is closely maintained within the narrow range of 1.7 to 2.6 mg/dL. There are no significant differences in magnesium concentration between men and women, nor with respect to age, and values in children are similar to those in adults (Table 2). The circadian variation in magnesium concentration is of low amplitude and not clinically significant.

Prolonged standing or hemolysis of the specimen can lead to a spurious increases in serum magnesium concentration. Concentrations expressed as mg/dL can be converted to mmol/L by dividing by 2.4, and to mEq/L by dividing by 1.2. (The atomic weight of magnesium is 24.31.)

REFERENCES

1. Moore EW: Ionized calcium in normal serum, ultrafiltrates, and whole blood determined by ion-exchange electrodes. *J Clin Invest* 49:318–334, 1970
2. Ladenson JH, Lewis JW, Boyd JC: Failure of total calcium corrected for protein, albumin, and pH to correctly assess free calcium status. *J Clin Endocrinol Metab* 46:986–993, 1978
3. Payne RB, Little AJ, Williams RB, Milner JR: Interpretation of serum calcium in patients with abnormal serum proteins. *Br Med J* 4:643–646, 1973
4. Markowitz M, Rotkin L, Rosen JF: Circadian rhythms of blood minerals in humans. *Science* 213:672–674, 1981
5. Halloran BP, Portale AA, Castro M, Morris RC Jr, Goldsmith

RS: Serum concentration of 1,25-dihydroxyvitamin D in the human: Diurnal variation. *J Clin Endocrinol Metab* 60:1104–1110, 1985

6. Jubiz W, Canterbury JM, Reiss E, Tyler FH: Circadian rhythm in serum parathyroid hormone concentration in human subjects: Correlation with serum calcium, phosphate, albumin, and growth hormone levels. *J Clin Invest* 51:2040–2046, 1972

7. Keating FR Jr, Jones JD, Elveback LR, Randall RV: The relation of age and sex to distribution of values in healthy adults of serum calcium, inorganic phosphorus, magnesium, alkaline phosphatase, total proteins, albumin, and blood urea. *J Lab Clin Med* 73:825–834, 1969

8. Arnaud SB, Goldsmith RS, Stickler GB, McCall JT, Arnaud CD: Serum parathyroid hormone and blood minerals: Interrelationships in normal children. *Pediatr Res* 7:485–493, 1973

9. Burritt MF, Slockbower JM, Forman RW, Offord KP, Bergstralh EJ, Smithson WA: Pediatric reference intervals for 19 biologic variables in healthy children. *Mayo Clin Proc* 65:329–336, 1990.

10. Pesce AJ, Kaplan LA (eds) *Methods in Clinical Chemistry.* CV Mosby, St. Louis, 1987

11. Bowers GN, Brassard C, Sena S: Measurement of ionized calcium in serum with ion-selective electrodes: A mature technology that can meet the daily service needs. *Clin Chem* 32:1437–1447, 1986

12. Loughead JL, Mimouni F, Tsang RC: Serum ionized calcium concentrations in normal neonates. *Am J Dis Child* 142:516–518, 1988

13. Nelson N, Finnstrom O, Larsson L: Neonatal reference values for ionized calcium, phosphate and magnesium. Selection of reference population by optimality criteria. *Scand J Clin Lab Invest* 47:111–117, 1987

14. Specker BL, Lichtenstein P, Mimouni F, Gormley C, Tsang RC: Calcium-regulating hormones and minerals from birth to 18 months of age: A cross-sectional study. II. Effects of sex, race, age, season, and diet on serum minerals, parathyroid hormone, and calcitonin. *Pediatrics* 77:891–896, 1986

15. Boink ABTJ, Buckley BM, Christiansen TF, Covington AK, Maas AHJ, Muller-Plathe O, Sachs C, Siggaard-Andersen O: IFCC recommendation: Recommendation on sampling, transport and storage for the determination of the concentration of ionized calcium in whole blood, plasma and serum. *Clin Chim Acta* 202: S13–S22, 1991

16. Marshall RW: Plasma fractions. In: Nordin BEC (ed) *Calcium, Phosphate and Magnesium Metabolism.* Churchill Livingston, London, pp 162–185, 1976

17. Portale AA, Halloran BP, Morris RC Jr: Dietary intake of phosphorus modulates the circadian rhythm in serum concentration of phosphorus: Implications for the renal production of 1,25dihydroxyvitamin D. *J Clin Invest* 80:1147–1154, 1987

18. Cam JM, Luck VA, Eastwood JB, de Wardener HE: The effect of aluminum hydroxide orally on calcium, phosphorus and aluminum metabolism in normal subjects. *Clin Sci Mol Med* 51:407–414, 1976

19. Mostellar ME, Tuttle EP: Effects of alkalosis on plasma concentration and urinary excretion of inorganic phosphate in man. *J Clin Invest* 43:138–149, 1964

20. Peraino RA, Suki WN: Influence of calcium on renal handling of phosphate. In: Massry SG, Fleisch H (eds) *Renal handling of phosphate.* Plenum, New York, pp 287–306, 1980

21. Brodehl J, Gellissen K, Weber HP: Postnatal development of tubular phosphate reabsorption. *Clin Nephrol* 17:163–171, 1982

22. Greenberg BG, Winters RW, Graham JB: The normal range of serum inorganic phosphorus and its utility as discriminant in the diagnosis of congenital hypophosphatemia. *J Clin Endocrinol Metab* 20:364–379, 1960

23. Meites S (ed) *Pediatric Clinical Chemistry.* The American Association for Clinical Chemistry, Washington, 1981

17. Parathyroid Hormone and Calcitonin

Lawrence E. Mallette, M.D., Ph.D., and *Robert F. Gagel, M.D.

Division of Endocrinology and Metabolism, Baylor College of Medicine, Houston, Texas
Section of Endocrine Neoplasia and Hormonal Disorders, University of Texas, M. D. Anderson Cancer Center, Houston, Texas

PARATHYROID HORMONE

Bedside clinical acumen can confirm the diagnosis of primary hyperparathyroidism with perhaps 95% certainty. Routine laboratory findings, such as elevated serum chloride values or radiographic visualization of subperiosteal bone resorption, can support the diagnosis, but these changes are either nonspecific or rare. Measurement of parathyroid hormone (PTH) in serum is the rational way to confirm the diagnosis. The ability to accurately measure circulating PTH has simplified the evaluation of this and other disorders of calcium metabolism.

To arrive at a diagnosis of presumptive primary hyperparathyroidism in the days before PTH could be measured, it was considered appropriate to exclude occult malignancy with numerous radiographic examinations, and perhaps to exclude granulomatous disease by administering a brief course of glucocorticoid. Today, when the serum PTH value is elevated in a well-validated assay, these other steps can usually be omitted. Ectopic production of authentic PTH does occur, but it is very rare and usually arises in a clinically obvious malignancy.

The improvements in PTH measurement methods over the last 20 years have arisen because of increased sensitivity and specificity of radioimmunoassay (RIA) and the adoption of techniques in addition to the RIA. This section will outline the basics of PTH secretion and catabolism as they apply to hormone measurement, review the methods currently available for PTH assay, discuss a few clinical situations in which PTH measurement may be useful, and make suggestions for timing of sampling to enhance diagnostic discrimination.

Background: PTH Secretion and Catabolism

The chief biologically active secretory form of PTH is an 84-amino-acid straight-chain polypeptide (1). Several quirks of PTH physiology complicated the task of developing an adequate immunological assay for PTH (Table 1). The first problem was that the hormone circulates at low

TABLE 1. *Facts about parathyroid hormone that made assay difficult*

Short circulating half-life with low circulating levels
Extensive catabolism with long-lived non-calcemic products
Multiple antigenic epitopes in the molecule

concentrations, the normal range for the intact PTH molecule being approximately 10 to 55 ng/L (1 to 5 pmol/L) (2,3). The intact, biologically active hormone has a short half-life (2 to 4 min), which helps account for its low concentration in serum (2). It is cleared by the kidney and liver (4,5).

The second problem was that PTH undergoes extensive catabolism, both in the parathyroid cell (before secretion) and in the liver. Some of the catabolic products enter the circulation and have a relatively long half-life in serum, accumulating to a level that is 5 to 20 times higher than that of the intact hormone. These catabolic products are missing the amino-terminal 27-amino-acid sequence of

intact PTH (5–7) that accounts for its hypercalcemic, hypocalciuric, and phosphaturic activities (8). The presence of these hormone fragments in serum tends to interfere with the immunologic measurement of the intact hormone (9).

In a simplified view, serum contains two classes of PTH fragments, those of hepatic origin and those of parathyroid gland origin (Fig. 1). The hepatic fragments are formed when enzymes on the surface of the Kupffer cells cleave the hormone at four sites in its 34–43 region (5). The amino-terminal fragment (that might have biologic activity) is either degraded within the liver or cleared rapidly from the circulation and is present only at vanishingly low concentrations in normal serum (10). The other class of PTH fragments, arising from the parathyroid cell itself, are abbreviated at each end of the molecule—they do not react in assays specific for either the 1–34 or 65–84 region (11). The amino-terminal fragment is degraded within the parathyroid cell and not secreted in significant amounts. At high calcium concentrations, the parathyroid cell suppresses the secretion of intact PTH to near zero, but PTH

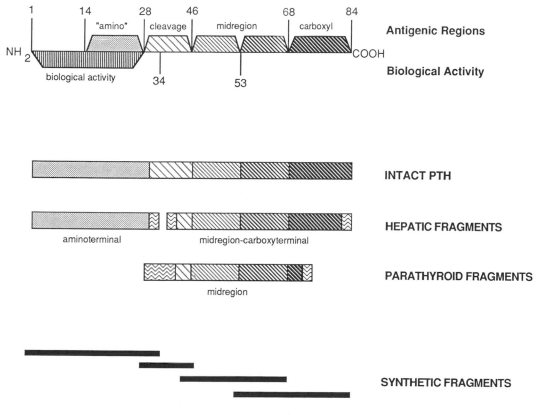

FIG. 1. Stylized diagram of antigenic and functional regions in the PTH molecule, circulating peptide fragments of the hormone, and available synthetic peptide fragments of PTH. Five antigenic regions may be differentiated **(top panel)**. Assays specific for each region have been developed. Biologic activity requires a major portion of the 1–28 region, but antibodies recognizing this region usually react with the more antigenic 14–28 portion. Four types of PTH peptides are present in serum **(middle panels)**, but the concentration of amino-terminal fragment in serum is very low. Wavy segments in the fragments indicate regions of uncertain or variable length. Four synthetic peptide fragments (*straight lines* in **bottom panel**) are widely available for establishing specificity or for use as radioligands.

fragments continue to be released (12,13) and are detectable in the serum of patients with nonparathyroid forms of hypercalcemia (14). Both classes of PTH fragments are cleared by the kidney and will accumulate in subjects with renal insufficiency.

The third quirk of nature that complicated measurement of PTH was the fact that the intact PTH molecule is large enough to possess at least five different antigenic epitopes (9). Antisera generated against the intact PTH molecule will contain several species of antibodies, each recognizing a different region of the molecule (Fig. 1). Different antisera will have different amounts of antibody for each epitope, each having its own affinity for that epitope.

These three problems made it advantageous to develop RIAs specific for a single epitope (or region) within the PTH molecule, to allow selection of a very high-affinity antibody species, and to simplify assay kinetics, as well as to develop later an assay that detects only molecules bearing two widely spaced epitopes (i.e., one that detects only the intact PTH molecule).

Measurement Methods

Two techniques for the measurement of PTH are currently widely available, the traditional RIA and the two-site immunologic assays, of which the most widely used is the immunoradiometric assay (IRMA). The RIA method uses an antibody against the target molecule and a radiolabeled version of the target molecule, called the radioligand or tracer (Fig. 2). Antibody and tracer are included in precisely the same amount (concentration) in every tube in the assay run, whereas the amount of unlabeled target molecule (added in the unknown sample or standard sample) varies from tube to tube. Tracer and unlabeled target molecules compete for binding to the antibody: higher concentrations of unlabeled target molecule cause less radioligand to be bound to the antibody. Measurement of the

fraction of tracer bound to antibody thus provides an estimate of the amount of unlabeled target molecule.

Early RIAs for human PTH were often not sensitive enough to detect normal levels of the hormone. Insufficient sensitivity made it impossible to discriminate low from normal PTH values and blurred the discrimination between normal and modestly elevated values. Newer reagents for RIA were developed to provide sufficient sensitivity: antibodies of higher affinity were generated using human PTH as antigen, rather than the heterologous PTHs (bovine or porcine) that had been used earlier (15–17). Fragments of PTH (Fig. 1) were synthesized for use as tracers (as well as to help determine regional specificity of the assay) (8). Unlike the native PTH-(1–84) molecule originally used as tracer, these fragments are relatively stable and show little nonspecific binding to serum proteins (18). Furthermore, their use as tracer establishes assay specificity by allowing only antibodies that recognize their epitope to participate in the assay.

Region-specific PTH RIAs of three types have been most widely used: the amino-terminal, midregion, and carboxy-terminal assays. Amino-terminal assays essentially detect only the intact hormone in serum, but these have mostly been supplanted by the more sensitive two-site assays for intact PTH, discussed below.

Midregion-specific RIAs employ PTH-(44–68) (tagged with tyrosine at position 43 to allow radioiodination) as radioligand. Depending on the anti-PTH antibody used, the assay may recognize the 44–53 region, the 53–68 region, or both (Fig. 1), but the distinction is clinically unimportant, because measurements with 44–53-specific and 53–68-specific assays correlate well on direct comparison (19). Midregion assays often have the advantage of great sensitivity. Those with the best sensitivity can distinguish even among varying degrees of hypoparathyroidism (20). Assay sensitivity is, of course, a property separate from specificity: sensitivity is determined by antibody–ligand affinity and tracer specific activity, whereas specificity is a function of the epi-

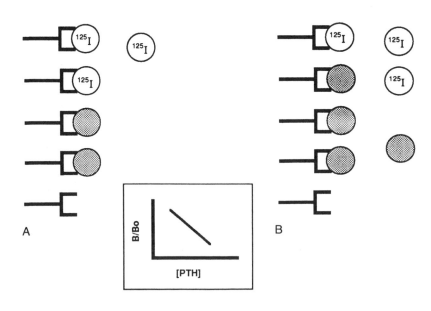

FIG. 2. Radioimmunoassay for PTH. Antibody *(stick figures)* and ^{125}I-labeled PTH fragment *(light circles)* are present at a constant concentration in each assay tube. Variable concentrations of unlabeled PTH *(dark circles)* compete with labeled PTH for binding to the available antibody sites. Moving from a lower concentration of unlabeled PTH **(A)** to a higher concentration **(B)** diminishes the number of counts bound to antibody **(inset)**. B/Bo, counts bound to antibody in the presence of the unknown or standard amount of unlabeled PTH, divided by antibody-bound counts without added unlabeled PTH.

tope being recognized. Midregion-specific assays that use lower-affinity antibodies may not be sensitive enough to discriminate low levels of PTH.

The ability of midregion-specific PTH assays to detect all three quantitatively important circulating PTH species, including the fragments of parathyroid origin, can offer one advantage. Some parathyroid adenomas release large amounts of PTH fragments relative to intact hormone (11), in which case the midregion PTH value will be more elevated than the intact PTH value.

Carboxy-terminal-specific assays, which detect the 69–84 region, perform differently from midregion-specific assays. They do not detect the PTH fragments of parathyroid origin. Thus they give lower values for total immunoreactivity and are not as useful for diagnosis of the parathyroid adenoma or for venous sampling studies for parathyroid tumor localization.

Terms indicating midregion and carboxy-terminal specificity, however, have sometimes been loosely applied. Certain midregion-specific assays (detecting only the 44–68 epitopes) have been named *midmolecule–carboxy-terminal* assays, a term that should imply recognition of the entire 44–84 region. Readers of the older literature should also be aware that RIAs originally were termed *carboxy-terminal specific* if they failed to detect synthetic PTH-(1–34), which for several years was the only synthetic PTH fragment available for testing. Some of the more useful of these assays were later found in fact to be midregion specific (21,22).

The development of two-site immunological assays allowed for the first time the specific measurement of the intact PTH molecule (3,23). This type of assay uses two different anti-PTH antibodies (or antibody pools), each recognizing epitopes in a separate region of the intact PTH molecule (Fig. 3). One antibody is bound to a solid phase to extract (capture) PTH from the serum sample. The second antibody is labeled and is used as a "probe" to detect captured molecules that bear both epitopes. Hormone fragments will not bind to both antibodies and will not be detected (Fig. 3).

In practice, the capture antibody is often a pool of antibodies against epitopes in the 44–84 region. Capture antibodies reading this region must be present in great excess so that their binding sites will not be swamped by the high levels of PTH fragments that are present in some serum samples (especially from renal failure patients), with a resulting failure to capture all of the intact PTH. The probe antibody is then directed against epitopes in the 1–33 region. Because antibody molecules are much larger than PTH itself, each probe antibody molecule can be radiolabeled at more than one site; this "hotter" labeling is one factor that enhances the sensitivity of the IRMA relative to the RIA.

Other methods have been described for measurement of PTH in serum. Two-site assays that use a probe antibody linked to an enzyme that can later generate a colored or fluorescent molecule have been developed (10) and will probably see greater use in the future as isotope technology becomes more expensive. Bioassays have been an invaluable research tool (2,24), but they are unlikely ever to be used routinely for clinical diagnosis, because adequate sensitivity requires the use of tissue slices and quantitative histochemical techniques.

Criteria for an Adequate PTH Assay

Several criteria define an adequate PTH assay. It should be sensitive enough to discriminate almost completely between normal subjects and patients with total hypoparathyroidism (denoted clinically by the requirement for the equivalent of at least 50,000 U/day of vitamin D to maintain adequate serum calcium values) (14). Between-assay and within-assay coefficients of variance should be below 10%, and samples should be run at least in duplicate.

Certain controls are necessary for PTH RIAs. A panel of sera from totally hypoparathyroid individuals should be included in each assay run to help define the zero value and detection limit (25). Assay buffer cannot be used for the zero reference, because nonspecific effects of serum proteins to decrease tracer binding will be interpreted as representing PTH immunoreactivity, thereby giving too high a normal range. Samples should also be assayed at two or more dilutions, to help in detecting false positives, which fail to "dilute out" in parallel with the standard curve. Up to 1% to 2% of human sera may produce such false-positive results in some RIAs (26). Multiple dilutions are not critical for the PTH IRMA.

The laboratory performing the assay should routinely provide the following information with their reports: the precise regional specificity of the assay, the expected ranges for totally hypoparathyroid patients and normal subjects, assay precision, and number of replicates and dilutions performed. Failure to follow these guidelines and to provide normative information in the past has led to false-positive or false-negative diagnoses.

Units

PTH assay results need not be expressed in SI units. PTH RIAs, even those with well-defined regional specificity, detect a mixture of peptides of varying molecular weight in serum. Thus, expression of results in molar units (pmol/L) is not appropriate. Results are often expressed in arbitrary units (μL-Eq or ng-Eq of an in-house standard, for example). Comparison of results between laboratories may be facilitated if the in-house standard is calibrated against the World Health Organization International Research Standard for Human Parathyroid Hormone for Immunoassay (27), with assay results expressed in units of ng-Eq/L. It is more appropriate to express the results of two-site assays for intact PTH in molar units, but there is still uncertainty about whether all species of PTH being measured have full biologic potency, because cleavage of even a single amino acid from the amino-terminal end of PTH will greatly reduce its biologic activity.

Influence of Renal Function on PTH Assay Results

Fragments of PTH are cleared largely by glomerular filtration. Midregion and carboxy-terminal RIAs are therefore sensitive to renal function. Glomerular filtration rates below 40 ml/min will cause an increase in midregion PTH values, even before significant parathyroid hyperplasia is thought to occur. Midregion PTH values also increase with aging, largely a result of the declining glomerular filtration rate,

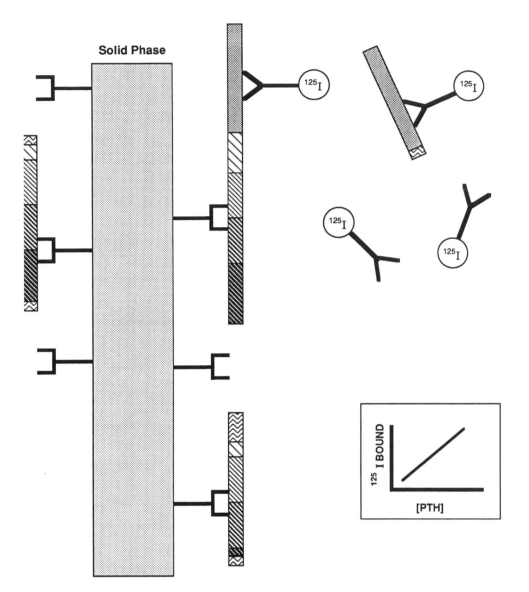

Solid Phase

FIG. 3. Two-site immunoradiometric assay for PTH. The capture antibody *(U-shaped stick figures)* is bound to a solid phase (plastic bead or test-tube wall) and is used to extract PTH from the serum sample. In this example, the capture antibody is midregion specific and captures the three types of PTH peptides. Intact PTH is completely captured, but an excess of unoccupied capture antibody remains. The bound intact PTH is the only captured species that will bind the ^{125}I-labeled "signal antibody" (amino-terminal specific in this example) *(Y-shaped stick figures)*. Any amino-terminal PTH fragments that are present will also bind the ^{125}I-labeled antibody, but they will be washed away when the solid phase is rinsed before counting. The number of counts bound to the solid phase after washing increases in direct proportion to the amount of intact PTH in the sample **(insert)**. Parathyroid hormone regions are coded here as in Fig. 1.

although a slight increase in parathyroid function may accompany aging (28).

Intact PTH is cleared in the kidney by peritubular uptake, a process that is better preserved during progressive renal failure than is glomerular filtration (4). Hepatic clearance of intact PTH also continues in renal insufficiency. For these reasons, intact PTH levels are less sensitive to declining glomerular filtration rates than are the values from midregion and carboxy-terminal assays that read hormone fragments. Renal failure does, however, prolong the half-life of bioactive PTH by a factor of roughly two (2), and it has been

shown that, in the first few minutes after parathyroidectomy, intact PTH values may fall less rapidly in those with renal insufficiency (29).

Specific Uses of PTH Assays

Differential Diagnosis of Hypercalcemia

Either type of PTH assay may be used for initial diagnosis, with the other performed selectively to confirm equivocal or unexpected results or to resolve diagnostic problems. The two-site assay for intact PTH is now run as the first choice in many centers, because of its relative independence of renal function and because it is easier to standardize and keep stable and is available as a reliable kit for local laboratory use.

PTH assays can help differentiate primary hyperparathyroidism from other (nonparathyroid-mediated) forms of hypercalcemia, such as malignancy, sarcoidosis, and thyrotoxicosis. Approximately 95% of patients with primary hyperparathyroidism have elevated values as measured with an adequate midregion-specific assay (14,21). The percentage with elevations in the two-site assay for intact PTH may be slightly less (30), perhaps because fragments are not being detected and perhaps because the upper limit of normal for intact PTH may be harder to define because of pulsatile hormone secretion (see later).

In patients with nonparathyroid hypercalcemia, midregion PTH values are depressed by 20% to 40%, but significant immunoreactivity is still detectable in the serum of 50% to 70% of the subjects (relative to hypoparathyroid subjects) (14,21). This immunoreactivity is thought to be derived from the parathyroid cell itself, which continues to release PTH fragments even at high ambient calcium concentrations (12,13). If the patient with nonparathyroid hypercalcemia also has significant renal insufficiency (creatinine clearance below 40 ml/min), these PTH fragments will accumulate and can even increase the midregion PTH value above the usual upper limit of normal (14). This increase will, of course, be far less than shown by a hyperparathyroid patient with the same degrees of hypercalcemia and renal dysfunction. Nevertheless, to avoid confusion, the assay for intact PTH should be used when serum creatinine values are above approximately 2.0 mg/dl.

Intact PTH values by IRMA are suppressed below the normal range in 70% to 80% of patients with nonparathyroid hypercalcemia and are in the lower half of the normal range in the remainder. In a group of 52 patients with malignancy hypercalcemia, all PTH values were below 25 pg/ml in an assay with an upper limit of normal of 55 pg/ml (31). This greater suppression in nonparathyroid hypercalcemias makes up for the slightly lower incidence of elevated values in primary hyperparathyroidism, and it produces a separation between diagnostic groups that is every bit as good as for the midregion assay. Decreased renal function in nonparathyroid hypercalcemia patients probably does have a small effect on the intact PTH value. In our hypercalcemic cancer patients, intact PTH values between 18 pg/ml and 25 pg/ml were associated with significant renal insufficiency (31).

Differential Diagnosis of Hypocalcemia

Measurement of PTH with either type of assay may help establish the cause of hypocalcemia. The PTH value should be undetectable in total hypoparathyroidism, but it may lie within the normal range if there is only a partial loss or inhibition of parathyroid function (partial hypoparathyroidism or magnesium deficiency, for example). The PTH value will be increased in pseudohypoparathyroidism, but one must be certain that an elevated PTH RIA value is not the result of interfering substances in patient serum, as discussed. Confirmation with more than one assay type is wise. The discrimination of type I from type II pseudohypoparathyroidism, of course, requires study of the phosphaturic and cyclic adenosine monophosphate (cAMP) excretory responses to infusion of synthetic PTH-(1–34) (32) (see Appendix vii).

Measurement of PTH can detect mild degrees of secondary hyperparathyroidism and is useful in situations that predispose to a deficiency of vitamin D or its action (intestinal malabsorption, dietary–environmental vitamin deficiency, resistance to vitamin D action). Serum 25-hydroxyvitamin D measurements can also be of value (see Chapter 19), but they may be a less sensitive means of detecting mild vitamin deficiency (28). PTH values can also be used to monitor the adequacy of treatment of secondary hyperparathyroidism. In mild degrees of secondary hyperparathyroidism, without overt hypocalcemia, the PTH value should return to normal with a few days of adequate treatment. If the deficiency of vitamin D action is chronic or severe enough to have caused symptomatic hypocalcemia, however, the PTH values may be markedly elevated (a reflection of parathyroid hyperplasia) and may take several weeks to return to normal after normocalcemia is restored (33).

Evaluation of Renal Osteodystrophy

One of the goals of managing patients in renal failure is to minimize the rate of parathyroid growth. A midregion PTH RIA may be used to assess the degree of parathyroid hyperfunction in renal failure once the assay system has been clinically validated in a set of patients well characterized as to severity of hyperparathyroid bone disease. One such assay was shown to give values from four- to 40-fold elevated in renal patients first entering dialysis and without clinical evidence of bone disease, whereas hemodialysis patients with radiographic and clinical evidence of significant hyperparathyroid bone disease showed values from 60- to 600-fold above normal (14). Hemodialysis patients with hypercalcemia not related to parathyroid hyperfunction showed midregion PTH values "only" four- to 20-fold elevated. In contrast, hemodialysis patients with autonomous (tertiary) hyperparathyroidism showed values more than 40-fold elevated.

The two-site assay for intact PTH can provide similar information, although the magnitude of the elevation of the intact PTH value will be much less for any degree of parathyroid hyperfunction, because the accumulating PTH fragments are not detected. Intact PTH values, however, show a greater day-to-day and minute-to-minute fluctuation than do midregion PTH values. Intact PTH values change quickly after a change in serum calcium concentration, and serum calcium fluctuates widely in renal failure patients as a result of changes in phosphate and calcium balance between and during dialyses. For example, intact PTH values have been shown to fall rapidly as serum calcium rises during hemodialysis (34). Values above 300 pg/mL are often associated with hyperparathyroid bone disease.

Use in Other Metabolic Bone Diseases

Measurement of PTH is indicated in other metabolic bone diseases. Patients with Paget's disease who develop primary or secondary hyperparathyroidism have an accelerated course of their bone disease, presumably because the pagetoid bone cells remain responsive to the effects of PTH. Furthermore, the incidence of hyperparathyroidism may be above 10% in Paget's disease (35). It thus may be wise to screen patients with symptomatic Paget's disease for occult hyperparathyroidism by measurement of PTH.

Measurement of PTH may also be useful in the assessment of normocalcemic hypophosphatemia. In the hereditary form of hypophosphatemic rickets/osteomalacia, serum PTH values are usually normal unless treatment with neutral phosphate has been instituted. Other forms of hypophosphatemia, however, may show parathyroid hyperfunction. Patients with mild vitamin D deficiency may present with hypophosphatemia and a slightly reduced but still normal serum calcium value, yet show a significant increase in PTH. Patients with the syndrome of hypophosphatemia related to prostate carcinoma or other malignancies show low serum 1,25-dihydroxyvitamin D values and may show increased PTH values. In the rare syndrome of masked primary hyperparathyroidism, a parathyroid adenoma is present but is unable to cause hypercalcemia because of concomitant vitamin D deficiency. These patients usually present with hypophosphatemia, elevated serum alkaline phosphatase values, bone pain, and markedly elevated PTH values. Their serum calcium values are, by definition, within or below the normal range.

Timing of the Sample: Influence of Ultradian Variation, Episodic Secretion, and Other Factors on PTH Assay Results

Secretion of PTH occurs episodically in normal subjects, with small secretory peaks of the intact hormone occurring several times a day and lasting several minutes. Because a normal range is presumably defined by a set of samples randomly obtained, episodic secretion makes the upper limit of normal for the intact PTH assay more difficult to define. An unexpectedly high intact PTH value in a normocalcemic subject should therefore be verified by obtaining a second sample or by measuring midregion PTH in the first sample. The midregion assay, because of the longer half-life of the peptides it detects, tends to integrate these secretory bursts over time and shows less minute-to-minute variation than does an assay for intact PTH.

When possible, midregion PTH values for diagnosis should be obtained before 1100 hr. In some normal subjects, midregion PTH values increase in the afternoon, the rise often beginning between 1130 and 1300 hr (36). Thus, a wider normal range must be used for afternoon samples, with the upper limit increased by perhaps 33%. An even greater increase in PTH values may occur at night (21), and nocturnal samples are not recommended for diagnosis. Fasting morning samples are also preferred for intact PTH measurements.

Like normal parathyroid glands, most parathyroid adenomas vary their secretion of PTH as an inverse function of the ambient serum calcium value. This fact can be used

to enhance the diagnostic discrimination of PTH assays. Values for PTH in those with primary hyperparathyroidism will often be higher if the sample is obtained after serum calcium has been lowered a bit (but not into the normal range) by the initial treatment (by dietary calcium restriction or hydration, for example). These maneuvers are unlikely ever to increase PTH values above normal in those with nonparathyroid forms of hypercalcemia, because they will not lower serum calcium into the normal range or below.

In hypocalcemic conditions, the differentiation of secondary hyperparathyroidism (vitamin D deficiency and pseudohypoparathyroidism) from hypoparathyroidism is enhanced if the PTH value is measured before treatment is instituted (33). Treatment of secondary hyperparathyroidism with calcium and/or vitamin D will tend to lower the PTH value, lessening the diagnostic separation between groups. In hypomagnesemic hypocalcemia, PTH values will increase within minutes after parenteral magnesium administration, a change that can be used to confirm the diagnosis of hypomagnesemia-induced parathyroid dysfunction.

For monitoring of renal failure patients, the optimal timing of intact PTH samples in relationship to hemodialysis has not been determined. Values obtained before dialysis might reflect the maximum hypocalcemic stress on the parathyroid glands, whereas values taken after dialysis when serum calcium has increased might give an estimate of parathyroid suppressibility. More study of this question is needed, but a consistent policy should probably be adopted at each unit for the timing of samples for long-term monitoring.

CALCITONIN MEASUREMENT

Measurement Methods

Measurement of serum calcitonin is useful in several clinical situations. It is the primary diagnostic tool for diagnosis of medullary thyroid carcinoma (37) and may be useful for diagnosis of other tumors in which ectopic production of calcitonin is observed (38). Serum calcitonin measurement has not proven diagnostically useful for any bone disease, although abnormalities of calcitonin secretion have been reported in Williams syndrome. It is now possible to measure normal circulating concentrations of calcitonin by utilizing one of several methods.

The first method is a standard RIA utilizing polyclonal antisera raised by injection of synthetic human calcitonin into rabbits (39–42) or goats (17). The sensitivity of these assays varies considerably, with the more sensitive assays capable of detecting normal circulating concentrations of calcitonin (2 to 10 pg/ml). Commercial kits are available that rival the sensitivity of the best research assays.

A second method utilizes a concentration technique. Calcitonin and other small peptides are adsorbed by passage of 10 to 50 ml of serum through a silica cartridge. The peptides are then eluted from the column. The eluate is dried and diluted in a small volume of assay buffer, to be assayed in a sensitive standard RIA (43–46). The advan-

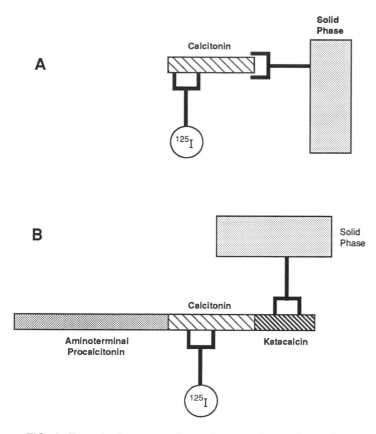

FIG. 4. Two-site immunoradiometric assay for calcitonin **(A)** or procalcitonin **(B)**. Calcitonin is extracted by antibody bound to a solid phase. This antibody recognizes an antigenic site that is present only after cleavage of the carboxyl-flanking peptide of the procalcitonin molecule (katacalcin), so procalcitonin is not extracted. The bound calcitonin is then quantitated with a second antibody labeled with ^{125}I. The assay for procalcitonin utilizes an extracting antibody against katacalcin and a labeled antibody against calcitonin.

tages of this technique include sensitivity (detection limit of 0.5 pg/ml) and elimination of other substances present in serum that may cause a false-positive elevation of the serum calcitonin (44). Disadvantages include the requirement for concentration of each sample and the exclusion of high-molecular-weight forms of calcitonin (procalcitonin) produced by lung carcinomas and other tumors (44,45,47, 48).

A third method for calcitonin measurement is the two-site IRMA, which uses affinity-purified polyclonal antibodies directed against two epitopes within the calcitonin monomer (49,50) to provide a specific and sensitive (10 pg/ml) assay for calcitonin monomer (Fig. 4). A similar technique has been applied to the development of a colorimetric ELISA for calcitonin using monoclonal antibodies (51). A two-site IRMA with specificity only for procalcitonin has also been developed (52). Its antisera are directed against an epitope in the sequence for calcitonin monomer and a second in the flanking region of calcitonin (katacalcin or carboxy-terminal-adjacent peptide) (Fig. 4). From the available reports, the sensitivity of the IRMA and ELISA techniques for calci-

tonin is less than that of the RIA or the concentration RIA, but no direct comparative studies have been performed. Chemiluminescent assays with even greater sensitivity are under development.

Specific Uses of Calcitonin Assays

Measurement of serum calcitonin is most frequently used for the diagnosis and management of medullary thyroid carcinoma. The best diagnostic accuracy is provided by use of a provocative stimulation technique such as the pentagastrin test (37,46,53) (Fig. 5), the combined calcium-pentagastrin test (54), or the short calcium infusion (see Appendix vii) (39). Interpretation of calcitonin values from these tests is usually straightforward. There are, however, diagnostic pitfalls. In 1% to 5% of tests, measurement of calcitonin with a standard RIA will give an elevated basal serum calcitonin with no additional increase after the provocative stimulation (Fig. 5) (37,44). This type of result is consistent with three possible explanations. First, the elevated serum calcitonin may represent a nonspecific RIA result. Such false-positive test results are usually assay specific, and re-assay of the samples with an RIA using a different antiserum or by the concentration technique will usually yield a normal result. A second possibility is that the elevated value represents a higher-molecular-weight form of calcitonin, ectopically produced by a tumor other than a medullary thyroid carcinoma; release of calcitonin from such tumors may not be increased by calcium or pentagastrin (38). A third, but rare, possibility is calcitonin production by a medullary thyroid carcinoma that responds poorly to a provocative stimulus.

The identification of mutations of the *RET* proto-oncogene that are causative for multiple endocrine neoplasia

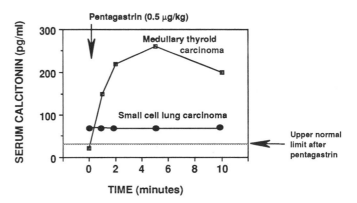

FIG. 5. Pentagastrin test for diagnosis of medullary carcinoma of the thyroid. Pentagastrin was injected intravenously, and serum calcitonin was measured by a standard calcitonin RIA at the indicated time points (see Appendix vii). The upper limit of normal after pentagastrin stimulation is indicated. The result with higher calcitonin values is consistent with C-cell hyperplasia or microscopic medullary thyroid carcinoma, whereas the elevated basal value with a flat response is consistent either with the ectopic production of calcitonin by a malignancy such as small-cell carcinoma of the lung or with an assay artifact.

(MEN) type IIA or hereditary medullary thyroid carcinoma now make it possible to perform a DNA-based analysis to determine gene carrier status (55). This analysis has largely replaced pentagastrin testing for family screening. This advance makes it less likely that pentagastrin testing will be used with the same frequency for the identification of hereditary medullary thyroid carcinoma in the future, although it remains useful for follow-up studies and the identification of sporadic medullary thyroid carcinoma.

In summary, measurement of circulating concentrations of calcitonin is easily performed by one of several techniques. Sensitive standard RIA kits and measurement of calcitonin by the concentration technique are commercially available. Measurement of calcitonin and procalcitonin by two-site IRMA is currently limited to the research laboratory.

REFERENCES

1. Keutmann HT, Sauer MM, Hendy GN, O'Riordan JLH, Potts JT Jr: Complete amino acid sequence of human parathyroid hormone. *Biochemistry* 17:5723–5729, 1978
2. Goltzman D, Gomolin H, DeLean A, Wexler M, Meakins JL: Discordant disappearance of bioactive and immunoreactive parathyroid hormone after parathyroidectomy. *J Clin Endocrinol Metab* 58:70–75, 1984
3. Nussbaum SR, Zahradnik RJ, Lavigne JR, et al.: Highly sensitive two-site immunoradiometric assay of parathyrin, and its clinical utility in evaluating patients with hypercalcemia. *Clin Chem* 33:1364–1367, 1988
4. Martin KJ, Hruska KA, Lewis J, Anderson C, Slatopolsky E: The renal handling of parathyroid hormone. Role of peritubular uptake and glomerular filtration. *J Clin Invest* 60:808–814, 1977
5. Segre GV, Perkins AS, Witters LA, Potts JT Jr: Metabolism of parathyroid hormone by isolated rat Kupffer cells and hepatocytes. *J Clin Invest* 67:449–457, 1981
6. Segre GV, Nial HD, Sauer RT, Potts JT Jr: Edman degradation of radioiodinated parathyroid hormone: Application to sequence analysis and hormone metabolism in vivo. *Biochemistry* 16:2417–2427, 1977
7. MacGregor RR, McGregor DH, Lee SH, Hamilton JW: Structural analysis of parathormone fragments elaborated by cells cultured from a hyperplastic human parathyroid gland. *Bone Miner* 1:41–50, 1986
8. Rosenblatt M: Parathyroid hormone: Chemistry and structure-activity relations. In: Ioachim HL (ed) *Pathobiology Annual.* Raven Press, New York, pp 53–86, 1981
9. Segre GV, Habener JF, Powell D, Tregear GW, Potts JT Jr: Parathyroid hormone in human plasma: Immunochemical characterization and biological implications. *J Clin Invest* 51:3163–3172, 1972
10. Klee GG, Preissner CM, Schryver PG, Taylor RL, Kao PC: Multisite immunochemiluminometric assay for simultaneously measuring whole-molecule and amino-terminal fragments of human parathyrin. *Clin Chem* 38:628–635, 1992
11. Marx SJ, Sharp ME, Krudy A, Rosenblatt M, Mallette LE: Radioimmunoassay for the middle region of human parathyroid hormone: Studies with a radioiodinated synthetic peptide. *J Clin Endocrinol Metab* 53:76–84, 1981
12. Hanley DA, Takatsuki K, Sultan JM, Schneider AB: Direct release of parathyroid hormone fragments from functioning bovine parathyroid glands in vitro. *J Clin Invest* 62:1247–1254, 1978
13. Mayer GP, Deaton JA, Hurst JG, Habener JF: Effects of plasma calcium concentration on the relative proportion of hormone and carboxyl fragments in parathyroid venous blood. *Endocrinology* 104:1778–1784, 1979
14. Mallette LE, Tuma SN, Berger RE, Kirkland J: Radioimmunoassay for the middle region of human parathyroid hormone using an

15. Fischer JA, Binswanger U, Dietrich FM: Human parathyroid hormone. Immunological characterization of antibodies against a glandular extract and the synthetic amino-terminal fragments 1–12 and 1–34 and their use in the determination of immunoreactive hormone in human sera. *J Clin Invest* 85:1382–1394, 1974
16. Manning RM, Hendy GN, Papapoulos SE, O'Riordan JLH: Development of homologous immunological assays for human parathyroid hormone. *J Endocrinol* 85:161–170, 1980
17. Mallette LE: General techniques for raising antisera against parathyroid hormone and calcitonin. In: Bikle DD (ed) *Assay of Calcium-Regulating Hormones.* Springer-Verlag, New York, pp 169–189, 1983
18. Sharp M, Marx SJ: Radioimmunoassay for the middle region of human parathyroid hormone: Comparison of two radioiodinated synthetic peptides. *Clin Chim Acta* 145:59–68, 1985
19. Mallette LE: Radioimmunoassays for the midregion of parathyrin. Characterization of 44–53 versus 53–68 specific assays *(abstract)*. *Clin Chem* 30:1041, 1984
20. Mallette LE, Cooper J, Kirkland JL: Transient congenital hypoparathyroidism. Possible association with lesions of the pulmonary valve. *J Pediatr* 101:928–931, 1982
21. Arnaud CD, Tsao HS, Littledike T: Radioimmunoassay of human parathyroid hormone in serum. *J Clin Invest* 50:21–34, 1971
22. Gallagher JC, Riggs BL, Jerpbak CM, Arnaud CD: The effect of age on serum immunoreactive parathyroid hormone in normal and osteoporotic women. *J Lab Clin Med* 95:373–385, 1980
23. Blind E, Schmidt-Gayk H, Scharla S, et al.: Two-site assay of intact parathyroid hormone in the investigation of primary hyperparathyroidism and other disorders of calcium metabolism compared with a midregion assay. *J Clin Endocrinol Metab* 67:353–360, 1988
24. Chambers DJ, Dunham J, Zanelli JM, et al.: A sensitive bioassay of parathyroid hormone in plasma. *Clin Endocrinol* 9:375–379, 1978
25. Habener JF, Potts JT Jr: Radioimmunoassay of parathyroid hormone. In: Antoniades HN (ed) *Hormones in Human Blood.* Harvard University Press, Cambridge, pp 551–558, 1976
26. Mallette LE, Nammour H: False elevation of the midregion PTH value. Inhibition of tracer binding by heterophilic antibody in patient serum *(abstract)*. *J Bone Miner Res* 2(suppl 1):102, 1987
27. Zanelli JM, Gaines Das RE: International collaborative study of N.I.B.S.C. Research Standard for human parathyroid hormone for immunoassay. *J Endocrinol* 86:291–304, 1980
28. Marcus R, Madvig P, Young G: Age-related changes in parathyroid hormone and parathyroid hormone action in normal humans. *J Clin Endocrinol Metab* 58:223–230, 1983
29. Ryan MF, Jones SR, Barnes AD: Clinical evaluation of a rapid parathyroid hormone assay. *Ann Clin Biochem* 29(pt 1):48–51, 1992
30. Endres DB, Villanueva R, Sharp CF Jr, Singer FR: Measurement of parathyroid hormone. *Endocrinol Metab Clin North Am* 18:611–630, 1989
31. Mallette LE, Beck P, VandePol C: Malignancy hypercalcemia: Evaluation of parathyroid function and response to treatment. *Am J Med Sci* 302:205–210, 1991
32. Mallette LE, Kirkland JL, Gagel RF, Law WM Jr, Heath H III: Synthetic human parathyroid hormone-(1–34) for the study of pseudohypoparathyroidism. *J Clin Endocrinol Metab* 67:964–972, 1988
33. Mallette LE, Wilson DP, Kirkland JL: Evaluation of hypocalcemia with a highly sensitive homologous radioimmunoassay for the midregion of parathyroid hormone. *Pediatrics* 71:64–69, 1983
34. Felsenfeld AJ, Ross D, Rodriguez M: Hysteresis of the parathyroid hormone response to hypocalcemia in hemodialysis patients with low turnover aluminum bone disease. *J Am Soc Nephrol* 2:1136–1143, 1991
35. Siris ES, Clemens TP, McMahon D, et al.: Parathyroid function in Paget's disease of bone. *J Bone Miner Res* 4:75–80, 1989
36. Mallette LE, Kirkland JL: Fine regulation of serum calcium. Acute midday decreases in calcium ion concentration trigger a

parathyroid response. In: Cohn DV, Fujita T, Potts J Jr (eds) *Endocrine Control of Bone and Calcium Metabolism.* Elsevier, New York, pp 268–271, 1984

37. Gagel RF, Tashjian AH Jr, Cummings T, et al.: The clinical outcome of prospective screening for multiple endocrine neoplasia type 2A. An 18-year experience. *N Engl J Med* 318:478–844, 1988

38. Samaan NA, Castillo S, Schultz PN, Khalil KG, Johnston DA: Serum calcitonin after pentagastrin stimulation in patients with bronchogenic and breast cancer compared to that in patients with medullary thyroid carcinoma. *J Clin Endocrinol Metab* 51:237–241, 1980

39. Parthemore JG, Bronzert D, Roberts G, Deftos LJ: A short calcium infusion in the diagnosis of medullary thyroid carcinoma. *J Clin Endocrinol Metab* 39:108–111, 1974

40. Parthemore JG, Deftos LJ: Calcitonin secretion in normal human subjects. *J Clin Endocrinol Metab* 47:184–188, 1978

41. Gagel RF, O'Briain DS, Voelkel EF, et al.: Pituitary immunoreactive calcitonin-like material: Lack of evidence for cross-reactivity with pro-opiomelanocortin. *Metabolism* 32:686–696, 1983

42. Heath H III, Sizemore GW: Plasma calcitonin in normal man: Differences between men and women. *J Clin Invest* 60:1135–1140, 1977

43. Body JJ, Heath H III: Estimates of circulating monomeric calcitonin: Physiological studies in normal and thyroidectomized man. *J Clin Endocrinol Metab* 57:897–903, 1983

44. Body JJ, Heath H III: "Nonspecific" increases in plasma immunoreactive calcitonin in healthy individuals: Discrimination from medullary thyroid carcinoma by a new extraction technique. *Clin Chem* 30:511–514, 1984

45. Heath H III, Body JJ, Fox J: Radioimmunoassay of calcitonin in normal human plasma: Problems, perspectives and prospects. *Biomed Pharmacother* 38:241–245, 1984

46. Gharib H, Kao PC, Heath H III: Determination of silica-purified plasma calcitonin for the detection and management of medullary thyroid carcinoma: Comparison of two provocative tests. *Mayo Clin Proc* 62:373–378, 1987

47. Deftos LJ, Roos BA, Bronzert D, Parthemore JG: Immunochemical heterogeneity of calcitonin in plasma. *J Clin Endocrinol Metab* 40:409–412, 1975

48. Lee JC, Parthemore JG, Deftos LJ: Immunochemical heterogeneity of calcitonin in renal failure. *J Clin Endocrinol Metab* 45:528–533, 1977

49. Motte P, Ait-Abdellah M, Vauzelle P, et al.: A two-site immunoradiometric assay for serum calcitonin using monoclonal antipeptide antibodies. *Henry Ford Hospital Medical J* 35:129–132, 1987

50. Motte P, Vauzelle P, Alberici G, et al.: Utilization of synthetic peptides for the study of calcitonin and biosynthetic precursors for calcitonin. *Int J Rad Appl Instrum B* 14:289–294, 1987

51. Seth R, Motte P, Kehely A, et al.: A sensitive and specific two-site enzyme-immunoassay for human calcitonin using monoclonal antibodies. *J Endocrinol* 119:351–357, 1988

52. Ghillani P, Motte P, Bohuon C, Bellet D: Monoclonal antipeptide antibodies as tools to dissect closely related gene products. A model using peptides encoded by the calcitonin gene. *J Immunol* 141:3156–3163, 1988

53. Wells SA Jr, Ontjes DA, Cooper CW, et al.: The early diagnosis of medullary carcinoma of the thyroid gland in patients with multiple endocrine neoplasia type II. *Ann Surg* 182:362–370, 1975

54. Wells SA Jr, Baylin SB, Linehan WM, et al.: Provocative agents and the diagnosis of medullary carcinoma of the thyroid gland. *Ann Surg* 188:139–141, 1978

55. Cote GJ, Wohllk N, Evans D, Goepfert H, Gagel R. *RET* proto-oncogene mutations in multiple endocrine neoplasia type 2 and medullary thyroid carcinoma. In: Thakker RV (ed) *Genetic and Molecular Biological Aspects of Endocrine Disease, Bailliere's Clinical Endocrinology and Metabolism* 9:609–630, 1995

18. Parathyroid-Hormone-Related Protein Assays

William J. Burtis, M.D., Ph.D.

Emerson Practice Associates, Concord, Massachusetts

Parathyroid-hormone-related protein (PTHrP) is a complex protein, recently purified from tumors of patients with humoral hypercalcemia of malignancy (HHM), which has amino acid sequence homology with parathyroid hormone (PTH) in the amino-terminal region (see Chapters 12,32) (1–5). The gene encoding PTHrP, unlike the gene for PTH itself, is expressed in many different tissues of the body (skin and other epithelia, the CNS, many endocrine glands, islet cells, breast, uterus, urinary bladder, and others). Even the non-PTH-like portion of the amino acid sequence of PTHrP is highly conserved across avian and mammalian species, suggesting that PTHrP probably plays important, although incompletely understood, roles in normal physiology.

Evidence is emerging that the cDNA-encoded protein undergoes complex posttranslational processing and is proteolytically cleaved into several smaller, biologically active fragments (6). For example, a midregion fragment, PTHrP(67–86)amide, has been shown to stimulate a placental calcium pump, whereas a carboxy-terminal region, PTHrP(107–111), may inhibit osteoclastic bone resorption

(7,8). Only the amino-terminal region [e.g., PTHrP (1–36)], having homology with PTH, is able to stimulate the recently cloned PTH/PTHrP receptor (9). In addition to classical PTH-like effects on bone and kidney, amino-terminal PTHrP also causes smooth muscle relaxation, vasodilatation, and complex tissue-specific effects on growth and differentiation (10–12). It is not clear whether all of these effects of amino-terminal PTHrP are mediated through the PTH/PTHrP receptor, or if there is a unique PTHrP receptor (9,13). In normal physiology, these biologically active peptides are in most situations acting at the local tissue level, with paracrine, autocrine, or possibly even intracellular or "intracrine" effects (14). When PTHrP is produced in an unregulated fashion by tumors, however, plasma levels of PTHrP rise and the protein begins to act systemically, in an endocrine manner. Thus, tumors expressing PTHrP cause hypercalcemia by secreting large amounts of PTHrP containing the amino-terminal region, which binds to and stimulates PTH/PTHrP receptors in bone and kidney. Whether there are more subtle endocrinologic effects of PTHrP in normal physiology (e.g., effects on calcium metabolism during lactation or pregnancy) is currently under investigation (15,16).

BIOASSAYS

Using a sensitive cytochemical bioassay, it was demonstrated over 10 years ago that circulating levels of PTH-like bioactivity are on average about tenfold elevated in patients with HHM compared with normal volunteers, despite normal levels of immunoreactive PTH (17). In retrospect, this was caused by elevated levels of PTHrP interacting with the PTH/PTHrP receptor. Because of the labor-intensive nature of this cytochemical bioassay, it is rarely performed today and is not clinically available.

Nephrogenous cyclic adenosine monophosphate (NcAMP) excretion represents a sort of *in vivo* bioassay for PTH-like activity. In fact, the existence of PTHrP was originally postulated largely because of the observation of increased NcAMP excretion in the urine of patients with HHM, despite normal serum levels of PTH (18) (see Appendix vii). The assay requires both plasma and (acidified) spot urine samples. A radioimmunoassay (RIA) is used to measure the urine cAMP (UcAMP) and plasma cAMP (PcAMP) concentrations. The cAMP produced in the kidney itself, NcAMP, is then calculated by subtracting the cAMP in the glomerular filtrate from the total UcAMP excretion:

$$NcAMP = [UcAMP \times (S_{Cr}/U_{Cr})] - PcAMP$$

where the units are nmol/100 ml of glomerular filtrate (19). Nephrogenous cAMP accounts for roughly half of the total UcAMP. Nephrogenous cAMP excretion results almost entirely from PTH-like stimulation of the proximal renal tubule; other hormones, such as vasopressin, whose action on the nephron is also mediated by intracellular cAMP, contribute relatively little NcAMP excretion.

Nephrogenous cAMP excretion is elevated in patients with hypercalcemia resulting either from hyperparathyroidism or from HHM. The NcAMP assay alone cannot be used to differentiate between these, the two most common causes of hypercalcemia, because both PTH and PTHrP are equipotent in stimulating renal adenylate cyclase in the proximal tubule and in raising NcAMP excretion. One approach is to measure both NcAMP and serum PTH, and if PTH is normal, to assume that an elevated NcAMP results from PTHrP. A more direct approach is to measure plasma PTHrP itself, using immunoassays that have recently become commercially available.

IMMUNOASSAYS

Within the past several years, a number of immunoassays have been developed that are capable of measuring circulating levels of PTHrP (20–34). These assays utilize antibodies directed at various regions of the protein. Because the proteolytic processing and metabolism of PTHrP is still incompletely worked out, the exact forms of PTHrP peptides existing in the circulation are unknown. There is no *a priori* reason to expect that all of these peptides would circulate at the same molar concentrations, or

that their levels would distinguish equally well between normal physiology and HHM, so each PTHrP assay must be validated with appropriate clinical controls. Furthermore, because the peptides are subject to proteolytic degradation after sample collection, specimens should in general be placed into tubes containing protease inhibitors and kept on ice, and the plasma should be separated and frozen promptly before being sent for assay (27).

The two most common types of immunoassays today are RIAs and immunoradiometric assays (IRMAs). There are several fundamental differences between the RIA and IRMA techniques (35). Radioimmunoassays utilize polyclonal antiserum raised against the peptide of interest. A given antiserum must be used at a specific, limited concentration such that it binds about 30% of trace amounts of ^{125}I-labeled peptide added to the assay tube. The RIA technique involves competition of cold and radiolabeled peptide for the limited number of antibody binding sites. Sensitivity is determined by the minimum concentration of cold peptide that will displace a significant amount of labeled peptide from these binding sites. IRMAs, in contrast, utilize two affinity-purified or monoclonal antibodies. These antibodies are used at high concentrations, as excess reagents in the chemical reaction. There is no radiolabeled tracer peptide, and no competition for limited binding sites. Cold peptide binds to the *capture antibody* (attached to a plastic surface) and also binds [125]I- labeled *signal antibody* (in solution, generally directed toward a second site on the peptide) (Fig. 1). Sensitivity is determined by the minimum concentration of cold peptide that will cause a statistically significant increase in counts of bound ^{125}I-labeled antibody above background. Often, IRMAs can be made more sensitive than RIAs because they are able to utilize much higher concentrations of antibody.

In our laboratory, we have developed RIAs for N-terminal PTHrP(1–36), midregion PTHrP(37–74), C-terminal PTHrP(109–138), "tail-region" PTHrP(141–173), and a two-site IRMA for N-terminal PTHrP(1–74) (21,31,33). Of these assays, only the PTHrP(1–74) IRMA and the C-terminal PTHrP(109–138) RIA are clinically useful at the present time. Other laboratories have also developed IRMAs and/or RIAs directed at various regions of PTHrP (20,22–30,32,34).

Our N-terminal PTHrP(1–74) IRMA utilizes affinity-purified anti-PTHrP(37–74) as the capture antibody, and ^{125}I-labeled, affinity-purified anti-PTHrP(1–36) as the signal antibody (21). Only peptides containing epitopes recognized by both of these antibodies are measured. Thus the assay is specific for fairly large forms of aminoterminal PTHrP; there is no cross-reactivity with PTH itself. Using this assay on plasma collected in tubes containing protease inhibitors, we found PTHrP(1–74) levels to average 21 pmol/L in patients with HHM, whereas most normal subjects had low (<5 pmol/L) or undetectable (<1 pmol/L) levels (Fig. 2). In contrast to patients with HHM, cancer patients with local osteolytic hypercalcemia (LOH) caused by direct bone involvement with low UcAMP excretion had low or undetectable PTHrP(1–74) levels. Patients with primary hyperparathyroidism or miscellaneous causes of hypercalcemia also had low or undetectable levels of

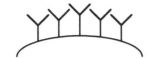

1. Coat Capture Antibody

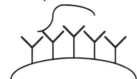

2. Add Sample

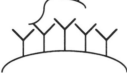

3. Add Signal Antibody

FIG. 1. Immunoradiometric assay methodology. *1*, Capture antibody, directed at one end of the protein of interest, is coated in excess on a solid plastic surface (e.g., a bead). *2*, Sample containing the protein of interest (assay standard or unknown) is added, incubated, and any unbound sample is then washed away. *3*, Signal antibody, directed at a second site on the protein and prelabeled with radioiodine *(asterisk)*, is added in excess, incubated, and then any unbound labeled antibody is washed away. The remaining bound signal antibody, measured in a gamma counter, is proportional to the amount of protein in the sample. For the PTHrP(1–74) IRMA (21), the capture antibody is affinity-purified anti-PTHrP(37–74), and the signal antibody is radiolabeled anti-PTHrP(1–36).

PTHrP. Patients with cancer and normal serum calcium levels occasionally had slightly elevated PTHrP(1–74) concentrations; some of these patients subsequently became hypercalcemic. In this series of 38 unselected patients with malignancy-associated hypercalcemia, about 80% had HHM with elevated plasma PTHrP levels, and 20% had LOH with low or undetectable PTHrP levels, confirming earlier observations suggesting that PTHrP is the most common cause of hypercalcemia in patients with cancer (18,36).

Our C-terminal PTHrP(109–138) RIA utilizes a rabbit polyclonal antiserum raised against tyrosine-labeled (Tyr[109])-PTHrP(109–138) (21). This assay is quite specific for short species of C-terminal PTHrP; PTHrP(107–138) and Tyr[109]-PTHrP(109–138) are recognized about equally well, but PTHrP(1–141) is only about 10% as potent (37). Using this assay on plasma collected in tubes containing protease inhibitors, we found PTHrP(109–138) levels to average 24 pmol/L is patients with HHM, levels similar to the molar concentrations of PTHrP(1–74) in these patients (21). The measured N- and C-terminal peptides must circulate in HHM as separate species, however, because an anti-PTHrP(1–36) antibody column removed PTHrP(1–74)

immunoactivity, but failed to remove PTHrP(109–138) immunoactivity from plasma. We found levels of C-terminal PTHrP to be undetectable (<2 pmol/L) in most normal subjects and in patients with hypercalcemia caused by hyperparathyroidism, vitamin D intoxication, or granulomatous diseases. In patients with renal insufficiency, however, C-terminal PTHrP levels are elevated. As creatinine clearance falls below about 20 ml/min, PTHrP(109–138) levels begin to rise, reaching on average 30 pmol/L in patients on dialysis (21,37). This finding suggests that a C-terminal PTHrP species is released into the circulation in patients without cancer, is renally cleared, and becomes measurable when it accumulates in patients with renal failure.

Our experience with a midregion PTHrP(37–74) and tail region PTHrP(141–173) RIA is more limited: it suggests the PTHrP species measured using these assays circulate at higher molar levels than those measured by the foregoing assays in normal subjects, but that concentrations do not increase significantly above normal levels in patients with HHM (31,33). Ratcliffe et al. reported a similar finding using their midregion PTHrP(37–67) RIA; molar concentrations were relatively high, but there was a large overlap between normal concentrations and those in

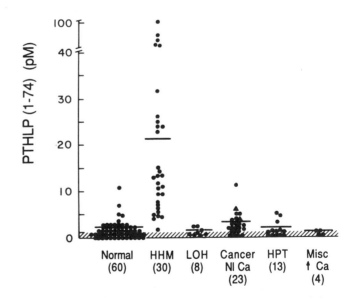

FIG. 2. Plasma concentrations of PTHrP(1–74) measured by IRMA. Normal volunteers (*n* = 60) usually had undetectable (<1 pmol/L) or low concentrations. Patients with malignancy-associated hypercalcemia (*n* = 38) were divided into two groups: those with elevated UcAMP excretion (HHM, *n* = 30) were found to have elevated PTHrP concentrations (mean, 21 pmol/L), whereas those with normal UcAMP excretion (LOH, *n* = 8) were found to have low or undetectable PTHrP concentrations. Patients with cancer and normal serum calcium (*n* = 23), hyperparathyroidism (*n* = 13), or miscellaneous causes of hypercalcemia (*n* = 4) also had low or undetectable PTHrP(1–74) concentrations. (From: Burtis WJ, Brady TG, Orloff JJ, et al.: Immunochemical characterization of circulating parathyroid hormone-related protein in patients with humoral hypercalcemia of cancer. *N Engl J Med* 322:1106–1112, 1990.)

patients with HHM (25). These investigators also reported unexpectedly disparate results in two N-terminal RIAs they developed: their direct RIA measured levels of 190 pmol/L but failed to differentiate patients with HHM from normal subjects, whereas their extraction RIA measured levels of only 11 pmol/L in patients with HHM and yet these low levels were clearly higher than those of normal subjects. A possible explanation is that the extraction RIA measures a large, intact-N-terminal, biologically active PTH-like species similar to that measured by IRMA, whereas the direct RIA measures a species inactivated by proteolytic cleavage at the arginine (Arg)19–21 residues (4). Whatever the explanation, the important point is that not all PTHrP assays measure peptides whose concentrations correlate closely with the HHM syndrome, so the track record of each assay in terms of its ability to diagnose HHM must be carefully scrutinized.

Circulating levels of aminoterminal PTHrP in normal subjects are still poorly defined, because they are below or just slightly above the detection limits of assays developed to date. The most sensitive IRMAs now have reported detection limits of about 0.1 pmol/L, yet most normal individuals still have undetectable levels in these assays. Midregion PTHrP RIAs, on the other hand, while less sensitive, are capable of detecting the higher concentrations of midregion species in normal subjects. It might be hoped that the ability to measure changes of PTHrP within the normal range would elucidate normal physiologic functions of the protein, but, to the extent that these actions are autocrine or paracrine in nature, circulating concentrations may poorly reflect events at the tissue or cellular level.

Elevated plasma concentrations of PTHrP, in contrast, are readily detectable with most current PTHrP assays in patients with HHM. When using the current PTHrP assays clinically for the differential diagnosis of hypercalcemia, several important points should be kept in mind (38,39). First, as discussed above, different assays provide different degrees of discrimination between patients with HHM and those without; IRMAs measuring large-N-terminal species of PTHrP seem to be best in this regard. Second, not all patients with hypercalcemia caused by malignancy will have elevated levels of PTHrP in even the best assay; about 20% will have LOH rather than HHM, so that PTHrP levels will be low. Third, not all patients with elevated plasma PTHrP concentrations will have a malignant tumor, because C-terminal levels of PTHrP are elevated in patients with renal insufficiency, and N-terminal levels may be elevated in patients with nonmalignant pheochromocytomas. In addition, rare patients with hypercalcemia due to mammary hypertrophy or lymphedema may also have elevated PTHrP levels (40,41).

The use of PTHrP as a tumor marker must still be considered investigational, although the expected variations in PTHrP levels have been seen after therapeutic intervention in a small number of patients with PTHrP-producing tumors (21–23). It is not yet clear how commonly elevations in PTHrP antedate the development of hypercalcemia. Clearly, the assays with the most potential in this regard would be those providing the largest separation between normal levels and concentrations in HHM. Open questions at the present time are whether tumors produce unique, abnormally processed forms of PTHrP, and indeed which tissues contribute to the normal circulating levels of the various PTHrP peptides.

ACKNOWLEDGMENTS

This work was supported by a Merit Review grant from the Department of Veterans Affairs. The author would like to gratefully acknowledge the expert secretarial assistance of Charleen Stewart.

REFERENCES

1. Strewler GJ, Nissenson RA: Hypercalcemia in malignancy. *West J Med* 153:635–640, 1990
2. Bilezikian JP: Parathyroid hormone-related peptide in sickness and in health. *N Engl J Med* 322:1151–1153, 1990
3. Mallette LE: The parathyroid polyhormones: New concepts in the spectrum of peptide hormone action. *Endocr Rev* 12:110–117, 1991
4. Burtis WJ: Parathyroid hormone-related protein: Structure, function, and measurement. *Clin Chem* 38:2171–2183, 1992
5. Broadus AE, Stewart AF: Parathyroid hormone-related protein: Structure, processing, and physiologic actions. In: Bilezikian JP (ed) *The Parathyroids*. Raven Press, New York, pp 259–294, 1994
6. Soifer NE, Dee KE, Insogna KL, Barri M, Drinkhill M, Findlay JBC, White IR, Caple IW: Parathyroid hormone-related protein: Secretion of a novel mid-region fragment by three different cell lines in culture. *J Biol Chem* 267:18236–18243, 1992
7. Care AD, Abbas SK, Pickard DW, et al.: Stimulation of ovine placental transport of calcium and magnesium by mid-molecule fragments of human parathyroid hormone-related protein. *J Exp Physiol* 75:605–608, 1990
8. Fenton AJ, Kemp BE, Hammonds RG, et al.: A potent inhibitor of osteoclastic bone resorption within a highly conserved pentapeptide region of parathyroid hormone-related protein; PTHrP (107–111). *Endocrinology* 129:3424–3426, 1991
9. Jueppner H, Abou-Samra A, Freeman M, et al.: A G protein-linked-receptor for parathyroid hormone and parathyroid hormone-related peptide. *Science* 254:1024–1026, 1991
10. Orloff JJ, Wu TL, Stewart AF: Parathyroid hormone-like proteins: Biochemical responses and receptor interactions. *Endocr Rev* 10:476–495, 1989
11. Yamamoto M, Harm SC, Grasser WA, Thiede MA: Parathyroid hormone-related protein in the rat urinary bladder: A smooth muscle relaxant produced locally in response to mechanical stretch. *Proc Natl Acad Sci USA* 89:5326–5330, 1992
12. Kaiser S, Laneuville P, Bernier SM, Rhim JS, Kremer R, Goltzman D: Enhanced growth of a human keratinocyte cell line induced by antisense RNA for parathyroid hormone-related peptide. *J Biol Chem* 267:13623–13628, 1992
13. Orloff JJ, Ganz MB, Ribaudo AE, et al.: Analysis of parathyroid hormone-related protein binding and signal transduction mechanisms in benign and malignant squamous cells. *Am J Physiol* 262 (Endocrinol Metab 25):E599–E607, 1992
14. Henderson JE, Amizuka N, Warshawsky H, et al.: Nucleolar localization of parathyroid hormone-related peptide enhances survival of chondrocytes under conditions that promote apototic cell death. *Mol Cell Biol* 15:4064–4075, 1995
15. Grill V, Hillary J, Ho PMW, et al.: Parathyroid hormone-related protein: a possible endocrine function in lactation. *Clin Endocrinol* 37:405–410, 1992
16. Bucht E, Rong H, Bremme K, et al.: Midmolecular parathyroid hormone-related peptide in serum during pregnancy, lactation, and in umbilical cord blood. *Eur J Endocrinol* 132:438–443, 1995
17. Goltzman D, Stewart AF, Broadus AE: Malignancy-associated hypercalcemia: Evaluation with a cytochemical bioassay for

parathyroid hormone. *J Clin Endocrinol Metab* 53:899–904, 1981

18. Stewart AF, Horst R, Deftos LJ, Cadman EC, Lang R, Broadus AE: Biochemical evaluation of patients with cancer-associated hypercalcemia: Evidence for humoral and nonhumoral groups. *N Engl J Med* 303:1377–1383, 1980

19. Broadus AE: Nephrogenous cyclic AMP. *Recent Prog Horm Res* 37:667–701, 1981

20. Budayr AA, Nissenson RA, Klein RF, et al.: Increased serum levels of a parathyroid hormone-like protein in malignancy-associated hypercalcemia. *Ann Intern Med* 111:807–812, 1989

21. Burtis WJ, Brady TG, Orloff JJ, et al.: Immunochemical characterization of circulating parathyroid hormone-related protein in patients with humoral hypercalcemia of cancer. *N Engl J Med* 322:1106–1112, 1990

22. Henderson JE, Shustik C, Kremer R, Rabbani SA, Hendy G, Goltzman D: Circulating concentrations of parathyroid hormone-like peptide in malignancy and in hyperparathyroidism. *J Bone Miner Res* 5:105–112, 1990

23. Kao PC, Klee GG, Taylor RI, Heath H: Parathyroid hormone-related peptide in plasma of patients with hypercalcemia and malignant lesions. *Mayo Clin Proc* 65:1399–1407, 1990

24. Ratcliffe WA, Norbury S, Heath DA, Ratcliffe JG: Development and validation of an immunoradiometric assay of parathyrin-related protein in unextracted plasma. *Clin Chem* 37:678–685, 1991

25. Ratcliffe WA, Norbury S, Stott RA, Heath DA, Ratcliffe JG: Immunoreactivity of plasma parathyrin-related peptide: Three region-specific radioimmunoassays and a two-site immunoaradiometric assay compared. *Clin Chem* 37:1781–1787, 1991

26. Grill V, Ho P, Body JJ, et al.: Parathyroid hormone-related protein: Elevated levels in both humoral hypercalcemia of malignancy and hypercalcemia complicating metastatic breast cancer. *J Clin Endocrinol Metab* 73:1309–1315, 1991

27. Pandian MR, Morgan CH, Carlton E, Segre GV: Modified immunoradiometric assay of parathyroid hormone-related protein: Clinical application in the differential diagnosis of hypercalcemia. *Clin Chem* 38:282–288, 1991

28. Blind E, Raue F, Gotzmann J, Schmidt-Gayk H, Kohl B, Ziegler R: Circulating levels of midregional parathyroid hormone-related protein in hypercalcemia of malignancy. *Clin Endocrinol* 37:290–297, 1992

29. Bucht E, Eklund A, Toss G, et al.: Parathyroid hormone-related peptide, measured by a midmolecule radioimmunoassay, in various hypercalcemic and normocalcemic conditions. *Acta Endocrinol* 127:294–300, 1992

30. Nakamura Y, Bando H, Shintani Y, Yokogoshi Y, Saito S: Serum parathyroid hormone-related protein levels in patients with hematologic malignancies or solid tumors. *Acta Endocrinol* 127:324–330, 1992

31. Burtis WJ, Debeyssey M, Philbrick WM, et al.: Evidence for the presence of an extreme carboxyterminal parathyroid hormone-related peptide in biological specimens. *J Bone Miner Res* 7(Suppl 1):S225, 1992

32. Fraser WD, Robinson J, Lawton R, et al.: Clinical and laboratory studies of a new immunoradiometric assay for parathyroid hormone-related protein. *Clin Chem* 39:414–419, 1993

33. Burtis WJ, Dann P, Gaich GA, Soifer NE: A high abundance midregion species of parathyroid hormone-related protein: Immunological and chromatographic characterization in plasma. *J Clin Endocrinol Metab* 78:317–322, 1994

34. Ikeda K, Ohno H, Hane M, et al.: Development of a sensitive two-site immunoradiometric assay for parathyroid hormone-related peptide: Evidence for elevated levels in plasma from patients with adult T-cell leukemia/lymphoma and B-cell lymphoma. *J Clin Endocrinol Metab* 79:1322–1327, 1994

35. Ekins R: More sensitive immunoassays. *Nature* 284:14–15, 1980

36. Godsall JW, Burtis WJ, Insogna KL, Broadus AE, Stewart AF: Nephrogenous cyclic AMP, adenylate cyclase-stimulating activity, and the humoral hypercalcemia of malignancy. *Recent Prog Horm Res* 42:705–750, 1986

37. Orloff JJ, Fodero JP, Debeyssey M, Burtis WJ: Accumulation of carboxyterminal fragment of the parathyroid hormone-related protein in plasma of patients with renal failure. *Kidney Int* 43:1371–1376, 1993

38. Gaich GA, Burtis WJ: The diagnosis and treatment of malignancy-associated hypercalcemia. *Endocrinologist* 1:371–379, 1991

39. Bilezikian JP: Clinical utility of assays for parathyroid hormone-related protein. *Clin Chem* 38:179–181, 1992

40. Khosla S, VanHeerden JA, Gharib H, et al.: Parathyroid hormone-related protein and hypercalcemia secondary to massive mammary hyperplasia. *N Engl J Med* 322:1157, 1990

41. Braude S, Graham A, Mitchell D: Lymphoedema/hypercalcemia syndrome mediated by parathyroid hormone-related protein. *Lancet* 337:140–141, 1991

19. Vitamin D Metabolites

Thomas L. Clemens, Ph.D., and *John S. Adams, M.D.

*Department of Endocrinology and Metabolism, University of Cincinnati, Cincinnati, Ohio; and *Department of Medicine, University of California, Los Angeles, Cedars-Sinai Research Institute, Los Angeles, California*

Assays for vitamin D metabolites in human serum or plasma have been improved greatly in recent years. Before 1971, when the first competitive protein binding assays for 25-hydroxyvitamin D (25OHD) were described (1,2), an estimate of the circulating concentration of active vitamin D metabolites was obtained solely by bioassay (3,4). Three significant technical advances have allowed accurate quantitation of the less plentiful metabolites of 25OHD: (i) the isolation of the vitamin D receptor protein (VDR); (ii) the introduction of sophisticated techniques for chromatographic purification of lipid extracts of serum; and (iii) the synthesis of radioligands of high specific activity. These advances have led to identification of a great number of vitamin D metabolites, but only measurements of serum concentrations of 25OHD and $1,25(OH)_2D$ have proven clinical utility. Therefore, in this chapter we will limit our discussion to a description of the methods and clinical significance of assaying these two metabolites in human serum.

ANALYTICAL METHODS

Sample Preparation for Measurement of 25-Hydroxyvitamin D and 1,25-Dihydroxyvitamin D

Most assays for vitamin D metabolites require solvent extraction to deproteinize the sample and free the metabolites from the vitamin D transport binding protein (DBP) and albumin (5). Ethanol, methanol, and acetonitrile effectively free 25OHD and 1,25(OH)$_2$D by deproteinization. Two-phase liquid-liquid partition with a variety of solvents, including chloroform-methanol, methylene chloride-methanol, ethylacetate-cyclohexane, hexane-isopropanol, and diethyl ether, provides a less contaminated extract (6). Of these, more selective solvents such as diethyl ether produce the cleanest extracts (7). Backwashing nonpolar organic extracts with weakly basic solutions removes acidic lipids. Extracts are then purified by preparative column chromatography to separate vitamin D metabolites and to eliminate lipid and other interfering substances extracted from serum. In particular, silicic acid or silica minicolumns have been recognized for their convenience and ability to separate D, 25OHD, and dihydroxylated metabolites (8,9). More recently, methods based on solid-phase extraction and preparative chromatography on a single octa decyl (C-18) silica reverse-phase cartridge have been reported for 25OHD and 1,25(OH)$_2$D (10–13). The original competitive radioreceptor assays for 1,25(OH)$_2$D required high-performance liquid chromatography (HPLC) to eliminate interfering compounds. The modern methods (Fig. 1) have significantly reduced the technical, instrumental, and specimen volume requirements for the measurement of 1,25(OH)$_2$D by competitive radioreceptor assay.

Methods requiring extraction and chromatography must be monitored for recovery of the analyte of interest and include solvent or column blanks. Recovery of each metabolite is estimated by adding tracer amounts of highly purified, tritiated 25OHD$_3$ or 1,25(OH)$_2$D$_3$ before the solvent extraction. If total 25OHD or 1,25(OH)$_2$D is to be measured by competitive protein-binding assay (CPBA), care must be taken to ensure that D$_2$ and D$_3$ metabolites are not separated and are recovered equally. Solvents, chromatographic media, and cartridges may contain substances that interfere with CPBA, especially with those using DBP. Undetectable levels of the vitamin D metabolites should be found when water blanks are treated identically to specimens.

Measurement of 25-Hydroxyvitamin D

Serum 25OHD is most often measured by CPBA or by direct quantitation by ultraviolet (UV) absorption on HPLC. CPBA has been most widely used because of the availability of reagents, modest specimen requirements, and ease of performance. Diluted rat serum, which contains a high-affinity DBP, is typically used as the specific binder, with tritiated 25OHD$_3$ of high specific activity (>100 Ci/mmol) as tracer. Because rat DBP recognizes both 25OHD$_2$ and 25OHD$_3$ (14), these assays measure the total 25OHD concentration. Methods using direct quantitation by UV absorption after separation by HPLC can quantitate 25OHD$_2$ and 25OHD$_3$ individually (15). However, because both vitamin D$_2$ and D$_3$ are found in serum as a consequence of ingestion of vitamin D (D$_2$ and D$_3$) supplemented, there is no benefit in differential measurement of 25OHD$_2$ and 25OHD$_3$ when assessing vitamin D status in clinical practice.

As described earlier, assays using DBP require extraction and chromatographic purification. Because DBP binds other circulating vitamin D metabolites, including 24,25(OH)$_2$D and 25,26(OH)$_2$D (14,16), methods that do not chromatographically separate 25OHD from these cross-reacting metabolites will overestimate its concentration. Other nonspecific substances can also be extracted from serum, even with selective solvents, and cross-react in nonchromatographic assays to falsely elevate the measured concentration of 25OHD (17,18). The practice of preparing standards in vitamin D–free serum to "blank out" nonspecific effects should be discouraged, because these effects undoubtedly vary between individuals in health and disease. Although most available assays can detect supranormal (toxic) levels of 25OHD, distinguishing between normal and subnormal

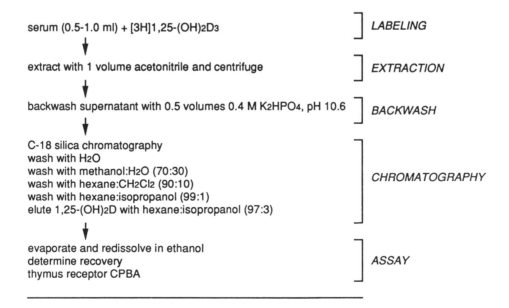

FIG. 1. Purification and quantitation of 1,25-(OH)$_2$D: the single silica cartridge system.

TABLE 1. *Serum 25-hydroxyvitamin D and 1,25-dihydroxyvitamin D in healthy individuals and normal relative variations*

	25OHD	1,25(OH)2D
Normal adults	10–50 ng/mL[a,b]	15–60 pg/mL[a,b]
Elderly	↓,→	↓,→,↑
Children	→	↑
Pregnancy	→	↑
Summer/fall	↑	→
Winter/spring	↓	→
Increasing latitude	↓	→

[a]SI units can be calculated as indicated below. The conversion factors are for 25OHD and 1,25(OH)$_2$D standards and assume that the D$_2$ and D$_3$ forms are measured in an equimolar basis. 25OHD ng/mL × 2.50 = nmol/L; 1,25(OH)$_2$D pg/mL × 2.40 = pmol/L.

[b]Both 25OHD and 1,25(OH)$_2$D are relatively stable in serum; however, samples should be frozen until assayed. Although serum and plasma yield similar results, serum is preferred because of its greater ease in handling. Interassay precision expressed as the coefficient of variation is typically 10% to 15% in the normal range.

levels can be problematic and requires well-validated chromatographic assays free of solvent, cartridge, and serum interference (19).

Radioimmunoassays (18,20) have also been reported for assay of 25OHD. However, because of the characteristics of the reported antisera, these methods also require chromatographic purification to eliminate nonspecific serum interference and often do not recognize 25OHD$_2$. In addition, vitamin D and other metabolites of D$_2$ and D$_3$ cross-react in this nonchromatographic assay. More recently, a radioimmunoassay has been developed that uses a more selective antibody and iodinated 25OHD as radioligand (21). Because of the ease and speed of performance, this assay should achieve widespread use in the near future.

HPLC coupled with direct UV quantitation can provide the most accurate measurement of 25OHD (25OHD$_2$ and 25OHD$_3$) (15,18,19). Unfortunately, the need for extraction and preparative chromatography of a relatively large sample volume (1–5 mL) and the expensive instrumental requirements have restricted the use of this method to research laboratories.

The normal range for 25OHD varies somewhat among laboratories and between the different methods. Because serum levels of 25OHD are influenced by sunlight, normal values are dependent on season and latitude (Table 1).

Measurement of 1,25-Dihydroxyvitamin D

Initial assays for 1,25(OH)$_2$D required extensive preliminary purification of the sample, usually by HPLC before radioreceptor assay (RRA). In 1984, introduction of a simplified method for assay of 1,25(OH)$_2$D (12,13), which did not require HPLC, substantially increased the availability of this analysis. This method combined solid-phase extraction with a novel RRA using a vitamin D receptor preparation from bovine thymus in a nonequilibrium assay (Fig. 1).

The bovine thymus vitamin D receptor has several advantages over the previously used chick intestinal receptor. The thymus receptor recognizes 1,25(OH)$_2$D$_2$ and 1,25(OH)$_2$D$_3$ equivalently, unlike the chick intestinal receptor (12,14), which underestimates 1,25(OH)$_2$D$_2$. In addition, the thymus receptor can be prepared in large quantities, providing a relatively unlimited and reproducible source of stable receptor. Also, the thymus receptor is less sensitive to lipid interference than the chick preparation, such that a more simple, non-HPLC pre-purification could be used. In this assay, extraction of 1 mL of serum yields a sensitivity of 2–5 pg/mL. An additional advantage of this assay is that it does not measure dihydrotachysterol (DHT) (22), which, when present in serum from patients receiving this analog, will interfere with the chick receptor assay.

The development of radioimmunoassays (RIAs) for 1,25(OH)$_2$D has been difficult because of the requirement for extremely specific antisera to detect relatively low circulating levels of the metabolite; the normal circulating concentration of 25-OHD is 500- to 1000-fold greater than that of 1,25(OH)$_2$D (23). Thus, antisera highly specific for 1,25(OH)$_2$D$_3$ frequently do not recognize 1,25(OH)$_2$D$_2$ (24). As a means to circumvent these problems, a novel immunoextraction method has been devised to selectively concentrate 1,25(OH)$_2$D before radioimmunoassays (25). Such improvements may eventually allow the development of RIAs that are more clinically useful.

The normal serum level of 1,25(OH)$_2$D varies with age and increases during pregnancy, as indicated in Table 1. Although there is a growing consensus that relative deficiency in vitamin D can exacerbate age-related bone loss, there is still controversy as to whether 1,25(OH)$_2$D levels go down (25), up (26), or do not change with aging. The serum 1,25(OH)$_2$D concentration is generally not affected by fluctuation in the circulating level of its natural substrate 25OHD. An exception is found in some patients with granuloma-forming diseases or in those with very low serum 25OHD levels who experience a rapid influx of vitamin D into the circulation (i.e., after sunlight exposure) (27).

Measurement of Vitamin D

Quantitation of vitamin D in serum is difficult because of its limited solubility, low concentration, and comigration with contaminating lipid. Existing methods require extraction, preparative chromatography, and one or more HPLC steps. Levels are measured with HPLC and UV absorption (15,28) or CPBA with DBP (16,29). Vitamin D binding protein from most species discriminates against vitamin D$_2$, which results in an underestimation of its concentration (29). Because of its rapid disappearance from the circulation after release from skin, vitamin D levels are of little value in determining vitamin D status. However, vitamin D assays have been used to assess its absorption in normal subjects and in patients with intestinal malabsorption after oral ingestion of a standard vitamin D$_2$ dose (30). In addition, vitamin D assays have been used to monitor the vitamin D content of foods and fortified dairy products. An interesting application was a study that found striking discrepancies in the reported and measured vitamin D values of randomly selected milk and infant formulas (31).

Measurement of 24,25-Dihydroxyvitamin D

The second most abundant vitamin D metabolite in serum, $24,25(OH)_2D$ has been measured with CPBA after extraction, preparative chromatography, and HPLC (16). As with vitamin D, DBP does not recognize $24,25(OH)_2D_2$ and $24,25(OH)_2D_3$ equally, resulting in underestimation of total $24,25(OH)_2D$ (14,16). Normal-phase HPLC on cyano-bonded silica or silica with methylene chloride–isopropanol separates $25OHD_2$-23,26-lactone, a metabolite not adequately resolved from $24,25(OH)_2D$ with previous systems (16,32). Because there is no known function for $24,25(OH)_2D$, its measurement in a clinical setting is not warranted.

Free 25-Hydroxyvitamin D and 1,25-Dihydroxyvitamin D

Circulating vitamin D and its metabolites are almost completely bound by serum proteins, primarily DBP but also by albumin. In normal individuals, approximately 0.4% of the $1,25(OH)_2D$ and 0.03% of the 25OHD are free (33,34). Under certain conditions, disturbances in the circulating concentrations of DBP and albumin alter the free levels of vitamin D metabolites. Consequently, several methods have been reported for the determination of free vitamin D metabolites (33,34), but these method are restricted to research settings.

CLINICAL UTILITY OF THE VITAMIN D METABOLITE ASSAYS

In general, there are four circumstances that prompt the clinician to investigate a patient's vitamin D status: (i) an abnormal serum calcium concentration; (ii) renal stone disease and hypercalciuria; (iii) metabolic bone disease; and (iv) the need to monitor a patient's response to vitamin D therapy. The most frequently encountered clinical states that result in disordered calcium and bone metabolism and that may present as an abnormal serum concentration of 25OHD or $1,25(OH)_2D$ are presented in Table 2. Recently, with the greater availability of the $1,25(OH)_2D$ assays, its use in clinical medicine has increased, and unfortunately the $1,25(OH)_2D$ assay is often ordered inappropriately. The following section outlines several clinical situations in which 25OHD and $1,25(OH)_2D$ determinations are recommended.

The Hypocalcemic Patient

When confronted with a hypocalcemic patient, it is useful to consider whether the reduction in the serum ionized calcium concentration is due to a deficiency in one or both of the classic calcemic hormones: $1,25(OH)_2D$ and parathyroid hormone (PTH). Vitamin D status is best assessed by assay of 25OHD. This metabolite, though less biologically active

TABLE 2. *Vitamin D metabolite concentrations in patients with disordered calcium homeostasis*

	25OHD	1,25(OH)2D
Hypocalcemia		
Vitamin D deficiency	D	D,I,N
Severe hepatocellular disease	D	D,N
Nephrotic syndrome	D	D,N
Renal failure	N	D
Hyperphosphatemia	N	D
Hypoparathyroidism	N	D,N
Pseudohypoparathyroidism	N	D,N
Hypomagnesemia	N	D,N
Vitamin D–dependent rickets, type I	N,I	D
Vitamin D–dependent rickets, type II	N,I	I
Hypercalcemia/hypercalciuria		
Vitamin D, 25OHD intoxication	I	N,D
1,25(OH)2D intoxication	N	I
Granuloma-forming diseases	N	I
Lymphoma	N	D,I
Hyperparathyroidism	N	D,I
Williams syndrome	N	I
Idiopathic hypercalciuria	N	I
Idiopathic osteoporosis	N	N,I
PTHrP-associated	N	D

D, decreased; I, increased; N, normal; PTHrP, parathyroid hormone–related protein.

than $1,25(OH)_2D$, has a long serum half-life (15–60 days) and most accurately reflects the body's total vitamin D stores. As vitamin D deficiency develops, increased PTH secretion (secondary hyperparathyroidism) can keep $1,25(OH)_2D$ levels within the normal range. In this situation, measurement of $1,25(OH)_2D$ alone would be misleading. In the hypocalcemic patient, a frankly low 25OHD level almost always indicates deficient cutaneous synthesis and dietary intake of vitamin D. These patients are rarer now in the United States because of the practice of supplementation of food with vitamin D. However, in elderly home-bound individuals, moderate to more severe vitamin D deficiency is now more widely recognized and is increasingly appreciated as a contributing factor to age-related bone loss (35). Patients with severe hepatocellular disease or nephrotic syndrome may have a low total serum calcium and 25OHD concentration owing to either a decrease in hepatic synthesis or urinary loss of proteins that bind calcium (albumin and prealbumin) and 25OHD (DBP, albumin) in the circulation. In such cases, a low serum ionized calcium concentration and a compensatory elevation in the circulating PTH concentration may aid in establishing the presence of true 25OHD deficiency. Hypocalcemia with a normal or elevated 25OHD concentration suggests either a deficiency or a decrease in the bioeffectiveness of PTH, an acquired abnormality in metabolism of 25OHD to $1,25(OH)_2D$ (i.e., renal failure, hyperphosphatemia), an inherited defect in $1,25(OH)_2D$ synthesis, or a defect in the action of $1,25(OH)_2D$ at its target tissue. Although both of these latter conditions are rare, they can usually be distinguished by assaying $1,25(OH)_2D$; values will be low or undetectable in patients with vitamin D–dependent rickets type I and often grossly elevated in patients with vitamin D–dependent rickets type II (see Chapter 60). In patients with hypocalcemia and diminished synthesis, release, or end-organ effectiveness of PTH (i.e., patients with hypoparathyroidism, pseudohyperparathyroidism, or magnesium deficiency), the $1,25(OH)_2D$ concentration will be inappropriately low. However, because of overlap of the serum $1,25(OH)_2D$ concentration into the normal range in such patients, measurement of this metabolite cannot be used to diagnose hypoparathyroidism.

The Hypercalcemic/Hypercalciuric Patient

The utility of the 25OHD assay in the evaluation of a hypercalcemic patient is limited. Only if 25OHD (or one its metabolites) is present in very high concentrations can it cross-react with the intestinal VDR to produce hypercalcemia. Thus, vitamin D intoxication may arise after ingestion of large amounts of vitamin D or $25OHD_3$. In this situation, the serum $1,25(OH)_2D$ concentration may be normal or even reduced, unless there is some additional abnormality in regulation of the 1-hydroxylation of 25OHD. Normal individuals do not become vitamin D intoxicated from endogenously synthesized vitamin D; the endogenous photosynthesis of vitamin D is regulated by the conversion of previtamin D to nonbiologically active photoisomers in the skin (36). However, in psoriatic patients receiving sequential whole-body UVB phototherapy, hypercalciuria accompanied by grossly elevated serum 25OHD levels has been observed (37).

As mentioned earlier, $1,25(OH)_2D$ levels are not always elevated in primary hyperparathyroidism, and therefore its assay is usually unnecessary for diagnosis or management. However, the $1,25(OH)_2D$ concentration may be helpful in detecting primary hyperparathyroidism in patients who are suspected to harbor the disease, but in whom confirmatory laboratory data are lacking; measurement of the serum $1,25(OH)_2D$ concentration, like measurement of the urinary cyclic adenosine monophosphate concentration, is an index of the bioactivity of circulating PTH. The finding of elevated $1,25(OH)_2D$ levels in the face of suppressed PTH concentrations in a patient with hypercalciuria with or without hypercalcemia is highly suggestive of the following: (i) exogenous intoxication with $1(OH)D_3$, DHT, or $1,25(OH)_2D$; (ii) endogenous overproduction of $1,25(OH)_2D$, as may occur in sarcoidosis, other granulomatous diseases, and lymphoma; (iii) idiopathic absorptive hypercalciuria (38); or (iv) idiopathic osteoporosis, a condition of premature bone loss observed principally, but not exclusively, in men (39). Hypercalcemia in patients with the syndrome of humoral hypercalcemia of malignancy, caused by tumor-derived parathyroid hormone–related protein (PTHrP), which activates the PTH receptor (40), is associated with low $1,25(OH)_2D$ levels. It is possible that these tumors release additional factors that suppress 25OHD–1-hydroxylase activity. Alternatively, other disease-related processes, such as severe hypercalcemia, might override any stimulatory effect of PTHrP.

Several new trends are likely to influence existing vitamin D applications and prompt new developments. First, the movement of health care from a fee-for-service toward a managed care environment can be expected to reduce the total numbers of vitamin D assays performed as providers seek to reduce costs. With this in mind, it will be important to use the most cost-effective assays and to apply them only where appropriate. In the research arena, the federal Women's Health Initiative is currently enrolling millions of American women in a study of the influence of dietary calcium and vitamin D supplementation on a number of end points, including bone density. Monitoring of circulating 25OHD in these women should ultimately lead to better guidelines on the impact of vitamin D supplementation on bone health in women. Finally, the discovery of analogs of $1,25(OH)_2D$ that are less calcemic than the parent metabolite but that retain selected biological actions (e.g., the ability to inhibit PTH secretion and inhibit cell proliferation) has spurred interest in their therapeutic application in a variety of disorders (41). Should any of these analogs find widespread therapeutic application, it may be necessary to develop new assays to monitor their serum levels during treatment. In addition, existing assays for circulating vitamin D metabolites will have to take into account potential interference by these analogues.

REFERENCES

1. Belsey RE, Deluca HF, Potts JT Jr: Competitive protein binding assay for vitamin D and 25-OH vitamin D. *J Clin Endocrinol Metab* 33:554–557, 1971
2. Haddad JG, Chyu KJ: Competitive protein binding radioassay for 25-hydroxy-cholecalciferol. *J Clin Endocrinol Metab* 33:992–995, 1971
3. McCollum FG, Simmonds N, Shipley PG, Park EA: Studies on experimental rickets. XVI. A delicate biological test for calcium depositing substances. *J Biol Chem* 54:41–50, 1922
4. Schacter D, Rosen SM: Active transport of Ca^{45} by the small intestine and its dependence on vitamin D. *Am J Physiol* 196: 357–365, 1959
5. Haddad JG Jr: Transport of vitamin D metabolites. *Clin Orthop* 142:249–261, 1979
6. Jones G, Seamark DA, Trafford DJH, Makin HLJ: Vitamin D: Cholecalciferol, ergocalciferol and hydroxylated metabolites. *Chromatogr Sci* 30:73–128, 1985
7. Taylor GA, Peacock M, Pelc B, Brown W, Holmes A: Purification of plasma vitamin D metabolites for radioimmunoassay. *Clin Chim Acta* 108:239–246, 1980
8. Koshy KT: Chromatography of vitamin D3 and metabolites. *Adv Chromatogr* 20:83–138, 1982
9. Adams JS, Clemens TL, Holick MF: Silica Sep-Pak preparative chromatography for vitamin D and its metabolites. *J Chromatogr* 226:198–201, 1981
10. Rhodes CJ, Claridge PA, Trafford DJH, Makin HLJ: An evaluation of the use of Sep-Pak C-18 cartridges for the extraction of vitamin D3 and some of its metabolites from plasma and urine. *J Steroid Biochem* 19:1339–1354, 1983
11. Hollis BW, Frank NE: Solid phase extraction system for vitamin D and its major metabolites in human plasma. *J Chromatogr* 343:43–49, 1985
12. Reinhardt TA, Horst RL, Orf JW, Hollis BW: A microassay for 1,25-dihydroxyvitamin D not requiring high performance liquid chromatography: Application to clinical studies. *J Clin Endocrinol Metab* 58:91–98, 1984
13. Hollis BW: Assay of circulating 1,25-dihydroxyvitamin D involving a novel single-cartridge extraction and purification procedure. *Clin Chem* 32:2060–2063, 1986
14. Jones G, Byrnes B, Palma F, Segev D, Mazur Y: Displacement potency of vitamin D2 analogs in competitive protein-binding assays for 25-hydroxyvitamin D3, 24,25-dihydroxyvitamin D3

and 1,25-dihydroxyvitamin D₃. *J Clin Endocrinol Metab* 50: 773–775, 1980

15. Jones G: Assay of vitamins D₂ and D₃ and 25-hydroxyvitamins D₂ and D₃ in human plasma by high-performance liquid chromatography. *Clin Chem* 24:287–298, 1978

16. Horst RL, Littledike ET, Riley JL, Napoli JL: Quantitation of vitamin D and its metabolites and their plasma concentrations in five species of animals. *Anal Biochem* 116:189–203, 1981

17. Dorantes LM, Arnaud SB, Arnaud CD: Importance of the isolation of 25-hydroxyvitamin D before assay. *J Lab Clin Med* 91: 791–796, 1978

18. Bouillon R, Van Herck E, Jans I, Tan BK, Van Baelen H, De Moor P: Two direct (nonchromatographic) assays for 25-hydroxyvitamin D. *Clin Chem* 30:1731–1736, 1984

19. Mayer E, Schmidt-Gayk H: Interlaboratory comparison of 25-hydroxyvitamin D determination. *Clin Chem* 30:1199–1204, 1984

20. Hollis BW, Napoli JL: Improved radioimmunoassay for vitamin D and its use in assessing vitamin D status. *Clin Chem* 31:1815–1819, 1985

21. Hollis BW, Kamerad JQ, Selvaag SR, Lorenz JD, Napoli JL: Determination of vitamin D status by radioimmunoassay using an [I¹²⁵]-labeled tracer. *Clin Chem* 39:529–533, 1992

22. Taylor A, Norman ME: 1,25(OH)₂D levels in dihydrotachysterol-treated patients: Influence on 1,25(OH)₂D assays. *J Bone Miner Res* 2:567–570, 1987

23. Bouillon R, De Moor P, Baggiolini EG, Uskokovic MR: A radioimmunoassay for 1,25-dihydroxycholecalciferol. *Clin Chem* 26:562–567, 1980

24. Jongen MJM, Van Ginkel FC, van der Vijgh WJF, Kuiper S, Netelenbos JC, Lips P: An international comparison of vitamin D metabolite measurements. *Clin Chem* 30:399–403, 1984

25. Quesada JM, Coopmans W, Ruiz B, Aljama P, Jans I, Bouillon R: Influence of vitamin D on parathyroid function in the elderly. *J Clin Endocrinol Metab* 75:494–501, 1992

26. Ebeling PR, Sandgren ME, DiMagno EP, Lane AW, DeLuca HF, Riggs BL: Evidence of an age-related decrease in intestinal responsiveness to vitamin D: Relationship between serum 1,25dihydroxyvitamin D3 and intestinal vitamin D receptor concentrations in normal women. *J Clin Endocrinol Metab* 75: 176–182, 1992

27. Adams JS, Clemens TL, Parrish JA, Holick MF: Vitamin D synthesis and metabolism after ultraviolet radiation of normal and vitamin D deficient subjects. *N Engl J Med* 306:722–725, 1982

28. Clemens TL, Adams JS, Nolan JM, Holick MF: Measurement of circulating vitamin D in man. *Clin Chim Acta* 121:301–308, 1982

29. Hollis BW, Roos BA, Lambert PW: Vitamin D in plasma: Quantitation by a nonequilibrium ligand binding assay. *Steroids* 37:609–619, 1981

30. Lo CW, Paris PW, Clemens TL, Nolan J, Holick MF: Vitamin D absorption in healthy subjects and in patients with intestinal malabsorption syndromes. *Am J Clin Nutr* 42:644–649, 1985

31. Holick MF, Shao Q, Liu WW, Chen TC: The vitamin D content of fortified milk and infant formula. *N Engl J Med* 326:1178–1181, 1991

32. Jones G: Chromatographic separation of 24(R), 25-dihydroxyvitamin D₃ and 25-hydroxyvitamin D₃-26,23-lactone using a cyano-bonded phase packing. *J Chromatogr* 276:69–74, 1983

33. Bikle DD, Gee E, Halloran B, Kowalski MA, Ryzen E, Haddad JG: Assessment of the free fraction of 25-hydroxyvitamin D in serum and its regulation by albumin and the vitamin D-binding protein. *J Clin Endocrinol Metab* 63:954–959, 1986

34. Bikle DD, Siiteri PK, Ryzen E, Haddad JG: Serum protein binding of 1,25-dihydroxyvitamin D: A re-evaluation by direct measurement of free metabolite levels. *J Clin Endocrinol Metab* 61: 969–975, 1985

35. Fraser DR, Vitamin D. *Lancet* 345:104–107, 1995

36. Holick MF, MacLaughlin JA, Doppelt SH: Factors that influence the cutaneous photosynthesis of previtamin D₃. *Science* 211:590–593, 1981

37. Prystowsky JH, Muzio PJ, Sevran S, Clemens TL. Effect of UVB phototherapy and oral calcitriol (1,25-dihydroxyvitamin D₃) on vitamin D photosynthesis in psoriasis patients. *J Amer Acad Derm* 1996 (in press)

38. Broadus AE, Insogna KL, Lang R, Mallette LE, Oren DA, Gertner JM, Kligor AS, Ellison AF: A consideration of the hormonal basis and phosphate leak hypothesis of absorptive hypercalciuria. *J Clin Endocrinol Metab* 58:161–169, 1984

39. Zerwekh JE, Sakhaee K, Breslau NA, Gottschalk F, Pak CYC: Impaired bone formation in male idiopathic osteoporosis: Further reduction in the presence of concomitant hypercalciuria. *Osteoporosis* Int 2:128–134, 1992

40. Martin TJ, Mosley JM, Gillespie MT: Parathyroid hormone-related protein: Biochemistry and molecular biology. *Crit Rev Biochem Mol Biol* 26:377–395, 1991

41. Brown AJ, Dusso A, Slatopolsky E: Selective vitamin D analogs and their therapeutic applications. *Semin Nephrol* 14: 156–174, 1994

20. Biochemical Markers of Bone Turnover

David R. Eyre, Ph.D.

Department of Orthopedics, University of Washington, Seattle, Washington

Reliable and convenient tests for quantifying bone turnover would aid in the clinical management of osteoporosis and other metabolic bone diseases. In recent years, immunoassays for novel bone metabolites have been reported in the research literature, with data indicating improved specificity and responsiveness to bone cell activity over traditional markers (1,2). Biochemical assays for monitoring bone turnover all rely on the measurement, in serum or urine, of enzymes or matrix proteins synthesized by osteoblasts or osteoclasts that spill over into body fluids, or of osteoclast-generated degradation products of the bone matrix itself. Serum levels of skeletal alkaline phosphatase and osteocalcin are currently the most convincing forma-

tion markers. The most useful resorption markers are all products of collagen degradation that for now are best measured in urine. Table 1 lists the more commonly explored biochemical markers of bone formation and resorption.

BONE FORMATION MARKERS

Total alkaline phosphatase activity in serum is still the most used index of bone formation in clinical use (e.g., to monitor Paget's disease of bone). Immunoassays for serum osteocalcin and bone-specific alkaline phosphatase have become the preferred tools in clinical research investiga-

TABLE 1. *Biochemical markers of bone remodeling*

Formation (osteoblast products)
  Propeptides of type I collagen (serum)
    C-propeptide
    N-propeptide
  Osteocalcin (serum)
  Alkaline phosphatase (serum)
    Total activity
    Bone-specific enzyme
Resorption (osteoclast products)
  Tartrate-resistant acid phosphatase (serum)
  Hydroxyproline (urine)
  Hydroxylysine glycosides (urine)
  Collagen cross-links (urine and serum)
    Total pyridinolines (Pyr and/or Dpy)
    Free pyridinolines (Pyr and/or Dpy)
    Cross-linked N- and C-telopeptides

tions where greater specificity is required. Propeptides of type I collagen have also proven to respond as expected as serum markers of bone formation (3,4), but they presumably reflect the sum of all type I collagen synthetic activity throughout the body and so are not bone specific.

Alkaline Phosphatase

The common form of alkaline phosphatase is a cell-membrane-associated enzyme expressed by liver, bone, kidney, and placenta from a single gene. Liver and bone are the primary sources of the serum enzymes, and the molecules differ posttranslationally in their glycosylation pattern. Alkaline phosphatase is a prominent product of osteoblasts and osteoblast precursors, and it plays a key role, as yet poorly defined, in mineralization. The development of monoclonal antibodies that can select for the osteoblast enzyme, bone-specific alkaline phosphatase (BAP), by recognizing a posttranslational characteristic, has provided the basis for a more specific index of bone formation activity (5,6). An immunoassay for the protein is more attractive than approaches that separate and measure the activities of the bone-derived and liver enzymes in serum (7,8). The measure of bone formation provided by alkaline phosphatase is indirect, depending presumably on a spillover of excess or spent enzyme from active osteoblasts and probably also pre-osteoblasts, lining cells, and perhaps osteocytes. Therefore, as with all bone-turnover assays, the quantitative relationship between serum levels of BAP and the actual rate of bone deposition may not be simple or constant within or between individuals.

Osteocalcin

Human osteocalcin (or bone Gla-protein, BGP) is a 49-residue polypeptide expressed under 1,25-dihydroxyvitamin D_3 control by osteoblasts as they actively deposit bone. Other calcified tissues, including dentin and calcified cartilage, also contain osteocalcin. Osteocalcin forms about 1% of the organic matrix of bone where it exists in close association with the surface of the mineral crystal-lites. Serum osteocalcin (9,10) seems to reflect primarily a spillover of osteoblast synthetic activity rather than degradation products of resorbed bone matrix. Osteocalcin in bone is probably degraded on resorption to fragments. These are probably not recognized by the latest immunoassays, which use specific monoclonal antibodies to measure only intact molecules and almost intact fragments that preserve the N-terminal sequence (e.g., in two-site assay formats) (11,12).

Although serum osteocalcin (the intact molecule) and bone-specific alkaline phosphatase immunoassays are emerging as the best indicators of bone formation activity, they do not always show parallel responses. For example, serum osteocalcin is not highly elevated and correlates poorly with either total serum alkaline phosphatase activity or levels of the bone-specific enzyme molecule in Paget's disease of bone (13). Osteocalcin levels are much lower than might be expected in this high-turnover condition. The relative lack of correlation between osteocalcin and serum alkaline phosphatase may reflect the expression of these proteins at different stages of osteoblast development and synthetic activity (14,15). Also, since serum osteocalcin is thought to represent only a fraction of the synthetic pool, which escapes incorporation into newly formed bone matrix, the amount of this spillover fraction may change under different conditions of osteoblast physiology and pathology.

Type I Collagen Propeptides

The common types of collagen, types I, II, and III, are synthesized as procollagen molecules which have their N- and C-propeptides removed extracellularly. Propeptides of all three collagen types can be found in serum as by-products of collagen synthesis, and all have seen use as indicators in clinical studies. Immunoassays for both N- and C-propeptides of type I collagen have been developed as markers of bone formation (1–4,16). Because bone is such a major organ of turnover of collagen type I, serum levels of these propeptides may reasonably reflect total bone-forming activity in the body. Data from clinical studies on various disease states support this concept, but they indicate a relatively low specificity and lack of responsiveness in conditions where changes in bone turnover are subtle (17). Furthermore, studies that compared N- and C-propeptide assay results showed poor correlation (16).

BONE RESORPTION MARKERS

Consistently, the most promising markers of bone resorption are urinary levels of collagen degradation products (Table 1).

Hydroxyproline

Total urinary hydroxyproline (after acid hydrolysis) is the traditional index, but its usefulness is blunted by contribution from the diet, lack of specificity to bone collagen, degradative losses of the free amino acid in the liver, and relatively tedious chemical assays. More precise assays for hydroxyproline by high-performance liquid chromatography (HPLC) appear to offer greater specificity for bone metabolism than the traditional colorimetric assay (18).

Hydroxylysine Glycosides

All collagens contain glycosylated hydroxylysine residues. There are two forms, glucosylgalactosylhydroxylysine (GGHyl) and galactosylhydroxylysine (GHyl). These are also excreted in urine as the free hydroxylysine glycosides, which presumably are derived from collagen catabolism (19). The degree of glycosylation and ratio of GGHyl/GHyl varies with collagen type and tissue type. For instance, human bone collagen type and contains mostly GHyl whereas skin contains mostly GGHyl (19), suggesting that analysis of GHyl in urine may be a useful index of bone resorption. Moro et al. (20) developed an HPLC assay for GGHyl and GHyl in urine and showed appropriate changes when applied to clinical conditions of high turnover such as metastatic bone disease (21). Although bone is clearly a significant source of the pool of GGHyl and GHyl in urine, other tissues also probably contribute. In addition, because the free amino acid glycosides, not peptides, are the primary forms in urine (19), the initial products of collagen degradation at the tissue level presumably become fully degraded in the liver and/or kidney.

Tartrate-Resistant Acid Phosphatase

Tartrate-resistant acid phosphatase (TRAP) is a prominent enzyme of osteoclasts that appears to be involved in bone matrix degradation. TRAP can dephosphorylate the protein osteopontin, for example (22). TRAP activity in serum is elevated in clinical conditions that cause increased bone turnover (23), but the degree of specificity to osteoclasts is not well defined, and it is known that other cell types produce TRAP activity (24). The development of immunoassays for the enzyme molecule (25,26) could prove more useful than enzyme activity measurements, but data are still few.

Pyridinoline Cross-links of Collagen

Urinary levels of pyridinoline have been the most studied bone resorption markers in the last decade (27,28). These complex amino acids appear not to be metabolized after tissue collagen is degraded and are excreted in urine, where they can be measured by HPLC using their natural fluorescence for detection (29). Usually, about two thirds are in the form of small peptides and the remaining are free amino acids. Two chemical forms exist: hydroxylysylpyridinoline (or simply pyridinoline, HP, or Pyr) and lysylpyridinoline (deoxypyridinoline, LP, or Dpy). These structures reflect posttranslational heterogeneity in the degree of hydroxylation of lysine residues at specific crosslinking sites in types I, II, III, and IX collagens (30).

The pyridinolines function as mature cross-links in collagen of most connective tissues other than skin. Because bone is such a major reservoir of type I collagen in the body and turns over faster than most major connective tissues, the pyridinolines in adult urine are primarily derived from bone resorption. This conclusion is supported by the observed similarity in the ratios of Pyr to Dpy in adult human bone (3.5:1) and urine (range, 2:1 to 7:1), compared with most nonbone connective tissues, in which Dpy is usually present at less than 10% of the content of Pyr (30,31). Urinary Dpy is therefore theoretically more specific than Pyr or total pyridinoline as a marker of bone degradation, and the clinical data from HPLC assay results support this (32).

However, it is important to recognize that even though the ratio of Pyr to Dpy is usually much higher in tissues other than bone, the concentration of Dpy can be as high as that in bone collagen, as it is, for example, in collagen of skeletal muscle and the vasculature (33,34). The ratio of Pyr to Dpy in vascular tissue and skeletal muscle collagen is also closer to that of bone at 6 to 8:1 (34). The absolute concentration of total pyridinolines in bone collagen is actually quite low (about 0.3 moles per mole of collagen) compared with other tissue collagens [1.5 moles/mole in cartilage; 0.5 to 1.0 moles/mole in vascular tissue, tendon, ligament, fascia, lung, intestine, liver, muscle, etc. (35)]. Therefore, because nothing is known about the turnover rates of collagen in these tissues relative to bone, it is still uncertain to what degree total pyridinolines or even Dpy can be relied on as specific markers of bone resorption. Half the total urinary pyridinolines could come from a nonbone source and still result in a ratio typically seen in urine (34).

Cross-linked N- and C-Telopeptide Assays

Figure 1 illustrates the two locations of pyridinoline cross-links in type I collagen, N-telopeptide-to-helix and C-telopeptide-to-helix. Pyridinoline-containing peptides (MW < 2 kDa) from both sites have been recovered from urine, that appear to resist further proteolysis (36). The

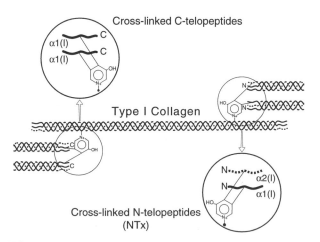

FIG. 1. Pyridinoline cross-links are located at two intermolecular sites in type I collagen fibrils, N-telopeptide-to-helix and C-telopeptide-to-helix. Both α1(I) and α2(I) N-telopeptides participate, but only α1(I) C-telopeptides. The α2(I) N-telopeptide is a favored participant in bone collagen cross-linking.

pool of cross-linked N-telopeptides from urine had a Pyr:Dpy ratio of about 2:1, indicating an origin in bone. Similar domains prepared from human bone collagen showed that two thirds of the Dpy in collagen is located at the N-telopeptide site and one third at the C-telopeptide site (36). The α2(I) N-telopeptide was also prominently involved in crosslinking in bone collagen, which appears to be a distinguishing property over nonmineralized collagens (36). The cross-linked N-telopeptides in urine were targeted, therefore, as a particularly promising marker of bone resorption. A monoclonal antibody, mAb 1H11, was prepared which recognized small cross-linked N-telopeptides that contained the α2(I) N-telopeptide sequence QYDGK̊GVG, where K̊ is involved in trivalent cross-linking (36). The antibody did not recognize synthetic, individual telopeptides alone, nor the pyridinoline cross-link structure itself. The latter property may be important because of potential photolytic and other destructive losses of the 3-hydroxypyridinium ring structure of pyridinolines in urine. Moreover, the peptide antigen (NTx) becomes recognizable by the antibody only when bone collagen is degraded to small peptides, for example by bacterial collagenase or by osteoclasts. Osteoclasts were shown to generate immunoreactive NTx, but not free pyridinolines, when cultured on human bone particles in vitro (37). The antigen, therefore, appears to embody conformational features and to be a proteolytic neoepitope. A microtiter-plate enzyme-linked immunosorbent assay (ELISA) was developed that can be applied directly to urine (36,38).

Assays for collagen type I cross-linked C-telopeptides (ICTP) have also been described. The ICTP assay uses a polyclonal antibody raised against a cross-linked C-telopeptide prepared from human bone collagen (39). It recognizes antigen in serum but not in urine. Clinical evidence in support of this assay as a specific indicator of bone-resorbing activity has been disappointing (40), and the entities being recognized in serum appear not to have been characterized. Another C-telopeptide assay for urine uses a polyclonal antiserum raised against a cross-linked synthetic octapeptide (EKAHDGGR) that matches the C-telopeptide domain of the α1(I) chain of type I collagen containing the cross-linking lysine residue (41,42). This sequence was selected with the anticipation that it would be protected from degradation when embodied in pyridinoline cross-linked structures (36,41).

Free Pyridinolines

Most reports on pyridinoline levels in urine have measured the total pools of Pyr and Dpy by HPLC after acid hydrolysis to convert peptides to free amino acids (33). The free fraction of Pyr and Dpy has also been targeted. This can be done by HPLC, but an immunoassay would be more convenient and would allow direct analysis without any pretreatment steps. A polyclonal antibody-based ELISA that recognizes free Pyr was originally described (43) and further developed into both polyclonal- and monoclonal-antibody based versions (44). More recently, a monoclonal antibody-based ELISA that is specific for free Dpy has also become commercially available (51).

Clinical Results

To date, most reports on the newer bone biomarkers have presented cross-sectional data showing statistically significant increases or decreases between different subject groups (e.g., postmenopausal, premenopausal, and Paget's disease). Performance data from longitudinal studies on individual subjects are few.

Bone formation markers (intact osteocalcin and alkaline phosphatase) generally give tighter overall coefficients of variance than urinary assays. This no doubt reflects in part the added error in having to normalize urinary values to a second analyte, creatinine. Serum formation markers, on the other hand, respond more slowly to changes in bone turnover rate that occur naturally [e.g., at menopause (46)], after surgical oophorectomy (47), or on intervention with the antiresorptive agents, estrogen (48) and bisphosphonate (40). In most clinical situations, resorption and formation are coupled, but the change in formation markers lags several months behind that of resorption markers, whether turnover activity goes up or down.

Studies comparing the newer formation and resorption markers have been reported (38,40,45,49). Based on the percentage increase in postmenopausal women over premenopausal women as a measure of increased turnover, BAP was the most responsive formation marker (40). Osteocalcin was a close second, but type I collagen C-propeptide was not significantly different (40). In response to the bisphosphonate, alendronate, the formation markers, BAP, osteocalcin, and type I C-propeptide all dropped 40% to 50%, but gradually, over 6 to 12 months (40). The most responsive resorption marker was the cross-linked N-telopeptide, NTx, in urine (40). This analyte showed the greatest increase at menopause (46) and the most rapid and greatest percentage drop from baseline in bisphosphonate intervention trials (38,40,49). Total Pyr and particularly total Dpy measured by HPLC after acid hydrolysis were also responsive, but quantitatively less so than NTx (38,40). In a separate study, the cross-linked C-telopeptide (CTx) in urine was also significantly elevated postmenopausally and suppressed by both estrogen and bisphosphonate therapy (45,50). Free pyridinolines (Pyr or Dpy) measured in urine by immunoassay turn out to be unresponsive to bisphosphonate intervention compared with the cross-linked N- or C-telopeptides, total Pyr, or total Dpy by HPLC (40,45,49). The exact reason is unclear, but it is notable that osteoclasts in vitro do not generate free pyridinolines but do produce the immunoreactive telopeptide analyte, NTx (37). Therefore, there may be other tissue sources of the free pyridinolines and a requirement for peptide breakdown in the liver or kidney (Fig. 2). Interestingly, free pyridinoline levels in urine, as well as total pyridinolines and telopeptide markers (45), were suppressed on long-term estrogen therapy, which might be explained by the systemic effects of estrogen on other tissues in contrast with bisphosphonates which specifically target osteoclasts. Further studies are clearly needed to understand better the tissue origins and metabolic handling in the liver and kidney of these various peptide and free amino acid degradation products of collagen. Conceptually, the ideal resorption marker would be a

OSTEOCLAST

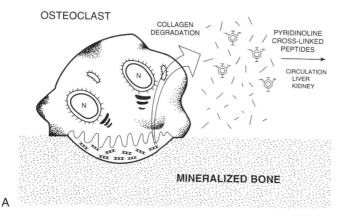

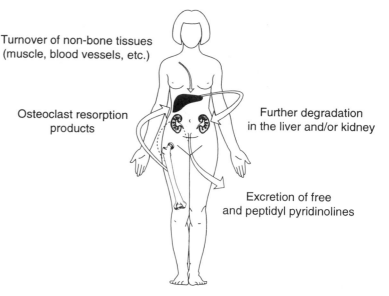

FIG. 2. Osteoclasts degrade bone collagen to peptides, including pyridinoline-containing structures **(A)**, but not to free pyridinolines, which are presumably generated from circulating peptides in the liver or kidney **(B)**.

unique product of the action of osteoclasts on bone that escapes further metabolism in the liver and is rapidly cleared by the kidney.

REFERENCES

1. Delmas PD: Clinical use of biochemical markers of bone remodeling in osteoporosis. *Bone* 13:517–521, 1992
2. Eriksen EF, Brixen K, Charles P: New markers of bone metabolism: Clinical use in metabolic bone disease. *Eur J Endocrinol* 132: 251–263, 1995
3. Parfitt AM, Simon LS, Villanueva AR, Krane SM: Procollagen type I carboxy-terminal extension peptide in serum as a marker of collagen biosynthesis in bone: Correlation with iliac bone formation rates and comparison with total alkaline phosphatase. *J Bone Miner Res* 2:427–436, 1987
4. Kraenzlin ME, Mohan S, Singer F, et al.: Development of a radioimmunoassay for the N-terminal type I procollagen: Potential use to assess bone formation. *Eur J Clin Invest* 19:A86, 1989
5. Hill CS, Wolfert RL: The preparation of monoclonal antibodies which react preferentially with human bone alkaline phosphatase and not liver alkaline phosphatase. *Clin Chim Acta* 186:315–320, 1990
6. Panigrahi K, Delmas PD, Singer F, Ryan W, Reiss O, Fisher R, Miller PD, Mizrahi I, Darte C, Kress BC, et al.: Characteristics of a two-site immunoradiometric assay for human skeletal alkaline phosphatase in serum. *Clin Chem* 40:822–828, 1994
7. Behr W, Barnert J: Quantification of bone alkaline phosphatase in serum by precipitation with wheat-germ lectin: A simplified method and its clinical plausibility. *Clin Chem* 32:1960–1966, 1986
8. Bouman AA, Scheffer PG, Ooms ME, Lips P, Netelenbos C: Two bone alkaline phosphatase assays compared with osteocalcin as a marker of bone formation in healthy elderly women. *Clin Chem* 41:196–199, 1995
9. Price PA, Nishimoto SK: Radioimmunoassay for the vitamin K-dependent protein of bone and its discovery in plasma. *Proc Natl Acad Sci USA* 77:2234–2238, 1980
10. Gundberg CM, Lian JB, Gallop PM, Steinberg JJ: Urinary γ-carboxyglutamic acid and serum osteocalcin as bone markers: Studies in osteoporosis and Paget's disease. *J Clin Endocrinol Metab* 57: 1221–1225, 1983
11. Garnero P, Grimaux M, Demiaux B, Preaudat C, Seguin P, Delmas PD: Measurement of serum osteocalcin with a human specific two-site immunoradiometric method. *J Bone Miner Res* 7:1389–1398, 1992
12. Deftos LJ, Wolfert RL, Hill CS, Burton DW: Two-site assays of bone GLA protein (osteocalcin) demonstrate immunochemical heterogeneity of the intact molecule. *Clin Chem* 38:2318–2321, 1992
13. Delmas PD, Demiaux B, Malaval L, Chapuy M.C, Meunier PJ: Serum bone GLA-protein is not a sensitive marker of bone turnover in Paget's disease of bone. *Calcif Tissue Int* 38:60–61, 1986
14. Deftos LJ, Wolfert RL, Hill CS: Bone alkaline phosphatase in Paget's disease. *Horm Metab Res* 23:559–561, 1991
15. Diaz-Diego EM, Diaz-Martin MA, de la Piedra C, Rapado A: Lack of correlation between levels of osteocalcin and bone alkaline phosphatase in healthy control and post-menopausal osteoporotic women. *Horm Metab Res* 27:151–154, 1995
16. Ebeling PR, Peterson JM, Riggs BL: Utility of type I procollagen propeptide assays for assessing abnormalities in metabolic bone diseases. *J Bone Miner Res* 7:1243–1250, 1992
17. Hassager C, Fabbri-Mabelli G, Christiansen C: The effect of the menopause and hormone replacement therapy on serum carboxyterminal propeptide of type I collagen. *Osteoporosis Int* 3:50–52, 1993
18. Pavori R, DeVecchi E, Fermo I, Arcelloni C, Diomede L, Magri F, Borini PA: Total urinary hydroxyproline determined with rapid and simple high-performance liquid chromatography. *Clin Chem* 38: 407–411, 1992
19. Segrest JP, Cunningham LW: Variation in human urinary O-hydroxylysyl glycoside levels and their relationship to collagen metabolism. *J Clin Invest* 49:1497–1509, 1970
20. Moro L, Modricky C, Stagni N, Vittur F, de Bernard B: High-performance liquid chromatographic analysis of urinary hydroxylysyl glycosides as indicators of collagen turnover. *Analyst* 109:1621–1622, 1984
21. Moro L, Gazzarini C, Crivellari D, Galligioni E, Talamini R, de Bernard B: Biochemical markers for detecting bone metastases in patients with breast cancer. *Clin Chem* 39:131–134, 1993
22. Ek-Rylander B, Flores M, Wendel M, Heinegård D, Andersson G: Dephosphorylation of osteopontin and bone sialoprotein by osteoclastic tartrate-resistant acid phosphatase. *J Biol Chem* 269: 14853–14856, 1994
23. Lau KHW, Orishi T, Wergedal JE, Singer FR, Baylink DJ: Characterization and assay of tartrate-resistant acid phosphatase activity in serum: Potential use to assess bone resorption. *Clin Chem* 33: 458–462, 1987
24. Hattersley G, Chambers TJ: Generation of osteoclastic function in mouse bone marrow cultures: Multinuclearity and tartrate-resistant acid phosphatase are unreliable markers for osteoclastic differentiation. *Endocrinology* 124:1689–1696, 1989
25. Kraenzlin ME, Lau K-HW, Liang L, Freeman TK, Singer FR, Stepan J, Baylink DJ: Development of an immunoassay for human serum osteoclastic tartrate-resistant acid phosphatase. *J Clin Endocrinol Metab* 71:442–451, 1990

26. Cheung CK, Panesar NS, Haines C, Masarei J, Swaminathan R: Immunoassay of tartrate-resistant acid phosphatase in serum. *Clin Chem* 41:679–686, 1995

27. Robins SP, Stewart P, Astbury C, Bird HA: Measurement of the cross-linking compound, pyridinoline, in urine as an index of collagen degradation. *Ann Rheum Dis* 45:969–973, 1986

28. Demers LM, Kleerekoper M: Recent advances in biochemical markers of bone turnover (editorial). *Clin Chem* 40:1994–1995, 1994

29. Black D, Duncan A, Robins SP: Quantitative analysis of the pyridinium cross-links of collagen in urine using ion-paired reverse-phase high-performance liquid chromatography. *Anal Biochem* 169:197–203, 1988

30. Eyre DR: Collagen cross-linking amino acids. *Methods Enzymol* 144:115–139, 1987

31. Beardsworth LJ, Eyre DR, Dickson IR: Changes with age in the urinary excretion of lysyl- and hydroxylysyl-pyridinoline: Two new markers of bone collagen turnover. *J Bone Miner Res* 5:671–676, 1990

32. Uebelhart D, Schlemmer A, Johansen JS, Gineyts E, Christiansen C, Delmas PD: Effect of menopause and hormone replacement therapy on the urinary excretion of pyridinium cross-links. *Clin Endocrinol Metab* 72:367–373, 1991

33. Seibel MJ, Robins SP, Bilezikian JP: Urinary pyridinium cross-links of collagen: Specific markers of bone resorption in metabolic bone disease. *Trends Endocrinol Metab* 3:263–270, 1992

34. Eyre DR: The specificity of collagen cross-links as markers of bone and connective tissue degradation. *Acta Orthop Scand Suppl* 266:166–170, 1995

35. Eyre DR, Van Ness K, Koob TJ: Quantitation of hydroxypyridinium crosslinks in collagen by high performance liquid chromatography. *Analyt Biochem* 137:380–388, 1984

36. Hanson DA, Weis M-A E, Bollen A-M, Maslan SL, Singer FR, Eyre DR: A specific immunoassay for monitoring human bone resorption: Quantitation of type I collagen cross-linked N-telopeptides in urine. *J Bone Miner Res* 7:1251–1258, 1992

37. Apone S, Fevold K, Lee M, Eyre D: A rapid method for quantifying osteoclast activity *in vitro*. *J Bone Miner Res* 9(suppl 1): S178, 1994

38. Gertz BJ, Shao P, Hanson DA, Quan H, Harris ST, Genant HK, Chesnut CH III, Eyre DR: Monitoring bone resorption in early post-menopausal women by an immunoassay for cross-linked collagen peptides in urine. *J Bone Miner Res* 9:135–142, 1994

39. Risteli J, Elomaa I, Niemi S, Novamo A, Risteli L: Radioimmunoassay for the pyridinoline cross-linked carboxy-terminal telopeptide of type I collagen: A new marker of bone degradation. *Clin Chem* 39:635–640, 1993

40. Garnero P, Shih WJ, Gineyts E, Karpf DB, Delmas PD: Comparison of new biochemical markers of bone turnover in late post-menopausal osteoporotic women in response to alendronate treatment. *J Clin Endocrinol Metab* 79:1693–1700, 1994

41. Bonde M, Qvist P, Fledelius C, Riis BJ, Christiansen C: Immunoassay for quantifying type I collagen degradation products in urine evaluated. *Clin Chem* 40:2022–2025, 1994

42. Bonde M, Qvist P, Fledelius C, Riis BJ, Christiansen C: Applications of an enzyme immunoassay for a new marker of bone resorption (CrossLaps): Follow-up on hormone replacement therapy and osteoporosis risk assessment. *J Clin Endocrinol Metab* 80: 864–868, 1995

43. Robins SP: An enzyme-linked immunoassay for the collagen cross-link pyridinoline. *Biochem J* 207:617–620, 1982

44. Seyedin SM, Kung VT, Daniloff YN, Hesley RP, Gomez B, Nielsen LA, Rosen HN, Zuk RF: Immunoassay for urinary pyridinoline: The new marker of bone resorption. *J Bone Miner Res* 8:635–641, 1993

45. Garnero P, Gineyts E, Arbault P, Christiansen C, Delmas PD: Different effects of bisphosphonate and estrogen therapy on free and peptide-bound bone cross-links excretion. *J Bone Miner Res* 10: 641–649, 1995

46. Ebeling PR, Atley LM, Guthrie JR, et al: Bone turnover markers and bone density across the menopausal transition. *J Clin Endocrinol Metab* (in press) 1996

47. Prior JC, Eyre DR, Ebeling PR, Wark JD: Trabecular bone loss after premenopausal oophorectomy is not prevented by conjugated estrogen or medroxyprogesterone—a double-blind, randomized 1-year study. *J Bone Miner Res* 9(suppl 1): S394, 1994

48. Prestwood KM, Pilbeam CC, Burleson JA, Woodiel FN, Delmas PD, Deftos LJ, Raisz LG: The short-term effects of conjugated estrogen on bone turnover in older women. *J Clin Endocrinol Metab* 79(2):366–371, 1994

49. Rosen HN, Dresner-Pollak R, Moses AC, Rosenblatt M, Zeind AJ, Clemens JD, Greenspan SL: Specificity of urinary excretion of cross-linked N-telopeptides of type I collagen as a marker of bone turnover. *Calcif Tissue Int* 54:26–29, 1994

50. Garnero P, Gineyts E, Riou JP, Delmas PD: *J Clin Endocrinol Metab* 79:780–785, 1994

51. Robins SP, Woitge H, Hesley R, et al: Direct enzyme-linked immunoassay for urinary deoxypyridinoline as a specific marker for measuring bone resorption. *J Bone Miner Res* 9:1643–1649, 1994

21. Radiologic Evaluation of Bone Mineral in Children

Richard M. Shore, M.D., and Andrew K. Poznanski, M.D.

Department of Radiology, Northwestern University Medical School, and Children's Memorial Hospital, Chicago, Illinois

Bone mineral evaluation in childhood is performed for different reasons than in adults, and the approaches used for this evaluation are consequently different. A major use of bone mineral evaluation in children is in the diagnosis and management of renal osteodystrophy and rickets. It is also useful in many other chronic conditions associated with bone loss, such as inflammatory bowel disease and juvenile rheumatoid arthritis. Bone mass evaluation is also of value in diverse congenital disorders, such as osteogenesis imperfecta and osteopetrosis. In premature infants, severe bone loss can occur, and radiologic evaluation may useful in determining its causes.

Bone mineral evaluation in childhood includes both quantitative and qualitative assessments. Because subjective assessment of bone density from skeletal radiographs is a poor indicator of bone mineral status, several techniques have been developed that are more useful in determining the amount of bone mineral present. These methods are essential in following bone mineralization longitudinally to evaluate the effects of therapy. Furthermore, children with mild bone mineral disorders often have skeletal radiographs that are within normal limits, and an abnormality can be recognized only with the quantitative techniques. Although these children are often asymptomatic, recognition of subtle mineral abnormalities is important because the disease process may lead to significantly reduced bone mineral mass at the completion of growth and thus predispose to an increased risk of symptomatic osteoporosis during adulthood. Quantitative evaluation alone is nonspecific, however, and should be used in conjunction with qualitative assessment of skeletal radiographs, as well as other clinical and laboratory data, to determine the mechanism and etiology of bone loss. Rickets, other vitamin deficiencies or poisonings, osteoporosis, hyperparathyroidism, and osteogenesis imperfecta may have typical radiographic appearances. There are also qualitative findings that indicate that bone mineral deficiency is present, and these are important to recognize because they may be the first clinical indication of a bone mineral abnormality.

QUANTITATIVE MEASUREMENTS OF BONE LOSS IN CHILDREN

Techniques to quantify bone loss in children may differ from those used in adults. One of the problems of many of the newer methods is the lack of normal values for young children. Another difference concerns the sites of bone mineral measurement that appear to be most useful. The methods that have pediatric applications include radiogrammetry (measurement of cortical dimensions) and multiple methods of quantifying photon absorption by bone, including single-photon absorptiometry (SPA), dual x-ray absorptiometry (DXA), and quantitative computed tomography (QCT).

Radiogrammetry

Measurements of cortical dimensions are usually performed on hand films, although the humerus is also useful in neonates. The second metacarpal is the bone that is most frequently used, and standards have been established for different populations (1). In the United States, the most commonly used standards are those of Garn et al. (2), with the cortical measurements performed at the midshaft of the second metacarpal. A high-detail film screen combination should be used, and the measurements are best made using a magnifying comparator scaled to measure one tenth of a millimeter. The outside and inside diameters of the cortex are measured. Based on these measurements, cortical thickness, cortical area, and percent cortical area can all be calculated. One difficulty is that the inside diameter may be poorly defined; this occurs primarily in conditions with rapid bone loss producing a permeative pattern with a ragged margin.

Cortical bone standards have also been developed for the humerus for neonates of varying gestational ages (3). These humeral measurements are obtained at the midshaft just above the level of the nutrient canal, which is profiled on the frontal view and seen *en face* on the lateral view. As for the second metacarpal, humeral cortical thickness is calculated from measurements of the outside and inside diameters. Premature infants can be followed longitudinally from birth to determine whether cortical bone mineral is growing along the normal growth curve as would have occurred *in utero,* or whether significant bone loss has occurred (Fig. 1). In

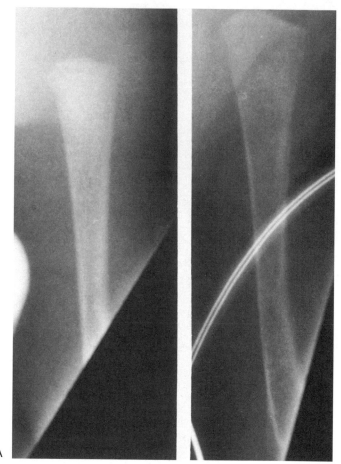

A   B

FIG. 1. Humerus of a premature infant at birth **(A)** and 6 weeks later **(B)**. Note the marked thinning of the cortex postnatally. Most of the loss has occurred by endosteal resorption. The outer diameter has shown little change, but the medullary diameter is considerably wider. Longitudinal humeral cortical thickness measurements for this patient are shown against the *in utero* growth curve for humeral cortical thickness at birth **(C)**.

severely ill premature infants, there is a rapid bone loss, which occurs mainly by endosteal resorption. This may predispose the infant to fractures, after even ordinary handling.

Virtama and Helela (4) have also developed cortical standards for a number of sites in other long bones in a Finnish population. Their values for the second metacarpal are reasonably close to the standards of Garn et al. (2).

Advantages

Radiogrammetry is the simplest, least expensive technique of measuring bone mineral. It is particularly useful in children because good standards are available that are age- and sex-specific and have been developed for several population groups in the United States, including Caucasians, African Americans, and Mexican Americans (1). In addition to calculation of cortical thickness, these measurements can be used to evaluate whether the bone loss is due to endosteal resorption or lack of periosteal surface apposition. In most

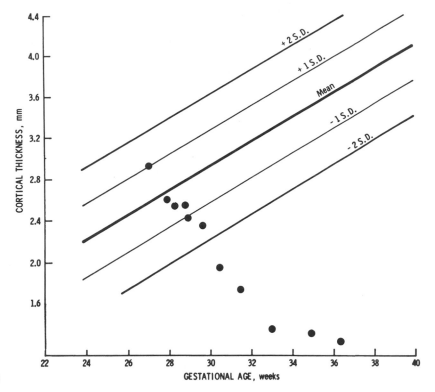

FIG. 1. *(continued)*. **(C):** At birth, the cortical thickness was 1 SD above the mean, but it decreased rapidly thereafter. At 10 weeks after birth, equivalent to just above 36 weeks' gestational age, the bone mineral was very low, much lower than that of even a 22-week gestational age infant. (From: Poznanski AK, Kuhns LR, Guire KE. *Radiology* 134:639–644, 1980.)

C

causes of pediatric osteoporosis, other than renal osteodystrophy, the usual mechanism of bone loss is increased resorption along the endosteal surface, resulting in a larger medullary space (5). There is also a lack of growth on the outer surface in osteogenesis imperfecta as well as in chronically ill children with poor nutrition, juvenile rheumatoid arthritis, or Crohn's disease (1,2,5). Because little or no bone can be lost from the outer surface, other than with subperiosteal resorption in hyperparathyroidism, a diminished outside diameter is indicative of lack of growth. Also, from the hand radiograph one can determine the presence or absence of subperiosteal resorption, indicating hyperparathyroidism, and intracortical resorption, indicating either hyperparathyroidism or other causes of rapid bone loss. These findings indicate that additional evaluation is needed to determine the mechanism and cause of bone loss. Another advantage of the hand radiograph in children is that skeletal age can be determined, allowing bone mineralization to be compared with either chronologic age or skeletal age-matched control values (5). The latter may be more realistic, particularly for disorders in which there is marked retardation of skeletal maturation or in delayed puberty.

Disadvantages

Radiogrammetry does not measure cancellous bone and does not recognize bone loss within the cortex. The inability to measure cancellous bone mass may seem to be less of a problem in children than in adults because osteoporotic fractures of the hip seldom occur in children. Trabecular bone accumulation during childhood is important, however, because it determines how much bone can be lost subse-

quently during adulthood before symptomatic osteoporosis develops. Intracortical bone loss is not recognized by measurement of cortical thickness, and thus if subperiosteal resorption or increased intracortical striations are seen on the hand radiograph, cortical measurements should not be used. This is seen most often in children with renal osteodystrophy, and in these cases, SPA or DXA is more accurate. Because radiogrammetry has lower precision than SPA or DXA, it is less sensitive than those techniques for recognizing changes over serial examinations.

Photon Absorption Methods

Single-Photon Absorptiometry

Single-photon absorptiometry (6) measures bone mass by the attenuation of a narrow photon beam, usually 27.5-keV x-rays from a ^{125}I source. Because soft tissue also attenuates photons, the amount of bone mineral can be calculated from total attenuation only if the body-part thickness is constant. This is achieved by placing the part being examined in a soft-tissue equivalent bath or bolus, and this limits the use of SPA to the extremities. The most frequently studied site is the radial diaphysis at the junction of the mid- and distal thirds of the forearm. This is called the "one-third site," and it contains primarily cortical bone. Because there is little variation in the radial shaft in that region, repositioning error is small and precision is quite high. The ultradistal radius has also been used as a site that contains a greater amount of trabecular bone. Repositioning error is more critical at the distal radius, however, which decreases precision. The calcaneus has also been used as a site containing a large amount of trabecular bone that can be measured by SPA. Bone mineral content (BMC) as measured by SPA is the amount of mineral per length of the bone that was scanned (g/cm). Dividing by bone width gives bone mineral density (BMD, g/cm^2), which is considered to be most indicative of the degree of bone mineralization. Because the bone thickness in the direction of the photon beam cannot be measured, BMD is a projectional area density (g/cm^2) rather than a true volume density (g/cm^3).

Advantages

SPA has high accuracy and precision and can identify intracortical bone loss that will not be detected by radiogrammetry. It is less expensive than DXA and QCT. The radiation dose from SPA is extremely low. Skin entrance doses have been estimated to be 60–180 μSv. More important, because only a very small part of the body is exposed, the effective dose equivalent is less than 1 μSv.

An important consideration for the use of SPA for bone mineral evaluation in children is the experience that has been gained with it. It has been used in children for more than two decades, there are well-established normal values for most children, and there is considerable clinical experience with interpreting the results of these studies. The largest set of normal data for children includes those at least 6 years of age (7), but there are data available for younger children (8,9). During most of childhood, BMC and BMD increase linearly with age for the radial and humeral diaphyses (10). SPA has proven useful for identifying osteopenia in many pediatric disorders, including renal disease, glucocorticoid therapy, anticonvulsant therapy, rheumatologic disease, cystic fibrosis, juvenile diabetes, and endocrine disorders (11).

Disadvantages

The major disadvantage of SPA is its limited versatility. The conventional one-third site provides a good sample of cortical bone, with only 5% trabecular bone. The distal radius includes a greater percentage of trabecular bone of approximately 25% (12), but even that region is still mostly cortical bone, and the precision of measurements at the distal radius is decreased. Another potential problem is that faulty readings may occur if the measures are done without taking radiographs of the forearm. If there is an old fracture, a bone island, or a cortical defect at the site of the measurement, these will be measured with the bone and result in a false estimate of overall bone mass. A potential disadvantage of SPA is lower long-term precision in children than in adults because the site of the measurement will not be the same each time. Because the distal end of the radius grows faster than the proximal, the one-third site will not be the same segment of bone on subsequent studies. Interpretation of SPA measurements in children may be faulty if the values are compared only with standards for the child's chronological age, whereas it would often be more appropriate to use the bone age. Therefore, if SPA is used in children, a radiograph of the hand and forearm should also be obtained. SPA has also been used in infants (13,14), but these data are very hard to reproduce. This difficulty is due to the rela-

tively small difference in attenuation between the radius and the soft tissues (15). The humerus and femur are more reliable in this population. Neonatal standards have been developed, but the data are limited, and it has not been established whether the results obtained in one laboratory are reproducible in another.

Dual-Photon and Dual X-Ray Absorptiometry

Dual-photon absorptiometry (DPA) and DXA are techniques that have been developed to measure bone mineral at multiple sites. By analyzing photon absorption at two different energies, one can calculate the amount of bone mineral, soft tissue, and fat without the need to have constant body-part thickness. This allows determination of whole-body composition as well as the BMC of multiple skeletal sites. The most frequently studied site is the lumbar spine, and the proximal femur and radius are often examined in addition. The first of these methods to be developed was DPA (16), which used a ^{153}Gd sealed source with photon energies of 44 and 100 keV. This required periodic replacement of expensive sources, and even 1-Ci sources had a relatively low photon flux. DXA (17) uses an x-ray tube instead of a radionuclide as a photon source. The dual-energy effect is achieved by either alternating the voltage across the tube or using alternating k-edge filtration. Although DPA and DXA are similar in concept, the higher photon flux from an x-ray tube has made DXA a much more effective clinical tool by decreasing the examination time and improving the spatial resolution. The time needed for examination of the lumbar spine is less than 5 minutes for DXA, compared with 20–45 minutes for DPA. The higher spatial resolution has improved selection of the region of interest and may assist in the identification of abnormalities that can invalidate the bone mineral determination. The accuracy and precision of DXA are also better than those of DPA. Therefore, DXA has replaced DPA, and the rest of this section will consider only DXA.

A major strength of DXA is its versatility. Its use for measuring cortical bone in the radius will be considered first, to compare it with SPA. Like SPA, DXA has been used at several sites in the forearm, with the most frequently used site being the radius at the junction of the mid- and distal thirds of the forearm. An image is generated that assists in accurate selection of the region of interest, and this may account for an even greater precision of DXA than of SPA for examination of the radius. The skin entrance dose for DXA of the forearm is 70 μSv, and because this is a limited area, the effective dose equivalent is less than 1 μSv. Normal values for several sites of the radius have been established in adults. However, published pediatric standards are not yet available. Several studies have compared DXA and SPA of the radial diaphysis, as summarized in the Table (18–24). All of these studies have shown that these measurements are highly correlated, although in most of these series there were small quantitative differences between DXA and SPA. Hence, "SPA-equivalent" values can be calculated from the DXA measurements and a derived regression formula. The error of this estimation is small relative to the normal range and its distribution. This suggests that SPA-equivalent val-

TABLE 1. *Correlation of dual x-ray absorptiometry (DXA) and single-photon absorptiometry (SPA) for radial bone mineral density*

	Weinstein (18)	Leboff (19)	Larcos (20)	Nieves (21)	Nelson (22)	Ilich (23)	Shore (24)
Subjects (N)	70	26	30	67	196	285	117
Age (yr)	12–86; mean 48	22–68	Adults	18–75; mean 51	Not stated	9–53; mean 21.8	2.6–17.8; mean 10.1
DXA	Hologic QDR-1000	Hologic QDR-1000	Hologic QDR-1000	Hologic QDR-1000	Hologic QDR-1000W	Lunar DPX-L	Hologic QDR-2000
SPA	Norland 2780	Lunar SP2	Non-commercial	Nuclear Data 1100A	Norland 2780a	Lunar SP2B	Lunar SP2
Site	Distal 1/3	Distal 1/3	Ultradistal	Distal diaphysis	Distal 1/3	Distal 1/3	Distal 1/3
Y-intercept[a]	−0.007	−0.127	−0.1	−0.162	−0.1025	+0.049	−0.119
Slope[a]	1.035	1.2107	1.19	1.140	1.206	0.928	1.0788
Correlation coefficient (r)	0.975	0.97	0.95	0.926	0.97	0.975	0.956

[a]Dependent variable (Y) = bone mineral density measured by SPA; independent variable (X) = bone mineral density measured by DXA. The regression formulas have been modified for those reports that used bone mineral density measured by DXA as the dependent variable and bone mineral density measured by SPA as the independent variable.

ues derived from DXA measurements can be used with SPA normal values. However, the error of SPA-equivalent values is relatively large compared with the precision of both DXA and SPA. Thus, interval changes in BMD cannot be evaluated adequately by comparing DXA with a previous SPA examination. In patients with previous SPA examinations who will subsequently be evaluated by DXA, the initial DXA study should be combined with a final SPA measurement for proper comparison with previous examinations and for the establishment of a new DXA baseline (20,21,24).

The major advantage of DXA over SPA is its ability to measure skeletal density at sites other than the extremities, especially the lumbar spine and proximal femur. Lumbar examinations typically include the first four lumbar vertebrae, usually studied in the frontal projection. For the lumbar spine, the skin entrance dose is 120 µSv and the effective dose equivalent is 1 µSv. Because DXA is a projectional rather than cross-sectional method, it includes both the cortical and trabecular components of the vertebra. A greater percentage of vertebral trabecular bone can be evaluated with DXA by using the lateral view and including only the vertebral bodies without the posterior elements. However, normal standards for the lateral view are not as well established as those for the frontal view in adults, and they are not available in children. Studies of normal lumbar bone mineral growth as measured by DXA (frontal view) have shown that BMD increases throughout childhood, with the greatest rate of increase during puberty (25–27). Similarly, weight and pubertal development were found to be the best clinical predictors of lumbar bone mineral during childhood and adolescence (26).

Although there are normal standards for DXA measurement of the lumbar spine in children, the clinical significance of lumbar BMD is not yet as well understood as that for the radial diaphysis. Several studies in adults have shown a poor correlation between those sites that contain mostly cortical bone and those that contain more trabecular bone, such as the spine and hip (12,28). Similarly, in children, most of the correlation between radial and lumbar BMD as measured by DXA is simply due to their individual correlations with age, height, and weight (24). The Z-scores (standard deviations from the mean) for radial and lumbar DXA examinations had no meaningful correlation. Thus, the conclusions regarding the normality or degree of abnormality of bone mineralization for one site were not related to those at another site. In particular, significant demineralization was demonstrated by radial DXA in many patients whose lumbar DXA measurements were within normal limits (24). This may be related to different factors that influence mineralization of cortical bone, as measured in the radius, and of trabecular bone, as measured in the lumbar spine. Evaluation of the effects of different disease states on cortical and trabecular bone will be important. The advent of DXA has made possible evaluation of the lumbar spine, and this is often the only site that is measured. Measurement of lumbar BMD alone, however, fails to provide the information on cortical bone status that had been measured previously by SPA. Therefore, DXA of the lumber spine should be combined with measurement of the radial diaphysis by either DXA or SPA for overall assessment of bone mineralization in children.

Quantitative Computed Tomography

Quantitative computed tomography is a method whereby computed tomography (CT) scanning is used to measure bone mineral, and this has been performed using both single-energy and dual-energy techniques. The attenuation numbers for specific regions of interest from the CT scan are compared with those for a phantom with several known concentrations of hydroxyapatite, which is scanned simultaneously. With QCT, the region of interest for bone mineral measurement is a well-defined volume, permitting examination of the trabecular bone within the vertebral bodies without including cortical bone. Furthermore, QCT defines the volume that is being measured rather than its two-dimensional projection, and thus, QCT measures bone mineral as a true volume density (g/cm³), which is less influenced by bone size. By analyzing the difference between regions of interest for the entire vertebra and the trabecular component, one can also determine vertebral cortical bone. Using these techniques, normal values for children have been established, and the factors that influence growth of the cortical and trabecular components of vertebrae in children have been studied (29,30). Cortical BMD increases throughout childhood and correlates well with height, weight, and muscle volume (30), which is similar to the linear growth of diaphyseal cortical bone as demonstrated by SPA (10). Trabecular BMD is relatively constant, however, in preadolescent children and then increases significantly with puberty (29,30). Although the ability of QCT to isolate specific regions within the vertebrae is useful, particularly in a research setting, there are several disadvantages, including the cost of the equipment and thus the cost of the examination, the need to compete with other examinations for scanner time, and the larger radiation dose. The skin entrance dose has been estimated to be 2–15 mSv, and the effective dose equivalent is approximately 50 µSv. QCT also does not have the ability to evaluate regional and whole-body composition, which can be studied by DXA.

QUALITATIVE EVALUATION OF RADIOGRAPHS FOR BONE LOSS

Overall Density

Subjective evaluation of radiographic density is a very inaccurate and inconsistent method for evaluation of bone loss (31). In the spine, more than 50% of bone can be lost without any evidence on the radiograph because it is mostly cortical bone that is seen on plain radiographs, and much loss of cancellous bone can occur before it is visualized. Also, the apparent density is very dependent on the radiographic technique used; the higher the kilovoltage, the more "washed out" the bone appears (Fig. 2). Similarly, not

using a high-ratio grid can make the bones look more osteopenic.

Appearance of the Cortex Compared With the Center of Bone

Although both cortical and trabecular bone are usually deficient in patients with osteopenia, there is often relative preservation of the thinned cortex, which stands out sharply against the very lucent trabecular region. This sign is sometimes useful in evaluation of the vertebrae (32), producing a "picture-frame vertebra" with the well-defined vertebral margins surrounding the lucent trabecular center. Similarly, relative cortical preservation in the epiphyses characterizes Wimberger's ring of scurvy, which is simply a manifestation of severe osteopenia. Sometimes focal areas of cortical lucency may be associated with endosteal scalloping (32). Although these findings are useful when present, they are technique dependent.

Appearance of Trabecular Pattern

A coarse trabecular pattern may be useful in evaluating the presence and type of osteopenia; however, it can also be quite inaccurate. Trabecular orientation is related to stress, and with osteopenia there is relative preservation of those trabeculae that are aligned in the direction of maximum stress. In the spine, the vertically oriented trabeculae are preserved, and thus, prominent vertical striations are usually a sign of osteoporosis. Similarly, in the hip, coarse trabeculation may be an indication of osteopenia; in adults, the degree of osteopenia can be graded by the number of trabecular patterns present (33). There is some difference in appearance between the coarse trabecular patterns in osteoporosis and hyperparathyroidism, but usually this is not a reliable differential sign.

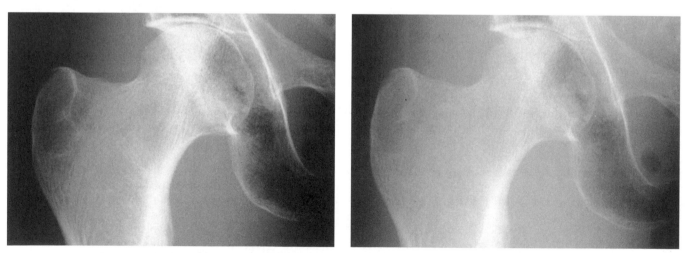

A

B

FIG. 2. Pelvic phantom. **A:** 70 kVp; **B:** 120 kVp. This is the same bone radiographed with two different techniques. Note how at the lower kVp the bones appear dense and well mineralized, with well-defined trabeculae, whereas at the higher kVp they appear much more osteopenic. Other factors, such as use of lower ratio grids and poor technique, can also change the appearance from that of good mineralization to poor mineralization.

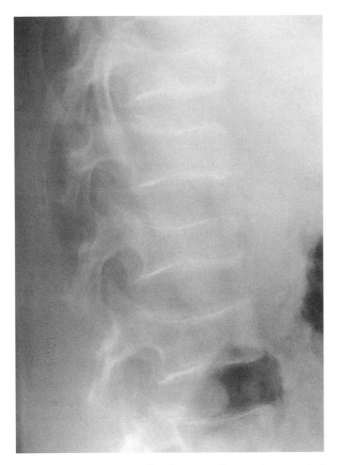

FIG. 3. Multiple compression fractures from osteoporosis in a boy with Crohn's disease. The vertebral bodies are flatter than normal, with indentations on the endplates. Compare with the vertebrae in Fig. 6, which show normal vertebral shape but are abnormally sclerotic.

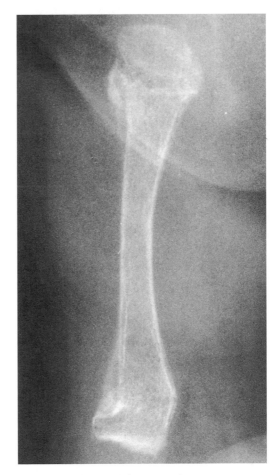

FIG. 4. Multiple femoral fractures in a premature neonate with bronchopulmonary dysplasia. There is callus around the upper femoral fracture. The lower fracture is angulated, with some callus on the lateral side. This is evidence of healing. The poorly mineralized bones in this infant fractured with no known trauma, but from normal handling in the nursery.

Presence of Compression Fractures of the Spine or Fractures of Other Bones

The appearance of anterior wedging or concave endplate deformities in the spine, seen best in the lateral projections, is a good sign of bone loss (32) (Fig. 3). In children, vertebral compression fractures may occur without any history of trauma in diseases associated with severe bone loss, such as osteogenesis imperfecta, rickets, juvenile rheumatoid arthritis, Crohn's disease, or corticosteroid therapy. Vertebral compressions may be the presenting sign of leukemia or neuroblastoma. Other disorders producing wedged vertebrae include Langerhans' cell histiocytosis, juvenile osteoporosis, Gaucher's disease, and Scheuermann's disease. A square impression on the endplate is seen characteristically in sickle cell disease.

Bone loss can be associated with a variety of fractures of the long bones as well as of the spine. In hyperparathyroidism, fractures through the growth plates and metaphyses are not uncommon. In osteogenesis imperfecta or in osteoporosis associated with neuromuscular abnormalities, particularly myelodysplasia, fracture healing with overabundant callus can be seen. In premature neonates on total parenteral nutrition, most fractures occur without a history of trauma (Fig. 4).

Presence of Bowing of the Bones in Children

A number of conditions with osteopenia in children will result in bowing of the long bones, particularly rickets (Fig. 5), osteogenesis imperfecta, and fibrous dysplasia. In some cases, there may be associated small cortical breaks on the convex surface. In children with rickets, the bowing is a manifestation of osteomalacia. After treatment for rickets, the bones tend to straighten with growth over time.

Presence of Subperiosteal Resorption and Other Signs of Hyperparathyroidism

Subperiosteal resorption is a pathognomonic manifestation of hyperparathyroidism (34,35). These resorptions are best seen on hand radiographs obtained with either industrial films or with mammography film screen combination, and they can be easily missed if ordinary screen exposures

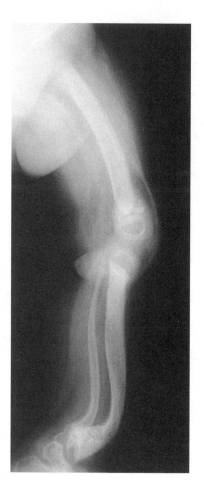

FIG. 5. Bowing of the lower extremity bones in a child with treated rickets. The legs may bend in any direction, depending on the stresses involved.

are obtained (36). To identify the resorptions properly, the radiographs may need to be examined with a magnifying glass. These findings are best seen along the radial aspect of the middle phalanges (Fig. 6A,B). The distal tufts may also be involved (Fig. 6A), but their involvement is not as specific as that of the phalanges because some irregularity of the tufts can occur normally. Thus, it is difficult to determine whether subtle tuft defects are due to normal variation or to hyperparathyroidism. Subperiosteal resorption may also be seen in other areas of the body. Commonly involved areas, particularly in infants and young children, include the medial aspects of the femoral neck, proximal humerus, and proximal tibia (Fig. 6C), as well as near the metaphyseal areas of many other bones. The growth plate and metaphysis can have a rickets-like appearance, with somewhat greater widening at the lateral and medial ends than in the center. Some of the other radiographic findings of hyperparathyroidism in children are those that are often considered to be more characteristic of secondary hyperparathyroidism from renal disease than of primary hyperparathyroidism, although they can be seen in both conditions. These findings include bone sclerosis, which can produce a "rugger jersey" appearance in the spine (Fig. 7) and a coarse trabecular pattern (36,37), and

arterial calcification (38). The rugger jersey appearance is not specific for hyperparathyroidism and may also be seen in osteopetrosis. In children, slipping of various epiphyses, particularly the proximal femoral and the proximal humeral, may be seen (39) (Figs. 8, 9). Avascular necrosis may also be present (Fig. 9A). Metaphyseal fractures can be symmetrical in various bones (Fig. 9C). Well-circumscribed lucent areas from brown tumors may be seen in any part of the skeleton (Figs. 6A, 8) and are often considered more characteristic of primary than of secondary hyperparathyroidism. However, in children they are seen more often with secondary hyperparathyroidism because it is much more common.

Presence of Linear Striations

Increased linear striations (40,41) in the cortex of the metacarpals as well as in other bones can be due to hyperparathyroidism, osteomalacia, and other causes of high bone turnover such as in hyperthyroidism. Some striation may be seen in normal children. Abnormal striations are usually not seen in slower forms of bone loss, such as that due to chronic diseases or juvenile rheumatoid arthritis. When intracortical resorption is present, cortical thickness measurements do not accurately represent the amount of cortical bone and thus are not useful in determining bone loss.

Metaphyseal Changes in Rickets

Rickets is a condition of inadequate mineralization of osteoid and cartilage at the growing ends of bones in children. The radiologic hallmarks of this disorder are apparent widening of the physis from accumulation of nonmineralized osteoid and cartilage, irregularity of the metaphysis, and loss of definition of the zone of provisional calcification (Fig. 10A). These changes are most severe in bones with the greatest growth, and thus are most pronounced in the distal femur and distal radius in most children. They are rarely seen in slow-growing bones, such as the tubular bones of the hand. Similarly, rachitic changes are greater during times of rapid growth, such as in infancy and adolescence, than during periods of slower growth. Widening of the anterior ribs, the rachitic rosary, may be seen radiographically (Fig. 10B). In osteitis fibrosa from hyperparathyroidism, accumulation of fibrous tissue in the metaphyses can produce lucencies that may appear similar to the nonmineralized osteoid of rickets. This may cause these disorders to be indistinguishable, although in some cases of hyperparathyroidism there is more erosion around the edge of the involved growth plate than is seen in rickets (37).

All types of rickets have similar changes at the growth plate, and the radiologic distinction among the various types of rickets may be difficult. Diagnosis is usually based on clinical and biochemical findings. Occasionally, differentiation by radiologic appearance is possible. For example, the radiologic appearance of X-linked hypophosphatemic rickets (XLH, vitamin D–resistant rickets) is unique in that one almost never sees secondary hyperparathyroidism in untreated cases. Furthermore, in older

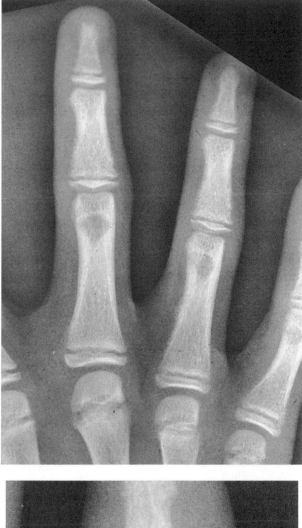

A

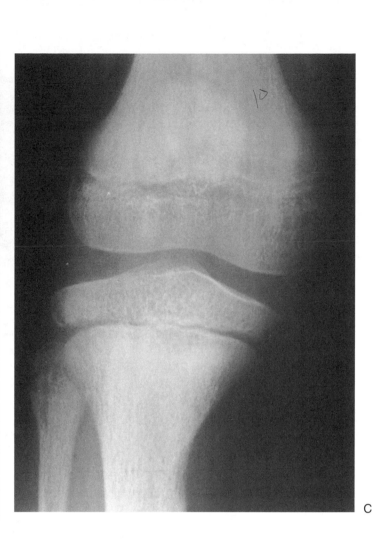

C

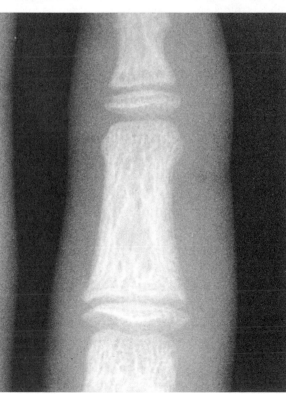

B

FIG. 6. Hyperparathyroidism. **A:** Moderately severe findings. Subperiosteal resorption is present, more prominent along the radial than the ulnar aspects of the middle phalanges, and there are also erosions of the terminal tufts. Lucent defects in the distal portions of the proximal phalanges are brown tumors of hyperparathyroidism. **B:** Child with more subtle findings of hyperparathyroidism. Subperiosteal erosion is more marked on the radial side of the finger. **C:** Erosion of the medial aspect of the proximal tibia in hyperparathyroidism due to renal osteodystrophy.

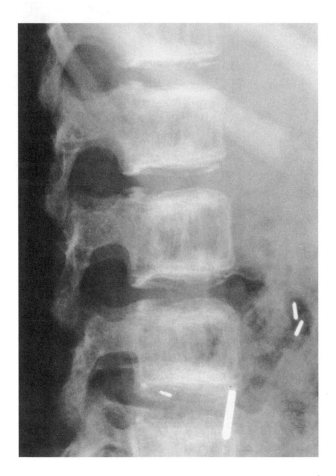

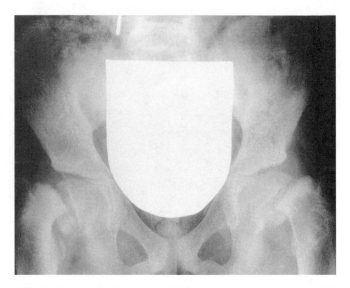

FIG. 8. Bilateral slipped capital femoral epiphyses in a child with renal osteodystrophy. Note the widened growth plates in the proximal femora and displacement of the femoral heads with respect to the neck. These are fractures through the growth plates. At the inferior margin of each growth plate, there is a small fragment of bone that probably broke from the metaphysis. The appearance is similar to that seen in developmental coxa vara. The lucency in the left femoral neck is a brown tumor, a manifestation of hyperparathyroidism.

FIG. 7. "Rugger jersey" spine in a child with renal osteodystrophy. The sclerotic bands on the upper and lower margins of each vertebra are characteristic of secondary hyperparathyroidism. Coarse trabeculae are seen in the vertebral bodies.

children with XLH, the long bones, particularly the femora, are usually thickened and bowed, and this is not seen in other forms of rickets. For comparison, in vitamin D–dependent rickets, usually due to absence of renal 1α-hydroxylase, the rachitic changes may be seen in younger infants than in other forms of rickets, and they are also associated with more severe findings of hyperparathyroidism. During the healing of rickets, initial calcification is usually at the zone of provisional calcification, leaving a lucent band between it and the irregular metaphysis, and this lucent band may be confused with leukemia or metaphyseal stress changes. During healing, apparent periosteal elevation may be present (Fig. 11).

Disorders Mimicking Rickets

There are a number of conditions that can mimic rickets (42), including copper deficiency, diphosphonate therapy, fluorosis, hypophosphatasia, primary and secondary hyperparathyroidism, Menkes' syndrome, Schwachman syndrome, and various forms of metaphyseal chondroplasia, particularly Jansen syndrome in the neonate and McKusick and Schmidt forms in older children. Mucolipi-

dosis II and osteopetrosis in infants may have manifestations similar to rickets. Among these conditions mimicking rickets, radiologic differentiation is often possible. For example, in Jansen syndrome, the epiphysis is markedly displaced from the metaphysis, much more so than in rickets (Fig. 12). Later on, bizarre chondroid calcifications are seen in metaphyseal regions, which are even more characteristic. The serum calcium level may be elevated in Jansen syndrome, which also differentiates it from rickets. Hypophosphatasia can usually be distinguished from rickets, with the metaphyseal defects appearing more punched-out as opposed to the more uniform involvement of the growth plate in rickets (Fig. 13). The rachitic-like changes of hyperparathyroidism can sometimes be differentiated by erosion along the edge of the growth plate. There are also a number of localized disorders that can mimic rickets. These include growth-plate fractures that have not been immobilized (Fig. 14), frostbite, radiation therapy, and chronic recurrent multifocal osteomyelitis.

Signs of Osteomalacia

Failure to mineralize osteoid seams adequately during the normal process of bone turnover defines osteomalacia. This process can occur in both children and adults, whereas rickets is limited to children before physeal closure. Radiologic differentiation of osteomalacia from other forms of osteopenia is difficult unless Looser zones, also called pseudofractures, are present. These are areas of cortical lucency with surrounding sclerosis that may not go completely through the cortex (Fig. 15). They are usually per-

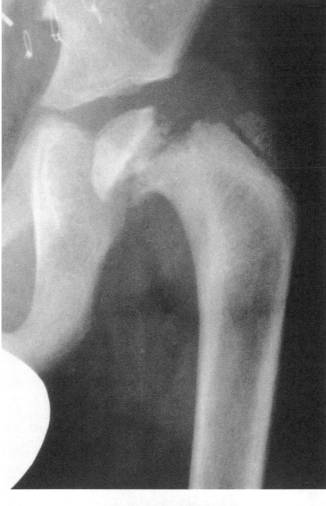

A

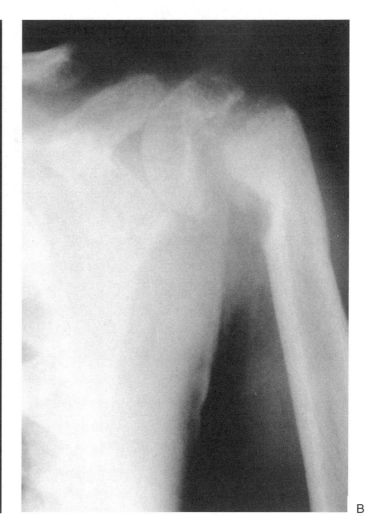

B

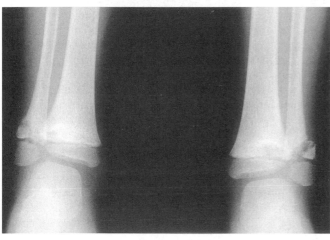

C

FIG. 9. Boy with tertiary hyperparathyroidism. **A:** Hip with widening of the growth plate and displacement of the capital femoral epiphysis. There is a small crescent of bone in the subcortical surface of the femoral head, which is a sign of avascular necrosis. **B:** Slipped epiphysis of the upper humerus. The growth plate is wide and irregular, and there is an erosion along the medial side of the upper humerus, indicating subperiosteal resorption from hyperparathyroidism. **C:** Bilateral growth plate and metaphyseal fractures (Salter II) of the fibulas. There are partially healed rachitic changes of the distal tibial growth plates.

pendicular to the cortex and are often seen along the medial side of the femoral neck and in the pubis or ischium, although they may also occur in other areas. The lucency represents nonmineralized osteoid, which accumulates at sites of increased bone turnover from stress. Although Looser zones are suggestive of osteomalacia, similar-appearing cortical lucencies may be seen in other disorders, including fibrous dysplasia and, in adults, Paget's disease.

Increased Bone Mineral with Sclerosis

Increased bone density on radiographs can be seen in a variety of bone dysplasias, the most classic of which is osteopetrosis. Although the bone appears dense and thick, it is very brittle and prone to fracture. Bands of density may also be seen and may mimic renal osteodystrophy in the spine.

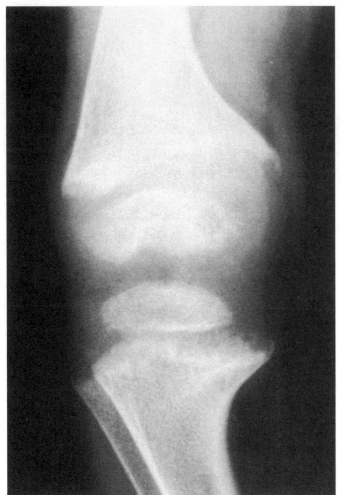

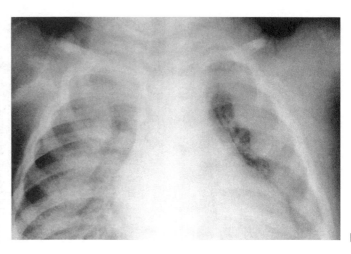

FIG. 10. Nutritional rickets. **A:** Characteristic rachitic findings at the knees, with widening and irregularity of the growth plate and marked fraying of the metaphyses of the distal femur and proximal tibia. The bone density is decreased, and there is some bowing. **B:** Chest x-ray shows widening of the ribs anteriorly, producing the rachitic rosary.

STRATEGIES TO EVALUATE BONE LOSS IN CHILDREN

Evaluation of the hand radiograph obtained with a high-detail film screen combination is probably the best initial method for evaluating suspected abnormalities of metabolic bone disease in children. The advantages include the availability of qualitative and quantitative data. From the hand radiograph, one can detect the presence of rickets in the distal radius and ulna. The bone age can be determined so that proper standards for bone mineralization can be used. The hand radiograph is useful for evaluating the periosteal and endosteal surfaces for the presence of subperiosteal resorption or cortical scalloping, and for determining whether cortical loss appears to be due to increased resorption or insufficient periosteal apposition. Good normative data for cortical measures are available not only for Caucasians, but also for other ethnic groups (1).

SPA or DXA is indicated for those conditions in which radiogrammetry is not a valid indicator of bone mineral status because of the presence of intracortical or subperiosteal bone loss, such as in renal osteodystrophy. SPA or DXA should be used when it is important to evaluate changes in bone mineralization in the most accurate and precise manner. There is considerable clinical experience with the use of SPA in children, and there are good standards for most age groups. When SPA is used in children, a radiograph of the hand and forearm should also be obtained. This permits the evaluation of qualitative signs of bone mineral abnormalities, skeletal maturation, and focal bone abnormalities that would invalidate the bone mineral study. DXA offers great versatility and is replacing SPA in many centers. DXA examinations should include the lumbar spine and the forearm because evaluation of the lumbar spine alone often fails to recognize cortical demineralization, which can be demonstrated by DXA or SPA studies of the radial diaphysis (24). Pending the development of normal values for DXA of the radius in children, DXA measurements can be converted to SPA-equivalent values and used with existing SPA standards. Although QCT is a useful research tool, it is not practical for standard clinical monitoring of children with bone mineral disorders.

Radiography of the knees is the best single view to determine the presence of rickets, because this is the site of most rapid growth. However, an anteroposterior view of the ankle or wrist may also be used. To detect the pseudofractures of osteomalacia, the best views are the hips or shoulders. Radiography of painful areas should be obtained because pseudofractures can occur in other areas.

Measurement of cortical thickness of the humerus is probably the simplest and best method for evaluation of bone loss in premature neonates. This is often readily

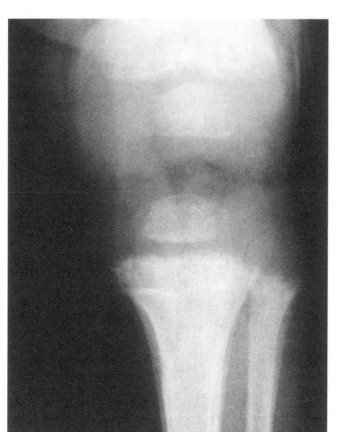

FIG. 11. Rickets with some healing. Apparent periosteal elevation of the shafts of the tibia and fibula is a sign of some degree of healing. Also, note that the distal portions of the metaphyses are more lucent than the rest. This is due to incomplete mineralization of the previously nonmineralized osteoid and is a sign of healing rickets.

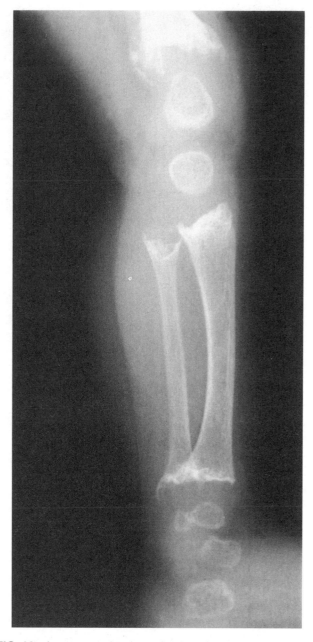

FIG. 12. Jansen syndrome, a dominantly inherited metaphyseal chondrodysplasia. Note the irregular, somewhat sclerotic metaphyseal ends reminiscent of rickets. However, there is marked separation between the peculiar round epiphyses of the distal femur and proximal tibia and their respective metaphyses. With further maturation, this wide space fills in with irregular calcification, giving the characteristic appearance of Jansen syndrome, which is then not confused with rickets.

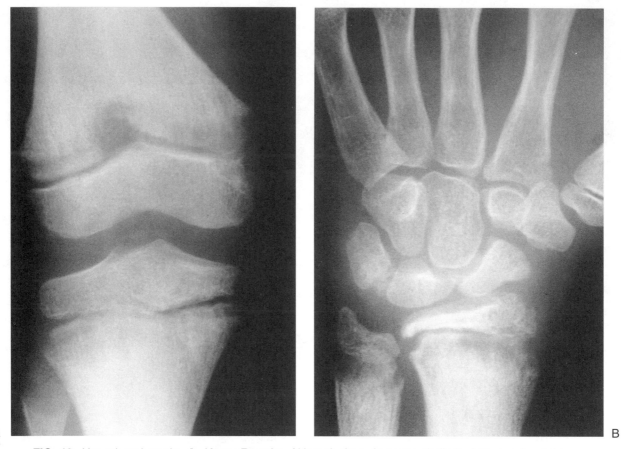

A

B

FIG. 13. Hypophosphatasia. **A:** Knee; **B:** wrist. Although there is some similarity between hypophosphatasia and rickets, the metaphyseal lucency is not the same as the fraying in rickets, which extends across the whole growth plate. The metaphyseal defects appear more focal than in rickets, and parts of the growth plate appear normal. In infants, the changes of hypophosphatasia may be similar to rickets but are usually more severe and occur at birth, whereas rickets is usually not seen before 3 months of age.

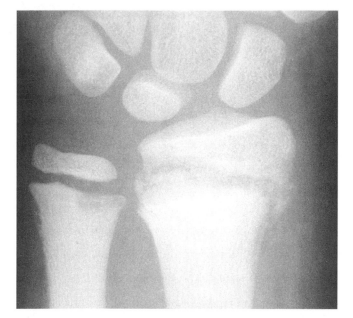

FIG. 14. Trauma mimicking rickets in a young football player who continued to play with a sore wrist for a few weeks. Widening and irregularity of the growth plates is due to unhealed growth-plate fractures of the radius and ulna, which had not been allowed to heal because of motion between the fragments. After casting, healing was complete.

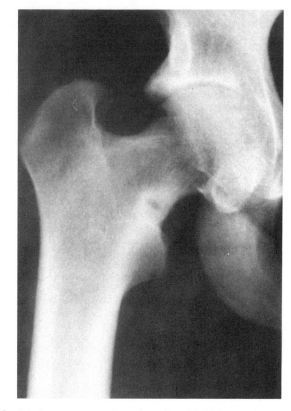

FIG. 15. Looser zone in a female with X-linked hypophosphatemic rickets and painful hips. The linear lucency in the medial portion of the femoral neck with sclerosis around it is a typical Looser zone (also called pseudofracture) and is indicative of osteomalacia.

obtained from available chest radiographs, so that additional films need not be taken. Because most of the bone loss appears to be due to endosteal resorption, this measure is an accurate means for evaluating appendicular bone loss. SPA has been used in infants; however, it is difficult to perform, and normal values for infants are also not as well established. DXA may be a potentially useful tool in neonates, but few data are currently available.

REFERENCES

1. Poznanski AK: *The Hand in Radiologic Diagnosis.* Philadelphia, WB Saunders, 1974
2. Garn SM, Poznanski AK, Nagy JM: Bone measurement in the differential diagnosis of osteopenia and osteoporosis. *Radiology* 100:509–518, 1971
3. Poznanski AK, Kuhns LR, Guire KE: New standards of cortical mass in the humerus of neonates: A means of evaluating bone loss in the premature infant. *Radiology* 134:639–644, 1980
4. Virtama P, Helela T (eds): *Radiographic Measurements of Cortical Bone.* Stockholm, Turku Auraprint Oy, 1969
5. Poznanski AK: Radiologic evaluation of growth. In: Davidson M (ed) *Growth Retardation Among Children and Adolescents With Inflammatory Bowel Disease: Report of Workshop Conducted in Reston, Virginia, March 6–8, 1981.* New York, National Foundation for Ileitis and Colitis, pp 53–81, 1983
6. Sorenson JA, Cameron JR: A reliable in vivo measurement of bone-mineral content. *J Bone Joint Surg* 49-A:481–497, 1967
7. Mazess RB, Cameron JR: Bone mineral content in US whites. In: Mazess RB (ed) *International Conference on Bone Mineral Measurement.* Publication 75-683. US Department of Health, Education, and Welfare. [Bethesda], pp 228–237, 1974
8. Runge H, Fengler F, Franke J, Koall W: Ermittlung des peripheren knochenmineralgehaltes bei normalpersonen und patienten mit verschiedenen knochenerkrankungen, bestimmt mit hilfe der photonenabsorptionstechnik am radius. *Radiologe* 20:204–214, 1980
9. Specker BL, Brazerol W, Tsang RC, Levin R, Searcy J, Steichen J: Bone mineral content in children 1 to 6 years of age: Detectable sex differences after 4 years of age. *Am J Dis Child* 141:343–344, 1987
10. Mazess RB, Cameron JR: Growth of bone in school children: Comparison of radiographic morphometry and photon absorptiometry. *Growth* 36:77–92, 1972
11. Chesney RW, Shore RM: The noninvasive determination of bone mineral content by photon absorptiometry (editorial). *Am J Dis Child* 136:578–580, 1982
12. Mazess RB, Pepper WW, Chesney RW, Lange TA, Lindgren U, Smith E Jr: Does bone measurement on the radius indicate skeletal status? *J Nucl Med* 25:281–288, 1984
13. Minton SD, Steichen JJ, Tsang RC: Decreased bone mineral content in small-for-gestational-age infants compared with appropriate-for-gestational-age infants: Normal serum 25-hydroxyvitamin D and decreasing parathyroid hormone. *Pediatrics* 71:383–388, 1983
14. Vyhmeister NR, Linkhart TA, Hay S, Baylink DJ, Ghosh B: Measurement of bone mineral content in the term and preterm infant. *Am J Dis Child* 141:506–510, 1987
15. Tyson JE, Maravilla A, Lasky RE, Cope FA, Mize CE: Measurement of bone mineral content in preterm neonates. *Am J Dis Child* 137:735–737, 1983
16. Wahner HW, Dunn WL, Mazess RB, Towsley M, Lindsay R, Markhard L, Dempster D: Dual-photon Gd-153 absorptiometry of bone. *Radiology* 156:203–206, 1985
17. Kellie SE: Diagnostic and therapeutic technology assessment: Measurement of bone density with dual-energy X-ray absorptiometry. *JAMA* 267:286–294, 1992

18. Weinstein RS, New KD, Sappington LJ: Dual-energy X-ray absorptiometry versus single photon absorptiometry of the radius. *Calcif Tissue Int* 49:313–316, 1991

19. Leboff MS, Fuleihan GE, Angell JE, Chung S, Curtis K: Dual-energy X-ray absorptiometry of the forearm: Reproducibility and correlation with single-photon absorptiometry. *J Bone Miner Res* 7:841–846, 1992

20. Larcos G, Wahner HW: An evaluation of forearm bone mineral measurement with dual-energy X-ray absorptiometry. *J Nucl Med* 32:2101–2106, 1991

21. Nieves JW, Cosman F, Mars C, Lindsay R: Comparative assessment of bone mineral density of the forearm using single photon and dual X-ray absorptiometry. *Calcif Tissue Int* 51:352–355, 1992

22. Nelson D, Feingold M, Mascha E, Kleerekoper M: Comparison of single-photon and dual-energy x-ray absorptiometry of the radius. *Bone Miner* 18:77–83, 1992

23. Ilich JZ, Hsieh LC, Tzagournis MA, Wright JK, Saracoglu M, Barden HS, Matkovic V: A comparison of single photon and dual X-ray absorptiometry of the forearm in children and adults. *Bone* 15:187–191, 1994

24. Shore RM, Langman CB, Donovan JM, Conway JJ, Poznanski AK: Bone mineral disorders in children: Evaluation with dual X-ray absorptiometry. *Radiology* 196:535–540, 1995

25. Glastre C, Braillon P, David L: Measurement of bone mineral content of the lumbar spine by dual energy X-ray absorptiometry in normal children: Correlations with growth parameters. *J Clin Endocrinol Metab* 70:1330–1333, 1990

26. Southard RN, Morris JD, Mahan JD, et al.: Bone mass in healthy children: Measurement with quantitative DXA. *Radiology* 179:735–738, 1991

27. Kröger H, Kotaniemi A, Kröger L, Alhava E: Development of bone mass and bone density of the spine and femoral neck—a prospective study of 65 children and adolescents. *Bone Miner* 23:171–182, 1993

28. Seldin DW, Esser PD, Alderson PO: Comparison of bone density measurements from different skeletal sites. *J Nucl Med* 29:158–173, 1988

29. Gilsanz V, Gibbens DT, Roe TF, et al.: Vertebral bone density in children: Effect of puberty. *Radiology* 166:847–850, 1988

30. Mora S, Goodman WG, Loro ML, Roe TF, Sayre J, Gilsanz V: Age-related changes in cortical and cancellous vertebral bone density in girls: Assessment with quantitative CT. *AJR* 162:405–409, 1994

31. Epstein DM, Dalinka MK, Kaplan FS, Aronchick JM, Marinelli DL, Kundel HL: Observer variation in the detection of osteopenia. *Skeletal Radiol* 15:347–349, 1986

32. Schneider R: Radiologic methods of evaluating generalized osteopenia. *Orthop Clin North Am* 15:631–651, 1984

33. Singh M, Nagrath AR, Maini PS: Changes in trabecular pattern of the upper end of the femur as an index of osteoporosis. *J Bone Joint Surg [Am]* 52:457–467, 1970

34. Meema HE, Oreopoulos DG: The mode of progression of subperiosteal resorption in the hyperparathyroidism of chronic renal failure. *Skeletal Radiol* 10:157–160, 1983

35. Debnam JW, Bates ML, Kopelman RC, Teitelbaum SL: Radiological pathological correlations in uremic bone disease. *Radiology* 125:653–658, 1977

36. Weiss A: Incidence of subperiosteal resorption in hyperparathyroidism studied by fine detail bone radiography. *Clin Radiol* 25:273–276, 1974

37. Parfitt AM: Clinical and radiographic manifestations of renal osteodystrophy. In: Davis DS (ed) *Calcium Metabolism in Renal Failure and Nephrolithiasis.* New York, John Wiley & Sons, pp 145–195, 1977

38. Meema HE, Oreopoulos DG, DeVeber GA: Arterial calcifications in severe chronic renal disease and their relationship to dialysis treatment, renal transplant, and parathyroidectomy. *Radiology* 121:315–321, 1976

39. Mehls O, Ritz E, Krempien B, Gilli G, Link K, Willich E, Scharer K: Slipped epiphyses in renal osteodystrophy. *Arch Dis Child* 50:545–554, 1975

40. Meema HE, Meema S: Comparison of microradioscopic and morphometric findings in the hand bones with densitometric findings in the proximal radius in thyrotoxicosis and in renal osteodystrophy. *Invest Radiol* 7:88–96, 1972

41. Meema HE, Oreopoulos DG, Meema S: A roentgenologic study of cortical bone resorption in chronic renal failure. *Radiology* 126:67–74, 1978

42. Frame B, Poznanski AK: Conditions that may be confused with rickets. In: DeLuca HJ (ed) *Pediatric Diseases Related to Calcium.* Holland/New York, Elsevier, pp 269–289, 1980

22. Scintigraphy in Metabolic Bone Disease

David C. Wang, M.D.,*Sambasiva R. Kottamasu, M.D., and Kastytis Karvelis, M.D.

*Division of Nuclear Medicine, Department of Diagnostic Radiology, Henry Ford Hospital, Detroit, Michigan; and
Wayne State University School of Medicine, and Department of Imaging, Children's Hospital of Michigan, Detroit, Michigan

Skeletal scintigraphy in clinical practice was greatly expanded with the development of bone-seeking technetium-99m (99mTc)-Sn compounds of polyphosphate and diphosphonate, which are easily prepared from readily available commercial kits. Technetium-99m is a gamma emitter with a physical half-life of 6 hours. It can be obtained from an inexpensive generator and has a gamma ray energy of 140 keV, which is well suited for gamma camera imaging. These characteristics make it an almost ideal agent for nuclear medicine imaging (1).

Bone scanning with radionuclides has gained wide clinical acceptance for evaluation of metastatic bone disease, primary bone tumors, osteomyelitis, and aseptic necrosis.

Metabolic bone disease has also been studied and detected by skeletal scintigraphy (1).

The factors that affect the rate and degree of skeletal uptake of radionuclides have not been clearly defined. Studies have shown that the initial uptake is predominantly related to blood flow; however, the following factors also play a role: capillary permeability, local acid-base relationships, the quality of mineralizable bone, bone turnover, hormones, and vitamins (2).

The rapid short-term uptake of the technetium phosphate compounds, which are analogs of calcium phosphate, is believed to occur by ion exchange (a chemical rather than a metabolic process) through replacement of hydroxyl groups at vascularized bone surfaces. Thus, periosteal, endosteal, trabecular, and haversian surfaces are the major sites of rapid ion exchange and will demonstrate increased uptake. The metaphyses of rachitic bones have been shown histologically to contain increased and dilated capillary networks, and it is likely that the increased uptake that is seen in the metaphyses is related to increased blood flow, despite the overall decreased rate of osteogenesis (1).

BONE SCANNING TECHNIQUE

Technetium-99m–labeled methylene diphosphonate or hydroxymethylene diphosphonate is administered intravenously. Dosages range from 10 to 25 mCi. The usual adult dose is 20 mCi, and 25 mCi is sometimes given when single-photon emission tomography is anticipated. The pediatric dosage is calculated based on body surface area (Table 1). Approximately 50% to 60% of the tracer is taken up by bone, with the remainder excreted by the kidneys (2). Total irradiation is ~0.7 rads to the bone and on average <0.4 rads to the ovaries or testes per 20-mCi dose of 99mTc (3).

No specific patient preparation is necessary; however, the patient should be encouraged to drink several large glasses of water (if not contraindicated) immediately after being injected to enhance renal clearance of tracer not bound to bone. This reduces the level of soft-tissue activity seen on the images as well as radiation dose to the patient.

Gamma camera imaging is performed at ~2–3 hours after injection. Scanning earlier than this may result in images that are degraded by significant blood pool activity. Anterior and posterior images of the entire body can be obtained with either a scanning whole-body camera or with multiple spot images.

Single-photon emission computed tomography imaging can provide additional spatial and contrast resolution and may be helpful in localizing areas of abnormality, especially in the hips, spine, knees, and skull. Sixty-four separate images (20–30 seconds each) are obtained with the camera head moving circumferentially about the patient. Computer reconstruction allows viewing of the images in the axial, sagittal, and coronal planes.

In addition to the standard delayed images, blood flow and blood pool images can be obtained. The three-phase scanning can demonstrate abnormally increased blood flow or soft-tissue perfusion in a specific area. The delayed static bone scan is performed at 2–3 hours. A fourth phase or further delayed images can be obtained at 16–24 hours if additional delineation between bone and soft tissue is needed.

FINDINGS ON BONE SCINTIGRAPHY

The scintigraphic diagnosis of metabolic bone disease begins with the recognition of generalized increased bone uptake. This generalized increase is often accompanied by localized uptake due to a superimposed focal pathologic process (4). Seven scintigraphic features of metabolic bone disease have been described by Fogelman et al. (Table 2). Metabolic bone disease is suggested if three or more of these findings are present. These findings, however, are not specific for a particular condition or group of disorders. Bone scintigraphy has low sensitivity and specificity for the diagnosis of most metabolic bone diseases compared with biochemical testing and bone biopsy (5). Attempts have been made to increase the specificity by quantification. Twenty-four–hour whole-body retention of tracer can distinguish Paget's disease, osteomalacia, and primary hyperparathyroidism from normal. This technique is technically demanding, and its accuracy is limited by the dependence of uptake not only on osteoblastic activity, but also on blood flow, kidney function, and other poorly understood factors (4). Although bone scanning may be of little use for early

TABLE 1. *Body surface area method for the calculation of radiopharmaceutical dosages for pediatric patients*

Patient weight (kg)	Body surface area (m2)	Fraction of adult dose
2	0.15	0.09
4	0.25	0.14
6	0.33	0.19
8	0.40	0.23
10	0.46	0.27
15	0.63	0.36
20	0.83	0.48
25	0.95	0.55
30	1.08	0.62
35	1.20	0.69
40	1.30	0.75
45	1.40	0.81
50	1.51	0.87
55	1.58	0.91

From: Chilton HM, Witcofski RL: Fundamentals of radiopharmaceuticals. In: Swanson DP, Chilton HM, Thrall JH (eds) *Pharmaceuticals in Medical Imaging.* New York, Macmillan, p 295, 1990.

TABLE 2. *Bone scan patterns in metabolic bone disease*

Generalized features
  Increased activity in axial skeleton
  Increased activity in long bones
  Increased activity in periarticular areas
  Prominent calvarium and mandible
  Beading of the costochondral junctions
  "Tie" sternum
  Faint or absent kidney images
Occasionally associated findings
  Focal tracer uptake involving one or more entire
    vertebrae (spinal compression fracture)
  Focal uptake in ribs or other skeletal areas (fractures,
    pseudofractures, stress microfractures)
  Abnormal tracer uptake in the kidneys (renal disease)
  Soft-tissue tracer uptake (soft-tissue calcification)

From: Wahner HW: Assessment of metabolic bone disease: Review of new nuclear medicine-procedures. *Mayo Clin Proc* 60:827–835, 1985.

detection of metabolic bone disorders, the recognition of abnormal image patterns may be helpful in the interpretation of atypical bone scans in patients who undergo screening for a variety of disease states (5).

Primary Hyperparathyroidism

Bone scintigrams are usually unremarkable in asymptomatic patients with primary hyperparathyroidism. Quantitation of skull uptake or measurement of the 24-hour total body retention may be helpful, and both are usually elevated. In more advanced cases of primary hyperparathyroidism, any or all of the common findings (Table 2) may be evident. Focal abnormalities such as collapsed vertebrae, cysts, or brown tumors may be seen. Cysts are generally photopenic, whereas brown tumors exhibit focal increased uptake. Increased lung or soft-tissue uptake may be present in patients with renal involvement. After parathyroidectomy, the elevated lung uptake will rapidly return to normal; however, abnormal bone uptake may persist for ~1 year (5).

Skeletal Scintigraphy in Osteoporosis

Skeletal scintigraphy with 99mTc diphosphonates frequently surpasses or complements radiographic findings in evaluating the focal complications of osteoporosis, including traumatic/insufficiency fractures, vertebral compressions, aseptic necrosis, and acute infarction. However, it is well known that routine skeletal radiographs have limited sensitivity in evaluating bone mineral content. As much as 30% to 40% of the bone mineral content may be lost before a decrease in bone density is evident radiographically. Most types of osteoporosis have no characteristic biochemical profile. Detection of osteoporosis is likewise imprecise when based on 99mTc diphosphonate skeletal imaging. Bone scans may demonstrate a normal or, rarely, a washed-out appearance with diffuse decreased skeletal uptake. Single- and dual-photon absorptiometry and quantitative computed tomography are sensitive techniques for measuring bone mineral content (see ref. 6 and Chapter 23).

Bone scintigraphy has a significant role in assessing the focal complications of osteoporosis. In patients with osteoporosis, back pain can occur as a result of microfractures without an obvious vertebral body collapse on radiographs. Bone scan, however, may show a localized increased uptake due to the microfractures. Total-body scans are useful in assessing the location and extent of the fractures throughout the skeleton, which commonly occur in the spine (Fig. 1), femoral neck, wrist, ribs, and pubis. In vertebral fractures, the radionuclide images, although initially demonstrating markedly increased uptake, usually are negative by 18–24 months, allowing some estimate of the age of the fractures to be made (6). Pinhole or single-photon emission tomography imaging, as well as magnetic resonance imaging, are useful for detecting early aseptic necrosis of the femoral heads when radiographs are equivocal or negative (6).

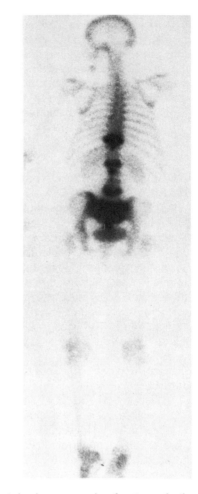

FIG. 1. Vertebral compression fractures in the thoracic and lumbar spine and sacral fracture in a patient with osteoporosis.

Osteoporotic patients receiving sodium fluoride treatment may develop insufficiency or "stress" fractures of the calcaneus, femur, or tibia because of an increased number of new resorption sites, before they are filled with new bone. Within the first few weeks, radiographs may be negative, but by 4–6 weeks, there is evidence of healing fractures. Radionuclide imaging will often show these lesions before they are radiographically evident (6).

Transverse fractures of the sacrum are often not apparent on radiographs, but are recognized on bone scan or computed tomography (Fig. 2B,C,D). Sacral fractures usually occur in patients with osteoporosis and other metabolic bone disease as the result of mild trauma. Clinical symptoms range from localized sacral tenderness to neurologic symptoms due to sacral nerve root irritation from cauda equina compression. The shape and anatomy of the sacrum, as well as coexistent osteopenia, make radiographic evaluation of this osseous structure very difficult. In the case of osteoporotic sacral fractures, the bone scan is very sensitive, and the characteristic H-shaped pattern of uptake across the sacrum and sacroiliac joints suggests the correct diagnosis (7).

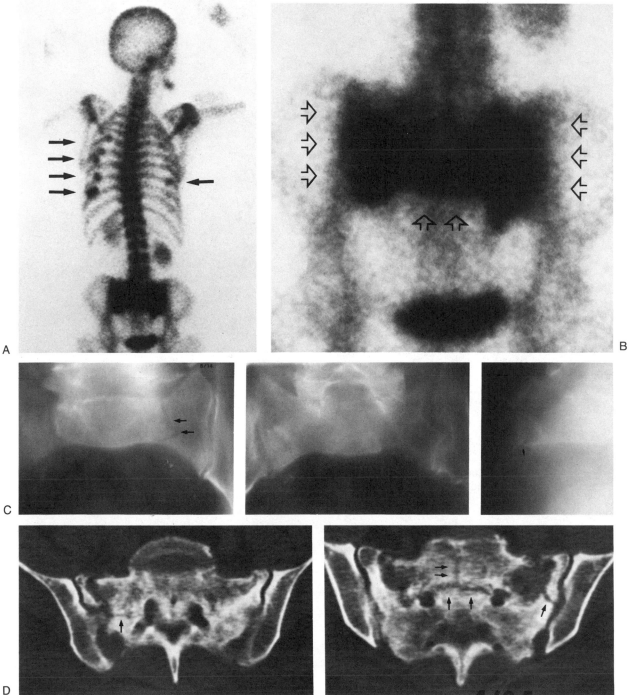

FIG. 2. Multiple insufficiency fractures with **(A)** increased uptake involving the ribs as well as **(B)** an "H"-type fracture of the sacrum, seen on linear tomography **(C)** and computed tomography **(D)** in this patient with osteoporosis.

Skeletal Scintigraphy in Osteomalacia and Rickets

Osteomalacia is a disorder in which mineral deposition in the newly formed osteoid is impaired. In addition, in growing children, impaired calcification of maturing cartilage at the zone of provisional calcification leads to the condition known as rickets. Common causes of osteomalacia include dietary deficiency, hepatic insufficiency, malabsorption, and renal insufficiency, which may be glomerular or tubular (see Section V).

In osteomalacia, radionuclide imaging with 99mTc diphosphonates often shows increased accumulation in the skeleton,

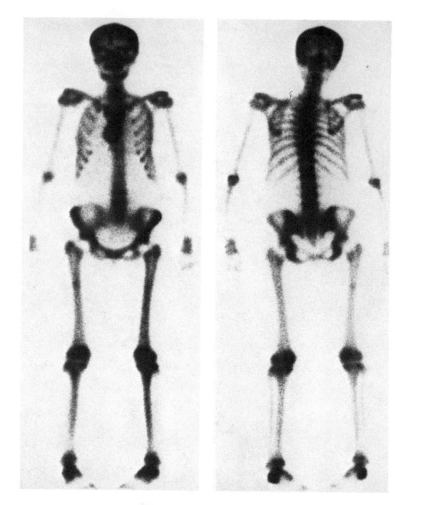

FIG. 3. *(Anterior, posterior)*: Diffuse increased uptake in the axial skeleton, calvarium, sternum, and ends of the long bones (bilateral hip prosthesis).

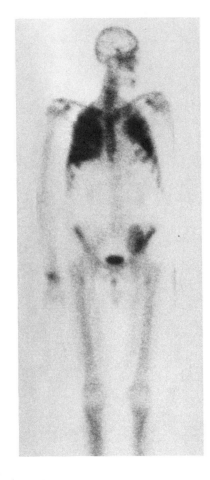

FIG. 4. Extensive pulmonary uptake in a patient with renal osteodystrophy. Note the transplanted kidney in the left pelvis.

which may involve either the entire skeleton or more prominent uptake in the axial skeleton, at the ends of the long bones and in the wrists. Increased uptake in the calvarium and at the costochondral junction is also frequently noted (Fig. 3). These findings are nonspecific and may be seen in other metabolic bone diseases (8). Focal areas of increased uptake due to multiple rib fractures, or Looser zones with or without insufficiency fractures, may be present (6).

Looser zones are often symmetrical and are oriented at right angles to the long axis of the involved bone. The common sites of Looser zones include the axillary aspect of the scapula, concave aspect of the long bones, pubic rami, ischium, ribs, and proximal ulna. These sites are often visualized on radionuclide images before becoming radiographically apparent (6).

Patients with renal osteodystrophy have a variable degree of osteomalacia and secondary hyperparathyroidism. Bone scintigraphy often demonstrates a nonspecific diffuse increased uptake involving the entire skeleton, or involving only the long bones with prominent calvarial uptake (6). Renal uptake is often faint or absent, which may reflect reduced excretion of the tracer by the kidneys because of increased skeletal uptake (8). Pulmonary uptake may be increased, usually when pulmonary calcification is severe

(Fig. 4) (4). Ectopic calcification may also demonstrate focal uptake (Fig. 5).

Skeletal uptake of the radionuclide, expressed as bone-to-soft tissue ratio, is significantly higher in osteomalacia patients than in controls. Fogelman (8) reported that the mean bone-to-soft tissue uptake ratio for the osteomalacia group was 6.57 ± 1.43, whereas that in the control patients was 4.05 ± 0.69 (8).

Other Metabolic Bone Diseases

Increased growth hormone secretion in acromegaly may result in diffuse increased uptake (5). A positive relationship between uptake and basal levels of growth hormone has been shown, and changes can be seen in response to therapy. However, assessment of activity is an unreliable indicator of severity, and the sensitivity and specificity of the scintigraphic changes are too low to be of practical clinical use (5).

Paget's disease is characterized by skeletal metaplasia and focal areas of intense uptake (Fig. 6). Diminished uptake can also be seen in the early lytic phase of the disease or in the late sclerotic phase, which no longer has active

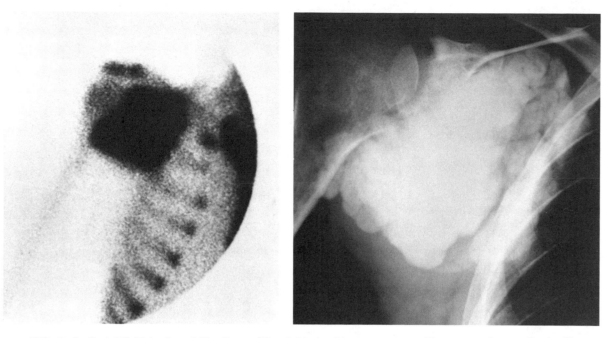

FIG. 5. *(Left, right)*: Ectopic calcifications of the right shoulder on x-ray and bone scan in a patient with severe renal osteodystrophy.

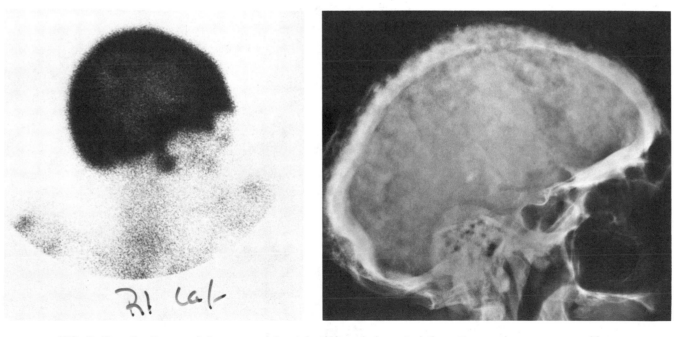

A

B

FIG. 6. Paget's disease. Intense cranial uptake **(A)** and characteristic cotton-wool appearance with widening of the diploe and basilar invagination **(B)**.

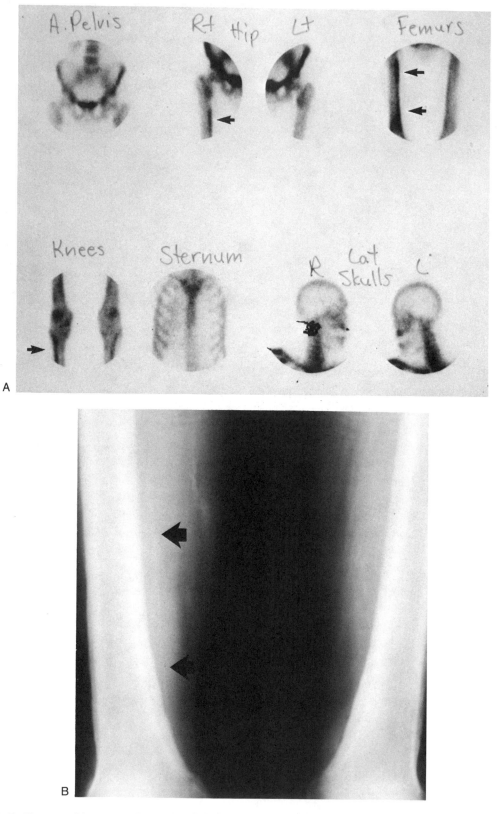

FIG. 7. Hypertrophic osteoarthropathy. **(A)** Increased periosteal uptake in the right femur and tibia on bone scan *(small arrows)*, and **(B)** periosteal calcification and cortical thickening on x-ray *(large arrows)*.

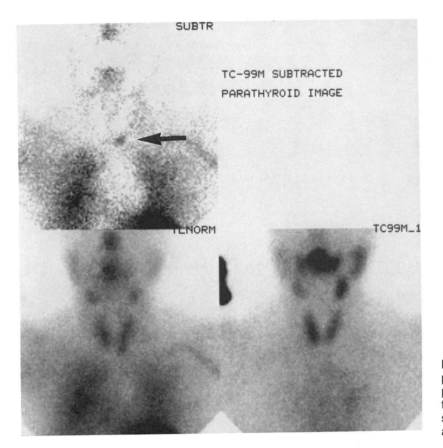

FIG. 8. Parathyroid subtraction scan. A small parathyroid adenoma is visible on the computer-subtracted image *(arrow)*. On their own, the 201Tl scan *(bottom left)* and the 99mTc scan *(bottom right)* are relatively unremarkable.

bone turnover (5). Fibrous dysplasia will also demonstrate focal areas of markedly increased uptake (5). Engelmann's disease and melorheostosis have characteristic patterns of increased uptake corresponding to well-recognized radiographic abnormalities (see ref. 9 and Chapter 68). Hyperthyroidism will cause a diffuse increase in uptake in the long bones, and elevated 24-hour total-body retention of tracer has been reported (5).

Hypertrophic osteoarthropathy exhibits a distinctive periosteal and periarticular uptake in the extremities, with early involvement of the distal third of the tibiae, fibulae, radii, and ulnae and later involvement of the femora, humeri, metacarpals, and metatarsals. The asymmetrical uptake seen in ~15% of patients with hypertrophic osteoarthropathy may give the appearance of metastatic disease (5) (Fig. 7).

PARATHYROID SCANNING

Primary hyperparathyroidism is most commonly due to a solitary parathyroid adenoma (10). Because of the 90% to 95% success rate of initial surgery, parathyroid scan has a limited role in preoperative evaluation; however, it is most useful before reoperation in patients with failed initial surgery. The scan can aid in locating an ectopic gland or an abnormal gland in a patient with surgically altered anatomy (11).

Imaging is performed using both 99mTc and 201Tl. Thallium is a potassium analog that distributes in relation-ship to blood flow and state of the Na+, K+-adenosine triphosphatase system (11). Because of their increased vascularity, both the thyroid and parathyroid glands exhibit increased uptake of thallium relative to surrounding tissue. By contrast, technetium is taken up only by the thyroid. An image of the parathyroid gland can be obtained by subtracting the 99mTc image from the 201Tl image. The sensitivity of the parathyroid subtraction scan (Fig. 8) ranges from 70% to 90%, depending on the size of the adenoma or area of hyperplasia. Adenomas <300 mg in size are difficult to identify (10).

An alternate method is the use of 99mTc sestamibi for parathyroid imaging. This technique exploits the differential washout characteristics of sestamibi. The blood pool image obtained 10 minutes after injection demonstrates uptake in both thyroid and parathyroid tissue. Delayed imaging at 2–3 hours after injection should show washout of activity from the thyroid tissue, with retention of activity in an adenoma. Some investigators attempt to increase the specificity of equivocal studies by performing a ^{123}I subtraction scan of the thyroid (11).

Palpation of the neck is necessary for correlating the scintigraphic findings. Adenomatous goiters, thyroid carcinoma, chronic thyroiditis, and lymphoma can give a false-positive appearance on a parathyroid subtraction scan (12).

REFERENCES

1. Genant HK: Bone-seeking radionuclides: An in vivo study of factors affecting skeletal uptake. *Radiology* 113:373–382, 1974

2. Mettler FA: *Essentials of Nuclear Medicine Imaging.* New York, Grune & Stratton, 1985
3. Snyder WS, et al: "S" Absorbed dose per unit cumulated activity for selected radionuclides and organs. MIRD Pamphlet No. 11. New York: The Society of Nuclear Medicine, 1975
4. Wahner HW: Assessment of metabolic bone disease. Review of new nuclear medicine procedures. *Mayo Clin Proc* 60:827–835, 1985
5. Siegel BA: *Nuclear Medicine: Self-Study Program 1.* New York, Society of Nuclear Medicine, 1988
6. McAfee JG: Radionuclide imaging in metabolic and systemic skeletal diseases. *Semin Nucl Med* 17:334–349, 1987
7. Reis T: Detection of osteoporotic sacral fractures with radionuclides. *Radiology* 146:783–785, 1983
8. Fogelman I: Role of bone scanning in osteomalacia. *J Nucl Med* 19:245–248, 1978
9. Shier CK: Ribbing's disease: Radiographic-scintigraphic correlation and comparative analysis with Engelmann's disease. *J Nucl Med* 28:244–248, 1987
10. Fine EJ: Parathyroid imaging: Its current status and future role. *Semin Nucl Med* 17:350–359, 1987
11. Taillefer R: Detection and localization of parathyroid adenomas in patients with hyperparathyroidism using a single radionuclide imaging procedure with technetium-99m-sestamibi (double-phase study). *J Nucl Med* 33:1801–1807, 1992
12. Winzelberg GG: Radionuclide imaging of parathyroid tumors: Historical perspectives and newer techniques. *Semin Nucl Med* 15:161–170, 1985

23. Bone Density Measurement and the Management of Osteoporosis

C. Conrad Johnston, Jr., M.D., Charles W. Slemenda, Dr.P.H., and *L. Joseph Melton III, M.D.

*Department of Medicine, Indiana University School of Medicine, Indianapolis, Indiana; and *Department of Health Sciences Research, Mayo Clinic and Foundation, Rochester, Minnesota*

All agree that osteoporosis is a major public health problem (see Chapter 49). Any amelioration of the impact of osteoporosis depends on a reduction of its attendant fractures. Many interventions depend, in turn, on bone density measurement, and appropriate clinical application of technologies for this purpose should be based on the following criteria: (i) bone density can be measured accurately and safely; (ii) fractures result at least in part from low bone mass; (iii) bone density measurements can estimate the risk of future fractures; (iv) such information cannot be obtained from other clinical evaluations; (v) clinical decisions can be based on information obtained from bone density measurements; and (vi) such decisions lead either to an intervention that would result in a reduction in future fractures or to avoidance of future diagnostic efforts and therapeutic interventions, which would reduce health care costs. These principles are reviewed in the following sections, concluding with a summary of clinical indications for bone density measurements devised by the Scientific Advisory Committee of the National Osteoporosis Foundation (1).

MEASUREMENT OF BONE DENSITY

Bone mass can be measured with good accuracy and excellent precision using a number of currently available techniques (Table 1), which are described in detail elsewhere (2–7). Single-photon absorptiometry (SPA) and, more recently, single-energy x-ray absorptiometry (SXA) have been used to measure the radius and os calcis, and dual-photon absorptiometry (DPA) or dual-energy x-ray absorptiometry (DXA) can measure bone mineral density (BMD) in the spine and proximal femur, as well as other regions. Quantitative computed tomography (QCT) can give information similar to DXA (an integral measurement of the vertebral body) or can assess cancellous bone of the spine alone, which might be preferable depending upon the relative contributions of cancellous and cortical bone to strength of the vertebral body. All of these methods are far superior to standard roentgenograms, which have an accuracy error rate of 30% to 50% for assessing bone mass. Moreover, the accuracy of bone density measurements compares favorably with that of many other accepted clinical tests, including screening tests such as serum cholesterol.

To this list of technologies can be added measurement of the phalanges by radiographic densitometry, a method for measuring bone mass at a peripheral site, usually the hand. An x-ray of the hand is made with an aluminum step wedge placed on the film as a standard, against which density can be determined. This method has been demonstrated to be accurate and precise, similar to SPA and SXA (8). Measurement in the phalanges correlates with other sites as well as other methods correlate between sites (9). More important, data from National Health and Nutritional Examination Survey I suggest that its prediction of hip fracture is as good as that of other peripheral measurements, with the relative risk approximating 2 (10,11). In addition, a prospective study in which bone mass measurements were made at the end of the study indicated good prediction of vertebral deformities (12). Thus, radiographic absorptiometry should be an adequate method for rank-ordering individuals based on their risk of subsequent osteoporotic fractures, but its use for prospective follow-up to determine changes or effects of therapy has not been demonstrated (13).

Ultrasound measurements (14) also correlate with bone density measurements (15), but may provide additional information regarding bone quality (16).

Methods for measuring bone mass are very safe, with low radiation exposure. Single-photon absorptiometry produces a dose of < 15 mRem, DPA and DXA < 5 mRem, and mod-

TABLE 1. *Comparison of bone densitometry techniques*

Technique	Site	Relative sensitivity	Precision (%)	Accuracy (%)	Duration of examination (min)	Absorbed dose (mRem)	Cost ($)
Standard techniques							
SPA	Proximal radius	1X	2–3	5	15	10	75
DPA	Spine, hip	2X	2–4	4–10	20–40	5	100–150
QCT	Spine	3–4X	2–5	5–20	10–20	100–1000	100–200
Newer developments							
SPA-R	Distal radius, calcaneus	2X	1–2	5	10–20	5–10	50[a]
DXA	Spine, hip	2X	1–2	3–5	5	1–3	75[a]
QCT-A	Spine, hip	3–4X	1–2	5–10	10	100–300	100[a]

[a]Projected cost.

DPA, dual-photon absorptiometry; DXA, DPA with a dual-energy x-ray source; SPA, single-photon absorptiometry; SPA-R, retilinear SPA; QCT, quantative computed tomography; QCT-A, QCT with advanced software and hardware capabilities. From: Genant HK, Block JE, Steiger P, Glueer CC, Ettinger B, Harris ST: *Radiology* 170:817–822, 1989.

ern QCT from 100 to 1000 mRem. These can be compared with the dose received from a chest x-ray of 20–50 mRem, full dental x-ray of 300 mRem, or abdominal computed tomography of 1–6 Rem (17,18).

RELATIONSHIP OF BONE DENSITY TO FRACTURES

There is considerable evidence that fractures result from low bone mass. Bone mineral density accounts for 75% to 85% of the variance in the ultimate strength of bone tissue (19), and such measurements also provide an accurate indication of the strength of whole bones (20–24). Because bone strength is an important determinant of fracture susceptibility, along with the likelihood of sustaining sufficient trauma, it follows that BMD is also correlated with fracture risk in patients (25). Indeed, there is a gradient of increasing fracture risk as bone mass falls that is independent of age (26), as illustrated in Fig. 1. On the left side of the figure, fracture risk is plotted against bone density for subjects of different ages, and it is clear that the risk increases with lower bone

mass within each age group. However, age is also an independent predictor of subsequent fracture risk, and the contribution of age increases as subjects grow older, as can be seen on the right side of the figure. Even after adjustment for the influence of age, though, most fractures among elderly women are due at least in part to low bone density (27).

There are, of course, other risk factors for these fractures. Bone density is a good *in vivo* measure of bone strength, but is not the only determinant of skeletal fragility. Age-related changes in bone composition or an accumulation of stress microfractures could impair bone quality (19), and bone loss is associated with changes in the architectural arrangement of bone tissue that lead to reduced bone strength (28,29). However, these factors cannot be measured directly by noninvasive means, and it remains to be shown that their contribution is greater than can be accounted for by bone loss alone (30). More recently, it was demonstrated that each standard deviation (SD) increase in femoral neck length was associated with a 1.8-fold increase in hip fracture risk, independent of bone mass (31). Even more important is the influence of trauma, especially in falls among the elderly. Falling is particularly important in the etiology of hip and distal forearm fractures

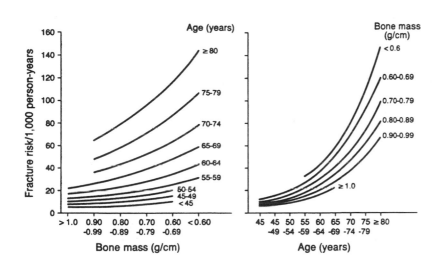

FIG. 1. Estimated incidence of fracture as a function of bone mass and age. (From: Hui SL, Slemenda CW, Johnston CC Jr: *J Clin Invest* 81:1804–1809, 1988.)

(32), but plays a role in vertebral fractures as well (33). The risk of falling increases with age (34), but not sufficiently to account for the exponential rise in hip fracture incidence, and most falls do not result in fracture (35). Although there is an age-related increase in the risk of falling directly on the hip, which is much more likely to result in hip fracture than other types of falls (36), bone density of the proximal femur is still an important determinant of the likelihood of fracture when a fall occurs (37). This situation is analogous to the etiology of coronary heart disease. As with heart disease, the causes of hip fractures are multifactorial. Measurement of any single risk factor (bone density, cholesterol) cannot completely explain the occurrence of the disease. Nonetheless, measurement of the factor identifies those who have the greatest risk of developing the disease and, thus, would benefit most from therapy.

BONE DENSITY MEASUREMENT PREDICTS FUTURE FRACTURES

There is ample evidence that bone mass measurements can stratify patients on the basis of fracture risk (25). Prospective studies show that bone density measurements in the radius, os calcis, spine, and femur can all predict the probability of fractures (38–49). More recently, ultrasound measurements were also shown to predict the incidence of vertebral fractures in a small prospective study (50). Bone density measurements at the lumbar spine or hip (two sites) with DPA and at the radius (two sites) with SPA performed comparably in predicting the risk of any moderate-trauma fracture for up to 10 years, with age-adjusted relative risks ranging from 1.4 to 1.6 per 1 SD decrease in bone mass (45). The long-term results from this small study are consistent with short-term results from much larger studies (42) and indicate that bone density measurements at any skeletal site are equally able to predict the risk of fractures in general (47). However, measurement at that particular site may be best for ascertaining the risk of a specific type of fracture, as considerable variation may be seen in bone mass assessed at one site compared with another in individual patients. Cummings et al. (44) demonstrated that bone density measured at the proximal femur was significantly better at predicting hip fractures than were measurements at other sites, as illustrated in Fig. 2.

Some confusion has resulted from the fact that bone density measurements do not clearly discriminate patients with fractures from those who have not yet experienced an osteoporotic fracture, i.e., there is overlap in the values for patients with spine, hip, and forearm fractures relative to controls (1). Because of this overlap in values, it has been argued that measuring bone mass is not helpful clinically. However, bone density measurements are not intended to be a diagnostic test for fractures—radiographs are needed instead. Rather, they measure a risk factor (reduced bone mass) for future fractures, and are properly used for risk stratification. This is again analogous to the measurement of other risk factors, such as cholesterol for coronary heart disease or blood pressure for stroke. Indeed, the relationship between bone density and the risk of fracture is as strong or stronger than the relationship between serum cholesterol and the risk of coronary heart disease (51).

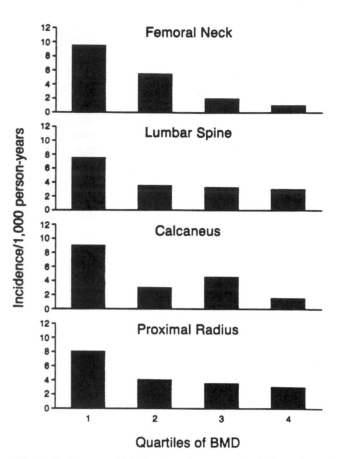

FIG. 2. Incidence of hip fracture by age-adjusted quartile of bone mineral density (BMD) measured at different skeletal sites. (From: Cummings SR, Black DM, Nevitt MC, Browner W, Cauley J, Ensrud K, Genant HK, Palermo L, Scott J, Vogt TM, for the Study of Osteoporotic Fractures Research Group: *Lancet* 341:72–75, 1993.)

FRACTURE RISK ASSESSMENT USING CLINICAL RISK FACTORS

It is commonly believed that osteoporosis-prone individuals can be identified through clinical observations, but this has never been demonstrated experimentally (52). For example, later age at menopause, estrogen or thiazide use, non-insulin-dependent diabetes, and greater height, weight, and strength were all positively associated with appendicular bone density among 9704 elderly women in the Study of Osteoporotic Fractures, whereas greater age, cigarette smoking, caffeine intake, prior gastric surgery, and a maternal history of fracture were negatively associated (53). However, models incorporating all of these independent predictors together explained only 20% to 35% of the variance in bone density at the radius or calcaneus. This low predictive power of known risk factors has been seen in other studies as well. Moreover, no one set of risk factors has been found consistently in all studies. In one evaluation of perimenopausal and early postmenopausal women (i.e., a population for whom estrogen therapy would be considered), age, height, weight, calcium and caffeine intake, alcohol and tobacco use, and a urinary marker of bone turnover were used to construct a model to predict bone density in the radius, lumbar spine, and hip (54). None of the models correctly identified more than 70% of the women with low bone mass at any site. This is not clinically acceptable, because most women with low bone mass can be correctly categorized by bone density measurements. Together, these studies demonstrate that various risk factors, although statistically significant, account for much less than half of the variability in bone mass and, therefore, do not provide adequate precision to classify individual patients (52).

An alternative approach might be to predict fractures directly and without reference to bone mass. A risk-factor score was able to discriminate those postmenopausal Dutch women who had fractures over 9 years of follow-up, but sensitivity and specificity were low (55). The lack of specificity was further revealed by the inability of various risk factors to predict vertebral fractures among a group of Japanese-American women (56). All of the women had at least two risk factors, and 91% had four or more of them. Likewise, the positive predictive value of an elevated risk-factor score was only 9% to 17% for identifying vertebral fractures among women in the United Kingdom, and most of this modest predictive power was contributed by a history of vertebral fracture per se (57). The most recent study found 16 independent risk factors for hip fracture, besides bone density, in a large population of elderly white women (58). Compared with 47% of the women who had two risk factors or fewer, the small group of women with five risk factors or more had a hip fracture incidence rate that was 17 times higher. Even in this group, however, os calcis bone density in the lowest third increased hip fracture risk by more than 40%. Thus, it appears that the assessment of some risk factors could be useful in conjunction with bone density measurements. It has been shown, for example, that the presence of fractures raises the risk of subsequent fracture above that attributable to bone mass alone (41), and combining several risk factors may have clinical utility. The individual who has slightly low bone mass, and is not at sufficient risk on that basis alone to justify an intervention, might be considered at higher risk if femoral neck length or a history of fracture were included in the assessment. However, no practical approach has yet been devised.

INDICATIONS FOR BONE DENSITY MEASUREMENTS

A task force of the National Osteoporosis Foundation has suggested the following clinical indications for bone mass measurements (1).

Estrogen-Deficient Women (Indication 1)

In estrogen-deficient women, bone density measurements can be used to diagnose significantly low bone mass to make decisions about hormone replacement or other therapy.

Rationale

Estrogen deficiency following menopause, oophorectomy, or prolonged amenorrhea from any cause is associated with accelerated bone loss. Bone loss, in turn, is associated with a greater risk of fractures. Bone loss and the associated risk of fractures can be prevented or slowed with estrogen replacement therapy (ERT). Bone density measurements are needed to determine which women have the lowest bone mass and will benefit most from treatment. Thus, measurement of bone mass will allow women to make rational decisions regarding long-term ERT for protection from osteoporosis. The same logic may apply to other treatments when estrogens are not indicated.

Background

It has been sufficiently demonstrated that there is a spectrum of bone mass in estrogen-deficient women, so that those with high or low bone density can be detected easily. As noted previously, bone mass measurements predict the risk of fractures. Therefore, decisions about ERT to prevent bone loss can be guided by measurement of bone density. A substantial proportion of postmenopausal women receive ERT for menopausal symptoms and other reasons that have little to do with osteoporosis, but treatment is typically for a limited time. It has been estimated that only 5% of postmenopausal women will get long-term ERT (10 years or more) for reasons independent of concerns about osteoporosis and, consequently, unaffected by potential bone mass measurements (1). Indeed, recent surveys indicate that only 3% to 8% of women with natural menopause are receiving ERT (59,60). Thus, the majority of postmenopausal women will have to weigh the costs and benefits of this therapy. Because ERT has side effects and potentially serious risks (61) and because patient acceptance may be a problem with the use of estrogen-progestin combinations, which often lead to cyclical bleeding, it is important to select those at greatest risk of future fracture for long-term ERT. This determination can be made reliably only by direct measurement of bone density.

Treatment with ERT will reduce future fractures. There is compelling evidence that long-term estrogen therapy prevents bone loss and fracture. In one clinical trial of three groups of patients followed for more than 6 years after oophorectomy, estrogen (mestranol) significantly retarded bone loss for as long as estrogens were prescribed, at least 10 years (62,63). These effects of estrogen were independent of the duration of ovarian insufficiency that preceded the onset of treatment (64), and recent data show ERT to be effective in slowing bone loss up to age 70 (65). However, because the effect of treatment is to slow the rate of bone loss, greater benefits are achieved with earlier treatment because bone mass is maintained at a higher level. Similar results have been found by other investigators, as reviewed elsewhere (66). There is also evidence that ERT prevents fractures. One randomized trial showed that 38% of oophorectomized women not on treatment experienced vertebral deformity, whereas 4% of the women taking ERT had such changes (63). Randomized trials of ERT for hip fracture prevention are less feasible because of the long delay between menopause and the average age at the time of fracture. However, numerous observational studies indicate that the use of ERT is associated with at least a 25% reduction in hip fractures (61). More recently, a retrospective cohort study of 245 long-term estrogen users vs. 245 controls found a 17% reduction in fractures (67). This result was largely due to prevention of wrist and spine fractures; the difference in hip fracture risk was not significant. Data from a large prospective study, on the other hand, indicated that current users who began ERT soon after menopause had a 70% reduction in hip fracture and a 50% reduction in all limb fractures combined (68). Thus, available data show that estrogen prescribed early after menopause for a minimum of 5–10 years will reduce the risk of osteoporotic fractures by up to 50%. There are, however, suggestions that the protective effect may begin to wane after ERT is stopped (68–71).

Bone density measurements should lead to an increase in appropriate outcomes (fewer fractures). It has been estimated that, in the absence of such measurements, 15% of women over age 50 would have long-term ERT and that 10% of the entire group of perimenopausal women would experience hip fracture during their lifetimes (1). In a program emphasizing bone mass measurements in the hip to identify high-risk women, it was estimated that 22% of women would have long-term ERT and that only 8% of all perimenopausal women would experience a hip fracture during their lifetimes. Bone mass measurements would result in treating 7% more women (from 15% to 22%) with ERT and might reduce the lifetime risk of hip fracture in all women (treated plus untreated) by as much as 2% (from 10% to 8%; a relative reduction of 20%). Another analysis suggested that long-term ERT treatment of 50-year-old women with hip BMD more than 1 SD below the young normal mean might reduce the lifetime fracture risk by about 15%, from 36% to 31% (61). This use of bone density measurement to direct ERT may be more (72) or less (73) cost-effective, depending on the assumptions made about outcomes and costs.

Protocol

Women should be measured to make a diagnosis of low bone mass when ERT is being considered specifically for the prevention of bone loss or treatment of osteoporosis (74). This could include women of any age who have amenorrhea of greater than 6 months' duration. The majority of these women would be perimenopausal. In addition, younger women with prolonged amenorrhea would be eligible if prevention of bone loss was of clinical concern and ERT (including oral contraceptives) was being considered. Women who are to be prescribed long-term ERT for reasons other than prevention of bone loss or treatment of osteoporosis need not be measured. Likewise, women in whom ERT is contraindicated or who refuse to consider estrogen or some other therapy to slow bone loss do not need bone mass measurements.

Although estrogen is the only drug approved in the United States for the prevention of osteoporosis, calcitonin is approved for the treatment of patients with established osteoporosis. Calcitonin has been shown to be effective in preventing bone loss in postmenopausal women (see Chapter 47), and this may lead eventually to its approval for the prevention of osteoporosis. Likewise, a number of bisphosphonates are currently under evaluation for the treatment and prevention of osteoporosis (see Chapter 47). Published data suggest that bone mass may be increased somewhat, at least in the short term, and fracture rates reduced. This class of drugs is also likely to be effective in preventing bone loss. Because all of these drugs have beneficial therapeutic effects only on the skeleton, they should be used only on those high-risk patients who are most likely to benefit, i.e., as assessed by bone density measurement.

Bone mass can be measured in the spine by QCT, DPA, or DXA; in the hip by DPA or DXA; or in the radius or os calcis by SPA or SXA. However, the specific level of bone mass at which an intervention should be undertaken is still somewhat uncertain (see Chapter 47). An ad hoc committee of the National Osteoporosis Foundation provisionally recommended that women be considered for ERT if they are amenorrheic and their bone density is more than 1 SD below the mean for young (age 30–35) normal women. At age 50, 1 SD below the mean is close to the empirical fracture threshold of approximately 1.0 g/cm^2 in the proximal femur and in the spine as assessed by DPA (1). The specific method of administration of estrogen or estrogen/progestin is discussed in Chapters 47 and 49. The length of time therapy should be continued is not certain, but a minimum of 10 years is suggested by the results of the studies reviewed earlier.

Patients whose bone mass is more than 1 SD above the mean for young normal subjects are relatively protected from osteoporosis and have a lower risk of fracture. They probably need no further measurement. If concern arises, measurement can be repeated in 5 or more years and ERT can be considered at that time. Estrogen replacement therapy is not usually indicated for patients within ± 1 SD of the mean, but they may benefit from measurements after 3–5 years to see if they have developed low bone mass (1). Further research may show that consideration of risk factors other than bone density will enhance the identification of high-risk patients within this group (48,58). For example, some have found evidence for a subgroup of postmenopausal women who lose bone at an accelerated rate (75), and it does appear that there are more vertebral fractures (but not forearm fractures) among those losing bone most rapidly (76). Should these data be confirmed, the most efficient way to identify those at highest fracture risk could be through a combination of biochemical markers of bone turnover and bone mass measurement (77).

Roentgenographic Abnormalities (Indication 2)

In patients with vertebral abnormalities or roentgenographic osteopenia, bone density measurements would be used to diagnose spinal osteoporosis before making decisions about further diagnostic evaluation and therapy.

Rationale

Patients commonly present with roentgenographic findings consistent with spinal osteoporosis. These are either a radiologist's diagnosis of spinal osteopenia or, often, abnormalities of the thoracic or lumbar vertebrae, including anterior wedging or endplate deformities. A diagnosis of osteoporosis should prompt an evaluation to exclude treatable causes of accelerated bone loss and should stimulate aggressive therapy to prevent further bone loss or to increase spinal bone mass. The complete clinical evaluation is potentially expensive, and therapy is associated with costs and health risks. Although indiscriminate treatment of such patients would lead to the maximum reduction of fracture risk, there is evidence that many individuals with vertebral abnormalities do not have significant osteoporosis. Consequently, the costs and risks associated with the clinical workup and long-term therapy cannot be justified for them, and it becomes essential to identify among those with roentgenographic vertebral abnormalities the smaller group with reduced bone mass.

Background

There is a spectrum of bone density in patients with vertebral deformities or apparent osteopenia on roentgenograms (78). Not all patients with findings suggestive of osteopenia actually have the condition, as the roentgenographic appearance of osteopenia is notoriously inaccurate. In addition to insensitivity in detecting bone loss (79), roentgenographic osteopenia is not correlated with vertebral fractures. For example, 29% of 218 ambulatory women aged 45 or older, seen as outpatients at Henry Ford Hospital, had roentgenographic osteopenia, but only one seventh of them had vertebral wedging or compression (80). Because the appearance of osteopenia can result from technical faults on the roentgenogram, normal individuals can be misclassified. Even vertebral fractures do not provide clear evidence of osteoporosis. Some true fractures are due to episodes of severe trauma earlier in life, whereas others are not fractures at all but represent old juvenile epiphysitis, positioning problems on the roentgenogram, or normal variations in vertebral body shape (81,82).

Although changes in vertebral shape indicate a fracture, change typically cannot be assessed because of the absence of baseline roentgenograms. Thus, fractures often must be diagnosed empirically, based on deviation from expected vertebral dimensions (83). The clinical picture provides little guidance, because vertebral fracture symptoms may be nonspecific (84). Inevitably, osteoporosis will be overdiagnosed in this clinical setting. Among an age-stratified random sample of women in Rochester, Minnesota, one fourth had vertebral abnormalities of one sort or another, but 21% of these women with apparent vertebral fractures had lumbar spine BMD values above the theoretical fracture threshold of 0.97 g/cm² (Fig. 3). As noted previously, vertebral fracture is related to bone mass, and bone density measurements reflect the probability of future fractures.

Bone density measurements will lead to an increase in appropriate outcomes (reduction in inappropriate evaluation and therapy for patients without osteoporosis). Practical savings to be derived from making bone mass measurements in this setting depend on the frequency with which vertebral abnormalities are encountered. It has been estimated that 5.6 million postmenopausal women have vertebral fractures (85). If as many as one fifth of them have bone density above the fracture threshold, there is a potential for evaluating or treating a large number of middle-aged women when they in fact have normal bone mass.

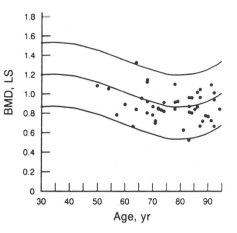

FIG. 3. Distribution of BMD of the lumbar spine (LS), by age, among Rochester, Minnesota women. The relation is best described by a cubic model: $\hat{\mu} = 0.517835 + 0.4922212 \times 10^{-1} \times age - 0.105822 \times 10^{-2} \times age^2 + 0.625726 \times 10^{-5} \times age^3$; $\sigma = 0.158749$, $r^2 = 0.33$. Values for women aged 50 years and older with one or more vertebral fractures are also indicated *(solid circles)*. (From: Melton LJ III, Kan SH, Frye MA, Wahner HW, O'Fallon WM, Riggs BL: *Am J Epidemiol* 129:1000–1011, 1989.)

Protocol

Any patient with a specific sign suggestive of spinal osteoporosis, including roentgenographic osteopenia or evidence of collapse, wedging, or ballooning of one or more thoracic or lumber vertebral bodies, should have a bone density measurement if that patient is a candidate for therapeutic intervention or extensive diagnostic evaluation. Such measurements are not indicated for patients whose workup or treatment will not be altered by the bone density result (e.g., patients previously evaluated and for whom no specific treatment was indicated). In this setting, bone mass should be measured in the spine by DPA, DXA, or QCT. Because the BMD of compressed vertebrae may be elevated (86), any fractures in the path of the scan should be eliminated from the analysis and only intact vertebrae evaluated.

Patients with vertebral abnormalities and spinal BMD above the fracture threshold would not be considered to have fractures on the basis of osteoporosis and, consequently, would not require a workup for metabolic bone disease and would not be treated for established osteoporosis, because all such therapy is aimed at preserving bone mass or increasing it. Women with vertebral abnormalities and spinal BMD below the fracture threshold would be considered to have osteoporotic fractures and would be evaluated further.

Glucocorticoid Therapy (Indication 3)

In patients receiving long-term glucocorticoid therapy, bone density measurements would be used to diagnose low bone mass (see Chapter 52).

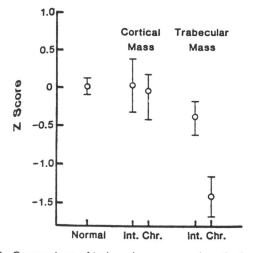

FIG. 4. Comparison of trabecular mass and cortical mass in normal controls and patients. The z-score is a function of the mean ± SD of age-adjusted and sex-adjusted values. Int., intermittent steroid use; Chr., chronic, or long-term, use. Trabecular mass in the long-term-use group was significantly smaller than in the normal ($p < 0.01$) and intermittent-use ($p < 0.03$) groups. *Bars* denote ± SEM. (From: Adinoff AD, Hollister JR: *N Engl J Med* 309:265–268, 1983.)

Rationale

Steroid therapy is required for a number of diseases, such as rheumatoid arthritis, chronic active hepatitis, inflammatory bowel disease, and asthma. This therapy has a number of serious side effects, including rapid bone loss leading to vertebral and other fractures (87). Some, but not all, steroid-treated patients experience this excessive bone loss (Fig. 4), and not all have fractures. The importance of assessment is increased because patients are frequently receiving long-term therapy. Moreover, unlike with involutional osteoporosis, patients may be children, and it must be determined whether skeletal development is lagging behind normal adolescent development patterns. Information about bone mass may permit improved patient management through more precise adjustments of dose and duration of therapy, to maximize therapeutic effects while minimizing skeletal complications.

Protocol

Patients who are to be placed on long-term (more than 1 month) glucocorticoid treatment (>7.5 mg of prednisone/day or equivalent) can have bone density measurements when it is possible to adjust the dose. Measurements of the spine using DPA, DXA, or QCT are advised because trabecular bone is primarily affected (87,88).

Primary Hyperparathyroidism (Indication 4)

In patients with asymptomatic primary hyperparathyroidism, bone density measurements would be used to diagnose low bone mass to identify those at risk of severe skeletal disease who may be candidates for surgical intervention (see Chapter 28).

Rationale

The clinical spectrum at presentation of primary hyperparathyroidism has changed with the advent of routine biochemical screening (89). Previously, patients presented with symptomatic bone disease, renal stones, or other complaints that alerted the physician and that led to surgical intervention. Now, many patients are asymptomatic and have no obvious complications when the diagnosis is made incidentally (89,90). The management of such asymptomatic individuals remains controversial (91). Primary hyperparathyroidism is associated with a decrease in bone mass in some patients (92), which can be detected by measurement of bone mass but not by the usual radiographic evaluation (Fig. 5). Such a reduction in bone mass may be accompanied by an increased frequency of fractures of the vertebrae, distal radius, and hip, as reviewed elsewhere (93). Thus, it can be argued that the finding of low bone mass in patients with otherwise asymptomatic hyperparathyroidism should be considered a possible indication for surgery (91). After successful surgery, bone density generally has been found to increase, although not to

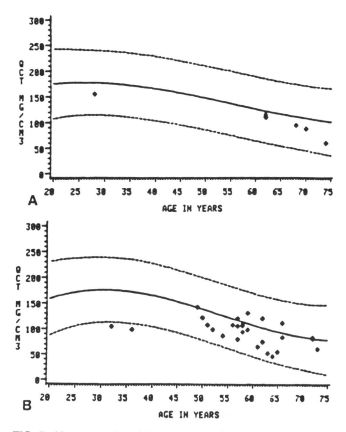

FIG. 5. Hyperparathyroid patients are plotted against normal curves as determined by QCT in males (**A**) and females (**B**). *Solid curves* indicate the cubic regression lines; *dashed lines* indicate the 95% confidence limits for the normal subjects. (From: Richardson ML, Pozzi-Mucelli RS, Kanter AS, Kolb FO, Ettinger B, Genant HK: *Skeletal Radiol* 15:85–95, 1986.)

normal values (93). Because low bone mass is related to fracture risk, an increase in bone density should reduce the risk of subsequent fractures.

Protocol

The diagnosis of primary hyperparathyroidism should be made using accepted clinical criteria (see Chapter 28). Those who have no symptoms that could be attributed to primary hyperparathyroidism that would lead to surgery should have measurements done. Bone mass may be measured in the radius by SPA or SXA or in the spine by DPA, DXA, or QCT.

Other Potential Indications

With the improvements in technology leading to better precision and accuracy of measurements, other indications for clinical application of bone density measurements may develop.

Universal Screening for Osteoporosis Prophylaxis

Bone mass measurement for osteoporosis prophylaxis meets some of the criteria for a screening test (i.e., the disease is common; screening tests are available; effective therapy is available for patients with abnormal tests; and treatment should reduce fracture incidence). However, some patients might be receiving effective treatment for reasons unrelated to osteoporosis, whereas others might decline therapy regardless of bone density measurement. In addition, optimal screening regimens have not been determined. Consequently, most authorities have recommended against universal (or unselective) screening (5,73,94,95). However, selective screening as outlined previously is justifiable (96).

Monitoring Bone Mass to Assess the Efficacy of Therapy

Therapeutic interventions to preserve bone mass are not always successful, and dose response may vary among patients (97). Because current methods for measuring bone density are quite precise (e.g., 1% for the spine with DXA and 1% to 2% for the radius with SPA), it may be possible to monitor responses to drugs and to alter the dose or type of drug used. Some have concluded that it is difficult to assess the true change in bone mass with two measurements taken closely enough together to provide relevant data for managing treatment (98–100). For example, two measurements of an individual 1 year apart, given a 2% SD of the difference between measurements and no actual bone loss, would yield a 95% confidence interval for the difference between the measurements extending from –5.6% to +5.6%. This results from the basic statistical fact that the variance of the difference between two measurements equals the sum of the two individual variances. Critics often note that bone loss over life is only approximately 1% per year in women and half that figure in men, and conclude that prospects are dim for monitoring changes in bone mass reliably. However, the issue is considerably more complex than this, for three rea-

sons: (i) recent changes in technology have improved the precision of longitudinal measurement; (ii) rates of bone loss around the time of menopause may be much greater than 1%, particularly in cancellous bone; and (iii) populations for whom such monitoring might be beneficial vary greatly. Considering ERT, the example given previously implies that, even with a precision error of 1% and bone loss at 3% per year, it would require a 2-year interval between measurements to identify accurately 85% of nonresponders to a therapy expected to prevent bone loss completely. Obviously, 2 years is an unsatisfactory length of time to wait before changing or reevaluating treatments. However, if the therapies being tried cause a short-term gain in bone mass (as is common with estrogen therapy and other regimens that act by slowing bone remodeling), then differences may be accentuated and shorter intervals between measurements may be possible. At present, however, insufficient data are available for approved drugs to suggest specific protocols for follow-up.

ACKNOWLEDGMENT

This chapter was adapted from a report of the Scientific Advisory Committee of the National Osteoporosis Foundation.

REFERENCES

1. Johnston CC Jr, Melton LJ III, Lindsay R, Eddy D: Clinical indication for bone mass measurement. *J Bone Miner Res* 4(Suppl 2):1–28, 1989
2. Mazess RB: Bone densitometry for clinical diagnosis and monitoring. In: DeLuca HF, Mazess R (eds) *Osteoporosis: Physiological Basis, Assessment, and Treatment.* New York, Elsevier Science Publishing Co., Inc., pp 63–85, 1990
3. Sartoris DJ, Resnick D: Current and innovative methods for noninvasive bone densitometry. *Radiol Clin North Am* 28:257–278, 1990
4. Lang P, Steiger P, Faulkner K, Glüer C, Genant HK: Osteoporosis. Current techniques and recent developments in quantitative bone densitometry. *Radiol Clin North Am* 29:49–76, 1991
5. Kanis JA and the WHO Study Group: Assessment of fracture risk and its application to screening for postmenopausal osteoporosis: Synopsis of a WHO report. *Osteoporosis Int* 4:368–381, 1994
6. Wahner HW, Fogelman I: *The Evaluation of Osteoporosis: Dual Energy X-Ray Absorptiometry in Clinical Practice.* London, Martin Dunitz Ltd, 1994
7. Johnston CC, Melton LJ III: Bone densitometry. In: Riggs BL, Melton LJ III (eds) *Osteoporosis: Etiology, Diagnosis and Management.* 2nd ed. Philadelphia, Lippincott-Raven Publishers, pp 275–297, 1995
8. Yang S-O, Hagiwara S, Engelke K, et al: Radiographic absorptiometry for bone mineral measurement of the phalanges: Precision and accuracy study. *Radiology* 192:857–859, 1994
9. Cosman F, Herrington B, Himmelstein S, Lindsay R: Radiographic absorptiometry: A simple method for determination of bone mass. *Osteoporosis Int* 2:35–38, 1991
10. Epstein RS, Lydick E, Suppapanya N, Ross PD, Yates AJ: Baseline measurement of bone mass from hand x-rays predicts hip fractures in a national sample of white women. *Osteoporosis Int* (in press)
11. Mussolino M, Looker A, Madans J, Edelstein D, Walker R, Lydick E, Epstein R: Phalangeal bone density and hip fracture risk. *J Bone Miner Res* 10(Suppl 1):S360, 1995
12. Ross P, Huang C, Davis J, Imose K, Yates J, Vogel J, Wasnich R: Predicting vertebral deformity using bone densitometry at various skeletal sites and calcaneus ultrasound. *Bone* 16:235–332, 1995
13. Yates AJ, Ross PD, Lydick E, Epstein RS: Radiographic absorp-

tiometry in the diagnosis of osteoporosis. *Am J Med* 98(Suppl 2A): 41S–47S, 1995

14. Kaufman JJ, Einhorn TA: Perspectives: Ultrasound assessment of bone. *J Bone Miner Res* 8:517–525, 1993

15. Ross P, Huang C, Davis J, Imose K, Yates J, Vogel J, Wasnich R: Predicting vertebral deformity using bone densitometry at various skeletal sites and calcaneus ultrasound. *Bone* 16:325–332, 1995

16. Heaney RP, Avioli LV, Chesnut CH III, Lappe J, Recker RR, Brandenburger GH: Osteoporotic bone fragility: Detection by ultrasound transmission velocity. *JAMA* 261:2986–2990, 1989

17. Kereiakes J, Rosenstein M: *Handbook of Radiation Doses in Nuclear Medicine and Diagnostic Radiology.* Boca Raton, Florida, CRC Press, 1980

18. Boshong SC: *Radiologic Science for Technologists: Physics, Biology and Protection.* 4th ed. St. Louis, CV Mosby Co., 1988

19. Melton LJ III, Chao EYS, Lane J: Biomechanical aspects of fractures. In: Riggs BL, Melton LJ III (eds) *Osteoporosis: Etiology, Diagnosis, and Management.* New York, Raven Press, pp 111–131, 1988

20. Eriksson SAV, Isberg BO, Lindgren JU: Prediction of vertebral strength by dual photon absorptiometry and quantitative computer tomography. *Calcif Tissue Int* 44:243–250, 1989

21. Lotz JC, Hayes WC: The use of quantitative computed tomography to estimate risk of fracture of the hip from falls. *J Bone Joint Surg* 72-A:689–700, 1990

22. Cody DD, Goldstein SA, Flynn MJ, Brown EB: Correlations between vertebral regional bone mineral density (rBMD) and whole bone fracture load. *Spine* 16:146–154, 1991

23. Myers ER, Sebeny EA, Hecker AT, Corcoran TA, Hipp JA, Greenspan SL, Hayes WC: Correlations between photon absorption properties and failure load of the distal radius in vitro. *Calcif Tissue Int* 49:292–297, 1991

24. Moro M, Hecker AT, Bouxsein ML, Myers ER: Failure load of thoracic vertebrae correlates with lumbar bone mineral density measured by DXA. *Calcif Tissue Int* 56:206–209, 1995

25. Ross PD, Davis JW, Vogel JM, Wasnich RD: A critical review of bone mass and the risk of fractures in osteoporosis. *Calcif Tissue Int* 46:149–161, 1990

26. Hui SL, Slemenda CW, Johnston CC Jr: Age and bone mass as predictors of fracture in a prospective study. *J Clin Invest* 81:1804–1809, 1988

27. Seeley DG, Browner WS, Nevitt MC, Genant HK, Scott JC, Cummings SR, and the Study of Osteoporotic Fractures Research Group: Which fractures are associated with low appendicular bone mass in elderly women? *Ann Intern Med* 115:837–842, 1991

28. Frankel VH, Pugh JW: Biomechanics of the hip. In: Tronzo RG (ed) *Surgery of the Hip Joint.* New York, Springer-Verlag, pp 115–131, 1984

29. Mosekilde LI: Sex differences in age-related loss of vertebral trabecular bone mass and structure—biomechanical consequences. *Bone* 10:425–432, 1989

30. McCalden RW, McGeough JA, Barker MB, Court-Brown CM: Age-related changes in the tensile properties of cortical bone. The relative importance of changes in porosity, mineralization, and microstructure. *J Bone Joint Surg* 75-A:1193–1205, 1993

31. Faulkner KG, Cummings SR, Black D, Palermo L, Glüer C-C, Genant HK: Simple measurement of femoral geometry predicts hip fracture: The study of osteoporotic fractures. *J Bone Miner Res* 8:1211–1217, 1993

32. Nevitt MC, Cummings SR: Type of fall and risk of hip and wrist fractures: The study of osteoporotic fractures. *J Am Geriatr Soc* 41:1226–1234, 1993

33. Cooper C, Atkinson EJ, O'Fallon WM, Melton LJ III: Incidence of clinically diagnosed vertebral fractures: A population-based study in Rochester, Minnesota, 1985–1989. *J Bone Miner Res* 7:221–227, 1992

34. Winner SJ, Morgan CA, Evans JG: Perimenopausal risk of falling and incidence of distal forearm fracture. *BMJ* 298:1486–1488, 1989

35. Gibson MJ: The prevention of falls in later life. *Dan Med Bull* 34(Suppl 4):1–24, 1987

36. Hayes WC, Myers ER, Morris JN, Gerhart TN, Yett HS, Lipsitz LA: Impact near the hip dominates fracture risk in elderly nursing home residents who fall. *Calcif Tissue Int* 52:192–198, 1993

37. Greenspan SL, Myers ER, Maitland LA, Resnick NM, Hayes WC: Fall severity and bone mineral density as risk factors for hip fracture in ambulatory elderly. *JAMA* 271:128–133, 1994

38. Wasnich RD, Ross PD, Heilbrun LK, Vogel JM: Prediction of postmenopausal fracture risk with use of bone mineral measurements. *Am J Obstet Gynecol* 153:745–751, 1985

39. Hui SL, Slemenda CW, Johnston CC Jr: Baseline measurement of bone mass predicts fracture in white women. *Ann Intern Med* 111:355–361, 1989

40. Cummings SR, Black DM, Nevitt MC, Browner WS, Cauley JA, Genant HK, Mascioli SR, Scott JC, Seeley DG, Steiger P, Vogt TM, and the Study of Osteoporotic Fractures Research Group: Appendicular bone density and age predict hip fracture in women. *JAMA* 263:665–668, 1990

41. Ross PD, Davis JW, Epstein RS, Wasnich RD: Pre-existing fractures and bone mass predict vertebral fracture incidence in women. *Ann Intern Med* 114:919–923, 1991

42. Black DM, Cummings SR, Genant HK, Nevitt MC, Palermo L, Browner W: Axial and appendicular bone density predict fractures in older women. *J Bone Miner Res* 7:633–638, 1992

43. Gärdsell P, Johnell O, Nilsson BE, Gullberg B: Predicting various fragility fractures in women by forearm bone densitometry: A follow-up study. *Calcif Tissue Int* 52:348–353, 1993

44. Cummings SR, Black DM, Nevitt MC, Browner W, Cauley J, Ensrud K, Genant HK, Palermo L, Scott J, Vogt TM: The Study of Osteoporotic Fractures Research Group: Bone density at various sites for prediction of hip fractures. *Lancet* 341:72–75, 1993

45. Melton LJ III, Atkinson EJ, O Fallon WM, Wahner HW, Riggs BL: Long-term fracture prediction by bone mineral assessed at different skeletal sites. *J Bone Miner Res* 8:1227–1233, 1993

46. Ross PD, Yhee Y-K, Davis JW, Wasnich RE: Bone density predicts fracture incidence among elderly men. In: Christiansen C, Riis B (eds) *Proceedings of the Fourth International Symposium on Osteoporosis and Consensus Development Conference, Hong Kong, March 27-April 2, 1993.* Aalborg, Denmark, Handelstrykkeriet Aalborg ApS, pp 190–191, 1993

47. Black DM, Cummings SR: How well can bone mineral density predict different types of fractures? In: Christiansen C, Riis B (eds) *Proceedings of the Fourth International Symposium on Osteoporosis and Consensus Development Conference, Hong Kong, March 27-April 2, 1993.* Aalborg, Denmark, Handelstrykkeriet Aalborg, ApS, pp 300–301, 1993

48. Nguyen T, Sambrook SP, Kelly P, Jones G, Lord S, Freund J, Eisman J: Prediction of osteoporotic fractures by postural instability and bone density. *BMJ* 307:1111–1115, 1993

49. Kröger H, Huopio J, Honkanen R, Tuppurainen M, Puntila E, Alhava E, Saarikoski S: Prediction of fracture risk using axial bone mineral density in a perimenopausal population: A prospective study. *J Bone Miner Res* 10:302–306, 1995

50. Heaney RP, Avioli LV, Chesnut CH III, Lappe J, Recker RR, Brandenburger GH: Ultrasound velocity through bone predicts incident vertebral deformity. *J Bone Miner Res* 10:341–345, 1995

51. Johnell O: Prevention of fractures in the elderly: A review. *Acta Orthop Scand* 66:90–98, 1995

52. Ribot C, Tremollieres F, Pouilles J-M: Can we detect women with low bone mass using clinical risk factors? *Am J Med* 98(Suppl 2A): 52S–55S, 1995

53. Bauer DC, Browner WS, Cauley JA, Orwoll ES, Scott JC, Black DM, Tao JL, Cummings SR, for the Study of Osteoporotic Fractures Research Group: Factors associated with appendicular bone mass in older women. *Ann Intern Med* 118:657–665, 1993

54. Slemenda CW, Hui SL, Longcope C, Wellman H, Johnston CC Jr: Predictors of bone mass in perimenopausal women: A prospective study of clinical data using photon absorptiometry. *Ann Intern Med* 112:96–101, 1990

55. van Hemert AM, Vandenbroucke JP, Birkenhäger JC, Valkenberg HA: Prediction of osteoporotic fractures in the general population by a fracture risk score: A 9-year follow-up among middle-aged women. *Am J Epidemiol* 132:123–135, 1990

56. Wasnich RD, Ross PD, MacLean CJ, Davis JW, Vogel JM: The relative strengths of osteoporotic risk factors in a prospective study of postmenopausal osteoporosis. In: Christiansen C, Johansen JS, Riis BJ (eds) *Osteoporosis 1987.* Copenhagen, Osteopress ApS, pp 394–395, 1987

57. Cooper C, Shah S, Hand DJ, Adams J, Compston J, Davie M, Woolf A (The Multicentre Vertebral Fracture Study Group): Screening for vertebral osteoporosis using individual risk factors. *Osteoporosis Int* 2:48–53, 1991

58. Cummings SR, Nevitt MC, Browner WS, Stone K, Fox KM, Ensrud KE, Cauley J, Black D, Vogt TM, for the Study of Osteoporotic Fractures Research Group: Risk factors for hip fracture in white women. *N Engl J Med* 332:767–773, 1995

59. Derby CA, Hume AL, Barbour MM, McPhillips JB, Lasater TM, Carleton RA: Correlates of postmenopausal estrogen use and trends through the 1980s in two Southeastern New England communities. *Am J Epidemiol* 137:1125–1135, 1993

60. Johannes CB, Crawford SL, Posner JG, McKinlay SM: Longitudinal patterns and correlates of hormone replacement therapy use in middle-aged women. *Am J Epidemiol* 140:439–452, 1994

61. Grady D, Rubin SM, Petitti DB, Fox CS, Black D, Ettinger B, Ernster VL, Cummings SR: Hormone therapy to prevent disease and prolong life in postmenopausal women. *Ann Intern Med* 117:1016–1037, 1992

62. Lindsay R, Hart DM, Aitken JM, MacDonald EB, Anderson JB, Clark AC: Long-term prevention of postmenopausal osteoporosis by oestrogen. Evidence for an increased bone mass after delayed onset of oestrogen treatment. *Lancet* 1:1038–1041, 1976

63. Lindsay R, Hart DM, Forrest C, Baird C: Prevention of spinal osteoporosis in oophorectomised women. *Lancet* 2:1151–1154, 1980

64. Abdalla H, Hart DM, Lindsay R: Differential bone loss and effects of long-term estrogen therapy according to time of introduction of therapy after oophorectomy. In: Christiansen C, Arnaud CD, Nordin BEC, Parfitt AM, Peck WA, Riggs BL (eds) *Osteoporosis 2.* Copenhagen, Aalborg Stifsbogtrykkeri, pp 621–624, 1984

65. Kohrt WM, Birge SJ Jr: Differential effects of estrogen treatment on bone mineral density of the spine, hip, wrist and total body in late postmenopausal women. *Osteoporosis Int* 5:150–155, 1995

66. Riggs BL, Melton LJ III: The prevention and treatment of osteoporosis. *N Engl J Med* 327:620–627, 1992

67. Maxim P, Ettinger B, Spitalny GM: Fracture protection provided by long-term estrogen treatment. *Osteoporosis Int* 5:23–29, 1995

68. Cauley JA, Seeley DG, Ensrud K, Ettinger B, Black D, Cummings SR, for the Study of Osteoporotic Fractures Research Group: Estrogen replacement therapy and fractures in older women. *Ann Intern Med* 122:9–16, 1995

69. Weiss NS, Ure CL, Ballard JH, Williams AR, Daling JR: Decreased risk of fractures of the hip and lower forearm with postmenopausal use of estrogens. *N Engl J Med* 303:1195–1198, 1980

70. Kiel DP, Felson DT, Anderson JJ, Wilson PWF, Moskowitz MA: Hip fracture and the use of estrogens in postmenopausal women: The Framingham Study. *N Engl J Med* 317:1169–1174, 1987

71. Paganini-Hill A, Chao A, Ross RK, Henderson BE: Exercise and other factors in the prevention of hip fractures: The leisure world study. *Epidemiology* 2:16–25, 1991

72. Tosteson AN, Rosenthal DI, Melton LJ III, Weinstein MC: Cost effectiveness of screening perimenopausal white women for osteoporosis: Bone densitometry and hormone replacement therapy. *Ann Intern Med* 113:594–603, 1990

73. U.S. Congress, Office of Technology Assessment: *Effectiveness and Costs of Osteoporosis Screening and Hormone Replacement Therapy, Volume I: Cost-Effectiveness Analysis.* OTA-BP-H-160. Washington, DC, U.S. Government Printing Office, August 1995

74. Rubin SM, Cummings SR: Results of bone densitometry affect women's decisions about taking measures to prevent fractures. *Ann Intern Med* 116:990–995, 1992

75. Christiansen C, Riis BJ, Rødbro P: Prediction of rapid bone loss in postmenopausal women. *Lancet* 1:1105–1108, 1987

76. Hansen MA, Overgaard K, Riis BJ, Christiansen C: Role of peak bone mass and bone loss in postmenopausal osteoporosis: 12-year study. *BMJ* 303:961–964, 1991

77. Riis BJ: Cost effective techniques for assessment of present and future bone mineral status: The practical integration of bone mass and biochemical markers. In: Christiansen C, Riis B (eds) *Proceedings of the Fourth International Symposium on Osteoporosis and Consensus Development Conference, Hong Kong, March 27-April 2, 1993.* Aalborg, Denmark, Handelstrykkeriet Aalborg ApS, pp 297–299, 1993

78. Melton LJ III, Kan SH, Frye MA, Wahner HW, O'Fallon WM, Riggs BL: Epidemiology of vertebral fractures in women. *Am J Epidemiol* 129:1000–1011, 1989

79. Epstein DM, Dalinka MK, Kaplan FS, Aronchick JM, Marinelli DL, Kundel HL: Observer variation in the detection of osteopenia. *Skeletal Radiol* 15:347–349, 1986

80. Smith RW Jr, Rizek J: Epidemiologic studies of osteoporosis in women of Puerto Rico and southeastern Michigan with special reference to age, race, national origin and to other related or associated findings. *Clin Orthop* 45:31–48, 1966

81. Doyle FH, Gutteridge DH, Joplin GF, Fraser R: An assessment of radiological criteria used in the study of spinal osteoporosis. *Br J Radiol* 40:241–250, 1967

82. Gallagher JC, Hedlund LR, Stoner S, Meeger C: Vertebral morphometry: Normative data. *Bone Miner* 4:189–196, 1988

83. Black DM, Palermo L, Nevitt MC, Genant HK, Epstein R, San Valentin R, Cummings SR, for the Study of Osteoporotic Fractures Research Group: Comparison of methods for defining prevalent vertebral deformities: The study of osteoporotic fractures. *J Bone Miner Res* 10:890–902, 1995

84. Ettinger B, Black DM, Nevitt MC, Rundle AC, Cauley JA, Cummings SR, Genant HK, and The Study for Osteoporotic Fractures Research Group: Contribution of vertebral deformities to chronic back pain and disability. *J Bone Miner Res* 7:449–456, 1992

85. Melton LJ III, Lane AW, Cooper C, Eastell R, O'Fallon WM, Riggs BL: Prevalence and incidence of vertebral deformities. *Osteoporosis Int* 3:113–119, 1993

86. Ryan PJ, Evans P, Blake GM, Fogelman I: The effect of vertebral collapse on spinal bone mineral density measurements in osteoporosis. *Bone Miner* 18:267–272, 1992

87. Lukert BP, Raisz LG: Glucocorticoid-induced osteoporosis: Pathogenesis and management. *Ann Intern Med* 112:352–364, 1990

88. Laan RF, Buijs WC, van Erning LJ, Lemmens JA, Corstens FH, Ruijs SH, van de Putte LB, van Riel PL: Differential effects of glucocorticoids on cortical appendicular and cortical vertebral bone mineral content. *Calcif Tissue Int* 52:5–9, 1993

89. Heath H III: Clinical spectrum of primary hyperparathyroidism: Evolution with changes in medical practice and technology. *J Bone Miner Res* 6(Suppl 2):S63–S70, 1991

90. Bilezikian JP: Primary hyperparathyroidism: Another important metabolic bone disease of women. *J Women's Health* 3:21–32, 1994

91. Anonymous: Consensus Development Conference Statement. *J Bone Miner Res* 6(Suppl 2):S9–S13, 1991

92. Richardson ML, Pozzi-Mucelli RS, Kanter AS, Kolb FO, Ettinger B, Genant HK: Bone mineral changes in primary hyperparathyroidism. *Skeletal Radiol* 15:85–95, 1986

93. Khosla S, Melton LJ III: Secondary osteoporosis. In: Riggs BL, Melton LJ III (eds) *Osteoporosis: Etiology, Diagnosis, and Management.* 2nd ed. Philadelphia, Lippincott-Raven Publishers, pp 183–204, 1995

94. Canadian Task Force on the Periodic Health Examination: The periodic health examination: 2. 1987 update. *Can Med Assoc J* 138:618–626, 1988

95. U.S. Preventive Services Task Force: Screening for postmenopausal osteoporosis. In: *Guide to Clinical Preventive Services: Report of the U.S. Preventive Services Task Force.* Baltimore, Williams & Wilkins, pp 239–243, 1989

96. Compston JE, Cooper C, Kanis JA: Bone densitometry in clinical practice. *BMJ* 310:1507–1510, 1995

97. Stevenson JC, Hillard TC, Lees B, Whitcroft SIJ, Ellerington MC, Whitehead MI: Postmenopausal bone loss: Does HRT always work? In: Christiansen C, Riis B (eds) *Proceedings of the Fourth International Symposium on Osteoporosis and Consensus Development Conference, Hong Kong, March 27-April 2, 1993.* Aalborg, Denmark, Handelstrykkeriet Aalborg ApS, pp 497–498, 1993

98. Heaney RP: En recherche de la différence (P < 0.05). *Bone Miner* 1:99–114, 1986

99. Cummings SR, Black D: Should perimenopausal women be screened for osteoporosis? *Ann Intern Med* 104:817–823, 1986

100. Davis JW, Ross PD, Wasnich RD, MacLean CJ, Vogel JM: Long-term precision of bone loss rate measurements among postmenopausal women. *Calcif Tissue Int* 48:311–318, 1991

24. Radiology of Osteoporosis and Other Metabolic Bone Diseases

Harry K. Genant, M.D.

Skeletal Section, Department of Radiology, University of California, San Francisco, San Francisco, California

Osteoporosis represents the most common form of metabolic bone disease, and its radiologic features are presented herein. The list of processes that are associated with or result in a generalized deficient quantity of bone (osteoporosis) is extensive (see Table 1). Histologically, the end result in each of these disorders is a deficient amount of osseous tissue, although different pathogenic mechanisms may be involved. In essence, the generalized osteoporoses represent a heterogeneous group of conditions encompassing many pathogenetic mechanisms, variably associated with low, normal, or increased bone-remodeling states.

Many terms have been used to describe the radiographic features of diminished bone density, such as "osteoporosis," "demineralization," "undermineralization," "deossification," and "osteopenia." The latter, osteopenia (meaning "poverty of the bone"), has become acceptable as a nonspecific, gross descriptive term for generalized or regional rarefaction of the skeleton.

The anatomic distribution of osteopenia or osteoporosis depends on the underlying cause. Osteopenia can be generalized, affecting the whole skeleton, or regional, affecting only a part of the skeleton, usually the appendicular skeleton. Typical examples of generalized osteopenias are involutional and postmenopausal osteoporosis, and osteoporosis caused by endocrine disorders such as hyperparathyroidism, hyperthyroidism, osteomalacia, and hypogonadism. Regional forms of osteoporosis result from factors affecting any part of the appendicular skeleton, such as disuse, reflex sympathetic syndrome, and transient osteoporosis of large joints. The distribution of osteopenia may vary considerably among different diseases and may be suggestive of a specific diagnosis. Focal osteopenia primarily reflects the underlying cause, such as inflammation, fracture, or tumor, and is not the subject of this chapter.

A number of characteristic radiographic features make the diagnosis of osteopenia or osteoporosis possible. However, the quantification of osteopenia by conventional radiography is inaccurate because it is influenced by many technical factors, such as radiographic exposure, film development, soft-tissue thickness of the patient, and others (1). It has been estimated that as much as 20% to 40% of bone mass must be lost before a decrease in bone density can be seen in lateral radiographs of the thoracic and lumbar spine (2,3). Finally, the diagnosis of osteopenia from conventional radiographs also depends on the experience of the reader and subjective interpretation (4). Therefore, the sensitivity of conventional radiography to detect early bone loss based on increased radiolucency is generally considered to be low (4–6).

In summary, a radiograph may reflect the amount of bone mass, histology, and gross morphology of the skeletal part examined. The principal findings of osteopenia are increased

TABLE 1. *Disorders associated with radiographic osteoporosis (osteopenia)*

I. Primary osteoporosis
    1. Involutional osteoporosis (postmenopausal and senile)
    2. Juvenile osteoporosis
II. Secondary osteoporosis
  A. Endocrine
    1. Adrenal cortex
      a. Cushing's disease
    2. Gonadal disorders
      a. Hypogonadism
    3. Pituitary
      a. Hypopituitarism
    4. Pancreas
      a. Diabetes mellitus
    5. Thyroid
      a. Hyperthyroidism
    6. Parathyroid
      a. Hyperparathyroidism
  B. Marrow replacement and expansion
    1. Myeloma
    2. Leukemia
    3. Metastatic disease
    4. Gaucher's disease
    5. Anemias (sickle cell, thalassemia)
  C. Drugs and substances
    1. Corticosteroids
    2. Heparin
    3. Anticonvulsants
    4. Immunosuppressants
    5. Alcohol
  D. Chronic disease
    1. Chronic renal disease
    2. Hepatic insufficiency
    3. Gastrointestinal malabsorption
    4. Chronic inflammatory polyarthropathies
    5. Chronic debility/immobilization
  E. Deficiency states
    1. Vitamin D
    2. Vitamin C (scurvy)
    3. Calcium
    4. Malnutrition
  F. Inborn errors of metabolism
    1. Osteogenesis imperfecta
    2. Homocystinuria

radiolucency and changes in bone microstructure (e.g., rarefaction of trabeculae, thinning of the cortices), eventually resulting in changes of the gross bone morphology, i.e., the recurrence of fractures. Further characteristics of osteopenic and osteoporotic disease conditions and specific techniques for their radiologic assessment are described in greater detail later.

PRIMARY OSTEOPOROSIS

Involutional, Postmenopausal, or Senile Osteoporosis

The term *involutional osteoporosis* has been used to describe the condition of gradual, progressive bone loss, often accompanied by fractures, seen in postmenopausal women and, with increasing age, in both men and women. It has been suggested that this broad category of involutional osteoporosis may represent two distinct syndromes—postmenopausal osteoporosis (type I) and senile osteoporosis (type II) (7–9). Gallagher (10) added a third type, meaning secondary osteoporosis. Even though the importance of estrogen deficiency for postmenopausal osteoporosis has been established, the distinction between the first two types of osteoporosis is not entirely accepted. Distinctions between postmenopausal and senile osteoporosis may sometimes be arbitrary, and the assignment of fracture sites to the different types of osteoporosis is uncertain.

Postmenopausal osteoporosis is believed to represent that process occurring in a subset of postmenopausal women, typically between the ages of 50 and 65 years. This group is characterized by accelerated trabecular bone resorption related to estrogen deficiency and is identified by a fracture pattern that involves predominantly the spine and wrist. Accelerated and disproportionate loss of trabecular bone in these areas structurally weakens the bone and predisposes these individuals to fractures. In senile osteoporosis, there is a proportionate loss of cortical and trabecular bone, in contrast to the disproportionate loss of trabecular bone in postmenopausal osteoporosis. Senile osteoporosis is characterized by fractures of the hip, proximal end of the humerus, tibia, and pelvis in elderly women and men, usually 75 years of age or older. The etiology of senile osteoporosis is speculative. However, factors that play a role include an age-related decrease in bone formation, diminished adrenal function, reduced intestinal calcium absorption, and secondary hyperparathyroidism.

Radiologic-Pathologic Findings

In the normal physiologic state in the adult, the rates of bone formation and bone resorption are roughly equal (i.e., coupled), allowing the total amount of osseous tissue to remain constant. In osteoporosis (11,12), this equilibrium is lost such that bone resorption predominates. This is reflected radiographically as various patterns of trabecular and cortical bone resorption, ultimately leading to osteopenia.

Trabecular bone resorption in the axial skeleton, particularly in postmenopausal osteoporosis, results in marked thinning and dissolution of transverse trabeculae, with relative preservation of the primary trabeculae or those aligned with the axis of stress. In areas in which trabecular bone predominates, such as the spine and pelvis, the combination of osteopenia and reinforcement of primary trabeculae may produce a striated bony appearance (Fig. 1). The reinforced primary trabeculae have a sharp appearance in osteoporotic bones, which occasionally aids in distinguishing osteoporosis from osteomalacia. In the latter, the trabeculae may appear indistinct or "fuzzy" as a result of irregular resorp-

tion from accompanying secondary hyperparathyroidism and from trabeculae that become coated by a layer of partially unmineralized osteoid. The loss of trabecular bone mass also accentuates the cortical outline, producing the so-called "picture framing" or "empty box" seen in osteoporosis of the vertebral bodies (Fig. 2). The vertebral bodies become weakened and the intervertebral disc may protrude into the adjacent vertebral body. The degree of protrusion varies, ranging from bending and buckling of the endplates (biconcave appearance) to herniation of disc material into the vertebral body (Schmorl's node formation) (Fig. 3). In more advanced cases, complete compression fractures of the vertebral bodies occur (Fig. 4).

Bone loss in the appendicular skeleton is initially most apparent radiographically at the ends of long and tubular bones, because of the predominance of cancellous bone in these regions. Endosteal resorption of bone has a prominent role, particularly in senile osteoporosis. The net result of this chronic process is widening of the medullary canal and thinning of the cortices, which is most pronounced in the appendicular skeleton (Fig. 5). In late stages of senile osteoporosis, the cortices are "paper thin" and the endosteal surfaces are smooth (Fig. 6). In rapidly evolving postmenopausal osteoporosis, on the other hand, accelerated endosteal and intracortical bone resorption may be seen and can be directly assessed by high-resolution radiographic techniques (Fig. 7).

When there is an overall loss of bone mass and progressive osteopenia, the skeletal system becomes weakened and fractures occur. These fractures are commonly seen in the vertebral bodies, femoral neck (Fig. 8), femoral intertrochanteric region (Fig. 9), distal radius, ribs, and pelvis. These may be the result of minor trauma or even normal stress on the abnormal bone (insufficiency fracture). Vertebral body and wrist fractures are generally seen at an earlier age than fractures of the femur (type II osteoporosis). Occasionally, these osteoporotic fractures are not identified on initial radiographs but are found by radionuclide bone scan, computed tomography (Fig. 10), magnetic resonance imaging, or by follow-up radiographic studies, as healing occurs. The radiologic appearance in the setting of partial healing may suggest a metastatic neoplastic process, particularly with fractures of the vertebrae, sacrum, hip, and pelvis (Fig. 11).

Idiopathic Juvenile Osteoporosis

The etiology of this rare disorder (13,14) is not known. Patients typically present before puberty with osteoporosis that is progressive initially and later stabilizes.

Radiologic-Pathologic Considerations

Bone formation is thought to proceed normally while, presumably, there is an increase in osteoclastic activity, yielding increased bone resorption (14). This causes a decrease in the quantity of bone (osteoporosis) while the quality of remaining bone is normal. This osteoporosis becomes most evident in the thoracic and lumbar spine with anterior wedging and biconcave deformities (Fig. 12) of the

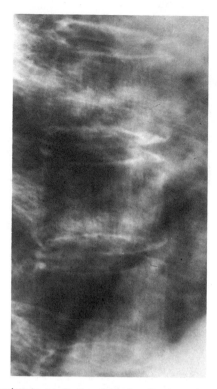

FIG. 1. Moderate postmenopausal osteoporosis of the thoracic spine with overall loss of bone density. The cortices are thinned and the vertebral bodies have a "striated" appearance due to loss of secondary trabeculae and reinforcement of sharply defined primary trabeculae.

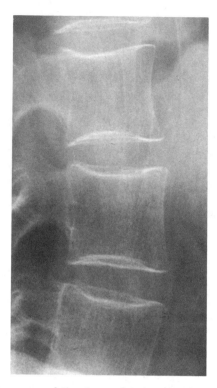

FIG. 2. Because of the loss of trabecular bone, there is accentuation of the cortices, resulting in the appearance of "picture framing" in this patient with postmenopausal osteoporosis.

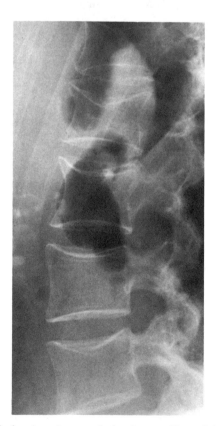

FIG. 3. Moderate osteoporotic fractures with endplate deformities of the lumbar spine due to involutional osteoporosis.

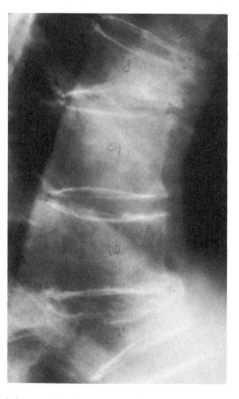

FIG. 4. Advanced osteoporotic fractures of the thoracic spine. Wedging and compression fractures have occurred as a result of involutional osteoporosis.

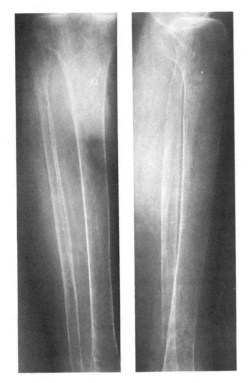

FIG. 5. Advanced involutional osteoporosis of the tibia and fibula producing marked thinning of the cortices due to chronic endosteal resorption and widening of the medullary space.

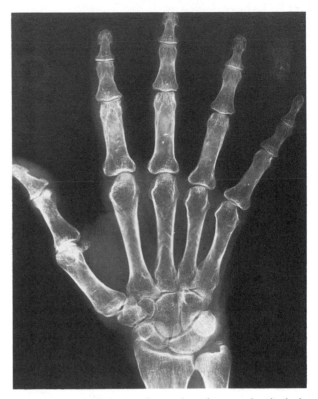

FIG. 6. High-resolution radiographs of a proximal phalanx showing endosteal scalloping and intracortical striation, indicating aggressive bone resorption in a recently (2 years previously) oophorectomized woman.

vertebral bodies are also found, and the condition should be distinguished from juvenile epiphysitis, or Scheuermann's disease (Fig. 13). Although fractures may be seen in the diaphysis of long bones, they occur more characteristically at the metaphysis. Presumably this is because the bony abnormality is more evident at sites of active bone turnover. Slipped capital femoral epiphyses may be seen.

The disorder is usually self-limited; however, if a large amount of osseous tissue is lost, the radiographic appearance may not return to normal. Laboratory values are typically normal, and diagnosis is made by exclusion.

SECONDARY OSTEOPOROSIS

Cushing's Disease (Endogenous and Exogenous)

Cushing's disease (7,13,15–20) is the result of an excess of adrenocortical steroids. This excess may be endogenous or exogenous. Endogenous Cushing's disease is caused by adrenal hyperplasia in the vast majority of cases, with other less frequent causes being tumors of the adrenal and pituitary glands. Exogenous Cushing's disease results from excessive corticosteroid medication and is far more common than the endogenous form.

Radiologic-Pathologic Considerations

As in osteoporosis, the equilibrium between bone formation and bone resorption is disrupted such that resorption

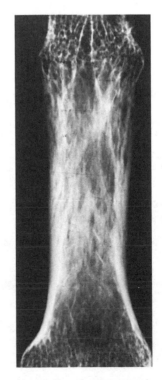

FIG. 7. Advanced involutional osteoporosis with generalized cortical thinning and uniform trabecular resorption.

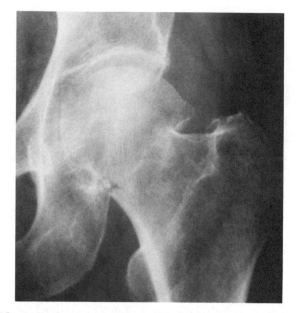

FIG. 8. Femoral neck fracture with mild valgus impaction in a patient with involutional osteoporosis.

predominates. Thus, the typical findings of osteoporosis are seen. Wedge, biconcave, and compression fractures are also seen. Histologically, exuberant endosteal callus formation is seen in compressed vertebrae and is manifested radiographically by increased density in the bony tissue adjacent to the vertebral endplate, referred to as "marginal condensation" (Fig. 14). This excessive callus formation is also evident in fractures involving other bones, including the ribs (which are commonly fractured in Cushing's disease).

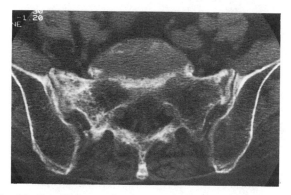

FIG. 10. Insufficiency fractures of the sacral ala due to advanced involutional osteoporosis.

Additional findings sometimes seen in Cushing's disease include a mottled appearance of the skull secondary to osteoporotic involvement. Osteonecrosis, particularly of the femoral heads (Fig. 15), is not uncommon in cases of exogenous steroid administration but occurs infrequently in the endogenous cases, for unknown reasons (7,21,22). Other less common findings seen only in exogenous Cushing's disease are joint infections, neuropathic-like joints, tendon rupture, delayed skeletal maturation, and decreased osteophyte formation (13,18).

Osteomalacia

Osteomalacia (13,23,24) is characterized by defective mineralization of osteoid in mature cortical and cancellous bone. It is a general term describing similar histopathologic and radiologic changes as are seen in a large group of diverse disorders. The etiology of osteomalacia in these disorders is also diverse, and may or may not be the result of a defect in vitamin D metabolism.

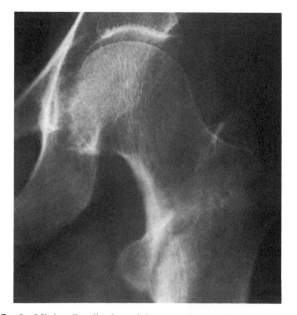

FIG. 9. Minimally displaced intertrochanteric fracture in a patient with late involutional osteoporosis.

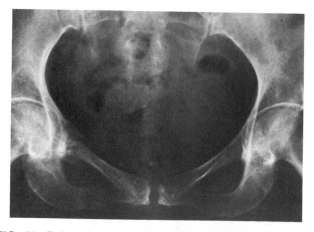

FIG. 11. Pelvic ring insufficiency fractures of the right pubic and ischial bones in a patient with involutional osteoporosis. Irregular resorption and reactive callus simulate a neoplastic process.

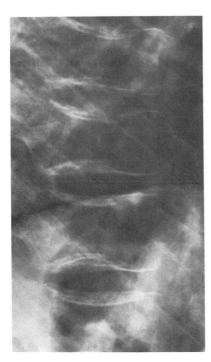

FIG. 12. Advanced idiopathic juvenile osteoporosis with biconcave vertebral deformities.

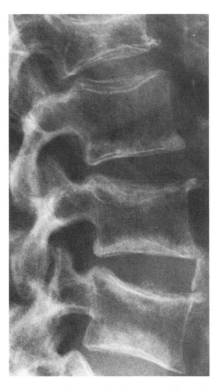

FIG. 14. Exogenous Cushing's disease. A lateral view of the lumbar spine demonstrates osteoporosis and biconcave vertebral bodies. The increased density adjacent to the vertebral endplates, called "marginal condensation," is the result of exuberant endosteal callus formation.

Radiologic-Pathologic Considerations

The primary abnormality in osteomalacia is the presence of excessive amounts of inadequately mineralized osteoid. This material is seen coating the trabeculae and thus accounts for the "fuzzy" appearance of these structures.

Focal accumulations of osteoid are seen to occur in compact bone at right angles to the long axis. Radiographically,

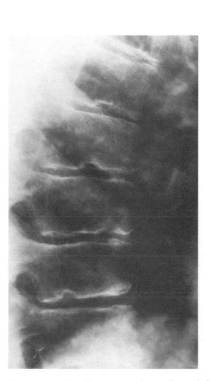

FIG. 13. Scheuermann's disease or juvenile epiphysitis with multiple discrete Schmorl's nodes and mild wedge deformities in the thoracic spine.

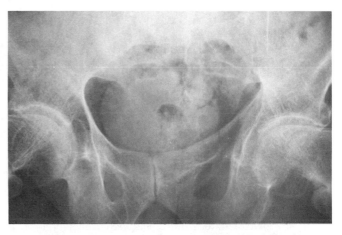

FIG. 15. Advanced osteomalacia showing generalized osteopenia, with bending deformities of the proximal femurs accompanied by medial pseudofractures of the femoral necks.

these are known as *Looser zones* or pseudofractures and are a distinguishing sign of osteomalacia, although they may occur in Paget's disease and, rarely, in simple osteoporosis (25). The exact etiology of Looser zones is unclear, although they probably represent partial insufficiency fractures. They are often symmetrical in distribution and are principally seen in the pubic rami, femoral necks (Fig. 15), scapulae, ribs, long bones, and metatarsals. Although they may remain unchanged for months or even years, true fractures may develop in these areas because they represent an area of weakened bone.

Intracortical bone resorption or cortical tunneling is observed in the tubular and long bones. High-resolution magnification techniques demonstrate these findings in the phalanges and metacarpals as a manifestation of the frequently associated secondary hyperparathyroidism (Fig. 16A). Intracortical resorption or tunneling is the most sensitive, although nonspecific, radiographic abnormality in osteomalacia, far more common than radiographic pseudofractures.

Radiologic thinning and loss of secondary trabeculae occur, resulting in decreased bone density and a coarsened appearance of the trabecular pattern, especially in the spine (Fig. 16B). Overall, the bones lose intrinsic strength, and bowing of long bones may occur. Scoliosis occasionally develops, and the vertebral bodies may assume a biconcave appearance (Fig. 17). Bone "softening" in other areas of the body may result in basilar invagination, protrusio acetabuli, and a triradiate appearance of the pelvis (13,24) (Fig. 15).

In some disorders causing osteomalacia, such as those associated with renal osteodystrophy, the massive amounts of osteoid present in the bones can become partially mineralized, typically in the presence of severe secondary hyperparathyroidism with a high serum calcium-phosphorus product. This results in increased bone density, particularly in the spine, giving the "rugger jersey" appearance (26,27) (Fig. 18). The exact mechanism of osteosclerosis in renal osteodystrophy, however, remains unclear.

Rickets

Like the term osteomalacia, rickets (13,24,28) is a general term used to describe the histopathologic and radiologic changes resulting from a group of diverse disorders. The final common pathway of these disorders is a loss of orderly maturation and mineralization of cartilage cells at the growth plate, resulting in similar pathologic and radiologic changes. Rickets represents osteomalacia in the growing skeleton.

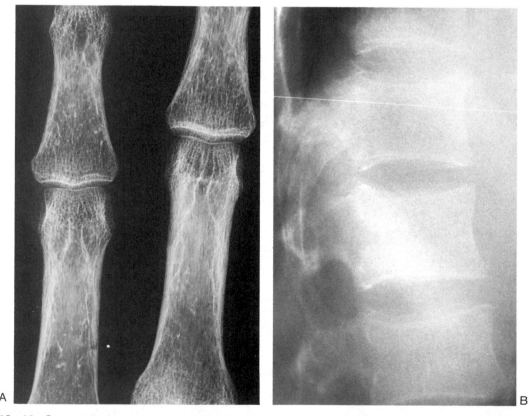

FIG. 16. Osteomalacia secondary to intestinal malabsorption. **A:** High-resolution radiograph of the hand demonstrates osteopenia accompanied by increased intracortical tunneling due to associated secondary hyperparathyroidism. **B:** Lateral view of the spine in this patient demonstrates osteopenia with indistinct cortical and trabecular outlines. Biconcave deformities of the vertebral bodies are also evident.

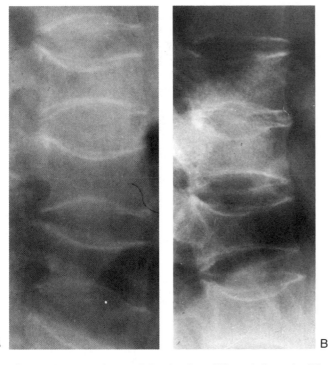

A   B

FIG. 17. Lateral views of the lumbar **(A)** and thoracic **(B)** spine in a patient with osteomalacia demonstrate moderate osteopenia involving the vertebral bodies. The trabeculae in the vertebral bodies appear indistinct, and there is evidence of bone softening with bowing of the endplates.

Radiologic-Pathologic Considerations

The radiologic findings at the physeal plate reflect the altered pathophysiology (29). The normal, ordered maturation and mineralization of cartilage cells become disrupted. This occurs predominantly in the hypertrophic zone, where the number of chondrocytes is seen to increase and the normal columnar formation of the cells is lost. There is a continued buildup of cells, resulting in the earliest radiographic finding of widening and lengthening of the growth plate (Fig. 19). Defective mineralization of the chondrocytes in the zone of provisional calcification yields the irregular metaphyseal margins seen on radiographs. Similar defective mineralization occurring in the zones of primary and secondary spongiosa produces a "frayed" appearance of the metaphyseal trabecular bone. As the cell mass in the hypertrophic zone continues to increase, it protrudes into the weakened metaphyseal region, causing cupping and widening of the metaphyses (Fig. 20). While this process is occurring on the metaphyseal side of the growth plate, similar processes are occurring on the epiphyseal side. The defective maturation and mineralization seen here result in an epiphysis that is osteopenic and has irregular, indistinct borders.

In the metaphysis and diaphysis, there is also defective mineralization of osteoid. In these areas, where mature bone is present, the radiographic findings of osteomalacia are produced.

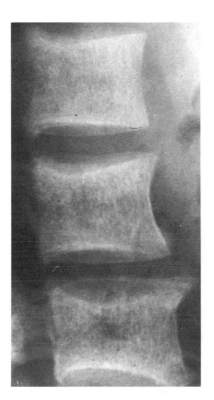

FIG. 18. Lumbar spine in renal osteodystrophy demonstrates mottled subchondral bands of sclerosis, the "rugger jersey" spine.

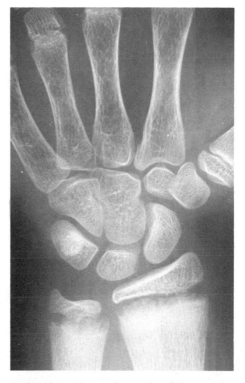

FIG. 19. Anteroposterior radiograph of the wrist in a child with rickets and osteopenia. Widening of the growth plates of the distal radius and ulna is evident. In addition, the zone of provisional calcification in both the radius and ulna is indistinct and the metaphyseal margins appear irregular. The cortices of the metacarpals are abnormally thin.

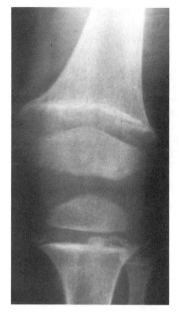

FIG. 20. Anteroposterior radiograph of the knee in rickets demonstrates diffuse osteopenia. The growth plates have widened and protrude into the weakened metaphyseal region, causing cupping and widening of the metaphyses. Note also the irregular, indistinct borders of the femoral epiphysis.

Additional radiographic findings include prominence of the growth plates at the costochondral junctions, producing the "rachitic rosary." The squared configuration of the skull seen occasionally results from excessive osteoid buildup in addition to abnormal remodeling. Because of the weakened nature of the bones, there is often bowing resulting from normal weight bearing and muscular stresses. Scoliosis, slipped capital femoral epiphyses, a triradiate configuration of the pelvis, and basilar invagination also may be seen.

Primary Hyperparathyroidism

This disorder stems from a primary defect in the parathyroid glands resulting in increased secretion of parathyroid hormone (PTH), causing an elevation of serum calcium and a reduction in serum phosphorus. The serum calcium becomes elevated, in part, by the action of PTH on bone by activation of the osteoclastic system and remodeling of osseous tissue. The resultant bony changes give the radiographic picture of primary hyperparathyroidism (13,26,30–32).

Radiologic-Pathologic Considerations

One of the effects of the elevated levels of PTH and a hallmark of this disorder is resorption of bone, or osteitis fibrosa. The resorption is believed to be the result primarily of stimulation of the osteoclast and occurs at many different sites (intracortical, endosteal, subchondral, subligamentous, and trabecular). Subperiosteal bone resorption,

which is most characteristic of hyperparathyroidism (13,31), is seen in approximately 10% of patients, most commonly on the radial aspect of the middle phalanges of the second and third digits (Fig. 21). Other sites commonly affected include the phalangeal tufts and the metaphyseal remodeling zones of the medial aspects of the proximal humerus, femur, and tibia.

Cortical striations and intracortical tunneling due to osteoclastic bone resorption (31) may be seen in more than half of the patients and are best detected in the tubular bones of the hands using magnification techniques (Fig. 22).

Erosions involving the sacroiliac joints, symphysis pubis, and ligamentous insertions; resorption of the distal or medial ends of the clavicle; and the development of "aggressive" Schmorl's nodes may all be attributed in part to subchondral resorption in these sites of high bone turnover.

In patients with primary hyperparathyroidism, the skull occasionally has a characteristic "pepper-pot" pattern, which results from trabecular resorption and remodeling of the space (13,31). Erosions of the calcaneus and inferior aspect of the distal clavicles are evidence of subligamentous resorption of these sites.

The combined effect of all these patterns of bone resorption is osteopenia in the majority of patients. Detection of this osteopenia by noninvasive bone mineral measurement becomes important for early diagnosis, as very few patients show diagnostic radiographic appearances of hyperparathyroidism on clinical presentation. Rarely, patients may demonstrate diffuse osteosclerosis (26).

Brown tumors (osteoclastomas) represent focal, bone-replacing lesions that occur most often in the metaphyses and diaphyses, though epiphyseal involvement may be seen (Fig. 23). They contain collections of giant cells that

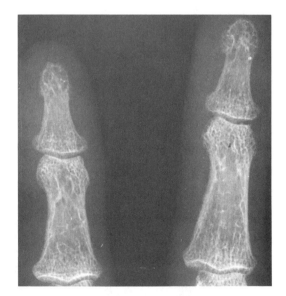

FIG. 21. Primary hyperparathyroidism with subtle subperiosteal bone resorption of the radial aspects of the middle phalanges, and irregular resorption of the tufts.

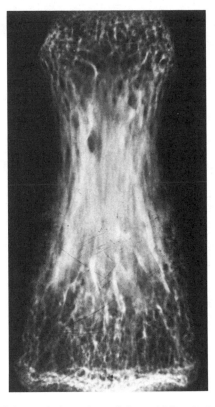

FIG. 22. High-resolution view of the middle phalanx shows marked subperiosteal and intracortical bone resorption in primary hyperparathyroidism.

are usually responsive to PTH, as the majority of lesions demonstrate healing with removal of the adenoma. They may occur as solitary lesions or involve multiple bones.

Osteogenesis Imperfecta

Osteogenesis imperfecta (13,33–35) is an inherited disorder of connective tissue that is usually transmitted in an autosomal dominant pattern. The defect in this disorder usually involves a mutation in the type I collagen gene. The classic clinical triad in this disease is (i) fragility of the bones, (ii) blue sclerae, and (iii) deafness. Two forms are recognized: the *congenita* form, in which life expectancy is usually short, and the *tarda* form, in which life expectancy is normal.

Radiologic-Pathologic Considerations

The abnormal collagen production seen in this disorder results in a primary defect in bone matrix. This and defective mineralization result in an overall loss of bone density involving both the axial and appendicular skeleton. The long bones may be either thin and gracile, as is usually the case in the tarda form, or they may be short and thick, as seen almost exclusively in the congenita form (Fig. 24). Multiple fractures (usually transverse) occur predominantly in the lower extremities, typically producing bowing deformities.

This bowing may indicate the severity of the disease, as it tends to correlate with the number of fractures. Avulsion fractures are also common.

Fracture healing is usually normal, but may demonstrate exuberant callus and pseudarthrosis. Inevitably, the extremities become shortened, which accounts in part for the short stature seen in most cases (33). Premature degenerative changes are often seen in the joints, primarily from intraarticular fractures and ligamentous laxity.

The skull and axial skeleton also show typical changes. Wormian bones (Fig. 25), enlargement of the paranasal sinuses, platybasia, and basilar impression are frequent findings. Severe kyphoscoliosis, biconcave vertebral bodies, wedge-shaped vertebral bodies, triradiate pelvis, and protrusio acetabuli may be present (Fig. 26).

Scurvy

Scurvy is the consequence of prolonged vitamin C deficiency. This deficiency causes a reduced formation of collagen and osteoid, and thus a reduced formation of bone (36,37). In contrast to rickets, calcification of the osteoid is not disturbed. Today in North America and Europe, scurvy is a rare disease that affects mainly young children and the elderly.

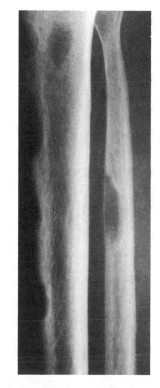

FIG. 23. Multiple brown tumors in primary hyperparathyroidism. Lateral radiograph of the leg in this patient with primary hyperparathyroidism demonstrates multiple brown tumors involving the tibia and fibula. The well-defined lytic appearance of these lesions is characteristic of brown tumors.

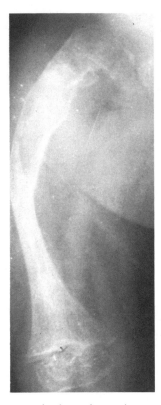

FIG. 24. Osteogenesis imperfecta (congenita form). An anteroposterior radiograph of the femur in this infant demonstrates bowing and thickening due to multiple fractures and exuberant callus formation.

Radiologic-Pathologic Considerations

In children, the decreased bone formation at the growth plates may produce characteristic radiographic findings. The zone of provisional calcification of the growth plate may be wide and dense, and therefore may be seen as a

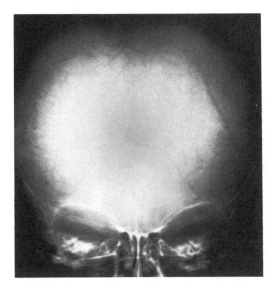

FIG. 25. Osteogenesis imperfecta. Typical skull findings in patients with osteogenesis imperfecta include numerous unfused ossification centers (wormian bones).

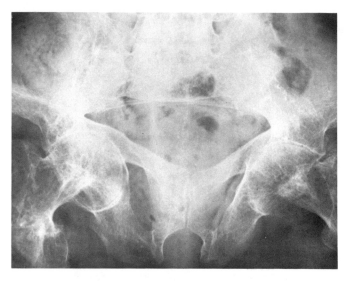

FIG. 26. A 50-year-old woman with osteogenesis imperfecta (tarda form). An anteroposterior pelvic radiograph demonstrates diffuse osteopenia. The pelvis has a triradiate configuration, and there is bilateral protrusio acetabuli.

transverse sclerotic line (white line of Frankl). Similar to the white line of Frankl, a zone of increased density may surround the ossification center in the epiphysis (Wimberger's sign). In addition to the characteristic findings at the growth plates, diffuse osteopenia and cortical thinning may be present (37,38). Elevation of the periosteum may be seen in long tubular bones of the lower extremities and generally indicates severe subperiosteal hemorrhage (Fig. 27). In adults, the radiographic signs of scurvy are less specific. These findings include diffuse osteopenia, thinned cortices, and insufficiency fractures of the spine and the appendicular skeleton.

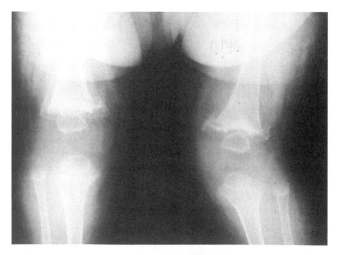

FIG. 27. Lower extremities of a child with scurvy demonstrate diffuse osteopenia, cortical thinning, transverse bands of dense calcifications adjacent to the growth plates, and periosteal new bone surrounding the diaphyses of the femur and tibia, indicating extensive subperiosteal hemorrhage.

ACKNOWLEDGMENT

Portions of this chapter have appeared in the following: Vogler JB, Genant HK: Metabolic and endocrine disease. In: Grainger RG, Allison DJ (eds) *Diagnostic Radiology—An Anglo-American Textbook of Imaging.* 2nd ed. London, Churchill Livingstone, 1992. Genant HK, Block JE: Postmenopausal and senile osteoporosis: Clinical epidemiology and detection. In: Viamonte M (ed) *Geriatric Radiology.* Baltimore, Williams & Wilkins, 1992. Genant HK, Vogler JB, Block JE: Radiology of osteoporosis. In: Riggs BL, Melton LJ (eds) *Osteoporosis: Pathogenesis, Diagnosis and Etiology.* New York, Raven Press, 1992.

REFERENCES

1. Heuck F, Schmidt E: Die quantitative Bestimmung des Mineralgehaltes des Knochens aus dem Röntgenbild. *Fortschr Röntgenstr* 93:523–554, 1960
2. Lachmann E, Whelan M: The roentgen diagnosis of osteoporosis and its limitations. *Radiology* 26:165–177, 1936
3. Virtama P: Uneven distribution of bone mineral and covering effect of non-mineralized tissue as reasons for impaired detectability of bone density from roentgenograms. *Ann Med Int Fenn* 49:57–65, 1960
4. Finsen V, Anda S: Accuracy of visually estimated bone mineralization in routine radiographs of the lower extremity. *Skeletal Radiol* 17:270–275, 1988
5. Epstein DM, Dalinka MK, Kaplan FS, Aronchick JM, Marinelli DL, Kundel HL: Observer variation in the detection of osteopenia. *Skeletal Radiol* 15:347–349, 1986
6. Williamson MR, Boyd CM, Williamson SL: Osteoporosis: Diagnosis by plain chest film versus dual photon bone densitometry. *Skeletal Radiol* 19:27–30, 1990
7. Steiner E, Jergas M, Genant HK: Radiology of osteoporosis. In: Marcus R (ed) *Osteoporosis.* San Diego, Academic Press, 1019–1054, 1995
8. Albright F: Osteoporosis. *Ann Intern Med* 27:861–882, 1947
9. Riggs BL, Melton LJ: Evidence for two distinct syndromes of involutional osteoporosis. *Am J Med* 75:899–901, 1983
10. Gallagher JC: The pathogenesis of osteoporosis. *Bone Miner* 9:215–227, 1990
11. Riggs BL, Melton LJ: Involutional osteoporosis. *N Engl J Med* 314:1676–1685, 1986
12. Parfitt MA: Morphologic basis of bone mineral measurements: Transient and steady state of effects of treatment in osteoporosis. *Miner Electrolyte Metab* 4:273–287, 1980
13. Resnick D, Niwayama G (eds): *Diagnosis of Bone and Joint Disorders.* 2nd ed. Philadelphia, WB Saunders, 1988
14. Jowsey J, Johnson KA: Juvenile osteoporosis: Bone findings in seven patients. *J Pediatr* 81:511–517, 1972
15. Bondy PK: The adrenal cortex. In: Bondy PK, Rosenberg LE (eds) *Metabolic Control and Disease.* 8th ed. Philadelphia, WB Saunders, p 1427, 1980
16. Jaffc HL: *Metabolic, Degenerative and Inflammatory Diseases of Bones and Joints.* Philadelphia, Lea & Febiger, 1972
17. Sissons HA: The osteoporosis of Cushing's syndrome. *J Bone Joint Surg* 38B:418–433, 1956
18. Bockman RS, Weinerman SA: Steroid-induced osteoporosis. *Orthop Clin North Am* 21:97–107, 1990
19. Rosenberg EF: Rheumatoid arthritis, osteoporosis, and fractures related to steroid therapy. *Acta Med Scand* 162(Suppl 34):211–224, 1958
20. Curtiss PH, Clark WS, Herndon CH: Vertebral fractures resulting from cortisone and corticotropin therapy. *JAMA* 156:467–469, 1954
21. Madell SH, Freeman LM: Avascular necrosis of bone in Cushing's syndrome. *Radiology* 83:1068–1070, 1964
22. Heimann WG, Freiberger RH: Avascular necrosis of the femoral and humeral heads after high-dosage corticosteroid therapy. *N Engl J Med* 263:672–675, 1969
23. Pitt MJ: Rachitic and osteomalacic syndromes. *Radiol Clin North Am* 19:581–599, 1981
24. Steinbach HL, Noetzli M: Roentgen appearance of the skeleton in osteomalacia and rickets. *AJR* 91:955, 1964
25. Perry GM, Weinstein RS, Teitelbaum SL, Avioli LV, Fallon MD: Pseudofractures in the absence of osteomalacia. *Skeletal Radiol* 8:17–19, 1982
26. Genant HK, Baron JM, Straus FH II, Paloyan E, Jowsey J: Osteosclerosis in primary hyperparathyroidism. *Am J Med* 59:104–113, 1975
27. Sundaram M: Renal osteodystrophy. *Skeletal Radiol* 18:415–426, 1989
28. Pitt MJ: Rickets and osteomalacia are still around. *Radiol Clin North Am* 29:97–118, 1991
29. Park EA: Observations on the pathology of rickets with particular reference to the changes at the cartilage-shaft junctions of growing bones. *Bull NY Acad Med* 15:495, 1939
30. Genant HK, Heck LL, Lanzl LH, Rossmann K, Horst JV, Paloyan JE: Primary hyperparathyroidism. A comprehensive study of clinical, biochemical and radiographic manifestations. *Radiology* 109:513–524, 1973
31. Steinbach HL, Gordan GS, Eisenberg E, et al: Primary hyperparathyroidism: A correlation of roentgen, clinical and pathologic features. *AJR* 86:329–343, 1961
32. Pugh DG: Subperiosteal resorption of bone; roentgenologic manifestation of primary hyperparathyroidism and renal osteodystrophy. *AJR* 66:577–586, 1951
33. King JD, Bobechko WP: Osteogenesis imperfecta. An orthopaedic description and surgical review. *J Bone Joint Surg* 53B:72–89, 1971
34. Kivirikko KI: Collagens and their abnormalities in a wide spectrum of diseases. *Ann Med* 25:113–126, 1993
35. Sillence DO, Senn A, Danks DM: Genetic heterogeneity in osteogenesis imperfecta. *J Med Genet* 16:101–116, 1979
36. Rosenberg AE: The pathology of metabolic bone disease. *Radiol Clin North Am* 29:19–35, 1991
37. Shamash R, Laufer D, Tulchinsky V: Scurvy—a disease not only of historical interest. *Br J Oral Maxillofac Surg* 26:258–260, 1988
38. Genant HK, Vogler JB, Block JE: Radiology of osteoporosis. In: Riggs BL, Melton LJ (eds) *Osteoporosis Etiology, Diagnosis and Management.* New York, Raven Press, pp 181–220, 1988

25. Bone Biopsy and Histomorphometry in Clinical Practice

Robert R. Recker, M.D.

Department of Internal Medicine, Creighton University; and St. Joseph's Hospital, Omaha, Nebraska

Bone modeling is the coordinated system of bone cell activity that shapes and sculpts the skeleton, and *bone remodeling* is the coordinated system of bone cell function that removes and replaces bone tissue with no net change in bone mass (1). Metabolic bone disease is manifest as derangement of one or both of these systems. They are directly examined by histomorphometric analysis of microscopic sections of trabecular bone from transilial bone biopsies. Fluorochromes must be given as tissue-time markers before biopsy, and the specimens must be processed without removal of mineral. Because the remodeling system is most prominent in adult metabolic bone disease, it is the focus of discussion here.

THE BONE REMODELING SYSTEM

The bone remodeling system has been characterized in numerous publications in the recent past (2). A brief summary is presented here. Remodeling occurs on trabecular and haversian bone surfaces. The first step is activation of osteoclast precursors to form osteoclasts, which then begin to excavate a cavity. After removal of about 0.05 mm^3 of bone tissue, the site remains quiescent for a short time. Then, activation of osteoblast precursors occurs at the site and the excavation is refilled (Figs. 1 and 2). In normal adults, there is no net change in the amount of bone after the work is finished. The average length of time required to complete the remodeling cycle is approximately 6 months (3), about 4 weeks for resorption and the rest for formation. This process serves several functions. It removes aged, microdamaged bone tissue and replaces it with new, mechanically competent bone tissue. It rearranges bone architecture to meet changing mechanical needs. Weakening of the skeleton by bone loss, abnormal accumulation of microdamage, or errors in geometry can come about only through defects in this system. Impediments of bone cell function, such as vitamin D deficiency, are manifest through this system.

Frost (4) has pointed out that population dynamics can be applied to the remodeling events that occur continuously in the skeleton. These dynamics can be examined by the use of histomorphometry of nondecalcified sections of trabecular bone from biopsy specimens taken after appropriate labeling with tissue-time markers.

THE BIOPSY PROCEDURE

The transilial approach is preferred over the vertical one by most workers because there is less discomfort to the patient and because most of the best-quality normal reference data from living subjects come from transilial biopsies

(3). The preferred site is approximately 2 cm posterior to the anterior superior spine, immediately inferior to the crest. With the patient supine and the hip slightly elevated on a folded sheet, the biopsy site is located by grasping the ala of the ilium immediately posterior to the anterior superior spine between the thumb and forefinger. The thumb then falls into the spot where the skin incision should be made and the trephine should be inserted.

After mild sedation of the patient with intravenous midazolam, the site of placement of the local anesthetic is marked with a felt-tipped pen. The surgeon performs a complete scrub; dons a cap, mask, gown, and gloves; and preps and drapes the operative site. He removes the core of bone through a 1.5-cm incision and closes the skin wound with two or three 5-0 monofilament sutures. The patient returns

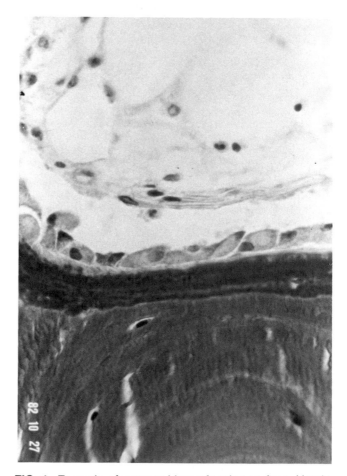

FIG. 1. Example of a normal bone-forming surface. Unmineralized osteoid is covered with plump osteoblasts.

164

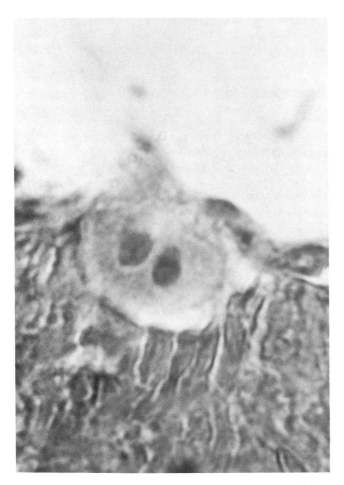

FIG. 2. Example of a normal bone-resorbing surface. Multinucleated osteoclasts are located in a Howship's lacuna.

to usual activities after 2 hours of quiet rest with instructions to keep the dressing dry and to avoid heavy physical activity for a few days. After 7 days, the sutures are removed.

It is most important for the surgeon to use very gentle pressure to advance the trephine through the ilium. This requires patience because the tendency is to hurry through the biopsy site, pressing ever harder as the trephine advances. Excessive pressure on the trephine will crush most osteopenic specimens and will create excessive artifact in others.

In a survey of 9131 biopsies (5,6), complications included 22 patients with hematomas, 17 with pain for more than 7 days, 11 with transient neuropathy, 6 with wound infection, 2 with fracture, and 1 with osteomyelitis, for a total incidence of complications of 0.7%. There were no deaths and no permanent disabilities. The procedure itself is nearly pain-free.

The Biopsy Instrument

The trephine should have an inner diameter of at least 7.5 mm, the dimension of the Bordier needle as modified by Meunier (Lepine a Lyon, Instruments de Chirurge, Lyon, France) or the Gauthier needle (Gauthier Medical Inc., Rochester, MN). The needle should always be very sharp. Sharpen (and recondition if necessary) after every three to five procedures.

Tetracycline Labeling

The ideal tissue-time bone fluorochrome label for use in humans is one of the tetracycline antibiotics. Demeclocycline fluoresces with an orange color, and all of the remainder fluoresce with a light lemon color. Most observers possess enough color acuity to distinguish between these labels. This difference in the color of fluorescence can be exploited to distinguish between pairs of labels given at different times. The author uses tetracycline hydrochloride, 250 mg four times daily, or demeclocycline, 150 mg four times daily. Tetracycline must be taken on an empty stomach. No dairy products or calcium supplements should be taken for 1 hour before and after the tetracycline.

There are practical limits for optimal timing of the labels. The minimum schedule is 2 days of label, 10 days free, and 2 days of label then 5 days before biopsy (2-10-2:5). The maximum schedule is 3-14-3:5. The author routinely uses 3-14-3:5. A thorough analysis of the optimal labeling schedule has been published (7). Longer labeling schedules will result in fewer surfaces taking the double label because of the "label escape" phenomenon, and shorter schedules will result in labels spaced too closely together for accurate inter-label width measurements (Fig. 3).

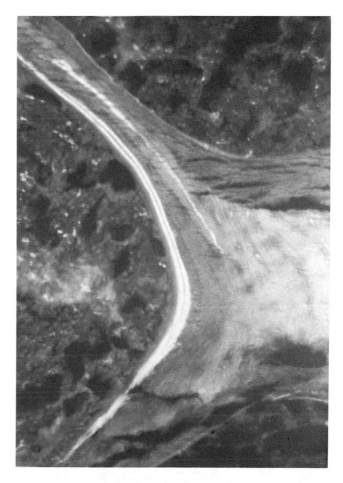

FIG. 3. Mineralizing surface containing two tetracycline labels given on a 3-14-3:5 schedule. One label is tetracycline hydrochloride and the other is demeclocycline.

Handling the Specimens

The biopsy core specimen should be placed in 70% ethanol immediately after removal. It can be stored for very long times in this solution without deterioration, but to ensure proper fixation, it should not be removed in less than 48 hours. The specimen is then dehydrated, defatted, embedded, and sectioned using one of the published methods (8). Methyl methacrylate is the preferred embedding agent in the author's laboratory, but several hard plastics are available and seem to work well. Five-micron sections are cut for light microscopy and 10-μm sections for fluorescence microscopy. A number of stains are used, as described previously (8), and unstained sections are used with epifluorescence to analyze the fluorochrome labels.

The basic microscope measurements (3,9) are trabecular bone volume (TV/BV), bone surface (BS), eroded surface (ES/BS), osteoid surface (OS/BS), mineralized surface (MS/BS), wall thickness (W.Th), osteoid thickness (O.Th), and mineral apposition rate (MAR). A microscope with integrating eyepiece reticule or with camera lucida and drawing tablet is used to obtain these data. Other important variables are calculated from these primary data (9).

INDICATIONS FOR BONE BIOPSY

The first criterion for choosing a diagnostic procedure in clinical medicine is to establish a diagnosis that will influence a treatment decision. The second is to establish information on prognosis. Further, the risk, discomfort, and expense of a diagnostic procedure should be appropriate to the importance of the information. Given these caveats, the number of clinical indications for transilial bone biopsy is small. The list below contains the most important ones (Table 1). This list may expand as more of the clinical disorders of bone metabolism become amenable to treatment. One impediment to widespread use of the biopsy is that availability of processing is limited. Most pathology laboratories cannot handle nondecalcified bone specimens or perform histomorphometry (Fig.2). The following list is offered with the expectation that clinicians will contact existing laboratories for processing of the specimens.

Postmenopausal Osteoporosis

There are certain situations in which bone biopsy is indicated in these patients, although it is not indicated in all of them. For example, in treatment trials, it is desirable to have

TABLE 1. *Indications for transilial bone biopsy*

Postmenopausal osteoporosis
Vitamin D–resistant rickets (various forms)
Renal osteodystrophy
Nutritional rickets and osteomalacia
Bone disease associated with chronic gastrointestinal
  disease
Bone disease associated with gastrointestinal surgery
Anticonvulsant osteomalacia
Primary hyperparathyroidism

baseline biopsy specimens to rule out confounding diagnoses and to compare with biopsies during treatment. With paired biopsies, we can learn whether remodeling characteristics at the beginning of treatment affected the outcome of treatment. We can obtain some understanding of the mechanism of a treatment response before waiting long enough to detect a positive bone mass effect or an antifracture effect. In some trials, bone biopsy is mandatory to determine the safety of a test drug that is suspected of suppressing remodeling or of producing abnormal bone tissue (Fig.3).

Every new treatment that is tested should be accompanied by bone biopsy in at least a subset of study subjects until safety and efficacy are assured. Some treatments can be predicted to fail based on the biopsy findings during treatment. An example would be continuous treatment with an agent that markedly inhibits activation of remodeling or impairs bone formation in those remodeling sites undergoing bone formation at the time the agent was introduced. Such an agent might harm the mechanical strength of the skeleton in the long term rather than improve it. This problem can be detected earlier by biopsy than with any other technology.

The incidence and prevalence of postmenopausal osteoporosis are very high in modern societies (10,11). Thus, it is clearly unrealistic and not necessary for every patient with postmenopausal osteoporosis to undergo transilial bone biopsy with tetracycline labeling, because confounding diagnoses are usually ruled out by noninvasive clinical methods.

Vitamin D–Resistant Rickets

There are many variants of this condition. Descriptions of the identifying characteristics of each are given in Chapters 60 and 61. Several recent reviews are available for the reader who is interested (12).

These patients present to the clinician with disordered growth and development. In patients with a negative family history who are presumed to have a new mutation, bone biopsy may be necessary to make the diagnosis. In addition, serial biopsies are valuable to judge the success of treatment and to evaluate the effect of changes in treatment in patients from families with a known diagnosis and in patients with nonfamilial varieties. The evaluation of new treatments requires the use of biopsy.

Renal Osteodystrophy

This condition represents the most important diagnostic use of transilial bone biopsy, because treatment decisions often depend on the results of the biopsy. The most dramatic example is the evaluation of hypercalcemia with bone pain and fractures in patients on chronic dialysis. If the biopsy shows predominantly osteitis fibrosa with brisk bone turnover, then partial parathyroidectomy may be indicated. On the other hand, if the biopsy shows little turnover (little or no fluorochrome label) and extensive aluminum deposits, then treatment with a chelating agent is indicated and parathyroidectomy is contraindicated. The biopsy can also help determine the extent of vitamin D deprivation and indicate the adequacy of vitamin D treatment.

Nutritional Rickets and Osteomalacia

These disorders are very uncommon in the developed world, and thus the call for biopsy to evaluate them is relatively rare. Nevertheless, the problem may be present in occult form among the elderly who reside in nursing homes, retirement centers, or in their own homes and thus do not get sufficient sunlight exposure. There has been uncertainty about the biochemical definition of nutritional vitamin D deficiency. The bone biopsy may be more sensitive than measurement of serum vitamin D to make the diagnosis (see Chapter 58). In the author's experience, careful histomorphometric analysis and comparison with a valid data base from age- and sex-matched normal subjects are surprisingly sensitive when the measurements of osteoid seam width, osteoid surface, and appositional rate are combined to calculate mineralization lag time (9). It is important to emphasize that simple measurement of osteoid seam width alone is not sufficient to determine whether osteomalacia or "hypovitaminosis D osteopathy" (13) is present.

Bone Disease Associated With Gastrointestinal Disease

The prototype is malabsorption syndrome of any type, such as with pancreatic insufficiency or celiac sprue (see Chapter 59). The predominant picture on bone biopsy is osteomalacia; however, the bone loss is greater than that seen in "pure" vitamin D deficiency. The bone lesion seems to be due to both vitamin D and calcium deficiency, the latter due to the combined effects of calcium malabsorption and excessive endogenous fecal calcium losses. Bone biopsy shows the presence and severity of osteomalacia and verifies the response to treatments.

Bone disease is a common complication of chronic bowel disease such as ulcerative colitis or regional enteritis. Bone biopsy may be the only reliable method of documenting bone disease in some patients before symptoms develop or before radiographic or biochemical findings develop.

Bone Disease Associated With Gastrointestinal Surgery

Many patients with a history of gastrointestinal surgery, including gastrectomy and bowel resection, can develop symptoms of musculoskeletal pain, reduced bone mass, and fracture (see Chapter 59). Bone biopsy can be used to document vitamin D deficiency and distinguish it from the joint and connective tissue disorders that may accompany gastrointestinal surgery.

Anticonvulsant Osteomalacia

Long-term anticonvulsant therapy, particularly in elderly patients, may cause musculoskeletal pain (14) and vertebral and hip fractures (see Chapter 65). In addition to osteopenia, patients may have a mineralization defect that produces prolonged mineralization lag time and accumulation of unmineralized osteoid. Transilial bone biopsy may be the only method of discovering this lesion, which may require changing the anticonvulsant therapy or adding treatment with one of the vitamin D preparations.

AVAILABILITY OF BONE HISTOMORPHOMETRY

Laboratory facilities that process transilial bone are scarce. However, the surgical procedure of obtaining the specimen is not difficult, and specimens can be mailed to one of the centers now performing bone histomorphometry. Physicians who contemplate performing the biopsy should contact a biopsy processing center ahead of time to obtain explicit instructions concerning the patient's history, the fluorochrome-labeling schedule, performance of the biopsy, fixing solution, mailing, and other procedures. Most centers require 4 weeks or more to report the results from a specimen.

REFERENCES

1. Frost HM: *Intermediary Organization of the Skeleton.* Boca Raton, Florida, CRC Press, 1986
2. Parfitt AM: Osteonal and hemi-osteonal remodeling: The spatial and temporal framework for signal traffic in adult human bone. *J Cell Biochem* 55:273–286, 1994
3. Recker RR, Kimmel DB, Parfitt AM, Davies KM, Keshawarz N, Hinders S: Static and tetracycline-based bone histomorphometric data from 34 normal postmenopausal females. *J Bone Miner Res* 3:133–144, 1988
4. Frost HM: Tetracycline-based histological analysis of bone remodeling. *Calcif Tissue Res* 3:211–237, 1969
5. Duncan H, Rao DS, Parfitt AM: Complications of bone biopsy. *Metab Bone Dis Relat Res* 2:475–481, 1980
6. Rao DS: Practical approach to biopsy. In: Recker RR (ed) *Bone Histomorphometry: Techniques and Interpretation.* Boca Raton, Florida, CRC Press, pp 3–11, 1983
7. Frost HM: Bone histomorphometry: Correction of the labeling "escape error." In: Recker RR (ed) *Bone Histomorphometry: Techniques and Interpretation.* Boca Raton, Florida, CRC Press, pp 133–142, 1983
8. Baron R, Vignery A, Neff L, et al: Processing of undecalcified bone specimens for bone histomorphometry. In: Recker RR (ed) *Bone Histomorphometry: Techniques and Interpretation.* Boca Raton, Florida, CRC Press, 13–36, 1983
9. Parfitt AM, Drezner MK, Glorieux FH, et al: Bone histomorphometry: Standardization of nomenclature, symbols, and units. *J Bone Miner Res* 2:595–610, 1987
10. Riggs BL, Melton L III: Involutional osteoporosis. *N Engl J Med* 314:1676–1686, 1986
11. Black DM, Cummings SR, Melton LJ: Appendicular bone mineral and a woman's lifetime risk of hip fracture. *J Bone Miner Res* 7:639–646, 1992
12. Peacock M: Osteomalacia and rickets. In: Nordin BEC (ed) *Metabolic Bone and Stone Diseases.* London, Churchill Livingstone, pp 71–111, 1986
13. Rao SD, Villanueva A, Mathews M, et al: *Histologic Evolution of Vitamin-D Depletion in Patients With Intestinal Malabsorption or Dietary Deficiency.* Amsterdam, Excerpta Medica, pp 224–226, 1983
14. Kragstrup J, Melsen F, Mosckilde L: Reduced wall thickness of completed remodeling sites in iliac trabecular bone following anticonvulsant therapy. *Metab Bone Dis Relat Res* 4:181–185, 1982

26. Molecular Diagnosis of Bone and Mineral Disorders

Robert F. Gagel, M.D., and Gilbert J. Cote, Ph.D.

Section of Endocrine Neoplasia and Hormonal Disorders, University of Texas M.D. Anderson Cancer Center, Houston, Texas

Discoveries during the past 5–10 years have greatly expanded our understanding of how genetic abnormalities cause bone and mineral disorders. Examples of such discoveries include the identification of mutations of type I collagen genes in osteogenesis imperfecta, vitamin D and estrogen receptor polymorphisms associated with osteoporosis, genes responsible for certain types of hereditary hypercalcemia, and point mutations of the *RET* proto-oncogene in multiple endocrine neoplasia type II (MEN II).

Diagnostic use of this type of information is very quickly making its way into clinical practice. For example, within 3 years of the description of point mutations in the *RET* proto-oncogene in MEN II, genetic testing for these mutations has replaced the pentagastrin stimulation test, the previous "gold standard" for diagnosing this condition (see Chapter 29). In the future, mutational analysis of the calcium receptor may be an important component in the differential diagnosis of hypercalcemia, especially in cases in which the diagnosis of hyperparathyroidism is equivocal (see Chapter 30). This rapid acquisition of new information and its application to disease management underscore the importance for clinicians in the bone and mineral field to acquire a fundamental knowledge of testing strategies and to understand the power and limitations of current approaches to genetic testing.

The single most important resource for up-to-date information related to specific genetic syndromes is provided by Online Mendelian Inheritance in Man (OMIM), available to all physicians without charge on the World Wide Web (details provided in Table 1). This concise but complete reference is an excellent starting point for genetic information relating to bone and mineral disorders and provides an intuitive, searchable textual data base that is updated on a regular basis. What follows is a description of the principles behind the most commonly used molecular genetic techniques and approaches.

POLYMERASE CHAIN REACTION (PCR)

A basic understanding of the principles underlying PCR is vital to molecular genetic diagnosis. The DNA used in

TABLE 1. *Summary of molecular defects in bone and mineral disorders*

Genetic disorder	Affected gene
Achondrogenesis-hypochondrogenesis	Collagen-2-a1
Achondroplasia	Fibroblast growth factor receptor 3
Albright osteodystrophy	Guanine nucleotide-binding alpha subunit-1
Apert syndrome	Fibroblast growth factor receptor 2
Crouzon syndrome	Fibroblast growth factor receptor 2
Ehlers-Danlos syndrome	Collagen-1-a2
Familial hypocalciuric hypercalcemia	Ca(2+)-sensing receptor 1 (PCAR 1)
Familial hypoparathyroidism	Parathyroid hormone
Hypophosphatasia	Alkaline phosphatase
Jackson-Weiss syndrome	Fibroblast growth factor receptor 2
Marfan syndrome	Fibrillin-1
McCune-Albright syndrome	Guanine nucleotide-binding alpha subunit-1
Metaphyseal chondrodysplasia, Murk-Jansen type	Parathyroid hormone receptor
Multiple endocrine neoplasia II	*RET* proto-oncogene
Osteogenesis imperfecta	Collagen-1-a2
Osteopetrosis	Carbonic anhydrase II
Otospondylomegaepiphyseal dysplasia	Collagen-11-a1
Pfeiffer syndrome	Fibroblast growth factor receptor 1 or 2
Pseudoachondroplasia	Cartilage oligomeric matrix protein (COMP)
Spondyloepiphyseal dysplasia	Collagen-2-a1
Stickler syndrome	Collagen-2-a1 or collagen-11-a1
Thanatophoric dysplasia	Fibroblast growth factor receptor 3
Vitamin D–resistant rickets, type IIA	Vitamin D receptor
Waardenburg syndrome	PAX3 or microphthalmia-associated transcription factor (MITF)
Williams syndrome	Elastin
X-linked hypophosphatemic rickets	X-linked endopeptidase

Information identifying the disorders and their respective affected genes was obtained by key word search of the Online Mendelian Inheritance in Man (OMIM), The Human Genome Data Base Project, Johns Hopkins University, Baltimore, Maryland. World Wide Web <URL:http://gdbwww.gdb.org/omim/docs/omimtop.html>, 1995.

diagnostic studies is most commonly extracted from peripheral white blood cells, and occasionally from other tissues. It is important, if possible, to obtain blood from an affected family member as well as the patient at risk. Occasionally, a DNA copy of mRNA from a specific tissue can be made by a technique called reverse transcription. The genomic DNA or the copy of the mRNA is used as a template for PCR, a method for amplification of a selected portion of a specific DNA sequence (1).

The specific portion of the gene of interest to be copied is targeted using small DNA fragments that are complementary to and flank the DNA sequence of interest (oligonucleotide primers). The addition of nucleotides and a thermostabile DNA polymerase, an enzyme that synthesizes new DNA, followed by heating and cooling through 20–30 cycles results in the formation of millions of copies of the targeted DNA (Fig. 1). Copies will be made of both parental alleles of the target DNA sequence (one derived from each parent). The sensitivity of the PCR reaction is so great that appropriate controls must be included in each amplification to exclude the possibility of DNA contamination. The amplified DNA serves as the starting material for all subsequent mutational analysis techniques.

GENERAL SCREENING TECHNIQUES TO DETECT MUTATIONS

There are many different strategies for identification of specific mutations. This summary will focus on the five most commonly used techniques and discuss the advantages and disadvantages of each (Fig. 2). Major factors for deciding which techniques to use include the size of the DNA sequence to be examined and the spectrum of mutations that cause the disease. For example, mutations affecting the collagen, type 1 alpha-1 gene in osteogenesis imperfecta (see Chapter 70) may affect any of the greater than 50 exons in the gene, and a broad screening approach (such as single-strand conformational polymorphism or denaturing gradient gel electrophoresis, discussed later) may provide the best approach to identify a mutation. Identification of a potential sequence abnormality would lead to the use of a more focused approach (such as DNA sequencing, restriction endonuclease analysis, or allele-specific hybridization).

The majority of the techniques for DNA analysis use gel electrophoresis. A sample containing the DNA molecules to be examined is applied to a gel (a thin layer of acrylamide or agarose), and an electrical current is applied to move the molecules along the long axis through the gel. Small differences in charge, size, or conformational state of an individual molecule can affect the mobility of the molecule (Fig. 2), making it possible to separate two pieces of DNA with as little as a single nucleotide difference.

Single-Strand Conformational Polymorphism (SSCP)

This technique relies on the theory that a denatured DNA molecule (one in which the two complementary strands of DNA that form the double helix are separated)

forms a unique single-stranded 3-dimensional structure (2). The major determinants of this structure are the specific DNA sequence and internal base pairing. A single nucleotide change may result in a conformation that differs from that of the normal sequence. In many genetic disorders, an affected individual will inherit one normal and one mutated copy of a gene, which can be detected by differences in DNA mobility on nondenaturing polyacrylamide gels (Fig. 2). This technique is particularly suited for analysis of large stretches of DNA sequence when the specific mutation is not known, such as the mutations described for osteogenesis imperfecta. DNA sequence analysis of the entire gene would be prohibitively expensive and time consuming. A disadvantage of SSCP is that it does not identify the specific mutation and generally cannot distinguish between mutations and nucleotide polymorphisms (a change in the DNA that does not alter the coding sequence of a protein). This technique cannot detect a mutation in which two copies of the mutated DNA (one from each parent) are inherited unless an external control from another patient is included in the analysis. More focused techniques, discussed later, are used to determine the nature of the DNA abnormality.

Denaturing Gradient Gel Electrophoresis (DGGE)

Like SSCP, this technique identifies mutations based on differences in DNA migration patterns (3). In this method, double-stranded DNA produced by PCR is applied to a gradient gel containing urea and formamide, which results in gradient-dependent denaturation (separation of the double helix into single strands) as gel electrophoresis proceeds. Separation of the DNA strands is responsible for altering the DNA mobility. DNA denaturation is sequence dependent. Therefore, a single nucleotide change will frequently generate a specific denaturation pattern. This effect is enhanced by the addition of "GC-clamps" or stretches of GCs to a single end of the PCR product to stimulate unidirectional DNA denaturation. This is a more complex technique, requiring a period of development for optimal results. The technique is, however, more sensitive than SSCP, more easily detects single base differences, and may be so specific that a characteristic electrophoretic pattern may be produced by a single base mutation. In most cases, however, the suspected mutation should be confirmed by a more specific technique.

SPECIFIC TECHNIQUES FOR DETECTION OF DNA SEQUENCE ABNORMALITIES

Direct DNA Sequencing

Direct DNA sequencing of PCR products is the most sensitive and specific method for detection of specific mutations (4). This technique is impractical to apply on a widespread basis, however, unless the region to be analyzed has been narrowed to several hundred to 1000 nucleotides. Direct DNA sequencing of a PCR product derived from genomic DNA permits analysis of both alleles or copies of the gene and the identification of new or

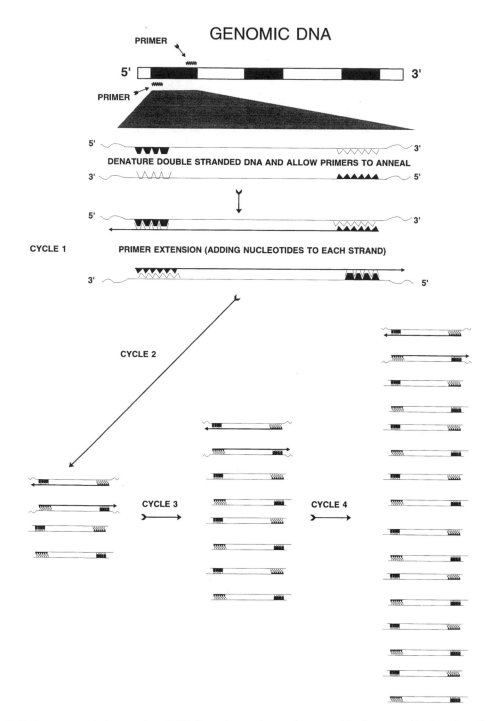

FIG. 1. Polymerase chain reaction. DNA from the patient to be tested is denatured by heating. Oligonucleotides, which complement a small sequence flanking the targeted piece of DNA, are added to the mixture. The oligonucleotides hybridize to the target DNA and serve as a template for extension of the DNA strand by a thermostabile polymerase. The DNA is again denatured by heating, followed by a new cycle of DNA synthesis (cycle 2). In subsequent cycles, there is a logarithmic increase in the number of copies of the targeted DNA. After 20–30 cycles, most of the DNA copies are of a single size.

unreported mutations. The disadvantages include its complexity and the difficulty of analyzing more than 200 nucleotides in a single sequencing reaction. In a disease such as multiple endocrine neoplasia type 2, in which more than 90% of known mutations are clustered in a small region of the *RET* proto-oncogene, this approach offers the

ability to detect most mutations in a single sequencing run (5).

One strategy used is to focus initially on the most common mutations and to extend sequencing to include other regions of the gene only in those individuals for whom the initial analysis does not identify a mutation.

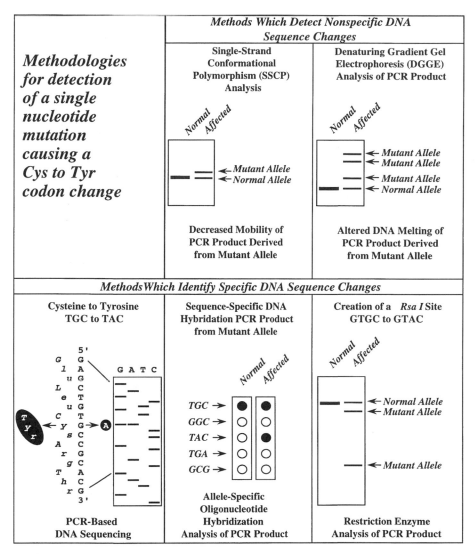

FIG. 2. Five different techniques for detecting a single nucleotide mutation. This figure schematically shows the results of five different methodologies to detect a single allele G to A DNA point mutation. The *upper panels* illustrate two nonspecific methods, single-strand conformational polymorphism analysis (SSCP) and denaturing gradient gel electrophoresis (DGGE). In the gel electrophoretic profiles of normal subjects, a single band (representing both parental alleles) is observed. In the sample from a patient with this mutation, two bands are noted in the SSCP analysis, one representing the normal and the other the mutant allele. The DGGE analysis of the patient sample with the mutation shows four bands. One band represents the denatured product of the normal allele, the other the mutated allele. The two additional mutant bands are formed as a result of double-stranded DNA composed of one normal strand and one mutant strand. In the *lower panels,* three additional methods are shown that identify specific DNA mutations. Direct DNA sequencing of the PCR product *(lower left panel)* shows the presence of two bands at the mutated codon (G and A, respectively), indicating that one allele (PCR product) contains the normal sequence and the other the mutated sequence. The *lower central panel* shows an allele-specific hybridization result. Five different oligonucleotides (using the DNA sequence shown in the *lower left panel*) containing the indicated mutations were dotted onto the filter. Hybridization of a PCR product from a patient with no mutation shows hybridization only to the oligonucleotide containing TGC, whereas the PCR product containing a normal and a mutated allele hybridizes to two different oligonucleotides. The G to A substitution creates an *Rsa*I restriction site. Addition of this endonuclease to the reaction mixture that contains the normal PCR product identifies only a single electrophoretic band *(lower right panel).* Addition of the same enzyme to a PCR product that contains one mutated allele results in the appearance of two new bands (indicated by mutant allele) as well as the band derived from the normal allele (normal allele).

Allele-Specific Hybridization

Short DNA sequences will hybridize (create a double-stranded piece of DNA by nucleotide pairing) most readily to a sequence with perfect complementarity (i.e., A's will hybridize best to T's, and G's to C's). In a disease caused by a single or finite number of nucleotide changes within a gene, it is possible to exploit complementarity to develop a detection system for a specific mutation (4).

There are several variations of this technique, but in its simplest form, oligonucleotides containing all possible disease-causing sequence changes are synthesized, dotted, and immobilized on a nylon membrane (Fig. 2). The complementary fragment of DNA from the patient is amplified by PCR and radiolabeled, and DNA/DNA hybridization is performed using conditions in which only a perfectly matched DNA sequence will hybridize. Only those DNA molecules from the patient that contain the mutant sequence will hybridize to the synthetic oligonucleotide. This method is rapid, technically easy to perform, and permits rapid analysis of large numbers of samples. The major drawback is its inability to detect mutations beyond those included in the dotted oligonucleotides, making it almost certain that a new or previously unidentified mutation will not be detected. This technique is best used for rapid screening of a family whose specific mutation is already known.

Restriction Endonuclease Analysis

This provides a simple and effective method for detecting the presence or absence of mutations at a single site and is useful when a mutation creates or destroys a restriction site. For example, a single nucleotide change in the sequence GTGC to GTAC would create a new restriction site for the endonuclease *Rsa*I. A PCR amplification product from a patient who inherited this mutation from a single parent would contain one normal DNA sequence and one containing the single nucleotide mutation. Addition of the restriction enzyme *Rsa*I to a PCR product from this patient would result in cleavage of the allele containing the mutant sequence into two fragments, whereas the allele containing the normal sequence would remain uncleaved. Separation of these fragments by gel electrophoresis (Fig. 2) would show one uncut fragment representing the normal sequence and two smaller fragments representing the cleaved mutant allele. Mutations that destroy an existing restriction site provide an additional analytic challenge because it is necessary to document that the enzyme is active before concluding that the failure to cleave the DNA fragment into two pieces is caused by a mutation. To establish the activity of the enzyme, a positive control (a piece of DNA that contains the normal restriction site) is included with each analysis. This technique is used most effectively when a single DNA sequence change causes all examples of the disease or in a family whose specific mutation is known.

SOURCES OF ERROR IN GENETIC TESTING

It is important that clinicians be aware of the frequency and nature of genetic testing errors (6). Sample mixup, espe-cially in the setting of family screening where many family members share a common last name, may occur in up to 5% of analyses. These errors may occur at the time of blood drawing or during subsequent analysis or recording. A second potential source of error is contamination by DNA from individuals who harbor a disease causing mutation. The funneling of large numbers of samples to a few laboratories for analysis of a single disease further increases the chance of contamination. The extreme sensitivity of PCR analysis makes it possible that a positive result could occur as a result of airborne contamination of a reaction tube. A third source of error is the failure to amplify both alleles, thereby resulting in the possibility of a false-negative result because only the normal allele is included in the analysis. The most common explanation for amplification failure is a random polymorphism (DNA sequence change) acting to reduce oligonucleotide primer hybridization during the PCR reaction.

If genetic testing is to be used as the sole determinant for decision making in disease management, it is important for the clinician to be aware of the possibility of errors and to take steps to minimize their impact on patient care. One simple approach that will eliminate the majority of these errors is to repeat each analysis, whether positive or negative, in a different laboratory on an independently obtained sample. This approach will identify most sample mixup, DNA contamination, and technical errors. Sending the sample to a separate laboratory that uses a different primer set for PCR amplification will also reduce the likelihood of a single allele amplification error.

INTEGRATION OF GENETIC INFORMATION INTO CLINICAL MANAGEMENT

Genetic testing has several important clinical uses. Identification of a specific disease-causing mutation may clarify and simplify patient management. For example, the identification of a mutation of the calcium receptor causative for familial hypercalcemic hypocalciuria (see Chapter 30) in an individual with an atypical clinical presentation may prevent unnecessary parathyroid surgery. In other situations, such as multiple endocrine neoplasia type II (see Chapter 29), the identification of a specific mutation may lead to a specific action (thyroidectomy) in a child (6).

In other situations, the benefits of genetic screening may be more ambiguous. The identification of a mutation in an individual with a severe and fatal form of osteogenesis imperfecta may not alter therapy for the patient; however, detection of the mutation may make prenatal genetic screening possible. Identification and categorization of these mutations are also important because gene therapy strategies, especially for single gene defects, are evolving rapidly. Table 1 provides a current summary of gene defects that cause bone and mineral diseases in humans.

An evolving area of genetic research implicates subtle DNA differences in the pathogenesis of disease. For example, reports now implicate vitamin D (7) and estrogen receptor polymorphisms (8) in the causation of osteoporosis. Although the role of these polymorphisms is currently controversial, there are examples in other systems that clearly point to population-based genetic differences that may influence disease expression. The techniques for identification of these polymorphisms are similar to those described for restriction analysis of a PCR product described in Fig. 2. Further characterization and clarification of the roles that these genetic polymorphisms play in disease genesis may permit us to identify high-risk populations for application of preventive strategies.

REFERENCES

1. Saiki RK, Gelfand DH, Stoffel S, et al: Primer-directed enzymatic amplification of DNA with a thermostable DNA polymerase. *Science* 239:487–491, 1988
2. Ainsworth PJ, Surh LC, Coulter-Mackie MB: Diagnostic single-strand conformational polymorphism (SSCP): A simplified non-radioisotopic method as applied to a Tay-Sachs B1 variant. *Nucleic Acids Res* 19:405–406, 1991
3. Fodde R, Losekoot M: Mutation detection by denaturing gradient gel electrophoresis (DGGE). *Hum Mutat* 3:83–94, 1994
4. Cotton RG: Current methods of mutation detection. *Mutat Res* 285:125–144, 1993
5. Khorana S, Gagel RF, Cote GJ: Direct sequencing of PCR products in agarose gel slices. *Nucleic Acids Res* 22:3425–3426, 1994
6. Cote GJ, Wohllk N, Evans D, Goepfert H, Gagel RF: RET proto-oncogene mutations in multiple endocrine neoplasia type 2 and medullary thyroid carcinoma. *Baillieres Clin Endocrinol Metab* 9:609–630, 1995
7. Morrison NA, Qi JC, Tokita A, Kelly PJ,Crofts L, Nguyen TV, Sambrook PN, Eisman JA: Prediction of bone density from vitamin D receptor alleles. *Nature* 367:284–287, 1994
8. Qi JC, Morrison NA, Nguyen CP, et al: Estrogen receptor genotypes and bone mineral density in women and men (abstract). *J Bone Miner Res* 10:S170, 1995

SECTION IV

Disorders of Serum Minerals

27. Hypercalcemia: Pathogenesis, Clinical Manifestations, Differential Diagnosis, and Management

Elizabeth Shane, M.D.

Department of Medicine, Columbia University, College of Physicians and Surgeons, New York, New York

The clinical presentation of hypercalcemia varies from a mild, asymptomatic, biochemical abnormality detected during routine screening, to a life-threatening medical emergency. In this chapter, pathogenesis, clinical manifestations, differential diagnosis, and management of hypercalcemia will be discussed.

PATHOGENESIS

The concentration of calcium in the extracellular fluid is critical for many physiologic processes. Under normal circumstances, the range is remarkably constant, between 8.5 to 10.5 mg/dl (2.1 to 2.5 mM). The exact normal range varies slightly, depending on the laboratory. Approximately half the total serum calcium is bound to plasma proteins, primarily albumin. A small component of the total calcium is complexed to anions such as citrate or sulfate. The remaining half circulates as the free calcium ion. It is only this ionized portion of the total serum calcium that is physiologically important, regulating neuromuscular contractility, the process of coagulation, and a variety of other cellular activities.

In a variety of chronic illnesses, a substantial reduction in the serum albumin concentration may lower the total serum calcium concentration, whereas ionized calcium concentrations remain normal. A simple correction for hypoalbuminemia may be made by adding 0.8 mg/dl to the total serum calcium concentration for every 1.0 g/dl by which the serum albumin concentration is lower than 4.0 g/dl. Thus, a patient with a total serum calcium of 10.5 mg/dl and a serum albumin level of 2.0 g/dl has a corrected total serum calcium of 12.1 mg/dl. Conversely, falsely elevated serum calcium levels may be observed, usually the result of an elevation of the serum albumin due to dehydration or hemoconcentration during venipuncture. A similar maneuver can be performed to correct the serum calcium in this situation, except that the correction factor must be subtracted from the serum calcium level.

In contrast to changes in the serum albumin concentration, which affect the total but not the ionized calcium level, alterations in pH affect the ionized but not the total calcium concentration. Acidosis increases the ionized calcium by decreasing the binding of calcium ions to albumin, whereas alkalosis decreases the ionized calcium by enhancing binding of calcium ions to albumin. Measurement of total serum calcium is usually adequate for most situations, but in complex cases (changes in both albumin and pH) a direct measurement of the ionized calcium should be performed.

Under normal circumstances, the plasma calcium concentration reflects a balance between the flux of calcium into the extracellular fluid from the gastrointestinal (GI) tract, the skeleton, and the kidney, and the flux of calcium out of the extracellular fluid into the skeleton and the urine. Hypercalcemia develops when the rate of calcium entry into the blood compartment is greater than its rate of removal. This occurs most commonly when accelerated osteoclastic bone resorption, or, less frequently, excessive GI calcium absorption, delivers quantities of calcium into the blood that exceed the capacities of the kidney to eliminate it and of the skeleton to reclaim it. Less commonly, normal rates of calcium entry into the extracellular fluid may result in hypercalcemia if the process of renal excretion or that of bone mineralization is impaired.

Accelerated bone resorption by osteoclasts, multinucleated bone-resorbing cells, is the primary pathogenetic mechanism in most instances of hypercalcemia (1). Osteoclasts may be stimulated to resorb bone by parathyroid hormone (PTH), PTH-related protein (PTHrP), and 1,25-dihydroxyvitamin D, all of which have been shown to cause hypercalcemia (2,3). A number of cytokines (interleukin-1α, interleukin-1β, tumor necrosis factor, lymphotoxin, and transforming growth factor-α) also stimulate osteoclastic bone resorption, but their ability to cause hypercalcemia in human disease has not been definitively established (4). Excessive GI absorption of calcium is a much less common cause of hypercalcemia, although it may play a role in hypercalcemic states characterized by excess vitamin D, such as lymphoma or vitamin D intoxication. Whether the primary cause of the hypercalcemia is accelerated bone resorption or excessive GI tract absorption of calcium, the kidney is the primary defender against a rise in the serum calcium. Thus, hypercalcemia is usually preceded by hypercalciuria, and it is only when the capacity of the kidney to excrete calcium has been exceeded that the patient becomes hypercalcemic (5).

Several other factors may contribute to the pathogenesis of hypercalcemia. In addition to stimulating osteoclast-mediated bone resorption, both PTH and PTHrP also increase reabsorption of calcium from the distal tubule, thus interfering with the ability of the kidneys to clear the filtered calcium load. Hypercalcemia interferes with the action of antidiuretic hormone on the distal tubule, causing a form of nephrogenic diabetes insipidus that results in polyuria. The thirst mechanism may not be fully operative because of the nausea and vomiting that frequently accompany hypercalcemia; thus urinary fluid losses may not be replaced, and dehydration may ensue. The resulting reduction in the extracellular fluid volume and associated reduction in the glomerular filtration rate exacerbate the hypercalcemia. Finally, immobilization may also contribute to hypercalcemia.

CLINICAL MANIFESTATIONS

The clinical presentation of the hypercalcemic patient (6) may involve several organ systems. The signs and symptoms tend to be similar regardless of the etiology of the hypercalcemia. Because an optimal extracellular calcium concentration is necessary for normal neurologic function, symptoms of neurologic dysfunction often predominate in hypercalcemic states. The patient (or family members) may notice subtle changes in the ability to concentrate or an increased sleep requirement. With increasing severity of the hypercalcemia, symptoms may gradually progress to depression, confusion, and even coma. Muscle weakness is common.

Gastrointestinal symptoms are often prominent, with constipation, anorexia, nausea, and vomiting present in varying degrees. Pancreatitis and peptic ulcer disease are unusual but have been reported. They may be somewhat more common if the hypercalcemia is due to primary hyperparathyroidism than to other causes of hypercalcemia.

Polyuria, resulting from the impaired concentrating ability of the distal nephron, is common, particularly during the early phases. Polydipsia is also usually present. The combination of polyuria and diminished fluid intake due to GI symptoms may lead to severe dehydration. Nephrolithiasis occurs in patients with primary hyperparathyroidism (15% to 20% in recent series), but along with nephrocalcinosis, it may also develop in patients with hypercalcemia due to other causes, particularly when the hypercalcemia is chronic.

Hypercalcemia increases the rate of cardiac repolarization. Thus shortening of the Q-T interval is observed commonly on the electrocardiogram. Bradycardia and first degree atrioventricular block, as well as other arrhythmias, may occur. Caution should be exercised when treating the hypercalcemic patient with digitalis, because increased sensitivity to this drug has been observed.

In general, the presence or absence of symptoms correlates with the degree of elevation of the serum calcium and with the rapidity of its rise. Most patients do not begin to show clinical features of hypercalcemia until the total calcium concentration exceeds 12 mg/dl, and patients are almost invariably symptomatic at levels above 14 mg/dl. However, there is much individual variation in this regard. Certain patients will be quite symptomatic with moderate hypercalcemia of 12.0 to 14.0 mg/dl, whereas others may show no overt symptomatology at a similar level. The latter situation occurs most often in the setting of chronic hypercalcemia. In other circumstances, the absence of symptoms in the severely hypercalcemic patient should prompt one to measure the ionized calcium level in order to be certain that hypercalcemia is not secondary to excessive binding of calcium to plasma proteins (Chapter 36).

DIFFERENTIAL DIAGNOSIS

Detection of an elevated serum calcium requires that the etiology be established. The many causes of hypercalcemia are listed in Table 1, and most will be covered separately in subsequent chapters. However, certain general principles that apply to the differential diagnosis of hypercalcemia are covered here.

Malignancy and primary hyperparathyroidism are by far the most common causes of hypercalcemia, accounting for more than 90% of hypercalcemic patients (6). Differentiating between these two diagnoses is generally not difficult on clinical grounds alone. The vast majority of patients with primary hyperparathyroidism have relatively mild hypercalcemia, within 1.0 mg/dl above the upper limits of normal and usually less than 12.0 mg/dl. They are often asymptomatic. Review of past medical records may reveal that the hypercalcemia has been present for months to years. When symptoms of hypercalcemia are present, they tend to be chronic, such as nephrolithiasis. In contrast, patients with hypercalcemia of malignancy are usually ill and are more likely to manifest the classic signs and symptoms of an elevated serum calcium. In general, the malignancy itself is readily apparent and presents little diagnostic challenge to the physician. Less commonly, occult malignancy may present with hypercalcemia, or the patient with primary hyperparathyroidism may present with moderate to severe elevation of the serum calcium that is associated with symptoms or with the acute onset of severe hypercalcemia (parathyroid crisis). Such cases pose a greater diagnostic problem.

The availability of reliable assays for intact PTH based upon double antibody techniques (two-site, immunoradiometric, or immunochemiluminescent assays) has been of great diagnostic value in the evaluation of the hypercalcemic patient. The majority of patients with primary hyperparathyroidism have intact PTH levels that are frankly elevated. Patients with hypercalcemia of malignancy virtually always demonstrate suppressed or undetectable levels of intact PTH. It is distinctly unusual for a patient with malignancy (excepting parathyroid cancer) to show elevated levels of PTH. When this occurs, two possibilities exist: the patient may have concomitant primary hyperparathyroidism, or the malignancy itself may be secreting PTH, an uncommon event.

In most patients with malignancy-associated hypercalcemia, the hypercalcemia is a reult of secretion of PTHrP by the tumor (2). Commercial assays for PTHrP are now available; when they show elevated calcium levels, they can prove helpful in the diagnosis of hypercalcemia of malignancy. However, a negative result does not exclude malignancy, particularly because certain tumors cause hypercalcemia by mechanisms independent of PTHrP, such as secretion of other bone resorbing cytokines, or extrarenal conversion of 25-hydroxyvitamin D to 1,25-dihydroxyvitamin D. Local bone-resorbing effects of tumors such as breast cancer also may be involved.

Hypercalcemia from causes other than malignancy or primary hyperparathyroidism may also occur. A thorough history and physical examination are invaluable in arriving at the correct diagnosis. Each of the etiologies listed in Table 1 is covered in one of the other chapters in this section.

MANAGEMENT

The decision to institute therapy for the hypercalcemic patient depends on the level of the serum calcium, and the

TABLE 1. *Differential diagnosis of hypercalcemia*

Most common
  Primary hyperparathyroidism
  Malignant disease
    Parathyroid hormone-related protein (carcinoma of lung, esophagus, head and neck, renal cell, ovary, and bladder)
    Ectopic production of 1,25-dihydroxyvitamin D (lymphoma)
    Lytic bone metastases (multiple myeloma and breast carcinoma)
    Other factor(s) produced locally or ectopically
Uncommon
  Endocrine disorders
    Thyrotoxicosis
  Granulomatous diseases
    Sarcoidosis
  Drug-induced
    Vitamin D
    Thiazide diuretics
    Lithium
    Estrogens and antiestrogens
    Androgens (breast cancer therapy)
    Aminophylline
    Vitamin A
    Aluminum intoxication (in chronic renal failure)
  Miscellaneous
    Immobilization
    Renal failure (acute and chronic)
    Total parenteral nutrition
Rare
  Endocrine disorders
  Pheochromocytoma
  Vasoactive intestinal polypeptide–producing tumor
  Familial hypocalciuric hypercalcemia
    Granulomatous diseases
      Tuberculosis
      Histoplasmosis
      Coccidioidomycosis
      Leprosy
  Miscellaneous
    Milk-alkali syndrome
    Hypophosphatasia

presence or absence of clinical manifestations of an elevated serum calcium. In general, patients with mild hypercalcemia (less than 12.0 mg/dl) do not have symptoms of hypercalcemia and do not derive significant clinical benefit from normalization of their serum calcium. Thus, immediate intervention is not usually necessary. In contrast, when the serum calcium is greater than 14.0 mg/dl, therapy should be initiated regardless of whether the patient has signs or symptoms of hypercalcemia. Moderate elevation of the serum calcium (12.0 to 14.0 mg/dl) should be treated aggressively if the patient demonstrates clinical signs or symptoms consistent with hypercalcemia. However, if such a patient is asymptomatic, a more conservative approach may be appropriate. It is also important to consider the underlying cause of the hypercalcemia when deciding whether therapy is necessary and the type of therapy to institute. For example, a patient with acute primary hyperparathyroidism, a completely curable condition, would warrant more aggressive treatment than a patient with diffuse metastatic cancer and a

poor prognosis. Another difficult situation arises in the patient whose serum calcium is about 12.0 mg/dl, not within the range one would usually treat aggressively, yet who has an altered mental status or other symptoms that could conceivably be ascribed to a hypercalcemic state. In such situations, it is important to consider other potential causes for the symptoms before instituting therapy.

The management of hypercalcemia is outlined in Table 2. When the serum calcium exceeds 12.0 mg/dl and signs and symptoms are present, a series of general measures should be instituted. Most of these therapeutic maneuvers tend to lower serum calcium by increasing urinary calcium excretion (7,8). Dehydration, resulting from the pathophysiologic events induced by the hypercalcemia (anorexia, nausea, vomiting, defective urinary concentrating mechanism, and polyuria) is very common. Hydration with normal saline, to correct the extracellular fluid deficit, is central to the early management of hypercalcemia from any cause. Restoration of the volume deficit can usually be achieved by the continuous infusion of 3 to 4 L of 0.9% sodium chloride over a 24- to 48-hr period. This maneuver generally lowers the serum calcium by 1.0 to 3.0 mg/dl. Hydration with saline enhances urinary calcium excretion by increasing glomerular filtration of calcium and decreasing both proximal and distal tubular reabsorption of sodium and calcium. However, saline hydration alone does not usually establish normocalcemia unless the calcium concentration is only modestly elevated. Moreover, this form of therapy must be used with caution in elderly patients or in others with compromised cardiovascular or renal function.

Under certain circumstances a loop diuretic, such as furosemide or ethacrynic acid, may be added to saline hydration in the therapy of hypercalcemia. Loop diuretics act on the thick ascending loop of Henle to inhibit both sodium and calcium reabsorption. Thus the use of such agents enhances urinary calcium losses, increases the likelihood of normalization of the serum calcium level, and mitigates the dangers of hypernatremia and volume overload that may accompany the use of intravenous saline. Only after extracellular fluid volume has been replenished should small doses of furosemide (10 to 20 mg) be administered as necessary to control clinical manifestations of volume excess. Overzealous use of loop diuretics before intravascular volume has been restored can

TABLE 2. *Management of hypercalcemia*

General
  Hydration
  Saline diuresis
  Loop diuretics
  Dialysis
  Mobilization
Specific
  Bisphosphonates
    Pamidronate
    Etidronate
    Clodronate
  Plicamycin (mithramycin)
  Calcitonin
  Gallium nitrate
  Therapy of underlying causes

worsen hypercalcemia by exacerbating volume depletion. Hypokalemia and other electrolyte abnormalities can ensue. Intensive therapy with large doses of furosemide (80 to 100 mg every 1 to 2 hours) and replacement of fluid and electrolytes based on measured urinary losses is rarely indicated. It must be emphasized that thiazide diuretics are contraindicated in this setting because they decrease renal calcium excretion and may worsen hypercalcemia.

Dialysis, another general measure, is usually reserved for the severely hypercalcemic patient. Peritoneal dialysis or hemodialysis with a low or zero calcium dialysate will lower serum calcium rapidly in those patients who are refractory to other measures or who have renal insufficiency. Finally, the patient should be mobilized as soon as clinically feasible to minimize the negative calcium balance that accompanies immobilization.

Specific approaches to the hypercalcemic patient are based on the underlying pathophysiology. Excessive mobilization of calcium from the skeleton resulting from an accelerated rate of bone resorption is the most common and important factor in the pathogenesis of hypercalcemia in the majority of patients. Numerous pharmacologic agents are available now that specifically block osteoclast-mediated bone resorption and effectively lower serum calcium in most hypercalcemic patients (Table 2).

Plicamycin, previously called mithramycin, is a cytotoxic antibiotic that blocks RNA synthesis in osteoclasts and therefore inhibits bone resorption. When administered intravenously in a dose of 15 to 25 µg/kg over a period of 4 to 6 hours, plicamycin effectively lowers elevated calcium levels in most patients. The serum calcium usually begins to decline within 12 hours of administration and generally reaches its nadir within 48 to 72 hours. Often a single dose may be sufficient to achieve normocalcemia. However, if necessary, the dose may be repeated several times at 24- to 48-hr intervals. The duration of the normocalcemia depends on the intensity of underlying bone resorption and may vary from days to weeks. Administration is commonly associated with nausea, which may be minimized by slow infusion rates. Plicamycin has considerable toxicity (bone marrow, renal, hepatic); it may be associated with transient elevation of transaminases and/or serum creatinine, with proteinuria, and with thrombocytopenia, particularly when repeated administrations (more than three or four) are required. These toxicities make this drug of limited usefulness in the setting of chronic hypercalcemia. Although bisphosphonates are replacing plicamycin as a less toxic first-line therapy in the severely hypercalcemic patient, when serum calcium requires rapid correction, plicamycin remains a reasonable choice.

Inorganic pyrophosphates are naturally occurring inhibitors of bone resorption. Bisphosphonates are analogs of pyrophosphate that are resistant to phosphatases. These drugs are bone-seeking compounds that bind to hydroxyapatite and prevent its dissolution. Osteoclast function is impaired after exposure to bisphosphonates, and these drugs have enjoyed increasing use in disorders characterized by excessive bone resorption. Gastrointestinal absorption of bisphosphonates is very poor, and therefore intravenous administration is usually necessary when they are used to treat hypercalcemia. Bisphosphonates should be administered in large volumes (>500 ml) over 4 hours to prevent nephrotoxity due to precipitation of calcium bisphosphonate. Two bisphosphonates, pamidronate and etidronate, are currently approved for use in the United States. Another effective bisphosphonate, clodronate, is widely available in Europe and the United Kingdom but is unavailable in the United States. A new generation of more potent bisphosphonates, including alendronate, risedronate, and aminobutane bisphosphonate, are currently under investigation.

Etidronate, a first-generation bisphosphonate, is administered by intravenous infusion at a daily dose of 7.5 mg/kg over 2 to 4 hours. Generally, the serum calcium begins to decline during the second day of therapy and reaches its nadir by the 7th day. If the serum calcium falls to near normal levels or into the normal range before completion of 3 days of therapy, the standard approved duration of therapy, the drug should be withheld. Etidronate, when administered intravenously at a dose of 7.5 mg/kg/day for 3 days, normalizes serum calcium in 30% to 40% of patients (9). Administration of the drug for up to 7 days (10) [either consecutive or interrupted] or as a single 24-hr infusion at a dose of 20 to 25 mg/kg (11) is more efficacious, but these approaches are not "officially" approved. Intravenous etidronate is safe and well tolerated. The oral use of etidronate to prevent recurrent hypercalcemia is of limited effectiveness and may be complicated by osteomalacia when administered in large doses (25 mg/kg) chronically.

Pamidronate is a potent bisphosphonate that is more effective than etidronate and comparable to plicamycin for the treatment of hypercalcemia. Although a variety of regimens have been reported, the recommended dose is 30 to 60 mg intravenously as a single infusion. When compared to 3 days of etidronate therapy (7.5 mg/kg), a single infusion of 60 mg of pamidronate has a more rapid onset of action and results in a greater decline in serum calcium and a longer duration of effect (9). Pamidronate may cause transient fever (20% of patients) and myalgias during the day following the infusion. Pretreatment with acetaminophen ameliorates these side effects in the majority of patients. Occasionally, transient leukopenia may develop. Mild, usually asymptomatic, hypocalcemia (10%) and hypophosphatemia (10% to 30%) may occur in some patients. At a dose of 90 mg, infusion reactions have been observed. Both pamidronate and clodronate have been reported to reduce the progression of skeletal metastases and prevent the onset of hypercalcemia in patients with breast cancer (9). The duration of the hypocalcemic effect of both etidronate and pamidronate is variable, ranging from several days to several weeks.

Calcitonin is a polypeptide hormone that is secreted by the parafollicular C-cells of the thyroid gland. Salmon calcitonin is the most potent and frequently used form of the drug. Calcitonin inhibits osteoclastic bone resorption, increases urinary calcium excretion, and is a very safe drug. Moreover, calcitonin has the most rapid onset of action of the available calcium-lowering drugs, causing the serum calcium to fall within 2 to 6 hours of administration. The usual dose ranges from 4 to 8 U/kg administered by intramuscular or subcutaneous injection every 6 to 8 hours. Unfortunately, the hypocalcemic effect of calcitonin is transient, not as pronounced as either plicamycin or the bisphosphonates, and rarely normalizes the serum calcium. The serum calcium concentration usually declines by a mean of

2 mg/dl and may begin to rise again within 24 hours, despite continued therapy. Calcitonin given in combination with bisphosphonates or plicamycin appears to achieve a more rapid and greater decrease in the serum calcium than when either drug is administered by itself. Used in this way, calcitonin has a role at the outset of therapy in severe instances of hypercalcemia, when it is desirable to lower the serum calcium more rapidly than can be accomplished with either plicamycin or a bisphosphonate alone (7).

Gallium nitrate, originally studied as a therapeutic agent for cancer, is also approved by the Food and Drug Administration for the therapy of hypercalcemia. Although its precise mechanism of action is uncertain, it appears to adsorb to hydroxyapatite crystals (1) and may inhibit bone resorption by reducing crystal solubility. A direct inhibitory effect upon the osteoclast has also been observed (12). When administered as a continuous 5-day infusion at a dose of 200 $mg/m^2/day$, it has been reported to normalize the serum calcium in a majority of patients. The rate of fall of the serum calcium was rather slow, in that a normal level was not reached until the end of the 5-day infusion, and the nadir was not achieved until 3 days later. Gallium nitrate causes elevation of the serum creatinine that may be potentiated by volume depletion and concomitant administration of other nephrotoxic drugs. Its use is contraindicated in renal insufficiency (i.e., serum creatinine greater than 2.5 mg/dl) and when other nephrotoxic agents are being used. It may also be associated with reduction in the serum phosphate and hemoglobin concentration. For these reasons, it is not the ideal agent for therapy of hypercalcemia.

Glucocorticoid therapy has been used for many years to treat hypercalcemia, particularly when due to hematologic malignancies such as lymphoma and multiple myeloma. Glucocorticoids are also effective in situations such as vitamin D toxicity or granulomatous diseases in which the hypercalcemia is mediated by the actions of 1,25-dihydroxyvitamin D. Glucocorticoids are seldom effective in patients with solid tumors or primary hyperparathyroidism. The usual dose is 200 to 300 mg of intravenous hydrocortisone, or its equivalent, daily for 3 to 5 days.

Intravenous phosphate was used in the past to lower serum calcium in hypercalcemic patients. However, intravenous phosphate is accompanied by a substantial risk of precipitation of calcium-phosphate complexes, leading to severe organ damage and even death. This form of therapy should rarely be necessary today and is not recommended.

Therapy for the underlying cause of the hypercalcemia should not be neglected, because specific therapy may be the most effective approach to the problem. However, patients with widespread metastatic disease, in whom no further specific antitumor chemotherapy is to be given, may be approached with the realization that reduction of the serum calcium per se will achieve little in the long run. In these circumstances, sometimes the best approach is to resist specific measures to reduce the serum calcium and to make the patient as comfortable as possible.

REFERENCES

1. Attie MF: Treatment of hypercalcemia. *Endocrinol Metab Clin North Am* 18:807–828, 1989
2. Halloran BP, Nissenson BA (eds): *Parathyroid Hormone-Related Protein: Normal Physiology and Its Role in Cancer.* CRC Press, Boca Raton, Florida, 1992
3. Adams JS, Fernandez M, Gacad MA, et al.: Vitamin-D metabolite-mediated hypercalcemia and hypercalciuria in patients with AIDS and non-AIDS associated lymphoma. *Blood* 73:235–239, 1989
4. Mundy GR: Hypercalcemic factors other than parathyroid hormone-related protein. *Endocrinol Metab Clin North Am* 18:795–805, 1989
5. Harinck HIJ, Bijvoet OLM, Plantingh AST, et al.: Role of bone and kidney in tumor-induced hypercalcemia and its treatment with bisphosphonate and sodium chloride. *Am J Med* 82:1133–1142, 1987
6. Bilezikian JP, Singer FR: Acute management of hypercalcemia due to parathyroid hormone and parathyroid hormone-related protein. In: Bilezikian JP, Marcus R, Levine MA (eds) *The Parathyroids.* Raven Press, New York, 1994
7. Bilezikian JP: Management of acute hypercalcemia. *N Engl J Med* 326:1196–1203, 1992
8. Grill V, Murray RML, Ho PWM, et al.: Circulating PTH and PTHrP levels before and after treatment of tumor induced hypercalcemia with pamidronate disodium (APD). *J Clin Endocrinol Metab* 74:1468–1470, 1990
9. Nussbaum SR: Pathophysiology and management of severe hypercalcemia. *Endocrinol Metab Clin North Am* 22:343–362, 1993
10. Jacobs TP, Gordon AC, Silverberg SJ, et al.: Neoplastic hypercalcemia: Physiologic response to intravenous etidronate disodium. *Am J Med* 82(suppl 2A):42–50, 1987
11. Flores JF, Singer FR, Rude RK: Twenty-four hour infusion of etidronate for hypercalcemia of malignancy. *Miner Elect Metab* 17:390–395, 1991
12. Hall TJ, Chambers TJ: Gallium inhibits bone resorption by a direct action on osteoclasts. *Bone Miner* 8:211–216, 1990

28. Primary Hyperparathyroidism

John P. Bilezikian, M.D.

Department of Medicine, Columbia University, College of Physicians and Surgeons, New York, New York

Primary hyperparathyroidism is one of the two most common causes of hypercalcemia and thus ranks high as a key diagnostic possibility in anyone with an elevated serum calcium concentration. The other most common cause of hypercalcemia is malignant disease. These two causes, primary hyperparathyroidism and hypercalcemia of malignancy, account for over 90% of all patients with hypercalcemia. A much longer, complete list of potential causes of hypercalcemia is considered after the first two are ruled out, or if there is reason to believe that a different cause is likely. The differential diagnosis of hypercalcemia as well as features of hypercalcemia of malignancy are considered elsewhere in this primer. In this chapter, the clinical presentation, evaluation, and therapy of primary hyperparathyroidism are covered.

Primary hyperparathyroidism is a relatively common endocrine disease with an incidence as high as 1 in 500 to 1 in 1000 (1). Among the endocrine diseases, perhaps only diabetes mellitus and hyperthyroidism are seen more frequently. The high visibility of primary hyperparathyroidism in the population today marks a dramatic change from several generations ago, when it was considered to be a rare disorder. The four- to fivefold increase in incidence since the early 1970s is primarily because of the widespread use of the autoanalyzer, which gratuitously provides serum calcium determinations when the test is ordered for other reasons (2). Thus, hypercalcemia is typically discovered when the patient is being evaluated for a set of complaints completely unrelated to hypercalcemia. Primary hyperparathyroidism occurs at all ages but is most frequent in the sixth decade of life. Women are affected more often than men by a ratio of 3:1. The majority of individuals are postmenopausal women. When found in children, an unusual event, it might be a component of one of several endocrinopathies with a genetic basis, such as multiple endocrine neoplasia type I or II (Chapter 29).

Primary hyperparathyroidism is a hypercalcemic state resulting from excessive secretion of parathyroid hormone from one or more parathyroid glands. The disease is caused by a benign, solitary adenoma 80% of the time. A parathyroid adenoma is a collection of chief cells surrounded by a rim of normal tissue at the outer perimeter of the gland. In the patient with a parathyroid adenoma, the remaining three parathyroid glands are normal. Less commonly, primary hyperparathyroidism is caused by a pathologic process characterized by hyperplasia of all four parathyroid glands. Four-gland parathyroid hyperplasia is seen in 15% to 20% of patients with primary hyperparathyroidism. It may occur sporadically or in association with multiple endocrine neoplasia, type I or II (Chapter 29). A very rare presentation of primary hyperparathyroidism is parathyroid carcinoma, occurring in fewer than 0.5% of patients with hyperparathyroidism (3). Pathologic examination of the malignant tissue might show mitoses, vascular invasion, and fibrous trabeculae, but it is often not definitive. Unless gross local or distant metastases are present, the diagnosis of parathyroid cancer can be exceedingly difficult to make.

The pathophysiology of primary hyperparathyroidism relates to the loss of normal feedback control of parathyroid hormone by extracellular calcium. Under virtually all other hypercalcemic conditions, the parathyroid gland is suppressed and parathyroid hormone levels are low. Why the parathyroid cell loses its normal sensitivity to calcium is unknown, but in adenomas this appears to be the major mechanism. In primary hyperparathyroidism due to hyperplasia of the parathyroid glands, the "set point" for calcium is not changed for a given parathyroid cell: it is the increase in the number of cells that gives rise to the hypercalcemia.

The underlying cause of primary hyperparathyroidism is not known. External neck irradiation in childhood, recognized in some patients, is unlikely to be causative in the majority of patients. The clonal origin of most parathyroid adenomas suggests a defect at the level of the gene control-

ling growth of the parathyroid cell or the expression of parathyroid hormone. Patients with primary hyperparathyroidism have been discovered in whom the parathyroid hormone gene is rearranged to a site adjacent to the *PRAD*-1 oncogene (4). This kind of gene rearrangement could be responsible for the altered growth properties of the abnormal parathyroid cell. Loss of one copy of a tumor suppressor gene located on chromosome 11 has also been seen in some parathyroid adenomas, but it seems to occur much more commonly in the multiple endocrine neoplasia syndrome, type I, than in sporadic primary hyperparathyroidism (5). Abnormalities in the p53 tumor suppressor gene have not been described in primary hyperparathyroidism (6). Finally, the recent discovery of the calcium-sensing receptor gene (7) and its role in the pathogenesis of familial hypocalciuric hypercalcemia (8) has led to attempts to implicate this gene in primary hyperparathyroidism. Recent studies, however, have not supported this concept (9–10). Thus, the molecular basis for primary hyperparathyroidism continues to be elusive.

SIGNS AND SYMPTOMS

Primary hyperparathyroidism is associated classically with skeletal and renal complications. At skeletal sites, excess parathyroid hormone can lead to a condition called *osteitis fibrosa cystica*. Subperiosteal resorption of the distal phalanges, tapering of the distal clavicles, a "salt and pepper" appearance of the skull, bone cysts, and brown tumors of the long bones are all overt manifestations of hyperparathyroid bone disease. The skeletal features are readily seen by conventional x-rays if they are present. Along with the major increase in incidence of primary hyperparathyroidism, however, overt hyperparathyroid bone disease has become most unusual. It is now seen in well under 5% of patients with primary hyperparathyroidism (11).

Like the skeleton, the kidney is also much less commonly involved in primary hyperparathyroidism than before. The incidence of kidney stones has declined from approximately 33% in the 1960s to 20% now. Nephrolithiasis, nevertheless, is still the most common complication of the hyperparathyroid process (12). Other renal features of primary hyperparathyroidism include diffuse deposition of calcium–phosphate complexes in the parenchyma (nephrocalcinosis). Hypercalciuria (daily calcium excretion of >250 mg for women or >300 mg for men) is seen in up to 30% of patients. In the absence of any other cause, primary hyperparathyroidism may be associated with a reduction in creatinine clearance.

The classic neuromuscular syndrome of primary hyperparathyroidism that is associated with a definable myopathy has virtually disappeared (13). In its place, however, is a less well defined syndrome characterized by easy fatigue, a sense of weakness, and a feeling that the aging process is advancing faster than it should. This is sometimes accompanied by an intellectual weariness and a sense that cognitive faculties are less sharp. In some studies, psychodynamic evaluation has appeared to reveal a distinct psychiatric profile (14). Whether these nonspecific features of primary hyperparathyroidism are truly part and parcel of the disease process, reversible upon successful parathyroid surgery, are issues that have not yet been settled by definitive studies (15).

Gastrointestinal manifestations of primary hyperparathyroidism have classically included peptic ulcer disease and pancreatitis. Peptic ulcer disease is not likely to be linked in a pathophysiologic way to primary hyperparathyroidism unless type I multiple endocrine neoplasia is present. Pancreatitis is virtually never seen anymore as a complication of primary hyperparathyroidism because the hypercalcemia tends to be so mild. Like peptic ulcer disease, the association between primary hyperparathyroidism and hypertension is tenuous. Although there may be an increased incidence of hypertension in primary hyperparathyroidism, it is rarely corrected or improved after successful surgery. Still other potential organ systems that in the past were affected by the hyperparathyroid state are now relegated to being archival curiosities. These include gout and pseudogout, anemia, band keratopathy, and loose teeth.

CLINICAL FORMS OF PRIMARY HYPERPARATHYROIDISM

The marked increase in incidence of hyperparathyroidism has led to the concomitant observation that its most common clinical form is asymptomatic hypercalcemia with serum calcium levels not higher than 1 mg/dl above the upper limits of normal. These patients do not have specific complaints and do not show evidence for any target organ complications. They have usually been discovered accidentally in the course of a routine multichannel screening test. Rarely, a patient will demonstrate serum calcium levels in the life-threatening range, so-called acute primary hyperparathyroidism or parathyroid crisis. These patients are invariably symptomatic of hypercalcemia (16). Although this is an unusual presentation of primary hyperparathyroidism, it should always be considered in any patient who presents with acute hypercalcemia of unclear etiology.

Unusual clinical presentations of primary hyperparathyroidism include the multiple endocrine neoplasias, types I and II, familial primary hyperparathyroidism not associated with any other endocrine disorder, familial cystic parathyroid adenomatosis, and neonatal primary hyperparathyroidism (Chapter 29).

EVALUATION AND DIAGNOSIS OF PRIMARY HYPERPARATHYROIDISM

The history and the physical examination rarely give any clear indications of primary hyperparathyroidism but are helpful because of the paucity of specific manifestations of the disease. The diagnosis of primary hyperparathyroidism is established by laboratory tests. There are two biochemical hallmarks of primary hyperparathyroidism: hypercalcemia and elevated levels of parathyroid hormone. Hypercalcemia is virtually always present. Occasionally, a patient with known mild hypercalcemia will have a normal serum calcium concentration. However, it is distinctly unusual for a patient with primary hyperparathyroidism to regularly show serum calcium levels within the normal range. The serum phosphorus tends to be in the lower range of normal. In approximately one third of patients, it is frankly low. The serum alkaline phosphatase activity may be elevated when bone disease is present. More specific markers of bone formation (bone-specific alkaline phosphatase, osteocalcin) and bone resorption (urinary pyridinoline, deoxypyridinoline, N-telopeptide of collagen) will be above normal when there is active bone involvement. The actions of parathyroid hormone to alter acid–base handling in the kidney will lead, in some patients, to a small increase in the serum chloride concentration and a concomitant decrease in the serum bicarbonate concentration. Urinary calcium excretion is elevated in approximately 30% of patients. The circulating 1,25-dihydroxyvitamin D concentration is elevated in some patients with primary hyperparathyroidism (17), although it is of little diagnostic value because 1,25-dihydroxyvitamin D levels are increased in other hypercalcemic states, such as sarcoidosis, other granulomatous diseases, and some lymphomas (18,19).

The lack of specific radiologic manifestations of primary hyperparathyroidism in the vast majority of patients means that x-rays are not cost effective in the evaluation of the patient with primary hyperparathyroidism. On the other hand, bone mineral densitometry has proved to be an integral component of the evaluation because of its great sensitivity to detect early changes in bone mass (Chapter 23). Patients with primary hyperparathyroidism tend to show a pattern of bone involvement that preferentially affects the cortical as opposed to the cancellous skeleton (20,21). The typical pattern is a reduction in bone density of the distal third of the forearm, a site enriched in cortical bone, and relative preservation of the lumbar spine, a site enriched in cancellous bone. The hip region, best typified by the femoral neck, tends to show values intermediate between the distal radius and the lumbar spine because its composition is a more equal mixture of cortical and cancellous elements. Bone densitometry has become an invaluable aspect of the evaluation of primary hyperparathyroidism because it gives a more accurate assessment of the degree of involvement of the skeleton than any other approach. This information is used to make recommendations for parathyroid surgery or for conservative medical observation (see following sections).

Measurement of the circulating parathyroid hormone concentration is the most definitive way to make the diagnosis of primary hyperparathyroidism. In the presence of hypercalcemia, an elevated level of parathyroid hormone virtually establishes the diagnosis. In over 90% of patients with primary hyperparathyroidism, the parathyroid hormone level will be elevated. Moreover, it is distinctly unusual for other causes of hypercalcemia to be associated with elevated concentrations of parathyroid hormone. Thus, the assay for parathyroid hormone helps also to rule out other causes of hypercalcemia. Certain radioimmunoassays that recognize the carboxy-terminal or mid-molecule portions of the parathyroid hormone molecule are useful (22). However, the immunoradiometric (IRMA) and immunochemiluminometric (ICMA) assays for parathyroid hormone that measure the intact molecule have replaced older radioimmunoassays as the gold standard (23). The utility of the parathyroid hormone measurement in the differential diagnosis of hypercalcemia is a result both of refinements in assay techniques and of the fact that the most common other cause of hypercalcemia, namely hypercalcemia of malignancy, is associated with suppressed levels of hormone. This is true even for the syndrome of humoral hypercalcemia of malignancy (Chapter 32) in which parathyroid-hormone-related peptide (PTHrP) is the major causative factor. There is no cross-reactivity with PTHrP in the IRMA and ICMA assays for parathyroid hormone. The only hypercalcemic disorders in which the parathyroid hormone concentration might be elevated are those related to lithium or thiazide diuretic use (Chapter 36). It is relatively easy to exclude either of these two possibilities by the history. If it is conceivable that the patient has drug-related hypercalcemia, the only secure way to make the diagnosis of primary hyperparathyroidism is to withdraw the medication and to confirm persistent hypercalcemia and elevated parathyroid hormone levels 2 to 3 months later.

TREATMENT OF PRIMARY HYPERPARATHYROIDISM

Surgery

Primary hyperparathyroidism is cured when the abnormal parathyroid tissue is removed. The decision to recommend surgery is tempered by the realization that the majority of patients with primary hyperparathyroidism are asymptomatic. Moreover, we lack predictive indices that indicate who among the asymptomatic are at risk for experiencing complications of this disease (24). In the absence of data that can predict who is at risk for the complications of this disease, a set of guidelines is used by many endocrinologists. If the serum calcium is more than 1 mg/dl above the upper limit of normal, it is the impression that the risks for developing the complications of primary hyperparathyroidism are greater. If the patient has any complications of primary hyperparathyroidism (e.g., overt bone disease, nephrolithiasis), surgery is generally considered even if the serum calcium may not be impressively high. Another surgical guideline is met by the patient who survives an episode of acute primary hyperparathyroidism with life-threatening hypercalcemia. Marked hypercalciuria (>400 mg daily excretion) is another general indication for surgery. If bone mass at the distal radius, as determined by bone densitometry, is more than two standard deviations below age- and sex-matched control subjects, surgery should be recommended. Finally, it is the impression that the relatively young patient with primary hyperparathyroidism (under 50 years old) is at greater risk over the long term simply because the younger patient is likely to live longer and be exposed for a greater period of time to the hyperparathyroid state. When one applies these guidelines, approximately 50% of patients with primary hyperparathyroidism will meet at least one criterion and thereby become a candidate for surgery.

These guidelines for surgery, however, are tempered by both the physician and the patient. Some physicians will recommend surgery for all patients with primary hyperparathyroidism; other physicians will not recommend surgery unless clear-cut complications of primary hyperparathyroidism are present. The patient enters into this dialogue as well. Some patients can not tolerate the idea of living with a curable disease and will seek surgery in the absence of any of the aforementioned guidelines. Other patients, with coexisting medical problems, may not wish to face the risks of surgery even though surgical indications are present.

Parathyroid surgery requires exceptional expertise and experience. The glands are notoriously variable in location, requiring the surgeon's knowledge of typical ectopic sites such as intrathyroidal, retroesophageal, the lateral neck, and the mediastinum. The surgeon must also be aware of the proper operation to perform. In the case of the adenoma, the other glands are ascertained to be normal and are not removed. In the case of multiglandular disease, the approach is to remove all tissue save for a remnant that is left *in situ* or autotransplanted in the nondominant forearm.

Postoperatively, the patient may experience a brief period of transient hypocalcemia, during which time the normal but suppressed parathyroid glands regain their sensitivity to calcium. This happens within the first few days after surgery (25), and it is usually not necessary to treat the postoperative patient aggressively with calcium when postoperative hypocalcemia is mild. In contrast, if overt skeletal disease is present, there may be a prolonged postoperative period of symptomatic hypocalcemia as a result of rapid deposition of calcium and phosphate into bones ("hungry bone" syndrome). These patients do require parenteral calcium for symptomatic hypocalcemia. In patients who have had previous neck surgery or who undergo subtotal parathyroidectomy (for multi-glandular disease), permanent hypoparathyroidism may ensue. Another long-term, but unusual complication of parathyroid surgery is damage to the recurrent laryngeal nerve, which can lead to hoarseness and reduced voice volume.

A number of localization tests are available to define the site of abnormal parathyroid tissue preoperatively. Among the noninvasive tests, ultrasonography, computed tomography (CT), magnetic resonance imaging (MRI), and scintigraphy are available (26). Radioisotopic imaging with thallium and technetium has been replaced by imaging with technetium-99m-sestamibi (27,28). Sestamibi is taken up both by thyroid and parathyroid tissue, but it persists in the parathyroid glands. Various approaches to the use of ^{99m}Tc-sestamibi include using the imaging agent alone, and thereby depending on a difference in uptake kinetics between thyroid and parathyroid tissue; or using it in combination with ^{99}Tc-pertechnetate or 123-iodine. The use of dual isotope methods is believed by some to provide better definition of the thyroid, from which the image obtained with sestamibi can be subtracted. Invasive localization tests with arteriography and selective venous sampling for parathyroid hormone in the draining thyroid veins are available when noninvasive studies have not been successful.

The value of preoperative localization tests in patients about to undergo parathyroid surgery is controversial. It has been claimed that localization of the parathyroid gland(s) prior to surgery leads to greater success in finding the gland(s) during the operation and that operating time is decreased. In considering this issue, it is helpful to compare patients who have had prior neck surgery with those who have not. In the latter group, these tests do not prevent failed operations or shorten operating time (29). Successful localization with any of these procedures is no better that 60% to 75%. Furthermore, an experienced parathyroid surgeon will find the abnormal parathyroid gland(s) well over 90% of the time in the patient who has not had previous neck surgery (30). Thus, it is hard to justify these tests in this group.

On the other hand, in patients who have had prior neck surgery, preoperative localization can be extremely helpful, even to the expert parathyroid surgeon. The general approach is to utilize the noninvasive studies first. Ultrasound and radioisotopic imaging are best for parathyroid tissue that is located in proximity to the thyroid, whereas CT and MRI testing are better for ectopically located parathyroid tissue. In view of the substantial incidence of false-positive studies with all the noninvasive localization procedures, confirmation with two is necessary to be confident of accurate localization. Arteriography and selective venous studies are reserved for those individuals in whom the noninvasive studies have not been successful (26). Marked elevation of parathyroid hormone in blood samples obtained from neck veins selectively draining abnormal parathyroid tissue can provide very useful information. When combined with arteriographic demonstration of the tumor, complete identification is established. Unfortunately, arteriography and selective venous catheterization are time consuming, expensive, and difficult procedures. Their success depends on the skill of the angiographer. When the need for these tests arises in a patient, referral is usually made to one of the few sites in the United States that do these studies on a regular basis.

In patients who undergo successful parathyroid surgery, the hyperparathyroid state is completely cured. Serum biochemistries normalize and the parathyroid hormone level returns to normal. In addition, bone mass improves substantially in the first 2 to 4 years after surgery (31). The increase is documented by bone densitometry. The cumulative increase in bone mass at each site (lumbar spine, femoral neck, and distal radius) is between 8% and 12%, a rather impressive improvement. It is particularly noteworthy that the lumbar spine, a site where parathyroid hormone appears to protect from age-related and estrogen-deficiency bone loss, is a site of rapid and substantial improvement.

Medical Management

If patients with primary hyperparathyroidism are not to undergo parathyroid surgery, a set of general medical guidelines is recommended (32). Adequate hydration and ambulation are always encouraged. Thiazide diuretics are to be avoided because they may lead to worsening hypercalcemia. Dietary intake of calcium should be moderate. There is no good evidence that patients with primary hyperparathyroidism show significant fluctuations of their serum calcium as a function of dietary calcium intake. High calcium intakes should be avoided, however, especially in patients whose 1,25-dihydroxyvitamin D level is elevated. Low calcium diets should also be avoided because they could theoretically lead to further stimulation of parathyroid hormone secretion.

We still lack an effective and safe therapeutic agent for the medical management of primary hyperparathyroidism. Oral phosphate will lower the serum calcium in patients with primary hyperparathyroidism by approximately 0.5 to 1 mg/dl. Phosphate appears to act by three mechanisms: interference with absorption of dietary calcium, inhibition of bone resorption, and inhibition of renal production of 1,25-dihydroxyvitamin D. Phosphate, however, is not used

widely as a therapy for primary hyperparathyroidism because of concerns related to ectopic calcification in soft tissues as a result of increasing the calcium–phosphate product. Moreover, oral phosphate leads to an undesirable further elevation of parathyroid hormone levels (33).

In postmenopausal women, estrogen therapy has been considered (34–36). The rationale for estrogen use in primary hyperparathyroidism is based upon the known antagonism by estrogen of parathyroid hormone–mediated bone resorption. Experience with estrogen therapy is still limited. Even though the serum calcium concentration does tend to decline after estrogen administration, parathyroid hormone levels and the serum phosphorous concentration do not change.

Bisphosphonates have also been considered as a possible medical approach to primary hyperparathyroidism. Two of the original bisphosphonates, etidronate and dichloromethylene bisphosphonate, have been studied. Although etidronate is not effective (37), dichloromethylene bisphosphonate was shown in early studies to reduce the serum calcium in primary hyperparathyroidism (38). However, it does not appear to lead to sustained reductions in the serum calcium concentration (39). The use of pamidronate in primary hyperparathyroidism has been rather exclusively as an intravenous preparation (40). Difficulties with oral formulations of pamidronate will restrict its use to only acute hypercalcemic states associated with primary hyperparathyroidism. It remains to be seen whether oral preparations of the new bisphosphonates currently being developed will be effective in primary hyperparathyroidism.

Finally, a more targeted approach to the medical therapy of primary hyperparathyroidism would be to interfere specifically with the production of parathyroid hormone. A new class of agents that alter the function of the extracellular calcium-sensing receptor (7) offers an exciting new approach to primary hyperparathyroidism. Such agents could conceivably reduce parathyroid hormone levels (41) and thereby control the hypercalcemic state. Clinical trials are currently ongoing with these calcimimetic agents in primary hyperparathyroidism.

Patients who are not surgical candidates for parathyroidectomy appear to do very well when they are managed conservatively (42–44). Routine medical follow-up usually includes visits twice yearly with serum calcium determinations. Yearly urinary calcium excretion tests and bone densitometry are also recommended. Biochemical data over 6 years of follow-up do not change. These include the serum calcium, phosphorus, parathyroid hormone, 25-hydroxyvitamin D, 1,25-dihydroxyvitamin D, and urinary calcium excretion. More specific markers of bone formation and bone resorption also do not appear to change. Several studies have confirmed, in addition, that bone mass as determined by bone densitometry at the lumbar spine, femoral neck, and distal radius does not change. It should be cautioned that the group of patients who appear to do well without surgery are preselected in that they do not meet accepted criteria for surgery. Such a benign course is shown thus for asymptomatic patients with primary hyperparathyroidism who do not meet any accepted criteria for surgery. Another cautionary note is that the longer-term longitudinal course of primary hyperparathyroidism, beyond the 6 years reported so far, is still to be established.

REFERENCES

1. Silverberg SJ, Fitzpatrick LA, Bilezikian JP: Hyperparathyroidism, In: Becker KL (ed) *Principles and Practice of Endocrinology and Metabolism,* 2nd ed. JB Lippincott, Philadelphia, 512–519, 1995
2. Heath H III, Hodgson SF, Kennedy MA: Primary hyperparathyroidism: Incidence, morbidity, and potential economic impact in a community. *N Engl J Med* 302:189, 1980
3. Wynne AG, Van Heerden J, Carney JA, Fitzpatrick LA: Parathyroid carcinoma: Clinical and pathological features in 43 patients. *Medicine* 71:197–205, 1992
4. Arnold A: Molecular genetics of parathyroid gland neoplasia. *J Clin Endocrinol Metab* 77:1108–1112, 1993
5. el-Deiry S, Levine MA: Molecular overtones of primary hyperparathyroidism. *J Clin Endocrinol Metab* 80: 3105–3106, 1995
6. Hakim JP, Levine MA: Absence of p53 point mutations in parathyroid adenomas and carcinoma. *J Clin Endocrinol Metab* 78: 103–106, 1994
7. Brown EM, Gamba G, Riccardi D, et al.: Cloning and characterization of an extracellular Ca^{2+}-sensing receptor from bovine parathyroid. *Nature* 366:575, 1993
8. Pollak MR, Brown EM, Chou Y-H W, Hebert SC, Marx SJ, Steinmann B, Levi T, Seidman CE, Seidman JG: Mutations in human calcium-sensing gene cause familial hypocalciuric hypercalcemia and neonatal severe hyperparathyroidism. *Cell* 75: 1297–1303, 1993
9. Hosokawa Y, Pollak MR, Brown EM, Arnold A: Mutational analysis of the extracellular calcium-sensing receptor gene in human parathyroid tumors. *J Clin Endocrinol Metab* 80, 3107–3110, 1995
10. Thompson DB, Samowitz WS, Odelberg S, Davis RK, Szabo J, Heath H III: Genetic abnormalities in sporadic parathyroid adenomas. Loss of heterozygosity for chromosome 3q markers flanking the calcium receptor locus. *J Clin Endocrinol Metab* 80: 3377–3380, 1995
11. Bilezikian JP, Silverberg SJ, Gartenberg F, Kim T-S, Jacobs TP, Siris ES, Shane E: Clinical presentation of primary hyperparathyroidism. In: Bilezikian JP, Marcus R, Levine MA (eds) *The Parathyroids,* Raven Press, New York, pp 457–470, 1994
12. Silverberg SJ, Shane E, Jacobs TP, Siris ES, Gartenberg F, Seldin D, Clemens TL, Bilezikian JP: Nephrolithiasis and bone involvement in primary hyperparathyroidism. *Am J Med* 89:327–334, 1990
13. Turken SA, Cafferty M, Silverberg SJ, de la Cruz L, Cimino C, Lange DJ, Lovelace RE, Bilezikian JP: Neuromuscular involvement in mild, asymptomatic primary hyperparathyroidism. *Am J Med* 87:553–557, 1989
14. Solomon BL, Schaaf M, Smallridge RC: Psychologic symptoms before and after parathyroid surgery. *Am J Med* 96:101–106, 1994
15. Kleerekoper M, Bilezikian JP. Parathyroidectomy for non-traditional features of primary hyperparathyroidism. *Am J Med* 96:99–100, 1994
16. Fitzpatrick LA. Acute primary hyperparathyroidism. In: Bilezikian JP, Marcus R, Levine MA (eds) *The Parathyroids* Raven Press, New York, pp 583–589, 1994
17. Broadus AE, Horst RL, Lang R, Littledike ET, Rasmussen H: The importance of circulating 1,25-dihydroxyvitamin D in the pathogenesis of hypercalciuria and renal-stone formation in primary hyperparathyroidism. *N Engl J Med* 302:421, 1980
18. Seymour JF, Gagel RF, Hagemesiter FB, Dimopoulous MA, Cabanillas F: Calcitriol production in hypercalcemic and normocalcemic Ptients with non-Hodgkin lymphoma. *Ann Intern Med* 121:633–640, 1994
19. Cox M, Haddad JG: Lymphoma, hypercalcemia and the sunshine vitamin. *Ann Intern Med* 121:709–712, 1994
20. Silverberg SJ, Shane E, de la Cruz L, Depmster DW, Feldman F, Seldin D, Jacobs TP, Siris ES, Cafferty M, Parisien MV, Lindsay R, Clemens TL, Bilezikian JP: Skeletal disease in primary hyperparathyroidism. *J Bone Miner Res* 4:283–291, 1989
21. Parisien MV, Silverberg SJ, Shane E, de la Cruz L, Lindsay R, Bilezikian JP, Dempster DW: The histomorphometry of bone in primary hyperparathyroidism: Preservation of cancellous bone structure. *J Clin Endocrinol Metab* 70:930–938, 1990
22. Nussbaum SR, Potts JT Jr: Advances in immunoassays for parathyroid hormone. In: Bilezikian JP, Marcus R, Levine MA (eds) *The Parathyroids.* Raven Press, New York, pp 157–169, 1994
23. Endres DB, Villanueva R, Sharp CR Jr, Singer FR: Immunochemiluminometric and immunoradiometric determinations of intact and total immunoreactive parathyrin: Performance in the differential diagnosis of hypercalcemia and hypoparathyroidism. *Clin Chem* 37:162–168, 1991
24. Kleerekoper M: Clinical course of primary hyperparathyroidism. In: Bilezikian JP, Marcus R, Levine MA (eds) *The Parathyroids.* Raven Press, New York, pp 471–484, 1994
25. Brasier AR, Wang C, Nussbaum SR: Recovery of parathyroid hormone secretion after parathyroid adenomectomy. *J Clin Endocrinol Metab* 61:495–500, 1988
26. Doppman JL: Preoperative localization of parathyroid tissue in primary hyperparathyroidism. In: Bilezikian JP, Marcus R, Levine MA (eds) *The Parathyroids.* Raven Press, New York, pp 553–566, 1994
27. Preoperative localization of parathyroid tissue with technetium-99m Sestamibi ^{123}I subtraction scanning. *J Clin Endocrinol Metab* 78:77–82, 1994
28. Mitchell BK, Kinder BK, Cornelius E, Stewart AF: Primary Hyperparathyroidism: Preoperative localization using technetium-sestamibi scanning. *J Clin Endocrinol Metab* 80:7–10, 1995
29. Roe SM, Burns RP, Graham LD, Brock WB, Russell WL: Cost-effectiveness of preoperative localization studies in primary hyperparathyroid disease. *Ann Surg* 219:582–586, 1994
30. Kaplan EL, Yoshiro T, Salti G: Primary hyperparathyroidism in the 1990s. *Ann Surg* 215:300–317, 1992
31. Silverberg SJ, Gartenberg F, Jacobs TP, Shane E, Siris E, Staron RB, McMahon D, Bilezikian JP: Increased bone density after parathyroidectomy in primary hyperparathyroidism. *J Clin Endocrinol Metab* 80:729–734, 1995
32. Consensus Development Conference Panel: Diagnosis and management of asymptomatic primary hyperparathyroidism: Consensus Development Conference Statement. *Ann Intern Med* 114: 593–597, 1991
33. Broadus AE, Magee JSI, Mallette LE, Horst RL, Lang R, Jensen RG, Gertner JM, Baron R: A detailed evaluation of oral phosphate therapy in selected patients with primary hyperparathyroidism. *J Clin Endocrinol Metab* 56:953–1961, 1983
34. Marcus R, Madvig P, Crim M, Pont A, Kosek J: Conjugated estrogens in the treatment of postmenopausal women with hyperparathyroidism. *Ann Intern Med* 100:633, 1984
35. Selby PL, Peacock M: Ethinyl estradiol and norethindrone in the treatment of primary hyperparathyroidism in postmenopausal women. *N Engl J Med* 314:1481, 1986
36. McDermott MT, Perloff JJ, Kidd GS: Effects of mild asymptomatic primary hyperparathyroidism on bone mass in women with and without estrogen replacement therapy. *J Bone Miner Res* 9:509–514, 1994
37. Kaplan RA, Geho WB, Poindexter C, Haussler M, Dietz GW, Pak CYC: Metabolic effects of diphosphonate in primary hyperparathyroidism. *J Clin Pharmacol* 17:410–419, 1977
38. Shane E, Baquiran DC, Bilezikian JP: Effects of dichloromethylene diphosphonate on serum and urine calcium in primary hyperparathyroidism. *Ann Intern Med* 95:23, 1981
39. Adami S, Mian M, Bertoldo F, et al.: Regulation of calcium-parathyroid hormone feedback in primary hyperparathyroidism: Effects of bisphosphonate treatment. *Clin Endocrinol* 33:391–397, 1990
40. Janson S, Tisell L-E, Lindstedt G, Lundberg P-A: Disodium pamidronate in the preoperative treament of hypercalcemia in patients with primary hyperparathyroidism. *Surgery* 110:480–486, 1991
41. Garrett JE, Steffey ME, Nemeth EF: The calcium receptor agonist NPS 568 suppresses PTH mRNA levels in cultured bovine parathyroid cells (abstract). *J Bone Miner Res* 10:M539, 1995
42. Christensson TAT: Primary hyperparathyroidism-pathogenesis, incidence and natural history. *Prog Surg* 18:34–44, 1990
43. Rao DS, Wilson RJ, Kleerekoper M, Parfitt AM: Lack of biochemical progression or continuation of accelerated bone loss in mild asymptomatic primary hyperparathyroidism: Evidence for a biphasic disease course. *J Clin Endocrinol Metab* 67:1294–1298, 1988
44. Silverberg SJ, Gartenberg F, Jacobs TP, Shane E, Siris E, Staron RB, Bilezikian JP: Longitudinal measurements of bone density and biochemical indices in untreated primary hyperparathyroidism. *J Clin Endocrinol Metab* 80:723–728, 1995

29. Familial Hyperparathyroid Syndromes

Hunter Heath III, M.D., and *Maurine R. Hobbs, Ph.D.

*Medical Division, Lilly USA, Eli Lilly and Company, Indianapolis, Indiana; and *Department of Human Genetics, University of Utah School of Medicine, Salt Lake City, Utah*

As described in Chapter 28, most cases of primary hyperparathyroidism (HPT) result from sporadic, benign parathyroid tumors (adenomas). However, up to 10% of cases may occur as hereditary forms of isolated HPT, or HPT associated with other genetically determined abnormalities. Recent genetic linkage and mutational analyses have confirmed the hereditary nature of these syndromes and, in some cases, have led to identification of specific genetic mutations responsible for parathyroid neoplasia or hyperfunction. The commonest variety of hereditary HPT occurs in the syndrome of multiple endocrine neoplasia type I (MEN I) (1), while the relative frequencies of the other disorders are poorly documented.

MULTIPLE ENDOCRINE NEOPLASIA TYPE I (WERMER SYNDROME)

The familial occurrence of parathyroid, anterior pituitary, and pancreatic tumors—today called MEN I (1)—was recognized as a distinct syndrome by Wermer in 1954 (Table 1). MEN I is transmitted in an autosomal dominant mode of inheritance with a high degree of penetrance. The most common feature of MEN I is HPT, which is almost always present. The clinical and biochemical presentation of HPT in MEN I resembles that of nonfamilial or sporadic HPT, except that MEN I occurs in both sexes equally, whereas

sporadic HPT occurs more frequently in women. In general, patients with MEN I are younger at the time of diagnosis than patients with sporadic HPT. In fact, childhood and neonatal cases have been reported.

The only definitive therapy for HPT in MEN I, as in sporadic cases, is surgical. The indications for surgery are also largely the same, including significant bone disease, active nephrolithiasis, change of mental status, or serum calcium above an arbitrary value, usually 11.0 to 11.5 mg/dl (2.75 to 2.88 mmol/L). Given the younger average age of MEN I patients, however, surgical intervention is generally undertaken fairly early.

The surgical approach to patients with HPT as part of the MEN-I syndrome is dictated by the underlying pathology of the parathyroid glands. Although solitary adenomas have been noted, HPT in MEN I is usually a multi-glandular disorder, with hyperplasia of all four parathyroids. The importance of recognizing hyperplasia in MEN I is that resection of a single gland or even less than three glands frequently leads to persistent or recurrent hypercalcemia. About 70% of patients with HPT and MEN I have remission of hypercalcemia after removal of three or more glands, whereas only about a third respond to resection of 2½ glands or less.

Most centers now perform a subtotal parathyroidectomy in hypercalcemic patients with MEN I, resecting 3½ glands

TABLE 1. *Characteristics of familial hyperparathyroid syndromes*

Feature	MEN I	MEN IIA	HPT-JT	Familial HPT	FBHH
Hyperparathyroidism	>95%	Histologically, up to 50%; about 10% hypercalcemic	>95%	100%	100%
Parathyroid carcinoma	Reported	Rare	4/10 families	Reported	—
Pancreatic tumors	30%–80%	—	—	—	—
Pituitary adenomas	15%–50%	—	—	—	—
Adrenocortical hyperplasia	<33%	—	—	—	—
Medullary CA thyroid	—	100%	—	—	—
Pheochromocytoma or adrenal medullary hyperplasia	—	Up to 50%	—	—	—
Lichen amyloidosis	—	Reported	—	—	—
Fibro-osseous jaw tumors	—	—	10/10 families	—	—
Wilms' tumor	—	—	3/10 families	—	—
Inheritance	AD	AD	AD	AD, AR (1 kindred)	AD
Genetic locus	11q12-q13	10q11.2	1q21-q31	Not mapped	3q13.3-q21, 19p, and unknown
Gene mutated	Unknown	*RET* proto-oncogene	Unknown	Unknown	Ca^{2+} receptor ($FBHH_{3q}$), others unknown

MEN, multiple endocrine neoplasia; HPT-JT, hyperparathyroidism–jaw tumor syndrome; FBHH, familial benign hypocalciuric hypercalcemia; CA, carcinoma; AD, autosomal dominant inheritance; AR, autosomal recessive inheritance.

and leaving about 50 mg of viable tissue. To avoid persistent hypercalcemia or permanent postoperative hypoparathyroidism, some surgeons perform total parathyroidectomy with autotransplantation of the abnormal parathyroid tissue into forearm muscles, reasoning that recurrent HPT will not require a second neck exploration. However, graft-dependent persistent or recurrent hypercalcemia may occur and be difficult to manage. Regardless of the approach, close follow-up and expert management of this frustrating condition is mandatory.

Patients with MEN I also frequently develop pancreatic and pituitary neoplasms. The pancreatic lesions are usually islet cell tumors, two thirds secreting excess gastrin, leading to Zollinger-Ellison syndrome, and about one third hypersecreting insulin, leading to fasting hypoglycemia. In a minority, a variety of other substances are secreted, including vasoactive intestinal peptide, prostaglandins, glucagon, pancreatic polypeptide, adrenocorticotropic hormone (ACTH), and serotonin.

The pituitary tumors in MEN I, thought initially to be largely nonfunctional, are now increasingly recognized as prolactinomas. These tumors may also secrete growth hormone, leading to acromegaly, or ACTH, resulting in Cushing's disease.

Up to one third of MEN I patients have enlargement of the adrenal glands. The histopathology includes diffuse and nodular cortical hypertrophy, cortical hyperplasia, adenomas, and, rarely, adrenocortical carcinoma. The cause(s) of the adrenal cortical hyperplasia are unknown.

The MEN I gene has been mapped to the long arm of chromosome 11 (11q13), but the specific gene mutated has not been identified (2). Offspring of MEN I patients have a 50% risk of inheriting the gene. MEN I–associated lesions may manifest as late as age 35 years in persons at genetic risk. Until molecular genetic diagnosis is possible, even extensive biochemical testing, including serum calcium, glucose, gastrin, and serum prolactin assays, may not identify all affected persons before overt symptoms develop (3). It is nonetheless important to screen first-degree relatives of affected individuals; serum calcium measurement alone will identify many cases. Genetic linkage testing is cumbersome, but sometimes it can be used for informed genetic counseling. Regrettably, the whole family must be sampled.

MULTIPLE ENDOCRINE NEOPLASIA TYPE IIA (SIPPLE SYNDROME)

Multiple endocrine neoplasia type IIA (MEN IIA) syndrome is characterized by medullary carcinoma of the thyroid, bilateral pheochromocytomas, and parathyroid hyperplasia (Table 1) (4). Originally described by Sipple in 1961, this syndrome is inherited as an autosomal dominant trait.

The dominant feature of the MEN IIA syndrome is medullary carcinoma of the thyroid, a calcitonin-secreting neoplasm derived from the thyroid C-cells, which occasionally leads to death from metastatic disease. Until recently, early detection was achieved primarily by the measurement of plasma calcitonin after infusion of calcium or pentagastrin. Once hypercalcitoninemia was detected in persons at

risk, early total thyroidectomy was generally performed. However, molecular genetic diagnosis is rapidly supplanting diagnosis by calcitonin assay (5).

The other major feature of MEN IIA is pheochromocytoma, present in up to 50% of patients, which may precede or follow detection of thyroid cancer. In contrast to sporadic pheochromocytoma, the tumor in MEN IIA is virtually always bilateral and often requires total adrenalectomy. Unrecognized pheochromocytoma can be lethal during surgical procedures, so this lesion should be diagnosed and treated before neck exploration. Indeed, patients with MEN IIA are far more likely to die from unrecognized pheochromocytoma than from medullary thyroid carcinoma.

Hyperparathyroidism is less common and milder in MEN IIA than in MEN I, but here also it is a result of diffuse parathyroid hyperplasia. However, the hyperplastic glands may be quite heterogeneous in size, leading to an erroneous diagnosis of adenomatous HPT. The surgical management is similar to that for HPT in MEN I.

Pruritic, pigmented cutaneous lesions localized to the upper back, and generally containing amyloid ("lichen amyloidosis"), have occurred in some MEN IIA families (6). The lesions are thought to be a form of dorsal neuropathy that could be an early clinical marker for MEN IIA.

The MEN IIA gene was localized by linkage analysis to the centromeric region of chromosome 10, and then identified as the *RET* proto-oncogene (8). MEN IIA results from a limited number of mutations in the *RET* proto-oncogene, and molecular genetic tests are now available commercially to permit presymptomatic diagnosis of MEN IIA in individuals (5). Persons at risk who are found to have a *RET* mutation may undergo appropriate testing and surgery electively, before complications have arisen (e.g., metastatic medullary thyroid carcinoma (MTC) renal damage from HPT). Affected persons may ultimately have total thyroidectomy, bilateral adrenalectomy, and subtotal parathyroidectomy.

THE HYPERPARATHYROIDISM–JAW TUMOR SYNDROME

The hyperparathyroidism–jaw tumor syndrome (HPT-JT) syndrome, first reported in 1958 by Jackson et al. (9,10), was recently localized to chromosome 1q21-q31 (Table 1). Affected families show autosomal dominant inheritance of a highly penetrant disorder encompassing early-onset parathyroid tumors that may recur, and fibro-osseous jaw tumors (10). Parathyroid carcinoma and a malignant renal neoplasm, Wilms' tumor, occur at lesser frequencies (44% and 33%, of families, respectively) (10).

Patients having HPT-JT may become severely hypercalcemic in childhood and up to the late teenage years. In contrast to the parathyroid hyperplasia found in other forms of inherited HPT, however, they usually have a solitary enlarged parathyroid gland (adenoma), sometimes cystic, and they become normocalcemic upon removal of the lesions. The severe HPT has resulted in crippling skeletal disease and death in several individuals.

The bone lesions of HPT-JT occur exclusively in the maxilla and mandible, appearing as punched-out "cystic" lesions on x-rays, and running a course independent from the HPT. Although often small and asymptomatic, the lesions may be large, destructive, persistent, or recurrent. The jaw tumors consist of trabeculae of woven bone set in a cytologically bland fibrocellular stroma; the original abnormal cell type is unknown. They differ strikingly from classic hyperparathyroid "brown tumors," which may occur anywhere in the skeleton, in their lack of osteoclasts. HPT-JT bone tumors occur mostly in adolescence or young adulthood. The malignant renal tumor, Wilms' tumor, is a rapidly progressive malignant mixed neoplasm with embryonal elements. Sporadic Wilms' tumor generally occurs before age 5, but Wilms' tumor has occurred at later ages in HPT-JT, up to age 53.

FAMILIAL ISOLATED PRIMARY HYPERPARATHYROIDISM

The existence of familial HPT as a disorder distinct from the MEN I, MEN IIA, and HPT-JT syndromes has been a subject of debate. Several kindreds with familial hypercalcemia and no other endocrine abnormalities have subsequently been reclassified as having MEN I or familial benign hypocalciuric hypercalcemia (FBHH) (Chapter 30). Isolated HPT in a Danish family followed for 20 years was mapped by genetic linkage analysis to 11q13 (the MEN I locus) (11). Thus, isolated HPT may sometimes represent an allelic variant of MEN I. One kindred has been described with apparent autosomal recessive inheritance of HPT and recurrent large parathyroid adenomas (12). Space does not permit detailed presentation here, but there appear to be many other variants of isolated familial HPT, some with adenomatous and some with hyperplastic parathyroid disease, and some in association with other disorders. We suspect that there are many genetically distinct forms of isolated familial HPT.

THE FAMILIAL BENIGN HYPOCALCIURIC HYPERCALCEMIAS

The familial benign hypocalciuric hypercalcemias (FBHH) comprise at least three distinct genetic variants, the most common of which is $FBHH_{3q}$ (mutations of the cell surface calcium receptor) (13). A chromosome 19p variant ($FBHH_{19p}$) has been reported, as well as one family in which the genetic locus is unknown ($FBHH_{OK}$) (Table 1). These functional (non-neoplastic) disorders of the parathyroids are described in more detail in Chapter 31.

SUMMARY AND CONCLUSIONS

Hereditary forms of HPT are increasingly recognized, and their genetic bases are becoming clearer; molecular genetic diagnosis is possible for some of them. Physicians should be aware of the characteristics of familial HPT syndromes, and seek clues to these diseases in newly diagnosed HPT patients. The implications of finding hereditary HPT are many, including the need for family screening, the necessity for special approaches to the parathyroid surgery, and the existence of serious concomitant diseases such as thyroid cancer, pheochromocytoma, or Wilms' tumor.

REFERENCES

1. Metz DC, Jensen RT, Bale AE, Skarulis MC, Eastman RC, Nieman L, Norton JA, Friedman E, Larsson C, Amorosi A, Brandi M-L, Marx SJ: Multiple endocrine neoplasia type I. In: Bilezikian JP, Marcus R, Levine MA (eds) *The Parathyroids: Basic and Clinical Concepts.* Raven Press, New York, pp 591–646, 1994
2. Thakker RV: The molecular genetics of the multiple endocrine neoplasia syndromes. *Clin Endcrinol* 38:1–14, 1993
3. Friedman E, Larsson C, Amorosi A, Brandi M-L, Bale AE, Metz DC, Jensen RT, Skarulis MC, Eastman RC, Nieman L, Norton JA, Marx SJ: Multiple endocrine neoplasia type I. Pathology, pathophysiology, molecular genetics, and differential diagnosis. In: Bilezikian JP, Marcus R, Levine MA (eds) *The Parathyroids: Basic and Clinical Concepts.* Raven Press, New York, pp 647–680, 1994
4. Gagel RF: Multiple endocrine neoplasia type II. In: Bilezikian JP, Marcus R, Levine MA (eds) *The Parathyroids: Basic and Clinical Concepts.* Raven Press, New York, pp 681–698, 1994
5. Ledger GA, Khosla S, Lindor NM, Thibodeaux SN, Gharib H: Genetic testing in the diagnosis and management of multiple endocrine neoplasia type II. *Ann Intern Med* 122:118–124, 1995
6. Gagel RF, Levy ML, Donovan DT, Alford BR, Wheeler T, Tschen JA: Multiple endocrine neoplasia type 2a associated with cutaneous lichen amyloidosis. *Ann Intern Med* 111:802–806, 1989
7. Chabre O, Labat-Moleur F, Berthod F, Tarel V, Stoebner P, Sobol H, Bachelot I: Atteinte cutanée associée à la neoplasie endocrinienne multiple de type 2A (syndrome de Sipple): Un marqueur clinique precoce. *La Presse Med* 21:299–303, 1992
8. Mulligan LM, Kwok JBJ, Healey CS, Elsdon MJ, Eng C, Gardner E, Love DR, Mole SE, Moore JK, Papi L, Ponder MA, Telenius H, Tunnacliffe A, Ponder BAJ: Germ-line mutations of the RET proto-oncogene in multiple endocrine neoplasia type 2A. *Nature* 363:458–460, 1993
9. Jackson CE, Norum RA, Boyd SB, Talpos GB, Wilson SD, Taggart RT, Mallette LE: Hereditary hyperparathyroidism and multiple ossifying jaw fibromas: A clinically and genetically distinct syndrome. *Surgery* 108:1006–1013, 1990
10. Szabo J, Heath B, Hill VM, Jackson CE, Zarbo RJ, Mallette LE, Chew SL, Besser GM, Thakker RV, Huff V, Leppert MF, Heath H III: Hereditary hyperparathyroidism-jaw tumor syndrome: The endocrine tumor gene HRPT2 maps to chromosome 1q21-q31. *Am J Hum Genet* 56:944–950, 1995
11. Kassem M, Xu C, Brask S, Eriksen EF, Mosekilde L, Kruse T: Familial isolated primary hyperparathyroidism. *J Bone Miner Res* 7(suppl 1):S249, 1992
12. Law WM Jr, Hodgson SF, Heath H III: Autosomal recessive inheritance of familial hyperparathyroidism. *N Engl J Med* 309:650–653, 1983
13. Heath H III, Odelberg S, Jackson CE, et al.: Clustered inactivating mutations and benign polymorphisms of the calcium receptor gene in familial benign hypocalciuric hypercalcemia suggest receptor functional domains. *J Clin Endocrinol Metab* 81:1312–1317,1996

30. Familial Hypocalciuric Hypercalcemia

Stephen J. Marx, M.D.

Genetics and Endocrinology Section, National Institute of Diabetes and Digestive and Kidney Diseases, National Institutes of Health, Bethesda, Maryland

Familial hypocalciuric hypercalcemia (FHH) [also termed familial benign hypercalcemia (FBH)] is an autosomal dominant trait characterized by moderate hypercalcemia and relative hypocalciuria (i.e., urine calcium that is low considering the simultaneous hypercalcemia) with high penetrance for both of these features throughout life (1,2).

CLINICAL FEATURES

Symptoms and Signs. Patients with FHH are usually asymptomatic. Occasionally they note easy fatigue, weakness, thought disturbances, or polydipsia. Although these symptoms are also common in typical primary hyperparathyroidism, they are less common and less severe in FHH. There seems to be an increased incidence of relapsing pancreatitis (1,3), and this can occasionally be severe and life threatening. There may be an increased incidence of gallstones, diabetes mellitus, and myocardial infarction (1,2). The rate of nephrolithiasis or of peptic ulcer disease is the same as in a normal population.

Radiographs and Indices of Bone Function. Radiographs are usually normal. Nephrocalcinosis has the same incidence as in a normal population. There is an increased incidence of chondrocalcinosis (usually clinically silent) and premature vascular calcification (1). Bone turnover measured by indices of bone formation (serum bone gla-protein and/or serum alkaline phosphatase) or by indices of bone resorption (ratio of urine hydroxyproline to creatinine) is mildly increased (4). Mean bone mass is normal, and there is not increased susceptibility to fracture (2,4).

Serum Electrolytes. Serum calcium in gene carriers is elevated throughout life. Typically, the degree of elevation decreases modestly from infancy to old age (1). The degree of elevation is similar to that in typical primary hyperparathyroidism. Both free and bound calcium are increased with a normal ratio of free to bound calcium (5). Serum magnesium is typically in the high range of normal or modestly elevated, and serum phosphate is modestly depressed.

Renal Function Indices. Creatinine clearance is generally normal. Urinary excretion of calcium is normal, with affected and unaffected family members showing a similar distribution of values. The normal urinary calcium in the face of hypercalcemia reflects increased renal tubular resorption of calcium (i.e., relative hypocalciuria). The renal tubular resorption of magnesium is also modestly increased. Because calcium excretion depends heavily on glomerular filtration rate, total calcium excretion is not a useful index to distinguish FHH from typical primary hyperparathyroidism. The ratio of calcium clearance to creatinine clearance,

$$ClCa/ClCr = [Ca_u \times V/Ca_s]/[Cr_u \times V/Cr_s]$$
$$= [Ca_u \times Cr_s]/[Cr_u \times Ca_s]$$

(where Cl is renal clearance, Ca is total calcium, Cr is creatinine, u is urine, V is volume, and s is serum) corrects for most of the variation from glomerular filtration. The clearance ratio in FHH is typically one third of that in typical primary hyperparathyroidism, and a cutoff value at 0.01 (note that the clearance ratio has no units) is helpful for this distinction in a patient with hypercalcemia.

Parathyroid Function Indices. Biochemical testing of parathyroid function, including serum PTH and 1,25-dihydroxyvitamin D [1,25(OH)$_2$D] is usually normal, with modest elevations in 5% to 10% of cases (6,7). The normal parathyroid function indices in the presence of lifelong hypercalcemia are inappropriate and indicative of a specific role for the parathyroids in maintenance of hypercalcemia. There is often mild parathyroid gland hyperplasia (evident only by careful measurement of gland size) (8,9).

Response to Parathyroidectomy. Subtotal parathyroidectomy results in only very transient lowering of serum calcium, with restoration of hypercalcemia within a week (2). Familial hypocalciuric hypercalcemia has been a common cause of unsuccessful parathyroidectomy, accounting for 10% of unsuccessful operations in several large series during the 1970s, before wider recognition of the implications of this diagnosis (10). Total parathyroidectomy in FHH leads to decreased production of 1,25(OH)$_2$D, hypocalcemia, and features of chronic hypoparathyroidism. In several FHH cases, deliberate total parathyroidectomy has been attempted without induction of hypocalcemia; presumably, small amounts of residual parathyroid tissue were sufficient to sustain hypercalcemia.

GENETICS OF FAMILIAL HYPOCALCIURIC HYPERCALCEMIA AND RELATION TO NEONATAL SEVERE PRIMARY HYPERPARATHYROIDISM

There is virtually 100% penetrance for hypercalcemia at all ages among heterozygotes for the FHH gene (1). The hypercalcemia has been documented in the first week of life (11). The degree of hypercalcemia shows clustering within kindreds, with several kindreds showing very modest hypercalcemia and several showing rather severe hypercalcemia (12.5 to 14 mg/dl) in all affected members (1,12). Genetic linkage analyses in eight families have indicated that a gene for FHH is on the long arm of chromosome 3 (13,14). In one large kindred, the FHH trait was linked to the short arm of chromosome 19 (14).

The prevalence of FHH has not been established, but it is probably similar to that for familial multiple endocrine neoplasia type I; each of these diseases may account for about 2% of cases with asymptomatic hypercalcemia.

190

Neonatal severe primary hyperparathyroidism is an unusual state of life-threatening, severe hypercalcemia with massive hyperplasia of all parathyroid glands. Most of these neonates have had FHH in one or both parents (12,15). Some cases clearly reflect a double dose of FHH genes (16). Other cases may result from an FHH heterozygote having gestated in a normocalcemic (i.e., FHH-negative) mother, which caused superimposed intrauterine secondary hyperparathyroidism (15,17,18). The maternal contribution to neonatal hyperparathyroidism in this latter setting may be self-limited.

PATHOPHYSIOLOGY

Biochemical testing has established that the parathyroid gland functions abnormally in FHH (see preceding sections). A surgically decreased gland mass can maintain the same calcium level by increasing hormone secretion rate per cell. Parathyroid function shows features expected from a selective and mild increase in glandular "setpoint" for calcium suppression of PTH secretion. Setpoint was measured in parathyroid cells from a neonate presumed to have a double-dose of FHH genes (19); these cells showed a setpoint higher than ever seen in any parathyroid adenoma. Depending on definition, FHH can therefore be labeled as a form of primary hyperparathyroidism. We prefer to consider it an atypical form of primary hyperparathyroidism in distinct contrast to the more typical form associated with hypercalciuria, nephrolithiasis, markedly increased gland mass, clear elevations of plasma PTH, and generally excellent response to subtotal parathyroidectomy.

In addition to the disturbance presumed to be intrinsic to the parathyroids in FHH, there is also a disturbance intrinsic to the kidneys. The tubular reabsorption of calcium, normally regulated by parathyroid hormone, remains strikingly increased even after total parathyroidectomy in FHH (20).

Most cases are probably caused by inactivating mutations in the calcium-ion-sensing receptor gene (21). The encoded product is predicted to be a seven transmembrane cell surface receptor (like adrenergic and many other receptors) that interacts with extracellular calcium ion, translating it into an intracellular signal through coupling to a cytoplasmic guanyl nucleotide binding protein. The unusual FHH kindreds not linked to the locus at chromosome 3q, such as that linked to 19p, represent mutation in other genes of unknown function.

MANAGEMENT

Intervention in the Typical Case of Familial Hypocalciuric Hypercalcemia. Because of the generally benign course and the lack of response to subtotal parathyroidectomy, virtually all patients should be advised against parathyroidectomy. Attempts to regulate serum calcium with medications (diuretics, estrogens, and phosphates) have not changed serum calcium. Familial hypocalciuric hypercalcemia is compatible with survival into the 1980s, and it is uncertain whether there is any decrease in average life expectancy.

Indications for Parathyroidectomy. In rare situations, such as (i) neonatal severe primary hyperparathyroidism resulting from a double dose of FHH gene, (ii) an adult with relapsing pancreatitis, and (iii) a child or an adult with serum calcium persistently above 14 mg/dl, parathyroidectomy may be necessary. Attempted total parathyroidectomy is recommended in these unusual situations. Several patients have had parathyroidectomy with fresh parathyroid autografts; most have developed graft-dependent recurrent hypercalcemia.

Sporadic Hypocalciuric Hypercalcemia. Without a positive family history, the decision about management of sporadic hypocalciuric hypercalcemia is difficult. Because there is a wide range of urine calcium values in patients with FHH and with typical primary hyperparathyroidism, an occasional patient with parathyroid adenoma will show a very low calcium-to-creatinine clearance ratio. Moreover, occasionally a patient with FHH may show a high ratio. Coexistent FHH and idiopathic hypercalciuria has been clearly documented in at least one case (1). Sporadic hypocalciuric hypercalcemia should generally be managed as typical FHH. In time, the underlying diagnosis may become evident; low morbidity in such patients should be anticipated for the same reasons that morbidity is low in FHH. Detection of a calcium-ion-sensing receptor mutation can be helpful. Failure to find one does not exclude FHH as there may be mutation outside the open reading frame or in other FHH genes.

Pregnancy. Pregnancy in an FHH carrier or in the spouse of an FHH carrier requires special understanding, because of possible antagonism between fetal and maternal calcium regulation. The affected offspring of a carrier should show asymptomatic hypercalcemia. The unaffected offspring of a carrier may show symptomatic hypocalcemia from fetal parathyroid suppression as a result of maternal hypercalcemia. The affected offspring of an unaffected mother may show rather severe neonatal hypercalcemia because of intrauterine secondary hyperparathyroidism; this will usually evolve into asymptomatic hypercalcemia without parathyroidectomy.

Family Screening. Because of the high penetrance for expression of hypercalcemia in FHH carriers, accurate genetic assignments can usually be made from one determination of total calcium (or preferably ionized or albumin-adjusted calcium). Family screening is particularly valuable to avoid unnecessary parathyroidectomy in those patients in whom hypercalcemia is initially recognized during blood testing for routine care. Genetic linkage testing and genomic analysis also have important roles.

CONCLUSIONS

Familial hypocalciuric hypercalcemia is a rather common cause of asymptomatic hypercalcemia, particularly when the hypercalcemia presents at early ages. The diagnosis requires alertness to urinary calcium. In the past, FHH was a common cause of unsuccessful parathyroidectomy. Although mild symptoms similar to those in typical primary hyperparathyroidism are quite common, virtually all patients should be followed without any intervention.

REFERENCES

1. Marx SJ, Attie MF, Levine MA, Spiegel AM, Downs RW Jr, Lasker RD: The hypocalciuric or benign variant of familial hypercalcemia: Clinical and biochemical features in fifteen kindreds. *Medicine* 60:397–412, 1981
2. Law WM Jr, Heath H III: Familial benign hypercalcemia (hypocalciuric hypercalcemia): Clinical and pathogenetic studies in 21 families. *Ann Intern Med* 102:511–519, 1985
3. Davies M, Klimiuk PS, Adams PH, Lumb GA, Anderson DC: Familial hypocalciuric hypercalcemia and acute pancreatitis. *Br Med J* 282:1029–1031, 1981
4. Kristiansen JH, Rødbro P, Christiansen C, Johansen J, Jensen JT: Familial hypocalciuric hypercalcemia. III. Bone mineral metabolism. *Clin Endocrinol* 26:713–716, 1987
5. Marx SJ, Spiegel AM, Brown EM, Koehler JO, Gardner DG, Brennan MF, Aurbach GD: Divalent cation metabolism. Familial hypocalciuric hypercalcemia versus typical primary hyperparathyroidism. *Am J Med* 65:235–242, 1978
6. Firek AF, Kao PC, Heath H III: Plasma intact parathyroid hormone (PTH) and PTH-related peptide in familial benign hypercalcemia: Greater responsiveness to endogenous PTH than in primary hyperparathyroidism. *J Clin Endocrinol Metab* 72:541–546, 1991
7. Kristiansen JH, Rødbro P, Christiansen C, Brochner MJ, Carl J: Familial hypocalciuric hypercalcemia. II. Intestinal calcium absorption and vitamin D metabolism. *Clin Endocrinol* 23:511–515, 1985
8. Thorgeirsson U, Costa J, Marx SJ: The parathyroid glands in familial hypocalciuric hypercalcemia. *Hum Pathol* 12:229–237, 1981
9. Law WM Jr, Carney JA, Heath H III: Parathyroid glands in familial benign hypercalcemia (familial hypocalciuric hypercalcemia). *Am J Med* 76:1021–1026, 1984
10. Marx SJ, Stock JL, Attie MF, Downs RW Jr, Gardner DG, Brown EM, Spiegel AM, Doppman JL, Brennan MF: Familial hypocalciuric hypercalcemia: Recognition among patients referred after unsuccessful parathyroid exploration. *Ann Intern Med* 92:351–356 1980
11. Orwoll E, Silbert J, McClung M: Asymptomatic neonatal familial hypercalcemia. *Pediatrics* 69:109–111, 1982
12. Marx SJ, Fraser D, Rapoport A: Familial hypocalciuric hypercalcemia. Mild expression of the gene in heterozygotes and severe expression in homozygotes. *Am J Med* 78:15–22, 1985
13. Chou Y-HW, Brown EM, Levi T, Crowe G, Atkinson AB, Arnqvist H, Toss G, Fuleihan GEH, Seidman JG, Seidman CE: The gene responsible for familial hypocalciuric hypercalcemia maps to chromosome 3q in four unrelated families. *Nature Genet* 1:295–300, 1992
14. Heath H III, Jackson CE, Otterud B, Leppart MF: Familial benign hypercalcemia (FBH) phenotype results from mutations at two distant loci on chromosomes 3q and 19p. *Clin Res* 41:270A, 1993
15. Marx SJ, Attie MF, Spiegel AM, Levine MA, Lasker RD, Fox M: An association between neonatal severe primary hyperparathyroidism and familial hypocalciuric hypercalcemia in three kindreds. *N Engl J Med* 306:257–264, 1982
16. Pollak MR, Chou YH-W, Marx SJ, et al.: Familial hypocalciuric hypercalcemia and neonatal severe hyperparathyroidism: Effects of mutant gene dosage on phenotype. *J Clin Invest* 93:1108–1112, 1994
17. Eftekhari F, Yousefzadeh DK: Primary infantile hyperparathyroidism: Clinical, laboratory, and radiographic features in 21 cases. *Skeletal Radiol* 8:201–208, 1982
18. Page LA, Haddow JE: Self-limited neonatal hyperparathyroidism in familial hypocalciuric hypercalcemia. *J Pediatr* 111:261–264, 1987
19. Marx SJ, Lasker RD, Brown EM, Fitzpatrick LA, Sweezey NB, Goldbloom RB, Gillis DA, Cole DE: Secretory dysfunction in parathyroid cells from a neonate with severe primary hyperparathyroidism. *J Clin Endocrinol Metab* 62:445–449, 1986
20. Attie MF, Gill JR Jr, Stock JL, Spiegel AM, Downs RW Jr, Levine MA, Marx SJ: Urinary calcium excretion in familial hypocalciuric hypercalcemia. Persistence of relative hypocalciuria after induction of hypoparathyroidism. *J Clin Invest* 72:667–676, 1983
21. Brown EM, Pollak M, Seidman CE, et al.: Calcium-ion-sensing cell-surface receptors. *N Engl J Med* 333:234–240, 1995

31. Tertiary Hyperparathyroidism and Refractory Secondary Hyperparathyroidism

Susan C. Galbraith, M.D., and *L. Darryl Quarles, M.D.

Department of Medicine, Division of Endocrinology, Yale University School of Medicine, New Haven, Connecticut
*Department of Medicine, Division of Nephrology, Duke University Medical Center, Durham, North Carolina

Hyperparathyroidism is characterized by elevated circulating levels of parathyroid hormone (PTH) that may be due to impaired sensitivity of PTH secretion to extracellular calcium (i.e., altered calcium sensing), augmented PTH production per cell (i.e., hypertrophy), and/or an expanded number of PTH-producing cells (i.e., hyperplasia). Differences in the underlying pathophysiology leading to PTH overproduction permit subclassification of hyperparathyroidism (HPT) into hereditary, primary, and secondary hyperparathyroidism. Familial hypocalciuric hypercalcemia and neonatal severe HPT (see Chapter 29) are characterized by impaired calcium sensing resulting from heterozygous and homozygous mutations, respectively, that inactivate the parathyroid cell surface calcium-sensing receptor (CaR).

Primary HPT (see Chapter 28) is characterized functionally by an insensitivity to calcium-mediated suppression of PTH secretion, and morphologically by glandular enlargement resulting from adenomatous transformation or diffuse hyperplasia of PTH-secreting cells. Secondary HPT, in contrast, is an acquired disorder representing an adaptive physiologic response to perturbations in calcium metabolism that, depending on its severity, may manifest variable degrees of abnormal calcium sensing, hypertrophy, and hyperplasia of the parathyroid gland. Prolonged abnormalities in calcium metabolism may eventually result in the evolution of secondary HPT to a state of apparent autonomous PTH secretion resembling primary HPT. Traditionally, *tertiary HPT* is a term used to describe patients with evolution of secondary HPT to autonomous PTH production, leading to elevated levels of serum calcium. *Refractory secondary HPT* defines another group of patients with severe secondary HPT without spontaneous hypercalcemia, who display nonsuppressible PTH secretion after correcting the inciting metabolic abnormalities [namely, hypocalcemia, hyperphosphatemia, and calcitriol deficiency (see following sections)]. In both tertiary and refractory secondary HPT, the parathyroid gland has reached a hyperfunctioning state that no longer responds appropriately to physiologic regulation.

PARATHYROID HORMONE–1,25-DIHYDROXYVITAMIN D AXIS

The hormonal actions of PTH increase serum calcium levels by mobilizing calcium from bone, enhancing reabsorption of calcium in the distal renal tubule, and increasing production of 1,25-dihydroxyvitamin D_3 [1,25(OH)$_2$D$_3$] in the kidney (see Chapters 9,11). 1,25(OH)$_2$D$_3$, in turn, enhances calcium uptake by the intestine, augments the osseous effects of PTH, and directly modulates parathyroid gland activity (see Chapter 13) (1). Overall, the amount of PTH released into the circulation by the parathyroid gland is determined by the rate of PTH secretion and synthesis, as well as by the number of PTH-producing cells. Calcium regulates parathyroid gland function through activation of the parathyroid cell surface G-protein-coupled calcium receptor (CaR) (2). Cation activation of CaR results in a parallel increase in intracellular calcium, which acts as a second messenger in control of PTH secretion and production. Changes in serum calcium levels also modulate cellular PTH synthesis at the level of pre-pro-PTH transcription (1) and may directly regulate parathyroid cell proliferation as well (3,4). In contrast, 1,25(OH)$_2$D$_3$ has no acute effects on PTH secretion but displays potent suppressive effects on PTH gene transcription and cell growth that are mediated by the vitamin D receptor, a classic nuclear steroid receptor. 1,25(OH)$_2$D$_3$ deficiency is sufficient to stimulate parathyroid gland hyperplasia in normocalcemic dogs, and administration of calcitriol can prevent parathyroid gland hyperplasia in animal models of secondary HPT (1,5–7). Vitamin D has a marked inhibitory effect on cellular proliferation in culture. Furthermore, vitamin D, but not calcium, downregulates expression of proto-oncogenes associated with cellular proliferation in parathyroid tissue and other cell models (8). The frequent association of vitamin D deficiency and hypocalcemia in many subjects with parathyroid hyperplasia (particularly those with uremia), however, makes separating the effects of vitamin D and calcium on glandular proliferation difficult to accomplish *in vivo*. 1,25(OH)$_2$D$_3$ also may have nongenomic effects on intracellular calcium concentrations, but the clinical significance of this pathway in the regulation of PTH secretion and synthesis is not clear. Finally, parathyroid-secreting cells display a basal, nonsuppressible component of PTH production that allows parathyroid hyperplasia to contribute significantly to increased circulating PTH levels in the absence of abnormalities in calcium and 1,25(OH)$_2$D$_3$ homeostasis.

PATHOGENESIS OF TERTIARY/REFRACTORY SECONDARY HYPERPARATHYROIDISM

There are several changes in the parathyroid gland at the tissue, cellular, and molecular levels that potentially explain the inability to restore PTH secretion to normal in some patients with secondary HPT. The most important factors appear to be an increased number of parathyroid cells, possible alterations in the calcium-sensing mechanism, and abnormalities of vitamin D receptor function. Additionally, end-organ resistance to PTH actions may contribute to persistent HPT in spite of calcium and vitamin D treatment.

Role of Increased Gland Size. An increased number of parathyroid cells having a nonsuppressible basal component of PTH secretion and a limited capacity to involute contribute to the genesis of tertiary/refractory secondary HPT. The idea that the parathyroid gland mass may be an important determinant of PTH hypersecretion is supported by several observations. Excessive amounts of normal parathyroid tissue implanted into rats produces hypercalcemia resulting from nonsuppressible basal circulating PTH levels (9–11), suggesting that an increase in the number of cells secreting basal amounts of PTH can overcome the normal homeostatic mechanisms controlling steady-state serum PTH levels. Clinical studies also illustrate that refractoriness to therapy correlates with the degree of parathyroid gland enlargement. In a series describing the histologic features of 128 parathyroid glands taken from patients with chronic renal insufficiency, the parathyroid glands of subjects with tertiary HPT were usually larger than those from patients with secondary HPT (12). The average weight of a single gland from patients with tertiary HPT was 25 times the weight of a normal parathyroid gland (12). Other studies have found a significant correlation between parathyroid gland size and the degree of PTH nonsuppressibility in chronic renal failure patients with refractory HPT (13). Moreover, PTH-secreting cells have a long life span with a limited ability to involute (undergo apoptosis), resulting in persistently increased cell numbers (11). A variety of clinical studies have found that unsuccessful treatment of uremic HPT is associated with a failure to reduce parathyroid gland size (13), whereas successful therapy correlates with a reduction in gland mass (14,15).

Phenotypic Alterations of the Parathyroid Gland in Tertiary Hyperparathyroidism. In addition to having an increased number of parathyroid chief cells, refractory/tertiary secondary HPT is often characterized by phenotypic alteration in the parathyroid gland that may contribute to refractoriness to therapy. In this regard, a nodular histologic pattern that is a marker of chief cell transformation is frequently found in patients with tertiary HPT. Nodular hyperplastic gland mass tends to be greater than diffusely hyperplastic glands, and nodules are more common in the glands of patients with tertiary than with secondary HPT (12). Furthermore, nodular hyperplastic tissue has altered regulation of PTH secretion compared with diffuse hyperplastic tissue, displaying a degree of insensitivity to calcium that resembles regulatory characteristics of primary adenomas (16–18). Autotransplantation of nodular hyperplastic glands may predispose to recurrent HPT following parathyroidectomy (see following). Immunohistochemical studies have provided evidence that cells within a nodule are derived from a monoclonal proliferation of a single parathyroid cell (19). Parathyroid nodules, which superficially resemble adenomatous transformation, may therefore represent clonal selection of abnormal PTH-secreting cells resulting from prolonged stimulus for parathyroid cell replication. Recent work using X-chromosome inactivation analysis to evaluate parathyroid tissue clonality in patients with end-stage renal disease and refractory secondary HPT showed that 64% of patients studied had at least one monoclonal parathyroid tumor (20). Acquired clonal transformation is also supported by recent studies showing molecular defects similar to those found in parathyroid adenomas and multiple endocrine neoplasia (MEN)-associated hyperplasia (20) in parathyroid tissues obtained from patients with tertiary HPT (21–23). Indeed, allelic loss of chromosome 11, which is the location of the MEN-I gene and is associated with primary parathyroid hyperplasia (22), is occasionally observed in glands from patients with tertiary HPT (21).

These abnormalities in cell number and control of proliferation may be linked to abnormalities in PTH secretory control. Ultrastructural studies of hyperplastic glands derived from patients with tertiary HPT reveal evidence of increased cellular machinery for production and secretion of hormone as well as an increased number of cells (10,24). Likewise, molecular studies in animal models note an increase in PTH mRNA content per cell consistent with increased PTH synthesis contributing to the hyperparathyroid state (25,26). Regardless, prolonged physiologic stimuli for polyclonal parathyroid hyperplasia may eventually result in monoclonal hyperplasia, possibly with the monoclonal cells displaying a more autonomous phenotype.

Role of Abnormal Calcium Sensing (Altered Setpoint). Impaired ability to sense changes in extracellular calcium plays a role in the pathogenesis of primary HPT and familial hypocalciuric hypercalcemia (FHH). Recently, workers have found mutations in the CaR gene in families with FHH, a condition in which elevated serum calcium is associated with an altered calcium setpoint and inappropriate PTH secretion (27,28) (see Chapter 30). Functionally, alterations in the CaR result in a rightward shift in the relationship between plasma PTH and ionized calcium (29). Similar shifts in the setpoint are also observed in primary HPT, though the molecular mechanisms underlying impaired calcium sensing remain to be established. To date, there have been no documented somatic mutations of CaR in either parathyroid adenomas or uremic secondary HPT. Indeed, the cloned CaR cDNA from a primary parathyroid adenoma lacks any coding-region mutation, and it was shown to have functional properties similar to that of normal parathyroid CaR cDNA when expressed in *Xenopus* oocytes (28). Recently, nonfunctional isoforms have been identified in glands derived from several patients with primary HPT (28), suggesting the possibility that modulation of CaR biosynthesis through alternative RNA processing may play a role in impaired calcium sensing.

Regardless, abnormalities in the calcium-sensing mechanism could be involved in the pathogenesis of tertiary/refractory secondary HPT. Studies of isolated parathyroid cells indicate that the calcium setpoint in parathyroid tissue derived from tertiary HPT is intermediate between that of normal and that of adenomatous glands (30,31). However, no differences in the parathyroid gland CaR mRNA levels were observed in animal models of secondary HPT (32). Moreover, the alteration in setpoint in patients with tertiary/secondary HPT is not uniform between patients with similar pathology, between glands removed from the same patient, or even between cells from the same gland (30). In this regard, analysis of the relationship between plasma PTH and ionized calcium in end-stage renal disease patients with secondary HPT of moderate severity failed to demonstrate a shift to the right of the curve, inconsistent with the notion of a simple setpoint error (33). Setpoint alterations, and abnormalities in CaR, in patients with secondary HPT may be limited to glands with adenomatous transformation. In addition, the possibilities that posttranscriptional processing, downstream signaling pathways, changes in CaR promoter activity, or other mechanisms could be responsible for abnormal CaR function have not been examined in secondary HPT. Further studies are needed to evaluate the role of abnormal calcium sensing in the genesis of tertiary/refractory HPT.

Role of Abnormal Vitamin D Receptor Function. Studies investigating the mechanism of calcium insensitivity and calcitriol resistance in secondary HPT have identified a possible role for persistent abnormalities in vitamin D homeostasis. The importance of vitamin D is reflected by the observation that vitamin-D-deficient rats are unable to modulate PTH mRNA levels in response to alterations of ambient calcium (25). Likewise, a change in calcium setpoint has been seen in a population of vitamin-D-deficient uremic patients with normal serum calcium levels (34). In patients with uremic HPT, down-regulation of the vitamin D receptor (VDR) number and impaired VDR binding to the vitamin D response element (35) likely contribute to calcitriol resistance. The concentration of VDR in the parathyroid tissue of dialysis patients is reduced (36). Uremia may also impair the ability of calcitriol to induce the expression of VDR (37,38). Moreover, decreased VDR density is associated with more severe forms of parathyroid hyperplasia in end-stage renal disease (being lower in nodular than diffuse hyperplasia) (39). A reduction of receptors could account for the decreased effect of vitamin D on direct PTH suppression and on the parathyroid cell's response to ambient calcium concentration. Abnormalities in vitamin D receptor number are not sufficient to explain refractory HPT, however, because correction of both vitamin D deficiency and abnormalities in vitamin D receptor number by renal transplantation fails to cure tertiary/refractory HPT in a significant percentage of patients (36). Indeed, recent *in vitro* studies have found that an unidentified uremic factor impairs the binding of VDR to the vitamin D response element (35), suggesting that impaired VDR–DNA interactions may also contribute to refractory HPT in some settings.

Although the exact molecular mechanisms of tertiary/refractory secondary HPT remain to be defined, a combination of hyperplasia, hypertrophy, and dysregulated control of PTH secretion and production by calcium and vitamin D combine to produce a state in which PTH production remains excessive in spite of adequate replacement of calcium and calcitriol and control of serum phosphorus.

CLINICAL CONDITIONS ASSOCIATED WITH TERTIARY/REFRACTORY SECONDARY HYPERPARATHYROIDISM

Refractory secondary HPT has been observed in many chronic disorders of calcium and $1,25(OH)_2D_3$ metabolism, including those that are associated with end-stage renal disease (ESRD), nutritional vitamin D deficiency, high-dose phosphate treatment of chronic hypophosphatemic disorders, various vitamin-D-resistant/dependent states, and certain hepatobiliary diseases.

End-stage Renal Disease

The uremic state presents multiple stimuli to the parathyroid gland that cause secondary HPT. These include hyperphosphatemia, $1,25(OH)_2D_3$ deficiency, down-regulation of $1,25(OH)_2D_3$ receptors, altered calcium sensing (or setpoint), and hypocalcemia. The presence of HPT is defined in end-stage renal disease (ESRD) by a circulating level of intact PTH of approximately 185 pg/ml—the value associated with histologic evidence of increased bone remodeling (40,41). This upper limit is roughly threefold greater than that of circulating PTH levels in normal individuals (65 pg/ml). The upper limit of PTH is likely higher in uremia because of the end-organ resistance to PTH.

Uremic secondary HPT is a heterogeneous disorder characterized by variable suppressible PTH levels that are likely related to the degree of parathyroid gland hyperplasia. Uremic HPT can be grouped according to the degree of PTH nonsuppressibility into responsive, refractory, and tertiary HPT. Responsive patients are able to normalize serum PTH levels in response to correction of hyperphosphatemia, hypocalcemia, and calcitriol deficiency. Responsive subjects have minimal parathyroid gland enlargement and appear to display normal sensitivity to calcium-mediated PTH suppression. The major abnormality identified by dynamic testing is an increased capacity to secrete PTH in response to hypocalcemic stimuli (42). Tertiary HPT is clinically manifested by the presence of markedly elevated PTH levels with characteristic, high-turnover metabolic bone disease and spontaneous hypercalcemia. Today, only a few patients with ESRD develop tertiary HPT (roughly 5% in most series) (43). Its development is related to the duration of ESRD requiring dialysis, and probably to adenomatous transformation and/or alterations in calcium-sensing mechanisms (see following sections) that occur as the result of extended periods of inadequate therapy. Refractory HPT, defined by the inability to normalize serum PTH in spite of optimal medical therapy, occurs in 12% to 55% of chronic maintenance hemodialysis patients (44). This range is consistent with the reported 30% of hemodialysis patients treated with vitamin D analogs that display progression of HPT (43). Refractory patients have markedly elevated PTH similar to tertiary HPT but without hypercalcemia. In general, patients with tertiary or refractory secondary HPT have intact PTH levels exceeding 1500 pg/ml, though there is no absolute circulating PTH threshold for establishing this diagnosis. Although patients with tertiary HPT may have abnormalities in ability to sense calcium, recent studies indi-

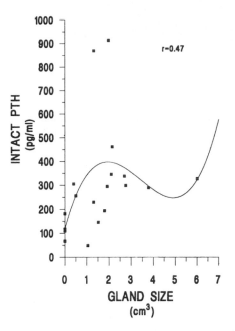

FIG. 1. Relationship between PTH suppression and estimated parathyroid gland size in chronic maintenance hemodialysis patients. Nineteen subjects with ESRD were maintained on thrice-weekly hemodialysis with 2.5 mEq/L calcium dialysate for 6 weeks before evaluating suppression of PTH by performing hemodialysis with a 3.5-mEq/L dialysis bath. The maximally suppressed serum PTH value (ending PTH expressed as percent of baseline) derived from such dynamic suppression was correlated with gland volume as estimated by magnetic resonance scanning or high-resolution ultrasound.

cate that most patients with refractory HPT do not have abnormalities of the calcium setpoint (33,40). Rather, the degree of PTH suppression in chronic hemodialysis patients is correlated with gland size as estimated by magnetic resonance imaging or high-resolution ultrasound (Fig. 1).

Renal transplantation may unmask tertiary/refractory HPT in patients with preexisting severe secondary HPT of long duration. Indeed, hypercalcemia has been reported to occur in as many as one third of successfully transplanted subjects (45,46). The restoration of $1,25(OH)_2D_3$ production by the renal allograft and amelioration of end-organ resistance to PTH may increase the susceptibility to hypercalcemia during the slow involution of hypersecreting parathyroid glands. Autopsy specimens taken from transplant patients without clinically evident HPT confirm that parathyroid gland hyperplasia does not rapidly resolve, even with the nearly normal metabolic milieu resulting from transplantation (47). In addition, the degree of elevation of PTH following hypocalcemic stimulation correlates with the residual parathyroid gland volume in renal transplant subjects (48).

Vitamin-D-Resistant/Dependent States

Large doses of oral phosphorous used to treat children with X-linked hypophosphatemic rickets can result in chronic stimulation of PTH secretion via lowering of the serum ionized calcium. A subset of these patients appear to develop tertiary HPT associated with diffuse parathyroid gland hyperplasia. Occasionally, parathyroid adenomas are observed. It is not clear whether these adenomas represent concurrence of primary HPT or monoclonal expansion derived from diffuse hyperplasia. In any event, subtotal parathyroidectomy and, more recently, total parathyroidectomy with autotransplantation have been effectively used to decrease functional parathyroid mass in these children (49).

Vitamin-D-Deficient States

Chronic vitamin D deficiency has been shown to result in refractory HPT. Detailed studies of a cohort of vitamin-D-deficient Asian vegetarians revealed inability to suppress PTH levels completely, even after a full year of therapy with calcium and calcitriol (48). The duration of parathyroid stimulation may be essential to development of a nonsuppressible state, because treatment of vitamin-D-deficient children with calcium and vitamin D typically results in rapid normalization of elevated PTH levels (51). Unlike that associated with ESRD and treatment of hypophosphatemic disorders, the HPT of chronic dietary vitamin D deficiency is mild to moderate.

Hepatobiliary Disorders

A similar cause of PTH hypersecretion has been postulated in patients with primary biliary cirrhosis, a disease state characterized by low $25(OH)D$ and $1,25(OH)_2D_3$ levels (secondary to inability of the liver to convert vitamin D effectively to $25(OH)D$ via vitamin D 25-hydroxylase). A group of patients with primary biliary cirrhosis who had been adequately supplemented with calcium and $1,25(OH)_2D_3$ were found to have an average PTH level significantly higher than normal controls. Thirty percent of the patients had a PTH level above the normal range (52). Again, severe hypercalcemia was absent, and other clinical manifestations of HPT were not severe enough to warrant parathyroidectomy in this group of patients.

THERAPY

Controversy exists over the role of $1,25(OH)_2D_3$ in the management of refractory HPT disorders. Although by definition these disorders are resistant to medical therapy, earlier studies suggested that high-dose intravenous calcitriol administration might effectively accomplish a "medical" parathyroidectomy (53). These initial results, however, have not been substantiated by controlled studies (13,44). Although there may be some advantage of the pulse administration of $1,25(OH)_2D_3$ by either the intravenous or the oral route (44), more recent studies suggest that pharmacologic calcitriol therapy, regardless of route of administration, is poorly tolerated (50% of subjects developed hypercalcemia and 75% developed hyperphosphatemia) and often ineffective in suppressing elevated PTH levels in chronic maintenance hemodialysis patients (44).

Cure of tertiary/refractory HPT requires surgical interventions designed to "debulk" the parathyroid gland. Surgical treatment is indicated in symptomatic patients with nonsuppressible serum PTH levels. Symptoms may include those related to hypercalcemia, hyperparathyroid bone disease, nephrocalcinosis, and nephrolithiasis. In ESRD patients, intractable pruritus, severe hyperphosphatemia, calciphylaxis, and soft-tissue calcification may be additional indications. In renal transplant patients with persistent HPT, serum calcium levels >12.5 mg/dl after 1 year, and progressive and unexplained renal insufficiency in the setting of hypercalcemia, are usual indications for parathyroidectomy. Patients with persistently elevated circulating PTH concentrations, but without hypercalcemia or symptoms, after intensive medical therapy are often managed expectantly, like patients with asymptomatic primary HPT. There are, however, no controlled studies that evaluate the relative benefit of conservative management of asymptomatic refractory HPT compared to parathyroidectomy.

Early approaches used subtotal parathyroidectomy that reduced parathyroid mass by approximately seven-eighths. With this procedure, some patients remained hyperparathyroid, requiring a second neck exploration for further tissue removal. Another alternative is total parathyroidectomy and autografting of parathyroid tissue fragments into the muscle of the forearm (54). The advantages of this procedure are lower failure rates and ability to reduce further parathyroid mass without further neck exploration. The disadvantages are the occasional induction of hypoparathyroidism and, rarely, continued tertiary HPT resulting from adenomatous growth of fragments reimplanted in the arm (55). Perhaps the ability to determine clonality in hyperplastic parathyroid tissue will someday enable a surgeon to avoid autotransplantation of potentially autonomous parathyroid tissue. The exception to the use of parathyroid autografting may be the renal transplant patient with HPT. In transplant patients, in order to minimize the risk of hypoparathyroidism, some clinicians prefer subtotal parathyroidectomy.

REFERENCES

1. Silver J: Regulation of parathyroid hormone synthesis and secretion. In: Coe FL, Favus MJ (eds) *Disorders of Bone and Mineral Metabolism.* Raven Press, New York, pp 83–105, 1992
2. Brown EM, Gamba G, Riccardi D, et al.: Cloning and characterization of an extracellular Ca^{2+}-sensing receptor from bovine parathyroid. *Nature* 366:575–580, 1993
3. Roth SK, Raisz LG: The course and reversibility of the calcium effect on the ultrastructure of the rat parathyroid gland in organ culture. *Lab Invest* 15:1187–1211, 1966
4. Brandi ML, Fitzpatrick LA, Coon HG, Aurbach GD: Bovine parathyroid cells: Cultures maintained for more than 140 population doublings. *Proc Natl Acad Sci* 83:1709–1713, 1986
5. Hendy GN, Stotland MA, Grunbaum D, Fraher LJ, Loveridge N, Goltzman D: Characteristics of secondary hyperparathyroidism in vitamin D-deficient dogs. *Am J Physiol* 256: E765–E772, 1989
6. Szabo A, Merke J, Beier E, Mall G, Ritz E: $1,25(OH)_2$ vitamin D_3 inhibits parathyroid cell proliferation in experimental uremia. *Kidney Int* 35:1049–1056, 1989
7. Nygren P, Larsson R, Johansson H, Ljunghall S, Rastad J, Akerstrom G: $1,25(OH)_2D_3$ inhibits hormone secretion and proliferation but not functional dedifferentiation of cultured bovine parathyroid cells. *Calcif Tissue Int* 43:213–218, 1988

8. Kremer R, Bolivar I, Goltzman D, Hendy GN: Influence of calcium and 1,25-dihydroxycholecalciferol on proliferation and proto-oncogene expression in primary cultures of bovine parathyroid cells. *Endocrinology* 125:935–941, 1989

9. Gittes RF, Radde IC: Experimental model for hyperparathyroidism: Effect of excessive numbers of transplanted isologous parathyroid glands. *J Urol* 95:595–603, 1966

10. Mayer GP, Habener JF, Potts JT Jr: Parathyroid hormone secretion in vivo: Demonstration of a calcium-independent, nonsuppressible component of secretion. *J Clin Invest* 57:678–683, 1976

11. Parfitt AM: Hypercalcemic hyperparathyroidism following renal transplantation: Differential diagnosis, management, and implications for cell population control in the parathyroid gland. *Miner Electrolyte Metab* 8:92–112, 1982

12. Krause MW, Hedinger CE: Pathologic study of parathyroid glands in tertiary hyperparathyroidism. *Hum Pathol* 16:772–784, 1985

13. Quarles LD, Yohay DA, Carroll BA, Spritzer CE, Minda SA, Bartholomay D, Lobaugh B: Prospective trial of pulse oral versus intravenous calcitriol treatment of hyperparathyroidism in ESRD. *Kidney Int* 45:1710–1721, 1994

14. Fukagawa M, Okazaki R, Takano K, et al.: Regression of parathyroid hyperplasia by calcitriol-pulse therapy in patients on long-term dialysis. *N Engl J Med* 323:421–422, 1990

15. Hoyodo T, Koumi T, Ueda M, et al.: Can oral 1,25(OH)$_2$D$_3$ therapy reduce parathyroid hyperplasia? *Nephron* 59:171–172, 1991

16. Rudberg C, Akerstrom G, Ljunghall S, et al.: Regulation of parathyroid hormone release in primary and secondary hyperparathyroidism—studies in vivo and in vitro. *Acta Endocrinol* 101:408–413, 1982

17. Rudberg C, Grimelius L, Johansson II, et al.: Alteration in density, morphology and parathyroid hormone release of dispersed parathyroid cells from patients with hyperparathyroidism. *Acta Pathol Microbiol Immunol Scand* 94:253–261, 1986

18. Wallfelt C, Larsson, R, Gylfe E, Ljunghall S, Rastad J, Akerstrom G: Secretory disturbance in hyperplastic parathyroid nodules of uremic hyperparathyroidism: Implication for parathyroid autotransplantation. *World J Surg* 12:431–438, 1988

19. Oka T, Yoshioka T, Shrestha GR, et al.: Immunohistochemical study of nodular hyperplastic parathyroid glands in patients with secondary hyperparathyroidism. *Virchows Archiv A Pathol Anat* 413:53–60, 1988

20. Arnold A, Brown MF, Urena P, Gaz RD, Sarfati E, Drueke TB: Monoclonality of parathyroid tumors in chronic renal failure and in primary parathyroid hyperplasia. *J Clin Invest* 95:2047–2053, 1995

21. Falchetti A, Bale AE, Amorosi A, et al.: Progression of uremic hyperparathyroidism involves allelic loss on chromosome 11. *J Clin Endo Metab* 76:139–144, 1993

22. Friedman E, Sakaguchi K, Bale AE, et al.: Clonality of parathyroid tumors in familial multiple endocrine neoplasia type I. *N Engl J Med* 321:213–218, 1989

23. Thakker RV, Bouloux P, Wooding C, et al.: Association of parathyroid tumors in multiple endocrine neoplasia type I with loss of alleles on chromosome 11. *N Engl J Med* 321:218–324, 1989

24. Svensson O, Wernerson A, Reinholt FP: Effect of calcium depletion on the rat parathyroids. *Bone Miner* 3:259–269, 1988

25. Naveh-Many T, Silver J: Regulation of parathyroid hormone gene expression by hypocalcemia, hypercalcemia, and vitamin D in the rat. *J Clin Invest* 86:1313–1319, 1990

26. Fukagawa M, Kaname S-Y, Igarashi T, Ogata E, Kurokawa K: Regulation of parathyroid hormone synthesis in chronic renal failure in rats. *Kidney Int* 39:874–881, 1991

27. Pollak MR, Brown EM, Chou Y-HC, et al.: Mutations in the human Ca^{2+}-sensing receptor gene cause familial hypo-calciuric hypercalcemia and neonatal severe hyperparathyroidism. *Cell* 75:1297–1303, 1993

28. Garrett JE, Capuano IV, Hammerland LG, et al.: Molecular cloning and functional expression of human parathyroid calcium receptor cDNAs. *J Biol Chem* 270:12919–12925, 1995

29. Kholsa S, Ebeling PR, Firek AF, Burritt MM, Kao PC, Heath H III: Calcium infusion suggests a set-point abnormality of parathyroid gland function in familial benign hypercalemia and more complex disturbances in primary hyperparathyroidism. *J Clin Endocrinol Metab* 76:715–720, 1993

30. Brown EM, Wilson RE, Eastman RC, Pallotta J, Marynick SP: Abnormal regulation of parathyroid hormone release by calcium in secondary hyperparathyroidism due to chronic renal failure. *J Clin Endocrinol Metab* 54:172–179, 1982

31. Wallfelt C, Gylfe E, Larsson R, Ljunghall S, Rastad J, Akerstrom G: Relationship between external and cytoplasmic calcium concentrations, parathyroid hormone release and weight of parathyroid glands in human hyperparathyroidism. *J Endocrinol* 116:457–464, 1988

32. Fox J, Brown EM, Hebert HC, Robers KV: Parathyroid gland calcium receptor gene expression is unaffected by chronic renal failure or low dietary calcium in rats *(abstract)*. *J Am Soc Nephrol* 5:879, 1994

33. Ramirez JA, Goodman WG, Gornbein J, Menezes C, Moulton L, Segre GV, Salusky IB: Direct in vivo comparison of calcium-regulated parathyroid hormone secretion in normal volunteers and patients with secondary hyperparathyroidism. *J Clin Endocrinol Metab* 76:1489–1494, 1993

34. Lopez-Hilker S, Galceran T, Chan Y-L, Rapp N, Martin KJ, Slatopolsky E: Hypocalcemia may not be essential for the development of secondary hyperparathyroidism in chronic renal failure. *J Clin Invest* 78:1097–1102, 1986

35. Patel SR, Ke H-Q, Vanholder R, Koenig RJ, Hsu CH: Inhibition of calcitriol receptor binding to vitamin D response elements by uremic toxins. *J Clin Invest* 96:50–59, 1995

36. Korkor AB: Reduced binding of [3H]1,25-dihydroxyvitamin D3 in the parathyroid glands of patients with renal failure. *N Engl J Med* 316:1573–1577, 1987

37. Hsu CH, Patel RS, Vanholder R: Mechanism of decreased intestinal calcitriol receptor concentration in renal failure. *Am J Physiol* 264:F662–F669, 1993

38. Naveh-Many T, Marx R, Keshet E, Pike JW, Silver J: Regulation of 1,25-dihydroxyvitamin D3 receptor gene expression by 1,25-dihydroxyvitamin D3 in the parathyroid in vivo. *J Clin Invest* 86:1968–1975, 1990

39. Fukuda N, Tanaka H, Tominaga Y, Fukagawa M, Kurokawa K, Seino Y: Decreased 1,25-dihydroxyvitamin D3 receptor density is associated with a more severe form of parathyroid hyperplasia in chronic uremic patients. *J Clin Invest* 92:1436–1443, 1993

40. Quarles LD, Lobaugh B, Murphy G: Intact parathyroid hormone overestimates the presence and severity of parathyroid-mediated osseous abnormalities in uremia. *J Clin Endocrinol Metab* 75:145–150, 1992

41. Salusky IB, Ramirez JA, Oppenheim W, Gales B, Segre GV, Goodman WG: Biochemical markers of renal osteodystrophy in pediatric patients undergoing CAPD/CCPD. *Kidney Int* 45:253–258, 1994

42. Messa P, Vallone C, Mioni G, Geatti O, Turrin D, Passoni N, Cruciatti A: Direct in vivo assessment of parathyroid hormone-calcium relationship curve in renal patients. *Kidney Int* 46:1713–1720, 1994

43. Mizumoto D, Watanabe Y, Fukuzawa Y, Yuzawa Y, Yamazaki C: Identification of risk factors on secondary hyperparathyroidism undergoing long-term haemodialysis with vitamin D3. *Nephrol Dial Transplant* 9:1751–1758, 1994

44. Indridason OS, Quarles LD: Oral versus intravenous calcitriol: Is the route of administration really important? *Current Opinion Neph Hyper* 1996 *(in press)*

45. David DS, Sakai S, Brennan BL, et al.: Hypercalcemia after renal transplantation: Long-term follow-up data. *N Engl J Med* 289:398–401, 1973

46. Cundy T, Kanis JA, Heynen G, Morris PJ, Oliver DO: Calcium metabolism and hyperparathyroidism after renal transplantation. *Quart J Med* 205:67–78, 1983

47. Diethelm AG, Edwards RP, Whelchel JD: The natural history and surgical treatment of hypercalcemia before and after renal transplantation. *Surgery* 154:481–490, 1982

48. McCarron DA, Muther RS, Lenfesty B, Bennet WM: Parathyroid function in persistent hyperparathyroidism: Relationship to gland size. *Kidney Int* 22:662–670, 1982

49. Kinder BK, Rasmussen H: New applications of total parathyroidectomy and autotransplantation: Use in proximal renal tubular dysfunction. *World J Surg* 9:156–164, 1985

50. Dandona P, Mohiuddin J, Weerakoon JW, Freedman DB, Fonseca V, Healey T: Persistence of parathyroid hypersecretion after vitamin D treatment in Asian vegetarians. *J Clin Endocrinol Metab* 59:535–537, 1984

51. Joffe BI, Hackeng WH, Seftel HC, Hartdegen RG: Parathyroid hormone concentrations in nutritional ricketts. *Clin Sci* 42:113–116, 1972

52. Fonseca V, Epstein O, Gill DS, et al.: Hyperparathyroidism and low serum osteocalcin despite vitamin D replacement in primary biliary cirrhosis. *J Clin Endocrinol Metab* 64:873–877, 1987

53. Slatopolsky E, Weerts C, Thielan J, Horst R, Harter M, Martin KJ: Marked suppression of secondary hyperparathyroidism by intravenous administration of 1,25-dihydroxy-cholecalciferol in uremic patients. *J Clin Invest* 74:2136–2143, 1984

54. Wells SA, Gunnells JE, Shelburne JD, Schneider AB, Sherwood LM: Transplantation of the parathyroid glands in man: Clinical indications and results. *Surgery* 78:34–44, 1975

55. Brennan MF, Brown EM, Marx SJ, et al.: Recurrent hyperparathyroidism from an autotransplanted parathyroid adenoma. *N Engl J Med* 299:1057–1059, 1978

32. Humoral Hypercalcemia of Malignancy

Andrew F. Stewart, M.D.

Department of Endocrinology, Yale University School of Medicine, New Haven, Connecticut; and Connecticut Veterans Affairs Medical Center, West Haven, Connecticut

The term *humoral hypercalcemia of malignancy* (HHM) describes, in broad terms, a clinical syndrome characterized by hypercalcemia which is caused by the secretion by a cancer of a circulating calcemic factor. The tumor typically has limited or no skeletal involvement. The term describes a classic endocrine system, with the "secretory gland" being the tumor and the "target organs" being the skeleton and the kidney. The term can be used in a general sense to describe the production by tumors of any humoral calcemic factor. For example, hypercalcemia resulting from the production of 1,25-dihydroxyvitamin D [$1,25(OH)_2D$] in patients with lymphoma, and hypercalcemia resulting from ectopic secretion of parathyroid hormone by an ovarian carcinoma, would both fulfill the literal criteria for being humoral forms of hypercalcemia. These examples are discussed further at the conclusion of this chapter. As currently used, however, the term *HHM* describes a very specific clinical syndrome that results from the production of parathyroid-hormone-related protein (PTHrP) (see Chapters 12,18). The large majority of patients with humorally mediated hypercalcemia have HHM. Several recent detailed reviews of the syndrome are listed at the end of this section.

The syndrome was first described in 1941, in a patient with a renal carcinoma and a solitary skeletal metastasis. Subsequent studies in the 1950s and 1960s documented the humoral nature of the syndrome by demonstrating that (i) typical patients had little or no skeletal tumor involvement, and (ii) the hypercalcemia and other biochemical abnormalities reversed when the tumor was resected or treated. Evidence provided in the 1960s and 1970s suggested that the responsible factor was either prostaglandin E_2, a vitamin-D-like sterol, or parathyroid hormone. It is now clear that none of these are responsible.

From a clinical standpoint, patients with HHM have advanced disease with tumors that are usually obvious clinically and, therefore, carry a poor prognosis. As a rule, by the time hypercalcemia occurs in a patient with cancer, survival can be measured in weeks to a few months. Exceptions to this rule include small, well-differentiated endocrine tumors such as a pheochromocytomas or islet cell tumors. In contrast

to patients with hypercalcemia due to skeletal involvement with cancer (see Chapter 33), who typically have breast cancer, multiple myeloma, or lymphomas, patients with HHM most often have squamous carcinomas (involving lung, esophagus, cervix, vulva, skin, or head and neck). Other tumor types commonly associated with HHM are renal, bladder, and ovarian carcinomas. Breast carcinomas may cause typical HHM or they may lead to hypercalcemia through skeletal metastatic involvement. Finally, the subset of hypercalcemic patients with lymphomas due to human T-cell leukemia virus I appear to have classic biochemical HHM. Patients with HHM account for up to 80% of patients with malignancy-associated hypercalcemia. Certain common tumors (e.g., colon, prostate, thyroid, oat cell, and gastric carcinomas) rarely cause hypercalcemia of any type.

Biochemically and histologically, patients with HHM share certain features with patients with primary hyperparathyroidism (HPT), and differ in other respects (Table 1) (Fig. 1). Both groups of patients have a humoral syndrome, both are hypercalcemic, and both are hypophosphatemic and display reductions in the renal tubular phosphorus threshold.

TABLE 1. *Similarities and differences between patients with primary hyperparathyroidism (HPT) and HHM*

	HPT	HHM
Humorally mediated hypercalcemia	+	+
Hypophosphatemia	+	+
Phosphaturia	+	+
Nephrogenous cAMP elevation	+	+
Increased osteoclastic bone resorption	+	+
Increased renal calcium reabsorption	+	±
Increased plasma $1,25(OH)_2D$	+	−
Increased osteoblastic bone formation	+	−
Increased circulating immunoreactive PTH	+	−
Increased circulating immunoreactive PTHrP	−	+
Hypercalcemia due primarily to effects on kidney and GI tract	+	−
Hypercalcemia due primarily to bone resorption	−	+

Both groups display increased nephrogenous or urinary cyclic AMP excretion, indicating an interaction of the respective humoral mediator with proximal tubular PTH receptors. Both groups display increases in osteoclastic bone resorption when bone is examined histologically (Fig. 2).

In contrast, patients with HHM differ from those with HPT in several important respects (Fig. 1) (Table 1). PTH is a potent stimulus for distal tubular calcium reabsorption, and patients with HPT therefore display only modest hypercalciuria. In contrast, most patients with HHM demonstrate marked increases in calcium excretion, perhaps reflecting a weaker effect of PTHrP on distal tubular calcium reabsorption. PTH is also a potent stimulus for the renal production of $1,25(OH)_2D$. Patients with HPT therefore often demonstrate increases in circulating $1,25(OH)_2D$ and a resultant increase in calcium absorption by the intestine. In contrast, patients with HHM display reductions in $1,25(OH)_2D$ values and in intestinal calcium absorption. The physiology underlying this observation is uncertain, because N-terminal

PTHrPs *in vitro* and *in vivo* stimulate renal 1α-hydroxylase, the enzyme that synthesizes $1,25(OH)_2D$. Osteoblastic bone formation is increased and coupled to the increased bone resorption rate in patients with HPT (Fig. 2). In patients with HHM, osteoblastic bone formation, however, is reduced and is therefore dissociated or uncoupled from the increased osteoclastic bone resorption (Fig. 2). The reasons for this uncoupling are also unclear, because synthetic N-terminal PTHrPs *in vitro* and *in vivo* in animals stimulate osteoblastic activity. Of course, immunoreactive PTH concentrations in plasma are elevated in patients with HPT, but they are normal or suppressed, depending primarily on the assay employed, in patients with HHM (Fig. 3). Conversely, immunoreactive PTHrP values are elevated in HHM, but they are normal in patients with HPT (Fig. 4). Preliminary studies have suggested that the immunoreactive PTHrP concentration may be useful in monitoring responses to surgery, chemotherapy, or radiotherapy in patients in whom levels are elevated prior to therapy.

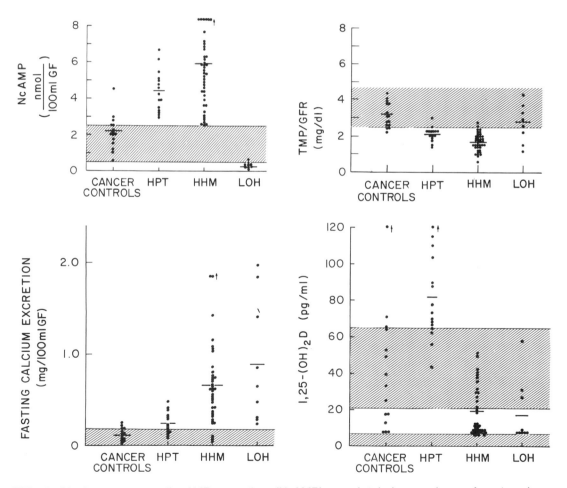

FIG. 1. Nephrogenous cyclic AMP excretion (NcAMP), renal tubular maximum for phosphorus (TmP/GFR), fasting calcium excretion, and plasma 1,25-dihydroxyvitamin D values in normocalcemic patients with cancer (cancer controls), and in patients with primary hyperparathyroidism (HPT), with humoral hypercalcemia of malignancy (HHM), and with hypercalcemia due to bone metastases or local osteolytic hypercalcemia (LOH). (Adapted from: Stewart AF, Horst R, Deftos LJ, Cadman EC, Lang R, Broadus AE. Biochemical evaluation of patients with cancer-associated hypercalcemia: Evidence for humoral and non-humoral groups. N Engl J Med 303:1377–1383, 1980, with permission.)

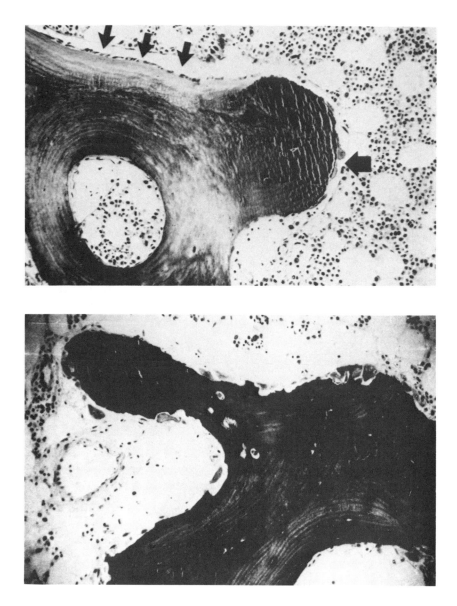

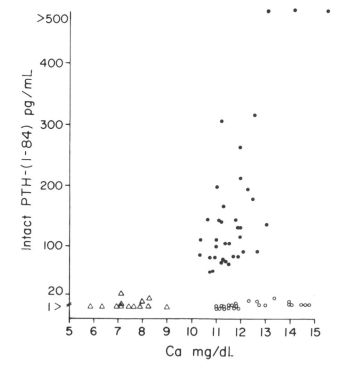

FIG. 2. Comparison of bone histology in a patient with HPT *(top panel)* and HHM *(bottom panel)*. In both groups, osteoclastic activity is accelerated, although it is higher in HHM than in HPT. In HPT, osteoblastic activity and osteoid are increased, but both are markedly decreased in HHM. It is this uncoupling of formation from resorption in HHM that plays the major role in causing hypercalcemia.

FIG. 3. Immunoreactive PTH concentration of PTH using a two-site immunoradiometric assay for PTH(1–84) in patients with primary hyperparathyroidism *(closed circles)*, in patients with hypoparathyroidism *(open triangles)*, and in patients with hypercalcemia of malignancy *(open circles)*. (From: Nussbaum S, Zahradnik RJ, Lavigne JR, et al. Highly sensitive two-site immunoradiometric assay of parathyrin and its clinical utility in evaluating patients with hypercalcemia. Clin Chem 33:1364–1367, 1987, with permission.)

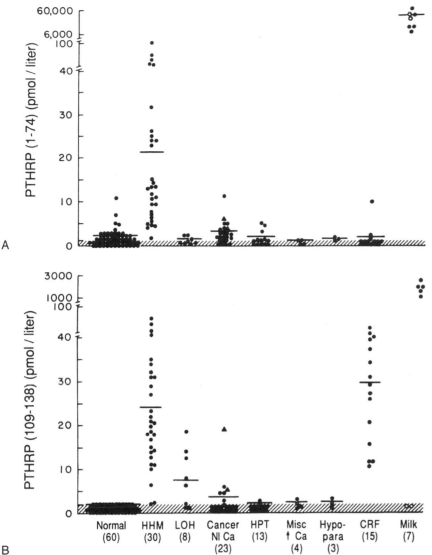

A

B

FIG. 4. Immunoreactive PTHrP values in patients with HHM and in various control groups. **A:** shows iPTHrP values obtained using a two-site immunoradiometric assay (IRMA) directed against PTHrP(1–74). **B:** shows iPTHrP values using a C-terminal PTHrP radioimmunoassay (RIA) directed against PTHrP(109–138). See Chapter 18 for a complete discussion. (From: Burtis WJ, Brady TG, Orloff JJ, et al. Immunochemical characterization of circulating PTH-related protein in patients with humoral hypercalcemia of malignancy. N Engl J Med 322:1106–1112, 1980, with permission.)

Hypercalcemia in patients with HHM has both skeletal and renal components. The skeletal component, as noted above, reflects increased osteoclast activity and uncoupling of osteoblasts from osteoclasts. The renal component reflects variable increases in distal tubular calcium resorption. Equally or more important, patients with HHM are usually volume depleted, partly as a result of their hypercalcemia, with resultant inability to concentrate the urine, and partly as a result of poor oral fluid intake. The volume depletion leads to a reduction in the filtered load of calcium and a reduction in the fractional excretion of calcium.

Therapy of HHM is discussed in more detail in Chapter 27; it should include measures aimed at (i) reducing the tumor burden, (ii) reducing osteoclastic bone resorption, and (iii) augmenting renal calcium clearance. Measures aimed at reducing tumor burden (surgery, radiotherapy, and chemotherapy) lead to a reduction in the circulating concentration of PTHrP. Measures aimed at inhibiting osteoclastic bone resorption (use of bisphosphonates, mithramycin, or calcitonin) may reverse hypercalcemia but have no effect on circulating PTHrP concentrations.

UNUSUAL FORMS OF HUMORAL HYPERCALCEMIA

The two broad categories of malignancy-associated hypercalcemia, described in this chapter (HHM) and in Chapter 33 (hypercalcemia due to hematologic malignancies and solid tumors associated with extensive skeletal involvement), comprise the vast majority of patients with cancer and hypercalcemia. It should, however, be clear that other mechanisms, although uncommon, may be encountered occasionally. For example, patients who clearly display humorally mediated hypercalcemic syndromes (i.e., hypercalcemia that is reversed by tumor resection) have been reported who do not fit into the HHM biochemical categorization described. The humoral mediator in these patients is unknown. Rare patients with renal carcinomas have been described who appear to have *bona fide* tumor secretion of prostaglandin E_2 as a cause.

Finally, it is important to emphasize that patients with cancer may develop hypercalcemia as a result of other coexisting conditions, such as primary hyperparathyroidism, tuberculosis, sarcoidosis, immobilization, and use of calcium-containing hyperalimentation solutions. These causes should be actively sought and corrected.

In addition to these poorly characterized syndromes, there are two types of malignancy-associated hypercalcemia which, although rare, have been well characterized and are interesting mechanistically.

1,25-Dihydroxyvitamin-D-Secreting Lymphomas

Breslau et al. and Rosenthal et al. in 1984 described six patients with malignant lymphomas, in whom circulating concentrations of 1,25(OH)$_2$D were found to be elevated, in some cases strikingly so. Seymour et al. presented a review and update of this syndrome in 1994. The elevation of plasma 1,25(OH)$_2$D is in contrast to findings in other types of malignancy-associated hypercalcemia (Fig. 1). No evidence for a role for either PTH or PTHrP production has been found. Resection or therapy of the lymphomas reversed the hypercalcemia and reversed the elevations in plasma 1,25(OH)$_2$D. No unifying histologic theme was present among the lymphomas. Rather, lymphomas of several different subcategories are included in this group. The 1,25(OH)$_2$D elevations and hypercalcemia are corrected with glucocorticoid therapy. This syndrome appears to be the malignant counterpart of sarcoidosis (Chapter 34) with malignant lymphocytes and/or macrophages converting diet- and sun-derived 25(OH)D to 1,25(OH)$_2$D.

Ectopic Hyperparathyroidism

From the 1940s through the 1970s, what is now called HHM was thought to be caused by ectopic secretion of parathyroid hormone by tumors. In the 1980s, it became clear that HHM was caused by PTHrP, and ectopic hyperparathyroidism was viewed as rare or nonexistent. At the time of this writing, four cases of what can be considered authentic ectopic hyperparathyroidism have been described, including small cell carcinomas of the lung and ovary, a clear cell carcinoma of the ovary, and a thymoma. Immunoreactive PTH was found to be elevated in modern, sensitive, specific immunoassays and returned to normal, together with hypercalcemia, after tumor resection. Parathyroid adenomas were not identified, but a gradient of PTH across one of the tumors was demonstrated. The tumors contained mRNA encoding PTH. In one case, ovarian tumor expression of PTH was shown to result from both gene amplification and a gene rearrangement in the upstream region of one allele of the PTH gene in tumor cells. PTHrP mRNA was absent in two of the three tumors but was present in the third. Thus, it is now clear that true ectopic hyperparathyroidism can occur, but that it is exceedingly rare.

SUGGESTED READINGS

Humoral Hypercalcemia of Malignancy

1. Bonjour J-P, Phillipe J, Guelpa G, Bisetti A, Rizzoli R, Jung A, Rosini S, Kanis JA: Bone and renal components of hypercalcemia in malignancy and responses to a single infusion of clodronate. *Bone* 9:123–130, 1988
2. Budayr AA, Nissenson RA, Klein RF, Pun KK, Clark OH, Diep D, Arnaud CD, Strewler GJ: Increased serum levels of a parathyroid hormone-like protein in malignancy-associated hypercalcemia. *Ann Intern Med* 111:807–812, 1989
3. Budayr AA, Zysset E, Jenzer A, Thiébaud D, Ammann P, Rizzoli R, Jaquet-Müller F, Bonjour JP, Gertz B, Burckhardt P, Halloran BP, Nissenson RA, Strewler GJ: Effects of treatment of malignancy-associated hypercalcemia on serum parathyroid hormone-related protein. *J Bone Miner Res* 9:521–526, 1994
4. Burtis WJ, Brady TG, Orloff JJ, Ersbak JB, Warrell RP, Olson BR, Wu TL, Mitnick MA, Broadus AE, Stewart AF: Immunochemical characterization of circulating PTH-related protein in patients with humoral hypercalcemia of malignancy. *N Engl J Med* 322:1106–1112, 1980
5. Case records of the Massachusetts General Hospital (Case 27461). *N Engl J Med* 225:789–791, 1941
6. Everhart-Caye M, Inzucchi SE, Guinness-Henry J, Mitnick MA, Stewart AF: Parathyroid hormone-related protein(1-36) is equipotent with parathyroid hormone(1-34) in humans. *J Clin Endocrinol Metab* 81: 199–208, 1996
7. Godsall JW, Burtis WJ, Insogna KL, Broadus AE, Stewart AF: Nephrogenous cyclic AMP, adenylate cyclase-stimulating activity, and the humoral hypercalcemia of malignancy. In: Greep RO (ed) *Recent Progress in Hormone Research*. San Diego, Academic Press, pp 705–750, 1986
8. Grill V, Ho P, Body JJ, Johanson N, Lee SC, Kukreja SC, Moseley JM, Martin TJ: Parathyroid hormone-related protein: Elevated levels in both humoral hypercalcemia of malignancy and hypercalcemia complicating metastatic breast cancer. *J Clin Endocrinol Metab* 73:1309–1315, 1991
9. Grill V, Murray RML, Ho PWM, Santamaria JD, Pitt P, Potts C, Jerums G, Martin TJ: Circulating PTH and PTHrP levels before and after treatment of tumor induced hypercalcemia with pamidronate disodium (APD). *J Clin Endocrinol Metab* 74:468–470, 1992
10. Ikeda K, Ohno H, Hane M, Yokoi H, Okad M, Honma T, Yamada A, Tatsumi Y, Tanaka T, Saitoh T, Hirose S, Mori S, Takeuchi Y, Fukumoto S, Terukina S, Iguchi H, Kiriyama T, Ogata E, Matsumoto T: Development of a sensitive two-site immunoradiometric assay for parathyroid hormone-related peptide: Evidence for elevated levels in plasma from patients with adult T-cell leukemia/lymphoma and B-cell lymphoma. *J Clin Endocrinol Metab* 79:1322–1327, 1994
11. Isales C, Carcangiu ML, Stewart AF: Hypercalcemia in breast cancer: A reassessment of the mechanism. *Am J Med* 82:1143–1147, 1987
12. Motokura T, Fukumoto S, Matsumoto T, Takahashi S, Fujita A, Yamashita T, Igarashi T, Ogata E: Parathyroid hormone-related protein in adult T-cell leukemia-lymphoma. *Ann Intern Med* 111: 484–488, 1989
13. Ralston SH, Gallacher SJ, Patel U, Campbell J, Boyle IT: Cancer-associated hypercalcemia: Morbidity and mortality. Clinical experience in 126 treated patients. *Ann Intern Med* 112:499–504, 1990
14. Rodman JS, Sherwood LM: Disorders of bone and mineral in malignancy. In: Avioli LV, Krane SM (eds) *Metabolic Bone Disease*, vol. 2. New York, Academic Press, pp 555–631, 1987
15. Skrabanek P, McPartlin J, Powell D: Tumor hypercalcemia and ectopic hyperparathyroidism. *Medicine* 59:262–282, 1980
16. Stewart AF, Horst R, Deftos LJ, Cadman EC, Lang R, Broadus AE: Biochemical evaluation of patients with cancer-associated hypercalcemia: Evidence for humoral and non-humoral groups. *N Engl J Med* 303:1377–1383, 1980
17. Stewart AF, Insogna KL, Broadus AE: Malignancy-associated hypercalcemia. In: DeGroot L (ed) *Endocrinology*, 3rd ed. WB Saunders, Philadelphia, pp 1061–1074, 1995
18. Stewart AF, Vignery A, Silverglate A, Ravin ND, LiVolsi V, Broadus AE, Baron R: Quantitative bone histomorphometry in humoral hypercalcemia of malignancy. *J Clin Endocrinol Metab* 55:219–227, 1982

1,25-Dihydroxyvitamin D and Lymphoma

19. Breslau NA, McGuire JL, Zerwekh JE, Frenkel ED, Pak CYC: Hypercalcemia associated with increased serum calcitriol levels in three patients with lymphoma. *Ann Int Med* 100:1–7, 1984
20. Rosenthal NR, Insogna KL, Godsall JW, Smalldone L, Waldron JA, Stewart AF: Elevations in circulating 1,25(OH)$_2$D in three patients with lymphoma-associated hyprecalcemia. *J Clin Endocrinol Metab* 60:29–33, 1985

21. Seymour JF, Gagel RF, Hagemeister FB, Dimopoulos MA, Cabanillas F: Calcitriol production in hypercalcemia and normocalcemia patients with non-Hodgkin lymphoma. *Ann Intern Med* 121:633–640, 1994

Ectopic Parathyroid Hormone Secretion

22. Nussbaum SR, Gaz RD, Arnold A: Hypercalcemia and ectopic secretion of parathyroid hormone by an ovarian carcinoma with

rearrangement of the gene for PTH. *N Engl J Med* 323:1324–1328, 1990
23. Rizzoli R, Pache J-C, Bidierjean L, Burger A, Bonjour J-P: A thymoma as a cause of true ectopic hyperparathyroidism. *J Clin Endocrinol Metab* 79:912–915, 1994
24. Yoshimoto K, Yamasaki R, Sakai H, Tezuka U, Takahashi M, Iizuka M, Sekiya T, Saito S: Ectopic production of PTH by small cell lung cancer in a patient with hypercalcemia. *J Clin Endocrinol Metab* 68:976–981, 1989

33. Hypercalcemia in Hematologic Malignancies and in Solid Tumors Associated with Extensive Localized Bone Destruction

Gregory R. Mundy, M.D.

Department of Medicine, Endocrinology and Metabolism, University of Texas Health Science Center, San Antonio, Texas

HYPERCALCEMIA AND BONE DESTRUCTION IN MYELOMA

Almost all patients with myeloma have extensive bone destruction. Bone destruction may occur either as discrete local lesions or as diffuse involvement throughout the axial skeleton. This increased bone resorption is responsible for a number of disabling features, including susceptibility to pathologic fracture, intractable bone pain, and, in some patients, hypercalcemia. Approximately 80% of patients with myeloma present with a chief complaint of bone pain. Hypercalcemia occurs in 20% to 40% of patients at some time during the course of the disease.

The bone destruction that occurs in myeloma is caused by an increase in the activity of osteoclasts. Myeloma cells in the marrow cavity produce cytokines that activate adjacent endosteal osteoclasts to resorb bone. This was first recognized by observations on cultured human myeloma cells, which were found to release local factors that stimulate osteoclast activity (1,2). Over the years, the identity of the cytokines responsible for stimulating osteoclasts has been sought, but it remains elusive. Established cultures of human myeloma cells produce lymphotoxin (3), and a major portion of bone-resorbing activity produced by these cells *in vitro* can be accounted for by lymphotoxin. Lymphotoxin is produced normally by activated T lymphocytes. It is a member of the same family of immune cell products as tumor necrosis factor (TNF) and interleukin-1, both of which are produced by cells in the monocyte–macrophage lineage. Lymphotoxin has overlapping biologic properties with those of TNF, and it binds to the same receptor. TNF is thought to be one of the major mediators of the systemic effects of endotoxic shock. In bone, these cytokines stimulate osteoclast precursors to replicate, but they also stimulate the differentiation of committed osteoclast precursors into mature cells. In addition to these actions, they act on mature multinucleated cells to cause them to form resorption lacunae (4,5). Lymphotoxin is not the only cytokine that has been

implicated in myeloma, however. Other studies show that interleukin-1 and interleukin-6 may be involved in the bone destruction (6,7). Studies showing interleukin-1 production have utilized freshly isolated collections of myeloma cells (which also contains normal bone marrow mononuclear cells). Myeloma cells are known to frequently produce interleukin-6, but interleukin-6 is not by itself a powerful bone-resorbing factor. The difficulties in interpreting these results is knowing whether the *in vitro* behavior of the myeloma cells is the same as their behavior *in vivo*. As a consequence, we cannot at this time be sure of the cytokine(s) responsible for bone destruction in myeloma.

Although essentially all patients with myeloma develop extensive bone destruction, less than 40% become hypercalcemic. Moreover, there is not a close correlation between the extent of bone destruction and the development of hypercalcemia (8). The explanation is that increased bone resorption is most likely to lead to hypercalcemia in those patients with impaired glomerular filtration, which decreases the kidney's capacity to excrete calcium and clear it from the circulation. Impairment of glomerular filtration is common in patients with myeloma (9) for a number of reasons. Probably the most important is the development of Bence Jones nephropathy, otherwise called "myeloma kidney." In this circumstance, free light-chain fragments of immunoglobulin molecules (Bence Jones proteins) are filtered by the glomerulus, but they impair both glomerular and tubular functions. Patients with myeloma may also develop azotemia due to recurrent infections, uric acid nephropathy, and amyloidosis.

Because the mechanisms responsible for hypercalcemia are different in patients with myeloma from the mechanisms in patients with other types of malignancy, there are subtle differences in laboratory tests at the time of diagnosis. Because renal function is impaired, many patients with myeloma have an increased serum phosphorus rather than the decreased serum phosphorus that is common with other types of malignancy. In addition, serum alkaline phosphatase, a marker of osteoblast activity, is usually not increased in patients with myeloma, because there is little active new bone formation. For similar reasons, bone scans may also be negative. The reason for the decrease in osteoblast activity in patients with myeloma is not known.

Treatment of myeloma patients with hypercalcemia may be difficult because of the impairment in glomerular filtration. Agents that are nephrotoxic should be avoided if possible. For example, plicamycin (also called mithramycin) is not an ideal therapeutic agent for hypercalcemia in myeloma because it is directly nephrotoxic and is dependent on the kidneys for its elimination. As a consequence, its use will often be associated with toxicity. Parenteral pamidronate (a bisphosphonate) and gallium nitrate are both extremely effective in this situation, although there is more experience with pamidronate. Pamidronate can be expected to reverse hypercalcemia in essentially all patients with myeloma. However, caution should be used with these agents in patients with severely impaired renal function. Hypercalcemia in many patients with myeloma responds well to treatment of the primary disease with alkylating agents and corticosteroids (10). Corticosteroids themselves are more frequently useful in the treatment of hypercalcemia in myeloma than they are in other malignancies. The combination of calcitonin and corticosteroids is usually effective in myeloma and may be particularly useful in those cases where glomerular filtration is impaired or other antihypercalcemic drugs are contraindicated, because neither agent is nephrotoxic. It is generally not advisable to treat an osteopenic patient with corticosteroids; however, once hypercalcemia has developed in a patient with myeloma, the prognosis is usually so poor that the objective of therapy may simply be to keep the patient free from hypercalcemia in the remaining months, and then corticosteroids may be very effective.

For patients with myeloma who have intractable bone pain, radiation therapy is recommended if the pain is localized. It can be dramatically effective in relieving symptoms.

HYPERCALCEMIA ASSOCIATED WITH LYMPHOMAS

Occasionally, patients with various lymphomas develop hypercalcemia (11). This can occur in Hodgkin's disease, in B-cell lymphomas, in T-cell lymphomas, and in Burkitt's lymphoma. In T-cell lymphomas, it is frequently associated with the human T-cell lymphotrophic virus type I (HTLV-I). This is a recently described oncogenic type C retrovirus that is related to the autoimmune deficiency syndrome (AIDS) virus, infects certain T cells, and results in a lymphoproliferative T-cell disorder (12). The cause of hypercalcemia and bone destruction in these lymphomas has been well characterized. In most cases, it is probably caused by a bone-resorbing factor produced by the neoplastic lymphoid cells. In Japan, where hypercalcemia associated with HTLV-lymphoproliferative disorders is common, serum 1,25-dihydroxyvitamin D is not increased, but production of the parathyroid hormone-related protein (PTHrP) by neoplastic cells has been clearly demonstrated (13). In a few patients, hypercalcemia may be due, at least in part, to increased 1,25-dihy-droxyvitamin D production by the lymphoid cells. Several patients with different types of lymphoma and hypercalcemia have been found to have an increased serum 1,25-dihydroxyvitamin D concentration (14). When measured, this has been associated with increased absorption of calcium from the intestine. Lymphoid cells transformed by inoculation with HTLV-I virus develop the capacity to synthesize 1,25-dihydroxyvitamin D (15). However, there has been controversy about the relative frequency of increased serum 1,25-dihydroxyvitamin D in patients with hypercalcemia associated with lymphoproliferative disorders. One group in California has reported that half of their patients have increased serum 1,25-dihydroxyvitamin D concentrations (16).

Hypercalcemia also occurs occasionally in other hematologic malignancies, such as chronic lymphocytic leukemia, acute leukemia, and chronic myelogenous leukemia, particularly during acute blast transformation. However, the association of hypercalcemia with these disorders is unusual enough that these patients should be carefully evaluated for another cause of hypercalcemia. In most patients, if another cause is present, this other cause will be primary hyperparathyroidism.

HYPERCALCEMIA IN SOLID TUMORS ASSOCIATED WITH EXTENSIVE LOCALIZED BONE DESTRUCTION

Solid tumors frequently spread to involve the skeleton, and when they do so, the bone lesions are usually destructive (osteolytic) (see ref. 17 for a review). Approximately one third to one half of all tumors spread to bone, the third most common site of metastasis of solid tumors (after the liver and the lung). However, there is a distinct pattern of tumor cell metastasis to bone. Common tumors such as lung, breast, and prostate cancer frequently metastasize to bone, and bone metastases are present in nearly all patients with advanced breast or prostate cancer.

There are two distinct types of tumor metastases, osteoblastic metastases and osteolytic metastases. Osteolytic metastases are much more common and more significant as a clinical problem. Lytic metastases are usually destructive and are much more liable to be associated with pathologic fracture and hypercalcemia.

Osteolytic bone metastasis is one of the most feared complications of malignancy. The consequences for the patient include intractable bone pain at the site of the metastasis, pathologic fracture following trivial injury, nerve compression syndromes as a result of obstruction of foramina (the most serious example is spinal cord compression), and hypercalcemia, when bone destruction is advanced. Once tumor cells are housed in the skeleton, curative therapy is no longer possible in most patients and only palliative therapy is available.

Tumor cells metastasize most frequently to the axial skeleton. It is clear that there are important properties of both the tumor cell (the seed), as well as the skeleton (the soil) that determine the likelihood that any particular tumor will metastasize to bone. These properties are only now being investigated, with the goal that understanding what

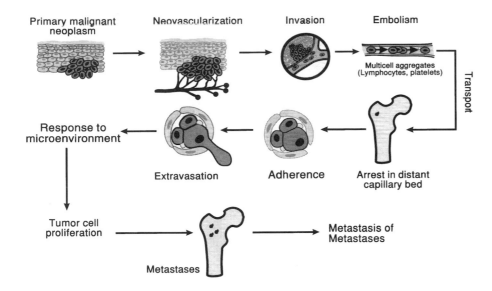

FIG. 1. Multiple steps involved in tumor migration from primary site in breast to bone. Each of these steps involves specific interactions between tumor cells and host cells, and each represents a potential target for drugs that may inhibit the process.

they are and how they affect tumor growth should lead to more effective treatments for metastatic cancer.

Because hypercalcemia of breast cancer is associated with extensive bone metastasis in the majority of patients, understanding the mechanism for tumor cell migration to bone should clarify the mechanisms by which breast cancer cells cause bone destruction (Fig. 1). Tumor cells spread to bone after being shed from the primary tumor. Release from the primary site is probably associated with the production of proteolytic enzymes by the cancer cells, which cause the cells to detach one from another. Once tumor cells enter the circulation, they traverse vascular organs including the red bone marrow. Within the bone marrow cavity, they migrate through wide-channeled sinusoids to the endosteal bone surface.

The migration of tumor cells from the bloodstream to the endosteal surfaces of bone is a multistep process that involves a number of distinct steps (18) (Fig. 2). These steps include (i) attachment to the basement membrane, probably via the basement membrane glycoprotein laminin and laminin receptors on the tumor cell surface; (ii) production of proteolytic enzymes (including matrix metalloproteinases) by tumor cells, which disrupt the basement membrane and allow tumor cells access to the organ stroma; (iii) directed migration of tumor cells via chemotactic processes through the basement membrane; and (iv) production of mediators that activate osteoclasts at the bone surface. These processes are now being unraveled by both *in vitro* and *in vivo* techniques. Some facts have recently become apparent:

1. Laminin receptors on tumor cells are important for a metastasis to form, and antagonists of laminin may block the metastatic process to bone (19).

2. Metastatic tumor cells in the bone microenvironment show properties that are different from those of the same tumor cells at the primary site (for example, they may produce PTHrP in bone but not at the primary site).

3. It is likely that the bone-derived factors stored in bone and released locally when bone is resorbed may alter the function of tumor cells in the bone microenvironment.

4. Tumor cells can be stimulated to migrate unidirectionally in response to the products of resorbing bone cultures (20), as well as in response to fragments of type 1 collagen (21), which is the most abundant protein in the bone matrix. Possibly, breast cancer cells are attracted by these mechanisms to sites of relatively active bone turnover, where they form a nidus that eventually becomes an osteolytic deposit.

5. Inhibitors of osteoclastic bone resorption can inhibit not only skeletal complications of cancer, but they can also impair tumor growth at the metastatic site (22).

Because bone metastasis is such an important complication of the most common tumors that affect humans (i.e., lung cancer and breast cancer), understanding the cellular

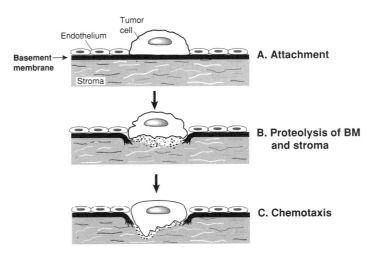

FIG. 2. Step-wise progression of tumor cells as they traverse basement membranes to migrate to the bone surface. Liotta (18) has proposed that this involves a multistep process including **(A)** attachment of the tumor cell to the basement membrane, **(B)** disruption of the basement membrane by tumor cell production of proteolytic enzymes, and **(C)** unilateral migration (chemotaxis) of tumor cells through the disrupted membrane to the underlying tissue stroma with eventual access to the bone surface.

events involved and devising therapeutic strategies to prevent new metastasis and to inhibit continued growth of established metastases is a very important therapeutic goal for cancer management.

The principles of treatment of hypercalcemic patients with metastatic bone disease and hypercalcemia are the same as those for other patients with hypercalcemia of malignancy (23).

REFERENCES

1. Mundy GR, Raisz LG, Cooper RA, Schechter GP, Salmon SE: Evidence for the secretion of an osteoclast stimulating factor in myeloma. *N Engl J Med* 291:1041–1046, 1974
2. Mundy GR, Bertolini DB: Bone destruction and hypercalcemia in plasma cell myeloma. *Semin Oncol* 13:291–299, 1986
3. Garrett RI, Durie BGM, Nedwin GE, et al.: Production of the bone resorbing cytokine lymphotoxin by cultured human myeloma cells. *N Engl J Med* 317:526–532, 1987
4. Thomson BM, Saklatvala J, Chambers TJ: Osteoblasts mediate interleukin-1 stimulation of bone resorption by rat osteoclasts. *J Exp Med* 164:104–112, 1986
5. Thomson BM, Mundy GR, Chambers TJ: Tumor necrosis factors alpha and beta induce osteoblastic cells to stimulate osteoclastic bone resorption. *J Immunol* 138:775–779, 1987
6. Bataille R, Jourdan M, Zhang Xue-Guang, et al.: Serum levels of interleukin-6, a potent myeloma cell growth factor, as a reflection of disease severity in plasma cell dyscrasias. *J Clin Invest* 84: 2008–2011, 1989
7. Cozzolino F, Torcia M, Aldinucci D, et al.: Production of interleukin-1 by bone marrow myeloma cells. *Blood* 74:387–390, 1989
8. Durie BGM, Salmon SE, Mundy GR: Relation of osteoclast activating factor production to the extent of bone disease in multiple myeloma. *Br J Haematol* 47:21–30, 1981
9. Harinck HIJ, Bijvoet OLM, Plantingh AST: Role of bone and kidney in tumor-induced hypercalcemia and its treatment with bisphosphonate and sodium chloride. *Am J Med* 82:1113–1142, 1987
10. Binstock ML, Mundy GR: Effects of calcitonin and glucocorticoids in combination with hypercalcemia of malignancy. *Ann Intern Med* 93:269–272, 1980
11. Canellos GP: Hypercalcemia in malignant lymphoma and leukemia. *Ann NY Acad Sci* 230:240–246, 1974
12. Bunn PA, Schechter GP, Jaffe E, et al.: Clinical course of retrovirus-associated adult T-cell lymphoma in the United States. *N Engl J Med* 309:247–264, 1983
13. Motokura T, Fukumoto S, Matsumoto T, et al.: Parathyroid hormone related protein in adult T-cell leukemia-lymphoma. *Ann Intern Med* 111:484–488, 1989
14. Breslau NA, McGuire JL, Zerwekh JE, Frenkel EP, Pak CYC: Hypercalcemia associated with increased serum calcitriol levels in three patients with lymphoma. *Ann Intern Med* 100:107, 1984
15. Fetchick DA, Bertolini DR, Sarin PS, Weintraub ST, Mundy GR, Dunn JD: Production of 1,25 dihydroxyvitamin D by human T-cell lymphotrophic virus-I transformed lymphocytes. *J Clin Invest* 78:592–596, 1986
16. Adams JS, Fernandez M, Gacad MA, et al.: Vitamin D metabolite-mediated hypercalcemia and hypercalciuria in patients with AIDS- and non-AIDS-associated lymphoma. *Blood* 73:235–239, 1989
17. Mundy GR, Martin TJ: Physiology and pharmacology of bone. In: *Handbook of Experimental Pharmacology*. Springer, 1993
18. Liotta LA: Tumor invasion: Role of the extracellular matrix. *Cancer Res* 46:1–7, 1986
19. Nakai M, Mundy GR, Williams PJ, Boyce B, Yoneda T: A synthetic antagonist to laminin inhibits the formation of osteolytic metastases by human melanoma cells in nude mice. *Cancer Res* 52:5395–5399, 1992
20. Orr W, Varani J, Gondek MD, Ward PA, Mundy GR: Chemotactic responses of tumor cells to products of resorbing bone. *Science* 203:176–179, 1979
21. Mundy GR, DeMartino S, Rowe DW: Collagen and collagen fragments are chemotactic for tumor cells. *J Clin Invest* 68:1102–1105, 1981
22. Sasaki A, Boyce BF, Story B, Wright KR, Chapman M, Boyce R, Mundy GR, Yoneda T: The bisphosphonate risedronate reduces metastatic human breast cancer burden in bone in nude mice. *Cancer Res* 55: 3551–3557, 1995
23. Mundy GR, Martin TJ: The hypercalcemia of malignancy: Pathogenesis and treatment. *Metabolism* 31:1247–1277, 1982

34. Hypercalcemia Due to Granuloma-Forming Disorders

John S. Adams, M.D.

Department of Medicine, University of California, Los Angeles, and Cedars-Sinai Research Institute, Los Angeles, California

PATHOGENESIS

The association of dysregulated calcium homeostasis and granuloma-forming disease was established in 1939 by the work of Harrell and Fisher (1). With the advent of automated serum chemistry testing, more recent studies indicate that mild to severe hypercalcemia is detected in 10% of patients with sarcoidosis, and up to 50% of patients will become hypercalciuric at some time during the course of their disease (2). Vitamin D was implicated in the pathogenesis of abnormal calcium metabolism after it was appreciated that patients with sarcoidosis who had hypercalcemia

or hypercalciuria (or both) absorbed high amounts of dietary calcium, and that normocalcemic patients were prone to hypercalcemia after receiving small amounts of vitamin D or ultraviolet light (3). It has been proposed that bone resorption is also an important contributor to the pathogenesis of hypercalciuria and hypercalcemia (4), based on the observations that a diet low in calcium seldom induces a normocalcemic state in sarcoidosis patients with moderate to severe hypercalcemia, and that urinary calcium excretion often exceeds dietary calcium intake. Recent studies (5,6) have demonstrated that generalized, accelerated trabecular bone loss occurs in patients with sarcoidosis before institu-

TABLE 1. *Human disease associated with 1,25-dihydroxyvitamin-D-mediated hypercalcemia/hypercalciuria*

Granuloma-forming diseases	
Sarcoidosis	Adams et al. (7)
Tuberculosis	Gkonos et al. (8)
Silicone-induced granulomatosis	Kozeny et al. (9)
Disseminated candidiasis	Kantarijian et al. (10)
Leprosy	Hoffman and Korzeniowski (11)
Wegener's granulomatosis	Edelson et al. (12)
Newborn subcutaneous fat necrosis	Cook et al. (13)
Malignant lymphoproliferative disease	
B-Cell lymphoma	Adams et al. (14)
Hodgkin's disease	Adams et al. (14) and Seymour and Gagel (15)
Lymphomatoid granulomatosis	Schienman et al. (16)

tion of steroid therapy. Rizzato et al. (6) showed that (i) bone mass was significantly decreased in patients with active sarcoidosis, (ii) bone loss was most marked in patients with hypercalcemia and/or hypercalciuria, and (iii) bone loss was most prominent in postmenopausal women with longstanding disease.

For many years, these and similar clinical observations suggested that hypercalcemia and/or hypercalciuria in patients with sarcoidosis resulted from a heightened sensitivity to the biologic effects of vitamin D. However, the discovery that a high proportion of these patients had elevated circulating concentrations of 1,25-dihydroxyvitamin D [1,25(OH)₂D] indicated that the endogenous overproduction of an active vitamin D metabolite was the etiology of disordered calcium regulation in this disease. More recently, high serum 1,25(OH)₂D concentrations have been reported in hypercalcemic patients with other granuloma-forming diseases and in patients harboring lymphoproliferative neoplasms (Table 1); in all of these disorders, there is a presumed extrarenal source for the hormone.

There are four major lines of clinical evidence suggesting that the endogenous extrarenal synthesis of 1,25(OH)₂D in some hypercalcemic/hypercalciuric patients with granulomatous disease and lymphoma is not subject to normal, physiologic regulatory influences (17). First, hypercalcemic patients possess a frankly high or inappropriately elevated serum 1,25(OH)₂D concentration, although their serum immunoreactive parathyroid hormone levels are suppressed and serum phosphorus concentrations are relatively elevated. If 1,25(OH)₂D synthesis were under the trophic control of parathyroid hormone and phosphorus, then 1,25(OH)₂D concentrations should be low. Second, unlike in normal individuals, whose serum 1,25(OH)₂D concentrations are not influenced by small to moderate increments of circulating 25-hydroxyvitamin D [25(OH)D] concentrations, the serum 1,25(OH)₂D concentration in patients with active sarcoidosis is exquisitely sensitive to an increase in the availability of substrate. Third, serum calcium and 1,25(OH)₂D concentrations are positively correlated to indices of disease activity; patients with sarcoidosis who

have widespread disease and high serum angiotensin-converting-enzyme activity are more likely to be hypercalciuric or frankly hypercalcemic (18–20). And fourth, the rate of endogenous 1,25(OH)₂D production, which is significantly increased in patients with sarcoidosis (21), is unusually sensitive to inhibition by factors (e.g., glucocorticoids) that do not influence the renal 1-hydroxylase.

CELLULAR SOURCE OF ACTIVE VITAMIN D METABOLITES

The sentinel report of Barbour et al. (22) proved the source of 1,25(OH)₂D to be extrarenal in sarcoidosis. These investigators described an anephric patient with sarcoidosis, hypercalcemia, and a high serum 1,25(OH)₂D concentration. The elevated 1,25(OH)₂D concentration in patients with sarcoidosis is now known to result from increased production of 1,25(OH)₂D by the macrophage (7), a prominent constituent of the sarcoid granuloma. Synthesis of 1,25(OH)₂D₃ from 25(OH)D₃ has been demonstrated *in vitro* by alveolar macrophages from hypercalcemic patients with sarcoidosis, and by granulomatous tissue. The salient properties of the macrophage 25(OH)D 1-hydroxylation reaction *in vitro* are depicted in Table 2. Although similar to the authentic renal 25(OH)D-1-hydroxylase in terms of kinetics and substrate specificity (23), the factors that exert a regulatory influence on the synthetic reaction in the kidney vary considerably from those that influence the sarcoid macrophage. The sarcoid macrophage 1-hydroxylation reaction is immune to the stimulatory effects of parathyroid hormone, but it is very sensitive to stimulation by interferon-gamma (IFN-γ), a lymphokine produced by activated lymphocytes, and sensitive to stimulation by modulators of this lymphokine's postreceptor signal transduction pathway, including nitric oxide (24,25). The macrophage hydroxylation reaction is very sensitive to inhibition by glucocorticoid, chloroquine and related analogs, and the cytochrome P450 inhibitor ketoconazole, but it is refractory to inhibition by 1,25(OH)₂D (23,26,27). The renal enzyme, on the other hand, is relatively insensitive to inhibition by glucocorticoids and is down-regulated by 1,25(OH)₂D. It is postulated that these differences are more a reflection of the cell in which the hydroxylase is expressed than a difference in the enzyme that catalyzes the reaction. This question cannot be resolved until the responsible enzymes from the macrophage and kidney are structurally characterized.

TABLE 2. *Characteristics of the sarcoid macrophage 25-hydroxyvitamin-D-hydroxylation reaction*

Side-chain-substituted secosteroid substrates preferred[a]
High affinity for substrate (50–100 nM)[a]
Not inhibited by product 1,25(OH)₂D₃
Not accompanied by a 24-hydroxylase
Stimulated by interferon-γ, calcium ionophore, leukotriene C₄, and nitric oxide
Inhibited by glucocorticoid, chloroquine, and ketoconazole

[a] Characteristic similar to that of the renal 1-hydroxylase.

IMMUNOACTIVITY OF 1,25-DIHYDROXYVITAMIN D

1,25-Dihydroxyvitamin D is known to exert a potent immunoinhibitory effect on activated human lymphocytes *in vitro*. These actions include inhibition of lymphocyte proliferation, lymphokine production, and immunoglobulin synthesis (28). It is suggested (29) that 1,25(OH)$_2$D produced by the macrophage in granulomatous diseases exerts a paracrine immunoinhibitory effect on neighboring, activated lymphocytes that express receptors for the hormone, and that this acts to slow an otherwise "over zealous" immune response that may be detrimental to the host. Despite the theoretical attractiveness of this model, there are few data to support a role for 1,25(OH)$_2$D as a paracrine immunoinhibitor *in vivo* (30).

TREATMENT OF HYPERCALCEMIA/HYPERCALCIURIA

The most important factor in the successful management of disordered vitamin D metabolism of sarcoidosis is recognition of patients at risk. Those at risk include patients with (i) indices of active, widespread disease (i.e., elevated serum angiotensin-converting-enzyme levels, diffuse infiltrative pulmonary disease); (ii) preexistent hypercalciuria; (iii) a previous history of hypercalcemia or hypercalciuria; (iv) a diet enriched in vitamin D and calcium; and (v) a recent history of sunlight exposure or treatment with vitamin D. All patients with active sarcoidosis should be screened for hypercalciuria. In a timed, fasting urine collection, a fractional urinary calcium excretion rate exceeding 0.16 mg calcium per 100 ml glomerular filtrate is considered hypercalciuria. If the fractional urinary calcium excretion rate is elevated, serum 25(OH)D and 1,25(OH)$_2$D concentrations should be determined as a disease marker and to judge the efficacy of therapy. Because hypercalciuria frequently precedes the development of overt hypercalcemia, the occurrence of either is an indication for therapy.

Glucocorticoids (40 to 60 mg prednisone or equivalent, daily) are the mainstay of therapy of disordered calcium homeostasis resulting from the endogenous overproduction of active vitamin D metabolites. Institution of glucocorticoid therapy results in a prompt decrease in the circulating 1,25(OH)$_2$D concentration (within 3 days), presumably by inhibition of the macrophage hydroxylation reaction. Normalization of the serum or urine calcium usually occurs within a matter of days (19). Failure to normalize the serum calcium after 10 days of therapy suggests the coexistence of another hypercalcemic process (e.g., hyperparathyroidism or humoral hypercalcemia of malignancy). Obviously, the dietary intake of calcium and vitamin D should be limited in such patients, as should sunlight (UV light) exposure. After a hypercalcemic episode, urinary calcium excretion rates should be monitored intermittently to detect recurrence. Glucocorticoids also appear to be effective in the management of vitamin-D-mediated hypercalcemia or hypercalciuria in other granuloma-forming diseases and lymphoma. It should be pointed out, however, that the number of patients so treated is few. Chloroquine, its hydroxy analog (hydroxy-chloroquine) (26,31), and ketoconazole (27) are also capable of reducing the serum 1,25(OH)$_2$D and calcium concentration in patients with sarcoidosis. Because of the limited experience with these drugs as antihypercalcemic agents, they should be limited to patients in whom steroid therapy is unsuccessful or contraindicated. The utility of the newer bisphosphonates in blocking bone resorption and decreasing serum and urine calcium levels in hypercalcemic/hypercalciuric patients with sarcoidosis is unknown.

REFERENCES

1. Harrell GT, Fisher S: Blood chemical changes in Boeck's sarcoid with particular reference to protein, calcium and phosphatase values. *J Clin Invest* 18:687–693, 1939
2. Studdy PR, Bird R, Neville E, James DG: Biochemical findings in sarcoidosis. *J Clin Pathol* 33:528–533, 1980
3. Bell NH, Gill JR Jr, Bartter FC: On the abnormal calcium absorption in sarcoidosis: Evidence for increased sensitivity to vitamin D. *Am J Med* 36:500–513, 1964
4. Fallon MD, Perry HM III, Teitelbaum SL: Skeletal sarcoidosis with osteopenia. *Metab Bone Dis Res* 3:171–174, 1981
5. Vergnon GM, Chappard D, Mounier D, et al.: Phosphocalcic metabolism, bone quantitative histomorphometry and clinical activity in 10 cases of sarcoidosis. In: Grassi C, Rizzato G, Pozzi E (eds) *Sarcoidosis and Other Granulomatous Disorders*. Elsevier, Amsterdam, pp 499–502, 1988
6. Rizzato G, Montemurro L, Fraioli P: Bone mineral content in sarcoidosis. *Semin Resp Med* 13:411–423, 1992
7. Adams JS, Singer FR, Gacad MA, et al.: Isolation and structural identification of 1,25-dihydroxyvitamin D3 produced by cultured alveolar macrophages in sarcoidosis. *J Clin Endocrinol Metab* 60:960–966, 1985
8. Gkonos PJ, London R, Hendler ED: Hypercalcemia and elevated 1,25-dihydroxyvitamin D levels in a patient with end stage renal disease and active tuberculosis. *N Engl J Med* 311:1683–1685, 1984
9. Kozeny GA, Barbato AL, Bansal VK, Vertuno LL, Hano JE: Hypercalcemia associated with silicone-induced granulomas. *N Engl J Med* 311:1103–1105, 1984
10. Kantarjian HM, Saad MF, Estey EH, Sellin RV, Samaan NA: Hypercalcemia in disseminated candidiasis. *Am J Med* 74:721–724, 1983
11. Hoffman VH, Korzeniowski OM: Leprosy, hypercalcemia, and elevated serum calcitriol levels. *Ann Intern Med* 105:890 891, 1986
12. Edelson GW, Talpos GB, Bone HG III: Hypercalcemia associated with Wegener's granulomatosis and hyperparathyroidism: Etiology and management. *Am J Nephrol* 13:275–277, 1993
13. Cook JS, Stone MS, Hansen JR: Hypercalcemia in association with subcutaneous fat necrosis of the newborn: Studies of calcium regulating hormones. *Pediatrics* 90:93–96, 1992
14. Adams JS, Fernandez M, Gacad MA, et al.: Vitamin D metabolite mediated hypercalcemia and hypercalciuria patients with AIDS and non-AIDS-associated lymphoma. *Blood* 73:235–239, 1989
15. Seymour JF, Gagel RF: Calcitriol: The major humoral mediator of hypercalcemia in Hodgkin's disease and non-Hodgkin's lymphomas. *Blood* 82:1383–1394, 1993
16. Schienman SJ, Kelberman MW, Tatum AH, Zamkoff KW: Hypercalcemia with excess serum 1,25-dihydroxyvitamin D in lymphomatoid granulomatosis/angiocentric lymphoma. *Am J Med Sci* 301:178–181, 1991
17. DeLuca HF, Schnoes HK: Vitamin D: Recent advances. *Ann Rev Biochem* 52:411–439, 1983
18. Sandler LM, Wineals CG, Fraher LJ, Clemens TL, Smith R, O'Riordan JLH: Studies of the hypercalcaemia of sarcoidosis: Effects of steroids and exogenous vitamin D3 on the circulating concentration of 1,25-dihydroxyvitamin D3. *Q J Med* 53:165–180, 1984
19. Meyrier A, Valeyre D, Bouillon R, Paillard F, Battesti JP,

Georges R: Resorptive versus absorptive hypercalciuria in sarcoidosis: Correlations with 25-hydroxyvitamin D3 and 1,25-dihydroxyvitamin D3 and parameters of disease activity. *Q J Med* 54:269–281, 1985

20. Adams JS, Gacad MA, Anders AA, et al.: Biochemical indicators of disordered vitamin D and calcium homeostasis in sarcoidosis. *Sarcoidosis* 3:1–6, 1986
21. Insogna KL, Dreyer BE, Mitnick M, Ellison AF, Broadus AE: Enhanced production rate of 1,25-dihydroxyvitamin D in sarcoidosis. *J Clin Endocrinol Metab* 66:72–75, 1988
22. Barbour GL, Coburn JW, Slatopolsky E, Norman AW, Horst RL: Hypercalcemia in an anephric patient with sarcoidosis: Evidence for extrarenal generation of 1,25-dihydroxyvitamin D. *N Engl J Med* 305:440–443, 1981
23. Adams JS, Gacad MA: Characterization of 1α hydroxylation of vitamin D3 sterols by cultured alveolar macrophages from patients with sarcoidosis. *J Exp Med* 161:755–765, 1985
24. Adams JS, Gacad MA, Diz MM, Nadler JL: A role for endogenous arachidonate metabolites in the regulated expression of the 25-hydroxyvitamin D-1-hydroxylation reaction in cultured alveolar macrophages from patients with sarcoidosis. *J Clin Endocrinol Metab* 70:595–600, 1990
25. Adams JS, Ren SY, Arbelle JE, Clemens TL, Shany S: A role for nitric oxide in the regulated expression of the 25 hydroxyvitamin D-1-hydroxylation reaction in the chick myelomonocytic cell line HD-11. *Endocrinology* 134:499–502, 1994
26. Adams JS, Diz MM, Sharma OP: Effective reduction in the serum 1,25-dihydroxyvitamin D and calcium concentration in sarcoidosis-associated hypercalcemia with short-course chloroquine therapy. *Ann Intern Med* 111:437–438, 1989
27. Adams JS, Sharma OP, Diz MM, Endres DB: Ketoconazole decreases the serum 1,25-dihydroxyvitamin D and calcium concentration in sarcoidosis-associated hypercalcemia. *J Clin Endocrinol Metab* 70:1090–1095, 1990
28. Rigby WFC: The immunobiology of vitamin D. *Immunol Today* 9:54–58, 1988
29. Adams JS: Hypercalcemia and hypercalciuria. *Semin Resp Med* 13:402–410, 1992
30. Barnes PF, Modlin RL, Bickle DD, Adams JS: Transpleural gradient of 1,25-dihydroxyvitamin D in tuberculous pleuritis. *J Clin Invest* 83:1527–1532, 1989
31. O'Leary TJ, Jones G, Yip A, et al.: The effects of chloroquine on serum 1,25-dihydroxyvitamin D and calcium metabolism in sarcoidosis. *N Engl J Med* 315:727–730, 1986

35. Hypercalcemic Syndromes in Infants and Children

Craig B. Langman, M.D.

Department of Pediatrics, Northwestern University, and Children's Memorial Hospital, Chicago, Illinois

Blood ionized calcium levels in normal infants and young children are similar to those of adults, with a mean ±2 SD = 1.21 ± 0.13 mM. In neonates, the normal blood ionized calcium level is dependent on postnatal age (1). In the first 72 hours after birth, there is a significant decrease in the blood ionized calcium level in term newborns, from 1.4 mM to 1.2 mM; the decrease is exaggerated in preterm neonates.

Chronic hypercalcemia in young infants and children may not be associated with the usual signs and symptoms described in this section. Rather, the predominant manifestation of hypercalcemia is "failure to thrive," in which linear growth is arrested and there is lack of appropriate weight gain. Additional features of chronic hypercalcemia in children include nonspecific symptoms of irritability, gastrointestinal reflux, abdominal pain, and anorexia. Acute hypercalcemia is very uncommon in infants and children; when it occurs, its manifestations are similar to those of older children and adults, with potential alterations in the nervous system, the conduction system of the heart, and kidney functions.

WILLIAMS SYNDROME

Williams et al. (2) described a syndrome in infants with supravalvular aortic stenosis and peculiar ("elfin-like") facies; hypercalcemia during the first year of life was also noted (3). However, the severe elevations in serum calcium initially described have failed to appear with equal frequency in subsequent series of such infants. Other series of children who have the cardiac lesion have failed to demonstrate the associated facial dysmorphism. It is thought that there exists a spectrum of infants with some or all of the above abnormalities, and a scoring system has been described to assign suspected infants as lying within or outside of the syndrome classification (4).

Two thirds of infants with Williams syndrome are small for their gestational age, and many are born past their expected date of birth. The facial abnormalities consist of structural asymmetry, temporal depression, flat malae with full cheeks, microcephaly, epicanthal folds, lacy or stellate irises, a short nose, long philtrum, arched upper lip with full lower lip, and small, maloccluded teeth. The vocal tone is often hoarse. Neurologic manifestations include hypotonia, hyperreflexia, and mild-to-moderate motor retardation. The personality of affected children has been described as "cocktail party," in that they are unusually friendly to strangers. Other vascular abnormalities have been described in addition to supravalvular aortic stenosis, including other congenital heart defects and many peripheral organ arterial stenoses (renal, mesenteric, and celiac). Hypertension may be present in infancy in a minority of children but increases in incidence after the first decade of life.

Hypercalcemia, if initially present, rarely persists to the end of the first year of life and generally disappears spontaneously. Despite the rarity of chronic hypercalcemia, persistent hypercalciuria is not uncommon. Additionally, many of the signs and symptoms of hypercalcemia mentioned previously and in the introduction to this section have been noted in these infants. The long-term prognosis for patients with Williams syndrome seems to depend on features other than the level of blood calcium, such as the level of mental retardation and the clinical significance of the cardiovascular abnormalities. Approximately 25% of patients may have radioulnar synostosis, which may impede normal developmental milestones of fine motor activities of the upper extremities if not recognized (5).

A search for the gene(s) responsible for Williams syndrome localized the cardiac component, supravalvular aortic stenois, to the long arm of chromosome 7 (6). It appears that translocations of the elastin gene may be responsible for isolated or familial supravalvular aortic stenosis, while deletion of the entire elastin locus produces Williams syndrome (7,8).

Despite the potential localization of the disorder to a deletion of the elastin locus on chromosome 7, the pathogenesis of the disorder remains unknown, although many studies have focused on disordered control of vitamin D metabolism. Previous studies of affected children have demonstrated increased circulating levels of 25-hydroxyvitamin D after vitamin D administration (9), increased levels of calcitriol (1,25-dihydroxyvitamin D) during periods of hypercalcemia (10) but not during normocalcemia (11,12), or diminished levels of calcitonin during calcium infusions (13). Although excess administration of vitamin D to pregnant rabbits may produce a clinical picture not dissimilar to Williams syndrome, the overwhelming majority of children with Williams syndrome are not the result of maternal vitamin D intoxication.

IDIOPATHIC INFANTILE HYPERCALCEMIA

In the early 1950s in England, Lightwood (14) reported a series of infants with severe hypercalcemia. Epidemiologic investigations have revealed that the majority of affected infants were born to mothers ingesting foods heavily fortified with vitamin D. The incidence of the disease declined dramatically with reduction of vitamin D supplementation. Other cases have been described without previous exposure to excessive maternal vitamin D intake, and the incidence of idiopathic infantile hypercalcemia (IIH) has remained fixed over the past 20 years. Affected infants have polyuria, increased thirst, and the general manifestations of hypercalcemia previously noted. Severely affected neonates may have cardiac lesions similar to those seen in Williams syndrome and may even manifest the dysmorphic features of those infants and children. The distinction between the two syndromes remains problematic (15). Other clinical manifestations include chronic arterial hypertension, strabismus, inguinal hernias, musculoskeletal abnormalities (disordered posture and mild kyphosis), and bony abnormalities (radioulnar synostosis and dislocated patella). Hyperacusis is present in the majority of affected children with IIH, but not Williams syndrome, and it is persistent.

As in Williams syndrome, disordered vitamin D metabolism with increased vitamin D sensitivity with respect to gastrointestinal transport of calcium has been posited as the cause of this disorder (16), although the data are conflicting.

We have recently identified seven consecutive children with IIH in whom the presence of an elevated level of N-terminal parathyroid-hormone-related protein (PTHrP) was demonstrated at the time of hypercalcemia (17). Further, in five of those children who achieved normocalcemia, the levels of PTHrP normalized or were unmeasurably low, and in one child with persistent hypercalcemia, the level of PTHrP remained elevated. No other nonmalignant disorder of childhood that we have examined, including two children with hypercalcemia from Williams syndrome, have had elevated levels of PTHrP.

In contrast to the hypercalcemia of Williams syndrome, the level of blood calcium in IIH remains elevated for a prolonged period in the most severely affected children. Therapy includes the use of glucocorticoids to reduce gastrointestinal absorption of calcium, as well as the avoidance of vitamin D and excess dietary calcium.

FAMILIAL HYPOCALCIURIC HYPERCALCEMIA

This disorder is also called familial benign hypercalcemia and has been recognized since 1972 (18) as a cause of elevated total and serum ionized calcium. The onset of the change in calcium is commonly before age 10 and has been described in newborns (19). However, in distinction to primary hyperparathyroidism, circulating levels of parathyroid hormone, phosphate, and calcitriol tend to be normal. Serum magnesium is also elevated. Renal clearances of calcium and magnesium are generally reduced. Overt clinical manifestations are generally uncommon and not those described for hypercalcemia, with the exception of fatigue and weakness. Renal function is preserved and there is a notable absence of either hypertension or nephrolithiasis (20,21). The hypercalcemia is lifelong in the majority of affected individuals. The hypercalcemia is not cured by parathyroidectomy, although abnormalities of parathyroid histology have been reported in patients with the disorder.

The gene responsible for sensing the level of extracellular ionized calcium has been cloned recently (22). Inheritance of one abnormal allele of the gene is associated with familial hypercalcemia with hypocalciuria (23), while inheritance of two abnormal alleles produces severe neonatal hyperparathyroidism (see following section) (24).

NEONATAL PRIMARY HYPERPARATHYROIDISM

Primary hyperparathyroidism is uncommon in neonates and children (25), with less than 100 cases reported to date. Additionally, only 20% of cases occur in children under 10 years of age. Hypercalcemia in the first decade of life may more likely be caused by the other disorders discussed previously. The presenting clinical manifestations are weakness, anorexia, and irritability, which are seen in a multitude of pediatric disorders. The association with other endocrine disorders occurs with decreased frequency in young children with primary hyperparathyroidism. Histologic examination of the parathyroid glands demonstrates that 20% to

40% of affected children may have hyperplasia rather than the more typical adenoma in older individuals.

Neonatal severe hyperparathyroidism is now known to result from inheritance of two mutant alleles associated with the calcium-sensing gene on chromosome 3 (24).

MISCELLANEOUS DISORDERS

Subcutaneous Fat Necrosis

Michael et al. (26) reported the association of significant birth trauma with fat necrosis in two small-for-gestational-age infants who subsequently developed severe hypercalcemia (serum calcium >15 mg/dl) and violaceous discolorations in pressure sites. Histologic examination of the affected pressure sites in such patients demonstrates both an inflammatory, mononuclear cell infiltrate and crystals that contain calcium. We have also noted hypercalcemia in several children with subcutaneous fat necrosis associated with major trauma or disseminated varicella. The mechanism of the hypercalcemia is unknown, but it may be related to mildly elevated levels of 1,25-dihydroxyvitamin D or excess prostaglandin E production. The prognosis for infants and children with subcutaneous fat necrosis depends on the duration of the hypercalcemia. Reductions in serum calcium have been noted with the use of exogenous corticosteroids, saline, and furosemide diuresis, and the avoidance of excess dietary calcium and vitamin D. Recurrence of hypercalcemia has not been seen.

Hypophosphatasia

This disorder is discussed in detail in Chapter 63 and is mentioned here, only for completeness. Severe infantile hypophosphatasia is associated with markedly elevated serum calcium levels and a reduction in circulating alkaline phosphatase, increase in urinary phosphoethanolamine, and elevated serum pyridoxal-5-phosphate concentrations.

Sarcoidosis

Thirty percent to 50% of children with the autoimmune disorder sarcoidosis (27) (see Chapter 34) manifest hypercalcemia, and an additional 20% to 30% demonstrate hypercalciuria with normocalcemia. Many of the presenting manifestations of children with sarcoidosis may be related to the presence of hypercalcemia.

Limb Fracture

Isolated weight-bearing limb fracture (28) (see Chapter 36) that requires immobilization for even several days, may be associated with elevated blood ionized calcium levels and hypercalciuria in young children and adolescents. Although prolonged immobilization itself commonly produces hypercalcemia and hypercalciuria, the occurrence after short-term bed rest in children probably reflects their more rapid skeletal turnover.

Vitamin D (Metabolite) Therapy

Children with renal osteodystrophy are commonly treated with calcitriol and develop hypercalcemia once every 12 to 15 treatment months (see Chapter 67). 25-Hydroxyvitamin D_3 therapy of children with renal osteodystrophy is associated with a slight decrease in the incidence of hypercalcemia. Children with hypocalcemic disorders treated with 1,25-dihydroxyvitamin D_3 therapy develop hypercalcemia at one third the frequency of children with renal osteodystrophy treated with any vitamin D metabolite (29). Treatment with the parent vitamin D compound is associated with the production of hypercalcemia similar to the rate produced with calcitriol. However, the hypercalcemia associated with vitamin D is prolonged four- to sixfold in comparison with hypercalcemia with metabolite therapy.

Jansen Syndrome

Jansen syndrome (30,31) presents in neonates with hypercalcemia and skeletal radiographs that resemble a rachitic condition. It is a form of metaphyseal dysplasia, and after infancy, the radiographic condition evolves into a more typical picture, with mottled calcifications in the distal end of the long bones. These areas represent patches of partially calcified cartilage protruding into the diaphyseal portion of bone. The skull and spine may be affected also.

The hypercalcemia appears to be lifelong. It has been shown recently to result from a gene defect that produces an amino acid substitution in the parathyroid hormone/parathyroid-hormone-like protein receptor, and that constitutively activates the receptor. This produces unopposed parathyroid hormone/parathyroid-hormone-like protein actions in such patients, and explains the absence of measurable levels of either hormone. Such patients appear to be at risk for the development of the complications of hyperparathyroidism in the adult years.

Incorrect Dosing of Human Milk with Vitamin D

An outbreak of hypercalcemia in eight patients was reported from the incorrect dosing of dairy milk with vitamin D, and, in addition, a defect was found in the concentrate used to fortify the milk (containing cholecalciferol rather than the expected ergocalciferol) (32,33). These same investigators extended their measurements of the vitamin D content to both commercial dairy milks and fortified infant formulas, and they found that only 29% of the milks and formulas contained within 20% of the stated vitamin D content. These studies suggest that improved monitoring of the fortification process is mandatory. Such studies may explain the rare finding of clinical vitamin D deficiency in children drinking "fortified" milk.

REFERENCES

1. Specker BL, Lichtenstein P, Mimouni F, Gormley C, Tsang RC: Calcium-regulating hormones and minerals from birth to 18

months of age: A cross-sectional study. II. Effects of sex, race, age, season, and diet on serum minerals, parathyroid hormone and calcitonin. *Pediatrics* 77:891–896, 1986

2. Williams JCP, Barratt-Boyes BG, Lowe JB: Supravalvular aortic stenosis. *Circulation* 24:1311–1316, 1961

3. Black JA, Bonham Carter RE: Association between aortic stenosis and facies of severe infantile hypercalcemia. *Lancet* 2:745–748, 1963

4. Preus M: The Williams syndrome: Objective definition and diagnosis. *Clin Genet* 25:422–428, 1984

5. Charvat KA, Hornstein L, Oestreich AE: Radio-ulnarsynostosis in Williams syndrome. A frequently associated anomaly. *Pediatr Radiol* 21:508–510, 1991

6. Ewart AK, Morris CA, Ensing GJ, Loker J, Moore C, Leppert M, Keating M: A human vascular disorder, supravalvular aortic stenosis, maps to chromosome 7. *Proc Natl Acad Sci USA* 90: 3226–3230, 1993

7. Curran ME, Atkinson DL, Ewart AK, Morris CA, Keppert MF, Keating MT: The elastin gene is disrupted by a translocation associated with supravalvular aortic stenosis. *Cell* 73:159–168, 1993

8. Ewart AK, Jin W, Atkinson D, Morris CA, Keating MT: Supravalvular aortic stenosis associated with a deletion disrupting the elastin gene. *J Clin Invest* 93:1071–1077, 1994

9. Taylor AB, Stern PH, Bell NH: Abnormal regulation of circulating 25OHD in the Williams syndrome. *N Engl J Med* 306:972–975, 1982

10. Garabedian M, Jacqz E, Guillozo H, Grimberg R, Guillot M, Gadnadoux M-F, Broyer M, Lenoir G, Balsan S: Increased plasma 1,25(OH)$_2$D$_3$ concentrations in infants with hypercalcemia and an elfin facies. *N Engl J Med* 312:948–952, 1985

11. Martin NDT, Snodgrass GJAI, Makin HLJ, Cohen RD: Letter to the editor. *N Engl J Med* 313:888–889, 1986

12. Chesney RW, DeLuca HF, Gertner JM, Genel M: Letter to the editor. *N Engl J Med* 313:889–890, 1986

13. Culler FL, Jones KL, Deftos LJ: Impaired calcitonin secretion in patients with Williams syndrome. *J Pediatr* 107:720–723, 1985

14. Lightwood RL: Idiopathic hypercalcemia with failure to thrive. *Arch Dis Child* 27:302–303, 1952

15. Martin NDT, Snodgrass GJAI, Cohen RD: Idiopathic infantile hypercalcemia—A continuing enigma. *Arch Dis Child* 59:605–613, 1984

16. Aarskog D, Asknes L, Markstead T: Vitamin D metabolism in idiopathic infantile hypercalcemia. *Am J Dis Child* 135:1021–1025, 1981

17. Langman CB, Budayr AA, Sailer DE, Strewler GJ: Nonmalignant expression of parathyroid hormone-related protein is responsible for idiopathic infantile hypercalcemia. *J Bone Miner Res* 7:593S, 1992

18. Foley TP Jr, Harrison HC, Arnaud CD, Harrison HE: Familial benign hypercalcemia. *J Pediatr* q81:1060–1067, 1972

19. Marx SJ, Attie MF, Spiegel AM, Levine MA, Lasker RD, Fox M: An association between neonatal severe primary hyperparathyroidism and familial hypocalciuric hypercalcemia. *N Engl J Med* 306:257–264, 1982

20. Marx SJ, Attie MF, Levine MD, Spiegel AM, Downs RW Jr, Lasker RD: The hypocalciuric or benign variant of familial hypercalcemia: Clinical and biochemical features in fifteen kindreds. *Medicine* 60:397–412, 1981

21. Law WM Jr, Heath H III: Familial benign hypercalcemia (hypocalciuric hypercalcemia) clinical and pathogenetic studies in 21 families. *Ann Intern Med* 102:511–519, 1985

22. Brown EM, Gamba G, Riccardi D, Lombardi M, Butters R, Kifor O, Sun A, Hediger MA, Lytton J, Hebert SC: Cloning and characterization of anextracellular Ca(2+)-sensing receptor from bovine parathyroid. *Nature* 366:575–580, 1993

23. Pollak MR, Brown EM, Chou YH, Hebert SC, Marx SJ, Steinmann B, Levi T, Seidman CE, Seidman JG: Mutations in the human Ca(2+)-sensing receptor gene cause familial hypocalciuric hypercalcemia and neonatal severe hyperparathyroidism. *Cell* 75:1297–1303, 1993

24. Pollak MR, Chou YH, Marx SJ, Steinmann B, Cole DE, Brandi ML, Papapoulos SE, Menko FH, Hendy GN, Brown EM: Familial hypocalciuric hypercalcemia and neonatal severe hyperparathyroidism. Effects of mutant gene dosage on phenotype. *J Clin Invest* 93(3):1108-1112, 1994

25. Bernulf J, Hall K, Sjogren I, Werner I: Primary hyperparathyroidism in children. *Acta Pediatr Scand* 59:249–258, 1970

26. Michael AF, Hong R, West CD: Hypercalcemia in infancy. *Am J Dis Child* 104:235–244, 1962

27. Jasper PL, Denny FW: Sarcoidosis in children. *J Pediatr* 73:499–512, 1968

28. Rosen JF, Wolin DA, Finberg L: Immobilization hypercalcemia after single limb fractures in children and adolescents. *Am J Dis Child* 132:560–564, 1978

29. Chan JCM, Young RB, Alon U, Manunes P: Hypercalcemia in children with disorders of calcium and phosphate metabolism during long-term treatment with 1,25(OH)$_2$D$_3$. *Pediatrics* 72:225–233, 1983

30. Frame B, Poznanski AK: Conditions that may be confused with rickets. In: Deluca HF, Anast CN (eds) *Pediatric Diseases Related to Calcium*. Elsevier, New York, pp 269–289, 1980

31. Schipiani E, Kruse K, Jüppner H: A constitutively active mutant PTH-PTHrp receptor in Jansen-type metaphyseal chondrodysplasia. *Science* 268:98–100, 1995

32. Jacobus CH, Holick MF, Shao Q, Chen TC, Holm IA, Kolodny JM, Fuleihan GE, Seely EW: Hypervitaminosis D associated with drinking milk. *N Engl J Med* 326:1173–1177, 1992

33. Holick MF, Shao Q, Liu WW, Chen TC: The vitamin D content of fortified milk and infant formula. *N Engl J Med* 326:1178–1181, 1992

36. Miscellaneous Causes of Hypercalcemia

Kai H. Yang, M.D., and Andrew F. Stewart, M.D.

Department of Endocrinology, Yale University School of Medicine, New Haven, Connecticut; and Connecticut Veterans Affairs Medical Center, West Haven, Connecticut

Hypercalcemia resulting from parathyroid disorders, from malignancies, and from granulomatous disorders make up the majority of cases of hypercalcemia. These have been discussed in the preceding chapters. In this chapter, attention is focused on less common causes of hypercalcemia. The references in the headings of ensuing sections are to articles that contain recent, more detailed reviews of the areas under discussion.

PROTEIN-BINDING ABNORMALITIES (1,2)

Hypocalcemia due to hypoalbuminemia is widely recognized. That hypercalcemia may result as a consequence of hyperproteinemia is less widely appreciated. This occurs in two settings. First, patients with dehydration and volume contraction may display hyperalbuminemia. Because albumin is the primary binding protein for calcium in blood, this hyperalbuminemia leads to an elevation in the total, but not the ionized, serum calcium. Because the ionized serum calcium concentration is normal, symptoms and signs of hypercalcemia are not present.

A second and far less common scenario has been described in patients with multiple myeloma who have an abnormal immunoglobulin that specifically binds calcium ions. As in patients with hyperalbuminemia, the globulin fraction, the total protein, and the total serum calcium concentrations are elevated, but the ionized serum calcium is normal. Symptoms and signs of hypercalcemia do not occur. Because elevations in ionized serum calcium can occur in multiple myeloma, hypercalcemia resulting from the binding to immunoglobulins may be inappropriately treated. Physicians may be alerted to artifactual hypercalcemia by the presence of moderate to severe hypercalcemia in the absence of symptoms, with normal Q-T intervals on electrocardiogram and normal urinary calcium excretion.

A number of formulae have been developed to predict or correct the serum calcium for reductions or elevations in serum albumin. In general, these are only moderately reliable. The firm diagnosis of a calcium–protein interaction requires direct measurement of ionized serum calcium concentration.

ENDOCRINE CAUSES OF HYPERCALCEMIA OTHER THAN HYPERPARATHYROIDISM

Thyrotoxicosis (3–8)

Mild hypercalcemia (10.5 to 11.5 mg/dl) frequently accompanies thyrotoxicosis. Although coexisting hyperparathyroidism has proved to be the cause of hypercalcemia in some of these patients, thyrotoxicosis alone can lead to hypercalcemia, a scenario that has been reported to occur in up to 50% of hyperthyroid patients. Renal calcium reabsorption and circulating 1,25-dihydroxyvitamin D (1,25(OH)$_2$D) values have been reported to be reduced in such patients, reflecting suppression of parathyroid function. Bone turnover and resorption are increased. Thus, hypercalcemia is believed to result from thyroxine- and triiodothyronine-induced bone resorption, a phenomenon that, over the long term, may account at least in part for the osteopenia associated with thyrotoxicosis. Hypercalcemia due to thyrotoxicosis may respond to therapy with β–adrenergic antagonists and, by definition, must reverse with therapy of the thyrotoxicosis.

Pheochromocytoma (9,10)

Hypercalcemia, at times severe, has been reported to occur in patients with pheochromocytoma. In most instances, hypercalcemia results from coexisting primary hyperparathyroidism as a manifestation of the multiple endocrine neoplasia syndrome type IIA (see Chapter 29). Occasionally, however, hypercalcemia reverses following adrenalectomy for the pheochromocytoma, an observation that suggests that the hypercalcemia resulted from the secretion by the pheochromocytoma of a circulating factor that stimulates bone resorption or induces hyperparathyroidism. Some evidence, albeit weak, suggests that catecholamines may play such a role. More recently, however, pheochromocytomas have been demonstrated to produce parathyroid-hormone-related protein (PTHrP) (see Chapters 12,32). Pheochromocytomas should be suspected and excluded prior to parathyroidectomy in all hypertensive patients with hyperparathyroidism.

Addison's Disease (11–13)

Hypercalcemia has been reported to occur in patients with primary adrenal insufficiency, typically during addisonian crisis. It has also been encountered in patients with secondary (pituitary) hypoadrenalism. The majority of reports are in the older literature, and the pathophysiology has not been thoroughly evaluated. Hypercalcemia may simply reflect hemoconcentration and volume contraction, with elevation in the serum albumin. In more recent studies, it has been shown that, at least in some patients, ionized calcium is elevated, and parathyroid hormone (PTH), PTHrP, and 1,25(OH)$_2$D are suppressed. Hypercalcemia responds to volume expansion and glucocorticoids.

Islet Cell Tumors of the Pancreas (14–17)

Islet cell tumors may secrete PTHrP (see Chapters 12,32), or they may occur with parathyroid gland hyperplasia as a feature of the multiple endocrine neoplasia type I syndrome (see Chapter 29). Interestingly, 90% of patients with islet cell tumors that secrete vasoactive intestinal polypeptide (VIP) develop hypercalcemia. These "VIP-omas" are manifested clinically by the WDHA syndrome: severe *w*atery *d*iarrhea ("pancreatic cholera"), *h*ypokalemia, and *a*chlorhydria. The mechanism responsible for hypercalcemia is unknown.

Growth Hormone Therapy (18)

Growth hormone has been used in surgical intensive care settings to prevent or reverse the catabolic consequences of chronic surgical illnesses. In one recent report, the use of growth hormone was associated with moderate hypercalcemia (11.5 to 12.5 mg/dl). This was most striking in patients being treated for thermal burns. PTH and 1,25(OH)$_2$ vitamin D were suppressed. The underlying mechanisms are unknown.

IMMOBILIZATION (19–22)

Weightlessness (as occurs in space flight) and complete, prolonged bed rest for orthopedic casting or traction, or because of spinal cord injury or other neurologic disorders, regularly lead to accelerated bone resorption and hypercalcemia in individuals with high underlying rates of bone turnover, including children, adolescents, and young adults, patients with primary or secondary hyperparathyroidism (as occurs in renal failure), patients with Paget's disease (see Chapter 75), and patients with early, mild, or "subclinical" instances of malignancy-associated hypercalcemia. Hypercalcemia develops within days to weeks of the onset of bed rest; it is associated with (i) increased osteoclastic bone resorption and decreased osteoblastic bone formation, (ii) hypercalciuria leading to nephrolithiasis, and (iii) if the condition is prolonged, osteopenia. The osteoclastic bone resorption, hypercalciuria, and hypercalcemia promptly reverse with the resumption of normal weight bearing. Passive range of motion exercises are ineffective. Circulating PTH and 1,25(OH)$_2$D levels are reduced, as is urinary cyclic AMP excretion. Preliminary evidence suggests that treatment with bisphosphonates may reverse or diminish immobilization-induced hypercalcemia and osteopenia. The mechanisms responsible for immobilization-induced bone resorption remain speculative.

THE MILK-ALKALI SYNDROME (23–25)

Excessive consumption of calcium and absorbable antacids may lead to a syndrome of hypercalcemia, metabolic alkalosis, and renal insufficiency known as the milk-alkali syndrome. This syndrome was first described in 1923 in a subset of patients treated for peptic ulcer disease with the Sippy diet (hourly milk or cream administration coupled with calcium, bismuth, and sodium bicarbonate salts). Two to 20 days later, patients developed headaches, a distaste for milk, nausea, and vomiting, associated with alkalosis and renal insufficiency. When serum calcium measurements became available, they were found to be elevated. With time, the syndrome may progress to include pruritis and band keratopathy.

The original milk-alkali syndrome developed in patients consuming excessive dairy calcium and absorbable antacids. As usage of histamine H$_2$ blockers and sucralfate has increased, the incidence of the milk-alkali syndrome has decreased. Recently, however, calcium carbonate has been prescribed with increasing frequency as an antacid or as prophylaxis for osteoporosis. Calcium carbonate, which contains both of the factors necessary for development of milk-alkali syndrome, may cause milk-alkali syndrome. Ingestion of from 2 to 8 g of elemental calcium per day is needed to produce the syndrome. Patients with preexisting renal insufficiency, thiazide use (and, thus, hypocalciuria), or preexisting hyperparathyroidism often require less calcium to develop the syndrome.

The pathophysiology of the milk-alkali syndrome is only partially understood. The administration of antacid contributes to the alkalosis. It also has been suggested that excessive calcium concentrations in the renal tubular lumen and the suppression of PTH enhance proximal tubular bicarbonate reabsorption. Volume depletion also stimulates proximal tubular bicarbonate reabsorption. Alkalosis may also inhibit renal calcium excretion. Dehydration from vomiting and hypercalcemia-induced nephrogenic diabetes insipidus, and interstitial renal calcification from hypercalcemia and hyperphosphatemia, all contribute to the development of renal insufficiency. Thus, a cycle is developed in which hypercalcemia is initiated by the ingestion of calcium and maintained by alkalosis. Alkalosis is induced by alkali ingestion and maintained by hypercalciuria and hypercalcemia.

Diagnosis requires a careful history, as most antacids are over-the-counter medications and may not be reported in a list of medications. Serum calcium and creatinine are elevated. Bicarbonate, phosphate, and magnesium levels are normal to high. Bone scans may show normal to increased uptake in the long bones and in areas of metastatic calcification.

Treatment consists of discontinuing the calcium and alkali, and saline infusion followed by loop diuretics. Severe cases have responded to dialysis. Azotemia may be irreversible in longstanding cases.

TOTAL PARENTERAL NUTRITION (26–28)

Hypercalcemia may occur in patients receiving total parenteral nutrition (TPN). In the early phases of therapy (days to weeks), hypercalcemia may result from excessive concentrations of calcium or vitamin D in the TPN fluid. In such cases, correction of hypercalcemia follows reformulation of the TPN solution by the pharmacy. Over the longer term (months to years), hypercalcemia associated with an osteomalacic osteodystrophy has been reported to occur in patients receiving TPN containing little or no calcium (see Chapter 66). This disorder has been ascribed to aluminum intoxication due to the inadvertent addition of aluminum to the TPN solution in the form of amino acid hydrolysates. With the removal of aluminum from TPN solutions in recent years, this syndrome has disappeared.

HYPERCALCEMIA RESULTING FROM MEDICATIONS

Vitamin D and Related Compounds (29–32)

Hypercalcemia is regularly encountered in patients receiving vitamin D or its analogs (25-hydroxyvitamin D, 1,25(OH)$_2$D, and dihydrotachysterol). Recently, an "outbreak" of hypercalcemia due to vitamin D intoxication has been described that resulted from the accidental oversupplementation of cow's milk with vitamin D by a commercial dairy. The recommended daily allowance for vitamin D is 400 U/day. The amount of vitamin D required to produce hypercalcemia is in excess of 50,000 U/week. Thus, hypercalcemia occurs not from over-the-counter multivitamin overdose but from prescribed doses of vitamin D or its analogs, usually used in the treatment of osteoporosis, hypoparathyroidism, malabsorption, or renal osteodystrophy. The hypercalcemia that occurs in this setting has gastrointestinal, renal, and skeletal components and responds to withdrawal of the vitamin D compound, to volume expansion, and to calciuresis. Occasionally, glucocorticoid treatment is required. The biologic half-life of vitamin D is very long (weeks to months), whereas that of its metabolites is relatively short (hours to days).

Vitamin A and Related Compounds (33,34)

Vitamin A in large doses (150,000 IU/day) may cause hypercalcemia. In the past, this was a medical curiosity limited to occasional intentional drug overdoses and to desperate Arctic explorers who consumed sled-dog and polar bear liver. More recently, however, the widespread use of vitamin A analogs, such as cis-retinoic acid for the treatment of acne and other dermatologic disorders and all-trans-retinoic acid for the treatment of hematologic malignancies, has been associated with the occasional occurrence of hypercalcemia. PTH, PTHrP, and plasma 1,25(OH)$_2$D are suppressed. The hypercalcemia appears to result from osteoclast-mediated bone resorption.

Estrogens and Antiestrogens (35,36)

Estrogens and antiestrogens cause hypercalcemia in approximately 30% of patients treated for breast cancer metastatic to the skeleton. The physiologic basis of this estrogen- or antiestrogen-"flare" is unknown. It has been associated with subsequent tumor regression when the offending drug can be continued. The hypercalcemia appears to be skeletal in origin, responsive to hydration and glucocorticoids, and self-limited.

Lithium (37)

Lithium carbonate in doses of 900 to 1,500 mg/day has been reported to cause hypercalcemia in approximately 5% of patients receiving the drug. There is no clear consensus as to the mechanism; some studies suggest an upward resetting of the parathyroid gland setpoint for calcium suppression of PTH secretion, whereas others indicate that the hypercalcemia is independent of parathyroid function. Except in patients with previously unrecognized coincidental primary hyperparathyroidism, the hypercalcemia will resolve if lithium therapy is discontinued.

Thiazide Diuretics (38)

Thiazide diuretics regularly cause hypercalcemia. The hypercalcemia appears to be largely renal in origin in that thiazide diuretics limit renal calcium excretion and enhance calcium reabsorption in the distal tubule. On the other hand, thiazide diuretics have been reported to cause hypercalcemia in anephric patients, suggesting that extrarenal effects also may be important. Hypercalcemia reverses rapidly with discontinuation of the offending drug. The thiazide effect on the kidney has been used in the treatment of hypoparathyroidism and nephrolithiasis due to renal calcium wasting.

Aminophylline (39)

Aminophylline and its derivatives have been reported to cause hypercalcemia. This has usually been observed after a loading dose of theophylline has raised serum theophylline levels above the therapeutic range. Serum calcium values become normal when patients are placed on maintenance therapy and serum theophylline levels fall into the therapeutic range. Theophylline-induced hypercalcemia is typically mild. Its mechanism is not known.

CHRONIC AND ACUTE RENAL FAILURE (40,41)

Hypercalcemia may occur in the settings of both acute and chronic renal failure. It develops in the recovery phase of acute tubular necrosis due to rhabdomyolysis. It has been postulated that the severe hyperphosphatemia that accompanies the early phases of acute renal failure in this syndrome exceeds the calcium phosphate solubility product and leads to the deposition of calcium phosphate complexes in soft tissues, as well as to hypocalcemia-mediated secondary hyperparathyroidism. As renal function recovers, the combination of excessive circulating PTH concentrations and reentry of calcium salts into the circulation from soft tissues leads to hypercalcemia.

In the setting of chronic renal failure, particularly in patients on hemodialysis, hypercalcemia is common and may result from vitamin D intoxication, calcium antacid overingestion, immobilization, aluminum intoxication, or combinations of the above (see Chapter 67).

MANGANESE INTOXICATION (42,43)

Manganese intoxication has been reported to produce severe hypercalcemia in workers exposed to toxic concentrations of manganese in contaminated industrial settings or wells. The mechanisms responsible for hypercalcemia are unknown.

ADVANCED CHRONIC LIVER DISEASE (44)

Patients with end-stage chronic liver disease awaiting liver transplantation have been reported to display hypercalcemia. The mechanisms underlying the hypercalcemia are unknown but are likely multifactorial.

SUBCUTANEOUS FAT NECROSIS (45,46)

Subcutaneous fat necrosis in neonates has been reported to cause hypercalcemia that is accompanied by increased circulating concentrations of $1,25(OH)_2D$ and reduced concentrations of PTH. It has been hypothesized that granulomas associated with fat necrosis secrete excessive quantities of $1,25(OH)_2D$ and cause hypercalcemia in a manner analogous to the hypercalcemia encountered in sarcoidosis and other granulomatous diseases (see Chapter 34).

REFERENCES

1. Ladenson JH, Lewis JH, McDonald JM, Slatopolsky E, Boyd JC: Relationship of free and total calcium in hypercalcemic conditions. *J Clin Endocrinol Metab* 48:393–397, 1978
2. Merlini G, Fitzpatrick LA, Siris ES, Bilezikian JP, Birken S, Beychok S, Osserman EF: A human myeloma immunoglobulin G binding four moles of calcium associated with asymptomatic hypercalcemia. *J Clin Immunol* 4:185–196, 1984
3. Peerenboom H, Keck E, Kruskemper GL, Strohmeye G: The defect in intestinal calcium transport in hyperthyroidism and its response to therapy. *J Clin Endocrinol Metab* 59:936–940, 1984
4. Burman KD, Monchick JM, Earll JM, Wartofski L: Ionized and total serum calcium and parathyroid hormone in hyperthyroidism. *Ann Intern Med* 84:668–671, 1976
5. Ross DS, Nussbaum SR: Reciprocal changes in parathyroid hormone and thyroid function after radioiodine treatment of hyperthyroidism. *J Clin Endocrinol Metab* 68:1216–1219, 1989
6. Britto JM, Fenton AJ, Holloway WR, Nicholson GC: Osteoblasts mediate thyroid hormone stimulation of osteoclastic bone resorption. *Endocrinology* 123:169–176, 1994
7. Rosen HN, Moses AC, Gundberg C, Kung VT, Seyedin SM, Chen T, Holick M, Greenspan SL: Therapy with parenteral pamidronate prevents thyroid hormone-induced bone turnover in humans. *J Clin Endocrinol Metab* 77:664–669, 1993
8. Rude RK, Oldham SB, Singer FR, Nicoloff JT: Treatment of thyrotoxic hypercalcemia with propranolol. *N Engl J Med* 294:431–433, 1976
9. Stewart AF, Hoecker J, Segre GV, Mallette LE, Amatruda T, Vignery A: Hypercalcemia in pheochromocytoma: Evidence for a novel mechanism. *Ann Intern Med* 102:776–779, 1985
10. Mune T, Katakami H, Kato Y, Yasuda K, Matsukura S, Miura K: Production and secretion of parathyroid hormone-related protein in pheochromocytoma: participation of an α–adrenergic mechanism. *J Clin Endocrinol Metab* 76:757–762, 1993
11. Muls E, Bouillon R, Boelaert J, Lamberigts G, Van Imschoot S, Daneels R, DeMoor P: Etiology of hypercalcemia in a patient with Addison's disease. *Calcif Tissue Int* 34:523–526, 1982
12. Vasikaran SD, Tallis GA, Braund WJ: Secondary hypoadrenalism presenting with hypercalcaemia. *Clin Endocrinol* 41:261–265, 1994
13. Diamond T, Thornley S: Addisonian crisis and hypercalcaemia. *Aust NZ J Med* 24:316, 1994
14. Mao C, Carter P, Schaefer P, Zhu L, Dominguez JM, Hanson DJ, Appert HE, Kim K, Howard JM: Malignant islet cell tumor associated with hypercalcemia. *Surgery* 117:37–40, 1994
15. Ratcliffe WA, Bowden SJ, Dunne FP, Hughes S, Emly JF, Baker JT, Pye JK, Williams CP: Expression and processing of parathyroid hormone-related protein in a pancreatic endocrine cell tumour associated with hypercalcaemia. *Clin Endocrinol* 40:679–686, 1994
16. Asa SL, Henderson J, Goltzman D, Drucker DJ: Parathyroid hormone-like peptide in normal and neoplastic human endocrine tissues. *J Clin Endocrinol Metab* 71:1112–1118, 1990
17. Verner JV, Morrison AB: Endocrine pancreatic islet disease with diarrhea. *Arch Intern Med* 133:492–500, 1974
18. Knox JB, Demling RH, Wilmore DW, Sarraf P, Santos AA: Hypercalcemia associated with the use of human growth mone in an adult surgical intensive care unit. *Arch Surg* 130:442–445, 1995
19. Stewart AF, Adler M, Byers CM, Segre GV, Broadus AE: Calcium homeostasis in immobilization: An example of resorptive hypercalciuria. *N Engl J Med* 306:1136–1140, 1982
20. Bergstrom WH: Hypercalciuria and hypercalcemia complicating immobilization. *Am J Dis Child* 132:553–554, 1978
21. Chappard D, Minaire P, Privat C, Berard E, Mendoza-Sarmiento J, Tournebise H, Basle MF, Audran M, Rebel A, Picot C, Gaud C: Effects of tiludronate on bone loss in paraplegic patients. *J Bone Miner Res* 10:112–118, 1995
22. Lueken SA, Arnaud SB, Taylor AK, Baylink DJ: Changes in markers of bone formation and resorption in a bed rest model of weightlessness. *J Bone Miner Res* 8:1433–1438, 1993
23. Beall DP, Scofield RH: Milk-alkali syndrome associated with calcium carbonate consumption. *Medicine* 74(2):89–96, 1995
24. McMillan DE, Freeman RB: The milk alkali syndrome: a study of the acute disorder with comments on the development of the chronic condition. *Medicine* 44(6):485–501, 1965
24. Orwoll ES. The milk-alkali syndrome: current concepts. *Ann Intern Med* 97:242–248, 1982
26. Ott SM, Maloney NA, Klein GL, Alfrey AC, Ament ME, Coburn JW, Sherrard DJ: Aluminum is associated with low bone formation in patients receiving chronic parenteral nutrition. *Ann Intern Med* 96:910–914, 1983
27. Klein GL, Horst RL, Norman AW, Ament ME, Slatopolsky E, Coburn JW: Reduced serum levels of 1a, 25-dihydroxyvitamin D during long-term total parenteral nutrition. *Ann Intern Med* 94:638–643, 1981
28. Shike M, Sturtridge WC, Tam CS, Harrison JE, Jones G, Murray TM, Husdan H, Whitwell J, Wilson DR, Jeejeebhoy KN: A possible role of vitamin D in the genesis of parenteral-nutrition-induced metabolic bone disease. *Ann Intern Med* 95:560–568, 1981
29. Haussler MR, McCain TA: Basic and clinical concepts related to vitamin D metabolism and action. *N Engl J Med* 297:1041–1050, 1977
30. Holick MF, Shao Q. Liu WW, Chen TC: The vitamin D content of fortified milk and infant formula. *N Engl J Med* 326:1178–1181, 1992
31. Jacobus CH, Holick MF, Shao Q, Chen TC, Holm IA, Kolodny JM, Guleihan GE-H, Seely EW: Hypervitaminosis D associated with drinking milk. *N Engl J Med* 326:1173–1177, 1992
32. Pettifor JM, Bikle DD, Cavalerso M, Zachen D, Kamdar MC, Ross FP: Serum levels of free 1,25-dihydroxyvitamin D in vitamin D toxicity. *Ann Intern Med* 122:511–513, 1995
33. Valente JD, Elias AN, Weinstein GD: Hypercalcemia associated with oral isotretinoin in the treatment of severe acne. *JAMA* 250:1899, 1983
34. Suzumiya J, Asahara F, Katakami H, Kimura N, Hisano S, Okumura M, Ohno R: Hypercalcaemia caused by all-trans retinoic acid treatment of acute promyelocytic leukaemia: Case report. *Eur J Haematol* 53:126–127, 1994
35. Legha SS, Powell K, Buzdar AU, Blumen-Schein GR: Tamoxifen-induced hypercalcemia in breast cancer. *Cancer* 47:2803, 1981
36. Valentin-Opran A, Eilon G, Saez S, Mundy GF: Estrogens and antiestrogens stimulate release of bone-resorbing activity in cultured human breast cancer cells. *J Clin Invest* 75:726, 1985
37. Speigal AM, Rudorfer MV, Marx SJ, Linnoila M: The effect of short-term lithium administration of suppressibility of parathyroid hormone secretion by calcium in vivo. *J Clin Endocrinol Metab* 59:354, 1984
38. Porter RH, Cox BG, Heaney D, Hostetter TH, Stinebaugh BJ, Suki WN: Treatment of hypoparathyroid patients with chlorthalidone. *N Engl J Med* 298:577, 1978

39. McPherson ML, Prince SR, Atamer E, Maxwell DB, Ross-Clunis H, Estep H: Theophylline-induced hypercalcemia. *Ann Intern Med* 105:52–54, 1986
40. Llach F, Felsenfeld AJ, Haussler MR: The pathophysiology of altered calcium metabolism in rhabdomyolysis-induced acute renal failure. *N Engl J Med* 305:117–123, 1981
41. Lane JT, Boudrea RJ, Kinlaw WB: Disappearance of muscular calcium deposits during resolution of prolonged rhabdomyolysis-induced hypercalcemia. *Am J Med* 89:523–525, 1990
42. Chandra SV, Seth PK, Mankeshwar JK: Manganese poisoning: Clinical and biochemical observations. *Environ Res* 7:374–380, 1974
43. Chandra SV, Shukla GS, Srivastava RS: An exploratory study of manganese exposure to welders. *Clin Toxicol* 18:407–416, 1981
44. Gerhardt A, Greenberg A, Reilly JJ, Van Thiel DH: Hypercalcemia. A complication of advanced chronic liver disease. *Arch Intern Med* 147:274–277, 1987
45. Finne PH, Sanderud J, Aksnes L, Bratlid D, Aarskog D: Hypercalcemia with increased and unregulated 1,25-dihydroxyvitamin D production in a neonate with subcutaneous fat necrosis. *J Pediatr* 112:792–794, 1983
46. Lewis HM, Ferryman S, Gatrad AR, Moss C: Subcutaneous fat necrosis of the newborn associated with hypercalcaemia. *J R Soc Med* 87:482–483, 1994

37. Hypocalcemia: Pathogenesis, Differential Diagnosis, and Management

Elizabeth Shane, M.D.

Department of Medicine, Columbia University, College of Physicians and Surgeons, New York, New York

Hypocalcemia is encountered commonly in medical practice. Like hypercalcemia, hypocalcemia varies in its clinical presentation from an asymptomatic biochemical abnormality to a severe life-threatening condition. The many causes of hypocalcemia are listed in Tables 1 and 2, and are also considered separately in subsequent chapters. Certain general principles that apply to the differential diagnosis and management of hypocalcemia are covered in this chapter.

PATHOGENESIS AND DIFFERENTIAL DIAGNOSIS

The concentration of calcium in the extracellular fluid is critical for many physiologic processes. Under normal circumstances, the range is kept remarkably constant, between 8.5 and 10.5 mg/dl (2.1 to 2.5 mM). The exact normal ranges vary slightly depending on the laboratory. Approximately half the total serum calcium is bound to plasma proteins, primarily albumin. A small component is complexed to anions such as citrate or sulfate. The remaining half circulates as free calcium ion. It is only this ionized portion of the total serum calcium that is physiologically important, regulating neuromuscular contractility, the activity of many enzymes, the process of coagulation, and a variety of other cellular activities.

In many chronic illnesses, substantial reductions may occur in the serum albumin concentration that may lower total serum calcium concentration while the ionized calcium concentration remains normal. A simple correction for hypoalbuminemia can be made by adding 0.8 mg/dl to the total serum calcium for every 1.0 g/dl by which the serum albumin is lower than 4.0 g/dl. Thus, a patient with a serum calcium of 7.8 mg/dl and a serum albumin of 2.0 mg/dl, has a corrected total serum calcium of 9.4 mg/dl. In contrast to changes in the serum albumin, which affect the total but not the ionized calcium level, alterations in pH affect the ionized calcium concentration without altering the total calcium level. Acidosis increases the ionized calcium by decreasing the binding of calcium ions to albumin, whereas alkalosis decreases the ionized calcium by enhancing binding of calcium ions to albumin. Measurement of total serum calcium is usually adequate for most clinical situations, but in complex cases, direct measurement of the ionized calcium should be performed.

The parathyroid glands are extremely sensitive to small changes in the serum ionized calcium level. Parathyroid hormone, through its acute effects on bone resorption and renal calcium reabsorption in the distal tubule, is responsible for the minute-to-minute regulation of the serum calcium level. Adjustments in intestinal calcium absorption via parathyroid-hormone-stimulated renal 1,25-dihydroxyvitamin D production require 24 to 48 hours to become maximal, and therefore they come into play only when the hypocalcemic stimulus is of a more chronic nature. Hypocalcemia occurs when there is a failure of, or incomplete compensation by, the parathyroid-hormone-controlled homeostatic mechanisms that defend against a hypocalcemic stimulus (see Chapter 9). The most common causes of hypocalcemia include hypoparathyroidism, deficiency or abnormal metabolism of vitamin D, hypomagnesemia, and acute or chronic renal failure. In general, hypocalcemic states may be classified according to whether they are associated with inappropriately low levels of parathyroid hormone (hypoparathyroid states) (Table 1) or whether parathyroid hormone levels are elevated, indicating normal parathyroid gland responsiveness to the low serum calcium (secondary hyperparathyroid states) (Table 2).

Idiopathic hypoparathyroidism is manifested by hypocalcemia and coexistent low or absent parathyroid hormone levels. It most often occurs as part of an autoimmune syndrome associated with deficient function of one or more endocrine glands (adrenals, thyroid, and ovaries), pernicious anemia, alopecia, vitiligo, and mucocutaneous candidiasis. This disorder is often familial, and its inheritance appears to be autosomal recessive. Familial hypoparathyroidism may also occur as an isolated defect, the mode of inheritance varying in each kindred. Rarely, congenital aplasia of the parathyroid glands may occur, usually in conjunction with defective development of the thymus (DiGeorge syndrome).

TABLE 1. *Hypoparathyroid states resulting in hypocalcemia*

Autoimmune
  Isolated
  End-organ deficiency syndrome
Postsurgical
Severe magnesium deficiency
Neck irradiation
Infiltrative
  Hemochromatosis
  Sarcoidosis
  Thalassemia
  Wilson's disease
  Amyloidosis
  Metastatic carcinoma
  DiGeorge syndrome
  Neonatal hypocalcemia
  Hungry bone syndrome (postparathyroidectomy)

TABLE 2. *Nonhypoparathyroid states resulting in hypocalcemia*

Vitamin D deficiency
  Lack of sunlight exposure
  Dietary lack
  Malabsorption
  Upper GI tract surgery
  Liver disease
  Renal disease
  Anticonvulsants
  Vitamin-D-dependent rickets, type I
    (1α–hydroxylase deficiency)
Parathyroid hormone resistance
  Pseudohypoparathyroidism
  Severe magnesium deficiency
Vitamin D resistance
  Vitamin-D-resistant rickets
  Vitamin-D-dependent rickets, type II (resistance to
    $1,25(OH)_2D$)
  Familial vitamin D resistance
Drugs
  Hypocalcemic agents
    Bisphosphonates
    Plicamycin
    Calcitonin
    Gallium nitrate
    Phosphate
  Anticancer agents
    Asparaginase
    Cisplatinum
    Cytosine arabinoside
    Doxorubicin
    WR 2721
  Other
    Ketaconazole
    Pentamidine
    Foscarnet
Miscellaneous
  Acute pancreatitis
  Massive tumor lysis
  Osteoblastic metastases
  Phosphate infusion
  Multiple citrated blood transfusions
  Toxic shock syndrome
  Acute rhabdomyolysis
  Acute severe illness

Postsurgical hypoparathyroidism, transient or permanent, may develop after neck surgery for thyroid disease as a result of inadvertent removal of or trauma to the parathyroid glands or their vascular supply. The widespread use of radioactive iodine to treat thyrotoxicosis has decreased the frequency of this occurrence. Neck exploration for primary hyperparathyroidism is now the most frequent situation in which postsurgical hypoparathyroidism occurs. Severe and prolonged hypocalcemia frequently develops after parathyroid surgery for osteitis fibrosis due to chronic renal insufficiency. In this situation, the relative hypoparathyroidism induced by the surgical procedure is complicated by deposition of available calcium into the healing bony lesions (hungry bone syndrome). Severe magnesium deficiency (see Chapter 42) is a rather common cause of hypocalcemia. The normal serum magnesium level is 1.8 to 3.0 mg/dl (0.8 to 1.2 mmol/L). In general, the serum magnesium is less than 1.0 mg/dl (0.4 mmol/L) when hypocalcemia is due to hypomagnesemia. At least two pathogenetic mechanisms have been implicated. Impaired secretion of parathyroid hormone resulting in absolute or relative hypoparathyroidism is present in the vast majority of patients with hypocalcemia secondary to hypomagnesemia. Increased resistance to the action of parathyroid hormone at bone and kidney has also been demonstrated in some patients with severe hypomagnesemia. A number of less common causes of hypoparathyroidism resulting from parathyroid hormone deficiency are listed in Table 1.

Hypocalcemia may also complicate a large number of primary disorders (Table 2) in patients who have intrinsically normal parathyroid glands. In these conditions, the fall in serum calcium caused by the underlying disease process results in a compensatory increase in parathyroid hormone secretion. This state of "secondary hyperparathyroidism" has the effect of raising the serum calcium, frequently into the low-normal range, by enhancing bone resorption, renal tubular calcium reabsorption and, where possible, gastrointestinal (GI) calcium absorption. The most common causes of hypocalcemia with normal parathyroid function (nonhypoparathyroid hypocalcemia) are related to the deficiencies in vitamin D and/or its active metabolites (see Chapters 58,59,67) that accompany a large number of GI or renal diseases. The syndromes of parathyroid hormone resistance (pseudohypoparathyroidism) and vitamin D resistance, also accompanied by secondary hyperparathyroidism, are reviewed in Chapters 39 and 61, respectively. Other causes of hypocalcemia include acute pancreatitis (Chapter 41), osteoblastic metastases, multiple transfusions of citrated blood, and acute rhabdomyolysis. In each of these situations, when the secondary hyperparathyroidism is insufficient to compensate for the hypocalcemic stimulus, hypocalcemia ensues.

CLINICAL FEATURES OF HYPOCALCEMIA

The signs and symptoms of acute hypocalcemia (Table 3) primarily result from enhanced neuromuscular irritability. Sensations of numbness and tingling involving the fingertips, toes, and circumoral region are early symptoms. Increased neuromuscular irritability may be demonstrated at the bedside by eliciting Chvostek's sign or Trousseau's sign. Chvostek's sign is twitching of the circumoral muscles in response to gently tapping the facial nerve just anterior to the ear. It should be noted that approximately 10% of normal individuals will demonstrate a slight twitch in response to this maneuver. Trousseau's sign is carpal spasm elicited by inflation of a blood pressure cuff to 20 mm Hg above the patient's systolic blood pressure for 3 min. The classic response—flexion of the wrist and metacarpophalangeal joints, extension of the interphalangeal joints, and adduction of the digits—reflects the heightened irritability of the nerves resulting from ischemia in the region of the cuff. A positive Trousseau's sign is rare in the absence of significant hypocalcemia.

Muscle cramps are often experienced by hypocalcemic patients. They most commonly involve the lower back, legs, and feet. In severe or acute hypocalcemia, the muscle cramps may progress to spontaneous carpopedal spasm (tetany). Laryngospasm or bronchospasm may also develop. Seizures of all types (syncopal episodes, petit mal, grand mal, and focal) may occur whether the hypocalcemia is acute or chronic. Other central nervous system manifestations include irritability, impaired intellectual capacity, and personality disturbances. Severe hypocalcemia may be accompanied by prolongation of the Q-T interval on the electrocardiogram and rarely, congestive heart failure; both cardiac manifestations are reversible with correction of the hypocalcemia. Although the presence of symptoms primarily reflects the degree of the hypocalcemia, a rapid rate of fall of the serum calcium and/or the concomitant presence of alkalosis, which enhances binding of ionized calcium to albumin, may also be associated with more severe signs and symptoms.

Patients with chronic hypocalcemia due to idiopathic hypoparathyroidism or pseudohypoparathyroidism may also have calcification of the basal ganglia and extrapyramidal neurologic symptoms. Subcapsular cataracts and abnormal dentition are also common in such patients (see Chapters 38, 39).

MANAGEMENT OF ACUTE HYPOCALCEMIA

Management of acute hypocalcemia will be considered in this chapter. Therapy of chronic hypocalcemia is discussed in Chapters 38, 39, 60, and 61.

TABLE 3. *Clinical features of hypocalcemia*

Neuromuscular irritability
   Paresthesias
   Chvostek's sign
   Trousseau's sign
   Laryngospasm
   Bronchospasm
   Tetany
   Seizures
   Prolonged Q-T interval on EKG

The decision to treat the hypocalcemic patient depends on the severity of the hypocalcemia, the rapidity with which it developed, and the presence or absence of clinical signs and symptoms. At one end of the spectrum, an asymptomatic patient with mild hypocalcemia (7.5 to 8.5 mg/dl, or 1.9 to 2.1 mmol/L) may warrant cautious observation and require only oral calcium supplements (500 to 1000 mg elemental calcium every 6 hr). In contrast, a patient with tetany, a sign of severe hypocalcemia, must be treated aggressively with intravenous calcium administration. Serum calcium levels of less than 7.5 mg/dl (1.9 mmol/L), or any level in a patient with symptoms, require parenteral calcium therapy.

The mainstay of therapy for acute symptomatic hypocalcemia is intravenous administration of calcium salts. Calcium should be administered with caution in digitalized patients, because sensitivity to the adverse effects of digitalis, particularly arrhythmias, is increased by hypercalcemia. Calcium gluconate (90 mg elemental calcium/10 ml ampule) is preferred over calcium chloride (272 mg elemental calcium/10 ml ampule), because it is less irritating to the veins. Initially, 1 to 2 ampules of calcium gluconate diluted in 50 to 100 ml of 5% dextrose (180 mg of elemental calcium) should be infused over 5 to 10 minutes. This procedure should be repeated as necessary to control symptomatic hypocalcemia. Persistent or less severe hypocalcemia may be managed by administration of more dilute calcium solutions over longer periods. In general, 15 mg/kg of elemental calcium infused over 4 to 6 hours will raise the serum calcium by 2 to 3 mg/dl (0.5 to 0.75 mmol/L). One practical approach is to initiate therapy with 10 ampules of calcium gluconate in 1 L of 5% dextrose infused at a rate of 50 ml/hr (45 mg of elemental calcium/hr); the rate of the infusion then may be titrated to maintain the serum calcium in the low normal range. When volume is a concern, the concentration of the solution may be increased. However, solutions of greater than 200 mg/100 ml of elemental calcium (more than 2 ampules of calcium gluconate/100 ml) should be avoided because of the propensity for irritation of veins and, in the event of extravasation, soft tissues. If hypocalcemia is likely to persist, therapy should be initiated early with oral calcium supplements (1 to 2 g elemental calcium) and 1,25-dihydroxyvitamin D ($1,25(OH)_2D$) (0.5 to 1.0 μg) daily.

The hypomagnesemic patient who is also hypocalcemic will require treatment of the hypomagnesemia before the hypocalcemia will resolve (Chapter 42). Moreover, in the acutely hypocalcemic patient in whom magnesium deficiency is clinically likely, it is appropriate to add magnesium to the treatment regimen while awaiting laboratory confirmation of hypomagnesemia.

SUGGESTED READINGS

1. Shane EJ, Bilezikian JP: Disorders of calcium, phosphate and magnesium metabolism. In: Askanazi J, Starker PM, Weissman C (eds) *Fluid and Electrolyte Management in Critical Care.* Butterworth, London, pp 337–353, 1986
2. Stewart AF, Broadus AE: Mineral metabolism. In: Felig P, Baxter JP, Broadus AE, Frohman LA (eds) *Endocrinology and Metabolism.* McGraw-Hill, New York, pp 1422–1433, 1987
3. Tohme JF, Bilezikian JP. Hypocalcemic emergencies. *Endocrinol Metab Clin North Am* 363–375, 1993

38. Hypoparathyroidism

David Goltzman and *David E.C. Cole

*Department of Medicine, McGill University and Royal Victoria Hospital, Montreal, Quebec, Canada and *Departments of Clinical Biochemistry, Medicine, and Genetics, University of Toronto, Toronto, Ontario, Canada*

Hypoparathyroidism is a clinical disorder that manifests when insufficient parathyroid hormone (PTH) is produced to maintain extracellular fluid (ECF) calcium within the normal range or when adequate circulating concentrations of PTH are unable to optimally function in target tissues to maintain ECF calcium within the normal range. The causes of hypothyroidism (Table 1) can be classified broadly as (i) failure of the parathyroid glands to develop, (ii) destruction of the parathyroid glands, (iii) reduced parathyroid gland function due to altered regulation, and (iv) impaired PTH action. The common aspect of these conditions is the presence of reduced, biologically active PTH. This results in common clinical and laboratory features, which may be influenced, however, by the specific pathogenesis of the hypoparathyroidism.

CLINICAL MANIFESTATIONS

The acute clinical signs and symptoms of hypoparathyroidism of any etiology include evidence of latent or overt increased neuromuscular irritability as a consequence of hypocalcemia (Chapter 37). The acute symptoms may occur more readily during times of increased demand on the calcium homeostatic system (pregnancy and lactation, the menstrual cycle, and states of alkalosis). Chronically, patients may manifest muscle cramps, pseudopapilledema, extrapyramidal signs, mental retardation, and personality disturbances, as well as cataracts, dry rough skin, coarse brittle hair, alopecia, and abnormal dentition. The dental abnormalities may include defects due to enamel hypoplasia, defects in dentin, shortened premolar roots, thickened lamina dura, delayed tooth eruption, and increased frequency of caries. Occasionally, patients may be edentulous. Finally, patients may sometimes be diagnosed only after a low serum calcium is detected during multiphasic blood screening as part of a routine examination.

TABLE 1. *Pathogenetic classification of hypoparathyroidism*

I. Failure of the parathyroid glands to develop
 Isolated hypoparathyroidism
 X-linked (#307700)[a]
 Autosomal recessive (#241400)
 DiGeorge sequence (#188400)
 Kenny–Caffey syndrome (#127000)
 Kearns–Sayre syndrome (#530000)
 Barakat syndrome (#146255/#256340)
 Hypoparathyroidism with short stature, mental retardation, and seizures (#241410)
II. Destruction of the parathyroid glands
 Surgical
 Polyglandular autoimmune disease (PGA type I, or HAM) (#240300)
 Radiation
 Metal overload (iron, copper)
 Granulomatous infiltration
 Neoplastic invasion
III. Reduced parathyroid gland function due to altered regulation
 Primary
  Autosomal dominant (#146200)
   Calcium sensor mutation (#145980)
   PTH mutation (#168450)
  Autosomal recessive
   PTH mutation (#168450)
 Secondary
  Maternal hyperparathyroidism
  Hypomagnesemia
IV. Impaired parathyroid hormone action
 Hypomagnesemia
 Pseudohypoparathyroidism

[a]Numbers refer to standardized entries in McKusick's genetic catalog, "Mendelian Inheritance in Man" (12), also available as a constantly updated on-line service (contact: help @ gdb.org).

LABORATORY ABNORMALITIES

The biochemical hallmarks of hypoparathyroidism are hypocalcemia and hyperphosphatemia in the presence of normal renal function. Serum calcium concentrations are often 6–7 mg/dl (1.50–1.75 mM) and serum phosphorus levels 6–9 mg/dl (1.93–2.90 mM). Serum concentrations of immunoreactive PTH are low or undetectable except in cases of PTH resistance where they are elevated or high normal. Serum concentrations of $1,25(OH)_2D_3$ are usually low and alkaline phosphatase is normal. Although the fractional excretion of calcium is increased, because of reduced intestinal calcium absorption and diminished bone resorption, the filtered load of calcium, and therefore the 24-hour urinary excretion of calcium is reduced. Nephrogenous cyclic AMP excretion is low and renal tubular reabsorption of phosphorus is elevated. Urinary cyclic AMP and phosphorus excretion both increase markedly after administration of exogenous bioactive PTH (Ellsworth–Howard test) except in PTH-resistant states (Chapter 39 and Appendix vii).

Basal ganglia and more widespread intracranial calcification may be detected on skull x-ray or CT scan and electroencephalographic changes may be present. Detection of limited parathyroid gland reserve may require an ethylenediaminetetraacetate (EDTA) infusion study, which should only be conducted under close supervision.

CAUSES OF HYPOPARATHYROIDISM

Failure of the Parathyroid Glands to Develop

Congenital agenesis or hypoplasia of the parathyroid glands can produce hypoparathyroidism that manifests in the newborn period. This may occur as isolated hypoparathyroidism (autosomal recessive or X-linked; the precise molecular genetic defects are unknown) in infants who also have thymic aplasia with immunodeficiency and congenital conotruncal cardiac anomalies. Genetic studies indicate that a wide range of etiologies—both genetic and environmental (Table 2)—may underlie the developmental abnormalities of the third and fourth branchial pouches that lead to this condition. Syndromologists have termed this condition the *DiGeorge sequence* to emphasize its etiologic heterogeneity and focus attention on other clinical findings that may suggest the primary cause. Hypoparathyroidism is a potential problem in any syndrome that includes the DiGeorge sequence. If the DiGeorge sequence of anomalies (now considered to include distinctive facial features, cleft lip/palate, and a wider variety of congenital heart disease) is not clearly part of another syndrome, it is likely the result of a microdeletion on the long arm of chromosome 22. Detection of the microdeletion by molecular cytogenetic analysis of chromosomal band 22q11.21-q11.23 using fluorescence *in situ* hybridization (FISH) is diagnostic. A negative result may suggest another cause of the hypoparathyroidism, although the possibility of as yet unknown deletions cannot be excluded. Individuals with the velocardiofacial (or Schprintzen) syndrome also have microdeletions of 22q and it is now believed that the two conditions overlap. The term "catch 22" has been applied to this cluster of disorders, as a mnemonic for the characteristic features (cardiac, abnormal facies, thymic aplasia, cleft palate, hypocalcemia with 22q deletion). All patients with otherwise unexplained persistent hypoparathyroidism

TABLE 2. *Conditions with DiGeorge sequence*

Chromosomal
dup(1q)
del(5p)
dup(8q)
del(10p)
del(22q)
Monogenic
Isolated autosomal dominant
Isolated autosomal recessive
Velocardiofacial syndrome or "CATCH 22"
Zellweger syndrome
Teratogenic
Diabetic embryopathy
Fetal alcohol syndrome
Retinoid embryopathy
Associational
Arhinencephalia/DiGeorge
CHARGE/DiGeorge
Cardiofacial/DiGeorge

CHARGE, Coloboma of the iris, heart disease, choanal atresia, retarded growth and development, genital anomalies, ear anomalies. Adapted from ref. 4.

in infancy should be karyotyped (± FISH for 22q11) and evaluated for other occult anomalies, including subclinical cardiac disease, renal dysplasia, and, occasionally, gastrointestinal maldevelopment. Although many cases of DiGeorge sequence are the result of *de novo* deletions, autosomal dominant inheritance is common. Demonstration of decreased parathyroid reserve in an otherwise healthy parent may require provocative testing, but evidence of inheritance may depend on other features (conotruncal cardiac anomalies, decreased cell-mediated immunity, etc.). As a rule, microdeletions are associated with a variable phenotype, even within a family.

The Kenny–Caffey syndrome, another congenital anomaly, is associated with absent parathyroid tissue, growth retardation, and medullary stenosis of tubular bones. Analysis of the PTH gene in this syndrome has revealed no defect. Hypoparathyroidism is also a component of several other single familial syndromes including Kearns–Sayre syndrome (a mitochondrial myopathy with ophthalmoplegia, retinal degeneration, and cardiac conduction defects), Barakat syndrome (nerve deafness and steroid-resistant nephrosis), and others (Table 1).

Destruction of the Parathyroid Glands

The most common cause of hypoparathyroidism is surgical excision of or damage to the parathyroid glands as a result of total thyroidectomy for thyroid cancer, radical neck dissection for other cancers, or repeated operations for primary hyperparathyroidism. Transient and reversible hypocalcemia following parathyroid surgery may be due to edema or hemorrhage into the parathyroids, "hungry bone syndrome" due to severe hyperparathyroidism, or postoperative hypomagnesemia. Prolonged hypocalcemia, which may develop immediately, or weeks or years after neck surgery, suggests permanent hypoparathyroidism. The incidence of this condition after neck exploration for primary hyperparathyroidism is usually less than 5% and often only 1% to 2%. In patients with a higher risk of developing permanent hypoparathyroidism, those with primary parathyroid hyperplasia or where repeated neck exploration is required to identify an adenoma, parathyroid tissue may be autotransplanted into the brachioradialis or sternocleidomastoid muscle at the time of parathyroidectomy or cryopreserved for subsequent transplantation if necessary.

Rarely, hypoparathyroidism has also been described in a small number of patients who receive extensive radiation to the neck and mediastinum; in metal overload diseases such as hemochromatosis (iron), thalassemia (iron), and Wilson's disease (copper); and in neoplastic or granulomatous infiltration of the parathyroid glands.

Hypoparathyroidism ("idiopathic") may also occur as a presumed autoimmune disorder either alone or in association with other endocrine deficiency states. It may be sporadic or familial. Antibodies directed against parathyroid tissue can be detected in 33% of patients with isolated disease and 41% of patients with hypoparathyroidism and other endocrine deficiencies, but may also be seen in some normals. It is uncertain as to whether the autoantibodies are of primary or secondary importance in the pathogenesis. In the polyglandular syndrome the most common associated manifestations are mucocutaneous candidiasis (moniliasis, 65% to 75%) and Addison's disease (55% to 60%). This has been termed the HAM (hypoparathyroidism, Addison's disease, moniliasis) syndrome. The etiology of this association is not understood. Adrenal insufficiency occurs in only 10% of all patients with hypoparathyroidism and moniliasis in only 15%, so that their presence should suggest polyglandular deficiency. Hypoparathyroidism, either as an isolated autoimmune disorder or as part of the HAM syndrome, may present between 6 months and 20 years of age (average age, 7–8 years). In the HAM syndrome, hypoparathyroidism manifests about 1–4 years after candidiasis occurs and before the onset of Addison's disease. Consequently, very few individuals with isolated Addison's disease will later develop hypoparathyroidism. Candidiasis may affect the skin, nails and mucous membranes of the mouth and vagina and is often intractable. Addison's disease can mask the presence of hypoparathyroidism or may manifest only in improvement of the hypoparathyroidism with a reduced requirement for calcium and vitamin D. The etiology of this association is not understood. Glucocorticoid therapy for the adrenal insufficiency, by diminishing gastrointestinal absorption of calcium and increasing renal calcium excretion, may worsen hypocalcemia and might be fatal if introduced before hypoparathyroidism is diagnosed.

In addition to Addison's disease and moniliasis, hypoparathyroidism in polyglandular autoimmune disease (PGA type I) may be associated with insulin-dependent diabetes mellitus, primary hypogonadism, autoimmune thyroiditis, keratoconjunctivitis, pernicious anemia, chronic active hepatitis, steatorrhea (malabsorption resembling celiac disease), alopecia (totalis or areata), and vitiligo. Pernicious anemia and diabetes mellitus usually develop after hypoparathyroidism. Most cases of PGA type I disease have been familial with an autosomal recessive pattern of inheritance.

Reduced Parathyroid Gland Function Due to Altered Regulation

Altered regulation of parathyroid gland function may be primary or secondary. Secondary causes include maternal hyperparathyroidism and hypomagnesemia. The infant of a mother with primary hyperparathyroidism generally develops hypocalcemia within the first 3 weeks of life but it may occur up to 1 year after birth (Chapter 40). Although therapy may be required acutely, the disorder is usually self-limited. Hypomagnesemia due to defective intestinal absorption or renal tubular reabsorption of magnesium may impair secretion of PTH and in this way contribute to hypoparathyroidism (Chapter by 42). Magnesium replacement will correct the hypoparathyroidism.

Primary causes of altered regulation of parathyroid gland function can have a genetic basis. To date, three rare genetic defects have been defined.

With the discovery of the parathyroid calcium sensor, new insights have been gained into the regulation of PTH secretion. A mutation in the sensor, resulting in constitutive activation, has been described in familial hypoparathyroidism inherited in an autosomal dominant manner. The activated parathyroid gland calcium receptor chronically suppresses PTH secretion. The activated kidney receptor induces hypercalciuria which also contributes to the hypocalcemia. A different genetic defect underlies the autosomal dominant isolated hypoparathyroidism described in one patient in whom a single base substitution (T → C) in exon 2 of the PTH gene was reported. This mutation in the signal sequence of PTH apparently impeded conversion of pre-pro-PTH to pro-PTH thereby reducing normal production of the hormone. In one family with autosomal recessive isolated hypoparathyroidism, exon slipping was demonstrated, i.e., exon 2 of the PTH gene was lost. This exon contains the initiation codon required for translation of mRNA encoding PTH and the signal peptide required for translocation of PTH. Consequently, reduced PTH production occurs. No doubt other molecular genetic abnormalities will be found in other families with both autosomal dominant and recessive isolated hypoparathyroidism.

Impaired PTH Action

Although in theory bio-inactive PTH may be synthesized and secreted by the parathyroid gland, this has not been documented. An early report suggesting this as a mechanism underlying hypoparathyroidism was not supported in a follow-up study. More commonly, ineffective PTH action appears to be due to peripheral resistance to the effects of PTH. Such resistance may occur secondary to hypomagnesemia (Chapter 42) or as a primary disorder (pseudohypoparathyroidism, Chapter 39).

THERAPY

The major goal of therapy in all hypoparathyroid states is to restore serum calcium and phosphorus as close to normal as possible. The main pharmacologic agents available are supplemental calcium and vitamin D preparations. Phosphate binders and thiazide diuretics may be useful as ancillary agents. The major impediment to restoration of normocalcemia is the development of hypercalciuria with a resulting predilection for renal stone formation. Since the renal calcium-retaining effect of PTH is lost, when treatment with vitamin D is initiated, the enhanced absorption of calcium from the gut results in an increased filtered load of calcium which is readily cleared through the kidney. Consequently urinary calcium may increase well before serum calcium is normalized. Frequently it is necessary to accept a low normal serum calcium concentration in order to prevent chronic hypercalciuria. If urine calcium concentrations reach high normal and the serum calcium is still less than 8 mg/dl (2 mM), addition of a thiazide diuretic may reduce urinary calcium and raise serum calcium into the normal range. If serum calcium is normalized and the serum phosphorus remains greater than 6 mg/dl (1.93 mM), a nonabsorbable antacid may be added to reduce the hyperphosphatemia and prevent metastatic calcification.

Dairy products, which are high in phosphate, should be avoided and calcium administered in the form of supplements. Generally at least 1 g/day of elemental calcium is required.

A variety of vitamin D preparations may be used including vitamin D_3 or D_2, 25,000–100,000 U (1.25–5 mg) per day; dihydrotachysterol, 0.2–1.2 mg per day; 1α hydroxyvitamin D_3, 0.5–2 µg per day; or $1,25(OH)_2D_3$, 0.25–1 µg per day. Although vitamin D_3 and D_2 are the least expensive forms of therapy, they have the longest durations of action and can result in prolonged toxicity. The remaining preparations listed above all have the advantage of shorter half-lives and no requirement for renal 1α hydroxylation which is impaired in hypoparathyroidism. Dihydrotachysterol is rarely used today, however, and $1,25(OH)_2D_3$ is probably the treatment of choice. In children, these preparations should be prescribed on a body weight basis.

Close monitoring of the patient's urine calcium and serum calcium and phosphorus are required initially but follow-up at 3- to 6-month intervals may be adequate once stable laboratory values are reached (generally within a month).

SUGGESTED READINGS

1. Arnold A, Horst SA, Gardella TJ, Baba H, Levine MA, Kronenberg HM: Mutation of the signal peptide-encoding region of the preproparathyroid hormone gene in familial isolated hypoparathyroidism. *J Clin Invest* 86:1084–1087, 1990
2. Barakat AY, D'Albora JB, Martin MM, Jose PA: Familial nephrosis, nerve deafness, and hypoparathyroidism. *J Pediatr* 191:61–64, 1977
3. Bergada I, Schiffrin A, Abu Srair H, et al: Kenny syndrome: description of additional abnormalities and molecular studies. *Hum Genet* 80:39–42, 1988
4. Cohen MM Jr, Cole DEC: Origins of recognizable syndromes: Etiologic and pathogenetic mechanisms and the process of syndrome delineation. *J Pediatr* 115:161–164, 1989
5. Gidding SS, Minciotti AL, Langman CB: Unmasking of hypoparathyroidism in familial partial DiGeorge syndrome by challenge with disodium edetate. *N Engl J Med* 319:1589–91, 1988
6. Glover TW: CATCHING a break on 22. *Nat Genet* 10:257–8, 1995
7. Harvey JN, Barnett D: Endocrine dysfunction in Kearns–Sayre syndrome. *Clin Endocrinol* 37:97–103, 1992
8. Herrera M, Grant C, van Heerden JA, Fitzpatrick LA: Parathyroid autotransplantation. *Arch Surg* 127:825–9, 1992
9. Hong R: The DiGeorge anomaly. *Immunodefic Rev* 3:1–14, 1991
10. Illum F, Dupont E: Prevalence of CT-detected calcification in the basal ganglia in idiopathic hypoparathyroidism and pseudohypoparathyroidism. *Neuroradiology* 27:32–37, 1985
11. Mallette L: Synthetic human parathyroid hormone 1-34 fragment for diagnostic testing. *Ann Intern Med* 109:800–802, 1988
12. McKusick VA: *Mendelian inheritance in man: Catalogs of autosomal dominant, autosomal recessive, and X-linked phenotypes.* 14th ed. Baltimore: The Johns Hopkins University Press, 1994
13. Neufeld M, MacLaren N, Blizzard RM: Autoimmune polyglandular syndromes. *Pediatr Ann* 9:154–162, 1980
14. Okano O, Furukawa Y, Morii H, Fujita T: Comparative efficacy of various vitamin D metabolites in the treatment of various types of hypoparathyroidism. *J Clin Endocrinol Metab* 55:238–243, 1982
15. Parkinson DB, Thakker RV: A donor splice site mutation in the parathyroid hormone gene is associated with autosomal recessive hypoparathyroidism. *Nat Genet* 1:149–152, 1992
16. Pollak MR, Brown EM, Estep HL, McLaine PN, Kifor O, Park J, Hebert SC, et al. Autosomal dominant hypocalcemia caused by a Ca^{2-}-sensing receptor gene mutation. *Nat Genet* 8:303–307, 1994
17. Sherwood LM, Santora AC: II. Hypoparathyroid states in the differential diagnosis of hypocalcemia. In: Bilezikian JP, Marcus R, Levine MA (eds) *The parathyroids.* Raven Press, New York, pp 747–752, 1994
18. Whyte MP, Kim GS, Kosanovich M: Absence of parathyroid tissue in sex-linked recessive hypoparathyroidism. *J Pediatr* 109:915, 1986

39. Parathyroid Hormone Resistance Syndromes

Michael A. Levine, M.D.

Division of Endocrinology and Metabolism, The Johns Hopkins University School of Medicine, Baltimore, Maryland

The term *pseudohypoparathyroidism* (PHP) describes a group of disorders characterized by biochemical hypoparathyroidism (i.e., hypocalcemia and hyperphosphatemia), increased secretion of parathyroid hormone (PTH), and target tissue unresponsiveness to the biological actions of PTH.

In the initial description of PHP, Fuller Albright and his associates focused on the failure of patients with this syndrome to show either a calcemic or a phosphaturic response to administered parathyroid extract (1). These observations provided the basis for the hypothesis that biochemical hypoparathyroidism in PHP was due not to a deficiency of PTH but rather to resistance of the target organs, bone and kidney, to the biological actions of PTH. Thus the pathophysiology of PHP differs fundamentally from true hypoparathyroidism, in which PTH secretion rather than PTH responsiveness is defective.

The initial event in the expression of PTH action is binding of the hormone to specific receptors located on the plasma membrane of target cells. Because the native and cloned receptors also bind parathyroid hormone-related protein with equivalent affinity, they are termed PTH/PTHrP receptors. The PTH/PTHrP receptor is coupled by heterotrimeric guanine nucleotide-binding regulatory proteins (G proteins) to signal effector molecules localized to the inner surface of the plasma membrane. Hormone binding is followed rapidly by the generation of a variety of second messengers, including cAMP, inositol 1,4,5-triphosphate and diacylglycerol, and cytosolic calcium, indicating that a single PTH/PTHrP receptor can couple not only to G_s to stimulate adenylyl cyclase, but also to G_q and G_{11} to stimulate phospholipase C. The best-characterized mediator of PTH action is cAMP, which rapidly activates protein kinase A. The relevant target proteins that are phosphorylated by protein kinase A, and the precise actions of these proteins, have not yet been fully characterized but include enzymes, ion channels, and proteins that regulate gene expression. In contrast to the well-recognized effects of the second messenger cAMP in bone and kidney cells, the physiologic importance of the phospholipase C signaling pathway in these PTH target tissues has not yet been established. For a complete discussion of the PTH/PTHrP receptor signaling system, the reader is referred to Chapters 11 and 12.

PATHOGENESIS OF PSEUDOHYPOPARATHYROIDISM

Characterization of the molecular basis for PHP commenced with the observation that cAMP mediates many of the actions of PTH on kidney and bone, and that administration of biologically active PTH to normal subjects leads to a significant increase in the urinary excretion of nephrogenous cAMP (2). The PTH infusion test remains the most reliable test available for the diagnosis of PHP and enables distinction between the several variants of the syndrome (Fig. 1). Thus, patients with PHP type I fail to show an appropriate increase in urinary excretion of both cAMP and phosphate (2), whereas subjects with the less common type II show a normal increase in urinary cAMP excretion but have an impaired phosphaturic response (3).

Pseudohypoparathyroidism Type Ia

Albright's original description of PHP emphasized PTH resistance as the biochemical hallmark of this disorder. Resistance to PTH alone would be consistent with a defect in the cell surface receptor specific for PTH. However, some patients with PHP type I display resistance to multiple hormones, including PTH, thyroid-stimulating hormone (TSH), gonadotropins, and glucagon, whose effects are mediated by cAMP (4). Cell membranes from most of these patients

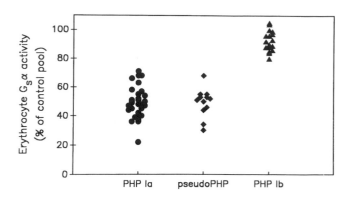

FIG. 2. $G_s\alpha$ activity in PHP type I and pseudoPHP. $G_s\alpha$ activity was measured in erythrocyte membrane extracts by complementation with membranes from S49 cyc- cells, which genetically lack $G_s\alpha$. The resultant adenylyl cyclase activity is expressed as a percentage of that of a control membrane preparation consisting of pooled erythrocyte membranes from several normal subjects.

show an approximate 50% reduction in expression or activity of $G_s\alpha$ protein (Fig. 2), a condition termed PHP type Ia. A generalized deficiency of $G_s\alpha$ may impair the ability of many hormones and neurotransmitters to activate adenylyl cyclase and thereby produce hormone resistance.

In addition to hormone resistance, patients with PHP type Ia also manifest a peculiar constellation of developmental and somatic defects that are collectively termed Albright's hereditary osteodystrophy (AHO) (1). The AHO phenotype consists of short stature, round facies, obesity, brachydactyly, and subcutaneous ossifications, but other abnormalities may also be present (5). The identification of individuals with AHO who lacked apparent hormone resistance led Albright to propose the rather awkward term *pseudopseudohypoparathyroidism* (pseudoPHP) to describe this normocalcemic variant of PHP (6). Subjects with pseudoPHP have a normal urinary cAMP response to PTH (2,7) (Fig. 1), which distinguishes them from occasional patients with PHP who maintain normal serum calcium levels without treatment (8). PseudoPHP is genetically related to PHP. Early clinical observations of AHO kindreds, in which several affected members had only AHO (i.e., pseudoPHP) while others had PTH resistance as well, (i.e., PHP) first suggested that the two disorders might reflect variability in expression of a single genetic lesion. Further support for this view derives from recent studies indicating that within a given kindred, subjects with either pseudoPHP or PHP type Ia have equivalent functional $G_s\alpha$ deficiency (Fig. 2) (7,9). It therefore seems reasonable to use the term AHO to simplify description of these two variants of the same syndrome and to acknowledge the common clinical and biochemical characteristics that patients with PHP type Ia and pseudoPHP share.

The identification of $G_s\alpha$ deficiency in patients with AHO (7,10) first led to the speculation that the primary defect in this disorder involves the $G_s\alpha$ gene. The human gene for $G_s\alpha$ (GNAS1) is a complex 20-kb gene (11) that maps to 20q13.2 (12). Molecular studies of DNA from subjects with AHO have disclosed a variety of GNAS1 gene

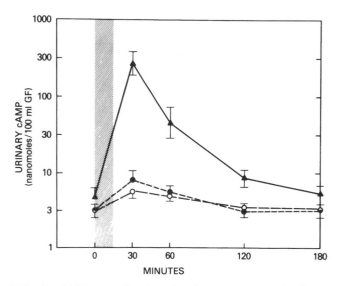

FIG. 1. cAMP excretion in urine in response to the intravenous administration of bovine parathyroid extract (300 USP units) from 9:00 a.m. to 9:15 a.m. The peak response in normals *(triangle)* is 50- to 100-fold times basal; patients with PHP type Ia *(solid circles)* or PHP type Ib *(open circles)* show only a two- to five-fold response.

mutations (13–19) that lead to decreased expression or function of G$_s\alpha$ protein. Although most gene mutations impair expression of G$_s\alpha$ mRNA (9,12), in some subjects abnormal forms of G$_s\alpha$ mRNA are produced (9,12) that encode dysfunctional G$_s\alpha$ proteins (11). Distinct G$_s\alpha$ mutations have been found in each kindred studied, implying that new and independent mutations must sustain the disorder. These observations provide molecular confirmation that inheritance of GNAS1 gene defects accounts for the autosomal dominant transmission of AHO.

These studies provide a molecular basis for G$_s\alpha$ deficiency but do not explain the striking variability in biochemical and clinical phenotype. Why do some G$_s\alpha$-coupled pathways show reduced hormone responsiveness (e.g., PTH, TSH, gonadotropins) whereas other pathways are clinically unaffected (ACTH in the adrenal and vasopressin in the renal medulla)? Perhaps even more intriguing is the paradox of why some subjects with G$_s\alpha$ deficiency have hormone resistance (PHP type Ia) whereas others may lack hormone resistance (pseudoPHP) or physical features of AHO altogether (18). The basis for the variable penetrance of these features in patients with G$_s\alpha$ deficiency remains unknown, but several observations suggest that complex mechanisms must be responsible for the variable expression of GNAS1 gene defects within members of a kindred. G$_s\alpha$ deficiency may be necessary but not sufficient to cause hormone resistance (or AHO). Perhaps variability in other components of the signal transduction pathway (e.g., there are multiple forms of adenylyl cyclase and phosphodiesterase that exhibit tissue-specific expression) may explain why identical defects in G$_s\alpha$ can have such variable consequences in different tissues or in different individuals.

In AHO, inherited G$_s\alpha$ gene mutations reduce expression or function of G$_s\alpha$ protein. By contrast, in the McCune–Albright syndrome, somatic mutations in the G$_s\alpha$ gene enhance activity of the protein (21,22). These mutations lead to constitutive activation of adenylyl cyclase and produce proliferation and autonomous hyperfunction of hormonally responsive cells. The clinical significance of G$_s\alpha$ activity as a determinant of hormone action is emphasized by the recent description by Iiri et al. (14) of two male patients with both precocious puberty and PHP type 1a. These two unrelated boys had identical GNAS1 gene mutations that resulted in a temperature-sensitive G$_s\alpha$ that is constitutively activated in the cooler environment of the testis while being rapidly degraded in other tissues at normal body temperature. Thus, different tissues in these two individuals could show hormone resistance (to PTH and TSH), hormone responsiveness (to ACTH), or hormone independence (to luteinizing hormone, LH).

Pseudohypoparathyroidism Type Ib

Subjects with PHP type I who lack features of AHO typically show hormone resistance that is limited to PTH target organs (Fig. 1) and have normal G$_s\alpha$ activity (Fig. 2) (4). This variant is termed PHP type Ib (23). Although patients with PHP type Ib fail to show a nephrogenous cAMP response to PTH, they often manifest skeletal lesions similar to those that occur in patients with hyperparathyroidism (24). These observations have suggested that at least one intracellular signaling pathway coupled to the PTH receptor may be intact in patients with PHP type 1b.

The molecular basis for PTH resistance in PHP type Ib has not been identified. Specific resistance of target tissues to PTH, and normal activity of G$_s\alpha$, has implicated decreased expression or function of the PTH/PTHrP receptor as the cause for hormone resistance, however. Evidence in favor of this hypothesis comes from studies of cultured skin fibroblasts from patients with PHP type Ib. These studies suggest that the mechanisms responsible for PTH resistance are likely to be heterogeneous. Fibroblasts from some, but not all, PHP type Ib patients accumulate less cAMP in response to PTH (23,25) and contain decreased levels of mRNA encoding the PTH/PTHrP receptor (26). Furthermore, in most cases, pretreatment of the cultured fibroblasts with dexamethasone normalizes the PTH-induced cAMP response and increases expression of PTH/PTHrP receptor mRNA (26). Taken in the context of recent molecular studies that have failed to disclose mutations in the coding exons of the PTH/PTHrP receptor gene (27), it is likely that defects that impair regulation or expression of the PTH/PTHrP receptor account for decreased receptor activity in patients with PHP type Ib.

Pseudohypoparathyroidism Type Ic

In a few patients with PHP type I, resistance to multiple hormones occurs in the absence of a demonstrable defect in G$_s$ or G$_i$ (4,28). The nature of the lesion in such patients is unclear, but it could be related to some other general component of the receptor–adenylyl cyclase system, such as the catalytic unit (29). Alternatively, these patients could have functional defects of G$_s$ (or G$_i$) that do not become apparent in the assays that are presently available.

Pseudohypoparathyroidism Type II

Pseudohypoparathyroidism type II is a heterogeneous disorder without a clear genetic or familial basis. In these patients renal resistance to PTH is manifested by a reduced phosphaturic response to administration of PTH, despite a normal increase in urinary cAMP excretion (3). These observations suggest that the PTH receptor–adenylyl cyclase complex functions normally to increase cAMP in response to PTH, and are consistent with a model in which PTH resistance arises from an inability of intracellular cAMP to initiate the chain of metabolic events that result in the ultimate expression of PTH action.

Although no supportive data are yet available, a defective cAMP-dependent protein kinase A has been proposed (3). Alternatively, the defect in PHP type II may not reside in the generation of an intracellular cAMP response but rather in other PTH-sensitive signal transduction pathways that lead to increased concentrations of other intracellular second messengers, i.e., inositol 1,4,5-triphosphate, diacylglycerol, and cytosolic calcium.

A PTH Inhibitor as a Cause of PTH Resistance

Several studies have reported an apparent dissociation between plasma levels of endogenous immunoreactive and bioactive PTH in patients with PHP type 1. Despite high circulating levels of immunoreactive PTH, the levels of bioactive PTH in many patients with PHP type I have been found to be within the normal range when measured with highly sensitive renal (30) and metatarsal (31) cytochemical bioassay systems. Furthermore, plasma from many of these patients has been shown to diminish the biological activity of exogenous PTH in these *in vitro* bioassays (32). Currently, the nature of this putative inhibitor or antagonist remains unknown. The observation that prolonged hypercalcemia can remove or reduce significantly the level of inhibitory activity in the plasma of patients with PHP has suggested that the parathyroid gland may be the source of the inhibitor. In addition, analysis of circulating PTH immunoactivity after fractionation of patient plasma by reversed-phase high performance liquid chromatography has disclosed the presence of aberrant forms of immunoreactive PTH in many of these patients (33). Although it is conceivable that a PTH inhibitor may cause PTH resistance in some patients with PHP, it is more likely that circulating antagonists of PTH action arise as a consequence of the sustained secondary hyperparathyroidism that results from the primary biochemical defect.

DIAGNOSIS OF PSEUDOHYPOPARATHYROIDISM

The biochemical hallmark of PHP is failure of the PTH target organ, the kidney, to respond to PTH. Accordingly, a diagnosis of PHP should be considered in an individual with biochemical hypoparathyroidism (i.e., hypocalcemia and hyperphosphatemia) who has an elevated plasma concentration of immunoreactive PTH. Because reduced serum concentrations of magnesium have been reported to impair target organ responsiveness to PTH, it is important first to exclude hypomagnesemia in these subjects.

The diagnosis of PHP (or pseudoPHP) may also be suspected on the basis of clinical features of AHO. However, several features of AHO, e.g., obesity, round face, brachydactyly, and mental retardation, are common to other disorders (Prader–Willi syndrome, acrodysostosis, Ullrich–Turner syndrome) that are often associated with chromosomal defects. A growing number of reports have described small terminal deletions of chromosome 2q in patients with variable AHO-like phenotypes. Terminal deletion of 2q37 [del(2)(q37.3)] is the first consistent karyotypic abnormality that has been documented in patients with an AHO-like syndrome (34,35). These patients have normal endocrine function and normal $G_s\alpha$ activity, however (35). Thus, high-resolution chromosome analysis, biochemical/molecular analysis, and careful physical and radiologic examination are essential in discriminating between these phenocopies and AHO.

The classical tests for PHP, the Ellsworth–Howard test and later modifications by Chase, Melson, and Aurbach (2), involved the administration of 200–300 USP units of purified bovine PTH or parathyroid extract. Although these preparations are no longer available, the synthetic human PTH(1-34) peptide has been approved for human use and several protocols for its use in the differential diagnosis of hypoparathyroidism have been developed. The patient should be fasting, supine except for voiding, and hydrated (250 ml of water hourly from 6 a.m. to noon). Two control urine specimens are collected before 9 a.m. Synthetic human PTH (1-34) peptide (5 U/kg body weight to a maximum of 200 U) is administered intravenously from 9 to 9:15 a.m., and experimental urine specimens are collected from 9 to 9:30, 9:30 to 10:00, 10:00 to 11:00, and 11:00 to noon. Blood samples should be obtained at 9 a.m. and 11 a.m. for measurement of serum creatinine and phosphorus concentrations. Urine samples are analyzed for cAMP, phosphorus, and creatinine concentrations, and results are expressed as nanomoles of cAMP per 100 ml GF and TmP/GFR. Normal subjects and patients with hormonopenic hypoparathyroidism usually display a ten- to 20-fold increase in urinary cAMP excretion, whereas patients with PHP type I (type Ia and type Ib), regardless of their serum calcium concentration, will show a markedly blunted response (Fig. 1). Thus, this test can distinguish patients with so-called normocalcemic PHP (i.e., patients with PTH resistance who are able to maintain normal serum calcium levels without treatment) from subjects with pseudoPHP (who will have a normal urinary cAMP response to PTH (2,7). The urinary cAMP and phosphate responses to PTH are dependent on the endogenous serum PTH and calcium levels (36), however, such that correction of hypocalcemia following treatment with vitamin D may normalize the phosphaturic response to PTH in patients with PHP type I.

Recent studies indicate that measurement of plasma cAMP (37) or plasma 1,25-dihydroxyvitamin D (38) after infusion of hPTH(1-34) may also differentiate PHP type I from other causes of hypoparathyroidism. Further testing (e.g., $G_s\alpha$ protein or gene analysis) is indicated only to confirm the diagnosis of PHP type Ia.

The diagnosis of PHP type II, a much rarer entity, is less straightforward. Documentation of elevated serum PTH and basal urinary (or nephrogenous) cAMP is a prerequisite for a definitive diagnosis of PHP type II (3). These subjects have a normal urinary cAMP response to infusion of PTH but characteristically fail to show a phosphaturic response. Unfortunately, interpretation of the phosphaturic response to PTH is often complicated by random variations in phosphate clearance, and it is sometimes not possible to classify a phosphaturic response as normal or subnormal regardless of the criteria employed. More perplexing yet is the observation that biochemical findings that resemble PHP type II have been found in patients with various forms of vitamin D deficiency. In these patients, marked hypocalcemia is accompanied by hyperphosphatemia due presumably to an acquired dissociation between the amount of cAMP generated in the renal tubule and its effect on phosphate clearance.

TREATMENT

The basic principles of treatment of hypocalcemia in PHP are essentially those outlined for the treatment of hormonopenic hypoparathyroidism. Therapy is directed at maintaining a low- to mid-normal serum calcium concentration and thereby controlling symptoms of tetany while avoiding hypercalciuria. Happily, the risk of treatment-related hypercalciuria is far less for patients with PHP than for individuals with hypoparathyroidism, as patients with PHP have a lower absolute calcium excretion and a higher setting of TmCa/GFR (36).

Patients with PHP type Ia will frequently manifest resistance to other hormones in addition to PTH and may display clinical evidence of hypothyroidism or gonadal dysfunction. The basic principles used in the treatment of primary hypothyroidism apply to therapy of hypothyroidism in patients with PHP type Ia, as do approaches for the evaluation and treatment of hypogonadism.

REFERENCES

1. Albright F, Burnett CH, Smith PH: Pseudohypoparathyroidism: an example of "Seabright-Bantam syndrome." *Endocrinology* 30: 922–932, 1942

2. Chase LR, Melson GL, Aurbach GD: Pseudohypoparathyroidism: defective excretion of 3′,5′-AMP in response to parathyroid hormone. *J Clin Invest* 48:1832–1844, 1969

3. Drezner MK, Neelon FA, Lebovitz HE: Pseudohypoparathyroidism type II: a possible defect in the reception of the cyclic AMP signal. *N Engl J Med* 280:1056–1060, 1973

4. Levine MA, Downs RW Jr, Moses AM, et al: Resistance to multiple hormones in patients with pseudohypoparathyroidism. Association with deficient activity of guanine nucleotide regulatory protein. *Am J Med* 74:545–556, 1983

5. Schwindinger WF, Levine MA: Albright hereditary osteodystrophy. *The Endocrinologist* 4:17–27. 1994

6. Albright F, Forbes AP, Henneman PH: Pseudopseudohypoparathyroidism. *Trans Assoc Am Physicians* 65:337–350, 1952

7. Levine MA, Jap TS, Mauseth RS, Downs RW, Spiegel AM: Activity of the stimulatory guanine nucleotide-binding protein is reduced in erythrocytes from patients with pseudohypoparathyroidism and pseudopseudohypoparathyroidism: biochemical, endocrine, and genetic analysis of Albright's hereditary osteodystrophy in six kindreds. *J Clin Endocrinol Metab* 62:497–502, 1986

8. Drezner MK, Haussler MR: Normocalcemic pseudohypoparathyroidism. *Am J Med* 66:503–508, 1979

9. Levine MA, Ahn TG, Klupt SF, et al: Genetic deficiency of the alpha subunit of the guanine nucleotide-binding protein Gs as the molecular basis for Albright hereditary osteodystrophy. *Proc Natl Acad Sci USA* 85:617–621, 1988

10. Van Dop C, Bourne HR, Neer RM: Father to son transmission of decreased Ns activity in pseudohypoparathyroidism type Ia. *J Clin Endocrinol Metab* 59:825–828, 1984

11. Kozasa T, Itoh H, Tsukamoto T, Kaziro Y: Isolation and characterization of the human Gsα gene. *Proc Natl Acad Sci USA* 85: 2081–2085, 1988

12. Levine MA, Modi WS, OBrien SJ: Mapping of the gene encoding the alpha subunit of the stimulatory G protein of adenylyl cyclase (GNAS1) to 20q13.2-q13.3 in human by in situ hybridization. *Genomics* 11:478–479, 1991

13. Lin CK, Hakakha MJ, Nakamoto JM, et al: Prevalence of three mutations in the Gsα gene among 24 families with pseudohypoparathyroidism type Ia. *Biochem Biophys Res Commun* 189: 343–349, 1992

14. Iiri T, Herzmark P, Nakamoto JM, Van Dop C, Bourne HR: Rapid GDP release from Gsα in patients with gain and loss of function. *Nature* 371:164–168, 1994

15. Luttikhuis ME, Wilson LC, Leonard JV, Trembath RC: Characterization of a de novo 43-bp deletion of the Gsα gene (GNAS1) in Albright hereditary osteodystrophy. *Genomics* 21:455–457, 1994

16. Patten JL, Johns DR, Valle D, et al: Mutation in the gene encoding the stimulatory G protein of adenylate cyclase in Albrightís hereditary osteodystrophy. *N Engl J Med* 322:1412–1419, 1990

17. Weinstein LS, Gejman PV, Friedman E, et al: Mutations of the Gsα-subunit gene in Albright hereditary osteodystrophy detected by denaturing gradient gel electrophoresis. *Proc Natl Acad Sci USA* 87:8287–8290, 1990

18. Miric A, Vechio JD, Levine MA: Heterogeneous mutations in the gene encoding the alpha subunit of the stimulatory G protein of adenylyl cyclase in Albright hereditary osteodystrophy. *J Clin Endocrinol Metab* 76:1560–1568, 1993

19. Schwindinger WF, Miric A, Zimmerman D, Levine MA: A novel Gsα mutant in a patient with Albright hereditary osteodystrophy uncouples cell surface receptors from adenylyl cyclase. *J Biol Chem* 269:25387–25391, 1994

20. Carter A, Bardin C, Collins R, Simons C, Bray P, Spiegel A: Reduced expression of multiple forms of the alpha subunit of the stimulatory GTP-binding protein in pseudohypoparathyroidism type Ia. *Proc Natl Acad Sci USA* 84:7266–7269, 1987

21. Schwindinger WF, Francomano CA, Levine MA: Identification of a mutation in the gene encoding the alpha subunit of the stimulatory G protein of adenylyl cyclase in McCune–Albright syndrome. *Proc Natl Acad Sci USA* 89:5152–5156, 1992

22. Weinstein LS, Shenker A, Gejman PV, Merino MJ, Friedman E, Spiegel AM: Activating mutations of the stimulatory G protein in the McCune–Albright syndrome. *N Engl J Med* 325:1688–1695, 1991

23. Silve C, Santora A, Breslau N, Moses A, Spiegel A: Selective resistance to parathyroid hormone in cultured skin fibroblasts from patients with pseudohypoparathyroidism type Ib. *J Clin Endocrinol Metab* 62:640–644, 1986

24. Kidd GS, Schaaf M, Adler RA, Lassman MN, Wray HL: Skeletal responsiveness in pseudohypoparathyroidism: A spectrum of clinical disease. *Am J Med* 68:772–781, 1980

25. Silve C, Suarez F, el Hessni A, Loiseau A, Graulet AM, Gueris J: The resistance to parathyroid hormone of fibroblasts from some patients with type Ib pseudohypoparathyroidism is reversible with dexamethasone. *J Clin Endocrinol Metab* 71:631–638, 1990

26. Suarez F, Lebrun JJ, Lecossier D, Escoubet B, Coureau C, Silve C: Expression and modulation of the parathyroid hormone (PTH)/PTH-related peptide receptor messenger ribonucleic acid in skin fibroblasts from patients with type Ib pseudohypoparathyroidism. *J Clin Endocrinol Metab* 80:965–970, 1995

27. Schipani E, Weinstein LS, Bergwitz C, et al: Pseudohypoparathyroidism type Ib is not caused by mutations in the coding exons of the human parathyroid hormone (PTH)/PTH–related peptide receptor gene. *J Clin Endocrinol Metab* 80:1611–1621, 1995

28. Farfel Z, Brothers VM, Brickman AS, Conte F, Neer R, Bourne HR: Pseudohypoparathyroidism: inheritance of deficient receptor-cyclase coupling activity. *Proc Natl Acad Sci USA* 78:3098–3102, 1981

29. Barrett D, Breslau NA, Wax MB, Molinoff PB, Downs RW,Jr.: New form of pseudohypoparathyroidism with abnormal catalytic adenylate cyclase. *Am J Physiol* 257:E277–E283, 1989

30. de Deuxchaisnes CN, Fischer JA, Dambacher MA, et al: Dissociation of parathyroid hormone bioactivity and immunoreactivity in pseudohypoparathyroidism type I. *J Clin Endocrinol Metab* 53: 1105–1109, 1981

31. Bradbeer JN, Dunham J, Fischer JA, Nagant de Deuxchaisnes C, Loveridge N: The metatarsal cytochemical bioassay of parathyroid hormone: validation, specificity, and application to the study of pseudohypoparathyroidism type I. *J Clin Endocrinol Metab* 67:1237–1243, 1988

32. Loveridge N, Fischer JA, Nagant de Deuxchaisnes C, et al: Inhibition of cytochemical bioactivity of parathyroid hormone by plasma in pseudohypoparathyroidism type I. *J Clin Endocrinol Metab* 54:1274–1275, 1982

33. Mitchell J, Goltzman D: Examination of circulating parathyroid hormone in pseudohypoparathyroidism. *J Clin Endocrinol Metab* 61:328–334, 1985

34. Wilson LC, Leverton K, Oude Luttikhuis ME, et al: Brachydactyly and mental retardation: an Albright hereditary osteodystrophy-like syndrome localized to 2q37. *Am J Hum Genet* 56: 400–407, 1995

35. Phelan MC, Rogers RC, Clarkson KB, et al: Albright hereditary

osteodystrophy and del(2)(q37.3) in four unrelated individuals. *Am J Med Genet* 58:1–7, 1995

36. Stone MD, Hosking DJ, Garcia-Himmelstine C, White DA, Rosenblum D, Worth HG: The renal response to exogenous parathyroid hormone in treated pseudohypoparathyroidism. *Bone* 14:727–735, 1993

37. Stirling HF, Darling JA, Barr DG: Plasma cyclic AMP response to intravenous parathyroid hormone in pseudohypoparathyroidism. *Acta Paediatr Scand* 80:333–338, 1991

38. Miura R, Yumita S, Yoshinaga K, Furukawa Y: Response of plasma 1,25-dihydroxyvitamin D in the human PTH(1-34) infusion test: an improved index for the diagnosis of idiopathic hypoparathyroidism and pseudohypoparathyroidism. *Calcif Tissue Int* 46:309–313, 1990

40. Neonatal Hypocalcemia

Thomas O. Carpenter, M.D.

Department of Pediatrics, Yale University School of Medicine, New Haven, Connecticut

CALCIUM METABOLISM IN THE PERINATAL PERIOD

Mineralization of the fetal skeleton is provided for by active calcium transport from mother to fetus across the placenta. The site of regulation of calcium transport is apparently a calcium pump in the basal membrane (fetus-directed side) of the trophoblast (1). Evidence in the pregnant ewe suggests that a midregion fragment of parathyroid hormone-related peptide (PTHrP) may play a role in the regulation of this function (2). At term the fetus is hypercalcemic, is likely to have elevated circulating calcitonin, and may have low levels of parathyroid hormone (PTH) compared to maternal circulation. An abrupt transition to autonomous regulation of mineral homeostasis occurs at partum. The abundant placental supply of calcium is removed and the circulating calcium level begins to fall, reaching a nadir within the first 4 days of life, and subsequently rising to normal adult levels in the second week of life.

HYPOCALCEMIC SYNDROMES IN THE NEWBORN PERIOD

Manifestations of neonatal hypocalcemia are variable and may not correlate with the magnitude of depression in the circulating ionized calcium level. As in older people, increased neuromuscular excitability (tetany) is a cardinal feature of newborn hypocalcemia. Generalized or focal clonic seizures, jitteriness, irritability, and frequent twitches or jerking of limbs are seen. Hyperacusis and laryngospasm may occur. Nonspecific signs include apnea, tachycardia, tachypnea, cyanosis, and edema; vomiting has also been reported. Neonatal hypocalcemia may be classified by its time of onset; differences in etiology are suggested by "early" occuring hypocalcemia as contrasted with that occurring "late" (3) (Table 1).

Early Neonatal Hypocalcemia

Hypocalcemia occurring during the first 3 days of life, usually between 24 and 48 hours postpartum, is termed "early neonatal hypocalcemia" and characteristically is seen in premature infants, infants of diabetic mothers, and asphyxiated infants. The premature infant normally has an exaggerated postnatal depression in circulating calcium, dropping lower and earlier than in the term infant. Total calcium levels may drop below 7.0 mg/dl, but the proportional drop in ionized calcium is less, and it may explain the lack of symptoms in many prematures with total calcium in this range.

TABLE 1. *Neonatal hypocalcemia*

	Characteristics	Mechanism
Early	Onset within first 3-4 days of life; seen in infants of diabetic mothers, perinatal asphyxia and preeclampsia	Uncertain; possible exaggerated postnatal calcintonin surge, possible decrease in parathyroid response
Late	Onset days 5-10 of life; seen in winter, in infants of mothers with marginal vitamin D intake; associated with dietary phosphate load	Possible transient parathyroid dysfunction; hypomagnesia in some cases; calcium malabsorption
Other congenital hypoparathyroidism	Usually present after first 5 days of life with overt tetany	
Late-late hypocalcemia	Present in prematures at 2-4 months; associated with skeletal hypomineralization and inadequate dietary mineral or Vitamin D intake	
Infants of hyperparathyroid mother	May be present as late as 1 year of age; mother possibly undiagnosed	
Ionized hypocalcemia	In exchange transfusion with citrated blood products, hypocalcemia infusions, or alkalosis	

Prematures have been variably reported to show normal, elevated, or impaired secretion of PTH during citrate-induced hypocalcemia. Conflict also exists regarding the action of PTH in the newborn. A several day delay in the phosphaturic effect of PTH in both term and preterm infants has been described; resultant hyperphosphatemia may decrease serum calcium. The premature infant's exaggerated rise in calcitonin may provoke hypocalcemia. A role for vitamin D and its metabolites in early neonatal hypocalcemia is less convincing.

The infant of the diabetic mother (IDM) also demonstrates an exaggerated postnatal drop in the circulating calcium level when compared with other infants of comparable maturity. As in premature infants, the decrease is not entirely explained by a fall in ionized calcium concentrations. The pregnant diabetic tends to have lower circulating PTH and magnesium levels; the IDM has lower circulating magnesium and PTH but normal calcitonin. Abnormalities in vitamin D metabolism do not appear to play a role in the development of hypocalcemia in the IDM. Strict maternal glycemic control during pregnancy results in a decreased incidence of hypocalcemia in the IDM.

Early hypocalcemia occurs in asphyxiated infants; calcitonin response is augmented and PTH levels are elevated. Infants of pre-eclamptic mothers and postmature infants with growth retardation develop early hypocalcemia and are prone to hypomagnesemia.

Late Neonatal Hypocalcemia

The presentation of hypocalcemic tetany between 5 and 10 days of life is termed "late" neonatal hypocalcemia. The incidence of this disorder is greater in full-term than in premature infants and is not correlated with birth trauma or asphyxia. Children affected are often being fed cow's milk or cow's milk formula, which may have 3–4 times the phosphate content of human milk. Hyperphosphatemia is associated with late neonatal hypocalcemia and may reflect (i) inability of the immature kidney to efficiently excrete phosphate; (ii) dietary phosphate load; or (iii) transiently low levels of circulating PTH. Others have noted an association between late neonatal hypocalcemia and modest maternal vitamin D insufficiency. An increased occurrence of late neonatal hypocalcemia in winter has also been noted.

Hypocalcemia associated with magnesium deficiency may present as late neonatal hypocalcemia (Chapter 41). Severe hypomagnesemia (circulating levels less than 0.8 mg/dl) may occur in congenital defects of intestinal magnesium absorption or renal tubular reabsorption. Transient hypomagnesemia of unknown etiology is associated with a less severe decrease in circulating magnesium (between 0.8 and 1.4 mg/dl). Hypocalcemia frequently complicates hypomagnesemic states due to impaired secretion of PTH. Impaired PTH responsiveness has also been demonstrated as an inconsistent finding in magnesium deficiency.

Other Causes of Neonatal Hypocalcemia

Symptomatic neonatal hypocalcemia may occur within the first 3 weeks of life in infants born to mothers with hyperparathyroidism (4). Presentation at 1 year of age has also been reported. Serum phosphate is often greater than 8 mg/dl; symptoms may be exacerbated by feeding with cow's milk or other high-phosphate formulas. The proposed mechanism for the development of neonatal hypocalcemia in the infant of the hyperparathyroid mother is as follows: maternal hypercalcemia occurs secondary to hyperparathyroidism resulting in increased calcium delivery to the fetus and fetal hypercalcemia, which inhibits fetal parathyroid secretion. The infant's suppressed parathyroid is not able to maintain normal calcium levels postpartum. Hypomagnesemia may be observed in the infant of the hyperparathyroid mother. Maternal hyperparathyroidism has been diagnosed as a result of the delivery of a hypocalcemic infants.

"Late-late" neonatal hypocalcemia has been used in reference to premature infants who develop hypocalcemia with poor bone mineralization within the first 3–4 months of life. These infants tend to have an inadequate dietary supply of mineral and/or vitamin D.

The previously discussed forms of neonatal hypocalcemia are generally found to be of a transient nature. More rarely, hypocalcemia which is permanent is detected in the newborn periods and due to congenital hypoparathyroidism (5) (Chapter 38). Isolated absence of the parathyroids may be inherited in X-linked or autosomal recessive fashion. Congenital hypoparathyroidism also occurs as the DiGeorge anomaly, classically the triad of hypoparathyroidism, T-cell incompetence due to a partial or absent thymus, and conotruncal heart defects (e.g., tetralogy of Fallot, truncus arteriosus) or aortic arch abnormalities. These structures are derived from the embryologic third and fourth pharyngeal pouches; the usual sporadic occurrence reflects developmental abnormalities of these structures. Other defects may variably occur in this broad-spectrum field defect. Familial occurrences have been reported; associations with abnormalities of chromosomes 22 and 10 have been reported. The Kenny–Caffey syndrome is another congenital anomaly associated with hypoparathyroidism, growth retardation, and medullary stenosis of tubular bones (6).

Decreases in the ionized fraction of the circulating calcium occur in infants undergoing exchange transfusions with citrated blood products or receiving lipid infusions. Citrate and fatty acids form complexes with ionized calcium, reducing the free calcium compartment. Alkalosis secondary to adjustments in ventilatory assistance may provoke a shift of ionized calcium to the protein-bound compartment.

TREATMENT OF NEONATAL HYPOCALCEMIA

Early neonatal hypocalcemia may be asymptomatic, and the necessity of therapy may be questioned in such infants. Most authors recommend that early neonatal hypocalcemia be treated when the circulating concentration of total serum calcium is less the 5–6 mg/dl (1.25–1.50 mmol/L) (or of ionized calcium less than 2.5–3 mg/dl, 0.62–0.72 mmol/L) in the premature infant and when total serum calcium is less than 6–7 mg/dl (1.50–1.75 mmol/L) in the term infant. Emergency therapy of acute tetany consists of intravenous (never intramuscular) calcium gluconate (10% solution) given slowly (less than 1 ml/min). A dose of 1–3 ml will usually arrest convulsions. Doses should generally not exceed 2 mg/kg body weight and may be repeated up to 4 times per 24 hours. After successful management of acute emergencies, maintenance therapy may be achieved by intravenous administration of 20–50 mg of elemental calcium per kg body weight per 24 hours. Calcium gluconate is a commonly used oral supplement. Management of late neonatal tetany should include a low-phosphate formula such as Similac PM 60/40, in addition to calcium supplements. A calcium/phosphate ratio of 4:1 has been recommended. Monitoring generally reveals that therapy can be discontinued after several weeks.

When hypomagnesemia is a causal feature of the hypocalcemia, magnesium administration may be indicated. Magnesium sulfate is given intravenously using cardiac monitoring or intramuscular as a 50% solution at a dose of 0.1–0.2 ml/kg. One or two doses may treat transient hypomagnesemia: a dose may be repeated after 12–24 hours. Patients with primary defects in magnesium metabolism require long-term oral magnesium supplements.

The place of vitamin D in the management of transient hypocalcemia is less clear. Daily supplementation of 400–800 U of vitamin D has been suggested for all premature infants as a preventive measure. Patients with normal intestinal absorption who develop late-late hypocalcemia with vitamin-D-deficienct rickets should respond within 4 weeks to 1000–2000 U of daily oral vitamin D. Such patients should receive a total of at least 40 mg of elemental calcium/kg body weight/day. In the various forms of persistent congenital hypoparathyroidism, long-term treatment with vitamin D (or its therapeutic metabolites) is used.

REFERENCES

1. Pitkin RM: Calcium metabolism in pregnancy and the perinatal period: a review. *Am J Obstet Gynecol* 151:99–109, 1985
2. Care AD: The placental transfer of calcium. *J Dev Physiol* 15: 253–257, 1991
3. Hillman LS, Haddad JG: Hypocalcemia and other abnormalities of mineral homeostasis during the neonatal period. In: Heath DA, Marx SJ (eds) *Calcium Disorders*. Butterworths, London, pp 248–276, 1982
4. Anast CS: Disorders of mineral and bone metabolism. In: Avery ME, Taeusch HW (eds) *Schaeffer's Diseases of the Newborn*. 5th ed. WB Saunders, Philadelphia, pp 464–479, 1984
5. Cole DEC, Carpenter TO, Goltzman D: Calcium homeostasis and disorders of bone and mineral metabolism. In: Collu R (ed) *Pediatric Endocrinology*. Raven Press, New York, pp 509–580, 1988
6. Fanconi S, Fischer JA, Wieland P, Atares M, Fanconi A, Giedion A, Prader A: Kenny syndrome: evidence for idiopathic hypoparathyroidism in two patients and for abnormal parathyroid hormone in one. *J Pediatr* 109:469–475, 1986

41. Miscellaneous Causes of Hypocalcemia

Karl L. Insogna, M.D., and *Andrew F. Stewart, M.D.

*Section of Endocrinology, Yale University School of Medicine, New Haven, Connecticut; and *Department of Endocrinology, Yale University School of Medicine, New Haven Connecticut, and Connecticut Veterans Affairs Medical Center, West Haven, Connecticut*

The list of disorders that may cause hypocalcemia is a long one. Several of these disorders (hypoparathyroidism, pseudohypoparathyroidism, hypocalcemic syndromes encountered in infants, and the hypocalcemia seen in patients with hyper- and hypomagnesemia) are described in the chapters immediately surrounding this chapter.

"FACTITIOUS" HYPOCALCEMIA DUE TO HYPOALBUMINEMIA

In the reverse of events described in Chapter 26 for "factitious" hypercalcemia, reductions in serum albumin encountered in patients with nephrotic syndrome, chronic illness, malnutrition, cirrhosis, and volume overexpansion will result in a reduction in the total, but not the ionized fraction, of the serum calcium. Such patients display none of the signs or symptoms of hypocalcemia (Q-T interval changes on electrocardiogram, paresthesias, tetany, cramping, Chvostek's or Trousseau's sign). The degree of hypocalcemia correlates roughly with the degree of hypoalbuminemia and a variety of formulas have been developed that permit one to calculate a total serum calcium that is corrected for the serum albumin. In general, however, these formulas are imprecise (1). If a question arises as to the "real" serum calcium in a given case, the ionized calcium should be measured.

HYPOCALCEMIA RESULTING FROM DISORDERS INVOLVING VITAMIN D

Hypocalcemia as an isolated finding resulting from disordered vitamin D metabolism is rare. Most individuals with abnormalities in either the production or the action of vitamin D metabolites present with other findings such as rickets or osteomalacia. The reader is therefore referred to Chapters 57–61, which deal with these two clinical entities for a more detailed consideration of the hypocalcemia seen with these disorders. The reader is also referred to Chapters 13 and 19 for more detailed reviews of vitamin D metabolism, chemistry, and serum assays.

Abnormalities in vitamin D metabolism can be divided into three broad categories: vitamin D deficiency, acquired or inherited disorders of vitamin D metabolism, and resistance to the actions of vitamin D.

Vitamin D deficiency is unusual in the United States because of the common practice of vitamin D supplementation of dairy products and other foods (see Chapter 58). It can only occur in patients in whom both exposure to ultraviolet (UV) light and dietary intake of vitamin D are inadequate.

However, certain subgroups, such as breast-fed infants of strictly vegetarian mothers, continue to be at risk for vitamin D deficiency (2). Recent immigrants from the Middle East to northern latitudes who continue to wear traditional dress—including long garments, hoods, and veils—represent another example. In more moderate stages of vitamin D deficiency, serum calcium concentrations are normal whereas hypophosphatemia due to secondary hyperparathyroidism may be apparent. In more severe disease, the clinical manifestations of rickets and/or osteomalacia are profound, and hypocalcemia is a more prominent biochemical finding. Serum 25-hydroxyvitamin D [25(OH)D] levels are important in the diagnosis of patients with nutritional vitamin D deficiency.

Vitamin D malabsorption leading to vitamin D deficiency may occur in patients with one of several gastrointestinal disorders (see Chapter 58). These include nontropical sprue, Crohn's disease, and pancreatic insufficiency. Osteomalacia and hypocalcemia may develop in these patients despite adequate nutritional intake and UV light exposure. The pathogenesis is not entirely clear; 25(OH)D and 1,25-dihydroxyvitamin D [1,25(OH)$_2$D] both undergo enterohepatic circulation, and it may be that losses due to interruption of this pathway lead to vitamin D deficiency (3). It is also possible that the diseased bowel may be incapable of absorbing vitamin D or responding to 1,25(OH)$_2$D. Circulating 25(OH)D concentrations are reduced, and hypocalcemia, when present, is usually modest.

Acquired or inherited abnormalities in vitamin D metabolism comprise the next broad group of disorders associated with hypocalcemia. Patients with cholestatic liver disease (Chapter 59) may develop osteomalacia and secondary hyperparathyroidism as a consequence of reduced hepatic hydroxylation of vitamin D to 25(OH)D or due to intestinal malabsorption of vitamin D metabolites. Circulating levels of 25(OH)D are reduced and may be aggravated by poor nutritional intake and inadequate UV light exposure. Hypocalcemia is usually modest in these patients as well.

Patients with advanced renal insufficiency often have hypocalcemia, which is due in part to the low production rates of 1,25(OH)$_2$D (Chapter 66). Other factors, including hyperphosphatemia and acidosis, contribute to the hypocalcemia in renal failure.

A variety of medications may be associated with acquired disorders of vitamin D metabolism (4) (Chapter 65). Of these, anticonvulsants are the most frequent medications causing mild hypocalcemia. Accelerated metabolism of 25(OH)D to more polar-inactive metabolites has been suggested as the cause of these abnormalities. Nutritional and other environmental factors may also contribute (5).

Vitamin-D-dependent rickets type I (VDDR I) is a rare autosomal recessive disorder presenting in children in which hypocalcemia is a prominent manifestation. Clinical features were initially described in 1961 and include profound rickets, hypocalcemia, marked secondary hyperparathyroidism, elevated alkaline phosphatase, and generalized aminoaciduria. The pathogenesis of this disorder appears to be a functional defect in 1α–hydroxylase activity with consequent inability to convert 25(OH)D to 1,25(OH)$_2$D (6). Thus, patients with this disorder are generally resistant to therapy with vitamin D, but physiologic doses of 1,25(OH)$_2$D3 lead to prompt healing of the rachitic lesions and correction of the hypocalcemia. Recently, the gene responsible for the disease was mapped to chromosome 12q14 (7). None of the currently identified components of the 1α-hydroxylase enzyme system appear to map to this location, so how the defect in VDDR I affects enzyme activity is unclear.

End-organ resistance to the action of 1,25(OH)$_2$D results in hypocalcemic vitamin D-dependent rickets type II (VDDR II; Chapter 60). In contrast to VDDR I, hypocalcemia in VDDR II is often (but not invariably) accompanied by dramatic elevations in circulating 1,25(OH)$_2$D. The classic phenotypic features of this autosomal recessive syndrome are similar to those of vitamin-D-resistant rickets type I with the additional findings of partial or complete alopecia and oligodontia. The relationship of this finding to the abnormalities in vitamin D function remains unknown. As might be anticipated, a number of molecular defects appear to result in the same phenotypic manifestations. The final common abnormality seems to be an inability of 1,25(OH)$_2$D to induce the usual intracellular events associated with binding to the vitamin D receptor and receptor–hormone complex binding to DNA. Thus, in most cases tested, the normal induction of the enzyme 25(OH)D 24-hydroxylase by 1,25(OH)$_2$D3 is absent. Point mutations in the DNA binding domain of the human vitamin D receptor gene have been demonstrated in skin fibroblasts from patients with this syndrome (8).

A spectrum of disease severity exists as reflected in patients' responses to therapy with vitamin D metabolites and oral calcium (9). Many patients can be successfully managed using these agents. It has been reported that patients with severe disease who are unresponsive to all vitamin D analogs may respond to prolonged intravenous infusions of calcium, which cures the rickets and corrects the secondary hyperparathyroidism.

HYPOCALCEMIA RESULTING FROM HYPERPHOSPHATEMIA

Since the 1930s it has been appreciated that oral or parenteral phosphorus may lower serum calcium levels. The mechanism whereby phosphorus administration lowers serum calcium remains unknown, however. Herbert et al. (10) showed that phosphate infusion lowered serum calcium in the presence and absence of the parathyroid glands, and changes in fecal and urinary calcium excretion during phosphate administration could not account for the fall in serum calcium. They suggested that the blood calcium phosphorus molar product, when exceeded, leads to spontaneous precipitation of calcium phosphate salts in soft tissues. The [Ca] × [P] product, when estimated from total serum calcium and phosphate concentrations (as mg/dl), normally is <60.

Hyperphosphatemia sufficient to cause hypocalcemia usually has an abrupt onset, is severe in magnitude, and often occurs in the setting of impaired renal function. Four clinical settings conducive to phosphate-induced hypocalcemia are recognized: excessive enteral or parenteral phosphate administration; the tumor lysis syndrome; rhabdomyolysis-induced acute renal failure; and the hypocalcemia of advanced renal insufficiency.

Excessive oral or parenteral phosphate administration may cause hypocalcemia by promotion of soft tissue calcification. Soft tissue calcification has been observed during the treatment of hypophosphatemia due to diabetic ketoacidosis and acute alcoholism (11). Adults receiving phosphate-containing enemas and infants fed "humanized" cow's milk rich in phosphate (12,13) may also become hypocalcemic. Discontinuation of phosphate usually leads to prompt correction of serum calcium, but chronic phosphate-induced hypocalcemia has been reported to cause secondary hyperparathyroidism.

Hypocalcemia caused by massive tumor lysis results from the release of intracellular phosphate during cell destruction. A common setting of the tumor lysis syndrome is during chemotherapy for rapidly proliferating neoplasms such as acute lymphoblastic leukemia in children (14). Under these conditions, hypocalcemia may persist beyond the hyperphosphatemia and may be aggravated by suppressed 1,25-dihydroxyvitamin D levels (15). Optimal management of patients with tumor lysis syndrome may include early use of phosphate-binding antacids and $1,25(OH)_2D3$, although these have not been tested by well-controlled clinical studies.

Rhabdomyolysis-induced acute renal failure may occur with trauma, or drug or alcohol abuse, and is frequently associated with marked hypocalcemia in the early oliguric phase and moderate to severe hypercalcemia in the subsequent polyuric phase (16). The mechanism of the hypocalcemia during rhabdomyolysis may be similar to the tumor lysis syndrome, as Llach et al. (16) have described hyperphosphatemia and suppressed serum $1,25(OH)_2D$ during the initial appearance of hypocalcemia. The appearance of hypercalcemia and high serum $1,25(OH)_2D$ levels during the diuretic phase of acute renal failure with rhabdomyolysis may result from the rapid development of secondary hyperparathyroidism during the initial hypocalcemia. Treatment goals include restriction of phosphate intake and absorption, and maintenance of normal serum calcium.

Hypocalcemia may develop during the course of chronic renal failure, and its severity may be aggravated by oral phosphate administration. The hypocalcemia may result from hyperphosphatemia due to reduced renal phosphate clearance by the failing kidney and phosphate-induced suppression of already reduced rates of $1,25(OH)_2D$ production. Prevention of secondary hyperparathyroidism may be achieved by early administration of phosphate-binding antacids and judicious use of $1,25(OH)_2D3$.

HYPOCALCEMIA RESULTING FROM PANCREATITIS

Hypocalcemia and tetany were first recorded in patients with pancreatitis in the early 1940s. Langerhans had observed in 1890 that the white deposits in the retroperitoneum ("fat necrosis") associated with pancreatitis were in fact insoluble calcium soaps or complexes of calcium and free fatty acids (FFAs). It is now believed that FFAs are generated by the action of pancreatic lipase, released from the damaged pancreas, on retroperitoneal and omental fat (triglyceride) to release their component FFAs into the peritoneum. These in turn avidly chelate calcium, removing it from extracellular fluid (17,18). Other mechanisms may be responsible for hypocalcemia in individual instances of pancreatitis-induced hypocalcemia. Hypoalbuminemia regularly occurs in patients with pancreatitis and leads to a reduction in total (but not ionized) serum calcium. Hypomagnesemia resulting from poor oral intake, alcohol use, and/or vomiting is common in pancreatitis and may lead to hypocalcemia (Chapter 41). It has also been postulated that hypocalcemia may result from excessive calcitonin secretion secondary to excessive pancreatic glucagon release. Support for this possibility is weak. Finally, it has been suggested that pancreatitis may liberate systemic factors, such as proteases that inhibit parathyroid hormone secretion and/or degrade circulating parathyroid hormone. There is no recent support for this possibility.

Clinically, patients with pancreatitis-induced hypocalcemia have severe pancreatitis, and hypocalcemia portends a poor outcome. Hypocalcemia is treated with parenteral calcium and magnesium replacement when indicated. Hypocalcemia due to vitamin D deficiency/malabsorption should be considered and excluded.

HYPOCALCEMIA DUE TO ACCELERATED SKELETAL MINERALIZATION.

Hypocalcemia occurs in settings where the rate of skeletal mineralization significantly outpaces the rate of osteoclastic bone resorption. Three examples of this type of hypocalcemia occur. The first is the hypocalcemia that follows the surgical correction of primary or secondary hyperparathyroidism. The abrupt cessation of PTH-mediated osteoclastic skeletal resorption in concert with continued mineralization of large quantities of previously formed osteoid lead to a hypocalcemic syndrome that has been termed "hungry bones" syndrome. This syndrome has also been described following thyroidectomy for hyperthyroidism. The key clinical issue is distinguishing postoperative hungry bones syndrome from postoperative hypoparathyroidism, a distinction that is not always easy. Hypocalcemia also occurs in patients with extensive osteoblastic metastases (19). As might be anticipated, this type of hypocalcemia occurs primarily in patients with prostate cancer and breast cancer metastatic to bone, but it has also been reported in patients with acute leukemia. Finally, hypocalcemia may worsen in patients with vitamin D deficiency following the institution of therapy with vitamin D. This type of hypocalcemia is confusing and alarming because one would expect the serum calcium to rise with vitamin D replacement in patients with rickets or osteomalacia. Hypocalcemia occurs in the early phases of vitamin D therapy as the large amounts of unmineralized osteoid are permitted to mineralize when vitamin D is provided.

HYPOCALCEMIA ENCOUNTERED IN ACUTE ILLNESSES

Hypocalcemia may be encountered in patients with acute sepsis. In one series (20), 12 of 60 patients with acute bacterial sepsis were hypocalcemic (displaying reductions in ionized serum calcium), and 6 of the 12 hypocalcemic patients died of their septic episode. In contrast, only 14 of 48 normocalcemic septic patients died, leading the authors to suggest that hypocalcemia confers an even graver prognosis on patients with sepsis. All of the patients had gram-negative sepsis. In contrast, none of 20 patients with staphylococcal sepsis became hypocalcemic. In addition, a reduction in total and ionized serum calcium has been reported to be a feature of the toxic shock syndrome (21). The mechanism responsible for hypocalcemia in gram-negative sepsis and in toxic shock syndrome is unknown. It has been suggested that hypocalcemia may result from interleukin-1 production during septic episodes because interleukin-1 injections cause hypocalcemia in mice (22). It has also been suggested that parathyroid "reserve" is subnormal in patients with acquired immunodeficiency syndrome (AIDS) (23).

Hypocalcemia in the setting of acute illness most often is multifactorial, reflecting combinations of hypoalbuminemia, hypomagnesemia, pancreatitis, chronic and/or acute renal failure, treatment with medications or transfusions that lower serum calcium, or cancer with osteoblastic metastases.

HYPOCALCEMIA ASSOCIATED WITH THE USE OF MEDICATIONS

Hypocalcemia may occur as the result of overzealous treatment with medications intended to reverse hypercalcemia and/or excessive bone resorption. Thus, *mithramycin* (plicamycin), *calcitonin, bisphosphonates,* and oral or parenteral *phosphate* preparations (Chapter 36) have all been reported to cause hypocalcemia. Hypocalcemia and osteomalacia may occur as the result of prolonged therapy with anticonvulsants such as *diphenylhydantoin* (phenytoin) or *phenobarbital* (Chapter 65). *Fluoride* overdosage has been associated with hypocalcemia, possibly due to excessive rates of skeletal mineralization and complexing of calcium by fluoride (24,25). Transfusion and plasmapheresis with *citrated blood* has been reported to cause hypocalcemia, particularly in patients receiving exchange transfusions (26). A recent addition to the list of drugs that may cause hypocalcemia is *radiographic contrast dyes* that may contain the calcium chelator ethylenediaminetetraacetate (EDTA), in conjunction with citrate (27). Chelation of calcium plus dilutional/osmotic effects of these agents are believed to be responsible for the mild hypocalcemia that has been observed. Finally, *foscarnet* (trisodium phosphonoformate), used in the treatment of patients with AIDS and opportunistic infections, has been reported to cause reductions in total and ionized serum calcium concentrations, perhaps through chelation or complexing of calcium in extracellular fluid (28).

REFERENCES

1. Ladenson JH, Lewis JH, McDonald JM, Slatopolsky E, Boyd JC: Relationship of free and total calcium in hypercalcemic conditions. *J Clin Endocrinol Metab* 48:393–397, 1978
2. Bachrach S, Fisher J, Parks J: An outbreak of vitamin D deficiency rickets in a susceptible population. *Pediatrics* 64:871–877, 1979
3. Kumar R: Hepatic and intestinal osteodystrophy and the hepatobiliary metabolism of vitamin D. *Ann Intern Med* 98:662–663, 1983
4. Frame B: Hypocalcemia and osteomalacia associated with anticonvulsant therapy. *Ann Intern Med* 74:294–295, 1971
5. Weinstien R, Bryce G, Sappington L, King D, Gallagher B: Decreased serum ionized calcium and normal vitamin D metabolite levels with anticonvulsant drug treatment. *J Clin Endocrinol Metab* 58:1003–1009, 1984
6. Fraser D, Kooh S, Kind P, Holick M, Tanaka Y, Deluca H: Pathogenesis of hereditary vitamin D-dependent rickets. *N Engl J Med* 289:817–822, 1973
7. Labuda M, Morgan K, Glorieux F: Mapping autosomal recessive vitamin D-dependency type I rickets to chromosome 12q14 by linkage analysis. *Am J Hum Genet* 47:28-36, 1990
8. Hughes M, Malloy P, Kieback D, Kesterson R, Pike J, Feldman D, O'Malley B: Point mutation in the human vitamin D receptor gene associated with hypocalcemic rickets. *Science* 242:1702–1705, 1988
9. Marx S, 1,25-dihydroxyvitamin D_3 receptors and resistance: Implications in rickets, osteomalacia, and other conditions in rickets. In: Glorieux FH (ed) *Nestle Nutrition Workshop Series* 21:167–184, 1991
10. Herbert L, Lemann J, Petersen J, Lennon E: Studies of the mechanism by which phosphate infusion lowers serum calcium concentration. *J Clin Invest* 45:1886–1894, 1966
11. Chernow B, Rainey T, Georges L, O'Brian J: Iatrogenic hyperphosphatemia: A metabolic consideration in critical care medicine. *Crit Care Med* 9:772–774, 1981
12. Biberstein M, Parker B: Enema-induced hyperphosphatemia. *Am J Med* 79:645–646, 1985
13. Venkaraman P, Tsang R, Greer F, Noguchi A, Laskarzewski P, Steichen J: Late infantile tetany and secondary hyperparathyroidism in infants fed humanized cow milk formula. *Am J Dis Child* 139:664–668, 1985
14. Zusman T, Brown D, Nesbit M: Hyperphosphatemia, hyperphosphaturia and hypocalcemia in acute lymphoblastic leukemia. *N Engl J Med* 289:1335–1340, 1973
15. Dunlay R, Camp M, Allon M, Fanti P, Malluche H, Llach F: Calcitriol in prolonged hypocalcemia due to the tumor lysis syndrome. *Ann Intern Med* 110:162–164, 1989
16. Llach F, Felsenfeld A, Haussler M: The pathophysiology of altered calcium metabolism in rhabdomyolysis-induced acute renal failure. *N Engl J Med* 305:117–123, 1981
17. Stewart AF, Longo W, Kreutter D, Jacob R, Burtis WJ: Hypocalcemia due to calcium soap formation in a patient with a pancreatic fistula. *N Engl J Med* 315:496–498, 1986
18. Dettelbach MA, Deftos LJ, Stewart AF: Intraperitoneal free fatty acids induce severe hypocalcemia in rats. *J Bone Min Res* 5:1249–1255, 1990
19. Abramson EC, Gajardo H, Kukreja SC: Hypocalcemia in cancer. *Bone Min* 10:161–169, 1990
20. Zaloga GP, Chernow B: The multifactorial basis for hypocalcemia during sepsis. Studies of the parathyroid hormone–vitamin D axis. *Ann Intern Med* 107:36–41, 1987
21. Chesney RW, McCarron DM, Haddad JG, Hawker CD, DiBella FP, Chesney PJ, Davis JP: Pathogenic mechanisms of the hypocalcemia of the staphylococcal toxic-shock syndrome. *J Lab Clin Med* 101:576–585, 1983
22. Boyce BF, Yates AJP, Mundy GR: Bolus injections of recombinant human interleukin-1 cause transient hypocalcemia in normal mice. *Endocrinology* 125:2780–2783, 1989
23. Jaeger P, Otto S, Speck RF, Villiger L, Horber FF, Casez J-P, Takkinen R: Altered parathyroid gland function in severely immunocompromised patients infected with human immunodeficiency virus. *J Clin Endocrinol Metab* 79:1701–1705, 1994
24. Arnow PM, Bland LA, Garcia-Houchins S, Fridkin S, Fellner SK: An outbreak of fatal fluoride intoxication in a long-term hemodialysis unit. *Ann Intern Med* 121:339–344, 1994
25. Gessner BD, Beller M, Middaugh JP, Whitford GM: Acute fluoride poisoning from a public water system. *N Engl J Med* 330:95–99, 1994

26. Tofalletti J, Nissenson RA, Endres D, McGarry E, Mogollon G: Influence of continuous infusion of citrate on responses of immuno-reactive PTH, calcium, magnesium components, and other electrolytes in normal adults during plasmapheresis. *J Clin Endocrinol Metab* 60:874–879, 1985

27. Mallette LE, Gomez LS: Systemic hypocalemia after clinical injection of radiographic contrast media: Amelioration by omission of calcium chelating agents. *Radiology* 147:677–679, 1982

28. Jacobson MA, Gambertoglio JG, Aweeka FT, Causey DM, Portale AA: Foscarnet-induced hypocalcemia and effects of foscarnet on calcium metabolism. *J Clin Endocrinol Metab* 72:1130–1135, 1991

42. Magnesium Depletion and Hypermagnesemia

Robert K. Rude, M.D.

Department of Medicine, University of Southern California, Los Angeles, California

HYPOMAGNESEMIA/MAGNESIUM DEPLETION

Magnesium (Mg) depletion appears to be more common than previously thought. Ten percent of patients admitted to city hospitals are hypomagnesemic and as many as 65% of patients in an intensive care unit have been reported to be hypomagnesemic (1,2). Hypomagnesemia and/or Mg depletion is usually due to losses of Mg from either the gastrointestinal tract or the kidney (3,4), as outlined in Table 1.

Causes of Magnesium Depletion

The Mg content of upper intestinal tract fluids is approximately 1 mEq/L. Vomiting and nasogastric suction therefore may contribute to Mg depletion. The Mg content of diarrheal fluids and fistulous drainage is much higher (up to

TABLE 1. *Common causes of Mg deficiency*

Gastrointestinal Disorders
  Prolonged nasogastric suction/vomiting
  Acute and chronic diarrheal states
  Intestinal and biliary fistulas
  Malabsorption syndromes
  Extensive bowel resection or bypass
Renal Loss
  Chronic parenteral fluid therapy
  Osmotic diuresis (glucose, urea)
  Hypercalcemia
  Alcohol/Drugs
  Diuretics (furosemide, ethacrynic acid)
  Aminoglycosides
  Cisplatin
  Cyclosporin
  Amphotericin B
  Pentamidine
  Metabolic acidosis
  Chronic renal disease
Endocrine and Metabolic
  Diabetes mellitus
  Phosphate depletion
  Primary hyperparathyroidism
  Hypoparathyroidism
  Primary aldosteronism
  Hungry bone syndrome

15 mEq/L), and consequently Mg depletion is common in acute and chronic diarrhea, regional enteritis, ulcerative colitis, and intestinal and biliary fistulas. Malabsorption syndromes due to nontropical sprue, radiation injury resulting from therapy for disorders such as carcinoma of the cervix, and intestinal lymphangiectasia may also result in Mg deficiency. Steatorrhea and resection or bypass of the small bowel, particularly the ileum, often results in intestinal Mg loss or malabsorption. Lastly, acute severe pancreatitis is associated with hypomagnesemia which may be due to the clinical problem causing the pancreatitis, such as alcoholism, or to saponification of Mg in necrotic parapancreatic fat.

Excessive excretion of Mg into the urine may be the basis of Mg depletion. Renal Mg reabsorption is proportional to tubular fluid flow as well as to sodium and calcium excretion (5). Therefore, chronic parenteral fluid therapy, particularly with saline, and volume expansion states, such as primary aldosteronism, may result in Mg depletion. Hypercalcemia and hypercalciuria have been shown to decrease renal Mg reabsorption and are probably the cause of renal Mg wasting and hypomagnesemia observed in many hypercalcemic states as well as in hypoparathyroid patients on vitamin D and calcium therapy. Osmotic diuresis due to glucosuria will result in urinary Mg wasting. Diabetes mellitus is probably the most common clinical disorder associated with Mg depletion (6).

An increasing list of drugs are becoming recognized as causing renal Mg wasting and Mg depletion. The major site of renal Mg reabsorption is at the loop of Henle; therefore diuretics such as furosemide and ethacrynic acid have been shown to result in marked Mg wasting (7). Aminoglycosides have been shown to cause a reversible renal lesion that results in hypermagnesuria and hypomagnesemia (8). Similarly, amphotericin B therapy has been reported to result in renal Mg wasting. Other renal Mg-wasting agents include cisplatin, cyclosporin, and pentamidine (8,9). A rising blood alcohol level has been associated with hypermagnesuria and is one factor contributing to Mg depletion in chronic alcoholism. Metabolic acidosis due to diabetic ketoacidosis, starvation, or alcoholism may also result in renal Mg wasting.

Hypomagnesemia may accompany a number of other disorders (3,4). Phosphate depletion has been shown experimentally to result in urinary Mg wasting and hypomagnesemia. Hypomagnesemia may also accompany the "hungry bone" syndrome, a phase of rapid bone mineral accretion in subjects with hyperparathyroidism or hyperthyroidism following surgical treatment. Finally, chronic renal tubular, glomerular, or interstitial diseases may be associated with renal Mg wasting.

Manifestations of Magnesium Depletion

Because Mg depletion is usually secondary to another disease process or to a therapeutic agent, the features of the primary disease process may complicate or mask Mg depletion. A high index of suspicion is therefore warranted (3,4).

Neuromuscular hyperexcitability may be the presenting complaint (10). Latent tetany, as elicited by positive Chvostek's and Trousseau's signs, or spontaneous carpal-pedal spasm may be present. Frank generalized seizures may also occur. Although hypocalcemia often contributes to the neurologic signs, hypomagnesemia without hypocalcemia has been reported to result in neuromuscular hyperexcitability. Other signs may include vertigo, ataxia, nystagmus, and athetoid and choreiform movements as well as muscular tremor, fasciculation, wasting, and weakness.

Electrocardiographic (ECG) abnormalities of Mg depletion in man include prolonged P-R interval and Q-T interval. Mg depletion may also result in cardiac arrhythmias (11–13). Supraventricular arrhythmias including premature atrial complexes, atrial tachycardia, atrial fibrillation, and junctional arrhythmias have been described. Ventricular premature complexes, ventricular tachycardia, and ventricular fibrillation are more serious complications. Recently, Mg administration to patients with acute myocardial infarction has been shown to decrease the mortality rate (14–16).

A common laboratory feature of Mg depletion is hypokalemia (17,18). During Mg depletion there is loss of potassium from the cell with intracellular potassium depletion as well as an inability of the kidney to conserve potassium. Attempts to replete the potassium deficit with potassium therapy alone are not successful without simultaneous Mg therapy. This biochemical feature may be a contributing cause of the ECG findings and cardiac arrhythmias discussed above.

Hypocalcemia is a common manifestation of moderate to severe Mg depletion (19,20). The hypocalcemia may be a major contributing factor to the increased neuromuscular excitability often present in Mg-depleted patients. The pathogenesis of hypocalcemia is multifactorial. In normal subjects, acute changes in the serum Mg concentration will influence parathyroid hormone (PTH) secretion in a manner similar to that of calcium. That is, an acute fall in serum Mg stimulates PTH secretion whereas hypermagnesemia inhibits PTH secretion. During chronic and severe Mg depletion, however, PTH secretion is impaired (21). The majority of patients will have serum PTH concentrations that are undetectable or inappropriately normal for the degree of hypocalcemia. Some patients, however, may have serum PTH levels above the normal range that may reflect early magnesium depletion. Regardless of the basal circulating PTH concentration, an acute injection of Mg

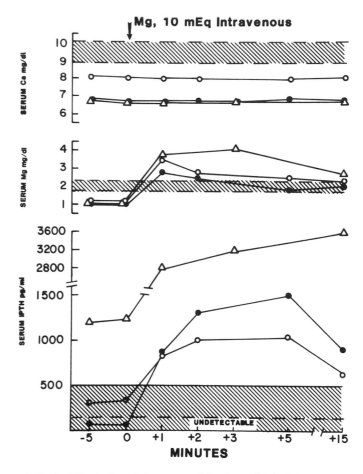

FIG. 1. Effect of an intravenous injection of 10 mEq magnesium on the serum concentration of calcium, magnesium, and iPTH in hypocalcemic magnesium-deficient patients with undetectable (o), normal (•), or elevated (△), levels of iPTH. *Shaded area* represents the range of normal for assay. *Broken line* for the iPTH assay represents the level of detectability. The magnesium injection resulted in a marked rise in PTH secretion within 1 minute in all three patients.

stimulates PTH secretion as illustrated in Fig. 1. Impaired PTH secretion therefore appears to be a major factor in hypomagnesemia-induced hypocalcemia. Hypocalcemia in the presence of normal or elevated serum PTH concentrations also suggests end-organ resistance to PTH (20). Patients with hypocalcemia due to Mg depletion have both renal and skeletal resistance to exogenously administered PTH as manifested by subnormal urinary cAMP and phosphate excretion and diminished calcemic response. This renal and skeletal resistance to PTH is reversed following several days of Mg therapy. The basis for the defect in PTH secretion and PTH end-organ resistance is not known. Because cAMP appears to be important in PTH secretion and mediating PTH effects in kidney and bone, it has been postulated that there may be a defect in the adenylate cyclase complex (22). Magnesium is necessary for cAMP formation as substrate (MgATP) as well as being an allosteric activator of adenylate cyclase.

Clinically, patients with hypocalcemia due to Mg depletion are resistant not only to PTH but to calcium and vitamin D therapy. The vitamin D resistance may be due to impaired metabolism of vitamin D, as serum concentrations of 1,25-dihydroxyvitamin D are low (23).

Diagnosis of Magnesium Depletion

Measurement of the serum Mg concentration is the most commonly used test to assess Mg status. The normal serum Mg concentration ranges from 1.5 to 1.9 mEq/L (1.8 to 2.2 mg/dl) and a value less than 1.5 mEq/L usually indicates Mg depletion (3,4). Mg is principally an intracellular cation and only approximately 1% of the body Mg content is in the extracellular fluid compartments. The serum Mg concentration therefore may not reflect the intracellular Mg content. Because vitamin D and calcium therapy are relatively ineffective in correcting the hypocalcemia, there must be a high index of suspicion for the presence of Mg depletion. Patients with Mg depletion severe enough to result in hypocalcemia are usually significantly hypomagnesemic. However, occasionally patients may have normal serum Mg concentrations. Magnesium deficiency in the presence of a normal serum Mg concentration has been demonstrated by measuring intracellular Mg (in lymphocytes or muscle biopsy), or by whole-body retention of infused Mg. Therefore, hypocalcemic patients who are at risk for Mg depletion but who have normal serum Mg levels should receive a trial of Mg therapy. The Mg tolerance test (or retention test) appears to be an accurate means of assessing Mg status (24). Correlations with skeletal muscle Mg content and Mg balance studies have been shown. A suggested protocol for the Mg tolerance test is shown in Table 2.

Therapy

Patients who present with signs and symptoms of Mg depletion should be treated with Mg (25). These patients will usually be hypomagnesemic and/or have an abnormal Mg tolerance test. The extent of the total body Mg deficit is impossible to predict, but it may be as high as 200–400 mEq. Under these circumstances parenteral Mg administration is usually indicated. An effective treatment regimen is the administration of 2 g $MgSO_4.7H_2O$ (16.2 mEq Mg) as a 50% solution every 8 hours intramuscularly. These injections can be painful; a continuous intravenous infusion of 48 mEq over 24 hours may therefore be preferred and is better tolerated. Either regimen will usually result in a normal to slightly elevated serum Mg concentration. Despite the fact that PTH secretion increases within minutes after beginning Mg administration, the serum calcium concentration may not return to normal for 3–7 days. This probably reflects slow restoration of intracellular Mg. During this period of therapy, serum Mg concentration may be normal but the total body deficit may not yet be corrected. Magnesium should be continued until the clinical and biochemical manifestations (hypocalcemia and hypokalemia) of Mg depletion are resolved.

Patients who are hypomagnesemic and have seizures or an acute arrhythmia may be given 8–16 mEq of Mg as an intravenous injection over 5–10 minutes followed by 48 mEq intravenously/day (10,25,26). Ongoing Mg losses should be monitored during therapy. If the patient continues to lose Mg from the intestine or kidney, therapy may have to be continued for a longer duration. Once repletion has been accomplished, patients usually can maintain a normal Mg status on a regular diet. If repletion is accomplished and the patient cannot eat, a maintenance dose of 8 mEq should be given daily. Patients who have chronic Mg loss from the intestine or kidney may require continued oral Mg supplementation. A daily dose of 300–600 mg of elemental Mg may be given in divided doses to avoid the cathartic effect of Mg.

Caution should be taken during Mg therapy in patients with any degree of renal failure. If a decrease in glomerular filtration rate exists, the dose of Mg should be halved, and the serum Mg concentration must be monitored daily. If hypermagnesemia ensues, therapy must be stopped.

HYPERMAGNESEMIA

Magnesium intoxication is not a frequently encountered clinical problem, although mild to moderate elevations in the serum Mg concentration may be seen in as many as 12% of hospitalized patients (1).

Symptomatic hypermagnesemia is virtually always due to excessive intake or administration of Mg salts (26,27). The majority of patients with hypermagnesemia have concomitant renal failure. Hypermagnesemia is usually seen in patients with renal failure who are receiving Mg as an antacid, enema, or infusion. Hypermagnesemia is also sometimes seen in acute renal failure in the setting of rhabomyolysis.

TABLE 2. *Suggested protocol for use of magnesium tolerance test*

I. Collect baseline 24-hour urine for magnesium/creatinine ratio.[a]
II. Infuse 0.2 mEq (2.4 mg) elemental magnesium per kg lean body weight in 50 ml 5% dextrose over 4 hours.
III. Collect urine (starting with infusion) for magnesium and creatinine for 24 hours.
IV. Percentage magnesium retained is calculated by the following formula:

$$\%Mg\ retained = 1 - \frac{[postinfusion\ 24\text{-}hr\ urine\ Mg - preinfusion\ urine\ Mg/creatinine \times postinfusion\ urine\ creatinine]}{} \times 100$$

V. Criteria for Mg deficiency:
>50% retention at 24 hr = definite deficiency
>25% retention at 24 hr = probable deficiency

[a]A fasting 2-hour spot or shorter-timed urine may be used.

Large amounts of oral Mg have rarely been reported to cause symptomatic hypermagnesemia in patients with normal renal function (27–29). The rectal administration of Mg for purgation may result in hypermagnesemia. Mg is a standard form of therapy for pregnancy-induced hypertension (preeclampsia and eclampsia) and may cause Mg intoxication in the mother as well as in the neonate. Ureteral irrigation with hemiacidrin (Renacidin) has been reported to cause symptomatic hypermagnesemia in patients with and without renal failure. Modest elevations in the serum Mg concentration may be seen in familial hypocalcemic hypercalcemia, lithium ingestion, and during volume depletion (3,4).

Signs and Symptoms

Neuromuscular symptoms are the most common presenting problem of Mg intoxication (27). One of the earliest demonstrable effects of hypermagnesemia is the disappearance of the deep tendon reflexes. This is reached at serum Mg concentrations of 4–7 mEq/L. Depressed respiration and apnea due to paralysis of the voluntary musculature may be seen at serum Mg concentrations in excess of 8–10 mEq/L. Somnolence may be observed at levels as low as 3 mEq/L and above.

Moderate elevations in the serum Mg concentration of 3–5 mEq/L result in a mild reduction in blood pressure. High concentrations may result in severe symptomatic hypotension. Mg can also be cardiotoxic. At serum Mg concentrations greater than 5 mEq/L ECG findings of prolonged P-R intervals as well as increased QRS duration and Q-T interval are seen. Complete heart block, as well as cardiac arrest, may occur at concentrations greater than 15 mEq/L.

Hypermagnesemia causes a fall in the serum calcium concentration. The hypocalcemia may be related to the suppressive effect of hypermagnesemia on PTH secretion or to hypermagnesemia-induced parathyroid hormone end-organ resistance (30,31). A direct effect of Mg on decreasing the serum calcium is suggested by the observation that hypermagnesemia causes hypocalcemia in hypoparathyroid subjects as well.

Other nonspecific manifestations of Mg intoxication include nausea, vomiting, and cutaneous flushing at serum levels of 3–9 mEq/L.

Therapy

The possibility of Mg intoxication should be anticipated in any patient receiving Mg, especially if the patient has a reduction in renal function. Mg therapy should merely be discontinued in patients with mild to moderate elevations in the serum Mg level. Excess Mg will be excreted by the kidney, and any symptoms or signs of Mg intoxication will resolve. Patients with severe Mg intoxication may be treated with intravenous calcium (27). Calcium will antagonize the toxic effects of Mg. This antagonism is immediate but transient. The usual dose is an infusion of 100–200 mg of elemental calcium over 5–10 minutes. If the patient is in renal failure, peritoneal dialysis or hemodialysis against a low-dialysis Mg bath will rapidly and effectively lower the serum Mg concentration.

REFERENCES

1. Wong ET, Rude RK, Singer FR. A high prevalence of hypomagnesemia in hospitalized patients. *Am J Clin Pathol* 79:348–352, 1983
2. Ryzen E, Wagers PW, Singer FR, Rude RK. Magnesium deficiency in a medical ICU population. *Crit Care Med* 13:19–21, 1985
3. Rude RK. Magnesium metabolism. In: Becker K (ed) *Principles and Practice of Endocrinology and Metabolism.* JB Lippincott, Philadelphia, pp 616–622, 1995
4. Rude RK, Singer FR. Magnesium deficiency and excess. *Annu Rev Med* 32:245–259, 1981
5. Quamme GA, Dirks JH. The physiology of renal magnesium handling. *Renal Physiol* 9:257–269, 1986
6. McNair P, Christensen MS, Christiansen C, Madsbad S, Transbol I: Renal hypomagnesaemia in human diabetes mellitus: its relation to glucose heomestasis. *Euro J Clin Invest* 12:81–85, 1982
7. Ryan AP. Diuretics and K/Mg depletion. Directions for treatment. *Am J Med* 82 (Suppl 3A):38–47, 1987
8. Shah GM, Hirschenbaum MA. Renal magnesium wasting associated with therapeutic agents. *Miner Electrolyte Metab* 17: 58–64, 1991
9. Shah GM, Alvarado P, Kirschenbaum MA. Symptomatic hypocalcemia and hypomagnesemia with renal magnesium wasting associated with pentamidine therapy in a patient with AIDS. *Am J Med* 89:380–382, 1990
10. Flink EB. Magnesium deficiency in human subjects–a personal historical perspective. *J Am Coll Nutr* 4: 17–31, 1985
11. Hollifield JW. Magnesium depletion, diuretics, and arrythmias. *Am J Med* 82: (Suppl 3A):30–37, 1987
12. Dyckner T, Wester PO. Magnesium deficiency contributing to ventricular tachycardia. *Acta Med Scand* 212:89–91, 1982
13. Iseri LT, Fairshter RD, Hardemann JL, Brodsky MA. Magnesium and potassium therapy in multifocal atrial tachycardia. *Am Heart J* 110:789–794, 1985
14. Rasmussen HS, McNair P, Norregard P, Backer V, Lindeneg O, Balslev S. Intravenous magnesium in acute myocardial infarction. *Lancet* 1:234–235, 1986
15. Kafka H, Langevin L, Armstrong PW. Serum magnesium and potassium in acute myocardial infarction: Influence on ventricular arrhythmias. *Arch Intern Med* 147:465–469, 1987
16. ISIS-4. A randomised factorial trial assessing early oral captopril, oral mononitrate, and intravenous magnesium sulphate in 58,050 patients with suspected acute myocardial infarction. *Lancet* 345: 669–685, 1995
17. Whang R, Flink EB, Dyckner T, Wester PO, Aikawa JK, Ryan MP. Magnesium depletion as a cause of refractory potassium repletion. *Arch Intern Med* 145:1686–1689, 1985
18. Ryan MP. Diuretics and potassium/magnesium depletion: directions for treatment. *Am J Med* 82(suppl 3A):38–47, 1987
19. Rude R.K. Magnesium deficiency in parathyroid function. In: Bilezikian JP (ed) *The Parathyroids.* Raven Press, New York, pp 829–842, 1994
20. Rude RK, Oldham SB, Singer FR. Functional hypoparathyroidism and parathyroid hormone end-organ resistance in human magnesium deficiency. *Clin Endocrinol* 5:209–224, 1976
21. Rude RK, Oldham SB, Sharp CF, Singer FR. Parathyroid hormone secretion in magnesium deficiency. *J Clin Endocrinol Metab* 47:800–806, 1978
22. Rude RK, Oldham SB: Hypocalcemia of Mg deficiency: Altered modulation of adenylate cyclase by Mg^- and Ca^- may result in impaired PTH secretion and PTH end-organ resistance. In: Altura BM, Aurbach J, Seelig JS (eds) *Magnesium in Cellular Processes and Medicine.* Karger, Basel, pp 183 195, 1987
23. Rude RK, Adams JS, Ryzen E, Endres DB, Niimi H, Horst RL, Haddad JG Jr, Singer FR. Low serum concentrations of 1,25-dihydroxyvitamin D in human magnesium deficiency. *J Clin Endocrinol Metab* 761:933–940, 1985

24. Ryzen E, Elbaum N, Singer FR, Rude RK. Parenteral magnesium tolerance testing in the evaluation of magnesium deficiency. *Magnesium* 4:137–147, 1985
25. Olerich MA, Rude RK. Should we supplement magnesium in our critically ill patients? *New Horizons* 2:186–192, 1994
26. Flink E. Magnesium deficiency: etiology and clinical spectrum. *Acta Med Scand* 647:125–137, 1981
27. Mordes JP. Excess magnesium. *Pharmacol Rev* 29:273–300, 1978
28. Fassler CA, Rodriguez RM, Badesch DB, Stone WJ, Marini JJ. Magnesium toxicity as a cause of hypotension and hypoventila-
tion: Occurrence in patients with normal renal function. *Arch Intern Med* 145:1604–1606, 1985
29. Zwanger ML. Hypermagnesemia and perforated viscus. *Ann Emerg Med* 15:1219–1220, 1986
30. Cholst IN, Steinberg SF, Trooper PJ, Fox HE, Segre GV, Bilezikian JP. The influence of hypermagnesemia on serum calcium and parathyroid hormone levels in human subjects. *N Engl J Med* 310:1221–1225, 1984
31. Slatopolsky E, Mercado A, Morrison A, Yates J, Klahr S. Inhibitory effects of hypermagnesemia on the renal action of parathyroid hormone. *J Clin Invest* 58:1273–1279, 1976

43. Hyperphosphatemia and Hypophosphatemia

Keith A. Hruska, M.D., and John Connolly, M.B., B.Ch., M.R.C.P.

Renal Division, Barnes-Jewish Hospital, St. Louis, Missouri

HYPERPHOSPHATEMIA

Serum inorganic phosphorus (Pi) concentrations are generally maintained at 2.5–4.5 mg/dl or 0.75–1.45 mM in adults, whereas hyperphosphatemia is not present in children unless serum Pi levels are greater than 6 mg/dl. Hyperphosphatemia most frequently results from renal insufficiency and the attendant inability to excrete Pi efficiently. Besides excretory deficiencies related to renal dysfunction, hyperphosphatemia may be the consequence of an increased intake of Pi or translocation of Pi from tissue breakdown into the extracellular fluid (1). Table 1 lists this and many of the other causes of hyperphosphatemia.

TABLE 1. *Causes of hyperphosphatemia*

Decreased renal phosphate excretion
    Renal insufficiency/failure
        Chronic
        Acute
    Hypoparathyroidism
    Pseudohypoparathyroidism
    Acromegaly
    Biphosphonates
    Tumoral calcinosis
    Children
Increased phosphate entrance to extracellular fluid
    Administration of IV, oral, or rectal phosphate salts
    Transcellular shifts
        Catabolic states
        Infections
        Fulminant hepatitis
        Hyperthermia
        Crush injuries
        Nontraumatic rhabdomyolysis
        Cytotoxic therapy
        Hemolytic anemia
        Acute leukemia
        Metabolic acidosis
        Respiratory acidosis
        Artifacts

Etiology and Pathogenesis

During the early and middle stages of *chronic renal insufficiency,* phosphate balance is maintained by a progressive reduction in tubular Pi transport leading to increased Pi excretion by the remaining nephrons and a maintenance of normal renal Pi clearance (2). In advanced renal insufficiency, the fractional excretion of Pi may be as high as 60% to 90% of the filtered load of phosphate. However, when the number of functional nephrons becomes too diminished (glomerular filtration rate usually <20 ml/min) and dietary intake is constant, Pi balance can no longer be maintained by reductions of tubular reabsorption, and hyperphosphatemia develops (2). When hyperphosphatemia develops, the filtered load of Pi per nephron increases and Pi excretion rises. As a result, Pi balance and renal excretory rate is reestablished, but at a higher serum Pi level.

Defects in renal excretion of Pi in the absence of renal failure may be primary, as in *pseudohypoparathyroidism* (see Chapter 39) or *tumoral calcinosis* (3,4). The latter is usually seen in young black males with ectopic calcification around large joints and is characterized by increased tubular reabsorption of calcium, Pi, and normal responses to parathyroid hormone (PTH) (5). Secondary tubular defects include *hypoparathyroidism* (see Chapter 38) (6) and high blood levels of growth hormone (7). Serum phosphorus values are normally elevated in children as compared with adults. Finally, bisphosphonates such as Didronel (disodium etidronate), Pamidronate, Aledronate, and so forth may cause hyperphosphatemia. The mechanisms of action are unclear, but they may involve cellular phosphate redistribution and decreased renal excretion (8).

Hyperphosphatemia can also be the consequence of an *increased intake* or administration of Pi. Intravenous administration of 1–2 g of Pi during the treatment of Pi depletion or hypercalcemia can cause hyperphosphatemia, especially in patients with underlying renal insufficiency. Hyperphosphatemia may also result from overzealous use of oral phosphates or of phosphate-containing enemas.

Administration of vitamin D and its metabolites in pharmacologic doses may be responsible for the development of hyperphosphatemia, although suppression of PTH and hypercalcemia-induced renal failure are important pathogenetic factors in this setting.

Transcellular shift of Pi from cells into the extracellular fluid compartment may lead to hyperphosphatemia, as seen in conditions associated with increased catabolism or tissue destruction (e.g., systemic infections, fulminant hepatitis, severe hyperthermia, crush injuries, nontraumatic *rhabdomyolysis,* and cytotoxic therapy for hematologic malignancies such as acute lymphoblastic leukemia and Burkitt's lymphoma) (1, for review). In this *"tumor lysis syndrome,"* serum Pi levels typically rise within 1–2 days after initiation of treatment. The rising serum Pi concentration often is accompanied by hypocalcemia, hyperuricemia, hyperkalemia, and renal failure.

Patients with *diabetic ketoacidosis* commonly have hyperphosphatemia at the time of presentation despite total body Pi depletion. Insulin, fluid, and acid–base therapy is accompanied by a shift of Pi back into cells and the development of hypophosphatemia. In lactic acidosis, hyperphosphatemia likely results from tissue hypoxia with a breakdown of ATP to AMP and Pi. Hyperphosphatemia may be *artifactual* when hemolysis occurs during the collection, storage, or processing of blood samples.

Clinical Consequences of Hyperphosphatemia

The most important short-term consequences of hyperphosphatemia are hypocalcemia and tetany, which occur most commonly in patients with an increased Pi load from any source, exogenous or endogenous. By contrast, soft tissue calcification and secondary hyperparathyroidism are long-term consequences of hyperphosphatemia that occur mainly in patients with renal insufficiency and decreased renal Pi excretion.

Hypocalcemia and Tetany

With rapid elevations of serum Pi, hypocalcemia and tetany may occur with serum Pi concentrations as low as 6 mg/dl, a level that, if reached more slowly, has no detectable effect on serum calcium. Hyperphosphatemia, in addition to its effect on the calcium × phosphate ion product with resultant calcium deposition in soft tissues, also inhibits the activity of 1α-hydroxylase in the kidney, resulting in a lower circulating level of 1,25-dihydroxyvitamin D_3. This further aggravates hypocalcemia by impairing intestinal absorption of calcium and inducing a state of skeletal resistance to the action of PTH.

Phosphate-induced hypocalcemia is common in patients with acute or chronic renal failure, and usually develops slowly. Tetany is uncommon unless a superimposed acid–base disorder produces an abrupt rise in plasma pH that acutely lowers the serum ionized calcium concentration. Profound hypocalcemia and tetany are occasionally observed during the early phase of the "tumor lysis" syndrome and rhabdomyolysis.

Soft Tissue Calcification

Ectopic calcification is usually seen in patients with chronic renal failure. Occasionally, an acute rise in serum Pi (e.g., during Pi treatment for hypercalcemia) may lead to ectopic calcification, especially when the calcium phosphate product exceeds 70. The blood vessels, skin, cornea ("band keratopathy") and periarticular tissues are common sites of calcium precipitation.

Secondary Hyperparathyroidism and Renal Osteodystrophy

Hyperphosphatemia due to renal failure also plays a critical role in development of secondary hyperparathyroidism and renal osteodystrophy (Chapter 67). In patients with advanced renal failure, the enhanced phosphate load from PTH-mediated osteolysis may ultimately become the dominant influence on serum phosphorus levels. This phenomenon may account for the correlation between serum phosphorus levels and the severity of osteitis fibrosa cystica in patients maintained on chronic hemodialysis.

Treatment

Correction of the pathogenetic defect should be the primary aim in the treatment of hyperphosphatemia. In most instances, however, the most effective way to treat hyperphosphatemia is to reduce dietary Pi intake. Because Pi is present in almost all foodstuffs, rigid dietary phosphate restriction requires a barely palatable diet that few patients can accept. However, dietary Pi can be reduced 600–1000 mg/day with modest protein restriction. A predialysis level of 4.5–5.0 mg/dl is reasonable and allows some room for removal of phosphorus with dialysis while avoiding severe postdialysis hypophosphatemia. To achieve this, most patients require the addition of phosphate binders to reduce intestinal absorption of dietary Pi.

Aluminum hydroxide or aluminum carbonate, when administered to patients with renal failure over the long term, has been shown to result in aluminum toxicity with encephalopathy, osteomalacia, proximal myopathy, and anemia. Therefore, calcium salts have replaced aluminum salts as first-line Pi binders (9–11). Calcium acetate and aluminum carbonate are equally potent and bind more Pi than equivalent amounts of calcium carbonate or citrate. In general treatment is started with 1 g of calcium carbonate with each meal and gradually increased up to 8–12 g daily. This regimen effectively controls serum Pi in about two thirds of patients on chronic dialysis (10). Calcium salts tend to increase serum calcium levels, and if hypercalcemia (>11 mg/dl) develops, calcium carbonate should not be increased further and reduction in dialysate calcium should be considered. If aluminum gels are used, calcium citrate must not be taken concomitantly because citrate markedly increases the absorption of aluminum. Maximal Pi binding occurs when phosphate binder is taken with a meal rather than 2 hours afterward.

The treatment of chronic hyperphosphatemia secondary to hypoparathyroidism occasionally requires that phosphate binders be added to the other therapeutic agents.

HYPOPHOSPHATEMIA

Hypophosphatemia is defined as an abnormally low concentration of inorganic phosphate in serum or plasma. Hypophosphatemia does not necessarily indicate total body Pi depletion because only 1% of the total body Pi is found in extracellular fluids. Conversely, serious Pi depletion may exist in the presence of a normal or even elevated serum Pi concentration. Moderate hypophosphatemia, defined as a serum Pi concentration between 2.5 and 1 mg/dl, is not uncommon and is usually not associated with signs or symptoms. Severe hypophosphatemia, defined as serum phosphorus levels below 1.0 mg/dl, is often associated with clinical signs and symptoms that require therapy. Approximately 2% of hospital patients have levels of serum Pi below 2 mg/dl according to some estimates. Hypophosphatemia is encountered more frequently among alcoholic patients and up to 10% of patients admitted to hospitals because of chronic alcoholism are hypophosphatemic.

Pathogenesis of Hypophosphatemia

Three types of pathophysiologic abnormalities can cause hypophosphatemia and total body Pi depletion: decreased intestinal absorption of Pi, increased urinary losses of this ion and a shift of Pi from extracellular to intracellular compartments. Combinations of these disturbances are common (12,13). The causes and mechanisms of moderate hypophosphatemia are shown in Table 2; the clinical conditions associated with severe hypophosphatemia are shown in Table 3.

Primary Hyperparathyroidism

This is a common entity in clinical medicine (14). Parathyroid hormone is secreted in excess of the physiologic needs for mineral homeostasis owing either to adenoma or hyperplasia of the parathyroid glands (Chapter 28). This results in decreased phosphorus reabsorption by the kidney, and the urinary losses of phosphorus result in hypophosphatemia. The degree of hypophosphatemia varies considerably because mobilization of phosphorus from stimulation of skeletal remodeling in part mitigates the hypophosphatemia.

Secondary hyperparathyroidism associated with normal renal function has been observed in patients with gastrointestinal abnormalities resulting in calcium malabsorption. Such patients may have low levels of serum calcium and phosphorus (15) (Chapter 41). In these patients, the hypocalcemia is responsible for increased release of PTH. Decreased intestinal absorption of phosphorus as a result of the primary gastrointestinal disease may contribute to the decrement in the levels of the serum phosphorus. In general, these patients have urinary losses of phosphorus that are out of proportion to the hypophosphatemia in contrast to patients with predominant phosphorus malabsorption and no secondary hyperparathyroidism in whom urinary excretion of phosphorus is low.

TABLE 2. *Causes of moderate hypophosphatemia*

Increased urinary losses
  Hyperparathyroidism
  Malabsorption
  Renal tubular defects
  Renal transplantation
  Abnormalities of vitamin D metabolism
    Vitamin D deficiency
    X-linked hypophosphatemic rickets
    Vitamin D-dependent rickets
  Oncogenic osteomalacia
  Alcohol abuse
  Poorly controlled diabetes mellitus
  Metabolic or respiratory acidosis
  Drugs: calcitonin, diuretics, glucocorticoids, bicarbonate
  Respiratory alkalosis
  Extracellular fluid volume expansion
Decreased intestinal absorption
  Antacid abuse
  Vitamin D deficiency
  Malabsorption
  Starvation, alcohol abuse
Shifts into cells
  Nutritional repletion
  Respiratory alkalosis
  Recovery from hypothermia
  Recovery from acidosis
  Acute gout
  Gram-negative bacteremia
  Salicylate poisoning
  Glucose
  Fructose
  Glycerol
  Insulin
  Blast crisis in leukemia

Renal Tubular Defects

Several conditions characterized by either single or multiple tubular ion transport defects have been characterized in which phosphorus reabsorption is decreased. In Fanconi syndrome, patients excrete not only an increased amount of phosphorus in the urine but also increased quantities of amino acids, uric acid, and glucose, resulting in hypouricemia and hypophosphatemia (16). There are other conditions in which an isolated defect in the renal tubular transport of phosphorus has been found, e.g., in fructose intolerance, an autosomal recessive disorder. Following renal transplantation, an acquired renal tubular defect may be responsible for the persistence of hypophosphatemia in some patients.

Vitamin D and its metabolites play an important role in phosphorus homeostasis (17,18). Vitamin D promotes intestinal absorption of calcium and phosphorus, and it is necessary to maintain the normal mineralization and remodeling processes of bone. In addition, vitamin D metabolites have important actions in the control of renal tubular ion transport.

Vitamin D-deficient rickets (when the deficiency occurs in children) or osteomalacia (when the deficiency occurs in adults) may result in severe deformities of the skeleton

(Chapter 58). Hypophosphatemia is the most frequent biochemical alteration associated with this metabolic abnormality.

X-Linked Hypophosphatemic Rickets

This X-linked dominant disorder is characterized by hypophosphatemia, decreased reabsorption of phosphorus by the renal tubule, decreased absorption of calcium and phosphorus from the gastrointestinal tract, and varying degrees of rickets or osteomalacia (Chapter 61). Patients with this disorder and the murine homologue (Hyp) exhibit normal levels of 1,25-dihydroxycholecalciferol and reduced Na-phosphate transport in the proximal tubule in the face of severe hypophosphatemia (19). Recent advances including the cloning of a phosphate-regulated Na-Pi transporter from rabbit kidney and the elucidation of defective 1,25-vitamin D catabolism in Hyp mouse proximal tubule have improved our understanding of the molecular basis for this disorder. The gene for X-linked hypophosphatemia is not the Pi transport protein itself, which maps to chromosome 5 (20), a gene encoding a neutral endopeptidase, termed PEX, has been described as responsible (21) (Chapters 61 and 62).

1,25-Dihydroxyvitamin D_3 therapy increases plasma phosphorus by pharmacologic stimulation of phosphorus absorption from the gastrointestinal tract. The defect in renal phosphorus reabsorption is unchanged despite treatment with 1,25-dihydroxyvitamin D_3. Therapeutically, the combination of neutral phosphate supplementation and 1,25-dihydroxycholecalciferol has led to an improvement in the bone disease of patients and an increase in their plasma phosphorus (22,23). However, episodes of hypercalcemia and secondary extraskeletal calcification have limited aggressive therapy.

Vitamin D-Dependent Rickets

This is a recessively inherited form of vitamin D-refractory rickets associated with hypophosphatemia, hypocalcemia, elevated levels of serum alkaline phosphatase, and, sometimes, generalized amino aciduria and severe bone lesions (Chapter 60). There are two main forms of the syndrome. Type I is an inborn error in conversion of 25-hydroxyvitamin D to 1,25-dihydroxyvitamin D due to deficiency of the renal 1-hydroxylase enzyme (24). This condition responds to very large doses of vitamin D_2 and D_3 but to normal doses of 1,25-dihydroxyvitamin D_3. Type II is characterized by an end-organ resistance to 1,25-dihydroxyvitamin D_3 due to an abnormal vitamin D receptor (25,26). Plasma levels of 1,25-dihydroxyvitamin D_3 are elevated. Large pharmacologic doses of 1,25-dihydroxyvitamin D_3 are required for treatment of this syndrome.

Oncogenic Osteomalacia

This entity is characterized by hypophosphatemia in association with malignant tumors (27,28) (Chapter 62). The patients exhibit osteomalacia on histomorphologic examination of bone biopsies, renal wasting of phosphorus, and markedly reduced levels of 1,25-dihydroxyvitamin D_3. The existence of a possible circulating humoral factor has long been suspected and is supported by the identification of tumor products from patients with sclerosing hemangioma that inhibit renal phosphate transport (Chapter 62) (29).

Alcohol and Alcohol Withdrawal

Alcohol abuse is a common cause of severe hypophosphatemia (Table 3) (30,31). Among the factors responsible for Pi depletion in the alcoholic are poor intake, the use of antacids, and vomiting. Patients with alcoholism have also been shown to have a variety of defects in renal tubular function, including a decrease in threshold for phosphate excretion, which are reversible with abstinence. Ethanol enhances urinary Pi excretion, and marked phosphaturia tends to occur during episodes of alcoholic ketoacidosis. Because such patients often eat poorly, ketonuria is common. Repeated episodes of ketoacidosis catabolize organic phosphates within cells and cause phosphaturia by mechanisms analogous to those seen in diabetic ketoacidosis. Chronic alcoholism may also cause magnesium deficiency and hypomagnesemia which may, in turn, cause phosphaturia and Pi depletion, especially in skeletal muscle (Chapters 42 and 55).

Nutritional Repletion: Oral, Enteral, and Parenteral Nutrition

Nutritional repletion of the malnourished patient implies the provision of sufficient calories, protein, and other nutrients to allow accelerated tissue accretion. In the course of this process, cellular uptake and utilization of Pi increase. When insufficient amounts of Pi are provided, an acute state of severe hypophosphatemia and intracellular Pi depletion with serious clinical and metabolic consequences can occur (32,33). This type of hypophosphatemia has been observed in malnourished patients receiving parenteral nutrition and following refeeding of prisoners of war.

Diabetes Mellitus

Patients with well-controlled diabetes mellitus do not have excessive losses of phosphate. However, in the presence of hyperglycemia, polyuria, and acidosis, Pi is lost through the urine in excessive amounts. In ketoacidosis,

TABLE 3. *Causes of severe hypophosphatemia*

Alcohol withdrawal
Nutritional repletion: oral, enteral, and parenteral nutrition
Diabetes/diabetic ketoacidosis
Respiratory alkalosis
Thermal burns
Leukemia
Increased urinary losses
Impaired gastrointestinal absorption

intracellular organic components tend to be broken down, releasing a large amount of Pi into the plasma, which is subsequently lost in the urine (34). This process, combined with the enhanced osmotic Pi diuresis secondary to glycosuria, ketonuria, and polyuria, may cause large urinary loses of Pi and subsequent depletion. The plasma Pi is usually normal or slightly elevated in the ketotic patient in spite of the excessive urinary losses because of the continuous large shift of Pi from the cells into the plasma. With insulin, fluids, and correction of the ketoacidosis, however, serum and urine Pi may fall sharply. Despite the appearance of hypophosphatemia during treatment, previously well-controlled patients with diabetic ketoacidosis of only a few days duration almost never have serious phosphorus deficiency. Serum Pi rarely falls below 1.0 mg/dl in these patients. Administration of Pi-containing salts does not improve glucose utilization; nor does it reduce insulin requirements or the time for recovery from ketoacidosis. Thus, Pi therapy should be reserved for patients with serum Pi concentration <1.0 mg/dl.

Respiratory Alkalosis

Intense hyperventilation for prolonged periods may depress serum Pi to values below 1.0 mg/dl (35). This is important in patients with alcoholic withdrawal because of attendant hyperventilation. A similar degree of alkalemia induced by infusion of bicarbonate depresses Pi concentration only mildly. The combined hypophosphatemic effects of respiratory and metabolic alkalosis may be pronounced.

Severe hypophosphatemia is common in patients with extensive burns. It usually appears within several days after the injury. Phosphorus is virtually undetectable in the urine. Hypophosphatemia may result from transductive losses, respiratory alkalosis, or other factors.

Increased Urinary Losses

Abnormalities in tubular handling of phosphate have been implicated in the genesis of severe hypophosphatemia induced by hypokalemia, hypomagnesemia, systemic acidosis, hypothyroidism, X-linked hypophosphatemic rickets (Chapter 61), hyperparathyroidism (Chapter 28), and humoral hypercalcemia of malignancy (Chapter 32). During the recovery phase from severe burns, hypophosphatemia may occur secondary to massive diuresis with phosphaturia. Renal transplantation may be followed by severe phosphaturia and hypophosphatemia due to tubular defects.

Impaired Gastrointestinal Absorption

Severe hypophosphatemia and phosphate depletion may result from vigorous use of oral antacids, which bind phosphate, usually for peptic ulcer disease (36). Patients so treated may develop osteomalacia and severe skeletal symptoms due to phosphorus deficiency.

Intestinal malabsorption can cause hypophosphatemia and phosphate depletion through malabsorption of Pi and vitamin D, and through increased urinary Pi losses resulting from secondary hyperparathyroidism induced by calcium malabsorption.

Leukemia

Advanced leukemia that is markedly proliferative ("blast crisis"), with total leukocyte counts above 100,000, has been associated with severe hypophosphatemia. This would appear to result from excessive phosphorus uptake into rapidly multiplying cells (37).

Clinical Effects of Severe Hypophosphatemia

Severe hypophosphatemia with phosphorus deficiency may cause widespread disturbances. There are at least eight well-established effects of severe hypophosphatemia (Table 4). The signs and symptoms of severe hypophosphatemia may be related to a decrease in 2,3-diphosphoglycerate in the red cell. This change is associated with increased affinity of hemoglobin for oxygen and therefore tissue hypoxia. There is also a decrease in tissue content of ATP and, consequently, a decrease in the availability of energy-rich phosphate compounds for cell function.

Central Nervous System

Some patients with severe hypophosphatemia display symptoms compatible with metabolic encephalopathy (38–40). They may display, in sequence, irritability, apprehension, weakness, numbness, paresthesia, dysarthria, confusion, obtundation, seizures, and coma. In contrast to delirium tremens, the syndrome does not include hallucinations. Patients with very severe hypophosphatemia may show diffuse slowing of their electroencephalogram.

Hematopoietic System

A decrease in the red cell content of 2,3-diphosphoglycerate and ATP leads to increased rigidity and, in rare instances, hemolysis (41). Hemolysis is usually provoked by unusual stress on the metabolic requirements of the red cell, such as severe metabolic acidosis or infection. When hemolysis has occurred, ATP content has invariably been

Leukocyte/macrophage dysfunction can be demonstrated *in vitro* using Pi-depleted cells (42). Suggestion that a predisposition to infection commonly seen in patients on intravenous hyperalimentation may be partly related to hypo-

TABLE 4. *Consequences of severe hypophosphatemia*

Red cell dysfunction
Leukocyte dysfunction
Platelet dysfunction
CNS dysfunction
Rhabdomyolysis
Osteomalacia/rickets
Metabolic acidosis
Cardiomyopathy

phosphatemia remains to be proven. Hypophosphatemia impairs granulocyte function by interfering with ATP synthesis.

In experimental hypophosphatemia there is an increase in platelet diameter, suggesting shortened platelet survival and also a marked acceleration of platelet disappearance from the blood. These lead to thrombocytopenia and a reactive megakaryocytosis. In addition, there is an impairment of clot retraction and a hemorrhagic tendency, especially involving gut and skin.

Musculoskeletal System

Myopathy and Rhabdomyolysis

Muscle tissue requires large amounts of high-energy bonds (ATP, creatine phosphate) and oxygen for contraction, for maintenance of membrane potential, and for other functions. Pi deprivation induces muscle cell injury characterized by a decrease in intracellular Pi and an increase in water, sodium, and chloride. An apparent relationship between hypophosphatemia and alcoholic myopathy has been observed in chronic alcoholism (43). The muscular clinical manifestations of Pi deficiency syndrome include myalgia, objective weakness, and myopathy with pathologic findings of intracellular edema and a subnormal resting muscle membrane potential on electromyography. In patients with preexisting Pi deficiency who develop acute hypophosphatemia, rhabdomyolysis might occur (44). Hypophosphatemia and phosphate deficiency may be associated with creatine phosphokinase elevations in blood.

Bone

Skeletal defects have been reported in association with Pi depletion of different causes. These are discussed in detail in Chapters 58–66. Suffice it to say here that phosphate depletion is associated with rickets in children and osteomalacia in adults (45,46).

Cardiovascular System

Severe hypophosphatemia has been associated with a cardiomyopathy characterized by a low cardiac output, a decreased ventricular ejection velocity, and an elevated left ventricular end-diastolic pressure (47). A decrease in myocardial content of inorganic phosphorus, ATP, and creatinine phosphate seems to underlie the impairment in myocardial contractility (48).

During phosphorus depletion, blood pressure may be low and the pressor response to naturally occurring vasoconstrictor agonists such as norepinephrine or angiotensin II is reduced.

Renal Effects of Hypophosphatemia and Phosphate Depletion

Severe hypophosphatemia and phosphate depletion affect the balance and serum concentrations of various electrolytes

TABLE 5. *Consequences of hypophosphatemia and phosphate depletion on renal function*

Glomerular filtration rate reduction
Metabolic abnormalities
    Reduced cellular Pi, ATP, phospholipid precursors
    Reduced gluconeogenesis
    Insulin resistance
    Hypoparathyroidism, reduced urinary cAMP
    Increased $1,25(OH)_2D_3$
Transport abnormalities
    Hypercalciuria
    Reduced proximal tubular Na^+ transport
    Hypermagnesiuria
    Pi retention
    Bicarbonaturia
    Metabolic acidosis
    Reduced glucose transport

(1, for review). It may produce changes in cardiovascular function as described above, renal hemodynamics affect renal tubular transport processes and induce marked changes in renal cell metabolism. These disturbances are listed in Table 5.

Tubular Transport

Calcium

A marked increase in urinary calcium excretion occurs during phosphate depletion proportional to the severity of phosphate depletion and the degree of hypophosphatemia (49).

Phosphate

Dietary Pi restriction and Pi depletion is associated with enhanced renal tubular reabsorption of Pi (39,50). Urinary excretion of Pi declines within hours after the reduction in its dietary intake, and Pi virtually disappears from the urine within 1–2 days. The changes in renal tubular reabsorption of Pi occur prior to detectable falls in the serum Pi. The adaptation to a reduction in Pi supply is a direct response of the proximal tubule. In addition, the ability of the kidney to conserve Pi produces a resistance to phosphaturic stimuli. Thus, the phosphaturic response to PTH is severely blunted during states of Pi depletion (50). However, it is also clear that the mechanism of Pi transport stimulated by Pi depletion does not share the regulatory pathways affected by PTH. The adaptation to reduced Pi supply is a separate system for the regulation of renal tubular Pi reabsorption. The details of how this system operates remain to be elucidated.

Metabolic Acidosis

Severe hypophosphatemia with Pi deficiency may result in metabolic acidosis through three mechanisms (51,52). First, severe hypophosphatemia is generally associated with a proportionate reduction of Pi excretion in the urine, thereby limiting hydrogen excretion as a titratable acid. Second, if Pi buffer is inadequate, acid secretion depends on production of ammonia and its conversion to ammonium ion. Ammonia production is severely depressed in Pi deficiency. The third mechanism is that of decreased renal tubular reabsorption of bicarbonate.

Treatment

The appropriate management of hypophosphatemia and Pi depletion requires identification of the underlying causes, treatment with supplemental Pi when necessary, and prevention of recurrence of the problem by correcting the underlying causes. The symptoms and signs of Pi depletion can vary, are nonspecific, and are usually seen in patients with multiple problems such as those encountered in intensive care unit settings. This makes it difficult to identify Pi depletion as the cause of clinical manifestations and Pi depletion is frequently overlooked.

Mild hypophosphatemia secondary to redistribution, with plasma Pi levels higher than 2 mg/dl, is transient and requires no treatment. In cases of moderate hypophosphatemia, associated with Pi depletion (serum Pi higher than 1.0 mg/dl in adults or 2.0 mg/dl in children), Pi supplementation should be administered in addition to treating the cause of hypophosphatemia. Milk is an excellent source of phosphorus, containing 1 g (33 mM) of inorganic phosphorus per liter. Skimmed milk may be better tolerated than whole milk, especially in children and malnourished patients because of concomitant lactose or fat intolerance. Alternatively, Neutraphos tablets (which contain 250 mg of Pi per tablet as a sodium or potassium salt) may be given. Oral Pi can be given in a dose up to 3 g/day (i.e., 3 tablets of Neutraphos every 6 hours). The serum Pi level rises by as much as 1.5 mg/dl, 60–120 minutes after ingestion of 1000 mg of Pi. A phosphosoda enema solution, composed of buffered sodium phosphate, may also be used in a dose of 15–30 ml 3 or 4 times daily.

Severe hypophosphatemia with serum levels lower than 0.5 mg/dl occurs only when there is cumulative net loss of more than 3.3 g of Pi. If asymptomatic, oral replacement with a total of 6–10 g of Pi (1–3 g of Pi per day) over a few days is usually sufficient. Symptomatic hypophosphatemia indicates that net Pi deficit exceeds 10 g. In these cases, 20 g of Pi is given spread over 1 week (up to 3 g/day). Patients with Pi deficiency tolerate substantially larger doses of oral Pi without side effects, such as diarrhea, than do normal subjects. However, patients with severe symptomatic hypophosphatemia who are unable to eat may be safely treated intravenously with 1 g of Pi delivered in 1 L of fluid over 8–12 hours. This is usually sufficient to raise serum Pi level to 1.0 mg/dl. It is unusual for hypophosphatemia to cause metabolic disturbances at serum Pi >1.0 mg/dl, so that full parenteral replacement is neither necessary nor desirable.

Treatment with phosphate can result in diarrhea, hyperphosphatemia, hypocalcemia, and hyperkalemia. These side effects can be prevented by paying careful attention to phosphorus dosages.

PREVENTION

The most effective approach to hypophosphatemia is prevention of predisposing conditions. Patients on total parenteral nutrition should receive a daily maintenance dose of Pi amounting to 1000 mg in 24 hours, with increases as required by the clinical and metabolic states. Alcoholic patients and malnourished patients receiving intravenous fluids, particularly those containing glucose, should receive Pi supplementation, particularly if hypophosphatemia is observed.

ACKNOWLEDGMENTS

This work was supported by NIH grants AR32087, AR39561, and DK09976 and a grant from the Shriner's Hospital for Crippled Children.

REFERENCES

1. Hruska K, Slatopolsky E: Disorders of phosphorus, calcium, and magnesium metabolism. In: Schrier RW, Gottschalk CW (eds) *Diseases of the Kidney.* 6th ed. Little, Brown, Boston, 1996, in press.
2. Slatopolsky E, Robson AM, Elkan I, Bricker NS: Control of phosphate excretion in uremic man. *J Clin Invest* 47:1865, 1968
3. Albright R, Burnett CH, Smith PH, et al: Pseudohypoparathyroidism—an example of Seabright Bantam syndrome. *Endocrinology* 30:922, 1942
4. Mitnick PD, Goldbarb S, Slatopolsky E, et al: Calcium and phosphate metabolism in tumoral calcinosis. *Ann Intern Med* 92:482, 1980
5. Lufkin EG, Wilson DM, Smith LH, et al: Phosphorus excretion in tumoral calcinosis: Response to parathyroid hormone and acetazolamide. *J Clin Endocrinol Metab* 50:648, 1980
6. Parfitt AJ: The spectrum of hypoparathyroidism. *J Clin Endocrinol Metab* 34:152, 1972
7. McConnell TH: Fatal hypocalcemia from phosphate absorption from laxative preparations. *JAMA* 216:147, 1971
8. Walton RJ, Russell RGG, Smith R: Changes in the renal and extrarenal handling of phosphate induced by disodium etidronate (EHDP) in man. *Clin Sci Mol Med* 49:45, 1975
9. Morniere PH, Roussel A, Tahira Y, et al: Substitution of aluminum hydroxide by high doses of calcium carbonate in patients on chronic hemodialysis: Disappearance of hyperalbuminemia and equal control of hyperparathyroidism. *Proc Eur Dial Transplant Assoc* 19:784, 1982
10. Slatopolsky E, Weerts C, Lopez S, et al: Calcium carbonate is an effective phosphate binder in dialysis patients. *N Engl J Med* 315:157, 1986
11. Slatopolsky E, Weerts C, Norwood K, et al: Long-term effects of calcium carbonate and 2.5 mEq/liter calcium dialysate on mineral metabolism. *Kidney Int* 36:897, 1989
12. Knochel JP: The pathophysiology and clinical characteristics of severe hyperphosphatemia. *Arch Intern Med* 137:203, 1977
13. Kreisberg RA: Phosphorus deficiency and hypophosphatemia. *Hosp Pract* 12:121, 1977
14. Arnaud CD, Clar OH: Primary hyperparathyroidism. In: Krieger DT, Bardin CW (eds) *Current Therapy in Endocrinology 1983–1984.* Decker/Mosby, Philadelphia/St Louis, p 277, 1983
15. Glikman RM: Malabsorption: Pathophysiology and diagnosis. In: Wyngaarden JB, Smith LH Jr (eds) *Cecil's Textbook of Medicine.* 17th ed. WB Saunders, Philadelphia, p 719, 1985
16. Roth KS, Foreman JW, Segal S: The Fanconi syndrome and mechanisms of tubular dysfunction. *Kidney Int* 20:705, 1981
17. Gray RW, Caldas AE, Wilz DR, et al: Metabolism and excretion of ^{3}H-1,25(OH)$_2$ vitamin D$_3$ in healthy adults. *J Clin Endocrinol Metab* 46:756, 1978
18. Gray RW, Wilz DR, Caldas AE, et al: The importance of phosphate in regulating plasma 1,25(OH)$_2$ vitamin D levels in humans: Studies in healthy subjects, in calcium-stone formers and in patients with primary hyperparathyroidism. *J Clin Endocrinol Metab* 45:299, 1977

19. Eicher EM, Southard JL, Scriver CR, et al: Hypophosphatemia: Mouse model for human familial hypophosphatemic (vitamin D-resistant) rickets. *Proc Natl Acad Sci USA* 73:4667, 1976
20. Kos CH, Lemieux N, Tihy F, Biber J, Murer H, Econs M, Tenenhouse HS: The renal specific Na$^+$-phosphate cotransporter cDNA maps to human chromosome 5q35 (Abstract). *J Am Soc Nephrol* 4:816, 1993
21. The Hyp Consortium. A gene (PEX) with homologies to endopeptidases is mutated in patients with x-linked hypophosphatemic rickets. *Nat Genet* 11:130–136, 1995
22. Glorieux FH, Marie PJ, Pettifor JM, Delvin EE: Bone response to phosphate salts, ergocalciferol, and calcitriol in hypophosphatemic vitamin D-resistant rickets. *N Engl J Med* 303:1023, 1980
23. Verge CF, Lam A, Simpson JM, Cowell CT, Howard NJ, Silink M: Effect of therapy in X-linked hypophosphatemic rickets. *N Engl J Med* 325:1843, 1991
24. Fraser D, Kooh SW, Kind HP: Pathogenesis of hereditary vitamin-D-dependent rickets. An inborn error of vitamin D metabolism involving defective conversion of 25-hydroxyvitamin D to 1,25-dihydroxyvitamin D. *N Engl J Med* 289:817, 1973
25. Liberman UA, Eil C, Marx SJ: Resistance of 1,25 dihydroxyvitamin D. Associated with heterogeneous defects in cultured skin fibroblasts. *J Clin Invest* 71:192, 1983
26. Malloy PJ, Hochberg Z, Pike JW, Feldman D: Abnormal binding of vitamin D receptors to deoxyribonucleic acid in a kindred with vitamin D-dependent rickets, type II. *J Clin Endocrinol Metab* 68:263, 1989
27. Parker MS, Klein I, Haussler MR, et al: Tumor-induced osteomalacia: Evidence of a surgically correctable alteration in vitamin D metabolism. *JAMA* 245:492, 1981
28. Sweet RA, Males JL, Hamstra AJ, et al: Vitamin D metabolite levels in oncogenic osteomalacia. *Ann Intern Med* 93:279, 1980
29. Cai Q, Hodgson SF, Kao PC, Lennon VA, Klee GG, Zinsmiester AR, Kumar R: Inhibition of renal phosphate transport by a tumor product in a patient with oncogenic osteomalacia. *N Engl J Med* 330:1645, 1994
30. Larsson K, Rebel K, Sorbo B: Severe hypophosphatemia—a hospital survey. *Acta Med Scand* 214:221, 1983
31. Ryback RS, Eckardt MJ, Pautler CP: Clinical relationships between serum phosphorus and other blood chemistry values in alcoholics. *Arch Intern Med* 140:673, 1980
32. Juan D, Elrazak MA: Hypophosphatemia in hospitalized patients. *JAMA* 242:163, 1979
33. Betro MG, Pain RW: Hypophosphatemia and hyperphosphatemia in hospital population. *Br Med J* 1:273, 1972
34. Seldin DW, Tarail R: The metabolism of glucose and electrolytes in diabetic acidosis. *J Clin Invest* 29:552, 1950
35. Mostellar ME, Tuttle EP: Effects of alkalosis on plasma concentration and urinary excretion of urinary phosphate in man. *J Clin Invest* 43:138, 1964
36. Shields HS: Rapid fall of serum phosphorus secondary to antacid therapy. *Gastroenterology* 75:1137, 1978
37. Zamkoff KW, Kirshner JJ: Marked hypophosphatemia associated with acute myelomonocytic leukemia: Indirect evidence of phosphorus uptake by leukemic cells. *Arch Intern Med* 140:1523, 1980.
38. Lotz M, Ney R, Bartter FC: Osteomalacia and debility resulting from phosphorus depletion. *Trans Assoc Am Physicians* 77:281, 1964
39. Lotz M, Zisman E, Bartter FC: Evidence for a phosphorus-depletion syndrome in man. *N Engl J Med* 278:409, 1968
40. Prins JS, Schriver M, Staghower JM: Hyperalimentation, hypophosphatemia and coma. *Lancet* 1:1253, 1973
41. Jacob HS, Amsden T: Acute hemolytic anemia and rigid red cells in hypophosphatemia. *N Engl J Med* 285:1446, 1971
42. Craddock PR, Yawta Y, Van Santen L: Acquired phagocyte dysfunction: A complication of the hypophosphatemia of parenteral hyperalimentation. *N Engl J Med* 290:1403, 1974
43. Knochel JP, Bilbrey GL, Fuller TJ, et al: The muscle cell in chronic alcoholism. The possible role of phosphate depletion in alcoholic myopathy. *Ann NY Acad Sci* 252:274, 1975
44. Knochel JP, Barcenas C, Cotton JR, et al: Hypophosphatemia and rhabdomyolysis. *J Clin Invest* 62:1240 1978
45. Baker, LRI Ackrill, P and Cattell, WR: Iatrogenic osteomalacia and myopathy due to phosphate depletion. *Br Med J* 3:150 1974
46. Cooke RS, Teitelbaum S, Avioli LV: Antacid induced osteomalacia and nephrolithiasis. *Arch Intern Med* 138:1007, 1978
47. Darsee JR, Nutter DO: Reversible severe congestive cardiomyopathy in three cases of hypophosphatemia. *Ann Intern Med* 89:867, 1978
48. Fuller TJ, Nichols WW, Brenner BJ, et al: Reversible depression in myocardial performance in dogs with experimental phosphorus deficiency. *J Clin Invest* 62:1194, 1978
49. Coburn JW, Massry SG: Changes in serum and urinary calcium during phosphate depletion: Studies on mechanisms. *J Clin Invest* 49:1073, 1970
50. Steele TH: Renal resistance to parathyroid hormone during phosphorus deprivation. *J Clin Invest* 58:1461, 1976
51. Dominguez JH, Gray RW, Lemann J Jr: Dietary phosphate deprivation in women and men: Effects on mineral and acid balances, parathyroid hormone and the metabolism of 25-OH-vitamin D. *J Clin Endocrinol Metab* 43:1056, 1976
52. O'Donovan DJ, Lotspeich WD: Activation of kidney mitochondrial glutaminase by inorganic phosphate and organic acids. *Nature* 212:930, 1966

Metabolic Bone Diseases

V. Introduction

Sundeep Khosla, M.D. and *Michael Kleerekoper, M.D., F.A.C.E.

*Department of Endocrinology, Mayo Clinic and Mayo Medical School, Rochester, Minnesota; and *Department of Internal Medicine, Wayne State University School of Medicine, and Harper Hospital, Detroit Michigan*

Metabolic bone diseases can be divided into two broad categories: osteoporosis, in which there is a decrease in bone mass and microarchitectural deterioration of the skeleton, and osteomalacia, where the primary defect is in the mineralization of bone. As the names imply, in osteoporosis the bones are porous and brittle, while in osteomalacia the bones are malacic or soft, but not particularly brittle. This section follows this classification, with Chapters 44 through 57 dealing with the problem of osteoporosis, and Chapters 58 through 66 with the various causes of osteomalacia. Chapter 67, on renal osteodystrophy in adults and children, is difficult to classify, because several different abnormalities may be present in this disease. This disorder also serves to remind us that while this classification is conceptually useful, more than one abnormality may exist in a given patient. For example, a patient who received steroid therapy after intestinal bypass surgery may have developed steroid-induced osteoporosis and may also have a mineralization defect as a result of vitamin D deficiency.

The term *osteoporosis* actually refers to a syndrome, with many causes and a number of clinical forms. Osteoporosis is generally categorized as primary or secondary, based on the absence or presence of associated medical diseases, surgical procedures, or medications known to be associated with accelerated bone loss. Describing the osteoporoses with a number of short, focused chapters has many practical advantages from the educational standpoint of this primer. However, the reader is reminded that most often patient care cannot be so neatly pigeon-holed. Thus, the chapters in the first part of this section deal separately with the different forms of primary and secondary osteoporosis, but information from several chapters may be relevant to any individual patient. Postmenopausal osteoporosis, the most common form of primary osteoporosis, is discussed in Chapters 44 through 50. These chapters review the epidemiology, pathogenesis, and prevention of this disease, including current concepts of the proper role of exercise and nutrition in preventing this disorder. Chapter 49 discusses the evaluation and management of osteoporosis. There, the reader is also referred to Chapters 23 and 24 of Section III, dealing more specifically with bone densitometry and radiology, as well as to Chapter 20 on biochemical markers of bone turnover. These earlier chapters deal more with the technical aspects of these diagnostic modalities, whereas Chapter 49 is intended to focus on the clinical evaluation of patients with osteoporosis. Because hip fracture represents a special problem and the most serious manifestation of this disease, it is dealt with separately (Chapter 50). It is also becoming clear that although osteoporosis may be more common in women, men also develop this disorder, as discussed in Chapter 53. Children and adolescents also develop an uncommon and relatively poorly understood form of primary osteoporosis, juvenile osteoporosis (Chapter 51). The remaining chapters in this part of the section deal with the secondary causes of osteoporosis, including steroid and drug-induced osteoporosis (Chapter 52) and bone loss related to excessive thyroid hormone (Chapter 54).

The second part of this section deals with the several causes of bone softening: rickets in children (before epiphyseal closure) and osteomalacia in adults. Vitamin D deficiency can result from inadequate intake (Chapter 58) or inadequate absorption (Chapter 59). Rickets or osteomalacia may also result from impaired metabolism or impaired action of vitamin D (Chapter 60). Inherited (Chapter 61) or acquired (Chapter 62) abnormalities of renal phosphate transport may also cause abnormal mineralization and soft bones. The remaining chapters deal with other causes of rickets and osteomalacia. As noted earlier, renal failure represents a somewhat unique and difficult-to-classify situation, because, although osteomalacia may be present, a variety of other skeletal abnormalities are also found in this disorder, as discussed in Chapter 67.

44. Epidemiology of Osteoporosis

Richard D. Wasnich, M.D.

Hawaii Osteoporosis Center, Honolulu, Hawaii

A recent consensus conference defined osteoporosis as a metabolic bone disease characterized by low bone mass and microarchitectural deterioration of bone tissue, leading to enhanced bone fragility and a consequent increase in fracture risk (1). Another distinguishing characteristic of osteoporosis is a normal mineral/collagen ratio, which distinguishes it from osteomalacia, a disease characterized by relative deficiency of mineral in relation to collagen.

Osteoporosis is the most prevalent metabolic bone disease in the United States and other developed countries. Fracture prevalence refers to the number of people in the population who at a given time have already had fractures related to osteoporosis. Vertebral fracture prevalence among women aged 65 has been estimated to be 27% in Minnesota (2) and 21% among Danish women at age 70 (3).

Incidence refers to the number of *new* fracture cases in a population within a specified time. For example, among Japanese–American women in Hawaii, 5% of 80-year-old women will experience a new vertebral fracture each year. In general, data concerning the prevalence and incidence of hip, wrist, and other nonvertebral fractures are more reliable than vertebral fracture data. That is because many vertebral fractures are not clinically evident; therefore only populations that have been surveyed by periodic spine x-rays yield accurate prevalence data.

Vertebral fracture data are further hampered by the absence of a clear radiographic definition of vertebral fracture (4).

Osteoporotic fractures increase with age; wrist fractures show a rising incidence in the 50s, vertebral fractures in the 60s, and hip fractures in the 70s (Fig. 1). There is at least a two fold higher incidence among women compared with men for all age-related fracture sites. Because life expectancy is longer for women, there are proportionately more older women than men, resulting in a greater fracture prevalence among women than would be predicted from the age-adjusted incidence ratio.

Interesting geographic and ethnic differences exist. For example, hip fracture rates are higher in white populations regardless of geographic location (5). In contrast, hip fracture rates are lower among blacks in the United States and South Africa, and also among Japanese both in Japan and in the United States (6,7).

Frequently, but not always, ethnic and geographic differences in fracture prevalence can be explained by differences in bone density. The strong relationship between diminishing bone density and the risk of fragility fractures is well established. The risk of new vertebral fractures increases by a factor of 2.0–2.4 for each standard deviation (SD) decrease of bone density, irrespective of the site of bone density measurement (8). Similar findings have been found for hip and other nonvertebral fractures. It has therefore been proposed by a World Health Organization (WHO) expert panel that women with bone density values more than 2.5 SD below the young adult mean value be considered as osteoporotic (9). If they also have one or more fragility fractures, they would be classified as severe, or established, osteoporosis. Those women with bone density values between 1 and 2.5 SD below the young adult mean values would be classified as osteopenic.

Because surveys of bone density are easier to obtain than are accurate fracture incidence data, they may provide better estimates of osteoporosis prevalence. Based on the WHO diagnostic categories, Melton has estimated that 54% of postmenopausal white women in the United States have osteopenia, and another 30% have osteoporosis (10). Thus white women alone account for 26 million people who are at risk for fracture. The addition of men and non-white women would increase the total considerably. This number compares to 30 million to 54 million Americans who have hypertension.

The aging of the world population, when combined with the exponential, age-related increases in fracture incidence, portend drastic increases in the costs of osteoporosis. Cummings et al. have estimated that the cost of hip fractures alone in the United States could reach $240 billion within 50 years (11). Although there is an increased mortality rate following both hip and vertebral fractures, the worst consequence of osteoporosis might not be the increased mortality but rather the fact that most patients must *live* with the disease for many years, with its associated loss of independence and impaired quality of life (12). This is particularly true for vertebral fractures, which begin at an earlier age than hip fractures and affect many more women and men.

RISK FACTORS

Major risk factors for osteoporosis, such as age and bone density, have been established by virtue of their direct and strong relationship to fracture incidence. These more potent risk factors might be categorized as clinical risk indicators (8). However, a majority of the suspected or established risk factors for osteoporosis are based on their relationship to bone density as a surrogate indicator of disease presence and are therefore only as valid as the surrogate indicator. This category of risk factors might be categorized as etiologic; the utility of these risk factors is more likely to be in the realm of public health than in the management of individual clinical patients.

Most risk factors fall into five major categories: age, or age-related; genetic; environmental; endogenous hormones and chronic diseases; and physical characteristics of bone (Table 1).

The relative contribution of individual risk factors is much influenced by the age at which they are expressed.

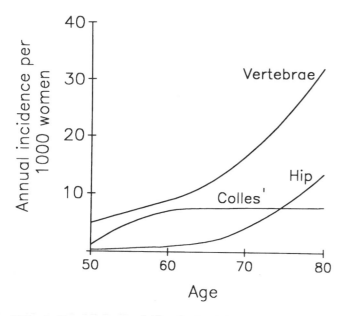

FIG. 1. Representation of the incidence rates for vertebral, Colles', and hip fractures in women.

TABLE 1. *Risk factors for osteoporosis*

Age, or Age-Related
  Each decade associated with 1.4–1.8-fold increased risk
Genetic
  Ethnicity: Caucasians and Oriental > blacks and
    Polynesians
  Gender: Female > male
  Family history
Environmental
  Nutrition; calcium deficiency
  Physical activity and mechanical loading
  Medications, e.g., corticosteroids
  Smoking
  Alcohol
  Falls (trauma)
Endogenous Hormones and Chronic Diseases
  Estrogen deficiency
  Androgen deficiency
  Chronic diseases, e.g., gastrectomy, cirrhosis,
    hyperthyroidism, hypercortisolism
Physical Characteristics of Bone
  Density (mass)
  Size and geometry
  Microarchitecture
  Composition

For example, estrogen deficiency during the adolescent years can be catastrophic to the growing skeleton. It also has a significant impact at age 50, but for some women the impact is negligible. After age 70 or 80, estrogen deficiency may be overshadowed by other risk factors. This concept is illustrated in Fig. 2. The clinical utility of bone density is derived from the fact that it is a composite, cumulative index of multiple other risk factors, both past and present, and including both genetic and lifestyle influences.

HETEROGENEITY

Because of its multifactorial etiology, it is not surprising that osteoporosis is a heterogeneous disorder. The relative contributions of age and estrogen deficiency have been emphasized in the past, but it is difficult to differentiate these two factors in most patients. It is also increasingly apparent that there are multiple, other contributing etiolo-

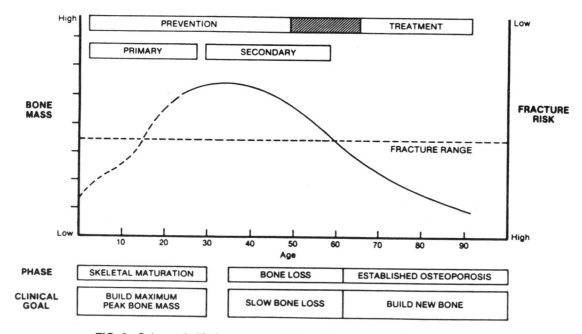

FIG. 2. Schematic lifetime representation of bone mass and fracture risk.

gies, including those that are unknown or poorly understood. Furthermore, the *predominant* etiology may vary substantially from patient to patient. Lastly, the major contribution of peak bone mass to ultimate fracture risk indicates that risk factors that are expressed during childhood and adolescence may contribute as much to lifetime fracture risk as do aging and menopause. In any case, *treatable* (and preventable) etiologies are of greater clinical and public health importance, particularly if they are also common, such as low bone density.

CLINICAL IMPLICATIONS

Ultimately, knowledge gained from epidemiologic studies should influence public health practice and clinical management of individual patients. These two applications are different, and are sometimes confused, perhaps because the correct interpretation and application of epidemiologic findings to clinical practice is not always intuitively apparent. For example, estrogen deficiency following menopause is a consistently demonstrated risk factor in population studies. However, there are many women who do not show significant bone loss in the years soon after menopause, and there are a minority, perhaps 25% to 30% of women, who never experience a fracture in their lifetime. These women generally have high bone density prior to the age of menopause and/or show less bone loss after menopause. For these women, estrogen deficiency is not a major risk factor and providing estrogen replacement to these women provides no demonstrable skeletal benefit. Thus, risk factors that apply to population groups may not necessarily apply to every (or any) individual. For example, black males have an increased risk of hypertension; however, it would not be considered prudent to treat all black men for hypertension in the absence of an objective indicator of disease.

THE MEANING OF A FRACTURE

Aside from the clinical and socioeconomic consequences of a fracture, there is another, crucial implication of a fragility fracture in an individual patient. The very presence of a fracture is a potent risk factor for future fractures, independent of bone density (13,14). Although the explanation for this finding is uncertain, in the spine it may be partially explained by altered load distribution on neighboring vertebral bodies. This would also help explain why vertebral fractures tend to cluster in the midthoracic and lower thoracic/upper lumbar spine.

However, one important implication is that the clinical goal of fracture risk management should be prevention of the first fracture. Because chronologically hip fractures are usually the last fracture to occur, more emphasis should be placed on early identification of women at high fracture risk and preventive measures initiated well prior to *any* fracture.

CUMULATIVE FRACTURE RISK

The concept of lifetime fracture risk has typically been applied to populations. Thus an average 50-year-old white woman has an approximate 17% lifetime risk of hip fracture (15). However, depending on levels of bone density and other risk factors, this figure will vary substantially between individuals.

The term "remaining lifetime fracture probability" (RLFP) has been used to describe an individual's fracture risk. RLFP is calculated from age, bone density, life expectancy, and anticipated future bone loss (16). The concept of cumulative fracture risk is important when deciding whether to employ pharmacologic agents to prevent future fractures. For such clinical decisions, measures of bone density alone are insufficient; current age must also be considered. The reason is that a woman whose bone density value is –1 SD (T score –1.0 and therefore osteopenic) at age 80 may not benefit from drug treatment because of her limited life expectancy and future bone loss. However, a 50-year-old with a similar, but normal, bone density, say –0.9 SD (T score –0.9), may gain a substantial benefit from drug intervention.

For this reason, the concept of RLFP may be a useful means of incorporating multiple risk factors into a single index of risk severity, which can better guide clinical decision making.

REFERENCES

1. Consensus development conference V, 1993. Diagnosis, prophylaxis, and treatment of osteoporosis. *Am J Med* 646–650, 1994
2. Melton, LJ III. Epidemiology of vertebral fractures in women. *Am J Epidemiol* 129:1000–1011, 1989
3. Jensen GF, Christiansen C, Boesen J, Hegedus V, Transbol I. Epidemiology of postmenopausal spinal and long bone fractures. *Clin Orthop* 166:75–81, 1982
4. Cooper C, O' Neill T, Silman A, on behalf of the European Vertebral Osteoporosis Study Group. *Bone* 14:589–597, 1993
5. Melton LJ, Riggs BL: Epidemiology of age-related fractures. In: Avioli LV (eds) *The Osteoporotic Syndrome: Detection, Prevention, and Treatment.* Grune and Stratton, New York, pp 45–72, 1983
6. Solomon L. Osteoporosis and fracture of the femoral neck in the South African Bantu. *J Bone Joint Surg* 50:B2–13, 1968
7. Ross PD, Norimatsu H, Davis JW, et al: A comparison of hip fracture incidence among native Japanese, Japanese-Americans, and American-Caucasians. *Am J Epidemiol* 133:801–809, 1991
8. Wasnich R. Bone mass measurement: prediction of risk. *Am J Med* 95:65–105, 1993
9. Kanis JA, Melton LJ III, Christiansen C, Johnston CC, Khaltaev N. The diagnosis of Osteoporosis. *J Bone Min Res* 9:1137–1141, 1994
10. Melton LJ III. How many women have osteoporosis now? *J Bone Miner Res* 10:175–177, 1995
11. Cummings SR, Rubin SM, Black D. The future of hip fractures in the United States. *Clin Orthop* 252:163–166, 1990
12. Barrett-Connor E. The economics and human costs of osteoporotic fracture. *Am J Med* 98:3–8, 1995
13. Ross PD, Davis JW, Epstein R, Wasnich RD. Pre-existing fractures and bone mass predict vertebral fracture incidence in women. *Ann Intern Med* 114:919–923, 1991
14. Wasnich RD, Davis JW, Ross PD. Spine fracture risk is predicted by non-spine fractures. *Ost Int* 4:1–5, 1995
15. Black D, Cummings S, Melton LJ. Appendicular bone mineral and a woman's lifetime risk of hip fracture. *J Bone Min Res* 7:639–646, 1992
16. Wasnich RD, Ross PD, Vogel JM, Davis JW. *Osteoporosis. Critique and Practicum.* Banyan Press, Honolulu, 1989

45. Pathogenesis of Postmenopausal Osteoporosis

Robert P. Heaney, M.D., F.A.C.P., F.A.I.N.

Creighton University, Omaha, Nebraska

Osteoporosis is defined elsewhere in this volume as a condition of skeletal fragility characterized by reduced bone mass and microarchitectural deterioration of bone tissue, with a consequent increase in risk of fracture. Decreased bone mass is thus visualized as a risk factor for fracture. The term osteoporosis is also used to designate a bone mass value more than 2.5 standard deviations below the young adult mean. Osteoporosis thus designates both one of the risk factors for fragility and the fragility condition itself. It is in this way analogous to hypertension, in which the term designates both the blood pressure level and the condition of increased risk of untoward vascular events.

It is useful to see both sides of this ambivalent definition because ultimately pathogenesis of osteoporosis involves the development not just of low bone mass but of the other causes of bony fragility as well. The interplay of the multiplicity of causal factors is illustrated well in Fig. 1, which sets forth age-specific fracture risk gradients for various values of forearm bone mass density (BMD). Three features stand out: (i) risk rises with declining bone mass; (ii) risk also rises with age, even when bone mass is held constant; and (iii) the gradients are steeper with advancing age, i.e., a given deficiency of bone makes a bigger difference in an older person than in a younger one. As Fig. 1 suggests, the age effect is, if anything, larger than the bone mass effect.

What does it mean to say that age increases fracture risk? This effect is a composite of other changes that accumulate with age: falling more often, falling in such a way as to strike vulnerable bony parts, loss of soft tissue protection over bony prominences, accumulation of unremodeled fatigue damage in the bony tissue, loss of critical trabecular connectivity, and possibly other factors. The pathogenesis

of falls is neurologic and pharmacotherapeutic, and is beyond the scope of this chapter. Similarly, the loss of soft tissue mass with advancing age is a nutritional problem and is covered in the chapter devoted to that topic. That leaves three contributors to osseous fragility: decreased bone mass, accumulated fatigue damage, and loss of trabecular connectivity. We will examine first how each makes bone fragile and then in turn will touch on what is known of the pathogenesis of each of these fragility components.

Before doing so it is necessary to mention yet another pathogenetic factor, i.e., bone geometry, which also has a major effect on fracture risk. One example is hip axis length, the distance from the lateral surface of the trochanter to the inner surface of the pelvis, along the axis of the femoral neck. Short hip axis length results in an architecturally stronger structure for any given bone density (2). This is probably the reason why Japanese and other Orientals have about half the hip fracture rate of Caucasians, despite similar bone density values. Likewise, large vertebral body endplate areas result in lower spine pressure values for individuals of the same body size. Those with small vertebral bodies are thus more likely to fracture. Finally, the force sustained by a bone when struck in falling is a function of body height. Other things being equal, a tall person striking the lateral surface of the hip in falling is more likely to sustain a fracture than a short person. Such geometric factors both contribute to individual fracture risk and explain a substantial portion of the population-level variance in fracture rate. In each situation, however, the ultimate pathogenesis of the fracture is the fall and the force sustained by the bone on impact.

DECREASED BONE MASS

For a given material density and bony architecture, bone strength rises as approximately the square of structural density. Thus, any factor decreasing bone mass will of necessity weaken bone: a 30% reduction, such as is common in osteoporosis, will decrease strength by about 50%. Bone mass and density are the most obvious of the bone strength factors, and certainly the best studied. It is often said that mass is the most important factor as well, but this is probably not correct. Simulations suggest that mass explains less than half of the observed fracture risk (3), and clinical studies have demonstrated that expressed fragility (e.g., in the form of a prior vertebral fracture) is a stronger predictor of future fracture than low bone mass by itself (4). The reasons for this non-mass-related fragility will be discussed later.

Low bone mass (or density) is plainly a multifactorial condition involving (i) genetic predisposition, (ii) failure to achieve genetic potential during growth, (iii) excessive leanness, (iv) disuse, (v) gonadal hormone deficiency, (vi) inadequate calcium and vitamin D intake, (vii) lifestyle and

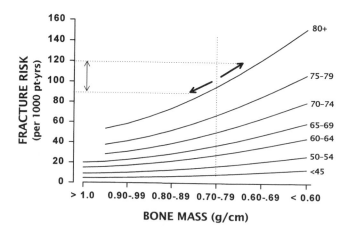

FIG. 1. Age-specific fracture risk gradients for forearm bone mineral density, redrawn from Hui et al. (1). Note that bone density declines to the right. (Copyright Robert P. Heaney, 1995. Reproduced with permission.)

medical factors (e.g., smoking, alcohol abuse, corticosteroids), (viii) remodeling errors, and (ix) miscellaneous factors. Several of these contributing causes are themselves related. For example, excessive leanness is frequently associated with both ovarian dysfunction and low calcium intake. Nevertheless, each appears to make a contribution in its own right. Most are covered in greater detail in other chapters.

Here it is necessary principally to recall that bone tissue is continually renewing itself, which means not just replacing tissue but seeking always to restore optimal mass density. This process is controlled by a classical negative feedback loop in which some cellular apparatus, most likely resident in the osteocytes, senses the degree of bending under routine loading of a part (typically on the order of 0.1% to 0.15% in any given dimension) and adjusts the local balance between bone formation and bone resorption so as to increase or decrease local bone stiffness and achieve that reference level of bending.

Failure to reach the genetic potential for bone density is most often a result of inadequate exercise and insufficient calcium intake (alone or in combination). In other words, suboptimal loading results in suboptimal stimulation of bone deposition. The result is that bone mass falls short of the genetic limit. Low calcium intake operates in a similar way: it limits how much bone density can be achieved within the envelope produced by growth and exercise (Chapter 48).

Weight is the single largest determinant of density in mature adults, explaining roughly half the population-level variance. It is not known how it operates. Almost certainly the effect involves more than just increased mechanical loading from carrying around the extra poundage, because lean mass is better correlated with bone density than is either fat mass or total body weight. The bone of heavy individuals behaves as if it had a lower setpoint for the reference level of bending under load. As a partial consequence of the increased bone density, fracture risk in obese women is about one third that of normal weight women.

By contrast, gonadal hormone loss, such as occurs in women at menopause, with anorexia nervosa or athletic amenorrhea, and gradually in aging men, appears to raise the setpoint of the bone mass regulatory system. After hormone loss, bone mass is sensed as being excessive. The relatively sharp drop across menopause is sufficient to result in remodeling carrying away about 15% of the bone over a period of 5+ years. (The quantity varies from region to region; 15% is what is typically found for the spine.) This loss is not specifically related to exercise or diet and would stop at the 15% quantum if diet and exercise were adequate. However, calcium requirement rises with age, food intake falls, and exercise usually decreases as well. As a result, bone loss typically continues and even accelerates with advancing age.

Smoking and alcohol abuse affect bone in uncertain ways. Alcohol is directly toxic to osteoblasts and is often associated with decreased calcium and vitamin D intakes and with excessive urinary loss of calcium. Calcium and vitamin D are covered in Chapter 48.

Remodeling errors are of two main types. First is excavation of overlarge haversian spaces in cortical bone. Radial

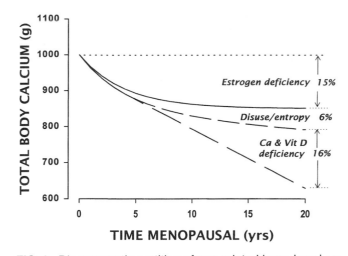

FIG. 2. Diagrammatic partition of age-related bone loss in a typical postmenopausal woman. The estrogen deficiency loss assumes no postmenopausal hormone replacement. The magnitude of the calcium deficiency loss is typical; it may be nonexistent in some individuals or substantially greater than shown in others. (Copyright Robert P. Heaney, 1991. Reproduced with permission.)

infilling is regulated by signals from the outermost osteocytes and is generally no more than 90 µM. Hence, large external diameters, which may simply occur randomly, lead to large central haversian canals, which then accumulate with age, leading to increased cortical porosity. In a similar way, osteoclast penetration of trabecular plates, or severing of trabecular beams, removes the scaffolding needed for osteoblastic replacement of resorbed bone. In both ways random remodeling errors (in addition to the other factors cited) tend to reduce both cancellous and cortical bone density and structural integrity. These remodeling errors represent a kind of entropy.

An illustrative partition of postmenopausal loss is set forth in Fig. 2, which superimposes entropic and nutritional losses on estrogen deficiency loss. The estrogen- and calcium-related losses are preventable. The entropic loss is not. Note that in the early menopausal years estrogen deficiency dominates. Note also that later, if calcium and vitamin D intakes are not adequate, nutritional loss can account, in the last analysis, for more bone loss than did menopausal estrogen loss.

BONE QUALITY AND ARCHITECTURE

We noted above that the strength of a bony structure rises roughly as the square of density, assuming constant intrinsic strength of the bony material. Here is where fatigue damage, trabecular connectedness, and other architectural factors enter into consideration. Fatigue damage weakens the material, changing its intrinsic strength, and trabecular disconnection weakens the structure. Both cause local volumes of bone to deform more under loading, thereby producing a signal greater than the reference level of bending.

Fatigue damage consists of ultramicroscopic rents in the basic bony material, resulting from the inevitable bending that occurs when a structural member is loaded. Fatigue damage is the principal cause of failure in mechanical engineering structures, and designers usually compensate by increasing the massiveness of a structure so that it bends little and thus has a larger margin of safety. Bones, by contrast, are designed to bend more and therefore have a relatively narrow margin of safety (about 2 times over peak physiologic loads). They solve the fatigue damage problem by the remodeling apparatus, which detects and removes fatigue-damaged bone. Fractures related to fatigue damage occur whenever the damage occurs faster than remodeling can repair it or whenever the remodeling apparatus is defective. March fractures and the fractures of radiation necrosis are well-recognized examples of fractures due to these two mechanisms. Fatigue damage definitely occurs in normal bone, under ordinary usage, though it is less certain as to precisely what role it may play in predisposing to osteoporotic fracture. It would, on the other hand, be surprising if bone were the only structural material known in which fatigue damage was not an important factor in failure. Furthermore, there is suggestive evidence for certain fractures (notably hip) that remodeling repair may be defective specifically at the site that ultimately fractures (5). Why remodeling surveillance or effectiveness might fail locally is not known. Nevertheless, it is clear that such failure would lead to accumulation of fatigue damage and, therefore, to local weakening of bone.

Bone structures loaded vertically, such as the vertebral bodies and femoral and tibial metaphyses, derive a substantial portion of their structural strength from a system of horizontal, cross-bracing trabeculae, which support the vertical elements and limit lateral bowing and consequent snapping under vertical loading. Severance of such trabecular connections is known to occur preferentially in postmenopausal women (6) and is considered to be a major reason for the large female/male preponderance of vertebral osteoporosis. That long, unsupported vertical trabeculae are susceptible to

fracture is reflected in the extraordinarily high prevalence of trabecular fracture callus sites in vertebral bodies examined at autopsy—typically 200–450 healing or healed fractures per vertebral body. While many of these will be well-enough healed at any given time to be structurally competent, others will be fresh and structurally weak. Such fractures are asymptomatic and their accumulation both reflects the impact of lost trabecular connections and greatly weakens the cancellous structure of the vertebral body. The incident fracture prediction ability of prior vertebral fractures (4) is probably due in part to the presence of such otherwise undetected trabecular defects. That is why prior fracture seems to predict future fracture even when bone density is relatively high. The reason for preferential osteoclastic severance of horizontal trabeculae is not known. It is sometimes attributed to overaggressive osteoclastic resorption, but that seems more descriptive than explanatory.

REFERENCES

1. Hui SL, Slemenda CW, Johnston CC Jr. Age and bone mass as predictors of fracture in a prospective study. *J Clin Invest* 81: 1804–1809, 1988
2. Faulkner KG, Cummings SR, Black D, Palermo L, Glüer C-C, Genant HK. Simple measurement of femoral geometry predicts hip fracture: the study of osteoporotic fractures. *J Bone Min Res* 8:1211–1217, 1993
3. Heaney RP. Is there a role for bone quality in fragility fractures? *Calcif Tissue Int* 53:S3–S5, 1993
4. Ross PD, Davis JW, Epstein RS, Wasnich RD. Pre-existing fractures and bone mass predict vertebral fracture incidence in women. *Ann Intern Med* 114:919–923, 1991
5. Eventov I, Frisch B, Cohen Z, Hammel I. Osteopenia, hematopoiesis and osseous remodeling in iliac crest and femoral neck biopsies: a prospective study of 102 cases of femoral neck fractures. *Bone* 12:1–6, 1991
6. Kleerekoper M, Villanueva AR, Stanciu J, Sudhaker R, Parfitt AM. The role of three-dimensional trabecular microstructure in the pathogenesis of vertebral compression fractures. *Calcif Tissue Int* 37:594–597, 1985

46. Physical Activity and Regulation of Bone Mass

Robert Marcus, M.D.

Department of Medicine, Stanford University, and Veterans Affairs Medical Center, Palo Alto, California

The primary function of bone is to provide a strong and resilient structure that permits resistance against gravitational and other forces while providing structural rigidity for locomotion. To accommodate both requirements, bone adapts to the mechanical demands that are placed on it. This principle, known as Wolff's law, may be paraphrased to state that bone accommodates the loads imposed on it by altering its mass and distribution of mass. When habitual loading increases, bone is gained; when loading decreases, bone is lost. What appears to be optimized by this adaptive response is the distribution of load-related strain, or deformation, within bones. As an example of how effective and broadly applicable this process is, it is remarkable that

when animals with diverse loading patterns engage in typical activities (running, jumping, and so forth), peak long bone strains consistently fall within a fairly narrow range of 2000–3500 microstrain (1 strain = 1% deformation; 3000 microstrain = 0.12% deformation) (1).

Habitual loading can be described as the sum of all individual daily loading events, with each event further characterized by its intensity and number of repetitions. Load magnitude seems to outweigh load repetitions as an influence on bone mass (2). The relationship between mechanical loading and bone mass is curvilinear, with a much steeper slope at very low levels of loading. Thus, the most easily demonstrable interaction between physical activity and bone mass is the substantial *loss* of bone that occurs with immobilizaton. Completely immobilized patients may lose 40% of their original bone mass in 1 year, whereas standing upright with postural shifting for 30 minutes each day may completely prevent the deleterious skeletal effects of bed rest. By contrast, the amount of bone that can be gained by active people who increase their level of exercise is very limited, accounting for only a few percent increase over a year's time.

BONE MASS IN ATHLETES

Trained athletes have higher bone mass than nonathletes (3), with the largest effect seen when the regimen includes strength training (4). Much of this literature may be confounded by the possibility that the musculoskeletal characteristics of athletes may differ from those of the general population even prior to training. This may explain why the results of exercise intervention studies have been relatively meager compared to differences reported in comparative studies. That there is certainly some skeletal effect of training emerges from the exaggerated increases in bone mineral density (BMD) that are observed in the racquet vs. the nonracquet forearms of elite tennis players (5).

PHYSICAL ACTIVITY AND BONE MASS IN NONATHLETES

A critical issue is whether the skeletal benefits enjoyed by elite athletes also extend to ordinary mortals. Bone *acquisition* by children (6), adolescents (7), and young women (8) seems clearly to reflect habitual physical activity. In contrast, a few (9,10), but certainly not all (11,12), cross-sectional studies in adults have shown a positive relationship of BMD to current or previous self-reported levels of physical activity. The validity of such studies is severely constrained by major difficulties in assessing a person's true physical activity level but is hampered even more when attempting to extrapolate rough indices of overall physical exertion to estimate skeletal loading. It may be that some of the most important daily loading events for the skeleton are not even recognized by a person who maintains an exercise record. This would be particularly true for such activities as pushing against a heavy door, lifting a box of canned goods, or some other occupational activity.

RESPONSE OF BONE TO EXERCISE

With one notable exception (13), well-controlled randomized exercise trials using strength (14–17) and endurance (15,16) activities have reported significant but modest positive effects of exercise on lumbar spine BMD of young women. Increases averaged 1% to 3% and were achieved during the first year, with few if any gains thereafter (16,17). Improvement in hip BMD was found in only one study, which continued for 2 years (17). Another study showed that strength training maintains lumbar spine BMD of recently menopausal women, but no such protection was found at other skeletal sites (18).

In older individuals, walking exercise has been correlated to BMD, but intervention studies have not found brisk walking either to increase BMD or to protect against loss (19). Some, but not all, intervention trials using resistance or mixed endurance/resistance exercise have shown significant gains in bone mass in older men and women (20–23). One intriguing report described an 8% gain in spine BMD for older women who participated in resistance exercise for 1 year and who were also taking estrogen replacement therapy (23). Other studies of older people, while not reporting significant *gains* in bone mass, do indicate that exercise may constrain the rate of bone *loss* (24).

SPECIAL ASPECTS OF EXERCISE AND BONE: AMENORRHEA, GYMNASTS, AND SWIMMERS

Optimal skeletal maintenance requires an adequate hormonal, mechanical, and nutritional milieu. Deficits in one sphere are not adequately compensated by overzealous attention to the others. Amenorrheic women athletes lose bone and have increased risk for fracture despite herculean training schedules (25,26). Despite initial views that cortical bone is spared in these women, recent data show significant deficits at all appendicular sites except the radius (27).

Competitive women gymnasts have a high prevalence of oligo- and amenorrhea. It would be expected that they would also suffer deficits in BMD. However, these athletes actually show higher than predicted BMD at all sites (28). One aspect of gymnastics training may explain this finding: whereas runners load their lumbar vertebrae with 3–5 body weights with each step, dismounting from parallel bars or other high-impact gymnastics activities gives vertebral loading of 15–20 body weights. Thus, the experience in gymnasts may provide insight to the type of mechanical loads that are most osteotrophic. By contrast, even though collegiate swimmers also participate in muscle strength training, they have lower bone mass than do other athletes or even sedentary individuals of similar age (29). This may be explained by the fact that elite swimmers spend ~25 buoyant hours per week, time taken from their possible weight bearing activity.

CONTRIBUTION OF EXERCISE TO BONE HEALTH OF OLDER PEOPLE

The modest BMD results with strength training should not trivialize the importance of exercise for protecting older people against falls. More than 90% of hip fractures follow as the immediate consequence of a fall onto the hip. Among the important risk factors for falls, muscle strength is perhaps most susceptible to improvement with strength training (30). Many older patients and their physicians ask about which exercise is best for the skeleton. One must realize that only one of five adult Americans exercises as little as once each week and that the 6-month attrition rate for people who start exercising is >50%. Thus, it serves no purpose to recommend a rigorous program to most people. Most important is to stimulate them to participate safely in any activity in a frequent, regular, and sustained manner. Therefore, for sedentary and/or frail elderly, a program of walking, low-impact or water aerobics, or other pleasant, nonthreatening, and safe activity is recommended. If after several months the patient wishes to do more rigorous activity, a referral to a physical therapy department for initiation of muscle strength exercise is warranted.

REFERENCES

1. Rubin CT, Lanyon LE: Dynamic strain similarity in vertebrates: an alternative to allometric limb bone scaling. *J Theoret Biol* 107: 321–327, 1984
2. Whalen RT, Carter DR, Steele CR: The relationship between physical activity and bone density. *Trans Orthop Res Soc 33rd Mtg* 12:464–470, 1987
3. Snow-Harter C, Marcus R: Exercise, bone mineral density, and osteoporosis. *Exercise Sport Sci Rev* 19:351–388, 1991
4. Block JE, Genant HK, Black D: Greater vertebral bone mineral mass in exercising young men. *West J Med* 145:39–42, 1992
5. Huddleston AL, Rockwell D, Kulund DN, et al: Bone mass in lifetime tennis players. *JAMA* 244:1107–1109, 1980
6. Slemenda CW, Miller JZ, Hui SL, Reister TK, Johnston CC Jr: Role of physical activity in the development of skeletal mass in children. *J Bone Min Res* 6:1227–1233, 1991
7. Ruiz JC, Mandel C, Garabedian M: Influence of spontaneous calcium intake and physical exercise on the vertebral and femoral bone mineral density of children and adolescents. *J Bone Min Res* 10:675–682, 1995
8. Recker RR, Davies KM, Hinders SM, Heaney RP, Stegman MR, Kimmel DB: Bone gain in young adult women. *JAMA* 268: 2403–2408, 1992
9. Aloia JF, Vaswani AN, Yeh JK, Cohn SH: Premenopausal bone mass is related to physical activity. *Arch Intern Med* 148:121–123, 1988
10. Snow-Harter C, Whalen R, Myburgh K, Arnaud S, Marcus R: Bone mineral density, muscle strength, and recreational exercise in men. *J Bone Min Res* 7:1291–1296, 1992
11. Sowers MR, Wallace RB, Lemke JH: Correlates of mid-radius bone density among postmenopausal women: a community study. *Am J Clin Nutr* 41:1045–1053, 1985
12. Mazess RB, Bardin HS: Bone density in premenopausal women: effects of age, dietary intake, physical activity, smoking, and birth-control pills. *Am J Clin Nutr* 53:132–142, 1991
13. Rockwell J, Sorensen A, Baker S, Leahey D, Stock J, Michaels J, Baran D: Weight training decreases vertebral bone density in premenopausal women: a prospective study. *J Clin Endocrinol Metab* 71:988–993, 1990
14. Gleeson PB, Protas EJ, LeBlanc AD, Schneider VS, Evans HJ: Effects of weight lifting on bone mineral density in premenopausal women. *J Bone Min Res* 5:153–158, 1990
15. Snow-Harter C, Bouxsein ML, Lewis BT, Carter DR, Marcus R: Effects of resistance and endurance exercise on bone mineral status of young women:a randomized exercise intervention trial. *J Bone Min Res* 7:761–769, 1992
16. Friedlander AL, Genant HK, Sadowsky S, Byl NN, Glüer C-C: A two year program of aerobics and weight training enhances bone mineral density of young women. *J Bone Min Res* 10:574–585, 1995
17. Lohman T, Going S, Pamenter R, et al: Effects of resistance training on regional and total bone mineral density in premenopausal women: a randomized prospective study. *J Bone Min Res* 10: 1015–1024, 1995
18. Pruitt LA, Jackson RD, Bartels RL, Lehnhard HJ: Weight-training effects on bone mineral density in early postmenopausal women. *J Bone Min Res* 7:179–185, 1992
19. Cavanaugh DJ, Cann CE: Brisk walking does not stop bone loss in postmenopausal women. *Bone* 9:201–204, 1988
20. Simkin A, Ayalon J, Leichter I: Increased trabecular bone density due to bone-loading exercises on postmenopausal osteoporotic women. *Calcif Tiss Int* 40:59–63, 1987
21. Dalsky G, Stocke KS, Eshani AA, et al: Weight-bearing exercise training and lumbar bone mineral content in postmenopausal women. *Ann Intern Med* 108:824–828, 1988
22. Menkes A, Mazel S, Redmond RA et al: Strength training increases regional bone mineral density and bone remodeling in middle-aged and older men. *J Appl Physiol* 74:2478–2484, 1993
23. Notelovitz M, Martin D, Tesar R, et al: Estrogen therapy and variable-resistance weight training increase bone mineral in surgically menopausal women. *J Bone Min Res* 6:583–590, 1991
24. Prince RL, Devine A, Dick I, et al: The effects of calcium supplementation (milk powder or tablets) and exercise on bone density in postmenopausal women. *J Bone Min Res* 10:1068–1075, 1995
25. Drinkwater BL, Nilson K, Chesnut CH III, Bremner WJ, Shainholtz, Southworth MB: Bone mineral content of amenorrheic and eumenorrheic athletes. *N Engl J Med* 311:277–281, 1984
26. Marcus R, Cann C, Madvig P, et al: Menstrual function and bone mass in elite women distance runners. Endocrine and metabolic features. *Ann Intern Med* 102:158–163, 1985
27. Myburgh KH, Bachrach LK, Lewis B, Kent K, Marcus R: Low bone mineral density at axial and appendicular sites in amenorrheic athletes. *Med Sci Sports Exerc* 25:1197–1202, 1993
28. Robinson TL, Snow-Harter C, Taaffe DR, Gillis D, Shaw J, Marcus R: Gymnasts exhibit higher bone mass than runners despite similar prevalence of amenorrhea. *J Bone Min Res* 10:26–35, 1995
29. Taaffe DR, Snow-Harter C, Connolly DA, Robinson TL, Brown MD, Marcus R: Differential effects of swimming versus weight-bearing activity on bone mineral status of eumenorrheic athletes. *J Bone Miner Res* 10:586–593, 1995
30. Cummings SR, Nevitt MC, Browner WS, et al: Risk factors for hip fracture in white women. *N Engl J Med* 332:767–773, 1995

47. Prevention of Osteoporosis

Robert Lindsay, Ph.D., M.B., Ch.B., F.R.C.P.

Department of Clinical Medicine, Columbia University, New York, New York; and Department of Medicine, Helen Hayes Hospital, West Haverstraw, New York

An ounce of prevention is worth more than any amount of treatment.

The definition of osteoporosis developed for the World Health Organization (WHO) is an operational one based on bone mass measurement. This definition is clearly stated to provide a diagnostic label and not necessarily provide an indication of the need for intervention. For the purposes of this chapter, "prevention" means intervention to prevent declining bone mass, irrespective of whether the patient can be classified as having osteoporosis by the WHO definition (below 2.5 standard deviation (SD) from the mean for young normal individuals). The assumption is that prevention of bone loss will reduce fracture risk the only benefit of intervention that is important to the patient. Strategies to prevent fracture in someone who already has osteoporotic fractures or to rebuild the skeleton are beyond the scope and dealt with as treatment.

The phenomenon of bone loss that precedes fractures in osteoporosis is associated in cancellous bone with disruption of the microarchitecture that includes complete loss of trabecular elements, a process that is considered mostly irreversible. It is clear, therefore, that the most efficient method of tackling these skeletal changes is by prevention. Both public health strategies and those that must be undertaken on an individual basis are important, with safety, at least as much as efficacy and low cost, determining those that might be instituted as public health priorities. Since, almost by definition, those individuals to be targeted for prevention are asymptomatic, the first priority is the identification of those at risk. Thus, the approach to osteoporosis is similar to that for hypertension or hypercholesterolemia.

IDENTIFICATION OF "AT-RISK" INDIVIDUALS

As in many other disorders of aging a large number of factors (Table 1) have been incriminated in the pathogenesis of fractures among the elderly (1). Some clearly change the onset, duration, or rate of bone loss in individuals, whereas others increase fracture risk by modifying the risk of injury. Yet others may be linked by association that is statistically significant without any demonstrable cause-and-effect relationship. A rough clinical evaluation of risk can be obtained by assessment of comparatively few such factors. The general factors include being female, Caucasian or Asian, and becoming postmenopausal (with surgical or early natural menopause probably conferring greater risk). For those fulfilling these criteria, a personal history of fracture after age 50 or a history of hip, wrist, or vertebral fracture in a first-degree relative, low-body-weight, and cigarette consumption adds to the risk (with each conferring additional risk). These features can easily be obtained by history and simple physical.

Superimposed on these are of course a wide variety of factors, including chronic illness, disuse, and drugs (steroids, diuretics, thyroid hormone, gonadotropin-releasing hormone

TABLE 1. *Proposed risk factors for osteoporosis*

Genetic
  Race
  Sex
  Familial prevalence
Nutritional
  Low calcium intake
  High alcohol
  High caffeine
  High sodium
  High animal protein
Lifestyle
  Cigarette use
  Low physical activity
Endocrine
  Menopausal age (oophorectomy)
  Obesity

agonists, Dilantin, tetracyclines, aluminum, and methotrexate).

In general, for each patient, the more risk factors present (1) and the longer the duration of their presence, the greater the risk of future problems (1,2). For example, a 55-year-old woman (postmenopausal) who has a family history, a prior fracture, is thin, and smokes has a relative risk of further fracture that is about 16 times the average for 55-year-old postmenopausal women. Physicians can use the presence of these factors in two ways. First, they can be used to sensitize the patient and the physician to the likelihood of osteoporosis and to target these individuals for further investigation and/or treatment. Second, those risk factors that are amenable to elimination or alteration should be discussed with the patient. Many risk factors (e.g., smoking, alcohol excess, physical inactivity) also contribute to development of diseases in organ systems other than bone and should be discussed in those terms.

Practically, menopause is the most common time when evaluation of the patient for osteoporosis begins, although nutritional and lifestyle habits should be changed as early in life as possible. No combination of these risk factors can indicate skeletal status for the individual patient, although they can be used to determine fracture risk. The analogy is hypertension for which there is also a list of risk factors, but no assemblage of these predicts an individual patient's blood pressure (although they may be predictive of risk of stroke). Nevertheless, risk factor review is a useful "initial" approach to the patient.

Skeletal Status

The best-documented risk factor to date is skeletal status. While on a population basis both the starting bone mass and the subsequent rate of loss of bone tissue must contribute to risk of fracture, for any individual we usually use bone mass at the time of consultation as the principal determinant of fracture risk. Fracture prevalence and incidence have been shown to be greater in those with low bone mass at any age and several studies indicate that low bone mass is predictive of an increased fracture risk (3,4). This suggests that a single measurement of bone mass will provide information that can be used clinically to determine risk of osteoporosis. Because hip measurements provide the best estimate of the most important osteoporotic fractures (hip and spine), this site is preferred if available. When required clinically, however, most would agree that any measurement is better than none. For a complete review of the techniques available for bone mass measurement, the reader is referred to Chapter 23. The clinician should learn the use of the techniques available in his or her area. The analogies in clinical practice are the measurement of blood pressure as a risk assessment for cerebrovascular accident, cholesterol, or lipoprotein fractionation as risk factors for coronary heart disease.

There is no absolute value of bone mass that indicates a need for treatment. Rather such information should be added to the entire clinical profile of any individual to establish the requirement to intervene. The presence of one or more risk factors would, for example, influence the decision to treat, as would the benefits, risks, and cost of intervention.

CLINICAL PROTOCOL

Prevention of bone loss in asymptomatic women is generally achieved using two complementary approaches: behavior modification (public health approach) and pharmacologic intervention. Again, this is similar to the management of hypertension and hypercholesterolemia.

The initial approach to the patient is based on modification of the risk factor profile. Elimination of secondary causes of osteoporosis is a mandatory part of this initial evaluation (Chapters 52, 54, 55, and 57). For prevention of primary (postmenopausal) osteoporosis, alterations in nutrition and lifestyle form the preliminary approach, on the assumption that a reduction in risk factor profile will be beneficial. Reductions in alcohol consumption and elimination of cigarette use are amenable to intervention and these measures are particularly beneficial to the patient's general health.

Calcium Supplementation

Although calcium is a nutrient and adequate intake should be obtained from nutritional sources (5), in practice it is difficult for many people to achieve a dietary intake >800 mg/day (the current recommended daily allowance). Self-imposed calorie restrictions and the avoidance of cholesterol results in limitation of dairy produce, the major source of dietary calcium in the Western world. Other sources of calcium include green vegetables, nuts, and certain fish. Bioavailability of calcium from foods is ~30%, with only calcium in spinach being unavailable for absorption.

In providing advice about calcium intake the intent is to ensure that the majority of the population obtain sufficient calcium to maintain calcium balance. Recommendations include an intake of 800 mg until age 10; 1200 mg during adolescence; and 1000 mg thereafter, increasing to 1200 mg during pregnancy and lactation, and 1500 mg if at increased risk of osteoporosis or if over age 65 (6). To achieve such intakes, it is commonly necessary to resort to calcium supplementation. Most individuals require only 500–1000 mg/day as a supplement to dietary sources to realize these intakes.

There are many forms of calcium available as supplement, and the advice to the patient should be as simple as possible. First, it is important that the calcium be bioavailable. Some studies suggest that name brands are in general more soluble than generic varieties, although most of the latter are clearly adequate. Because calcium absorption is better in an acid environment for the carbonate, we recommend that the supplement be taken with food (for carbonate), although there is a school of thought that argues for the supplement to be taken at night to reduce the proposed nocturnal surge in bone resorption. The addition of a modest calcium supplement to each meal is a regimen to which the patient can easily adhere. Both calcium carbonate and citrate offer the highest calcium content per unit tablet weight (40% and 30%, respectively). Absorption of calcium as the citrate is slightly more efficient and not dependent on gastric acidity. However, this may not be biologically important for most patients, and citrate is generally more expensive.

At the recommended dietary intakes, calcium supplementation is virtually free of side effects. If eructation, intestinal colic, and constipation occur with the carbonate, then citrate is a useful alternative. Care should be taken in prescribing calcium supplements to patients with a history of renal stones. If urine calcium excretion is not increased, the citrate salt may be used.

Several clinical trials have demonstrated the effect of calcium supplementation on bone mass. In general, the results confirm a weak "antiresorptive" effect with some prevention of loss. The effects are most obvious in the elderly but can be seen in some premenopausal populations. The effect is more modest in the years immediately following menopause, when estrogen loss is driving bone loss. The consequences of an adequate calcium intake are reductions in the risk of fracture that are modest but consistent. The modest effectiveness, inexpensiveness, freedom from side effects, and prevalence of inadequate intake all argue for increased calcium intake as a public health measure.

Vitamin D

Some studies indicate a modest effect of supplemental vitamin D on bone mass in at-risk populations, such as the elderly, the institutionalized, and those with disorders likely to impair vitamin D supply or metabolism. Intakes of 400–800 U/day of vitamin D_3 are easy to obtain (many multivitamin preparations have 400 U of D) and are safe. High doses (>1000 U/day) are not recommended. The effect of vitamin D supplementation by itself on fracture frequency is not known, as it is usually supplied with calcium and combinations have been shown to reduce the risk of hip fracture. Vitamin D metabolites and analogs are currently not recommended for prevention of osteoporosis.

Physical Activity

It has long been assumed that adequate physical activity is associated with the prevention of osteoporotic fractures, but the evidence is sparse, largely because of the difficulty in conducting good-quality controlled trials in this area. There is no doubt that at the extremes of activity effects on bone and fracture are evident, but it is within the range of normal activity that the doubts persist. However, because physical activity is associated with a number of health benefits and well-being, it remains an important feature of osteoporosis prevention.

Changing the pattern of physical activity may be difficult, especially for patients who are less positively motivated. This is especially true when discussing prevention with patients, who are, by definition, asymptomatic. Most of the patients seen in our clinic are at a relatively low level of fitness and may require formal cardiovascular evaluation before beginning an exercise program. We suggest that the exercise activity chosen be fun to improve compliance. In the absence of proven benefit for any specific exercise for prevention of osteoporosis, any weight-bearing activity suffices (6). Recreational therapy, which has a social component, may serve to improve patient compliance. However, even simple activities such as walking are useful and can be added to the daily routine with minimal difficulty. Back-strengthening exercise is probably also of value, and patients may be referred to a trainer for specific instructions because there may be limitations of exercises that force spinal flexion. In addition to any potential beneficial effects on the skeleton, continued activity in patients' daily lives reduces the risk of falls, trauma from falls, and fracture.

Pharmacologic Therapy to Prevent Bone Loss

A considerable body of data supports the concept that estrogen administration to postmenopausal women reduces skeletal turnover and reduces the rate of bone loss (7). Epidemiologic data indicate that estrogen use is associated with a reduction in the risk of fracture, especially fractures of the hip and wrist (Colles' fracture). Risk reduction averaged over several studies appears to be on the order of 50%. For vertebral fractures the interpretation of the few prospective data available suggest that estrogens also reduce the risk of vertebral fracture by as much as 75%.

Several general guidelines can be given for the use of estrogen for this indication. Because estrogens primarily reduce the rate of bone loss, the earlier therapy is begun, the more likely the bone mass and structure will be preserved. However, recent data suggest that estrogen therapy reduces the rate of bone loss in estrogen-deficient women independent of age, with reduction in bone loss among older individuals, at least up to the eighth decade (8). The minimum effective dose of estrogen for most individuals is 0.625 mg conjugated equine estrogen or its equivalent (9). Efficacy has been demonstrated for several other estrogens, including estradiol and estrone sulfate. It is also apparent that the route of administration is not important, and several studies have demonstrated that transdermal estrogen is effective (10).

The effects of estrogen continue for as long as treatment is provided, whereas bone loss ensues when treatment is discontinued at a rate comparable to the rate of bone loss that occurs immediately after ovariectomy. Prospective controlled clinical trials have confirmed the long-term efficacy of estrogen for bone loss prevention for at least 10 years. It appears, however, that long-term administration—possibly lifelong—is required to reduce fracture risk, perhaps because of the bone loss that occurs when treatment is stopped (11).

Practical Aspects of Estrogen Administration

Although menopausal symptoms remain the most frequent indication for estrogen therapy, prevention of osteoporosis is becoming a more widely recognized indication for therapy for postmenopausal women. Treatment of menopause is accompanied by an excellent symptomatic response to therapy. For control of bone loss, however, the majority of patients are in the asymptomatic phase of bone loss. The physician always faces problems of acceptance and compliance in providing therapy for an asymptomatic phase of a disease whether it be hypertension, hypercholesterolemia, or osteoporosis. The epidemiologic data that indicate that estrogens may reduce the risk of ischemic heart disease add another benefit for estrogen use. The more recent suggestion

that estrogens improve cognitive function and reduce the risk of Alzheimer's disease among aging women is preliminary and requires more detailed study. The potential complications of endometrial and breast malignancies must also be discussed with each patient.

When the patient presents for an assessment of the risk of osteoporosis we begin with evaluation of the risk factors. The presence of enough risk factors may be sufficient to precipitate both patient and physician into treatment, especially above 60 years of age where there is more imminent risk of fracture. For most individuals, when therapy is being considered specifically for osteoporosis prevention a bone mass measurement should be performed. This allows determination of the future risk of fracture for the individual patient. The lower the bone mineral density, the greater the likelihood that therapy is required. The level of bone mass that requires intervention varies with age and the presence or absence of risk factors. Nomograms that allow treatment decisions based on age, Z or T scores, and risk factors are being developed at present. However, when bone mass falls into the diagnostic range for osteoporosis, after evaluation for secondary causes of bone loss, treatment with hormone replacement therapy should be considered. When bone mass is above this level, a wait-and-see approach can be proposed, especially for younger individuals with no risk factors. With increasing age and presence of risk factors a more aggressive approach can be recommended.

In our clinic we include a discussion about the other effects of estrogen. Estrogens, given unopposed by progestins, increase the risk of endometrial hyperplasia and carcinoma. There is more doubt about the effect of estrogen on breast cancer, but long-term therapy (>15 years) may increase the risk slightly (10% to 30%) (12). On the other hand, estrogens alleviate menopausal symptoms, improve urogenital atrophy, and appear to reduce the risk of ischemic heart disease by as much as 50% (13). In addition, they may reduce the risk of thrombotic stroke modestly, and more recently have been suggested to reduce the risk of Alzheimer's disease. Estrogens have been associated with improved overall mortality. Thus, the implications of estrogen use are considerably more complex than simply effects on the skeleton.

The specific protocol for estrogen use remains a subject of considerable discussion and controversy. Some general recommendations can be made. All patients should have a mammography and be taught breast self-examination before therapy is initiated. The schedule for mammography in this age range should be based on the National Cancer Institute's guidelines and be independent of the decision to treat, but treatment certainly mandates it. If the patient has gone through a natural menopause and still has her uterus, combination or sequential therapy with a progestin is used to protect the endometrium (14). There is no rationale at present for progestin in patients who have undergone hysterectomy. There is no evidence that addition of a progestin will negatively impact on the estrogen effect on the skeleton. One study using norethindrone acetate, a 19-nortestosterone derivative, suggested that there may be an additive effect when given along with estrogens (15). For younger women just after menopause, we favor a sequential regimen. Estrogen is given every day, with rest periods at the end of each month only for those who have significant mastalgia with therapy, whereas the progestin is given from the first of each calendar month for at least 12 days (2 weeks is often simpler). Most patients will have some endometrial shedding, which may be fairly light, between the 11th and 21st of each month (16). Recurrent bleeding not on that schedule requires investigation. The progestin dose should be the minimum required for endometrial protection. For medroxyprogesterone acetate, the most commonly used progestin in the United States, 5 mg/day is the minimum, but it must be increased to 10 mg if bleeding is out of schedule. Norethindrone is available in 5 mg tablets in the United States, but this is an excessive dose. If there are symptoms with medroxyprogesterone acetate, norethindrone [one-half tablet a day (2.5 mg)] may be tried, or two tablets a day of a progestin only oral contraceptive containing 0.35 mg norethindrone per tablet. The latter is an expensive regimen even when used for only 2 weeks each month. The estrogen dose required to reduce bone loss in most individuals is 0.625 mg conjugated equine estrogen or its equivalent (9). The 0.05-mg estradiol patch also appears sufficient (10). Because some patients will continue to lose bone on these doses (perhaps as much as 5% to 15%), measurement of bone mass after 1 year with the highly precise dual-energy x-ray absorptionmetry (DXA) technique may be advantageous. It is not clear if those individuals who lose bone on estrogen therapy are nonresponders or partial responders who will subsequently respond to an increase in the daily dose.

Older women and those who wish to avoid monthly vaginal bleeding may consider a combined continuous regimen. In this regimen the estrogen and progestin are both given each day of the month. The estrogen dose is similar to that recommended above, but the progestin dose may be reduced by half. This regimen is associated with some irregular, unheralded bleeding in the first 2–6 months of treatment in ~50% of patients, but close to 80% will become amenorrheic thereafter. Because the early bleeding is often light and may just be spotting, many patients will suffer this temporary inconvenience in return for the promise of no further bleeding. Long-term endometrial safety data using the combined regimen are sparse.

Side effects of therapy include occasional weight gain and, rarely, an idiosyncratic increase in blood pressure. Therefore, blood pressure should be measured in all patients after 3 months of therapy. Progestin side effects include irritability and mood swings, often described as being premenstrual, which may become sufficiently troublesome to require the progestin dose to be reduced to the minimum. Increased risks of deep vein thrombosis and gallstones are recorded as side effects but rarely seen. The relationship between estrogen use and breast cancer has been outlined above.

For prevention of osteoporosis, treatment should be continued for as long as feasible, at least 5–10 years, and possibly lifelong. As a practical issue we review each patient on at least an annual basis and evaluate with her the benefits and her concerns regarding treatment. Modifications can be made at this time. We now use repeat measurements of bone mass by DXA to monitor patients to ensure that bone loss is not progressing. This can also be used as an aid to compliance, which is notably poor with estrogens, primarily because of bleeding and the perceived risk of cancer. An alternative to bone mass measurement is to measure the biochemical indices of bone remodeling before and at some time, often 3 months, after the institution of treatment. Estrogens are associated with a reduction in alkaline phosphatase (especially the bone-specific isoenzyme), osteocalcin, and urinary hydroxyproline, deoxypyridinoline, and pyridinoline crosslinks (17). A biochemical response usually indicates a skeletal response but may not be absolutely predictive.

The high rate of poor compliance noted by some authors appears most often associated with failure to educate the patient adequately about the expected results of therapy and the potential problems. In practice, once patients are established on therapy for 6 months to 1 year, they usually are comfortable remaining on treatment for many years thereafter.

The main contraindication to estrogen therapy is the presence or history of an estrogen-dependent tumor, especially breast malignancy. Other relative contraindications include undiagnosed vaginal bleeding, a prior history of endometrial malignancy (3 years posthysterectomy), active thromboembolic disease, and grossly abnormal liver or renal function. Hypertension and diabetes are not contraindications but must be controlled before therapy is begun.

Alternatives to Estrogen

Calcitonin

Salmon calcitonin is a Food and Drug Administration (FDA)–approved alternative to estrogen for the treatment but not prevention of osteoporosis (17). Salmon calcitonin can be delivered by an intranasal spray, which obviates the problems of parenteral administration. The indication for its use is osteoporosis as a second-line therapy for those who cannot or should not take estrogens. The recommended dose is 200 U/day as a single nasal administration (18). However, larger doses may be required for prevention, especially in the immediate postmenopausal period (probably 400 U/day). Controlled data documenting the effect of calcitonin on fractures are somewhat sparse. Side effects of nasal administration are usually mild with local nasal irritation being the most frequent. Flushing and nausea are more usually associated with parenteral administration but may occur especially with higher doses by intranasal route. With long-term use antibody formation occurs in a significant proportion of patients and has been suggested to be responsible for reduced long-term efficacy, although with no definitive proof that this is so. The major advantages to calcitonin are its safety, its specificity to bone, and the fact that it can be used in male patients.

Bisphosphonates

These agents are derivatives of pyrophosphate but are not metabolized by the body (19). The bisphosphonates are potent inhibitors of bone remodeling; however, the mode of action of these drugs is still not entirely clear, and each of the bisphosphonates may affect remodeling with subtle but important differences. The agents appear to be well tolerated and to date are without significant side effects, apart from upper gastrointestinal distress that is related to their irritant effect on the mucosa, and some generalized aches that occur in some individuals in the early weeks of treatment. The major advantages of bisphosphonates include the oral route of administration and their specificity for the skeleton. One bisphosphonate, alendronate, is approved by the FDA for treatment of osteoporosis (designated in the package insert as a *T* score below –2.0), but not prevention. Clinical trials suggest a reduction in the risk of vertebral fracture of 48% and a 30% (20) reduction in the risk of peripheral fractures, although the latter was not statistically significant. Because of their ease of use and their low level of side effects, bisphosphonates may become important therapies in the prevention of osteoporosis of all types. The concerns with these agents is their poor intestinal absorption (generally less than 1% of ingested dose) and their long residence time in bone. Long-term data will be required to determine if the latter is problematic. The former requires dosing on an empty stomach. The recommendations for alendronate dosing are that it should be given first thing in the morning with 6–8 ounces of water (not coffee or juice) and that a minimum of one-half hour be allowed before any additional food or drink is taken. The recommended dose is 10 mg/day.

Since both calcitonin and bisphosphonates are agents that affect the skeleton specifically and are more expensive than estrogens (cost of drug), guidelines for their use differ, and both at present should probably be reserved for the highest risk groups.

Certain progestins by themselves appear to have bone-sparing effects but are unlikely to be used in prevention. The addition of a progestin to estrogen, as previously noted, does not negatively impact on the skeletal effect of the estrogen, and certain progestins may enhance the bone-sparing effects of estrogens (15). For postmenopausal patients with a history of breast cancer, there is some evidence that the so-called antiestrogen tamoxifen in doses usually used to prevent cancer recurrence (20–30 mg/day) (20,21) may reduce the rate of bone loss and prevent osteoporosis, a potentially serious problem for this group of patients. Tamoxifen is not FDA-approved for osteoporosis prevention, and patients who are on tamoxifen should have bone mass carefully monitored so that a bone-specific agent can be added early should bone loss occur.

CONCLUSIONS

The initial approach to osteoporosis prevention consists of identification of those subjects likely to be at risk; behavior modification to eliminate risk factors and improved nutrition and lifestyle; and estrogen intervention, which remains the cornerstone of prevention for the postmenopausal patient. Calcitonin (nasal spray) and oral bisphosphonates are alternatives available for those at greatest risk or those who cannot or will not take hormone replacement therapy.

REFERENCES

1. Riggs BL, Melton LJ III: Involutional osteoporosis. *N Engl J Med* 314:1676–1686, 1986
2. Consensus Development Conference: Prophylaxis and treatment of osteoporosis. *Osteo Int* 1:114–126, 1991
3. Hui SL, Slemenda CW, Johnston CC Jr: Baseline measurement of bone mass predicts fracture in white women. *Ann Intern Med* 111:355–361, 1989
4. Johnston CC Jr, Melton LJ III, Lindsay R, et al: Clinical indications for bone mass measurement. *J Bone Min Res* 4:1–28, 1989
5. Heaney RP: Effect of calcium on skeletal development, bone loss, and risk of fractures. *Am J Med* 91:23S–28S, 1991
6. Dalsky GP, Stocke KS, Ehsani AA, et al: Weight-bearing exercise training and lumbar bone mineral content in postmenopausal women. *Ann Intern Med* 108:824–828, 1988
7. Lindsay R: Sex steroids in the pathogenesis and prevention of osteoporosis. In: Riggs BL (ed) *Osteoporosis: Etiology, Diagnosis and Management.* Raven Press, New York, pp 333–358, 1988
8. Lindsay R, Tohme J: Estrogen treatment of patients with established postmenopausal osteoporosis. *Obstet Gynecol* 76:290–295, 1990
9. Lindsay R, Hart DM, Clark DM: The minimum effective dose of estrogen for prevention of postmenopausal bone loss. *Obstet Gynecol* 63:759–763, 1984
10. Stevenson JC, Cust MP, Gangar KF, Hillard TC, Lees B, Whitehead MI: Effects of transdermal versus oral hormone replacement therapy on bone density in spine and proximal femur in postmenopausal women. *Lancet* 336:265–269, 1990
11. Cauley JA, Seeley DG, Ensrud K, Ettinger B, Black D, Cummings SR: Estrogen replacement therapy and fractures in older women. *Ann Intern Med* 122:9–16, 1995
12. Hulka BS: Hormone-replacement therapy and the risk of breast cancer. *Cancer* 40:289–296, 1990
13. Barrett-Connor E, Bush TL: Estrogen and coronary heart disease in women. *JAMA* 265:1861–1967, 1991
14. Voight LF, Weiss NS, Chu J, et al: Progestogen supplementation of exogenous estrogens and the risk of endometrial cancer. *Lancet* 338:274–277, 1991
15. Christiansen C, Riis BJ: 17β-Estradiol and continuous norethisterone: a unique treatment for established osteoporosis in elderly women. *J Clin Endocrinol Metab* 71:836–841, 1990
16. Padwick ML, Pryse-Davies J, Whitehead MI: A simple method for determining the optimal dosage of progestin in postmenopausal women receiving estrogen. *N Engl J Med* 315:930–934, 1986
17. Uebelhart D, Schlemmer A, Johansen JS, Gineyts E, Christiansen C, Delmas PD: Effect of menopause and hormone replacement therapy on the urinary excretion of pyridinoline cross-links. *J Clin Endocrinol Metab* 72:367–373, 1991
18. Overgaard K, Hansen MA, Jensen SB, Christiansen C. Effect of salcatonin given intranassaly on bone mass and frature rates in established osteoporosis: a dose–response study. *Br Med J* 305:556–561, 1992
19. Fleisch H: The possible use of bisphosphonates in osteoporosis. In: DeLuca HF, Mazess R (eds) *Osteoporosis: Physiological Basis, Assessment and Treatment.* Elsevier, New York, pp 323–330, 1990
20. Turken S, Siris E, Seldin D, Lindsay R: Effects of tamoxifen on spinal bone density. *JNCI* 81:1086–1088, 1989
21. Love RR, Mazess RB, Barden HS, et al: Effects of tamoxifen on bone mineral density in postmenopausal women with breast cancer. *N Engl J Med* 326:852–856, 1992

48. Nutrition and Osteoporosis

Robert P. Heaney, M.D., F.A.C.P., F.A.I.N.

Creighton University, Omaha, Nebraska

Nutrition plays a role in pathogenesis, prevention, and treatment of osteoporosis (1). The nutrients known with certainty to be important are calcium, vitamin D, protein, and calories. Phosphorus, certain trace minerals (manganese, copper, and zinc), and vitamins C and K, while involved in bone health generally, are less certainly involved in osteoporosis. Bone cells, of course, are as dependent on total nutrition—including all the vitamins and trace minerals—as any other cell or tissue types. However, current bone mass and bone strength are dependent on cell activity over a many year period, and hence acute nutrient deficiencies, while undoubtedly impairing current cellular competence, tend to have less effect on overall bone strength, which is our concern here in a primer on osteoporosis. The major exceptions to this generalization are the nutrients calcium and vitamin D.

CALCIUM

Calcium is the principal cation of bone mineral. Bone constitutes a very large nutrient reserve for calcium which, over the course of evolution, acquired a secondary, structural function that dominates our concern with respect to osteoporosis. As noted elsewhere (see "Pathogenesis" Chapter 45), bone strength varies as the approximate second power of bone density. While reserves are designed to be used in times of need, it nevertheless must be recognized that any decrease in bone mass produces a corresponding decrease in bone strength.

Bone mass is limited both by the genetic program and by experienced mechanical loading. However, neither limit can be reached if calcium intake is insufficient. Bone resorption, as noted elsewhere in this volume, is controlled by parathyroid hormone, which in turn is concerned with maintenance of extracellular fluid calcium ion levels. Whenever absorbed calcium intake is insufficient to meet either the demands of growth or the drain of dermal and excretory losses, resorption will increase and bone mass will be reduced.

The intake of calcium that is optimal for growth and adult maintenance has been estimated at a National Institutes of Health (NIH) Consensus Conference in 1994 (2) to be 800–1000 mg/day during childhood, 1200–1500 mg/day from age 12 to 24, 1000 mg/day from age 25 to time of estrogen deprivation or age 65 (whichever comes first), and 1500 mg/day thereafter. These intakes are mostly above 1989 Recommended Dietary Allowances (RDAs) and are specific for the United States (and probably Canada as well). The difference is larger than the numbers alone indicate. An RDA is a value for a population and is intended to be an intake at or above the actual requirement of 90% to 95% of the individuals making up the population. (Thus many individuals could have intakes below the RDA which would still be fully adequate for their own needs. Conventionally, nutritionists have considered as cause for concern only individual values less than two thirds of the RDA.) An optimal intake value, by contrast, applies to individuals.

The specific applicability of the National Institutes of Health (NIH) values to North America is a function of the effect of other nutrients on the calcium requirement. High intakes of both protein and sodium, such as are typical of the United States, increase urinary calcium loss and thereby increase the calcium intake requirement. On low intakes of both nutrients, such as might be found in certain Third World environments, the adult requirement can be less than 500 mg/day. This is part of the reason why requirements seem to vary across different countries and cultures.

Low calcium intakes in childhood are associated with increased risk of osteoporosis later in life as well as increased fracture risk even in adolescents (1,3). Calcium intakes are positively correlated with bone mass at all ages, but most especially in old age when the requirement rises and the calcium intake tends to drop (thereby widening the gap between need and supply). Calcium supplementation reduces both bone loss and fracture rate in the elderly (4–8). Only in the few years immediately following estrogen withdrawal at menopause is calcium without much effect (9). (This is largely because bone loss then is due mainly to estrogen deficiency, not to nutrient deficiency.) The abnormal parathyroid secretory physiology, high circulating parathyroid hormone (PTH) levels, and elevated biomarkers for bone resorption typical of the elderly are all reversible with a high calcium intake (10). These hallmarks of the aging calcium economy, once considered due to aging itself, are now recognized as manifestations of calcium privation. Thus, at one and the same time, low calcium intakes are pathogenetic for osteoporosis and high intakes are prophylactic.

Prophylaxis is provided by meeting the NIH recommendations, either by natural foods (principally low-fat dairy products, tofu, a few greens, and a few crustaceans) or by calcium-fortified foods (such as fortified fruit juices, bread, yogurt, breakfast cereals, potato chips, rice, and so forth). Calcium-rich foods, especially milk, tend to be less expensive per calorie than the calcium-poor foods they would displace in the diet. Hence calcium administered in this way has a negative cost and such dietary change has a very favorable cost–benefit relationship.

Supplements may also be indicated. Calcium carbonate is the salt most widely used in the United States. Like all calcium sources (including food), supplements should be taken with meals to ensure optimal absorption. Even for relatively less soluble salts such as the carbonate, gastric acid is not necessary if the supplement is taken with food. Brand name or chewable products have proved over the years to be the most reliable.

Calcium is also of critical importance as cotherapy in the treatment of established osteoporosis. Agents capable of increasing bone mass (such as fluoride and the newer bisphosphonates) cannot achieve their full effect if calcium intake is limiting. Certain agents, such as fluoride (and possibly PTH) with a preferential trophic effect for axial cancellous bone, will actually take bone from other regions of the skeleton to meet the needs of new bone formation in the central skeleton when ingested calcium is not adequate. Because of poor absorption efficiency in the elderly in general and in many osteoporotics in particular, therapeutic intakes must be well above the NIH maintenance figure of 1500 mg/day, probably 2000–2500 mg/day. Unless the number and variety of calcium-fortified foods increases substantially, supplements will be the obvious choice here.

Vitamin D

Vitamin D is important for bone, certainly for its role in facilitating calcium absorption, but probably for other reasons as well. (One of the best attested effects of $1,25(OH)_2D$ is the prompt rise in serum osteocalcin that follows administration of the hormone.) Vitamin D also facilitates PTH-mediated bone resorption.

Serum $25(OH)D$ levels decline with age. This is partly due to decreased solar exposure. Intestinal calcium absorption also decreases with age due to decreased 1α-hydroxylation of $25(OH)D$, and decreased responsiveness of the intestinal mucosa to circulating $1,25(OH)_2D$. Vitamin D supplementation in the elderly reduces fractures of all types (11). It takes about 600 IU/day to maintain $25(OH)D$ levels in healthy young males (which is more than the Recommended Daily Allowance, or RDA, of 200 IU), and the vitamin D requirement is probably higher still in the elderly. Hence it seems prudent to recommend intakes of 800 IU in all elderly individuals with or without osteoporosis. If individuals succeed in raising their calcium intakes through increased milk consumption, they will at the same time improve their vitamin D status because fluid milks in the United States are fortified with vitamin D at a level of 100 IU per serving.

Protein and Calories

Total nutrition, and specifically adequacy of protein and energy intake, is important in several ways. First, malnutrition predisposes to falls. Second, soft tissue mass over bony prominences (e.g., lateral hip) distributes the energy sustained in falls and thereby reduces point loads on bone. Finally, adequacy of protein intake is a major factor in determining outcome after hip fracture. Patients with hip fracture are commonly malnourished, enter the hospital with low serum albumin levels, and typically become more severely hypoproteinemic during hospitalization. Serum albumin levels are the single best predictor of survival or death following hip fracture (12). Protein supplementation of hip fracture patients has been shown to improve outcome dramatically (fewer deaths, less permanent institutionalization, more return to independent living) (13,14). Unfortunately, most hospital standards of care for hip fracture patients lack a nutritional component.

Phosphorus

Phosphorus intake is generally above the RDA in North Americans; hence phosphorus depletion is not common. (There has even been some concern expressed that there is too much phosphorus in the American diet. That is probably not the case.) However, low phosphorus intakes are relatively common among the elderly (i.e., 25% of individuals over 65 ingest under two thirds of the RDA). Whether such low intakes contribute to the problem of osteoporosis is not known. Nevertheless, phosphate is just as important a component of bone mineral as is calcium. When serum phosphorus levels are low, bone mineralization will be limited by phosphate depletion in the immediate environment of the mineralizing front before calcium depletion occurs. It is probable that osteoblast function is severely compromised by low ambient phosphate concentrations even sooner.

Vitamins and Trace Minerals

Vitamins C and K and the minerals manganese, copper, and zinc are necessary cofactors for enzymes involved in the synthesis or post translational modification of various constituents of bone matrix; when these micronutrients are deficient in the diets of growing animals various bone lesions develop (15). Bone fragility has been reported with manganese deficiency in one human patient, and a bony lesion resembling osteoporosis occurs in sheep with copper deficiency. However, it is not known as to whether acquired adult deficiencies of any of these minerals in humans play a role in pathogenesis or treatment of osteoporosis. One randomized trial involving supplementation with manganese, copper, and zinc produced suggestive, but not conclusive, evidence of some benefit when these minerals were added to a calcium supplementation regimen (16).

Vitamin C is necessary for collagen crosslinking, and bony defects are well recognized as a part of the scurvy syndrome. However, apart from general nutritional considerations, there is no known role for vitamin C in osteoporotic bony fragility.

Vitamin K is necessary for the γ carboxylation of three bone matrix proteins, a step necessary for their binding to hydroxyapatite. Osteocalcin is the best studied of these. Circulating serum osteocalcin is commonly undercarboxylated in patients with osteoporosis, especially those with hip fracture, and the defect responds to modest doses of vitamin K (17). There is also suggestive evidence that vitamin K may reduce urinary calcium loss in patients with osteoporosis. What is not known is the extent to which these changes are causal or are instead simply markers for the general debility and global malnutrition common in elderly patients with osteoporosis. Vitamin K deficiency is, however, easily treatable and, if some component of the fragility of the elderly is due to inadequate intakes or colonic synthesis of vitamin K, that component of the fracture burden could be inexpensively eliminated.

REFERENCES

1. Heaney RP. Nutrition and risk for osteoporosis. In: Marcus R, Feldman D, Kelsey J (eds) *Osteoporosis*. Academic Press, San Diego, 483–505, 1996.
2. NIH Consensus Conference: Optimal Calcium Intake. *JAMA* 272: 1942-1948, 1994
3. Chan GM, Hess M, Hollis J, Book LS: Bone mineral status in

childhood accidental fractures. *Am J Dis Child* 138:569–570, 1984

4. Chapuy MC, Arlot ME, Duboeuf F, Brun J, Crouzet B, Arnaud S, Delmas PD, Meunier PJ: Vitamin D₃ and calcium to prevent hip fractures in elderly women. *N Engl J Med* 327:1637–1642, 1992

5. Chevalley T, Rizzoli R, Nydegger V, Slosman D, Rapin C-H, Michel J-P, Vasey H, Bonjour J-P: Effects of calcium supplements on femoral bone mineral density and vertebral fracture rate in vitamin D-replete elderly patients. *Osteoporosis Int* 4:245–252, 1994

6. Recker RR, Hinders S, Davies KM, Heaney RP, Stegman MR, Kimmel DB, Lappe JM: Correcting calcium nutritional deficiency prevents spine fractures in elderly women. *J Bone Min Res* 1995 (submitted)

7. Reid IR, Ames RW, Evans MC, Gamble GD, Sharpe SJ: Effect of calcium supplementation on bone loss in postmenopausal women. *N Engl J Med* 328:460–464, 1993

8. Aloia JF, Vaswani A, Yeh JK, Ross PL, Flaster E, Dilmanian FA: Calcium supplementation with and without hormone replacement therapy to prevent postmenopausal bone loss. *Ann Intern Med* 120:97–103, 1994

9. Dawson-Hughes B, Dallal GE, Krall EA, Sadowski L, Sahyoun N, Tannenbaum S: A controlled trial of the effect of calcium supplementation on bone density in postmenopausal women. *N Engl J Med* 323:878–883, 1990

10. McKane WR, Khosla S, O'Fallon WM, Robins SP, Burritt MF, Riggs BL: Role of calcium intake in modulating age-related increases in parathyroid function and bone resorption. *J Clin Endocrinol Metab* 81:1699–1703, 1996

11. Heikinheimo RJ, Inkovaara JA, Harju EJ, Haavisto MV, Kaarela RH, Kataja JM, Kokko AM-L, Kolho LA, Rajala SA: Annual injection of vitamin D and fractures of aged bones. *Calcif Tissue Int* 51:105–110, 1992

12. Rico H, Revilla M, Villa LF, Hernandez ER, Fernandez JP: Crush fracture syndrome in senile osteoporosis: a nutritional consequence. *J Bone Min Res* 7:317–319, 1992

13. Delmi M, Rapin CH, Bengoa JM, Delmas PD, Vasey H, Bonjour JP: Dietary supplementation in elderly patients with fractured neck of the femur. *Lancet* 335:1013–1016, 1990

14. Bastow MD, Rawlings J, Allison SP: Benefits of supplementary tube feeding after fractured neck of femur. *Br Med J* 287:1589–1592, 1983

15. Heaney RP: Nutritional factors in osteoporosis. *Annu Rev Nutr* 13:287–316, 1993

16. Strause L, Saltman P, Smith K, Andon M: The role of trace elements in bone metabolism. In: Burckhardt P, Heaney RP (eds) *Nutritional Aspects of Osteoporosis*. Raven Press, New York, pp 223–233, 1991

17. Vermeer C, Jie K-S G, Knapen MHJ: Role of vitamin K in bone metabolism. *Annu Rev Nutr* 15:1–22, 1995

49. Evaluation and Treatment of Postmenopausal Osteoporosis

Michael Kleerekoper, M.D., F.A.C.E., and *Louis V. Avioli, M.D., F.A.C.E.

*Department of Internal Medicine, Wayne State University School of Medicine, and Harper Hospital, Detroit, Michigan; and *Departments of Medicine and Orthopedic Surgery, Washington University Medical Center, Barnes-Jewish Campus, St. Louis, Missouri*

Osteoporosis is a disease characterized by low bone mass and the development of nontraumatic or atraumatic fractures as a direct result of the low bone mass. A nontraumatic fracture has been arbitrarily defined as one occurring from trauma equal to or less than that of a fall from a standing height. In the preclinical state, the disease is characterized simply by a low bone mass without fractures. This totally asymptomatic state is often termed osteopenia. Osteoporosis and osteopenia are the most common metabolic bone diseases in the developed countries of the world, whereas osteomalacia may be more prevalent in underdeveloped countries where nutrition is suboptimal. To be able to evaluate more fully the prevalence and incidence of osteoporosis worldwide, the World Health Organization (WHO) recently convened an expert panel to define osteoporosis on the basis of bone mass measurement (1). Table 1 provides the diagnostic categories for women that were established by that panel. Osteoporotic fractures may affect any part of the skeleton except the skull. Most commonly, fractures occur in the distal forearm (Colles' fracture), thoracic and lumbar vertebrae, and proximal femur (hip fracture).

The epidemiology of osteoporosis is detailed in Chapter 44 and is only briefly summarized here. The incidence of osteoporotic fractures increases with age, is higher in whites than in blacks, and is higher in women than in men. The female to male ratio is 1.5:1 for Colles' fractures, 7:1 for vertebral fractures, and 2:1 for hip fractures. Because most osteoporotic fractures do not require admission to the hospital, it is difficult to obtain precise figures on the true prevalence of this disease. Almost without exception, a hip fracture requires admission to a hospital, and current estimates indicate that there are 275,000 new osteoporotic hip fractures each year in the United States. It has been estimated that after menopause, a woman's lifetime risk of sustaining an osteoporotic fracture is one in three. Regrettably, despite improvements in surgical techniques and anesthesiology, most hip fractures require surgical intervention on a nonelective basis, and there is a 15% to 20% excess mortality after an osteoporotic hip fracture. Perhaps more important, after such fractures, less than one third of the patients are restored to their prefracture functional state within 12 months of the fracture. Most patients require some form of ambulatory support, and many require institutional care. Current estimates indicate that each new case of osteoporotic hip fracture costs $40,000, and the annual expenditure for short-term care after an osteoporotic hip fracture already exceeds $8 billion. Chapter 50 provides more details on the special problems posed by osteoporotic fractures of the hip.

PATHOGENESIS

Once peak adult bone mass has been attained in the third, possibly fourth, decade of life, bone mass at any point in

TABLE 1. *Diagnostic criteria for osteoporosis[a]*

Normal	Bone mineral density (BMD) or bone mineral content (BMC) within 1 SD of young adult reference mean
Low bone mass (osteopenia)	A value for BMD or BMC between −1.0 and −2.5 SD below young adult reference mean
Osteoporosis	A value for BMD or BMC −2.5 or more SD below the young adult reference mean
Severe (established) osteoporosis	Osteoporosis with one or more fragility fractures

SD, standard deviation
[a]From Ref. 1 with permission.

TABLE 2. *Factors commonly associated with osteopenic and/or osteoporotic syndrome(s)*

Genetic
  White or Asiatic ethnicity
  Positive family history
  Small body frame
Lifestyle
  Smoking
  Inactivity
  Nulliparity
  Excessive exercise (producing amenorrhea)
  Early natural menopause
  Late menarche
Nutritional factors
  Milk intolerance
  Life long low dietary calcium intake
  Vegetarian dieting
  Excessive alcohol intake
  Consistently high protein intake
Medical disorders
  Anorexia nervosa
  Thyrotoxicosis
  Hyperparathyroidism
  Cushing syndrome
  Type I diabetes
  Alterations in gastrointestinal and hepatobiliary function
  Occult osteogenesis imperfecta
  Mastocytosis
  Rheumatoid arthritis
  "Transient" osteoporosis
  Prolonged parenteral nutrition
  Prolactinoma
  Hemolytic anemia
Drugs
  Excessive dose of thyroid hormone
  Glucocorticoid drugs
  Anticoagulants
  Chronic lithium therapy
  Chemotherapy (breast cancer or lymphoma)
  Gonadotropin-releasing hormone agonist or antagonist therapy
  Anticonvulsants
  Chronic phosphate-binding antacid use
  Extended tetracycline use[a]
  Diuretics producing calciuria[a]
  Phenothiazine derivatives[a]
  Cyclosporin A[a]

[a]Not yet associated with decreased bone mass in humans, although identified as either toxic to bone in animals or as inducing calciuria or calcium malabsorption in humans.

time is the difference between peak adult bone mass and the loss of bone mass that has occurred since this was attained. Because age-related bone loss is a universal phenomenon in humans, any circumstance that limits an individual's ability to maximize peak adult bone mass increases the likelihood of developing osteoporosis later in life. Strategies for maximizing peak adult bone mass have been described in Chapters 46–48.

The excessive bone loss that characterizes the pathogenesis of osteoporosis results from abnormalities in the bone remodeling cycle (see Chapters 5, 25). In brief, bone remodeling is a mechanism for keeping the skeleton "young" by a process of removal of old bone and replacement with new bone. The cycle is initiated by resorption of old bone, recruitment of osteoblasts, deposition of new matrix, and mineralization of that newly deposited matrix. It appears that with each cycle there is a slight, imperceptible deficit in bone formation. The total bone loss is, therefore, a function of the number of cycles in process at any one time. Conditions that increase the rate of activation of the bone remodeling process thus increase the proportion of the skeleton undergoing remodeling at any one time and increase the rate of bone loss. In this circumstance, which is called high-turnover osteoporosis, the deficit per unit of remodeling is apparently constant. Most of the secondary causes of osteoporosis (Table 2) are associated with this increased rate of activation of the remodeling cycle. In the normal aging process, there appears to be a progressive impairment of the signaling between bone resorption and bone formation, such that with every cycle of remodeling, there is an increase in the deficit between resorption and formation because osteoblast recruitment is inefficient. Thus, excessive bone loss can occur even when activation of the skeleton is not increased and, in fact, when activation of the skeleton might be decreased. This gives rise to the concept of low- or normal-turnover osteoporosis.

CLASSIFICATION OF OSTEOPOROSIS

In addition to describing osteoporosis as being of the high- or low-turnover type, there are several other classification systems. The first is the classification into primary and secondary, the latter being osteoporosis for which a clearly identifiable etiologic mechanism is recognized. Primary osteoporosis is further characterized into postmenopausal and senile. In postmenopausal osteoporosis, there is an apparent excess loss of cancellous bone with relative sparing of cortical bone, and the clinical syndromes involve Colles' fracture and vertebral fracture. In senile osteoporosis, there is a more concordant loss of both cortical and cancellous bone. The pathogenesis of senile osteoporosis is uncertain, but it is postulated to result from an age-related decline in renal production of 1,25-dihydroxyvitamin D and calcium malabsorption, with subsequent secondary hyperparathyroidism. It is the hyperparathyroidism that is largely responsible for the excess cortical bone loss. The fracture syndrome often seen in the patient with senile osteoporosis involves hip fracture.

CLINICAL MANIFESTATIONS OF OSTEOPOROSIS

As mentioned previously, osteoporosis without fracture is entirely without symptoms. This does not lessen its importance, because the aim of all therapies should be to prevent even the first fracture, let alone subsequent fractures. When osteoporosis is complicated by the development of an osteoporotic fracture, the symptoms and signs are those related to the fracture itself. Osteoporotic vertebral fractures may represent a unique situation, and this will be discussed separately. Primary orthopedic management of peripheral fractures should not be influenced by the fact that the fracture results from osteoporosis. Management consists of immobilization and analgesia. There does not appear to be anything about an osteoporotic fracture that results in delayed fracture union. If delayed fracture union or fracture nonunion complicates an osteoporotic fracture, one needs to look for conditions other than osteoporosis, such as osteomalacia, hyperparathyroidism, or occult forms of osteogenesis imperfecta. Immobilization should be for only a limited period of time, sufficient to ensure primary fracture healing. Longer immobilization will lead to accelerated bone loss and must be avoided. The brittleness of the osteoporotic skeleton may complicate open surgical repair of osteoporotic fractures, with limited purchase for pins, plates, screws, or nails. Restoration of the prefracture anatomic and functional state is the goal in the management of osteoporotic fractures of the appendicular skeleton. Regrettably, with respect to osteoporotic hip fractures, this is not often the outcome that is attained, given the excess morbidity and mortality already discussed. In general, this is because surgical repair of an osteoporotic hip fracture is usually a nonelective procedure. Circumstances that appear to increase mortality after a hip fracture are related to the overall medical health and nutritional status of the subject sustaining the fracture. Frail, elderly subjects taking large numbers of medications and with mental impairment have the greatest mortality, and this is particularly so in men compared with women. Of those patients who survive the early operative intervention for an osteoporotic hip fracture, less than one third are restored to their prefracture functional state, and either require institutionalized care or some form of ambulatory support.

Osteoporotic vertebral fractures are quite different from other osteoporotic fractures. Surveys of spine radiographs in older subjects suggest that many vertebral fractures have occurred in the absence of acute symptoms. If acute symptoms do occur at the time of fracture, these will be manifest as intense pain and limitation of motion. Operative intervention is infrequently required for stabilization of these fractures. However, the principles of immobilization for a short time should still hold. The concept of placing the patient with an osteoporotic fracture in a back brace for years is to be decried. Similarly, the acute skeletal pain after an osteoporotic vertebral fracture should dissipate within 4–6 weeks. If skeletal tenderness persists much beyond this, other causes for the fracture (e.g., metastatic disease, multiple myeloma) should be considered. Osteoporotic fractures of the vertebral bodies rarely result in "referred nerve pain syndrome" or long tract symptoms or signs. Again, if a fracture is complicated by these symptoms or signs, causes other than osteoporosis should be considered.

Once a vertebral body has been fractured, restoration of normal anatomy is not possible. In fact, refracture of the same vertebra with further abnormalities of shape and size is often the outcome. Thus, even those vertebral fractures that are not associated with any acute symptoms at the time of fracture give rise to chronic pain, disability, and often obvious deformity. All vertebral fractures are associated with loss of stature; in the thoracic spine this is associated with a progressive increase in the degree of kyphosis, and in the lumbar spine this is associated with a progressive flattening of the lordotic curve and scoliosis in some individuals. As the number of vertebrae involved increases and the severity of individual vertebral deformities progresses, these anatomic changes become more pronounced. There is gradual loss of the waistline contour and protuberance of the abdomen, and in severe cases the lower ribs approximate the pelvic rim and ultimately lie within the pelvis. Each of these progressive anatomic deformities is associated with symptoms. The progressive loss of stature results in progressive "shortening" of the paraspinal musculature, that is, the paraspinal muscles are actively contracting, resulting in the pain of muscle fatigue. This is the major cause of the chronic back pain in spinal osteoporosis. Careful clinical examination reveals that the skeleton (spine) itself is not tender, and most patients indicate that the pain is paraspinal. The pain is worse with prolonged standing and is often relieved by walking. After an acute fracture, there may be associated paraspinal muscle spasm, but this dissipates with time. The loss of height and the protuberant abdomen are usually not associated with direct symptoms per se, but do give the patient the emotional discomfort of the altered body image. Many patients attempt to wear abdominal flattening girdles or go on weight-reduction diets, both of which will be of limited benefit and potential harm. It is important that the patient be advised of the irreversible nature of these anatomic changes. One common complaint of patients with advanced disease is vague gastrointestinal distress aggravated by eating. This can be alleviated somewhat by having the patient consume frequent smaller meals. This is a particularly vexing problem for patients with chronic airway disease who have osteoporosis as a result of therapy with corticosteroids. In these patients, the flattened diaphragm coupled with the shortened spinal column results in marked diminution of the size of their abdominal cavity.

There are several important approaches to the long-term management of patients with these chronic deformities from spinal osteoporosis. Of particular importance is educating the patient to understand the nature of the deformity so that he or she can have realistic expectations concerning body image and the anticipated goals of therapy (relief of pain, restoration of function, maintenance of a reasonable quality of life, and prevention of further fractures). The major focus of therapy should be rehabilitation and analgesia aimed at lessening the chronic back pain. However, caution must be used with analgesics and nonsteroidal anti-inflammatory agents, many of which cause significant constipation. Straining of the stool to relieve constipation from narcotic analgesics tends to aggravate back pain substantially. In this regard, it is worth noting that many generic calcium preparations also tend to cause vague gastrointestinal symptoms, including constipation in some patients. It is equally important to instruct the patient adequately in activities of daily living so that he or she bends, lifts, and stoops in a manner that does not increase strain on the brittle skeleton. Nurses, physical therapists, and occupational therapists become important partners in the management of the patient with spinal osteoporosis. In many respects, this nonpharmacologic approach to these patients is far more important than the pharmacologic therapy.

DIAGNOSTIC STUDIES IN OSTEOPOROSIS

The same diagnostic approach should be taken with patients suspected of having osteoporosis whether or not they have already sustained an osteoporotic fracture. These studies should only be undertaken once an appropriate history and physical examination have been completed. The history, physical examination, and studies should all be conducted with the aim of determining the extent and severity of disease, pathogenesis of the bone loss, and physiology of the skeleton at the time of presentation. Although postmenopausal and senile osteoporosis are the most prevalent forms of the disease, it must be remembered that as many as 20% of women who otherwise appear to have postmenopausal osteoporosis can be shown to have additional etiologic factors above and beyond their age, gender, and ethnic background. Many of these secondary causes of osteoporosis (Table 2) can be suggested from the history and physical examination so that appropriate investigations can be ordered.

If an osteoporotic fracture is suspected, it is imperative that radiographs be taken of the appropriate part of the skeleton. However, there is no clear indication for radiographs of the skeleton if fracture is not suspected. All patients suspected of having osteoporosis, with or without fracture, should have measurement of bone mass (see Chapter 23 for details). The one possible exception is the patient with far advanced disease clinically and radiographically. Because osteoporosis may be the only manifestation of many of the secondary causes listed earlier, it is appropriate to perform simple screening studies looking for these causes in each patient. A biochemical profile will provide information about renal and hepatic function, primary hyperparathyroidism, and possible malnutrition. A hematologic profile might also provide clues to the presence of myeloma and malnutrition. The precise role of hyperthyroidism, particularly exogenous, in the pathogenesis of accelerated bone loss and osteoporosis remains unresolved. Nonetheless, for the time being at least, it seems prudent to obtain a sensitive thyroid-stimulating hormone assay in all patients with documented bone loss. A 24-hour urine collection for measurement of calcium (which should always be accompanied by measurement of creatinine and sodium) will detect patients with hypercalciuria, which may be the end result of excess skeletal loss or may contribute to excess skeletal loss. In contrast, a very low urine calcium level (50 mg or less for 24 hours) may provide a clue to the presence of vitamin D malnutrition or malabsorption (2). It is our practice to obtain a 24-hour urine collection in all osteoporotic subjects. A 24-hour urine-free cortisol determination should be considered as the only test that can document occult Cushing's disease, which may have osteoporosis as the only presenting feature. The yield from using the urinary-free cortisol test is quite small, but it is probably the only way to detect this uncommon disorder. In general, the intensity with which one looks for occult secondary causes of accelerated bone loss should be related to any unusual features of the clinical presentation, such as bone loss in a premenopausal woman, in a woman very early in menopause, or in a man without obvious hypogonadism. One should also pay particular attention to patients whose fractures occur at unusual sites.

CALCITROPIC HORMONES AND BIOCHEMICAL MARKERS OF BONE REMODELING

In most cases of osteoporosis, there is no need to measure the calcitropic hormones (parathyroid hormone, calcitriol, or calcitonin) unless there is a specific indication for these measurements based on the history, physical examination, and biochemical screening. Although there are reports of abnormalities in some of these measurements when compared with published reference ranges, this is not the case when the reference values are appropriately adjusted for age, gender, and ethnic background.

In contrast, it is becoming increasingly important to monitor the biochemical markers of bone remodeling that are discussed in detail in Chapter 20. The control of bone remodeling is detailed in Chapter 5, and the role of abnormalities in the remodeling cycle in the pathogenesis of osteoporosis has been described briefly. It may be useful to make an analogy between turnover abnormalities leading to osteoporosis and abnormalities in the red cell life cycle leading to anemia. High-turnover bone loss with increased resorption and increased, but insufficient, formation would be analogous to hemolytic anemia with increased red cell destruction and increased (but insufficient) red cell formation, characterized by the increased reticulocyte count in this type of anemia. Low-turnover bone loss with normal resorption and subnormal formation would be analogous to anemia of chronic disease.

There is increasing evidence that biochemical markers of bone formation and resorption are a useful adjunct in predicting the rate of bone loss and the response to therapy. Table 3 lists the biochemical markers of bone resorption and formation that were available through commercial diagnostic laboratories at the time of this writing (December 1995). The reader should remain aware that this is a rapidly changing field and that other markers are available in laboratories of individual investigators. Table 3 also provides details of the reference intervals for these tests in healthy premenopausal white women.

Theoretically, patients with high-turnover osteoporosis should have increased levels of resorption and formation markers, should be experiencing bone loss at an accelerated rate, and should respond best to therapy with drugs that inhibit bone resorption. In contrast, those with low- or normal-turnover osteoporosis should have normal or low levels of the markers, should not be losing bone at an accelerated rate, should respond less well to antiresorptive therapy, and

TABLE 3. *Biochemical markers of bone remodeling*[a]

Marker	Reference interval[b]
Bone resorption	
Lysylpyridinoline (LP)	24–52 nM Pyd/mM Cr
Deoxylysylpyridinoline (DPD)	2.5–6.2 nM Dpd/mM Cr
N-telopeptide of the cross-links of collagen (NTX)	5–65 nM/mM creatinine based upon 95% CI
C-telopeptide of the cross-links of collagen (PICP)	13–96 nM/mM Cr
Bone formation	
Osteocalcin (OCN) [bone Gla protein (BGP)]	1.6–9.2 ng/ml
Bone specific alkaline phosphatase (BSAP)	11.6–30.6 BAP, U/L
Carboxy-terminal extension peptide of type I procollagen (PICP)	45–190 µg/L

[a]All resorption markers are based on urine collected after an overnight fast. Usually a spot sample of the first or second voided urine is analyzed. Data are normalized for creatinine excretion. All formation markers are based on random serum samples. CI, confidence interval.

[b]Reference interval is for premenopausal women.

should be treated preferentially with drugs that primarily enhance bone formation. To date, only a small fraction of these theoretical scenarios has been formally documented in prospective studies. This is mainly because the studies are not yet complete, and not necessarily because the theory is defective. The biggest difficulty has been demonstrating that the markers can be used to select therapy for individual patients, principally because the only therapies available are all antiresorptive. As therapeutic options broaden over the next several years, the usefulness of biochemical markers in this fashion will become more apparent.

At present, the most practical use of these markers is to monitor the response to therapy. It has been demonstrated that changes in markers after just 3 months of therapy are significantly related to changes in bone mass after 24 months of therapy (3). This is of considerable practical importance, particularly with respect to patient compliance with treatment, as changes in bone mass in response to therapy may not become apparent within 12 months of treatment. The markers may also provide confidence for dose adjustment, allowing the clinician to use a smaller than recommended dose of therapy if that proves sufficient to restore biochemical markers of remodeling to the normal premenopausal range.

In summary, the current approach to evaluation of the osteoporotic patient involves documentation of bone mass, documentation of fractures if present, a diligent search for secondary causes, and then an evaluation of the biochemistry of skeletal remodeling.

MEDICAL THERAPY

At the time of this writing, the only drugs approved by the Food and Drug Administration (FDA) for treatment of postmenopausal osteoporosis are estrogen, calcitonin, and the bisphosphonate alendronate. The FDA is evaluating a request for approval of a sustained-release sodium fluoride preparation. Although calcitriol and etidronate are both approved by the FDA for use in the United States, osteoporosis is currently not an approved indication. Oral calcium supplements are not subject to FDA regulation, and sodium fluoride as a supplement is also not subject to FDA regulation. In the following sections, we will discuss what is known about each of these possible therapies for postmenopausal osteoporosis.

The primary role for estrogen in the prevention of early postmenopausal bone loss and the subsequent development of osteoporotic fractures has been discussed in detail in Chapter 47. A definitive role for the use of estrogen in established osteoporosis with fractures is much less well established. Estrogen is an "antiresorptive" agent in that it inhibits bone resorption by decreasing the frequency of activation of the bone remodeling cycle. Estrogen would be expected to be most efficient if bone remodeling or bone turnover were increased. This is why it is so effective in the early stages of menopause. If an individual patient with established osteoporosis can be shown to have increased bone remodeling, estrogen will be effective in inhibiting remodeling, no matter how long it has been since the patient had her menopause. Thus, estrogen therapy will slow down the rate of bone loss in any estrogen-deficient woman so treated. However, the ability of estrogen to result in any net gain in bone mass is limited, with the best results being a 2% to 4% annual increase for 2 years. Recent studies have suggested that older women may also receive benefit from estrogen of similar magnitude (4). There are some studies showing that estrogen reduces the rate of occurrence of new vertebral fractures in patients with established osteoporosis. The usual starting dose is 0.625 mg of conjugated equine estrogen (Premarin®) or 0.05 mg of transdermal estrogen (Estraderm®). Short-term complications of estrogen therapy in women with established osteoporosis include breast tenderness and vaginal bleeding (5). If estrogens are given without progesterone, there is an increased likelihood of endometrial hyperplasia. The relationship between estrogen therapy and breast cancer is not well established, but most studies suggest that there is little, if any, increased risk of breast cancer during the first 10–15 years of therapy. Such long-term studies in established osteoporosis have not been conducted, and as long as therapy is tolerated, estrogen therapy, once indicated, should be continued indefinitely.

Synthetic salmon calcitonin (Calcimar® and Miacalcin®) is available in the United States as a subcutaneous injection or nasal spray formulation. Like estrogen, calcitonin inhibits bone resorption and slows down the rate of bone loss. The ability of calcitonin to increase bone mass is a function of the rate of bone remodeling at the time calcitonin therapy is initiated. The response is better in patients with increased bone turnover than in patients with low turnover (6). Again, a beneficial effect is observed as long as the medication is used, especially in intermittent-pulse regimens (6–11). There is increasing evidence that calcitonin has inherent analgesic properties, and many physicians recommend its use in the early postfracture period because of this effect (11). The major side effects of calcitonin are transient flushing of the face and nausea. These side effects are all dose dependent and virtually disappear with nasal spray formulations. The recommended dose is 100 U subcutaneously daily, but few patients tolerate this large dose initially. We have found that starting with a dose as low as 25 U subcutaneously three times per week is tolerated by most patients, and the dose can be increased gradually over a period of 2–3 months if needed. Intermittent-pulse dose regimens have also been used, with documentation of increased bone mass and decreased fracture incidence (12). Calcitonin is dispensed in a concentration of 200 U/ml. Because most patients use insulin syringes calibrated for a dose of 100 U/ml, it is important that they receive adequate instruction on the amount of solution to inject to achieve the desired dosage. Therapy should be continued for as long as the drug is tolerated (12). The recommended dose of nasal spray calcitonin is 200 U daily, with limited opportunity for dose adjustment.

As discussed earlier, use of the biochemical markers may assist in finding a suitable dose of estrogen or calcitonin for individual patients, particularly if side effects or other concerns limit the recommended starting dose. For example, breast tenderness on estrogen is less likely in older women if initiated in a dose of Premarin 0.3 mg/d. If this dose can be demonstrated to have reduced the rate of resorption, dose adjustment might not be indicated. Similarly, if the markers of resorption have not changed appropriately (arbitrarily a 40% to 50% reduction from baseline after 8–12 weeks of therapy), the patient might be more willing to consider a higher dose of therapy. This is equally appropriate when trying to minimize the gastrointestinal side effects of calcitonin.

Alendronate (Fosamax®) is an amino-bisphosphonate for which extensive clinical trials have been completed worldwide; it was recently approved by the FDA for the treatment of osteoporosis. In the clinical trials, there was a progressive increase in spine and hip bone mineral density during 3 years of daily therapy at a dose of 10 mg once a day (13–15). There were fewer and less severe spinal fractures in patients receiving therapy compared with those on placebo. The drug was well tolerated with few side effects, and more than 80% of those on therapy responded with an increase in bone mass. The major potential problem with this therapy is that, in common with other bisphosphonates, oral absorption of alendronate is very poor, with less than 1% of an orally administered dose being absorbed. This poor absorption is further impaired if the medication is taken with food, any liquid except water, or with calcium supplements. These problems can be avoided if patients are advised to take the medication first thing in the morning with water and to delay breakfast for at least 30 minutes. The major side effect is esophagitis in a small proportion of patients.

Etidronate (Didronel®), the first bisphosphonate to become clinically available, has been used in several clinical trials to stabilize or increase bone mass and also to possibly reduce the vertebral fracture rate (14,16–18). However, the effect on the vertebral fracture rate is still controversial and by no means well established. The major short-term effect of bisphosphonate is nausea (14,16–18). The treatment regimen for etidronate is 400 mg orally daily for 2 weeks followed by a 10–12-week etidronate-free period, with a repeat of this 3-month cycle for 2 years. Because this bisphospho-

nate is poorly absorbed orally and because its absorption is obliterated when given concurrently with calcium, it is important to advise the patient not to ingest any calcium, either as a supplement or in food, for 4 hours before or after ingestion of each tablet. Clinical trials of this therapy used 1500 mg calcium as a daily supplement during the etidronate-free periods. It is imperative that etidronate be used in this rigorous treatment cycle and that the dose not be exceeded in amount or duration. There is evidence from long-term treatment of Paget's disease that large doses or longer duration of therapy with etidronate may result in a mineralization defect and an increased risk of developing osteomalacia and hip fractures. This drug is not an FDA-approved therapy for osteoporosis. As noted earlier for calcitonin and estrogen, etidronate is an antiresorptive drug. There is very little formal evidence that its effectiveness is a function of remodeling activity at the time therapy is initiated. One can anticipate a gain of 2% to 4% annually in spinal bone mass.

Although calcitriol (Rocaltrol®) in a dose of 0.25 μg/d has been shown in one study to reduce the vertebral fracture rate compared with a group of patients taking calcium alone (19), other clinical trials have not found calcitriol to be effective in this regard. However, because calcitriol is the most potent metabolite (17) of vitamin D, it does increase intestinal calcium absorption, often resulting in hypercalciuria or hypercalcemia. Patients should be cautioned to monitor their calcium intake to avoid excessive amounts and should also be monitored every 6–8 weeks for development of hypercalciuria or hypercalcemia, because clinical symptoms and signs of these conditions may be very subtle and not evident until irreversible renal damage has occurred. It is unclear what specific effect calcitriol has on bone mass, although in some instances, increments in bone mass of 1% to 2% per annum have been recorded.

The effect of calcium supplementation on bone mass and vertebral fracture rate in established osteoporotic syndromes is not well studied. Studies that are available suggest that calcium supplementation in postmenopausal women does decrease the rate of bone loss when administered in doses of 1000–1500 mg/d, especially in individuals with histories of marginally low calcium intake (5,20–24). A combination of calcium supplements and exercise has also proven effective in stabilizing skeletal bone loss rates in postmenopausal female populations. Obviously, it is important to maintain adequate calcium supplement in addition to the active drug during estrogen, calcitonin, or alendronate therapeutic interventions, because it is difficult to mineralize newly formed matrix fully in the absence of adequate calcium. However, calcium should be taken at least 1 hour after alendronate.

Sodium fluoride is widely used as a therapy for postmenopausal osteoporosis. In doses of 50–75 mg/d, the increase in spinal bone mass achieved with sodium fluoride approximates 8% per year, twice that seen with either estrogen, calcitonin, or bisphosphonates. However, there is little evidence from properly conducted clinical trials that this increase in bone mass translates into a reduction in vertebral fractures. Moreover, sodium fluoride is associated with a significant degree of gastrointestinal distress and also a painful lower-extremity syndrome believed to represent stress fractures induced by fluoride. Recently reported studies with a lower dose of a slow-release sodium fluoride preparation administered cyclically have indicated a beneficial effect on vertebral fracture rates (25). The best results were reported in those osteoporotic patients with the highest bone mass (>65% of peak adult bone mass). Therapy was most effective in preventing fractures in previously nonfractured vertebrae; there was no significant effect on the progression of fractures in vertebra that were already fractured before initiation of treatment. It should be emphasized that these patients were also subjected to estrogen therapy. An FDA advisory panel recently recommended that a slow-release sodium fluoride preparation be approved for treatment of osteoporosis (26).

There are reports that the prevalence of osteoporotic hip fractures decreases in hypertensive patients receiving long-term therapy with hydrochlorothiazide (13,16,18). This has not been confirmed in all studies. To our knowledge, there are no formal prospective studies of thiazide diuretic therapy in osteoporotic or postmenopausal normotensive populations. Until such studies are reported and shown to be effective, thiazide diuretics should not be used as therapy for osteoporosis. However, a case could be made for selecting thiazides as the diuretic of choice in patients with osteoporosis, should diuretic therapy be otherwise indicated. Because thiazides decrease renal excretion of calcium and, uncommonly, may lead to mild hypercalcemia, extreme caution should be used when considering calcitriol therapy in a patient taking thiazides, or thiazide therapy in a patient taking calcitriol. Side effects such as hypomagnesemia, hyperglycemia, hypercholesterolemia, and hypokalemia preclude advocating this drug as potentially therapeutic for osteoporotic patients who are not hypertensive (27,28).

Newer generations of bisphosphonates, synthetic parathyroid hormone, selective estrogen receptor modulators (SERMs), and various combinations and treatment regimens of these experimental drugs, as well as the drugs listed earlier, are currently undergoing extensive clinical trials. At present, the safety and efficacy of these various drugs and their potential combinations are not well established. Consequently, their use cannot be recommended. One exception is the antiestrogen tamoxifen. This drug is widely prescribed for women with breast cancer to minimize the likelihood of recurrence. Tamoxifen inhibits bone resorption in the same manner as estrogen and is effective in preserving bone mass. However, because of reported side effects, not the least of which is endometrial carcinoma, its use should be restricted to women for whom it is prescribed as adjunctive therapy for breast cancer. Table 4 lists the several therapies that are currently under active investigation in the United States. It is anticipated that some of these therapies will become available for clinical use by the year 2000.

SELECTING A THERAPY AND MONITORING THE RESPONSE TO THERAPY

At a minimum, every patient with established osteoporosis, with or without fractures, should be given supplemental calcium at 1000–1500 mg/d. Specific therapy for osteoporosis should be restricted to estrogen, calcitonin, and alendronate, given that these drugs are approved by the FDA for

TABLE 4. *Pharmacologic therapies for osteoporosis*

Approved by the FDA with an osteoporosis indication
Estrogen
Calcitonin, subcutaneous or nasal spray
Alendronate
Approved by the FDA without an osteoporosis indication
Calcitriol
Etidronate
Thiazide
Approval pending for an osteoporosis indication
Sodium fluoride, slow-release
In clinical trial
I. SERM
Droloxifene
Roloxifene
II. Bisphosphonate
Ibandronate
Risedronate
Tiludronate
III. Parathyroid hormone

FDA, Food and Drug Administration; SERM, selective estrogen receptor modulator.

an osteoporosis indication. Bone mass, which should always be measured at baseline, should be monitored at the end of 12 months of therapy. A decrease in bone mass of 2% or greater should prompt a change in therapy—either a change in dose or a change in medication. After a patient has experienced 1 full year of successful therapy, that is, 1 year of therapy with either an increase in bone mass or a 2% decrease, monitoring can be restricted to biannual measurement of bone mass. At present, there is no indication that therapy should be discontinued as long as the patient is tolerating the medication and there is no progressive decrement in bone mass. It should be noted that the antifracture efficacy of each of these drugs during the early therapeutic phase is not well established, and the occurrence of an osteoporotic fracture within the first 6–12 months of therapy should not be taken as an indication of failed therapy. The patient should be made completely aware of this before initiation of therapy. We recommend that each patient have a baseline measurement of biochemical markers of bone remodeling before initiating therapy. The patient should be seen and clinically evaluated 6–8 weeks later to ascertain compliance and possible side effects from therapy. It would also be appropriate to repeat the biochemistry at this time to determine that there is indeed a decrease in the rate of bone remodeling. If there is no satisfactory change in the biochemistry, one should consider increasing the dose. If the dose of medication is changed for whatever reason, clinical and biochemical evaluation should be repeated in 6–8 weeks until a satisfactory response is achieved. If there is no response to 3 months of therapy, one should consider a change in medication. Studies confirming the scientific rationale for monitoring biochemical markers of bone remodeling have not been fully completed. However, available data suggest that the anticipated early (3 months or less) change in several of the markers, in response to successful therapy, is greater than the precision error of the biochemical measurement. This is in contrast to serial measurement of bone mineral density, for which even a good response to therapy cannot be detected within 1 year in most patients because the anticipated change is close to the precision limits of the methods. Furthermore, there is evidence that early (3 months) changes in biochemical markers reliably predict later (24 months) changes in bone mass. Most patients and their treating physicians are reluctant to take therapy for 12 months before measurable feedback is available, and this practical consideration may dictate the frequency with which biochemical markers are monitored. As far as is known, there are no ill effects of long-term use of calcitonin or alendronate in the treatment schedules described previously. Cost and convenience become important factors in long-term patient acceptance of these drugs. Because of the potential association between long-term estrogen therapy and development of endometrial and breast cancer, appropriate monitoring for these complications must be continued. Patients must be instructed in the technique of monthly breast self-examination and must undergo an annual examination by a clinician and an annual mammogram. All episodes of unexplained vaginal bleeding must be fully evaluated by a gynecologist. In women with an intact uterus, progesterone should be given along with estrogen; most patients will soon develop either amenorrhea or a stable, recognizable bleeding pattern, which should not give rise to concern or investigation.

It is important to reemphasize that drug therapy should never be substituted for the common-sense approaches to daily living discussed in some detail in earlier sections. This includes emphasizing safety and fall prevention and avoiding drugs such as sedatives, hypnotics, and antihypertensives, which might predispose to sedation, ataxia, or postural hypotension. Patients should all be encouraged to become involved in a regular active exercise/rehabilitation program. With appropriate medical, nursing, and rehabilitation care, most patients, except for those with the most advanced disease with multiple vertebral compression fractures, can be expected to be restored to reasonable functional health with a good quality of life. Likewise, an anticipated goal of therapy should be to prevent even the first osteoporotic fracture in patients whose therapy is initiated early.

REFERENCES

1. World Health Organization: Assessment of fracture risk and its application to screening for postmenopausal osteoporosis. Report of a WHO Study Group. *World Health Organ Tech Rep Ser* 843: 1–129, 1994
2. Villarcal DT, Civitelli R, Chines A, Avioli LV: Subclinical vitamin D deficiency in postmenopausal women with low vertebral bone mass. *J Clin Endocrinol Metab* 72:628–634, 1991
3. Garnero P, Shih WJ, Gineyts E, Karpf DB, Delmas PD: Comparison of new biochemical markers of bone turnover in late postmenopausal women in response to alendronate treatment. *J Clin Endocrinol Metab* 79:1693–1700, 1994
4. Lufkin EG, Wahner HW, O'Fallon WM, et al: Treatment of postmenopausal osteoporosis with transdermal estrogen. *Ann Intern Med* 117:1–9, 1992
5. Prince RL, Smith M, Dick IM, et al: Prevention of postmenopausal osteoporosis. Comparative study of exercise, calcium supplementation, and hormone replacement therapy. *N Engl J Med* 325:1189–1195, 1991

6. Civitelli R, Gonnelli S, Zacchei F, et al: Bone turnover in postmenopausal osteoporosis. *J Clin Invest* 82:1268–1274, 1988
7. Avioli LV: Heterogeneity of osteoporotic syndromes and the response to calcitonin therapy. *Calcif Tissue Int* 49(Suppl 2):S16–19, 1991
8. Rico H, Hernandez ER, Diaz-Mediaville J, et al: Treatment of multiple myeloma with nasal spray calcitonin: A histomorphometric and biochemical study. *Bone Miner* 8:231–237, 1990
9. Mazzuoli GF, Passeri M, Gennari C, et al: Effects of salmon calcitonin in postmenopausal osteoporosis: A controlled double-blind clinical study. *Calcif Tissue Int* 38:3–8, 1986
10. Overgaard K, Riis BJ, Christiansen C, et al: Effect of calcitonin given intranasally on early postmenopausal bone loss. *BMJ* 299: 477–479, 1989
11. Lyritis GP, Tsakalabos S, Magiasis B, et al: Analgesic effect of salmon calcitonin on osteoporotic vertebral fractures. Double-blind, placebo-controlled study. *Calcif Tissue Int* 49:369–372, 1991
12. Rico H, Hernandez ER, Revilla M, Gomez-Castresana F: Salmon calcitonin reduces vertebral fracture rate in the postmenopausal crush fracture syndrome. *Bone Miner* 16:131–138, 1992
13. Jones G, Nguyen T, Sambrook PN, Eisman JA: Thiazide diuretics and fractures: can meta-analysis help? *J Bone Miner Res* 10:106–111, 1995
14. Storm T, Thamsborg G, Steiniche T, Genant HK, Sorensen OH: Effect of intermittent cyclical etidronate therapy on bone mass and fracture rate in women with postmenopausal osteoporosis. *N Engl J Med* 322:1265–1271, 1990
15. Leiberman UA, Weiss SR, Broll J, et al: Effect of all alendronate on bone mineral density and the incidence of fracture in postmenopausal osteoporotic women. *N Engl J Med* 333:1437–1443, 1995
16. LaCroix AZ, Wienpahl J, White LR, et al: Thiazide diuretic agents and the incidence of hip fracture. *N Engl J Med* 322:286–290, 1990
17. Ott SM, Chesnut CH III: Calcitriol treatment is not effective in postmenopausal osteoporosis. *Ann Intern Med* 110:267–274, 1989
18. Watts NB, Harris ST, Genant HK, et al: Intermittent cyclical etidronate treatment of postmenopausal osteoporosis. *N Engl J Med* 323:73–79, 1990
19. Tilyard MW, Spears GFS, Thompson J, Dovey S: Treatment of postmenopausal osteoporosis with calcitriol or calcium. *N Engl J Med* 326:357–361, 1992
20. Overgaard K, Hansen MA, Nielsen V-AH, Riis BJ, Christiansen C: Discontinuous calcitonin treatment of established osteoporosis: Effects of withdrawal of treatment. *Am J Med* 89:1–6, 1990
21. Dawson-Hughes B, Dallal GE, Krall EA, Sadowski L, Sahyoun N, Tannenbau S: Controlled trial of the effect of calcium supplementation on bone density in postmenopausal women. *N Engl J Med* 323:878–883, 1990
22. Dawson-Hughes B: Calcium supplementation and bone loss: A review of controlled clinical trials. *Am J Clin Nutr* 54:274S–280S, 1991
23. Elders PJM, Netelenbos JC, Lips P, et al: Calcium supplementation reduces vertebral bone loss in perimenopausal women: A controlled trial in 248 women between 46 and 55 years of age. *J Clin Endocrinol Metab* 73:533–540, 1991
24. Licata AA, Jones-Gall DJ: Effect of supplemental calcium on serum and urinary calcium in osteoporotic patients. *J Am Coll Nutr* 11:164–167, 1992
25. Pak YC, Sakhaee K, Adams-Huet B, Piziak V, Peterson RD, Poindexter JR: Treatment of postmenopausal osteoporosis with slow-release sodium fluoride. Final report of a randomized controlled trial. *Ann Intern Med* 123:401–408, 1995
26. Hedlund LR, Gallagher JC: Increased incidences of fractures in osteoporosis patients treated with sodium fluoride. *J Bone Miner Res* 4:223–225, 1989
27. Martin BJ, Milligan K: Diuretic associated hypomagnesemia in the elderly. *Arch Intern Med* 147:1768–1771, 1987
28. Ray WA: Thiazide diuretics and osteoporosis: Time for a clinical trial? (Editorial). *Ann Intern Med* 115:64–65, 1991

50. The Special Problem of Hip Fracture

Eric S. Orwoll, M.D.

Department of Endocrinology and Metabolism, Portland Veterans Affairs Medical Center; and Department of Medicine, Oregon Health Sciences University, Portland, Oregon

Metabolic skeletal disorders are commonly generalized and may cause fracture of virtually any bone. Fractures of the proximal femur are unique. They are devastating both to the health of the affected individual as well as to society, and have been the focus of intense study. The understanding of their causation is more complete than for other complications of metabolic skeletal disease. They justifiably deserve special comment.

THE IMPORTANCE OF HIP FRACTURE

The public health impact of hip fracture is enormous. In 1990, there were more than 350,000 hip fractures in North America, more than 400,000 in Europe, and almost 600,000 in Asia (1). As the population increases and ages, these numbers will rise dramatically. The economic implications are obvious (2,3).

The effects of osteoporosis on individuals are equally impressive. In elderly women, there is a 12% to 30% reduction in expected survival after hip fracture (4), and the mortality rate is even greater in men (5). Age and prefracture condition are important indicators of outcome, as the increased mortality after hip fracture is probably the result of an interaction between preexisting conditions and the fracture itself (6,7). In addition to acute morbidity and mortality, hip fracture is commonly the precedent to prolonged or permanent dependency. Fifty percent of patients who survive the acute care of hip fracture are discharged to nursing homes, and 25% remain institutionalized 1 year later (8,9). Essentially permanent nursing home care is needed in an important fraction of patients (10). Not surprisingly, the determinants of function after recovery from hip fracture are complex, and include comorbid conditions as well as social context (11).

EPIDEMIOLOGY

Hip fracture is uncommon below the age of 50. When it occurs at younger ages, it is frequently the result of intense trauma or the presence of conditions known to affect skeletal health (12). Most hip fractures occur in the elderly, at a median age of approximately 80 years (6,13,14). In middle age, the incidence of hip fracture begins to rise rapidly, so that by age 50, the lifetime risk of hip fracture is 17% among U.S. women. The rise in the incidence of hip fracture is also dramatic in men, but it begins about a decade later, resulting in a fairly consistent male to female incidence ratio of roughly 1:2 in most developed countries (15,16). However, there is considerable geographic variation in the male to female ratio, with a complete reversal observed in some areas (14). Finally, there are pronounced racial effects on hip fracture rates, with blacks and Asians having lower fracture rates than whites (17–19).

CAUSATION

Skeletal Fragility

A convincing body of evidence links proximal femoral bone mass to the subsequent risk of hip fracture in women. An older woman with hip bone mineral density (BMD) 1 standard deviation (SD) below the mean is about seven times more likely to suffer a hip fracture than a woman with BMD 1 SD above the mean (20) (Fig. 1). Interestingly, BMD measures of the femoral neck do not predict femoral neck fracture risk in very elderly women (>80 years) (21), suggesting that in older age, factors other than bone mass become more prominent in the causation of fracture. Bone mineral density measures at other skeletal sites (spine, radius, calcaneus) also predict hip fracture risk, but with slightly less power (20) (Fig. 1).

Proximal femoral BMD is influenced by a wide variety of factors. Density increases rapidly during childhood and adolescence, and several variables have been found to influence the accumulation of peak bone mass (22), including heredity, gender, nutrition, mechanical forces, and hormonal factors. In turn, peak femoral bone mass appears to influence lifetime fracture risk. For instance, gender- and race-related differences in fracture risk can be traced in part to differences in adolescent skeletal development (22,23).

Bone mineral loss occurs from the proximal femur in adults of both sexes. There is presumed to be an accelerated phase of bone loss during the early postmenopausal period, and femoral BMD is higher in women who receive estrogen replacement (24). The rate of bone loss is similar in men and women after the age of 60 (25,26), and actually appears to accelerate in the oldest segment of the population (26,27). The determinants of femoral bone mass in adults are numerous, including body weight, gonadal status, activity and strength, nutrition (calcium, vitamin D), lifestyle (alcohol, caffeine, tobacco), and a variety of medications and medical conditions (7,21,26).

Although measures of bone mass provide valuable insight into skeletal fragility, other factors may also be important. This is an area of considerable research attention, but already it is apparent that several aspects of gross femoral structure (hip axis length, cortical thickness, trochanteric width, trabecular structure) independently influence fracture risk (28–33) (Fig. 2).

The likelihood of hip fracture appears to be related to the history of previous fragility fractures. For instance, a woman who has a prevalent vertebral fracture is about twice as likely to experience a subsequent hip fracture (34). To

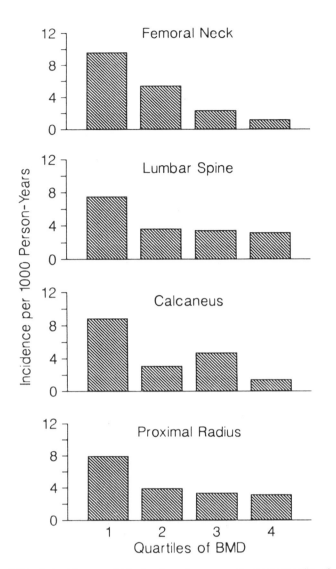

FIG. 1. Incidence of hip fracture by age-adjusted quartile of bone mineral density (BMD) (20).

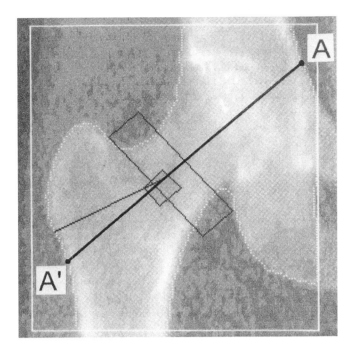

FIG. 2. Definition of the hip axis length (A-A′) from a dual-energy x-ray absorptiometry scan of the proximal femur (29).

some extent, this is the result of reduced bone mass, but there appears to be added risk independent of BMD, suggesting that other factors (skeletal structure, trauma propensity) may also be important.

The two major subtypes of hip fracture (femoral neck and trochanteric) have somewhat distinct epidemiologic patterns and clinical character (35,36), suggesting different etiologies (Table 1). In general, trochanteric fractures occur relatively more frequently in older women, are associated with lower trochanteric and higher femoral neck BMD, are less strongly associated with a maternal history of femoral fracture, and occur more frequently in patients who have experienced other osteoporotic fractures. On the other hand, fall characteristics, body habitus, and hip axis length have been found to be similar in the two kinds of fractures (35,37).

Osteoporosis is the major metabolic disorder underlying skeletal fragility, but osteomalacia also has been found in a minority of patients with hip fracture. This is particularly true in the elderly with restricted nutrition and sunlight exposure. For unclear reasons, in the last 10–15 years the prevalence of osteomalacia in patients with hip fracture appears to have declined (38).

Trauma

As opposed to vertebral fractures, the vast majority of hip fractures in the elderly occur as a direct result of falls (7). Even an uncomplicated fall from a standing height generates enough force to fracture an elderly femur (39). Factors that increase the likelihood of falls are important determinants of hip fracture risk (7,21,40), including drugs or medications (sedatives, alcohol, antidepressants), muscle weakness, disorders of gait and balance (neuromuscular impairment, visual dysfunction), cognitive impairment, and environmental hazards. The contribution of fall propensity to the risk of hip fractures is as important as that of skeletal fragility, and may be more important in the most elderly.

TABLE 1. *Fracture type*

Characteristic	Trochanteric	Femoral neck
More likely in older women	X	
Lower trochanteric bone mineral density	X	
Osteoporotic fractures common	X	
Maternal hip fracture		X
Falling increases risk	X	X
More likely in thin subjects	X	X
Greater hip axis length	X	X

In addition to the frequency of falls, the character of the fall is crucial in defining fracture risk. Whereas approximately one third of the elderly fall each year, only a small fraction experience hip fracture. A fall to the side, particularly in tall and thin individuals, is much more likely to cause a fracture (7,31). Falls associated with fractures most often occur in frail individuals, with little ability to protect themselves from direct impact on the trochanter. Women are more likely to fall on a hip than are men (41).

TREATMENT

Virtually all proximal femoral fractures require surgical fixation and an intense (and often prolonged) period of rehabilitation. During this time, there is considerable risk of additional bone loss (42) and other complications. Delayed union and femoral head avascular necrosis are notorious, especially in femoral neck fractures, and osteoporotic bone is particularly susceptible to added problems (43). During the immediate postoperative period, attention to factors that promote the rehabilitation process is important. For instance, many elderly who experience a hip fracture are not well nourished, a problem that can be exacerbated during the postoperative inpatient stay. Nutritional supplementation during this time has reduced hospital-associated complications and mortality (44). This regimen should include adequate vitamin D and calcium supplementation (45). Early restoration of mobility is preferred to preserve as much function as possible.

PREVENTION

Current efforts to prevent hip fracture have focused on maximizing proximal femoral biomechanical strength and reducing fall propensity. In both areas, there are as yet insufficient long-term data. In men, there have been no trials of strategies to prevent fracture.

In women, postmenopausal estrogen replacement has been shown reliably to reduce the risk of hip fracture (24). Other drugs are less well demonstrated as effective (46). Dietary calcium and vitamin D supplementation have reduced hip fracture risk dramatically in some frail older women (47). The effectiveness of some other potentially useful interventions (calcitonin, anabolic steroids, bisphosphonates, parathyroid hormone) has not been adequately documented (48).

The prevention of falls in the elderly is also important. Strength and balance can be improved quickly and dramatically in the elderly with appropriate exercise regimens, and successful programs for the reduction of falls in the elderly have been described (49). Such mundane apparatus as hip pads and cushioned floors in high-risk environments (e.g., nursing homes) may be quite effective (50). It is important to identify those at highest risk, to whom the most intensive preventive interventions should be directed.

REFERENCES

1. Cooper C, Campion G, Melton LJ III: Hip fractures in the elderly: A world-wide projection. *Osteoporosis Int* 2:285–289, 1992
2. Norris RJ: Medical costs of osteoporosis. *Bone* 13:S11–S16, 1992
3. Barrett-Connor E: The economic and human costs of osteoporotic fracture. *Am J Med* 98:2A-3S–7S, 1995
4. Cummings SR, Kelsey JL, Nevitt MC, O'Dowd KJ: Epidemiology of osteoporosis and osteoporotic fractures. *Epidemiol Rev* 7:178–208, 1985
5. Jacobsen SJ, Goldberg J, Miles TP, Brody JA, Stiers W, Rimm AA: Race and sex differences in mortality following fracture of the hip. *Am J Public Health* 82:1147–1150, 1992
6. Keene GS, Parker MJ, Pryor GA: Mortality and morbidity after hip fractures. *BMJ* 307:1248–1250, 1993
7. Nevitt MC: Epidemiology of osteoporosis. *Rheum Dis Clin North Am* 20:535–559, 1994
8. Ray WA, Griffin MR, Baugh DK: Mortality following hip fracture before and after implementation of the prospective payment system. *Arch Intern Med* 150:2109–2114, 1990
9. Palmer RM: The impact of the prospective payment system on the treatment of hip fractures in the elderly. *Arch Intern Med* 149:2237–2241, 1989
10. Chrischilles EA, Butler CD, Davis CS, Wallace RB: A model of lifetime osteoporosis impact. *Arch Intern Med* 151:2026–2032, 1991
11. Weatherall M: Case mix and outcome for patients with fracture of the proximal femur. *N Z Med J* 106:451–452, 1993
12. Gray AJR, Parker MJ: Intracapsular fractures of the femoral neck in young patients. *Injury* 25:667–669, 1994
13. Cummings SR: Are patients with hip fractures more osteoporotic? *Am J Med* 78:487–494, 1985
14. Elffors I, Allander E, Kanis JA, Gullberg B, Johnell O, Dequeker J, Dilsen G, Gennari C, Lopes Vaz AA, Lyritis G, Mazzuoli GF, Miravet L, Passeri M, Perez Cano R, Rapado A, Ribot C: The variable incidence of hip fracture in southern Europe: The MEDOS Study. *Osteoporosis Int* 4:253–263, 1994
15. Jones G, Nguyen T, Sambrook PN, Kelly PJ, Gilbert C, Eisman JA: Symptomatic fracture incidence in elderly men and women: The Dubbo Osteoporosis Epidemiology Study (DOES). *Osteoporosis Int* 4:277–282, 1994
16. Jacobsen SJ, Goldberg J, Miles TP, Brody JA, Stiers W, Rimm AA: Hip fracture incidence among the old and very old: A population-based study of 745,435 cases. *Am J Public Health* 80:871–873, 1990
17. Farmer ME, White LR, Brody JA, Bailey KR: Race and sex differences in hip fracture incidence. *Am J Public Health* 74:1374–1380, 1984
18. Ross PD, Norimatsu H, Davis JW, Yano K, Wasnich RD, Fujiwara S, Hosoda Y, Melton LJ III: A comparison of hip fracture incidence among native Japanese, Japanese Americans, and American Caucasians. *Am J Epidemiol* 133:801–809, 1991
19. Cummings SR, Cauley JA, Palermo L, Ross PD, Wasnich RD, Black D, Faulkner KG: Racial differences in hip axis lengths might explain racial differences in the rates of hip fracture. *Osteoporosis Int* 4:226–229, 1994
20. Cummings SR, Black DM, Nevitt MC, Browner W, Cauley J, Ensrud K, Genant HK, Palermo L, Scott J, Vogt TM, S.O.F. Research Group: Bone density at various sites for prediction of hip fractures. *Lancet* 341:72–75, 1993
21. Cummings SR, Black D: Bone mass measurements and risk of fracture in Caucasian women: A review of findings from prospective studies. *Am J Med* 98:2A-24S–28S, 1995
22. Bonjour JP, Theintz G, Law F, Slosman D, Rizzoli R: Peak bone mass. *Osteoporosis Int* 1:S7–S13, 1994
23. Gilsanz V, Roe TF, Mora S: Changes in vertebral bone density in black girls and white girls during childhood and puberty. *N Engl J Med* 325:1597–1600, 1991
24. Cauley JA, Seeley DA, Ensrud K, Ettinger B, Black D, Cummings SR: Estrogen replacement therapy and fractures in older women. *Ann Intern Med* 122:9–16, 1995
25. Hannan MT, Felson DT, Anderson JJ: Bone mineral density in elderly men and women: Results from the Framingham osteoporosis study. *J Bone Miner Res* 7:547–553, 1992
26. Jones G, Nguyen T, Sambrook P, Kelly PJ, Eisman JA: Progressive loss of bone in the femoral neck in elderly people: Longitudinal findings from the Dubbo osteoporosis epidemiology study. *BMJ* 309:691–695, 1994
27. Orwoll ES, Oviatt SK, McClung MR, Deftos LJ, Sexton G: The rate of bone mineral loss in normal men and the effects of calcium and cholecalciferol supplementation. *Ann Intern Med* 112:29–34, 1990
28. Gluer CC, Cummings SR, Pressman A, Li J, Gluer K, Faulkner

KG, Grampp S, Genant HK: Prediction of hip fractures from pelvic radiographs: The Study of Osteoporotic Fractures. *J Bone Miner Res* 9:671–677, 1994

29. Faulkner KG, McClung M, Cummings SR: Automated evaluation of hip axis length for predicting hip fracture. *J Bone Miner Res* 9:1065–1070, 1994

30. Reid IR, Chin K, Evans MC, Jones JG: Relation between increase in length of hip axis in older women between 1950s and 1990s and increase in age specific rates of hip fracture. *BMJ* 309:508–509, 1994

31. Hayes WC, Piazza SJ, Zysset PK: Biomechanics of fracture risk prediction of the hip and spine by quantitative computed tomography. *Radiol Clin North Am* 29:1–18, 1991

32. Genant HK, Gluer C-C, Lotz JC: Gender differences in bone density, skeletal geometry, and fracture biomechanics. *Radiology* 190:636–640, 1994

33. Mazess RB: Fracture risk: A role for compact bone. *Calcif Tissue Int* 47:191–193, 1990

34. Kotowicz MA, Melton LJ III, Cooper C, Atkinson EJ, O'Fallon WM, Riggs BL: Risk of hip fracture in women with vertebral fracture. *J Bone Miner Res* 9:599–605, 1994

35. Greenspan SL, Myers ER, Maitland LA, Kido TH, Krasnow MB, Hayes WC: Trochanteric bone mineral density is associated with type of hip fracture in the elderly. *J Bone Miner Res* 9:1889–1894, 1994

36. Baudoin C, Fardellone P, Sebert J-L: Effect of sex and age on the ratio of cervical to trochanteric hip fracture. *Acta Orthop Scand* 64:647–653, 1993

37. Mautalen CA, Vega EM: Different characteristics of cervical and trochanteric hip fractures. *Osteoporos Int* 3 (Suppl 1):102–105, 1993

38. Robinson CM, McQueen MM, Wheelwright EF, Gardner DL, Salter DM: Changing prevalence of osteomalacia in hip fractures in southeast Scotland over a 20-year period. *Injury* 23:300–302, 1992

39. Greenspan SL, Myers ER, Maitland LA, Resnick NM, Hayes WC: Fall severity and bone mineral density as risk factors for hip fracture in ambulatory elderly. *JAMA* 271:128–133, 1994

40. Grisso JA, Kelsey JL, Strom BL, O'Brien LA, Maislin G, LaPann K, Samelson L, Hoffman S: Risk factors for hip fracture in black women. *N Engl J Med* 330:1555–1559, 1994

41. O'Neill TW, Varlow J, Silman AJ, Reeve J, Reid DM, Todd C, Woolf AD: Age and sex influences on fall characteristics. *Ann Rheum Dis* 53:773–775, 1994

42. McCarthy CK, Steinberg GG, Agren M, Leahey D, Wyman E, Baran DT: Quantifying bone loss from the proximal femur after total hip arthroplasty. *J Bone Joint Surg* 73-B:774–778, 1991

43. Cornell CN: Management of fractures in patients with osteoporosis. *Orthop Clin North Am* 21:125–141, 1990

44. Delmi M, Rapin CH, Bengoa JM, Delmas PD, Vasey H, Bonjour JP: Clinical practice: Dietary supplementation in elderly patients with fractured neck of the femur. *Lancet* 335:1013–1016, 1990

45. Ng K, St John A, Bruce DG: Secondary hyperparathyroidism, vitamin D deficiency and hip fracture: Importance of sampling times after fracture. *Bone Miner* 25:103–109, 1994

46. Kanis JA, Johnell O, Gullberg B, Allander E, Dilsen G, Gennari C, Lopes Vaz AA, Lyritis GP, Mazzuoli G, Miravet L, Passeri M, Perez Cano R, Rapado A, Ribot C: Evidence for efficacy of drugs affecting bone metabolism in preventing hip fracture. *BMJ* 305:1124–1128, 1992

47. Chapuy MC, Arlot ME, Duboeuf F, Brun J, Crouzet B, Arnaud S, Delmas PD, Meunier PJ: Vitamin D₃ and calcium to prevent hip fractures in elderly women. *N Engl J Med* 327:1637–1642, 1992

48. Kanis JA: Treatment of osteoporosis in elderly women. *Am J Med* 98:2A-60S–66S, 1995

49. Tinetti ME, Baker DI, McAvay G, Clasu EB, Garrett P, Gottschalk M: A multifactorial intervention to reduce the risk of falling among elderly people in the community. *N Engl J Med* 331:821–827, 1994

50. Lauritzen JB, Petersen MM, Lund B: Effect of external hip protectors on hip fractures. *Lancet* 341:11–13, 1993

51. Juvenile Osteoporosis

Michael E. Norman, M.D.

Department of Pediatrics, University of North Carolina School of Medicine, Chapel Hill, North Carolina

The diagnosis of osteoporosis in children is usually made when skeletal radiographs reveal a generalized decrease in mineralized bone (e.g., osteopenia) in the absence of rickets or excessive bone resorption (e.g., osteitis fibrosa). Juvenile osteoporosis occurs typically before the onset of puberty, but it may also be seen in younger children, especially when they are growing rapidly. It may be due to an inherited condition that is clinically evident from birth or early infancy, or it may be acquired during childhood. There are a primary or idiopathic form and a number of secondary forms of juvenile osteoporosis. The condition is uncommon; between 1939 and 1991, ~60 cases of idiopathic juvenile osteoporosis (IJO) were reported in the literature. However, the onset of osteoporosis just before or after the onset of puberty can have far-reaching effects, because one half of skeletal mass is acquired during the adolescent years.

PATHOPHYSIOLOGY

True osteoporosis is defined histomorphometrically by a decreased total amount of normally formed bone. During bone formation (modeling) and bone remodeling, two fundamental defects may occur, singly or in combination: (i) a defect in bone-forming cells leading to decreased or defective matrix formation; and (ii) abnormalities in the coupling of bone formation and resorption, in which an imbalance develops between matrix formation (mineralization) and bone resorption. An inherited group of disorders known as osteogenesis imperfecta usually represents defects in bone-forming cells, in which mutations in one of the two genes encoding type I procollagen produce defective matrix (see Chapter 70). IJO and the secondary causes of osteoporosis represent various expressions of the latter type of defect. IJO and chronic corticosteroid therapy are the most important forms of acquired juvenile osteoporosis. Early reports of calcium balance have suggested that IJO changes, with initially negative or inappropriately neutral balances (1,2), progressing to positive balance during the healing phase (2,3) and in response to vitamin D administration. Jowsey and Johnson (4) and Hoekman et al. (5) presented histologic evidence of increased bone resorption, whereas Smith (6) and Reed et al. (7) found decreased bone formation as the major pathophysiologic event in IJO. Evans et al. (8) and Marder et al. (9) suggested a role for 1,25-dihydroxyvitamin D deficiency in the pathogenesis of IJO. Several reports have also suggested a role for calcitonin deficiency in some patients (10). The bone loss noted in astronauts undergoing prolonged periods of weightlessness in space may be analogous to IJO, with rapid resorption of weight-bearing bones and suppressed bone formation. Both weightlessness and IJO appear to be reversible (6). Some have speculated that IJO, like weightlessness, consists of some fundamental disturbance in the mechanical forces that stimulate new bone formation in the growing and young adult skeleton. Finally, recent data in adult osteoporotic patients suggest impaired bone formation related in part to reduced insulin-like growth factor 1 secretion (7).

CLINICAL FEATURES

The typical child presenting with IJO is immediately prepubertal and healthy. Symptoms begin with an insidious onset of pain in the lower back, hips, and feet, and difficulty walking. Knee and ankle pain and fractures of the lower extremities may be present. IJO affects both sexes equally; family and dietary histories are negative. Physical examination may be entirely normal or reveal thoracolumbar kyphosis or kyphoscoliosis, pigeon chest deformity, crown-pubis to pubis-heel ratio of less than 1.0, loss of height, deformities of the long bones, and limp. Generally, these physical abnormalities are reversible, although several of the original patients subsequently developed crippling deformities that left them wheelchair bound with cardiorespiratory abnormalities (1).

The history and physical examination of children with secondary forms of osteoporosis reflect the primary disease more than the osteoporosis (Table 1). There is usually a family history of osteoporosis or of the primary disease, evidence of failure to thrive, immobilization, or administration of corticosteroid or anticonvulsant drugs.

BIOCHEMICAL FEATURES

There are no known biochemical abnormalities characteristic of IJO, and no known endocrine disorder has been identified. In some children (1,2,5), calcium balance is markedly negative or inappropriately neutral, and serum calcium levels are normal. Urine calcium excretion may be normal or elevated. Serum phosphorus, bicarbonate, magnesium, and alkaline phosphatase levels are also normal. The disease eventually resolves with time and the onset of puberty, and can be detected by improvement in calcium balance. Increased urinary hydroxyproline excretion, an indirect indicator of increased bone resorption, as well as hypercalcemia and suppressed parathyroid hormone secretion have been observed in some patients. Suppression of parathyroid hormone secretion reduces 1,25-dihydroxyvitamin D synthesis and decreases intestinal calcium absorption, contributing to the negative calcium balance (5).

In secondary forms of osteoporosis, biochemical and clinical clues to diagnosis depend on the underlying primary disease (2,8).

TABLE 1. *Differential diagnosis of juvenile osteoporosis*

I. Primary
   Calcium deficiency
   Idiopathic juvenile osteoporosis
   Osteogenesis imperfecta
      Multiple subtypes
II. Secondary
   Endocrine
      Cushing syndrome
      Diabetes mellitus
      Glucocorticoid therapy
      Thyrotoxicosis
   Gastrointestinal
      Biliary atresia
      Glycogen storage disease, type I
      Hepatitis
      Malabsorption
   Inborn errors of metabolism
      Homocystinuria
      Lysinuric protein intolerance
   Miscellaneous
      Acute lymphoblastic leukemia
      Anticonvulsant therapy
      Cyanotic congenital heart disease
      Immobilization

RADIOLOGIC FEATURES

Conventional radiography is a relatively insensitive method for detecting bone loss; ~30% of skeletal mineral must be lost before osteopenia can be appreciated. In the absence of fractures or rickets, osteomalacia may be difficult to distinguish from osteoporosis as the cause of osteopenia. Looser lines or changes of secondary hyperparathyroidism favor rickets or osteomalacia, whereas biconcave vertebral deformities favor osteoporosis (see Chapter 24). Children with fully expressed IJO present with generalized osteopenia, fractures of the weight-bearing bones, and collapsed or misshapen vertebrae. Disc spaces may be widened asymmetrically because of wedging of the vertebral bodies (Fig. 1). Sclerosis may be noted. Long bones are usually normal in length and cortical width, unlike the thin, gracile bones of children with osteogenesis imperfecta (see Chapter 70). The pathognomonic x-ray finding of IJO is neo-osseous osteoporosis, an impaction-type fracture occurring at sites of newly formed weight-bearing metaphyseal bone. Typically, such fractures are seen at the distal tibiae, adjacent to the ankle joint and adjacent to the knee and hip joints (2,6). Using photon absorptiometry and computed tomography for detection of decreased bone mineral density, childhood osteoporosis may be diagnosed much earlier.

BONE BIOPSY

Few qualitative or quantitative studies of bone tissue have been performed in childhood osteoporosis. From microradiographs of bone, Cloutier et al. (3) and Jowsey and Johnson (4) reported increased bone resorption in IJO. They speculated that excessive dietary phosphorus intake may have stimulated parathyroid-mediated bone resorption. In contrast, Smith (6), using quantitative static histology of iliac

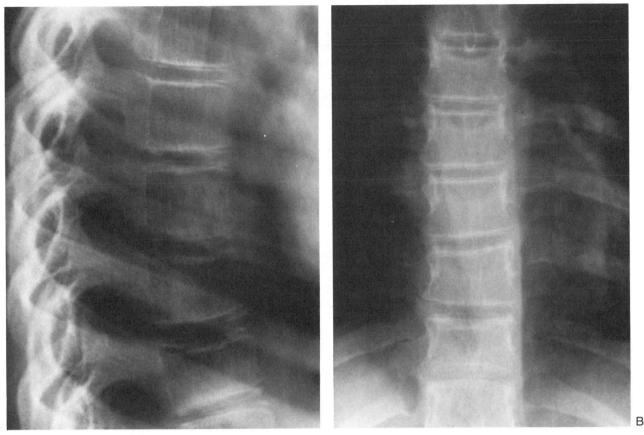

A   B

FIG. 1. A 10-year-old white female with back pain. **A:** Lateral view of thoracolumbar spine reveals wedge compression fracture of T8 and T9 with patchy sclerosis of T7. There was generalized osteopenia of the skeleton, confirmed by computed tomography. **B:** Anterior view of the same patient reveals loss of height of T8 on the right side. The vertebral bodies are osteopenic.

bone, found indirect evidence of decreased bone formation. Evans et al. (8) found no abnormalities of endosteal bone formation by histomorphometry (using double tetracycline labeling) in a 12-year-old boy with severe IJO. They suggested that the major evidence for impaired periosteal new bone formation in IJO would come from careful study of skeletal radiographs and not from bone biopsy material.

DIFFERENTIAL DIAGNOSIS

Osteogenesis imperfecta is the most important entity to consider in the differential diagnosis of IJO (12). Comparisons with IJO are listed in Table 2 (see Chapter 70). Osteogenesis imperfecta can usually be differentiated from IJO by clinical characteristics, radiologic findings, and a positive family history. Diseases resulting in osteoporosis in childhood that must be differentiated from IJO are outlined in Table 1. Secondary causes of osteoporosis must be excluded in those children who present without the typical features of IJO. As a result, the diagnosis of IJO is reached by excluding secondary causes of osteoporosis and osteogenesis imperfecta.

THERAPY

Prompt and definitive diagnosis early in the course of the disease is important, although there is no specific medical or surgical therapy. Supportive care is instituted promptly (non-weight-bearing, crutch walking, and physical therapy) in anticipation of spontaneous recovery with the onset of puberty. There may be a role for supplemental calcitriol therapy in selected patients (8,9). Sodium fluoride increases bone mass and has been reported to reduce fracture rates in primary vertebral osteoporosis (13). Fluoride treatment has been associated with a number of toxicity symptoms and musculoskeletal complaints in adults, and it remains unclear whether the hyperosteoidosis associated with this therapy produces increased bone strength. The author has used long-term fluoride therapy with a positive clinical response in one patient with IJO *(unpublished observations)*. Based on findings of decreased bone resorption on bone biopsy in one child, Hoekman et al. (5) reported dramatic clinical, biochemical, and radiologic responses with bisphosphonate, which inhibits bone resorption. Osteoporosis in most patients is reversible. Treatment of secondary causes of osteoporosis requires careful management of the underlying disease to minimize bone loss.

PROGNOSIS

With the exception of a few patients who develop progressive lower-extremity, spine, and chest-wall deformities and require confinement to wheelchairs or bed, the progno-

TABLE 2. *Differential diagnosis: osteogenesis imperfecta (OI) vs. idiopathic juvenile osteoporosis (IJO)*

Characteristic	OI	IJO
Family history	Often positive	Negative
Age at onset	Birth	2–3 yr before puberty
Duration of signs/symptoms	Lifelong (intermittent)	1–4 yr
Physical findings	Thin gracile bones, short stature	Upper-lower segment ratio <1.0
	Multiple deformities and contractures	Dorsal kyphoscoliosis
	Blue sclerae[a], deafness	Pectus carinatum
	Lax joints, hernias	Abnormal gait
	Abnormal dentition	
Calcium balance	Positive	Negative in acute phase
Radiologic findings	Narrow long bones	Long bones with thin cortices
	Thin ribs	Wedge compression fractures of spine
	Pathologic fractures, rarely metaphyseal in location	Metaphyseal fractures common
	Wormian skull bones	
Molecular studies (dermal fibroblasts)	Abnormal collagen	Normal collagen

[a]Classic dominant inherited form, with associated nerve deafness.

sis of IJO is generally excellent. Distinguishing features have been recognized that identify the subgroup of children with poor prognosis. The prognosis of osteogenesis imperfecta is dependent on the inherited subtype and is discussed in Chapter 70. The most effective treatment of secondary osteoporosis is successful therapy of the underlying disease. Failing this, supportive care should be provided as with IJO.

REFERENCES

1. Dent CE, Friedman M: Idiopathic juvenile osteoporosis. *Q J Med* 34:177–210, 1965
2. Brenton DP, Dent CE: Idiopathic juvenile osteoporosis. In: Bickel JH, Stern J (eds) *Inborn Errors of Calcium and Bone Metabolism.* Baltimore, University Park Press, pp 223–238, 1976
3. Cloutier MD, Hayles AB, Riggs BL, Jowsey J, Bickel WH: Juvenile osteoporosis: Report of a case including a description of some metabolic and microradiographic studies. *Pediatrics* 40: 649–655, 1967
4. Jowsey J, Johnson KA: Juvenile osteoporosis: Bone findings in seven patients. *J Pediatr* 81:511–517, 1972
5. Hoekman K, Papapoulos SE, Peters ACB, Bijvoet OL: Characteristics and bisphosphonate treatment of a patient with juvenile osteoporosis. *J Clin Endocrinol Metab* 61:952–956, 1985
6. Smith R: Idiopathic osteoporosis in the young. *J Bone Joint Surg* 62-B:417–427, 1980
7. Reed BY, Zeswekh JE, Sakhaee K, Breslau N, Gottschalk F, Pak CYC: Serum IGF-I is low and correlated with osteoblastic surface in idiopathic osteoporosis. *J Bone Miner Res* 10:1218–1224, 1995
8. Evans RA, Dunstan CR, Hills E: Bone metabolism in idiopathic juvenile osteoporosis: A case report. *Calcif Tissue Int* 35:5–8, 1983
9. Marder HK, Tsang RC, Hug G, Crawford AC: Calcitriol deficiency in idiopathic juvenile osteoporosis. *Am J Dis Child* 136: 914–917, 1982
10. Saggese G, Bertelloni S, Baroncelli GI, Perri G, Calderazzi A: Mineral metabolism and calcitriol therapy in idiopathic juvenile osteoporosis. *Am J Dis Child* 145:457–461, 1991
11. Jackson EC, Strife CF, Tsang RC, Marder HK: Effect of calcitonin replacement therapy in idiopathic juvenile osteoporosis. *Am J Dis Child* 142:1237–1239, 1988
12. Teotia M, Teotia SPS, Singh RK: Idiopathic juvenile osteoporosis. *Am J Dis Child* 133:894–900, 1979
13. Harrison JE: Fluoride treatment for osteoporosis. *Calcif Tissue Int* 46:287–288, 1990

52. Glucocorticoid and Drug-Induced Osteoporosis

Barbara P. Lukert, M.D., F.A.C.P.

Department of Medicine, University of Kansas Medical Center, Kansas City, Kansas

Glucocorticoid-induced bone loss has been recognized since Cushing described osteoporosis as a component of the constellation of findings in patients with hypercortisolism due to adrenocorticotropic hormone–producing pituitary tumors. The problem received little attention until cortisone was used to treat rheumatoid arthritis. These patients showed dramatic improvement in the inflammatory component of their disease, but within a year a striking percentage developed vertebral compression fractures. We are now very familiar with the rapid bone loss that occurs in patients taking glucocorticoids for the management of a number of diseases.

Glucocorticoids have a greater effect on trabecular bone than on cortical bone, hence bone loss is most rapid and fractures are most likely in vertebrae, ribs, and the ends of long bones. Bone is lost at a very rapid rate during the first year of therapy, with reports of losses as great as 20% in 1 year (1).

The true incidence of osteoporosis-related fractures in patients taking steroids for more than 6 months is unknown, but available data suggest that the incidence is between 30% and 50% (2). Even low doses of steroids, including inhaled steroids, cause bone loss, but the precise dose below which bone is not affected remains unclear. It appears that doses of prednisone exceeding 7.5 mg/day (or equivalent doses of other steroids) cause significant loss of trabecular bone in most people.

All patients—young and old, men and women, and all races—are susceptible to steroid-induced bone loss. Young people who have a high rate of bone remodeling appear to be particularly susceptible. Deceleration of growth and reduced total body calcium have been reported in children treated with glucocorticoids, even when only inhaled steroids are used. Although longitudinal studies are not available, children treated with glucocorticoids are not likely to achieve an optimum peak bone mass, thus becoming at greater risk for osteoporosis-related fractures in adulthood. Postmenopausal women are at greater risk for fractures, presumably because they have preexisting age-related and menopause-related bone loss.

EFFECTS OF GLUCOCORTICOIDS

A multitude of systemic and local effects of glucocorticoids on bone and mineral metabolism lead to a very rapid acceleration of bone loss (Fig. 1).

Histomorphometry

Bone histomorphometry shows a reduction in mean wall thickness of trabecular bone packets, low mineral apposition rate, elevation of parameters of bone resorption, suppression of osteoblastic recruitment, and depression of mature osteoblast function. The total amount of bone replaced in each remodeling cycle is reduced by 30%. There appears to be a shortening of the life span of the active osteoblast population in each basic multicellular unit (3).

Effect on Osteoblasts and Bone Formation

Physiologic concentrations of glucocorticoids enhance the function of differentiated osteoblasts and increase collagen synthesis (4). However, prolonged exposure to supraphysiologic concentrations inhibits synthetic processes (5). Cell replication is decreased after 48 hours of exposure; thus, prolonged inhibition of bone formation may be due in part to a decrease in proliferation of periosteal precursor cells (6). There is an additional direct inhibitory effect on differentiation of osteoblasts for collagen synthesis and on osteocalcin production (7,8).

Effect on Bone Resorption

Glucocorticoids have a biphasic effect on osteoclasts. Physiologic concentrations are required for the late stages of differentiation and function, whereas the generation of new osteoclasts involving cell replication is inhibited by high doses and prolonged exposure. Resorption is stimulated by glucocorticoids in fetal rat parietal bones *in vitro* (9). Glucocorticoids can enhance the attachment of macrophages to bone by altering cell surface oligosaccharides.

Glucocorticoid-induced enhanced resorption observed *in vivo* may be due in large part to secondary hyperparathyroidism. Secondary hyperparathyroidism increases the birth rate of bone-remodeling units and probably also increases the amount of bone resorbed at each site. Animal experiments have shown that the increase in resorption can be prevented by parathyroidectomy.

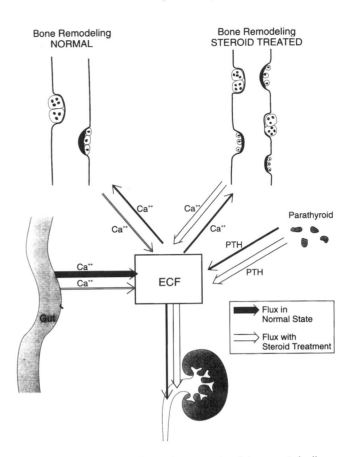

FIG. 1. Effect of steroids on bone and calcium metabolism. Glucocorticoids inhibit gastrointestinal absorption and increase renal excretion of calcium. Negative calcium balance and perhaps failure to transport calcium into the parathyroid cell cause an increase in secretion of PTH. PTH increases the number of sites undergoing bone remodeling. Glucocorticoids inhibit osteoblastic bone formation at each site. The combination of an increased number of sites undergoing remodeling and a decrease in bone formation at each site causes rapid bone loss.

Effect on Sex Hormones

Glucocorticoids inhibit pituitary secretion of gonadotropins, ovarian and testicular secretion of estrogen and testosterone, and adrenal secretion of androstenedione and dehydroepiandrosterone (10,11). Because these hormones decrease bone resorption, their absence accelerates glucocorticoid-induced bone loss.

Intestinal Absorption and Renal Excretion of Calcium

Most patients taking pharmacologic doses of glucocorticoids have impaired active transcellular transport of calcium. The exact mechanisms are poorly understood, but are partially independent of vitamin D. Intestinal absorption and renal tubular reabsorption of calcium are significantly impaired in patients taking glucocorticoids, and these abnormalities may play an important role in the development of secondary hyperparathyroidism (12,13). Fasting urinary calcium excretion and parathyroid hormone (PTH) levels are elevated in normal subjects receiving glucocorticoids for only 5 days. The origin is probably twofold: increased skeletal mobilization and decreased tubular reabsorption that occurs despite elevated parathyroid hormone (PTH). The transport defect is made worse by high sodium intake and is decreased by sodium restriction and thiazide diuretics (14).

Effect on Parathyroid Hormone and Vitamin D Metabolism

The effects of glucocorticoids on serum concentrations of PTH and the vitamin D metabolites remain controversial. Both high and low levels of 25-hydroxyvitamin D (25(OH)D) have been reported. The discrepancies are probably due to variations in dietary intake and sunlight exposure rather than to steroid-induced changes in absorption or metabolism of vitamin D. Both PTH and 1,25-dihydroxyvitamin D [1,25(OH)$_2$D] levels in serum are higher in glucocorticoid-treated patients with asthma than in age-matched controls, despite higher calcium levels (15). This suggests that there may be a change in cell calcium receptors resulting in altered transport of calcium.

Glucocorticoids enhance the sensitivity of osteoblasts to PTH, and PTH-mediated inhibition of alkaline phosphatase activity, collagen synthesis, and citrate decarboxylation are all potentiated by glucocorticoids. The sensitivity to renal tubule effects of PTH are also increased by glucocorticoids.

Many of the actions of 1,25(OH)$_2$D are inhibited by glucocorticoids even though 1,25(OH)$_2$D levels are elevated. The inhibition may be mediated by both alterations in membrane response to vitamin D and receptor changes. The effect of glucocorticoids on calcitriol receptors depends on the species and growth phase of cell cultures. Glucocorticoids down-regulate the receptor in mouse osteoblasts but up-regulate the receptor in rats. The expression by osteoblasts of osteocalcin, the major noncollagenous bone protein, is stimulated by 1,25(OH)$_2$D and inhibited by glucocorticoids (16).

Effect of Glucocorticoids on Prostaglandins, Cytokines, and Growth Factors

Prostaglandins

Glucocorticoids inhibit the production of prostaglandins, particularly PGE$_2$, in bone (17). The major long-term effect of PGE$_2$ on bone in organ culture is to stimulate collagen and noncollagen protein synthesis. When PGE$_2$ is added to bones treated with glucocorticoids, the glucocorticoid-induced decrease in cell replication and collagen synthesis is partially reversed. Glucocorticoid effects cannot be explained entirely on the basis of low prostaglandin levels because the effect cannot be reproduced by inhibition of prostaglandin synthesis with nonsteroidal drugs such as indomethacin.

Cytokines

Interleukin-1 (IL-1) and interleukin-6 (IL-6) induce bone resorption and inhibit bone formation. It is unlikely that these cytokines play a major role in glucocorticoid-induced bone loss because their production by T-lymphocytes is inhibited by glucocorticoids, and both the bone-resorbing activity and the inhibitory effect of IL-1 on collagen synthesis are partially inhibited by cortisol.

Growth Factors

The growth hormone–dependent peptide, insulin-like growth factor 1 (IGF-1) or somatomedin C, is synthesized by bone cells and stimulates bone cell replication and collagen synthesis (18). Pharmacologic doses of cortisol inhibit synthesis of IGF-1 by fetal rat calvaria. Glucocorticoids also affect IGF-binding proteins (IGFBP), which inhibit or enhance IGF activity (19). The composite effect of glucocorticoids is to decrease IGFBP-5, which enhances the anabolic effect of the IGF system, and to increase IGFBP-3 and IGFBP-4, which inhibit anabolic effects.

Transforming growth factor beta (TGF-ß) enhances osteoblast replication and bone matrix protein synthesis. Glucocorticoids decrease these anabolic effects by redistributing the binding of TGF-ß1 toward extracellular matrix storage sites and away from receptors involved in intracellular signal transduction.

Osteonecrosis

Osteonecrosis (also known as aseptic or avascular necrosis) is a serious complication of steroid therapy. It occurs in 4% to 25% of patients receiving glucocorticoid therapy. The hip, head of the humerus, and distal femur are most frequently affected. Possible mechanisms for etiology include a vascular theory, proposing that ischemia is caused by microscopic fat emboli; a mechanical theory that attributes ischemic collapse of the epiphysis to osteoporosis and the accumulation of unhealed trabecular microcracks, resulting in fatigue fractures; and the theory that increased intraosseous pressure due to fat accumulation as part of Cushing syndrome leads to mechanical impingement on the sinusoidal vascular bed and decreased blood flow.

Management of Glucocorticoid-Induced Osteoporosis

It is important to be aggressive and to maintain a positive attitude in the prevention and treatment of steroid-induced bone loss. Patients who are losing bone rapidly are unlikely to manifest any clinical or biochemical signs or symptoms of abnormalities of bone metabolism until bone loss is so severe that atraumatic fractures occur. Awareness of potential problems and prior planning can prevent and even reverse bone loss to some degree.

Patients who will be taking either high- or low-dose glucocorticoids for more than 2 months should be considered at risk. The major components of management are listed in Table 1. It is important to use a short-acting steroid in the lowest effective dose and to use topical steroids when possible, remembering, however, that even inhaled steroids cause bone loss. Secondary hyperparathyroidism should be prevented by controlling urinary loss of calcium with salt restriction and, if necessary, a thiazide diuretic, and by maintaining an oral intake of calcium of 1500 mg/day. An exercise program should be prescribed to prevent myopathy and reduce bone resorption. Estrogen/progesterone replacement in women and testosterone replacement in men should be used when there are no contraindications (20). Even mild degrees of vitamin D insufficiency should be treated and monitored with serum 25(OH)D levels. Bone density should be measured every 6 months during the first 2 years of therapy to assess adequacy

TABLE 1. *Management of patients taking glucocorticoids*

General measures
Use lowest effective dose of glucocorticoid with shortest half-life.
Encourage weight-bearing and isometric exercises.
Maintain good nutritional status.
Prevent secondary hyperparathyroidism
Restrict sodium intake to 3 g/d to decrease hypercalciuria and improve absorption of calcium. Add thiazide and potassium-sparing diuretic if necessary.
Maintain a calcium intake of 1500 mg/d.
Maintain serum 25(OH)D level at upper limits of normal.
Replace gonadal hormones
Begin estrogen/progesterone replacement therapy in postmenopausal women and women whose menses become irregular.
Give Depo-Testosterone to men if serum free testosterone is low.
Assess bone density every 6 months for first year.
If bone mass continues to fall in spite of conservative measures, consider treatment with a bisphosphonate or calcitonin.

25(OH)D, 25-hydroxyvitamin D.

of the treatment program. If rapid bone loss continues, treatment with calcitonin (21), a bisphosphonate (22), or sodium fluoride (23) should be considered.

Deflazacort, an oxazoline derivative of prednisone, may prove to have fewer adverse effects on the skeleton while maintaining approximately 80% of the anti-inflammatory effects of prednisone. Although deflazacort inhibits gastrointestinal absorption of calcium and bone formation, these inhibitory effects are less than those of prednisone.

CYCLOSPORINE

Cyclosporine is frequently given with prednisone to suppress the immune response, particularly in organ transplant recipients. This combination of drugs causes rapid bone loss. The effects of cyclosporine on bone and calcium metabolism are not as well understood as those of glucocorticoids, but its effects on bone differ. Serum osteocalcin levels are elevated in patients taking cyclosporine, whereas they are depressed in patients taking prednisone (24). Synthesis of $1,25(OH)_2D$ is elevated by cyclosporine, but not by glucocorticoids (25). This may explain the differences in osteocalcin levels.

EXCHANGE RESINS

Exchange resins such as cholestyramine, which are used to lower cholesterol by binding bile salts in the intestine, can decrease the absorption of fat-soluble vitamins A, D, and K and result in deficiency of these vitamins. If cholestyramine is given for long periods of time, levels of these vitamins should be monitored and supplemented when indicated.

ANTICONVULSANT-INDUCED ABNORMALITIES IN BONE METABOLISM

The anticonvulsant drugs diphenylhydantoin (DPH), phenobarbital, and carbamazepine, and combinations of these drugs, cause alterations in calcium metabolism. In patients taking these particular anticonvulsant drugs, serum levels of calcium and 25OHD are significantly lower and alkaline phosphatase levels are higher than in control subjects. Frank hypocalcemia has been reported in 3% to 30%, elevated alkaline phosphatase in 10% to 70%, and low serum 25(OH)D in 8% to 33%. Serum $1,25(OH)_2D$ may be high early in treatment and low later in treatment. Valproate has not been shown to induce any of the changes in calcitropic hormones or in other bone-related biochemical parameters.

Changes in calcium homeostatic mechanisms associated with anticonvulsant drugs have been ascribed to treatment-induced vitamin D deficiency, which leads to poor calcium absorption and secondary hyperparathyroidism. All of the commonly used anticonvulsant agents induce the liver cytochrome P 450 system. This system mediates drug oxidation reactions and enhances the hepatic conversion of steroid hormones, including vitamin D metabolites, to polar, biologically inactive products, which are excreted in urine and bile (26). These changes increase the requirement for vitamin D, and a state of vitamin D insufficiency or deficiency ensues unless the supply of vitamin D is increased. The dose of vitamin D required to maintain serum 25(OH)D in the normal range is between 400 and 4000 IU/day. The majority of patients appear to maintain normal levels on 2400 IU/day (27).

Susceptibility to the adverse effects of anticonvulsant drugs on calcium and vitamin D metabolism is increased by poor dietary intake of vitamin D, limited ultraviolet light exposure, multidrug therapy, prolonged therapy, and combination with other drugs that induce the hepatic P 450 enzyme system (28).

Anticonvulsant drugs also have direct effects on cellular metabolism unrelated to vitamin D. Diphenylhydantoin inhibits calcium transport in the gut and suppresses osteoblastic and osteoclastic activity in bone *in vitro* (29), and both phenobarbital and DPH inhibit the resorptive response to PTH and vitamin D metabolites. Paradoxically, elevated serum levels of osteocalcin, bone-specific alkaline phosphatase, and C-terminal extension peptide of type I procollagen, all markers of bone formation; and cross-linked carboxyl-terminal telopeptide of type I collagen, a marker of bone matrix resorption, reflect high rates of remodeling in patients taking anticonvulsant drugs (30). This apparent paradox is most likely due to a composite of opposing effects of anticonvulsants on cellular metabolism and the effect of an anticonvulsant-induced decrease in vitamin D metabolites and increase of PTH secretion. The ultimate effect of anticonvulsants on bone is quite variable, as is the frequency of anticonvulsant-related bone disease. The bone disease may present as full-blown osteomalacia; however, the patient is more often asymptomatic but has low serum 25(OH)D levels, mild hypocalcemia, and slightly elevated alkaline phosphatase and PTH.

Early measurements of bone density of the mid-radius using single-photon absorptiometry demonstrated a 10% to 30% decrease when compared with normal age-matched controls (31). A more recent study using dual-photon absorptiometry failed to show significant bone loss in the femoral neck in a group aged 5–20 years who were taking anticonvulsants but were otherwise healthy (32). Adult women taking DPH were found to have decreased bone density in the femoral neck. Bone densities were normal for men even though biochemical markers of bone remodeling showed increased turnover (30).

TABLE 2. *Management of patients taking anticonvulsant drugs*

Beginning of therapy
Maintain good nutritional status and level of physical activity.
Assure intake of 1500 mg of calcium and 800 IU vitamin D daily.
After 6 or more months of therapy
1. Measure serum calcium, alkaline phosphatase, 25(OH)D
2. If 25(OH)D is low, begin vitamin D 50,000 IU once a week.
3. Measure 25(OH)D 3 months after beginning high dose of vitamin D.
4. Adjust dose to maintain 25(OH)D in normal range.
5. Measure 24-hr urine calcium. If low, increase calcium intake.
6. Assess serum 25(OH)D yearly once it is normal.

25(OH)D, 25-hydroxyvitamin D.

Diagnosis and Treatment

Alterations in calcium and bone metabolism should be suspected in all patients who are taking DPH, phenobarbital, or carbamazepine. All patients should be encouraged to remain physically active and to consume 800 IU of vitamin D and 1500 mg of calcium daily (Table 2). Serum calcium, phosphorous, and 25(OH)D levels should be measured. If the 25(OH)D level is below normal, vitamin D 50,000 IU once weekly should be prescribed. The serum 25(OH)D level should then be assessed 3 months after starting this dose, and the dose should be adjusted as needed to maintain a level in the normal range. Assessment should be repeated yearly. When the 25(OH)D level is normal, 24-hour excretion of calcium should be measured, and if this is low, calcium supplementation should be increased, as a low level is indicative of impaired intestinal absorption.

REFERENCES

1. Gennari C, Imbimbo B, Montagnani M, Bernini M, Nardi P, Avioli LV: Effects of prednisone and deflazacort on mineral metabolism and parathyroid hormone activity in humans. *Calcif Tissue Int* 36:245–252, 1984
2. Adinoff AD, Hollister JR: Steroid-induced fractures and bone loss in patients with asthma. *N Engl J Med* 309:265–268, 1983
3. Dempster DW: Bone histomorphometry in glucocorticoid-induced osteoporosis. *J Bone Miner Res* 4:137–141, 1989
4. Wong GL: Basal activities and hormone responsiveness of osteoblastic activity. *J Biol Chem* 254:6337–6340, 1979
5. Dietrich JW, Canalis EM, Maina DM, Raisz LG: Effect of glucocorticoids on fetal rat bone collagen synthesis in vitro. *Endocrinology* 104:715–721, 1979
6. Canalis EM: Effect of cortisol on periosteal and nonperiosteal collagen and DNA synthesis in cultured rat calvariae. *Calcif Tissue Int* 36:158–166, 1984
7. Lukert B, Mador A, Raisz LG, Kream BE: The role of DNA synthesis in the responses of fetal rat calvariae to cortisol. *J Bone Miner Res* 6:453–460, 1991
8. Morrison N, Eisman J: Role of the negative glucocorticoid regulatory element in glucocorticoid repression of the human osteocalcin promoter. *J Bone Miner Res* 8:969–975, 1993
9. Gronowicz G, McCarthy MB, Raisz LG: Glucocorticoids stimulate resorption in fetal rat parietal bones in vitro. *J Bone Miner Res* 5:1223–1230, 1990
10. Crilly RG, Cawood M, Marshall DH, Nordin BE: Hormonal status in normal, osteoporotic and corticosteroid-treated postmenopausal women. *J R Soc Med* 71:733–736, 1978
11. MacAdams MR, White RH, Chipps BE: Reduction of serum testosterone levels during chronic glucocorticoid therapy. *Ann Intern Med* 104:648–651, 1986
12. Suzuki Y, Ichikawa Y, Saito E, Homma M: Importance of increased urinary calcium excretion in the development of secondary hyperparathyroidism of patients under glucocorticoid therapy. *Metabolism* 32:151–156, 1983
13. Lukert BP, Stanbury SW, Mawer EB: Vitamin D and intestinal transport of calcium: Effects of prednisolone. *Endocrinology* 93:718–722, 1973
14. Adams JS, Wahl TO, Lukert BP: Effects of hydrochlorothiazide and dietary sodium restriction on calcium metabolism in corticosteroid treated patients. *Metabolism* 30:217–221, 1981
15. Bikle DD, Halloran B, Fong L, Steinbach L, Shellito J: Elevated 1,25-dihydroxyvitamin D levels in patients with chronic obstructive pulmonary disease treated with prednisone. *J Clin Endocrinol Metab* 76:456–461, 1993
16. Price PA, Otsuka AA, Poser JW, Kristaponis J, Raman N: Characterization of gamma-carboxyglutamic acid containing protein form bone. *Proc Natl Acad Sci USA* 73:1447–1451, 1976
17. Raisz LG, Pilbeam CC, Fall PM: Prostaglandins: Mechanisms of action and regulation of production in bone. *Osteoporosis Int* 3(Suppl 1):136–140, 1993
18. Canalis E, McCarthy T, Centrella M: Isolation of growth factors from adult bovine bone. *Calcif Tissue Int* 43:346–351, 1988
19. Kream BE, LaFrancis PM, Fall PM, Feyen JHM, Raisz LG: Insulin-like growth factor binding protein-2 blocks the stimulatory effect of glucocorticoids on bone collagen synthesis. *J Bone Miner Res* 7(Suppl 1):5100, 1992
20. Lukert BP, Johnson BE, Robinson RG: Estrogen and progesterone replacement therapy reduces glucocorticoid-induced bone loss. *J Bone Miner Res* 7:1063–1069, 1992
21. Luengo M, Picado C, Del Rio L, Guanabens N, Monsterrat JM, Setoain J: Treatment of steroid-induced osteopenia with calcitonin in corticosteroid-dependent asthma: A one-year follow-up study. *Am Rev Respir Dis* 142:104–107, 1990
22. Mulder H, Smelder HAA: Effect of cyclical etidronate regimen on prophylaxis of bone loss of glucocorticoid (prednisone) therapy in postmenopausal women. *J Bone Miner Res* 7:S331, 1992
23. Meunier PJ, Birancon D, Chavassieux P, et al: Treatment with fluoride: Bone histomorphometric findings. In: Christiansen C, Johansen JS, Riis BJ (eds) *Osteoporosis 1987*. Copenhagen, Osteopress, pp 824–828, 1987
24. Shane E, Rivas MDC, Silverberg SJ, Kim TS, Staron RB, Bliezikian JP: Osteoporosis after cardiac transplantation. *Am J Med* 94:257–264, 1993
25. Stein B, Halloran BP, Reinhardt T, et al: Cyclosporin-A increases synthesis of 1,25-dihydroxyvitamin D_3 in the rat and mouse. *Endocrinology* 128:1369–1373, 1991
26. Hahn TJ, Hendin BA, Scharp CR, Haddad JG Jr: Effect of chronic anticonvulsant therapy on serum 25-hydroxycalciferol levels in adults. *N Engl J Med* 287:900–904, 1972
27. Collins N, Maher J, Cole M, Baker M, Callaghan N: A prospective study to evaluate the dose of vitamin D required to correct low 25-hydroxyvitamin D levels, calcium, and alkaline phosphatase in patients at risk of developing antiepileptic drug-induced osteomalacia. *Q J Med* 78:113–122, 1991
28. Gough H, Goggin T, Bissessar A, Baker M, Crowley M, Callaghan N: A comparative study of the relative influence of different anticonvulsant drugs, UV exposure and diet on vitamin D and calcium metabolism in out-patients with epilepsy. *Q J Med* 59:569–577, 1986
29. Dietrich JW, Duffield R: Effects of diphenylhydantoin on synthesis of collagen and non-collagen protein in tissue culture. *Endocrinology* 106:606–610, 1980
30. Valimiaki MJ, Tiihonen M, Laitinen K, Tahtela R, Karkkainen M, Lamberg-Allardt C, Makela P, Tunninen R: Bone mineral density measured by dual-energy x-ray absportiometry and novel markers of bone formation and resorption in patients on antiepileptic drugs. *J Bone Miner Res* 9:631–367, 1994
31. Barden HS, Mazess RB, Chesney RW, Rose PG, Chun R: Bone status in children receiving anticonvulsant therapy. *Metab Bone Dis Relat Res* 4:43–47, 1982
32. Timperlake RW, Cook SD, Thomas KA, Harding AF, Bennett JT, Haller JS, Anderson RM: Effects of anticonvulsant drug therapy on bone mineral density in a pediatric population. *J Pediatr Orthop* 8:467–470, 1988

53. Osteoporosis in Men

Jeffrey A. Jackson, M.D.

Division of Endocrinology, Scott & White Clinic, Texas A & M University Health Science Center, Temple, Texas

Osteoporosis in men has received much less attention and study than its counterpart in women. Recent studies suggest that vertebral fractures in men occur more commonly than previously appreciated, with an incidence in men up to one half of that in women (1,2). The greatest morbidity, mortality (actually greater in men than women), and societal expense, however, are caused by hip fractures in men, which account for 25% to 30% of all hip fractures. This constitutes a significant public health problem, predicted to increase considerably in the next 30 years. The lower incidence of osteoporosis in men is due to higher peak bone cross-sectional area and size; lower rate of age-related cortical bone loss; a different pattern of trabecular bone loss with age, with predominant thinning rather than perforation; the absence of a distinct menopause equivalent with associated acceleration of bone loss; shorter life expectancy; and reduced propensity to fall.

The differential diagnosis of osteopenia, or moderately reduced bone mass (not strictly defined yet in men) without fractures, and osteoporosis in men is shown in Table 1.

TABLE 1. *Differential diagnosis of osteopenia and osteoporosis in men[a]*

Endocrinopathies	Hypogonadism, Cushing syndrome, hyperthyroidism, primary hyperparathyroidism, hyperprolactinemia, acromegaly, and idiopathic hypercalciuria
Osteomalacia	Vitamin D deficiency, phosphate-wasting syndromes, metabolic acidosis, and inhibitors of mineralization
Neoplastic disease	Multiple myeloma, systemic mastocytosis, diffuse bony metastases, vertebral metastases, myelo- and lymphoproliferative disorders
Drug-induced	Glucocorticoids, ethanol, excessive thyroid hormone, heparin, anticonvulsants, and tobacco smoking
Hereditary disorders	Osteogenesis imperfecta, Ehlers-Danlos and Marfan syndromes, and homocystinuria
Other disorders	Immobilization, chronic disease (rheumatoid arthritis, liver/kidney failure), malnutrition, skeletal sarcoidosis, Gaucher's disease, hypophosphatasia, and hemoglobinopathies
Idiopathic Age-related	Juvenile and adult

[a]Adapted from: Jackson JA, Kleerekoper M: *Medicine* 69:139–152, 1990.

This list also applies to other groups of patients, such as black and premenopausal women. Detailed discussions of bone loss associated with endocrinopathies other than hypogonadism, osteomalacia, neoplastic diseases, glucocorticoids and other drugs, and other disorders such as osteogenesis imperfecta, immobilization, and rheumatoid arthritis are presented elsewhere in this book.

HYPOGONADISM

Long-standing testosterone deficiency is typical of up to 30% of men presenting with spinal osteoporosis (3). These men most commonly present in the sixth decade and in retrospect, most have had hypogonadal symptoms of impotence and decreased libido in excess of 20–30 years. Virtually any cause of hypogonadism (primary or secondary) may be associated with osteoporosis in men, including Klinefelter syndrome, hypogonadotropic hypogonadism, hyperprolactinemia, hemochromatosis, mumps orchitis, and castration (4). Testosterone deficiency may be a significant risk factor for hip fracture in elderly men (5) and may contribute to bone loss associated with aging in general, malignancy and other systemic diseases (see Chapters 55 and 57), malnutrition, ethanol abuse, and glucocorticoid excess (see Chapter 52).

Detection of hypogonadism in osteoporotic men may be quite challenging. Pitfalls include lack of palpably abnormal testes (not uncommon in secondary hypogonadism occurring after puberty), denial of hypogonadal symptoms (testosterone-deficient men may be capable of adequate sexual function), and presence of "normal" serum total testosterone levels despite clear elevations in serum luteinizing hormone (sometimes due to associated increases in sex hormone-binding globulin). Every osteopenic or osteoporotic man should have routine measurement of serum testosterone (total or free) and of luteinizing hormone.

Histomorphometric heterogeneity in hypogonadal osteoporotic men (similar to that of postmenopausal osteoporosis, except for lack of subnormal bone formation rates) (3) may reflect a gradual transition from osteoclast- to osteoblast-dependent bone loss over time. The increased remodeling activation and bone turnover in such men appear to be correctable by testosterone replacement (3) or calcitonin (4). Testosterone deficiency may reduce calcitonin secretion, and synthesis of calcitriol may be impaired, particularly when substrate (calcidiol) is deficient (3,6). Parallels between the bone effects of gonadal hormone deficiency in men and women may be due to similar direct effects on bone; both estrogen and androgen receptors have been demonstrated *in vitro* in human osteoblasts and osteoblast-like cells as well as in bone marrow stromal cells and osteoclast-like multinucleated cells (7). The recent finding of markedly reduced bone mineral density in a man with severe estrogen resistance (8) suggests that local aromatization of testosterone to estradiol may be necessary for normal bone homeostasis.

Study of the effects of testosterone replacement therapy on bone mineral density has been quite limited. Significant increases in radial and spinal bone mineral densities have been reported in patients with hypogonadotropic hypogonadism and initially open epiphyses after testosterone treatment for up to 2 years, but those with initially closed epiphyses showed minimal improvement (9). Restoration of gonadal function after successful treatment of hyperprolactinemic hypogonadal men resulted in significant increases in only cortical bone density (10). Spine and forearm bone mineral densities increased in hypogonadal men with hemochromatosis treated by testosterone replacement and venesection (11).

IDIOPATHIC OSTEOPOROSIS

The diagnosis of idiopathic osteoporosis should be made only after all other causes have been excluded (1,12). Idiopathic juvenile osteoporosis is discussed in Chapter 51. In adults, men predominate by a 10:1 ratio, although some investigators have reported more equal representation by women (13). Idiopathic osteoporosis accounts for at least 30% to 40% of osteoporosis in adult men. These men usually present with vertebral compression fractures in the third to sixth decades. The trend toward early recognition of radiographic osteopenia and measurement of bone mineral density will likely detect more of these patients in the future before fracture occurrence. This would be vastly preferable to the current practice of delayed diagnosis until after three or four vertebral fractures have occurred, followed by a lengthy (although necessary) workup for secondary causes before therapeutic decisions are made.

Performance of dynamic bone histomorphometry on these patients is generally unnecessary with the clinical availability of improved biochemical markers of bone turnover (14). However, bone histomorphometry has been useful in exploring the pathophysiology of bone homeostasis in idiopathic osteoporosis. Most studies have shown defective osteoblast function with low bone-formation rates (3,13), correlated with reduced levels of insulin-like growth factor 1 in one study (13). There appears to be considerable heterogeneity, however, with at least one subgroup of men having hypercalciuria and increased bone turnover (15), perhaps related to excessive interleukin-1 or other humoral growth factors. Alterations in calcitriol synthesis may also contribute to bone loss in some of these patients.

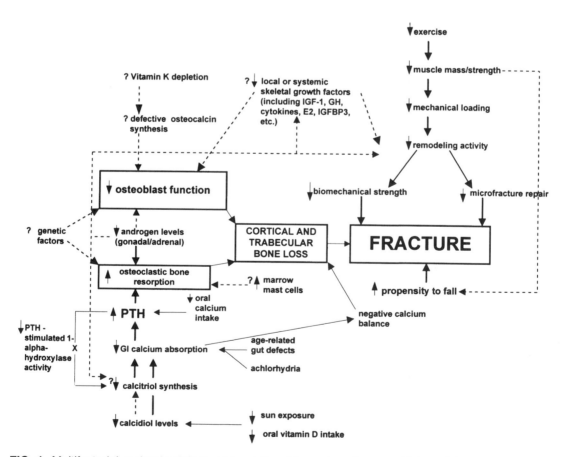

FIG. 1. Multifactorial pathophysiology of involutional bone loss in men. (Adapted from: Jackson JA, Kleerekoper M: *Medicine* 69:139–152, 1990.)

The utility of bone-turnover assessment in selection of treatment modalities (i.e., therapies stimulating bone formation in patients with low bone-turnover and antiresorptive agents for those with increased bone turnover), though intuitively gratifying, has not yet been confirmed in clinical studies of osteoporosis. At present, because there is a void in approved pro-osteoblastic agents, it appears reasonable to use antiresorptive agents (bisphosphonates or calcitonin) combined with oral calcium and low-dose vitamin D (for patients with low urinary calcium) or thiazides (for those with urinary calcium >200 mg/d) and to follow biochemical markers of turnover and serial bone densitometry. Physical therapy and counseling on osteoporotic precautions and safe exercises also are essential, as in all osteoporotic patients.

INVOLUTIONAL BONE LOSS IN MEN

Cross-sectional studies of bone mass and density in aging men have shown a gradual decline in bone mineral content at cortical sites (3% to 4% loss per decade after age 40), although recent longitudinal studies suggested a higher rate of loss (5% to 10% per decade). There may be a more rapid decline in men after age 50 (much less than menopausal losses in women). Periosteal bone formation in men appears to compensate for endosteal resorption, with no reduction in bending strength with age (16). Cancellous bone loss appears similar in both sexes (7% to 12% loss per decade), with only a slightly greater rate of loss in women. Quantitative computed tomography shows greater trabecular decline, as bone densitometric techniques measure integral bone density including cortical shell, posterior processes, and extravertebral calcifications. Qualitative differences in trabecular microarchitecture between the sexes may be quite distinct: men appear to have more reduction in trabecular width with age, whereas women have a greater fall in trabecular number (17), which may disproportionately reduce biomechanical strength in women.

Figure 1 summarizes the current understanding of the multifactorial pathophysiology of involutional bone loss in men (1,2,12). The major factor appears to be reduction in osteoblast function with age, possibly due to decreased osteoblast longevity or impaired regulation of osteoblast activity and recruitment or formation-resorption coupling by systemic or local skeletal growth factors. Decreased mechanical loading, exercise, and muscle mass in the elderly may impair remodeling activity. Negative calcium balance in aging men is due to insufficient oral calcium intake and decreased gastrointestinal calcium absorptive efficiency, which may partly relate to subnormal calcitriol levels reported by some investigators. An age-related increase in bone resorption appears less prominent and may relate to several hormonal factors. Increases in serum parathyroid hormone with age have been reported by most investigators. Calcitonin levels measured by monomeric assays do not fall with age in either sex. A fall in gonadal function with age (18) may contribute significantly to involutional bone loss in men. Increased propensity to fall

TABLE 2. *Prevention of osteoporosis in men: general measures*[a]

Routine maintenance of adequate calcium intake throughout life
1000 mg/d elemental calcium in younger men and preadolescent boys
1500 mg/d in adolescent boys and men > ages 60–65
Routine maintenance of adequate vitamin D intake throughout life
Low-dose vitamin D supplementation to push total intake to 600–800 IU/d in men > ages 60–65
Lifelong regular physical exercise
Recognize and treat testosterone deficiency early
Limit ethanol use and avoid tobacco smoking
Recognize other high-risk men (Table 3); consider specific prophylactic treatment regimens
Postgastric surgery (oral calcium ± vitamin D)
Chronic glucocorticoid therapy (oral calcium ± vitamin D and thiazides)
Avoidance of falls

[a]Adapted from: Jackson JA, Kleerekoper M: *Medicine* 69:139–152, 1990.

also plays a major role in involutional fractures; elderly women fall two to four times more often than men.

PREVENTION

Because current therapy of established osteoporosis is inadequate and no therapeutic agent has yet been convincingly proven effective in preventing osteoporotic fractures in men, emphasis must be placed on prevention of bone loss (Table 2). Specific measures may include routine calcium and vitamin D supplementation in men after ages 60–65, lifelong regular exercise, prompt recognition and treatment of testosterone deficiency, moderation of ethanol intake, and avoidance of tobacco smoking. Recognition of risk factors for osteoporosis in men (19) (listed roughly in order of importance in Table 3) is also important. In the future, specific programs for prevention of falls (and selective use of hip padding) will likely yield beneficial results for the elderly.

TABLE 3. *Risk factors for osteoporosis in men*[a]

Caucasian (? Asiatic) ancestry
Impaired gonadal function
Significant ethanol use
Cigarette smoking
Drugs, particularly glucocorticoids
Chronic illness/immobilization
Inactive lifestyle
Postgastric surgery or intestinal resection
Low dietary calcium intake
Lean body build
? Family history of osteoporotic fractures
? Chronic excess sodium, caffeine, protein, and phosphorus intake

[a]Adapted from: Jackson JA, Kleerekoper M: *Medicine* 69:139–152, 1990.

REFERENCES

1. Orwoll ES, Klein RF: Osteoporosis in men. *Endocr Rev* 16:87–116, 1995
2. Seeman E: The dilemma of osteoporosis in men. *Am J Med* 98(Suppl 2A):76S–88S, 1995
3. Jackson JA, Kleerekoper M, Parfitt AM, Rao DS, Villanueva AR, Frame B: Bone histomorphometry in hypogonadal and eugonadal men with spinal osteoporosis. *J Clin Endocrinol Metab* 65:53–58, 1987
4. Stepan JJ, Lachman M, Zverina J, Pacovsky V, Baylink DJ: Castrated men exhibit bone loss: Effect of calcitonin treatment on biochemical indices of bone remodeling. *J Clin Endocrinol Metab* 69:523–527, 1989
5. Jackson JA, Riggs MW, Spiekerman AM: Testosterone deficiency as a risk factor for hip fractures in men: A case-control study. *Am J Med Sci* 304:4–8, 1992
6. Francis RM, Peacock M, Aaron JE, et al.: Osteoporosis in hypogonadal men: Role of decreased plasma 1,25-dihydroxyvitamin D, calcium malabsorption and low bone formation. *Bone* 7:261–268, 1986
7. Vanderscheueren D, Bouillon R: Androgens and bone. *Calcif Tissue Int* 56:341–346, 1995
8. Smith EP, Boyd J, Frank GR, et al.: Estrogen resistance caused by a mutation in the estrogen-receptor gene in a man. *N Engl J Med* 331:1056–1061, 1994
9. Finkelstein JS, Klibanski A, Neer RM, et al.: Increases in bone density during treatment of men with idiopathic hypogonadotropic hypogonadism. *J Clin Endocrinol Metab* 69:776–783, 1989
10. Greenspan SL, Oppenheim DS, Klibanski A: Importance of gonadal steroids to bone mass in men with hyperprolactinemic hypogonadism. *Ann Intern Med* 110:526–531, 1989
11. Diamond T, Stiel D, Posen S: Effects of testosterone and venesection on spinal and peripheral bone mineral in six hypogonadal men with hemochromatosis. *J Bone Miner Res* 6:39–43, 1991
12. Jackson JA, Kleerekoper M: Osteoporosis in men: Diagnosis, pathophysiology, and prevention. *Medicine* 69:139–152, 1990
13. Reed BY, Zerwekh JE, Sakhaee K, Breslau NA, Gottschalk F, Pak CYC: Serum IGF 1 is low and correlated with osteoblastic surface in idiopathic osteoporosis. *J Bone Miner Res* 10:1218–1224, 1995
14. Garner P, Shih WJ, Gineyts E, Karpf DB, Delmas PD: Comparison of new biochemical markers of bone turnover in late postmenopausal osteoporotic women in response to alendronate treatment. *J Clin Endocrinol Metab* 79:1693–1700, 1994
15. Perry HM, Fallon MD, Bergfield M, Teitelbaum SL, Avioli LV: Osteoporosis in young men: A syndrome of hypercalciuria and accelerated bone turnover. *Arch Intern Med* 142:1295–1298, 1982
16. Ruff CB, Hayes WC: Sex differences in age-related remodeling of the femur and tibia. *J Orthop Res* 6:886–896, 1988
17. Aaron JE, Makins NB, Sagreiya K: The microanatomy of trabecular bone loss in normal aging men and women. *Clin Orthop* 215:260–271, 1987
18. Vermeulen A: Clinical review 24: Androgens in the aging male. *J Clin Endocrinol Metab* 73:221–224, 1991
19. Seeman E, Melton LJ III, O Fallon WM, Riggs BL: Risk factors for spinal osteoporosis in men. *Am J Med* 75:977–983, 1983

54. Hyperthyroidism, Thyroid Hormone Replacement, and Osteoporosis

Daniel T. Baran, M.D.

Departments of Medicine, Orthopedics, and Cell Biology, University of Massachusetts Medical Center, Worcester, Massachusetts

Thyroid hormone increases bone remodeling (1). Although both osteoblast and osteoclast activities are increased by elevated levels of thyroid hormone, osteoclast activity predominates, with a resultant loss of bone mass. It appears that thyroid hormones stimulate osteoclastic bone resorption by an indirect effect mediated by osteoblasts. The presence of osteoblasts is required for thyroid hormones to increase bone resorption (2,3). Osteoblasts possess thyroid hormone receptors, based on biochemical binding studies and detectable messenger ribonucleic acid (mRNA) levels for thyroid hormone receptor (4). Bone cell–specific triiodothyronine responses appear to be associated with differing patterns of receptor gene expression and stages of osteoblast phenotype expression.

Thyroid hormone directly stimulates osteoblast production of alkaline phosphatase (5), osteocalcin (6), and insulin-like growth factor (7). Thyrotoxicosis is associated with increased serum levels of osteocalcin (8) and alkaline phosphatase (9). Despite increased osteoblastic activity, the enhanced bone formation cannot compensate for thyroid hormone–induced increments in bone resorption. The increased bone resorption is detected by increased urinary levels of hydroxyproline and collagen cross-links in thyrotoxic patients (1,10,11). The lev-els of these biochemical markers of bone turnover appear to correlate with circulating levels of thyroid hormone.

Abnormalities in serum calcium concentrations are also observed in patients with hyperthyroidism. Mild hypercalcemia has been reported in 20% of patients with thyrotoxicosis (12), but the modest degree of hypercalcemia rarely causes symptoms. Serum parathyroid hormone (PTH) levels and bioactivity (13), serum 1,25-dihydroxyvitamin D_3 [$1,25(OH)_2D_3$] (14), and intestinal calcium absorption (15) are decreased in patients with thyrotoxicosis, suggesting that thyroid hormone–induced increases in bone resorption explain the occurrence of hypercalcemia.

Hypercalciuria also is common in patients with thyrotoxicosis. The increased calcium excretion normalizes after treatment of thyrotoxicosis (12).

In thyrotoxicosis, the surface area of unmineralized matrix (osteoid) is increased. In contrast to osteomalacia, mineralization rates are increased. The increased bone turnover in the presence of excessive levels of thyroid hormone is characterized by an increase in the number of osteoclasts, the number of resorption sites, and the ratio of resorptive to formative surfaces. In contrast to the normal bone-remodeling cycle, which lasts about 200 days, in hyperthyroid patients the cycle is shortened, primarily because of a decrease in the length of the formation period, with failure to replace resorbed bone completely (1) (Fig. 1). The histologic changes in cortical bone in hyperthyroidism are characterized by increased porosity (1). In hyperthyroidism, there are also changes in the gene expression markers in cortical bone.

In summary, thyroid hormone effects on osteoblasts and osteoclasts result in alterations in mineral metabolism and in the remodeling cycle, manifested by histologic and molecular changes in bone. These changes appear to be reflected in altered bone mineral density.

BONE MASS AND FRACTURE RISK IN THYROID DISEASE

Bone mass is reduced in patients with thyrotoxicosis (16,17). The detrimental effects of thyroid hormone on the skeleton appear to occur more frequently in female patients. As a result of the decrease in bone density, individuals with a history of thyrotoxicosis have an increased risk of fracture (18) and sustain fractures at an earlier age than individuals who have never been thyrotoxic (19).

The decreased bone density noted in thyrotoxic patients is reversible after effective treatment. Normalization of the thyroid function tests results in significant increases in axial and appendicular bone density compared with pretreatment values (16,17). If the detrimental skeletal effects of supraphysiologic levels of thyroid hormone were restricted to individuals with thyrotoxicosis, therapy would be expected to prevent any further skeletal damage and in fact restore at least a portion of the bone mass that was lost before effective treatment.

Administration of high doses of thyroid hormone to suppress thyroid-stimulating hormone (TSH) secretion in patients with differentiated thyroid carcinoma and nontoxic goiter is considered appropriate therapy for those conditions. In patients prone to osteoporosis, however, this therapy may aggravate fracture risk. TSH-suppressive doses of thyroid hormone have been reported to decrease or to have no effect on bone mineral density (BMD) in women. A metanalysis of the reports in which BMD was assessed in women receiving TSH-suppressive doses of thyroxine concluded that treatment led to a 1% increase in annual bone loss in postmenopausal women (20). In contrast, thyroid hormone replacement therapy in the absence of TSH sup-

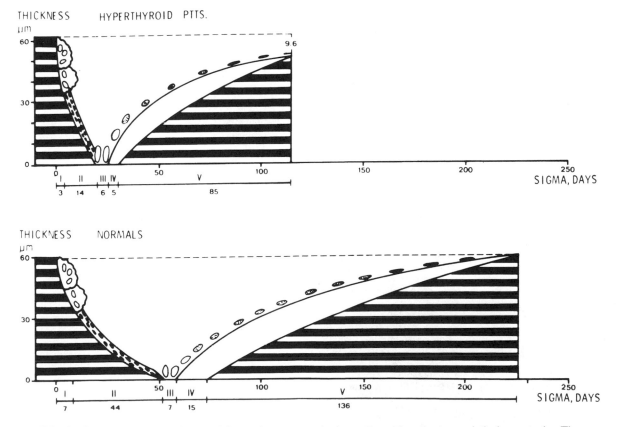

FIG. 1. Smoothed resorption and formation curves in hyperthyroid patients and their controls. The durations of the different resorption and formation periods are given below the curves. I, osteoclastic function period; II, mononuclear function period; III, preosteoblast-like cell function period; IV, initial mineralization lag time; V, mineralization period. For the hyperthyroid group, the negative balance between resorption depth and formation thickness is indicated (-9.6 μM). (Reprinted from: Eriksen EF, Mosekilde L, Melsen F. *Bone* 6:421–428, 1985, with kind permission from Elsevier Science, Ltd, The Boulevard, Langford Lane, Kidlington OX5 1GB, UK.)

pression does not appear to be associated with detrimental effects on BMD (21).

PREVENTION OF THYROID HORMONE–INDUCED BONE LOSS

Treatment of thyrotoxic patients increases bone density compared with pretreatment values (16,17). A more difficult situation is presented by the patient who requires TSH-suppressive doses of thyroid hormone. Bone mass measurements at 1- to 2-year intervals will detect those patients with accelerated rates of bone loss. In animal models of thyroid hormone–induced TSH suppression, bisphosphonates appear to prevent the detrimental effects of thyroid hormone on the skeleton (22), whereas calcitonin does not inhibit thyroid hormone–induced bone loss in these animal models (23). Bisphosphonates also prevent the increases in the biochemical markers of osteoblast and osteoclast activity that occur after thyroid hormone administration in humans (24). In a cross-sectional study, estrogen appeared to negate the thyroid hormone–associated loss of bone density in postmenopausal women taking replacement doses of thyroid hormone (25). Women taking suppressive doses of thyroid hormone who were also taking estrogen had significantly higher BMD values than women who were taking suppressive doses of thyroid hormone alone, and similar values to those women taking neither thyroid hormone nor estrogen. Bone density values did not differ by estrogen status in women taking replacement doses of thyroid hormone (25). Thus, current evidence suggests that estrogen or bisphosphonate therapy should be considered for those individuals requiring TSH-suppressive doses of thyroid hormone who demonstrate accelerated rates of bone loss or who already manifest decreased bone mass.

REFERENCES

1. Mosekilde L, Eriksen EF, Charles P: Effects of thyroid hormone on bone and mineral metabolism. *Endocrinol Metab Clin North Am* 19:35–63, 1990
2. Allain TJ, Chambers TJ, Flanagan AM, McGregor AM: Triiodothyronine stimulates rat osteoclastic bone resorption by an indirect effect. *J Endocrinol* 133:327–331, 1992
3. Britto JM, Fenton AJ, Holloway WR, Nicholson GC: Osteoblasts mediate thyroid hormone stimulation of osteoclastic bone resorption. *Endocrinology* 134:169–176, 1994
4. Williams GR, Bland R, Sheppard MC: Characterization of thyroid hormone (T₃) receptors in three osteosarcoma cell lines of distinct osteoblast phenotype: Interactions among T₃, vitamin D₃, and retinoid signaling. *Endocrinology* 135:2375–2385, 1994
5. Sato K, Han DC, Fujii Y, Tsushima T, Shizume K: Thyroid hormone stimulates alkaline phosphatase activity in cultured rat osteoblastic cells (ROS 17/2.8) through 3,5,3′-triiodo-L-thyronine nuclear receptors. *Endocrinology* 120:1873–1881, 1987
6. Rizzoli R, Poser J, Burgi U: Nuclear thyroid hormone receptors in cultured bone cells. *Metabolism* 35:71–74, 1986
7. Schmid C, Schlapfer I, Futo E, et al.: Triiodothyronine (T₃) stimulates insulin-like growth factor (IGF)-1 and IGF binding protein (IGFBP)-2 production by rat osteoblasts in vitro. *Acta Endocrinol (Copenh)* 126:467–473, 1992
8. Garrel DR, Delmas PD, Malaval L, Tourniaire J: Serum bone Gla protein: A marker of bone turnover in hyperthyroidism. *J Clin Endocrinol Metab* 62:1052–1055, 1986
9. Cooper DS, Kaplan MM, Ridgway EC, Maloof F, Daniels GH: Alkaline phosphatase isoenzyme patterns in hyperthyroidism. *Ann Intern Med* 90:164–168, 1979
10. Harvey RD, McHardy KC, Reid IW, et al.: Measurement of bone collagen degradation in hyperthyroidism and during thyroxine replacement therapy using pyridinium cross-links as specific urinary markers. *J Clin Endocrinol Metab* 72:1189–1194, 1991
11. Krakerauer JC, Kleerekoper M: Borderline low serum thyrotropin level is correlated with increased fasting urinary hydroxyproline excretion. *Arch Intern Med* 152:360–364, 1992
12. Baxter JD, Bondy PK: Hypercalcemia of thyrotoxicosis. *Ann Intern Med* 65:429–442, 1966
13. Mosekilde L, Christensen MS: Decreased parathyroid function in hyperthyroidism: Interrelationships between serum parathyroid hormone, calcium-phosphorus metabolism and thyroid function. *Acta Endocrinol (Copenh)* 84:566–575, 1977
14. Bouillon R, Muls E, DeMoor P: Influence of thyroid function on the serum concentration of 1,25-dihydroxyvitamin D₃. *J Clin Endocrinol Metab* 51:793–797, 1980
15. Haldimann B, Kaptein EM, Singer FR, Nicoloff JT, Massry SG: Intestinal calcium absorption in patients with hyperthyroidism. *J Clin Endocrinol Metab* 51:995–997, 1980
16. Rosen CJ, Alder RA: Longitudinal changes in lumbar bone density among thyrotoxic patients after attainment of euthyroidism. *J Clin Endocrinol Metab* 75:1531–1534, 1992
17. Diamond T, Vine J, Smart R, Butler P: Thyrotoxic bone disease in women: A potentially reversible disorder. *Ann Intern Med* 120:8–11, 1994
18. Cummings SR, Nevitt MC, Browner WS, Stone K, Fox KM, Ensrud KE, Cauley J, Black D, Vogt TM: Risk factors for hip fracture in white women. Study of Osteoporotic Fractures Research Group. *N Engl J Med* 332:767–773, 1995
19. Solomon BL, Wartofsky L, Burman KD: Prevalence of fractures in postmenopausal women with thyroid disease. *Thyroid* 3:17–23, 1993
20. Faber J, Galloe AM: Changes in bone mass during prolonged subclinical hyperthyroidism due to L-thyroxine treatment: A meta-analysis. *Eur J Endocrinol* 130:350–356, 1994
21. Duncan WE, Chung A, Solomon B, Wartofsky L: Influence of clinical characteristics and parameters associated with thyroid hormone therapy on the bone mineral density of women treated with thyroid hormone. *Thyroid* 4:183–190, 1994
22. Ongphiphadhanakul B, Jenis LG, Braverman LE, et al.: Etidronate inhibits the thyroid hormone-induced bone loss in rats assessed by bone mineral density and messenger ribonucleic acid markers of osteoblast and osteoclast function. *Endocrinology* 133:2502–2507, 1993
23. Ongphiphadhanakul B, Alex S, Braverman LE, Baran DT: TSH-suppressive L-thyroxine therapy decreases bone density in the rat: Effect of hypogonadism and calcitonin. *J Bone Miner Res* 7:1227–1231, 1992
24. Rosen HN, Moses AC, Gundberg C: Therapy with parenteral pamidronate prevents thyroid hormone-induced bone turnover in humans. *J Clin Endocrinol Metab* 77:664–669, 1993
25. Schneider DL, Barrett-Connor EL, Morton DJ: Thyroid hormone use and bone mineral density in elderly women: Effects of estrogen. *JAMA* 271:1245–1249, 1994

55. Miscellaneous Causes of Osteoporosis

Socrates E. Papapoulos, M.D.

Department of Endocrinology and Metabolic Diseases, University Hospital, Leiden, The Netherlands

The title of this chapter encompasses a collection of heterogeneous conditions that can be associated with increased bone loss, low bone mass, and fractures. In some of these conditions a causal relation to osteoporosis is established; in others there may be more than one link to osteoporosis, and in some the etiology is unknown. The first category includes endocrinopathies such as Cushing's disease; thyrotoxicosis; severe primary hyperparathyroidism and hypogonadism of varying etiologies (e.g., hypothalamic amenorrhea, prolactin secreting pituitary adenomas, treatment of endometriosis with synthetic luteinizing hormone-releasing hormone analogs), drugs such as glucocorticosteroids, anticonvulsants, and cyclosporin A; or genetic disorders such as osteogenesis imperfecta. These subjects are discussed elsewhere in this volume. In the second category belong conditions thought to adversely affect bone metabolism and/or structure through multiple disease- and therapy-related mechanisms such as rheumatoid arthritis (see Chapter 57), gastrointestinal diseases (see Chapter 59), organ transplantation (see Chapter 52), and prolonged immobilization (see Chapter 46). Finally, in the third category belong conditions the pathogeneses of which are still ill defined such as, for example, pregnancy-associated osteoporosis. This chapter focuses on this third category and on disorders that have as common pathogenetic mechanism the definite or possible interaction between the bone tissue and its bone marrow microenvironment.

In recent years the role of the bone marrow microenvironment in the regulation of bone metabolism has attracted considerable attention. It becomes increasingly clear that these two compartments cannot be considered separately, and better understanding of the bone marrow physiology and pathology may enhance our knowledge of bone pathology. Although examination of bone tissue by sophisticated morphometric techniques provides invaluable information about bone remodeling and its disturbances, for the elucidation of the driving forces for the observed changes, concurrent examination of the bone marrow may be essential. This approach is gaining popularity but we currently lack the necessary knowledge and tools to interpret or recognize all important pathology that may be related to osteoporosis. Identification of such relations not only is essential for understanding the mechanisms of bone loss and the pathogenesis of bone destruction but may also lead to more rational therapeutic interventions. For some bone marrow disorders, however, the link to bone pathology is clear. These include mainly disorders in which the bone marrow is infiltrated by malignant cells.

MULTIPLE MYELOMA

Multiple myeloma is typically associated with bone pathology. Nearly 80% of patients have bone pain at presentation and pathologic fractures have been reported in up to 60% of patients. Bone lesions are usually focal and lytic but diffuse osteopenia can also be present. In rare cases osteosclerotic lesions may also be seen. The prevalence of vertebral fractures, assessed morphometrically in x-rays of the spine of 250 patients with multiple myeloma was 56%, and there was a relation between the presence of vertebral fractures and the severity and prevalence of bone pain (1). This high prevalence together with the fact that the incidence of multiple myeloma is highest in the seventh decade of life, a period when the incidence of fractures due to primary osteoporosis is also high, makes this disease an important cause of secondary osteoporosis, which may not be recognized unless appropriate investigations are performed.

In our unit last year we encountered three women with vertebral fractures and multiple myeloma who had been diagnosed with primary osteoporosis and were treated accordingly by their physicians. With the greater awareness of osteoporosis and the wider availability of means to diagnose and treat it, we may be confronted with more cases like these unless major efforts are taken to inform the medical profession about the need to carefully assess patients presenting with vertebral fractures.

Bone destruction in multiple myeloma is due to increased osteoclastic activity induced by bone-acting cytokines, which are produced by the malignant cells. These have been named in the past, collectively, osteoclast-activating factor (OAF) and probably include interleukin-6, tumor necrosis factor, interleukin-1β, and macrophage colony stimulating factor (M-CSF). In multiple myeloma there is an uncoupling between bone resorption and bone formation and this is reflected in the generally normal serum alkaline phosphatase activity, normal to low serum osteocalcin concentrations, and in the increased urinary excretion of biochemical indices of bone resorption. In addition, bone scans show usually no abnormalities, which contrasts the findings in patients with metastatic bone disease from solid tumors. In patients with multiple myeloma bone complaints respond generally well to chemotherapy but bone destruction may progress. Because this is due to increased bone resorption bisphosphonates have not only been used in the treatment of hypercalcemia, which occurs in about one third of the patients, but also for the prevention of the other skeletal complications.

Evidence is accumulating that newer bisphosphonates can reduce significantly, skeletal morbidity in patients with multiple myeloma, especially those on second-line chemotherapy (1). The doses of bisphosphonates used are, however, substantially higher than those used in the treatment of primary osteoporosis. Positive results have been obtained in large clinical trials with oral clodronate and intravenous pamidronate leading to registration of these compounds for this indication in various countries.

Apart from multiple myeloma, leukemia may also be associated with diffuse osteopenia and vertebral fractures especially in children (adolescents) with acute lymphoblastic leukemia (2) and may be due to local release of osteotropic factors by the malignant cells. Convincing evidence for that is, however, lacking. Development of osteopenia and fractures after treatment of the leukemia is most probably multifactorial and therapeutic interventions appear to play a major role in that (3). With improving survival of patients with this common childhood malignancy, osteoporosis may become an important clinical issue in such patients.

BREAST CANCER

Breast cancer is the most frequent malignant tumor and the most common cause of death due to cancer among women in industrialized countries. Breast cancer metastasizes frequently to the skeleton and about 70% of patients with advanced cancer develop symptomatic skeletal disease (4). Metastases are usually localized in bone that is rich in red marrow, particularly at sites of active hematopoiesis, and the axial skeleton (spine, ribs, pelvis) is most frequently affected.

In a placebo-controlled trial to evaluate the effect of the bisphosphonate clodronate on skeletal complications in patients with breast cancer and bone metastases, the rate of new vertebral fractures in the placebo group was 124 per 100 patient-years (5). This incidence exceeds by far published incidences of vertebral fractures in patients with primary osteoporosis.

Skeletal complications in patients with breast cancer are a major cause of morbidity and deterioration of the quality of life. Furthermore, patients with first metastasis to the skeleton live longer and if the disease remains confined to the skeleton survival may be even longer, but requires efficient preventive and/or palliative interventions.

The reason for the strong preference of breast cancer cells (and of other osteotropic tumors) for the skeleton is not known. There is, however, general agreement that bone destruction involves mainly the activation of the normal osteoclastic pathway (6). Breast cancer cells in the direct vicinity of bone release factors which stimulate the formation and/or the activity of osteoclasts leading to increased bone resorption.

Current evidence suggests that bone resorption may also be systemically stimulated by parathyroid hormone-related protein (PTHrP). Bone components (e.g., growth factors, cytokines, collagen fragments) that are released during bone resorption may in turn stimulate the chemotaxis and attachment of new cancer cells to bone, thus amplifying the process. Inhibition of bone resorption may therefore not only decrease bone destruction but may also disrupt this cycle.

Ample evidence in support of the first notion has been obtained in human studies with the use of bisphosphonates. Clodronate and pamidronate were shown in controlled studies to significantly decrease skeletal morbidity in patients with breast cancer and bone metastases and to decrease the frequency of new vertebral fractures (clodronate) (5,7). Evidence for the second notion was recently obtained in an ani-

mal model of metastatic breast cancer. It was shown that inhibition of cancer-induced bone resorption by the bisphosphonate risedronate induced a significant reduction in the tumor burden in the bone marrow (8). Thus, although the differential diagnosis of vertebral fractures in patients with breast cancer presents usually no difficulties, their pathogenesis as well as their management are a challenge to physicians involved in the care of patients with skeletal disorders.

For completeness, it should also be mentioned that anticancer treatment of premenopausal women can lead to early menopause and bone loss. As estrogen therapy is contraindicated in these but also in postmenopausal patients with breast cancer, other therapeutic options need to be considered. Compounds antagonizing the effects of estrogens on breast (and uterus) while acting agonistically on bone and lipid metabolism are gaining popularity. Such compounds are currently named SERMs (selective estrogen receptor modulators). Up until now results have been obtained with the use of tamoxifen, which is used in the treatment of patients with breast cancer but may increase the risk of uterine carcinoma. Tamoxifen has been also shown to reduce bone loss in women with breast cancer (9). However, in a recent study of healthy late postmenopausal women given tamoxifen (20 mg/day) there was only a small protective effect on bone mineral density of the axial skeleton. This was comparable in magnitude to that of calcium supplements and less than that of estrogens or bisphosphonates (10). Other SERMs are currently under clinical development but it is too early to derive any conclusions about their effectiveness.

CHRONIC ANEMIAS

Homozygous β-thalassemia is usually described as an example of chronic anemia predisposing to osteoporosis. Evidence for that has been obtained by skeletal radiographs, by bone density measurements, and by bone histology (11,12). In patients with thalassemia there is expansion of the bone marrow space, due to hyperplasia of the marrow, with thinning of the adjacent trabeculae. In addition, iron deposits have been described in the bone marrow, the bone marrow–bone interface at the mineralization front, but also in osteoblasts due to frequent blood transfusions as in patients with hemochromatosis. Apart from these potential mechanisms for the development of osteoporosis, patients with thalassemia have also a multiplicity of other metabolic disturbances that may predispose to osteoporosis such as, for example, hepatic and gonadal dysfunction. Hypogonadism appears to be a major contributing factor as suggested recently in cross-sectional as well as in longitudinal studies of thalassemic patients on different transfusion and iron chelation regimens with or without hormonal replacement (13). Thus, all the evidence collected so far suggests multiple causes for the low bone mass with hypogonadism perhaps being the predominant cause. However, Greep et al. (14) reported reduced bone mass in patients with thalassemia trait (thalassemia minor). These patients have a mild hemolytic anemia, do not need blood transfusions, have no endocrine or hepatic dysfunction, and have a normal life expectancy. These clearly preliminary observations, if confirmed, can have a significant impact on our understanding of the role of the bone marrow microenvironment in the regulation of bone metabolism and further studies in this area are certainly worth undertaking.

MASTOCYTOSIS

Mastocytosis, a multiorgan disease of unknown etiology, is characterized by abnormal mast cell proliferation limited to the skin (urticaria pigmentosa) or involving, in addition, lymph nodes, the bone marrow, the liver, the spleen, and the gastrointestinal tract. Because of the multiorgan involvement and the biologic potential of the mast cells, the disease has heterogeneous manifestations and variable prognosis.

Skeletal symptoms are present in about 60% to 75% of the patients with systemic mast cell disease, being the presenting clinical manifestation in about 5% (15). Skeletal changes are usually confined to the axial skeleton and include, among others, generalized osteopenia and vertebral fractures. Bone biopsies from patients with mast cell infiltration of the bone marrow and osteoporosis show increased bone turnover but imbalance in the remodeling activity in favor of resorption has also been reported (16,17).

The mechanism of bone destruction in mastocytosis is not known and is thought to be due to increased heparin production by the mast cells (see further) and/or to bone-acting cytokines that are produced in excess by these cells. Of particular interest are reports of patients with vertebral osteoporosis and bone marrow mast cell lesions without any other manifestation of mast cell disease (16). These patients would have been classified as primary osteoporosis if a bone biopsy had not been taken.

The prevalence of mast cell lesions in the bone marrow of patients with symptomatic spinal osteoporosis is about 3% to 4%. This is admittedly low but such patients tend to have more severe and progressive osteoporosis. At present the diagnosis of mast cell lesions can only be established by bone marrow histology but the diagnostic value of measurements of products of the mast cells, such as histamine metabolites, in biological fluids needs to be properly assessed. The relevant question is whether the increase in mast cells in the bone marrow of these patients is causally related to osteoporosis. Mast cells may be increased in the bone marrow of patients with primary osteoporosis (18) but their number is less than that observed in mast cell disease. In addition, the pattern of mast cell infiltration of the bone marrow as well as cell morphology in patients with osteoporosis as the sole manifestation of mastocytosis appears to differ from those seen in the marrow of patients with systemic mast cell disease. The condition may thus represent part of the spectrum of primary osteoporosis or, alternatively, a variant of mast cell disease. There is no specific treatment for osteoporosis associated with mast cell disease and only case studies have reported variable success with the use of histamine antagonists or bisphosphonates (19–21).

HEPARIN TREATMENT

Heparin is an effective treatment for thromboembolic disorders. It is usually given for a few days and if long-term treatment with antithrombotic agents is indicated this is done with the use of oral anticoagulants, mainly coumarin derivatives. There are, however, instances when heparin therapy may be prolonged and these include, first, contraindications to oral anticoagulant therapy and, second, prevention and treatment of thromboembolic episodes during pregnancy as vitamin K antagonists may carry increased risks for the fetus.

Early studies have already reported increased incidence of osteoporotic fractures in heparin-treated patients (22). A number of subsequent reports supported this observation and it was suggested that development of osteoporosis during heparin therapy depends on the dose of the drug and the duration of treatment.

Recently, two relatively large studies examined the relation between heparin therapy and osteoporosis in clinically relevant groups of patients. In the first study occurrence of symptomatic vertebral fractures was assessed in 184 pregnant women who received a mean dose of 19,000 IU/day of heparin for an average period of 25 weeks (23). Spinal fractures occurred in 4 (2.2%) women postpartum and there was a suggestion of a relation to the amount of heparin given. This is a low incidence but it should be noted that it occurred in young women and that x-rays were made only in women with sudden severe back pain, which may have underestimated the number of incident vertebral fractures. In addition, this study provided no information about a possible effect of heparin on bone mass that may be of significance later in life.

The second study assessed the skeletal effects of heparin treatment given subcutaneously to 80 patients with venous thromboembolic episodes and contraindications to oral coumarin therapy (24). Half of the patients received unfractionated heparin 10,000 IU twice daily whereas the other half received low-molecular-weight heparin 5000 IU twice daily for a period of 3–6 months. Both treatments had similar antithrombotic effects. In total, 7 of the 80 patients (8.8%) developed symptomatic vertebral fractures and 6 of them were treated with unfractionated heparin. Patients with fractures were older (mean 79 ± 6 years vs. 67 ± 15 years in the nonfracture group) and had significantly lower baseline bone mineral density of the femur but not of the lumbar spine. Bone mineral density decreased with treatment, on average by 4% at the spine and 2% at the femur. This study suggested, in addition, that the osteopenic effects of heparin therapy may be less pronounced with the use of low-molecular-weight heparin preparations, a conclusion that was also supported by animal studies (25).

The mechanism responsible for the skeletal effects of heparin is unknown and may involve the same pathway as in mast cell disease. Various hypotheses have been proposed to explain the action of heparin on bone including stimulation of osteoclastic activity by enhancement of parathyroid hormone (PTH) dependent bone resorption or stimulation of collagenase synthesis, suppression of osteoblastic activity, and/or interference with the parathyroid–vitamin D axis.

A recent study with bone cultures from rat fetuses showed stimulation of osteoclastic resorption by unfractionated heparin to a level similar to that induced by PTH or calcitriol; low-molecular-weight heparin appeared to be less effective in stimulating resorption (26). The authors concluded that heparin promotes bone resorption and that the size and the sulfation of the molecule are major determinants of this action. On the other hand, van der Wiel et al. (27) failed to detect any changes in biochemical indices of bone resorption in healthy volunteers given heparin 5000 IU twice daily subcutaneously for 10 days. Thus, although the pathogenesis of heparin-induced osteoporosis remains to be resolved and its true clinical significance to be determined, caution is needed when treating older patients with heparin for long, as this may predispose to symptomatic spinal osteoporosis.

PREGNANCY-ASSOCIATED OSTEOPOROSIS

Osteoporosis occurring during pregnancy is an intriguing syndrome first described about 40 years ago (28). In the following years reports of sporadic cases supported the view that this is a rare condition, but recent evidence suggests that it may not be that uncommon (29). Pregnancy-associated osteoporosis presents during the third trimester or postpartum usually with back pain, loss of height, and vertebral fractures, but pain in the hips and femoral fractures have also been described in a few patients. The primary involvement of the axial skeleton is further supported by bone densitometry measurements. In bone biopsies taken from patients 2 weeks to 5 years after the affected pregnancy, histologic features of osteoblast failure have been reported (30). In two thirds of the cases the disease occurs during the first pregnancy and does not generally recur in subsequent pregnancies. Isolated cases of recurrence, however, have also been described. Clinical recovery is rapid and the long-term prognosis is usually good.

During pregnancy there is a stress on maternal calcium stores to meet the needs of the fetus that is compensated by alterations in maternal calcium and bone metabolism, particularly by the marked increases in estrogen production. This has led to the hypothesis that pregnancy-associated osteoporosis occurs at an already pathologic background rather than being a separate entity. However, analysis of published cases reveals possible risk factors for osteoporosis in a minority of patients. For example, Smith et al. (30) reported that in only 4 of 24 patients a preexisting disorder known to decrease bone mass was present; this was also the case in 6 of 35 patients with pregnancy-associated osteoporosis evaluated by postal questionnaire (29). In these two studies preexisting conditions included heparin therapy (3), glucocorticoid treatment (2), mild osteogenesis imperfecta (1), history of anorexia nervosa and of thyroid disease (2), celiac disease (1), and antiepileptic treatment (1). In an analysis of 72 cases (mainly from the literature but also own), Saraux et al. (31) reported the use of heparin as a potential risk factor in 6 patients. It is also of interest that in the above-mentioned postal survey it was found that the mothers of patients with pregnancy-associated osteoporosis had a significantly higher prevalence of fractures compared

with controls (29), suggesting that genetic factors may also be involved in the pathogenesis of the disease. On the other hand, the rapid clinical improvement, the densitometric evidence of recovery, and the nonoccurrence in subsequent pregnancies led to the suggestion that the disease may be related to a particular pregnancy (or to a particular fetus) for reasons not yet clear (30).

Elucidating the pathogenesis of pregnancy-associated osteoporosis is not easy. Apart from the rarity of the disease, its delayed recognition, when alterations in bone metabolism have already occurred, contribute to this difficulty. The inability of radiologic investigations during pregnancy and the difficulty in interpreting changes in biochemical indices of bone metabolism, especially during the third trimester, complicate the evaluation of such patients further. Finally, back complaints are common in pregnant women and it has been hypothesized that some of them may in fact have unrecognized milder forms of pregnancy-associated osteoporosis (32). Designing strategies to approach this intriguing syndrome may provide some clues of its real prevalence and its possible consequences for the skeletal integrity of such patients later in life.

REFERENCES

1. McCloskey E. Bisphosphonates in multiple myeloma. In: Bijvoet OLM, Fleisch HA, Canfield RE, Russell RGG (eds) *Bisphosphonate on Bons*. Amsterdam, Elsevier Science, pp 391–402, 1995
2. Newman AJ, Melhorn DK. Vertebral compression in childhood leukemia. *Am J Dis Child* 125:863–865, 1973
3. Atkinson SA, Fraher L, Gundberg CM, Andrew M, Pai M, Barr RD. Mineral homeostasis and bone mass in children treated for acute lymphoblastic leukemia. *J Pediatr* 114:793–800, 1989
4. Rubens RD. Bone involvement in solid tumours. In: Bijvoet OLM, Fleisch HA, Kanfield RE, Russell RGG (eds) *Bisphosphonate on Bons*. Amsterdam, Elsevier Science, pp 337–347, 1995
5. Paterson AHG, Powels TJ, Kanis JA, McCloskey E, Hanson J, Ashley S. Double-blind controlled trial of oral clodronate in patients with bone metastases from breast cancer. *J Clin Oncol* 11:59–65, 1993
6. Guise TA, Mundy GR. Breast cancer and bone. *Cur Opin Endocrinol Diab* 2:548–555, 1995
7. van Holten-Verzantvoort ATM, Kroon HM, Bijvoet OLM, et al. Palliative pamidronate treatment in patients with bone metastases from breast cancer. *J Clin Oncol* 11:491–498, 1993
8. Sasaki A, Boyce BF, Story B, et al. Bisphosphonate risedronate reduces metastatic human breast cancer burden in bone in nude mice. *Cancer Res* 55:3551–3557, 1995
9. Love RR, Mazess RB, Barden HS, et al. Effects of tamoxifen on bone mineral content in postmenopausal women with breast cancer. *N Engl J Med* 326:852–856, 1991
10. Grey AB, Stapleton JP, Evans MC, Tatnell MA, Ames RW, Reid IR. The effect of the antiestrogen tamoxifen on bone mineral density in normal late postmenopausal women. *Am J Med* 99:636–641, 1995
11. Orvietto R, Leichter I, Rachmilewitz EA, Margulies JY. Bone density, mineral content and cortical index in patients with thalassemia major and the correlation to their bone fractures, blood transfusion and treatment with desferioxamine. *Calcif Tissue Int* 50:397–399, 1992
12. Vernejoul MC de, Girot R, Geuris J et al. calcium phosphate metabolism and bone disease in patients with homozygous thalassemia. *J Clin Endocrinol Metab* 54:276–281, 1982
13. Anapliotou MLG, Kastanias IT, Psara P, Evangelou EA, Liparaki M, Dimitriou P. The contribution of hypogonadism to

the development of osteoporosis in thalassaemia major: new therapeutic approaches. *Clin Endocrinol* 42:279–287, 1994

14. Greep N, Anderson AL, Gallaher JCh. Thalassemia minor: a risk factor for osteoporosis? *Bone Miner* 16:63–72, 1992
15. Travis WD, Li C, Bergstrahl EJ, Yam LT, Swee RG. Systemic mast cell disease: analysis of 58 cases and literature review. *Medicine* 67:345–368, 1988
16. Chines A, Pacifici R, Avioli LV, Teitelbaum SC, Korenblat PE. Systemic mastocytosis presenting as osteoporosis. A clinical and histomorphometric study. *J Clin Endocrinol Metab* 72:140–144, 1991
17. de Gennes C, Kuntz D, de Vernejoul MC. Bone mastocytosis. *Clin Orth Rel Res* 279:281–291, 1992
18. Frame B, Nixon R. Bone marrow mast cells in osteoporosis and aging. *N Engl J Med* 279:626–630, 1968
19. Cundy T, Beneton MHC, Darby AJ, Marshall WJ, Kanis JA. Osteopenia in systemic mastocytosis: natural history and response to treatment with inhibitors of bone resorption. *Bone* 8:149–155, 1987
20. Graves L, Stechschulte DJ, Morris DC, Lukert BP. Inhibition of mediator release in systemic mastocytosis is associated with reversal of bone changes. *J Bone Miner Res* 5:1113–1119, 1990
21. Watts RA, Scott DGI, Crisp AJ. Mastocytosis and osteoporosis. *Br J Rheum* 31:715, 1992
22. Griffith GC, Nichols G, Asher JD, Flanagan B. Heparin osteoporosis. *J Am Med Assoc* 193:85–88, 1965
23. Dahlman TC. Osteoporotic fractures and the recurrence of thromboembolism during pregnancy and the purperium in 184 women undergoing thromboprophylaxis with heparin. *Am J Obst Gynecol* 168:1265–1270, 1993
24. Monreal M, Lafoz E, Olive A, del Rio L, Vedia C. Comparison of subcutaneous unfractionated heparin with low molecular weight heparin (Fragmin) in patients with venous thromboembolism and contraindications to coumarin. *Thromb Haem* 71:7–11, 1994
25. Monreal M, Vinas L, Monreal L, Lavin S, Lafoz E, Angles AM. Heparin-related osteoporosis in rats. A comparative study between unfractonated heparin and low molecular weight heparin. *Haemostasis* 20:204–207, 1990
26. Shaughnessy SG, Young E, Deschamps P, Hirsh J. The effects of low molecular weight and standard heparin on calcium loss from fetal rat calvaria. *Blood* 86:1368–1373, 1995
27. van der Wiel HE, Lips P, Huijgens PC, Netelenbos JC. Effects of short-term low-dose heparin administration on biochemical parameters of bone turnover. *Bone Miner* 22:27–32, 1993
28. Nordin BEC, Roper A. Postpregnancy osteoporosis - a syndrome. *Lancet* 1:431–434, 1995
29. Dunne F, Walters B, Marshall T, Heath DA. Pregnancy associated osteoporosis. *Clin Endocrinol* 39:487–490, 1993
30. Smith R, Athanasou NA, Ostlere SJ, Vipond SE. Pregnancy-associated osteoporosis. *Q J Med* 88:865–878, 1995
31. Saraux A, Bourgeais F, Ehrhart A, Baron D, Le Goff P. Osteoporose de la grossesse: Quatre observation. *Rev Rhum Ed Fr* 60:596–600, 1993
32. Khastgir G, Studd J. Pregnancy-associated osteoporosis. *Br J Obst Gynecol* 101:836–838, 1994

56. Orthopedic Complications of Osteoporosis

Thomas A. Einhorn, M.D.

Department of Orthopedics, Mount Sinai School of Medicine, New York, New York

Most osteoporosis-related complications in orthopedics relate to problems associated with fractures and fracture management, and how the osteoporotic skeleton responds to joint reconstructive procedures. Specific attention to the quality of fracture fixation and the use of implants in weak bone is required. Control of the metabolic condition, including treatment of the underlying cause of the osteoporosis (if known), and pharmaceutical management of the condition may improve surgical results. It may be necessary to alter the surgeon's usual preference for specific fixation devices to meet the anatomic and physiologic needs of the deformed or qualitatively impaired bone. In certain osteoporotic conditions in which bone remodeling is affected, a prolonged period of fracture healing may be anticipated and this period of healing may exceed the rate of healing in normal nonosteoporotic bone.

The orthopedist must be aware that the osteoporotic skeleton may suffer unusual types of injuries because of the fragile quality of the bone. For example, patients with osteoporosis who are engaged in athletic events may experience injuries in which their soft tissue structures have a greater ability to withstand mechanical loads than the bones that support them. As an example, a common skiing injury, rupture of the anterior cruciate of the knee, usually occurs when an anterior displacement force is applied to the knee and the ligament becomes stretched rupturing in its midsubstance. However, since the ligament is anchored in the joint to the bone of the femur and tibial plateau, if the cross-sectional area and strength of the ligament exceeds the bone's resistance to tensile loading, an avulsion fracture may occur in osteoporotic bone instead of a failure (tear) occurring in the ligament. Not only must the orthopedist be aware of the possibility of this type of problem, but the method of operative repair and the rehabilitation program must take into consideration the limited capacity of the bone to support a tensile force in the ligament. Other complications of osteoporosis relate to the reconstruction of the diseased or deformed skeleton during treatments such as osteotomy, arthrodesis, and arthroplasty. In each case, the ability of the osteoporotic skeleton to respond to mechanical conditions, implant devices, or cementation techniques must be recognized and addressed. This chapter will review some of these situations.

MANAGEMENT OF FRACTURES IN PATIENTS WITH OSTEOPOROSIS

Skeletal fractures are the most common orthopedic condition associated with osteoporosis. The goals of treatment are rapid mobilization and a return to normal activities; prolonged immobilization through the use of conservative fracture management is generally discouraged because it places the patient at risk of pulmonary decompensation, thromboembolic disease, decubitus formation, and further skeletal deterioration from disuse. Although the treatment of each fracture must be addressed individually, the following are general guidelines for the management of osteoporotic fractures:

1. Elderly patients are best treated by rapid, definitive fracture management aimed at early restoration of mobility and function. In general, these patients are considered to be at their healthiest on the initial day of injury and thus are in the best condition to undergo an operation at that time (1,2). In some cases, survival is benefited by judicious preoperative management to reverse medical decompensation causing or resulting from the injury. In addition, the extent and scope of the operative intervention should be minimized in order to reduce operative time, blood loss, and physiologic stress to the patient.

2. The goal of operative intervention is to achieve stable fracture fixation and permit early return of function. For the lower extremity, this is dictated by the ability of the patient to return to a weight bearing status early in the treatment period. Although anatomic restoration is important for intraarticular fractures, metaphyseal and diaphyseal fractures require early stabilization and perfect anatomic reduction is less important.

3. The primary mode of failure of internal fixation is due to the inability of the osteoporotic bone to support fixation devices. Since the strength of bone is directly related to the square of its mineral density (3), osteoporotic bone may lack the strength to support rigid fixation devices such as plates and screws. Moreover, comminution is generally more extensive in osteoporotic fractures and fixation devices should be chosen to allow compaction and settling of fracture fragments into stable patterns that minimize stresses at the bone–implant interface. Finally, implants should be chosen that minimize stress shielding in order to avoid further regional bone loss. For these reasons, sliding nail-plate devices, intramedullary systems, and tension band wiring constructs that allow load sharing and compaction are generally preferred over rigid systems.

4. Although the events of fracture healing proceed normally in almost all osteoporotic patients, an inadequate calcium intake could result in deficits in callus mineralization or remodeling (4). Since it has been shown that many elderly patients are malnourished, fracture healing may be enhanced when nutritional deficiencies are corrected (4,5). Therefore, for optimal results, nutritional assessment should be included in patient evaluation and in certain cases protein supplementation, physiologic doses of vitamin D (400–800 IU/day) and calcium (1.5 g elemental calcium/day) should be administered in the perioperative and postoperative periods.

Hip Fractures

A number of factors influence the occurrence of hip fractures. The medical and epidemiologic issues relating to hip

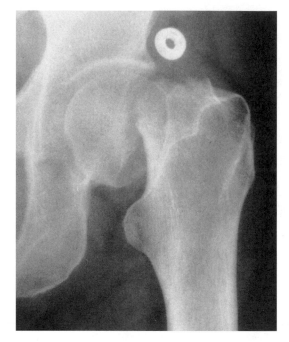

FIG. 1. Anteroposterior view of a typical intracapsular (femoral neck) fracture. Since the hip capsule inserts just above the greater and lesser trochanters of the femur, this fracture is anatomically located within the hip joint. As such, it is referred to as an intracapsular fracture.

fracture incidence are reviewed in Chapter 50. Although hip fractures have been classified according to several systems, patients with osteoporosis generally sustain one of two types of hip fractures, intracapsular or intertrochanteric. In intracapsular fractures, the fracture occurs within the hip capsule and frequently results in an interruption of the blood supply to the femoral head. These fractures are also known as cervical fractures, transcervical fractures, or femoral neck fractures (Fig. 1). Intertrochanteric fractures are extracapsular fractures that occur in an area in which biomechanical forces are only moderately high. The name "intertrochanteric" is derived from the fact that the fracture is anatomically propagated between the greater and lesser trochanters of the femur (Fig. 2).

Intracapsular fractures are problematic because of the high incidence of nonunion and avascular necrosis that occurs in spite of adequate treatment. These complications are related to the retrograde blood supply to the femoral head and the fact that the branches of the medial femoral circumflex artery, which nourish the femoral head within the hip capsule, are apposed to the femoral neck and are usually interrupted when intracapsular fractures are displaced. Closed reduction and pin and screw fixation using a variety of implants are consistently associated with a 14% incidence of nonunion and a 15% incidence of avascular necrosis (Fig. 3) (2).

The treatment options for intracapsular fractures are reduction and internal fixation vs. hemiarthroplasty. Since the degree of displacement of an intracapsular fracture may predict its prognosis, the decision of operative treatment is dictated by the extent of displacement of the fracture. The classification system used to help make these assessments is known as the Garden classification (Fig. 4). This is a four-stage classification system in which stage I fractures are those that are incomplete, nondisplaced, and frequently

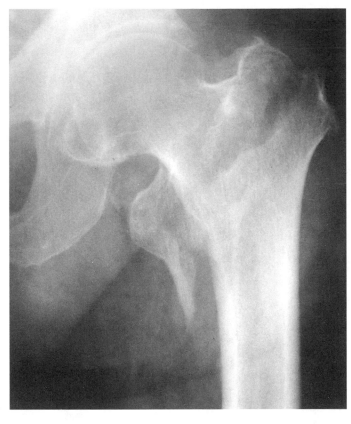

A

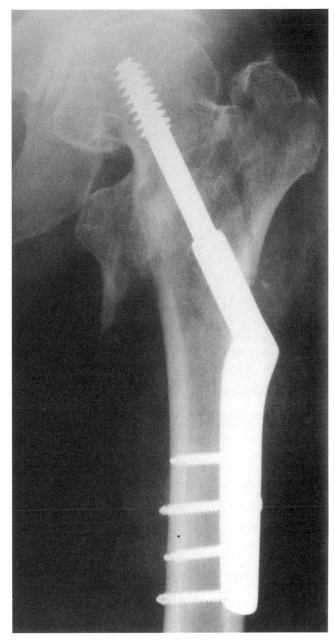

B

FIG. 2. A: Anteroposterior view of a typical intertrochanteric fracture. Note that the fracture line is propagated between the greater and lesser trochanters, and the lesser trochanter is actually displaced from the femur being pulled medially by the iliopsoas muscle insertion. **B:** Anteroposterior view of the same fracture 2 months after operative treatment. Note that with the use of a sliding hip screw the fracture fragments have settled or compacted into a stable configuration.

angled into a valgus position; stage II fractures are those that are complete, nondisplaced, but potentially unstable; stage III fractures are completely displaced, but a portion of the capsule remains intact; and in stage IV fractures, the fracture is completely displaced and the capsule is completely disrupted. Studies have shown that stage III and IV fractures have the highest rates of nonunion. Therefore, reduction and fixation with pins is generally preferred in stage I and II fractures while hemiarthroplasty is often used in the treatment of stage III and IV injuries (Fig. 5). The advantages of internal fixation are that the anatomy is restored, the patient undergoes a normal period of fracture healing, and if the joint has not been injured, the patient can expect normal service from the hip after the fracture has healed. The advantage of hemiarthroplasty is the immediate return to function because the replaced joint does not need to undergo a period

of healing. However, hemiarthroplasty is associated with its own set of complications including loosening and breakage of implants, and the risk of infection. Most authors agree that treatment by hemiarthroplasty is associated with a higher perioperative morbidity.

Intertrochanteric fractures have received less attention than femoral neck fractures because nonunion and avascular necrosis are uncommon in intertrochanteric fractures. However, the prevalence of malunion with resulting varus, shortening, and external rotational deformity is significant and can be disabling. In addition, when bone quality is particularly poor, the use of fixation devices may be beset with problems such as loss of fixation and screw penetration into the hip joint (2). Telescoping or sliding hip screw devices are an improvement over fixed nail devices in that they allow controlled compaction of the fracture until a stable fracture pat-

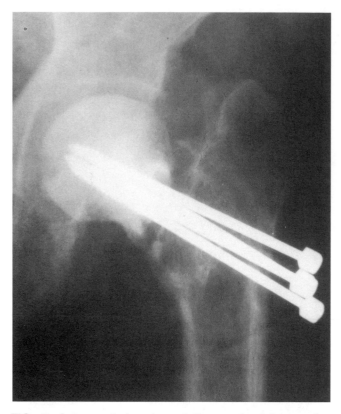

FIG. 3. Anteroposterior view of the proximal femur of a patient 3 months after open reduction and internal fixation of a displaced intracapsular fracture. Note that there is a diastasis at the fracture site, the pins have begun to migrate laterally, and the femoral head is radiodense, suggesting osteonecrosis.

tern is achieved. However, it is still necessary for the surgeon to obtain an adequate reduction before using such a device. When used properly, a load-sharing device will result in a decrease in the stresses between the implant and the bone and a more favorable biomechanical situation (Fig. 2B).

In some situations, the bone in the trochanteric region of the femur is so osteoporotic that any type of fixation system is at risk of failure. In these situations, orthopedists have resorted to the use of methyl methacrylate cement to enhance the purchase of implant devices in the bone and prevent penetration or cutting out of the device. More

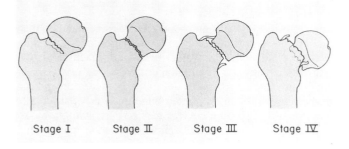

FIG. 4. Schematic of the Garden classification of intracapsular hip fractures.

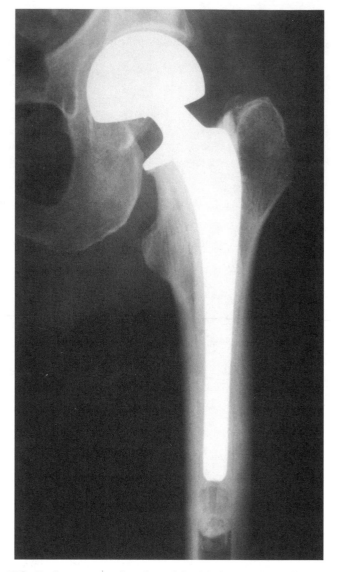

FIG. 5. Anteroposterior view of the hip in a patient who has undergone a hemiarthroplasty for the treatment of a displaced (stage IV) intracapsular hip fracture.

recently, a calcium phosphate-based material has been developed that may prove effective when injected into the site of a fracture or used with a fixation device at the time of fracture management. This material is presently experimental but current investigations on its use in the treatment of hip fractures have yielded encouraging results (6).

Fractures About the Knee

Osteoporotic bone that supports the knee joint is susceptible to supracondylar fractures of the distal femur and fractures of the tibial plateau. Because both of these fractures may be associated with comminution and intraarticular extension, they carry a high risk for postoperative degenerative joint disease and arthrofibrosis. Treatment protocols are therefore aimed at early knee rehabilitation and strengthening of the quadriceps mechanism.

Management of fractures about the knee in patients with osteoporosis can be difficult. Frequently, the degree of comminution is so extensive that choices of internal fixation are limited. Occasionally, special imaging techniques such as computed tomography (CT) scanning and plain tomography can help delineate the size and position of the fracture fragments. Because these fractures can be immobilized in a well-padded long leg cast or brace, the urgency for operative treatment is usually not as great as for the hip or the femoral shaft. However, long-term immobilization of these fracture not only limits a patient's activity but can lead to joint stiffness particularly in the elderly population.

In supracondylar fractures, the objectives of operative treatment are anatomic restoration and rigid fixation to allow immediate rehabilitation. Although good results have been obtained with one-piece blade plates and 90° telescoping screw plates, the recent advent of short locked intramedullary nails (GSH Nail®, Richards Manufacturing Company, Memphis, Tennessee) has aided in the management of these injuries. The advantage of this rigid type of fixation is that the patient's knee can be immediately moved in rehabilitation protocols.

Tibial plateau fractures generally result from a valgus stress to the knee in conjunction with falling and twisting. The degree of compromise that occurs as a result of tibial plateau fractures depends on the degree of instability and angular deformity. Minimally displaced fractures, i.e., those with less than 5 mm of depression, can be treated with immobilization of the knee followed by active motion. Nonweightbearing of the injured limb should be maintained until fracture healing has occurred at approximately 6–8 weeks. The use of continuous passive motion (CPM) has been found to be extremely helpful and the use of a hinge knee brace between CPM sessions enhances recovery. Fractures displaced by more than 8 mm, or those with associated varus or valgus instability of 5–10° or greater, require open reduction and internal fixation. Postoperatively, a varus molded cast brace followed by CPM is used. Weight bearing is delayed for a period of 8–10 weeks posttreatment.

Fractures of the Humerus

Three types of humeral fractures occur in osteoporotic patients: fractures of the proximal humerus, the humeral diaphysis, and the supracondylar region of the elbow. Generally, these fractures result from minor falls and usually occur with minimal displacement.

Fractures of the proximal humerus are common and account for approximately 5% of fractures in this patient population. Eighty percent of these fractures occur through the cancellous bone of the surgical neck and are impacted without significant displacement (2). These fractures are considered stable and can be treated by immobilization in a sling or sling like system. Range of motion activities including pendulum exercises can be started to avoid shoulder stiffness. Generally, 3–4 weeks is sufficient to allow for early healing prior to full passive range of motion with active range of motion taking place by 5–6 weeks. Unimpacted fractures can be treated with a sling or sling like device. Occasionally, closed reduction and percutaneous pin

fixation are required to achieve stable reduction. Comminuted fractures involving three- or four-part displacement are best treated by prosthetic replacement followed by early vigorous physical therapy. Open reduction and internal fixation can be used when the fragments are sufficiently large and there is less than extensive comminution. Open reduction and internal fixation using screws and tension band wires have been shown to work well. However, if difficulty is encountered in obtaining adequate purchase of screws, pins, or wires in bone, hemiarthroplasty is recommended.

Humeral shaft fractures in most cases are treated by nonoperative means. Occasionally, intramedullary nailing is needed to control angulation; however, because of the large amount of soft tissue in the arm, more angulation is acceptable with humeral shaft fractures than with fractures of other long bones.

Fractures of the distal humerus, especially those with an intraarticular component, present a particular challenge to orthopedic treatment. The potential for chronic disability is high and hence anatomic reduction and stable fixation is required. These fractures are associated with a high degree of morbidity and elbow stiffness is not uncommon. Early operative intervention followed by carefully planned physical therapy is needed.

Fractures of the Distal Radius

Fractures of the distal radius, most notably Colles' fractures, are a common complication of osteoporosis. Although it is generally held that substantial deformity of the distal radius can be acceptable when associated with relatively normal function, complications arise from this injury including loss of reduction, radial shortening, and painful prominence of the ulna (2). Many of these complications can be avoided by accurate reduction that restores the normal length and orientation of the distal radioulnar joint followed by early mobilization of the hand and upper extremity. Closed reduction and casting under local or regional anesthesia are generally successful in restoring the length of the distal radius. Healing is usually rapid and return to function occurs in about 6 weeks. Adequate reduction implies no radial shortening and at least a neutral angulation of the distal radial articular surface in the anterior–posterior plane. Unstable and severely comminuted fractures are best treated with internal or external fixation. External fixation is frequently difficult in osteopenic bone due to loosening of the pins in bone of poor quality. Therefore, the goal of treatment in these types of injuries is to obtain adequate reduction and control over the fracture fragments and immobilization long enough for early healing to take place. Once this has occurred, conversion to a cast or a splint is recommended. Current investigations using a calcium phosphate-based bone paste suggest that this material may enhance the fixation of these fragments and allowing for early conversion from a full-length arm cast to a short arm volar splint (6).

Spinal Fractures

Fractures of the spinal column are common in patients with osteoporotic bone. Vertebral fractures are grouped according to fracture type (wedge, biconcavity, or compression) and by degree of deformity (7). However, the vast majority of fractures of the osteoporotic spine are considered stable because the posterior spinal elements remain intact. Therefore, operative intervention is rarely required in spinal osteoporosis.

Symptomatic relief of spinal pain is often difficult to achieve because the causes are related not only to microcracks or fractures within the bone but also to stresses placed on the interspinous ligaments, facet joint capsules, and paraspinal muscles. Although narcotic medications are sometimes effective, their use should be discouraged or at least limited because the abuse potential is high. In many instances, significant symptomatic relief can be achieved through physical therapy, rehabilitation, and bracing. External support in the form of a bivalved custom polypropylene body jacket is useful during the acute painful phase of a fracture but should be discontinued when symptoms subside. These devices may cause paraspinal muscles to undergo atrophy with prolonged use, and it is those paraspinal muscles that are ultimately needed for support in maintaining the integrity of the spinal column complex. In those patients who upon careful evaluation are deemed able to withstand some low-level spinal stresses, a program of back extension and deep breathing exercises should be prescribed (8). In addition, counseling and instruction should be provided to all patients on the subjects of correct posture and body mechanics to prevent further pathologic fractures and the propensity to fall.

Operative management of osteoporotic spinal fractures is rarely indicated and should be reserved for the patient who has a fracture that is causing gross deformity resulting in pulmonary or neurologic impairment. The ability of the surgeon to obtain adequate purchase in bone is the main problem affecting any type of spinal fixation system. The recent development of the calcium phosphate-based materials may lead to the availability of new, fast-setting cements that could be effective in this application.

PROBLEMS ASSOCIATED WITH RECONSTRUCTIVE OPERATIVE PROCEDURES

Patients with osteoporosis are more prone to develop skeletal deformities as a result of physiologic bowing of qualitatively impaired bone or malunions of previous fractures. Correction of these deformities involves osteotomy, fixation, and bone healing. Planning of the osteotomy site and the placement of the bone cuts follow the same principles used in reconstructive surgery of the normal skeleton. Fixation, however, follows the principles outlined above for fracture management. In general, load-sharing devices such as intramedullary nails are preferred to rigid fixation systems. In addition, a very popular and effective method of osteotomy correction, small pin external fixation, is not suitable for patients with severe osteoporosis because of the propensity of small pins to cut out of qualitatively impaired bone.

Patients with diseased joints such as degenerative osteoarthritis are candidates for arthrodeses or total joint arthroplasties. While there are no special problems associated with arthrodeses in patients with osteoporosis, the types

of fixation systems used in conjunction with these procedures follow the same principles described for fractures. With respect to total joint arthroplasty, surgeons should follow the same principles used in the management of joints supported by normal bone; however, special care should be taken during reaming and component insertion. When reaming the acetabular socket, reamers should be used at lower speeds and the results of the reaming should be checked more frequently so that penetration of the acetabulum does not occur. This is particularly relevant in patients who use corticosteroids. When reaming the femoral canal, special attention should be paid to the positioning of all reamers and guide wire systems because it is easy to penetrate the cortex.

Insertion of cement under pressure in patients with osteoporotic bone can lead to unusual complications. For example, even when there are no breaks in the cortices of the femoral canal, highly pressurized cement and implant insertion can result in a blow out of the cortical wall. Similarly, once an implant has been seated in the joint and the cement cured, settling or subsidence of the implant–cement composite may occur leading to increased joint laxity.

Fractures occur more frequently around total joint prostheses in osteoporotic bone and the surgeon must be prepared to handle these complications. A common example occurs in the patient who has a total knee replacement and subsequent supracondylar fracture. Although controversy exists concerning the management of these injuries in patients with normal bone, the prolonged period of healing associated with osteoporotic bone and the limited amount of trabecular bone in this area dictates that the best method of management is fixation. The use of a short intramedullary nail can be very useful in this setting. Finally, although most fractures occur from traumatic events, the surgeon must be aware that resistance encountered intraoperatively in the process of reduction or dislocation of the joint can lead to an increased risk of iatrogenic fracture. For this reason, particular care must be taken in the gentle intraoperative manipulation of the limbs of osteoporotic patients who are undergoing total joint arthroplasty.

SUMMARY

Patients with osteoporosis present a special challenge to the orthopedist. While most issues relate to the management of fractures sustained in fragile bone, special problems associated with reconstructive orthopedic procedures must also be addressed. The goal of any treatment is the rapid restoration of mobility and function and a return of the patient to a level of activity which supports their general health. Long-term immobilization should be avoided. In situations where it is possible to reduce the effects of an offending agent, such as corticosteroids, all efforts should be made to do so. Recently, several new pharmacologic agents have been approved by the U.S. Food and Drug Administration for the treatment of osteoporosis. These agents carry the hope of reducing the morbidity of this disease. Hopefully, they will also lead to an improvement in bone quality such that the response of the skeleton to operative interventions will also be improved. The combined approach of general health maintenance, the judicious use of pharmacologic agents, and a program of regular exercise should reduce the orthopedic complications associated with this disease.

REFERENCES

1. Villar RN, Allen SM, Barnes SJ: Hip fractures in healthy patients: operative delay vs. prognosis. *BMJ* 293:1203–1204, 1986
2. Cornell CN: Management of fractures in patients with osteoporosis. *Orthop Clin N Am* 21:125–141, 1990
3. Carter DR, Hayes WC: The compressive behavior of bone as a two-phase porous structure. *J Bone Joint Surg* 59:954–962, 1977
4. Einhorn TA, Bonnarens F, Burstein AH: The contributions of dietary protein and mineral to the healing of experimental fractures: A biomechanical Study. *J Bone Joint Surg* 68A:1389–1395, 1986
5. Jensen JE, Jensen TG, Smith TK, Johnston DA, Dudrick SJ: Nutrition in orthopaedic surgery. *J Bone Joint Surg* 64A:1263–1272, 1982
6. Constantz BR, Ison IC, Fulmer MT, Poser RD, Smith ST, Van Wagoner M, Ross J, Goldstein SA, Jupiter JB: Skeletal repair by in situ formation of the mineral phase of bone. *Science* 267:1796–1799, 1995
7. Eastell R, Cedel SI, Wahner HW, Riggs BL, Melton LJ III: Classification of vertebral fractures. *J Bone Min Res* 6:207–214, 1991
8. Sinaki M, Mikkelesen BA: Postmenopausal spinal osteoporosis: flexion versus extension exercises. *Arch Phys Med Rehabil* 65:593–596, 1984

57. Osteoporosis and Rheumatic Diseases

Steven R. Goldring, M.D.

Department of Medicine, Harvard Medical School; Division of Rheumatology, Deaconess and New England Baptist Hospitals, Boston, Massachusetts

The rheumatic diseases include a diverse group of disorders that have in common their propensity to affect articular structures. The most commonly involved joints are the so-called diarthrodial joints, which consist of two articulating surfaces lined by hyaline cartilage. Arthritic processes most often affect the cartilage surfaces and the synovial lining but may also involve the subchondral bone and joint capsule. Amphiarthroses that are characterized by fibrocartilaginous union, e.g., the intervertebral disks, are also frequently affected in rheumatic disorders.

Osteoarthritis is a prototypical example of a rheumatic disease in which the pathologic events are restricted almost entirely to the joint structures. Many of the rheumatic diseases, however, may affect extraarticular organ systems and these conditions are often accompanied by significant systemic symptoms that may dominate the clinical picture. These illnesses, which include, for example, conditions such as rheumatoid arthritis (RA), systemic lupus erythematosus (SLE), and the spondyloarthropathies, are believed to be initiated by disturbances in immune regulation that involve complex interactions between unique host genetic susceptibility and specific environmental factor(s). In these disorders, not only may skeletal tissues be involved at juxtaarticular and subchondral sites, but in addition there is evidence that many of these conditions may produce generalized effects on bone remodeling that affect the entire skeleton.

Among the rheumatic disorders, RA represents an excellent model for gaining insights into the effects of local as well as systemic consequences of inflammatory processes on skeletal tissue remodeling. Three principal forms of bone disease have been described in RA. The first is that characterized by a focal process that affects the immediate subchondral and juxtaarticular bone. The synovial lesion of RA is characterized by the proliferation of the synovial lining cells and infiltration of the tissue by inflammatory cells, including lymphocytes, plasma cells, and activated macrophages (1,2). The proliferative synovial tissue (pannus) invades the immediately adjacent bone resulting in progressive focal osteolysis that gives rise to the characteristic cystic bone "erosions" that can be detected radiographically. Analysis of the immediate bone–pannus interface reveals the frequent presence of multinucleated cells with phenotypic features of osteoclasts (3,4), suggesting that the focal osteolytic lesions of RA are mediated at least in part by authentic osteoclasts. The origin of these cells is not clear, but some authors have speculated that they are derived from mononuclear cell precursors present within the inflamed synovium and that they are induced to differentiate into osteoclasts by the cytokines that are produced locally within the inflamed synovial tissue (5–7). There is also evidence that the macrophages and macrophage polykaryons associated with this lesion can also contribute to the bone resorption (6).

A second form of bone disease observed in patients with RA is the presence of juxtaarticular osteopenia adjacent to inflamed joints. Histologic examination of this bone tissue reveals the presence of frequent osteoclasts and increased osteoid and resorptive surfaces consistent with increased bone turnover (3,8). Local aggregates of inflammatory cells, including macrophages and lymphocytes, are often detected in the marrow space. It has been suggested that these cells are derived from the synovial lining and that they migrate into the marrow where they release local products that affect bone remodeling (3). Decreased joint motion and immobilization in response to the joint inflammation likely represent additional contributing factors to this local bone loss.

The third form of bone disease associated with RA is the presence of generalized axial and appendicular osteopenia at sites that are distant from inflamed joints (9–11). Although there are conflicting data concerning the effects of RA on skeletal mass, the presence of a generalized reduction in bone mass has been confirmed using multiple different techniques and there is compelling evidence that this reduction is associated with an increased risk of hip and vertebral fracture (12–15). The conflicting data are in part related to the fact that most observations have been based on cross-sectional studies and have focused on patients late in the evolution of their disease when factors such as disability, or corticosteroid and other treatments, may confound the analyses. Histomorphometric analysis of bone biopsies from patients with RA indicate that in the absence of corticosteroid use the cellular basis of the generalized reduction in bone mass is related to a decrease in bone formation rather than an increase in bone resorption (16–18). More recently, biochemical markers of bone turnover have been used to study patients with RA and the results of these studies indicate that in patients receiving corticosteroids there is an increase in bone resorption (19,20).

Several factors have emerged as important determinants of bone mass in patients with RA. These include age and menopausal status, reduced mobility, disease activity, influence of antirheumatic therapy (especially corticosteroids), and disease duration (21–28). A recent study by Gough and coworkers (21) in a large longitudinal prospective study concluded that significant amounts of generalized skeletal bone was lost early in RA and that this loss was associated with disease activity. These findings support the previous observations of Als et al. (29), who also noted a significant decrease in bone mass during the early phases of RA.

There is still considerable controversy regarding the effects of corticosteroids in affecting the progression of bone loss in RA. In part this is related to the tendency to use these medications in patients with more severe disease. Some authors suggest that if steroids satisfactorily suppress inflammation and maintain mobility, the deleterious effects of corticosteroids may be outweighed (21,22). It is premature, however, to generally advocate the use of corticosteroids in patients with RA since there is considerable evidence that their chronic use is associated with many potentially serious extraskeletal complications (30). This cautionary note is supported by the recent findings of Saag and coworkers who noted that low-dose long-term prednisone use, ≥5 g/day, was correlated in a dose-dependent fashion with the development of several different adverse reactions, including fracture (31).

Although not associated with focal bone erosions, generalized bone loss is also a significant clinical problem in patients with SLE. Reductions in both cortical as well as trabecular bone mass have been reported, even in the absence of corticosteroid treatment (32–34). As in patients with RA, the effects of systemic inflammation, decreased physical activity, nutritional factors, sex steroid influences, and drug treatments all likely contribute to the adverse effects on generalized bone mass. Similar factors contribute to the reduced bone mass and increased incidence of fractures in patients with a history of juvenile chronic (rheumatoid) arthritis (35,36). In addition, there is evidence of delayed skeletal linear growth.

Ankylosing spondylitis is characterized by inflammation at the entheses in the spine and peripheral skeleton. Although local bone erosions may be detected early in the course of the disease, new bone formation and ankylosis of the spine eventually develop in many patients. Several studies have documented an increased incidence of spinal compression fractures in patients with this disorder (37–39). Because of the chronic back pain experienced by many patients with ankylosing spondylitis and the high incidence of paraspinal calcifications and syndesmophytes, many of these fractures are not detected. Although not well studied, the decrease in axial bone density has been attributed to the effects of immobilization of the spine associated with the progressive ankylosis. It is interesting that appendicular bone appears to be normal in these individuals.

In contrast to the observations in individuals with inflammatory arthropathies, several authors have suggested that there is a reduced frequency of osteoporosis in patients with osteoarthritis (40–43). In a recent study, Hart et al. (44) examined the relationship between osteoarthritis of the hand, knee, and spine and bone density using dual x-ray absorptiometry of the spine and femoral neck. Their results suggest that the two conditions are inversely related. Adjustments for age, physical activity, and obesity as well as smoking and hormone replacement therapy did not affect results. The mechanisms that account for this observed relationship are not clearly defined.

REFERENCES

1. Harris ED Jr.: Rheumatoid arthritis. Pathophysiology and implications for therapy. *N Engl J Med* 322:1277–1289, 1990
2. Krane SM, Conca W, Stephenson ML, Amento EP, Goldring MB: Mechanisms of matrix degradation in rheumatoid arthritis. *Ann NY Acad Sci* 580:340–354, 1990
3. Bromley M, Woolley DE: Chondroclasts and osteoclasts at subchondral sites of erosion in the rheumatoid joint. *Arthritis Rheum* 27:968–975, 1984
4. Harada Y, Wang JT, Gorn AH, Gravallese EM, Thornhill TS, Jasty M, Harris WH, Juppner H, Goldring SR: Identification of the cell types responsible for bone resorption in rheumatoid arthritis. *Arthritis Rheum* 37:1994
5. Ashton BA, Ashton IK, Marshall MJ, Butler RC: Localization of vitronectin receptor immunoreactivity and tartrate resistant acid phosphatase activity in synovium from patients with inflammatory and degenerative arthritis. *Ann Rheum Dis* 52:133–137, 1993
6. Chang JS, Quinn JM, Demaziere A, Bulstrode CJ, Francis MJ, Duthie RB, Athanasou NA: Bone resorption by cells isolated from rheumatoid synovium. *Ann Rheum Dis* 51:1223–1229, 1992
7. Firestein GS, Alvaro-Garcia JM, Maki R: Quantitative analysis of cytokine gene expression in rheumatoid arthritis. *J Immunol* 144: 3347–3353, 1990
8. Shimizo S, Shiozawa S, Shiozawa K, Imura S, Fujita T: Quantitative histological studies on the pathogenesis of peri-articular osteoporosis in rheumatoid arthritis. *Arthritis Rheum* 28:25–31, 1985
9. Joffe I, Epstein S: Osteoporosis associated with rheumatoid arthritis: pathogenesis and management. *Semin Arthritis Rheum* 20:256–272, 1991
10. Peel NF, Eastell R, Russell RG: Osteoporosis in rheumatoid arthritis—the laboratory perspective. *Br J Rheum* 30:84–85, 1991
11. Woolf AD: Osteoporosis in rheumatoid arthritis—the clinical viewpoint. *Br J Rheum* 30:82–84, 1991
12. Spector TD, Hall GM, McCloskey EV, Kanis JA: Risk of vertebral fracture in women with rheumatoid arthritis. *BMJ* 306:558, 1993
13. Hooyman JR, Melton LJ, Nelson AM, O'Fallon WM, Riggs BL: Fractures after rheumatoid arthritis. *Arthritis Rheum* 27:1353–1361, 1984
14. Beat AM, Bloch DA, Fries JF: Predictors of fractures in early rheumatoid arthritis. *J Rheumatol* 18:804–808, 1991
15. Verstraeten A, Dequeker J: Vertebral and peripheral bone mineral content and fracture incidence in postmenopausal patients with rheumatoid arthritis: effect of low dose corticosteroids. *Ann Rheum Dis* 45:852–857, 1986
16. Kroger H, Arnala I, Alhava EM: Bone remodeling in osteoporosis associated with rheumatoid arthritis. *Calcif Tissue Int* 49:S90, 1991

17. Compston JE, Vedi S, Croucher PI, Garrahan NJ, O'Sullivan MM: Bone turnover in non-steroid treated rheumatoid arthritis. *Ann Rheum Dis* 53:163–166, 1994
18. Mellish RWE, O'Sullivan MM, Garrahan NJ, Compston JE: Iliac crest trabecular bone mass and structure in patients with non-steroid treated rheumatoid arthritis. *Ann Rheum Dis* 46:830–836, 1987
19. Hall GM, Spector TD, Delmas PD: Markers of bone metabolism in postmenopausal women with rheumatoid arthritis. Effects of corticosteroids and hormone replacement therapy. *Arthritis Rheum* 38:902–906, 1995
20. Gough AK, Peel NF, Eastell R, Holder RL, Lilley J, Emery P: Excretion of pyridinium crosslinks correlates with disease activity and appendicular bone loss in early rheumatiod arthritis. *Ann Rheum Dis* 53:14–17, 1994
21. Gough AK, Lilley J, Eyre S, Holder RL, Emergy P: Generalized bone loss in patients with early rheumatoid arthritis. *Lancet* 344:23–27, 1994
22. Kirwan JR: The effect of glucocorticoids on joint destruction in rheumatoid arthritis. *N Engl J Med* 333:142–146, 1995
23. Kroger H, Honkanen R, Saarikoski S, Alhava E: Decreased axial bone mineral density in perimenopausal women with rheumatoid arthritis —a population based study. *Ann Rheum Dis* 53:18–23, 1994
24. Laan RF, van Riel PL, van de Putte LB: Bone mass in patients with rheumatoid arthritis. *Ann Rheum Dis* 51:826–832, 1992
25. Laan RF, van Riel PL, van Erning LJ, Lemmens JA, Ruijs SH, van de Putte LB: Vertebral osteoporosis in rheumatoid arthritis patients: effect of low dose prednisone therapy. *Br J Rheumatol* 31:91–96, 1992
26. Sambrook PN, Eisman JA, Champion D, Yeates MG, Pocock NA, Eberl S: Determinants of axial bone loss in rheumatoid arthritis. *Arthritis Rheum* 30:721–728, 1987
27. Sambrook P, Birmingham J, Champion D, Kelly P, Kempler S, Freund J, Eisman J: Postmenopausal bone loss in rheumatoid arthritis: effect of estrogens and androgens. *J Rheumatol* 19:357–361, 1992
28. Sambrook P, Nguyen T: Vertebral osteoporosis in rheumatoid arthritis patients: effect of low dose prednisone therapy. *Br J Rheumatol* 31:573–574, 1992
29. Als OS, Gotfredsen A, Riis BJ, Christiansen C: Are disease duration and degree of functional impairment determinants of bone loss in rheumatoid arthritis? *Ann Rheum Dis* 44:406–411, 1985
30. Fries JF, Williams CA, Ramsey DR, Bloch DA: The relative toxicity of disease-modifying antirheumatic drugs. *Arthritis Rheum* 36:297–306, 1993
31. Saag KG, Koehnke R, Caldwell JR, Brasington R, Burmeister LF, Zimmerman B, Kohler JA, Durst DE: Low dose long-term corticosteroid therapy in rheumatoid arthritis: an analysis of serious adverse events. *Am J Med* 6:115–123, 1994
32. Dykman TR, Gluck OS, Murphy WA, Hahn TJ, Hahn BH: Evaluation of factors associated with glucocorticoid-induced osteopenia in patients with rheumatic diseases. *Arthritis Rheum* 28:361–368, 1985
33. Kalla AA, Fataar A, Jessop SJ, Bewerunge L: Loss of trabecular bone mineral density in systemic lupus erythematosus. *Arthritis Rheum* 36:1726–1734, 1993
34. Dhillon VB, Davies MC, Hall ML, Round JM, Ell PJ, Jacobs HS, Snaith ML, Isenberg DA: Assessment of the effect of oral corticosteroids on bone mineral density in systemic lupus erythematosus: a preliminary study with dual energy x-ray absorptiometry. *Ann Rheum Dis* 49:624–626, 1990
35. Loftus J, Allen R, Hesp R, David J, Reid DM, Wright DJ, Green JR, Reeve J, Ansell BM, Woo PM: Randomized, double-blind trial of deflazacort versus prednisone in juvenile chronic (or rheumatoid) arthritis: a relatively bone-sparing effect of deflazacort. *Pediatrics* 88:428–436, 1991
36. Varonos S, Ansell BM, Reeve J: Vertebral collapse in juvenile chronic arthritis: its relationship with glucocorticoid therapy. *Calcif Tissue Int* 41:75–78, 1987
37. Hanson CA, Shagrim JW, Duncan H: Vertebral osteoporosis in ankylosing spondylitis. *Clin Orthop* 74:59–64, 1971
38. Will R, Palmer R, Bhalla AK, Ring F, Calin A: Osteoporosis in early ankylosing spondylitis: a primary pathological event? *Lancet* 2:1483–1485, 1989
39. Ralston SH, Urquhart GD, Brzeski M, Sturrock RD: Prevalence of vertebral compression fractures due to osteoporosis in ankylosing spondylitis. *BMJ* 300:563–565, 1990
40. Dequeker J: The relationship between osteoporosis and osteoarthritis. *Clin Rheum Dis* 11:271–296, 1985
41. Cooper C, Cook PL, Osmond C, Fisher L, Cawley MID: Osteoarthritis of the hip and osteoporosis of the proximal femur. *Ann Rheum Dis* 50:540–542, 1991
42. Price T, Hesp R, Mitchell R: Bone density in generalized osteoarthritis. *J Rheumatol* 14:560–562, 1987
43. Nevitt MC, Lane NE, Scott JC, Hochberg MC, Pressman AR, Genant HK, Cummings SR: Radiographic osteoarthritis of the hip and bone mineral density. *Arthritis Rheum* 38:907–916, 1995
44. Hart DJ, Mootoosamy I, Doyle DV, Spector TD: The relationship between osteoarthritis and osteoporosis in the general population: the Clingford study. *Ann Rheum Dis* 53:158–162, 1994

58. Nutritional Rickets and Osteomalacia

Gordon L. Klein, M.D., M.P.H.

Department of Pediatrics, University of Texas Medical Branch, Galveston, Texas

Recommended dietary intakes of vitamin D and minerals for infants, children, and adults are listed elsewhere (see Appendix IV). Intakes of vitamin D, calcium, or phosphorus substantially below these recommendations may result in rickets or osteomalacia. Rickets is a disorder of mineralization of the bone matrix, or osteoid, in growing bone; it involves both the growth plate (epiphysis) and newly formed trabecular and cortical bone. Osteomalacia is also a defect in bone matrix mineralization, but it occurs after the cessation of growth and involves only the bone and not the growth plate. The mineralization defects in rickets, resulting from inadequate calcium and/or phosphate deposition in the matrix, has an uncertain etiology. However, there is a common finding of low calcium and phosphate concentration in the extracellular fluid surrounding rachitic cartilage and bone, suggesting that local factors may be responsible for the undermineralization (1).

Deficiencies of vitamin D, calcium, or phosphorus due to inadequate nutritional intake (Table 1) can result in defective bone mineralization. We will consider each separately.

VITAMIN D DEFICIENCY

The main natural sources of vitamin D in foods are the fish liver foods. Otherwise, fortification of foods such as

TABLE 1. *Causes and recommended management of nutritional rickets and osteomalacia*

Condition	Causes	Recommended management (ref.)
Vitamin D deficiency	Lack of adequate sunlight	Ultraviolet lamp or increased sunlight exposure (2)
	Consumption of diet low in fortified foods	Vitamin D_2 treatment. Variable: usually 1500–5000 IU/day orally (3); 10,000–50,000 IU/month intramuscular (3); 600,000 IU (15 mg) in 6 doses orally (7) in 1–2 hours
	Unsupplemented breast-fed infant	Prevention: vitamin D_2 400 IU/day orally (3) for premature infants
	Total parenteral nutrition	400–800 IU/day orally (10, 14); 20–25 IU/kg/day in total parenteral nutrition (9)
Calcium deficiency	Lack of dietary calcium	Treatment: 700 mg/day orally (11); 1–2 g/day orally (13)
	High phytate diet	30 mg/kg/day orally in breast-fed infants (17)
	Inadequate calcium in total perenteral nutrition	Prevention: in premature infants, 200 mg/kg/day orally (14); 20–60 mg/dl (5–15mM) in parenteral nutrition (9)
Phosphate deficiency	Breast-fed infants, inadequate phosphate in total parenteral nutrition-premature infants	Treatment: 25 mg/kg/day in breast-fed infants (17); withdrawl of aluminium-containing antacids (18); 115–120 mg/kg/day orally in premature infants (14); 15–47 mg/dl (5–15 mM) in parenteral nutrition (9)

milk and eggs has been necessary to prevent the occurrence of vitamin D deficiency in the United States (2,3). However, consumption of unfortified foods in an environment with reduced exposure to sunlight can lead to vitamin D deficiency in many developing countries (2,3). This is especially true of Asian women who wear veils, consume unfortified foods when pregnant, and nurse their infants. Another group at risk for vitamin D deficiency is breast-fed infants who do not receive vitamin D supplementation. Breast milk has been shown to be low in vitamin D, and cases of rickets in breast-fed infants have been reported (3).

Rickets can also develop in infants receiving total parenteral nutrition (TPN) solution exclusively from which vitamin D and calcium were inadvertently omitted (4).

However, it is unclear as to whether absence of vitamin D alone would have been sufficient to produce bone disease. Adults who received TPN devoid of vitamin D for up to 1 year did not develop osteomalacia although their serum levels of 25-hydroxyvitamin D (25(OH)D) were very low (5).

Pathogenesis

A diagram illustrating the steps in the pathogenesis of vitamin D-deficient rickets is shown in Fig. 1. The most biologically active vitamin D metabolite, 1,25-dihydroxyvitamin D [1,25(OH)$_2$D], is made in the kidney by hydroxylation of 25(OH)D that comes from the liver (see Chapter 13). 1,25-Dihydroxyvitamin D enhances calcium and phosphate absorption from the small intestine. During vitamin D deficiency, intestinal calcium and phosphate absorption are reduced, causing hypocalcemia. The hypocalcemia in turn stimulates the parathyroid glands to secrete increased quantities of parathyroid hormone (PTH). Parathyroid hormone acts indirectly on osteoclasts to pro-

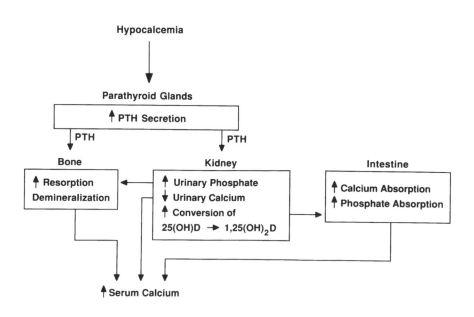

FIG. 1. Body's reaction to hypocalcemia with the consequent resorption of bone.

mote bone resorption and increase calcium and phosphorus available to the blood. In addition, PTH acts on the kidney to promote tubular calcium reabsorption and increase phosphate excretion. Parathyroid hormone also stimulates the renal conversion of 25(OH)D to 1,25(OH)$_2$D. 1,25-Dihydroxyvitamin D stimulates the small intestine to absorb more calcium and phosphorus (3).

Clinical and Laboratory Manifestations

Clinical manifestations of rickets include hypotonia, muscle weakness, and, in severe cases, tetany. Weight-bearing produces a bowing deformity of the long bones.

Prominence of the costochondral junction, the so-called rachitic rosary, can also be seen (Fig. 2), as can an indentation of the lower ribs, Harrison's groove, due to softening. Occasionally there is indentation of the sternum in response to the force exerted by the diaphragm and intercostal muscles. Deformities of the back, including kyphosis and lordosis, along with limb bowing, can contribute to a waddling gait. There is also an increased frequency of fractures.

Abnormalities of the skull, especially in younger infants, include a softened calvarium (craniotabes), parietal flattening, and frontal bossing. There is delayed eruption of permanent dentition and enamel defects can occur (3).

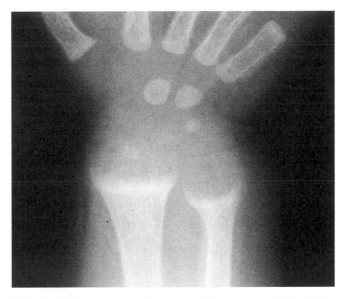

FIG. 3. Wrist demonstrating typical findings of rickets in the radius and ulna. Note widening of the metaphyses, irregularity of the metaphyses, widening of the epiphyseal line, and cupping of the metaphyses. In addition, note that the bones in general are demineralized. (x-ray and interpretation provided courtesy of Leonard Swischuk, M.D., Department of Radiology, University of Texas Medical Branch, Galveston, Texas.)

Diffuse bone pain is the most common manifestation of osteomalacia, although there is some tendency for localization of pain in the hip area. Pelvic deformities and a waddling gait may also be present.

Roentgenographically the long bones are the earliest and most common sites of change. Typically there is thinning of the cortex and rarefaction of the shaft with widening, fraying, and cupping of the distal ends of the shaft and disappearance of the zone of provisional cartilaginous calcification (Fig. 3). Thin cortical radiolucent lines (stress fractures) at right angles to the bone shaft may be seen in osteomalacia as well as other metabolic bone disorders. These are most often symmetric and bilateral. Decreased bone density is also seen. The pelvis and ribs are the most frequently affected areas (3).

Biochemical findings, as expected, include low or normal serum levels of calcium, low serum levels of phosphorus, and markedly elevated serum alkaline phosphatase levels. This enzyme elevation probably reflects increased bone turnover. Serum PTH levels are elevated when hypocalcemia is present. Serum levels of 25(OH)D are low in vitamin D deficiency; secondary hyperparathyroidism and low serum phosphorus stimulate renal production of 1,25(OH)$_2$D so that levels of this hormone are either normal or high if adequate vitamin D is present (3). Serum osteocalcin concentrations are within the normal range, although insufficient data are available to be definitive. Iliac crest bone biopsies of two Indian children, ages 36 and 69 months, revealed increased osteoid seams and reduced mineralization when compared with normal, though only semiquantitative data were published (6).

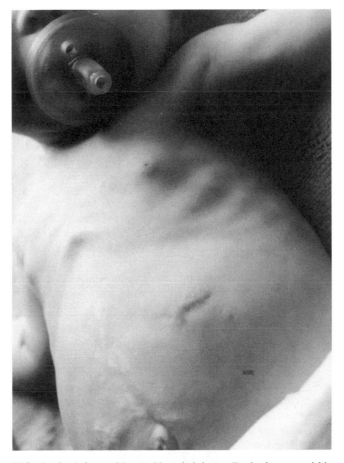

FIG. 2. An infant with nutritional rickets displaying a rachitic rosary at the costochondral junction.

Treatment and Prevention

Recommended doses of vitamin D for treatment and prevention of vitamin D deficiency rickets are given in Table 1. In vitamin D deficiency due to fat malabsorption, use of a more polar compound, such as 25(OH)D, 20–30 μg/day, or 1,25(OH)$_2$D, 0.15–0.5 μg/day, may be more efficacious. Alternatively, ergocalciferol (vitamin D$_2$ in oil) given intramuscularly may be effective (4). The dose and frequency of administration must be adjusted depending on the serum levels of calcium, phosphorus, alkaline phosphatase, and 25OHD. In infants doses have ranged from 10,000 to 50,000 IU (250–1250 μg) per month. Complications of vitamin D$_2$ therapy include hypercalcemia and hypercalciuria (3). Alternatively, for patients whose rickets or osteomalacia results from lack of exposure to sunlight, either increased exposure to sunlight or ultraviolet lamp treatment may prove beneficial (2). Alternatively, recent data suggest that single-day large-dose therapy with vitamin D (600,000 IU, 15 mg) will result in improvement in nutritional rickets within 4–7 days and can serve as a useful diagnostic test to differentiate nutritional rickets from other forms (7).

Rickets of prematurity is generally considered a disease of calcium and/or phosphate deficiency rather than vitamin D deficiency. When long-term TPN therapy is involved, aluminum accumulation may also be a contributing factor (8). Currently, doses of vitamin D$_2$ for parenteral use in TPN-fed infants are 20–25 IU (0.5 μg/kg/day) (9). The oral dose of vitamin D$_2$ is between 400 and 800 IU (10 and 20 μg) daily (10–14).

For prevention of vitamin D deficiency not due to malabsorption or prematurity, daily exposure to adequate sunlight, consumption of fortified milk, or dietary supplementation of 400 IU (10 μg) is recommended.

CALCIUM DEFICIENCY

Decreased calcium intake or intestinal absorption has been associated with rickets. Kooh and colleagues (11) described rickets in an infant receiving prolonged nutrition with lamb-based formula, which provided adequate phosphorus but only 180 mg/day of calcium. Vitamin D supplements were provided to give this child up to 800 IU (20 μg) per day. With the provision of 700 mg calcium/day there was marked biochemical and roentgenographic improvement after 1 month (11).

Similarly, Pettifor and coworkers (12) identified a population of children in South Africa who consumed no milk or dairy products and whose daily calcium intake was estimated to be only 125 mg, whereas phosphate intake was adequate. Biochemical and roentgenographic evidence of rickets was present. Moreover, bone histology in three children revealed increased unmineralized osteoid (matrix) and decreased bone turnover, diagnostic of osteomalacia (12,13). Calcium supplementation led to both biochemical and histologic improvement (13).

Reduction in calcium absorption may contribute to calcium deficiency rickets. Consumption of cereals and other grain products high in phytate could lead to intraluminal calcium phytate complexation and consequent calcium malabsorption. This has been postulated by Stamp (2) and colleagues in Asian populations living in London. However, they subsequently demonstrated in two children that despite continued consumption of a high phytate diet, rickets improved with ultraviolet light therapy (2). Thus, it is possible that lack of sunlight rather than phytate-induced calcium malabsorption was responsible for the rickets in these children.

Another source of calcium deficiency-induced bone disease is total parenteral nutrition. Early in the development of TPN therapy, inadvertent omission of calcium led to rickets that was reversed by addition of calcium (4). Today relative lack of calcium in the TPN solutions may be in part responsible for the osteopenia and rickets of prematurity (10).

Pathogenesis

The pathogenesis of calcium deficiency rickets is similar to that of vitamin D-deficiency rickets in that hypocalcemia causes secondary hyperparathyroidism. Parathyroid hormone increases bone resorption and enhances the renal conversion of 25(OH)D to 1,25(OH)$_2$D to increase intestinal calcium and phosphorus absorption. Alkaline phosphatase also reflects elevated osteoblastic bone cell activity. Both the patients of Kooh et al. (11) and those of Pettifor and colleagues (12,13) had normal serum 25(OH)D levels, demonstrating that they were not vitamin D-deficient. The patient of Kooh et al. were hypophosphatemic, whereas those from South Africa were not.

Clinical manifestations of calcium-deficiency rickets are similar to those described for vitamin D deficiency.

Treatment and Prevention

In the cases described from Canada and South Africa, oral calcium treatment was given (11–13) as shown in Table 1. Response to treatment was assessed by reduction in serum alkaline phosphatase levels and improvement in roentgenographic and histologic abnormalities. Special premature formulas now contain 75–150 mg calcium/dL. Currently, approximately 200 mg/kg/day is the goal for daily oral calcium intake (14). Parenteral solutions contain from 20 to 60 mg calcium/dL (9). Use of solutions containing 20 mg/dL of calcium resulted in a 20% incidence of rickets and osteopenia among premature infants in an intensive care nursery (15). Experience with 60 mg calcium/dL has been too limited to determine whether it reduces the incidence of rickets.

PHOSPHATE DEFICIENCY

Phosphate deficiency has been reported to cause rickets and osteomalacia. During the early development of TPN, omission of phosphate resulted in rickets that resolved with appropriate phosphate supplementation (4). However, premature infants may still receive inadequate phosphate relative to their needs (10). The calcium and phosphate added to parenteral nutrition solutions are limited by the possibility of calcium phosphate precipitation. According to Mierzwa (16), the following equation may serve as a guide to determining whether calcium and phosphate will precipitate in solutions:

$$\frac{\text{Phosphate (mmol)} \times 1.8}{\text{Volume (L)}} = A$$

$$\frac{\text{Calcium gluconate (mg)} \times 4.6/1000}{\text{Volume (L)}} = B$$

If $A \times B$ is <300 the parenteral nutrition solution is not likely to precipitate. Preliminary reports indicate that newer amino acid formulations supplemented with the sulfur-containing amino acids taurine and cysteine allow greater quantities of calcium and phosphate to remain in solution in TPN formulations (16).

Nutritional hypophosphatemic rickets has also been reported in a premature infant who was breast-fed without calcium or phosphate supplements (17).

Others at risk for hypophosphatemic osteomalacia include those who have been taking antacids for long periods of time (18) and those patients receiving dialysis who have osteomalacia (see Chapter 67). Antacid-induced osteomalacia results from aluminum complexation with dietary phosphate in the intestinal lumen that prevents phosphate absorption. Aluminum itself does not become deposited in bone in significant quantities (18).

Pathogenesis

The pathogenesis of phosphate-deficiency rickets differs from that of vitamin D and calcium deficiency in that neither hyperparathyroidism nor vitamin D deficiency is present. Patients become phosphate deficient, causing a reduction in serum phosphorus. Phosphate deficiency and hypophosphatemia increase renal production of $1,25(OH)_2D$. 1,25-Dihydroxyvitamin D increases bone resorption *in vitro*, and it is possible but not proven that elevated serum levels of $1,25(OH)_2D$ cause bone resorption in these patients (17), although there is evidence that it may do so in adults (19).

Treatment and Prevention

Recommended parenteral phosphate intake for premature infants and phosphate and calcium supplementation regimens for breast-fed prematures are given in Table 1. Roentgenographic changes of rickets resolved in one breast-fed infant after 3 months of calcium and phosphate supplementation (17). However, these recommendations may not be sufficient to ensure optimal bone mineral content (14). The phosphate available in specialized premature infant formulas is approximately 75 mg/dl (14). Long-term evaluation must be completed before one can conclude that this supplementation is effective in reducing the incidence of osteopenia and rickets in prematures.

For patients requiring long-term antiulcer therapy, use of nonaluminum-containing medications such as cimetidine or ranitidine should be considered.

REFERENCES

1. Klein GL, Simmons DJ: Nutritional rickets: thoughts on pathogenesis. *Ann Med* 25:379–386, 1993
2. Stamp TCB: Factors in human vitamin D nutrition and in the production and cure of classical rickets. *Proc Nutr Soc* 34:119–130, 1975
3. Sandstead HH: Clinical manifestations of certain classical deficiency diseases. In: Goodhart RS, Shils ME (eds) *Modern Nutrition in Health and Disease.* 6th ed. Philadelphia, Lea and Febiger, pp 693–696, 1980
4. Klein GL, Chesney RW: Metabolic bone disease associated with total parenteral nutrition. In: Lebenthal E (ed) *Total Parenteral Nutrition: Indication, Utilization, Complications, and Pathophysiological Considerations.* 1st ed. New York, Raven Press, pp 431–443, 1986
5. Shike M, Sturtridge WC, Tam CS, Harrison JE, Jones G, Murray TM, Husdan H, Whitwell J, Wilson DR, Jeejeebhoy KN. A possible role of vitamin D in the genesis of parenteral nutrition, induced metabolic bone disease. *Ann Intern Med* 95:560–568, 1981.
6. Mukherjee A, Battacharyya AIG, Barkar PC. Kwashiorkor, marasmus syndrome and nutritional rickets–a bone biopsy study. *Trans Royal Soc Trop Med Hyg* 85:688–689, 1991.
7. Shah BR, Finberg L. Single day therapy for vitamin D–deficiency rickets: a preferred method. *J Pediatr* 1125:487–490, 1994.
8. Sedman AB, Klein GL, Merritt RJ, Miller NL, Weber KO, Gill WL, Anand H, Alfrey AC: Evidence of aluminum loading in infants receiving intravenous therapy. *N Engl J Med* 312:1337–1343, 1985
9. Koo WWK, Kaplan LA, Bendon R, Succop P, Tsang RC, Horn J, Steichen D: Response to aluminum in parenteral nutrition during infancy. *J Pediatr* 109:877–883, 1986
10. Hillman LS: Neonatal osteopenia-diagnosis and management. In: Frame B, Potts JT Jr (eds) *Clinical Disorders of Bone and Mineral Metabolism.* Amsterdam, Excerpta Medica, pp 427–430, 1983
11. Kooh SW, Fraser D, Reilly BJ, Hamilton JR, Gall DG, Bell L: Rickets due to calcium deficiency. *N Engl J Med* 297:1264–1266, 1977
12. Pettifor JM, Ross FP, Travers R, Glorieux FH, DeLuca HF: Dietary calcium deficiency: A syndrome associated with bone deformities and elevated serum 1,25-dihydroxyvitamin D concentrations. *Metab Bone Dis Rel Res* 2:301 -306, 1981
13. Marie PJ, Pettifor JM, Ross FP, Glorieux FH: Histological osteomalacia due to dietary calcium deficiency in children. *N Engl J Med* 307:584–588, 1982
14. Greer FR, Steichen JJ, Tsang RC: Effects of increased calcium, phosphorus and vitamin D intake on bone mineralization in very low birth weight infants fed formulas with polycose and medium chain triglycerides. *J Pediatr* 100:951–955, 1982
15. Koo WWK, Oestreich A, Tsang RC, Sherman R, Steichen J: Natural history of rickets and fractures in very low birth weight (VLBW) infants during infancy. *J Bone Min Res* 1:123(abstract 255), 1986
16. Mierwza MW: Stability and compatibility in preparing TPN solution. In: Lebenthal E (ed) *Total Parenteral Nutrition: Indications, Utilization, Complications, and Pathophysiological Considerations.* 1st ed. New York, Raven Press, pp 219–230, 1986
17. Rowe JC, Wood DH, Rowe DW, Raisz LG: Nutritional hypophosphatemic rickets in a premature infant fed breast milk. *N Engl J Med* 300:293–296, 1979
18. Carmichael KA, Fallon MD, Dalinka M, Kaplan FS, Axel L, Haddad JG: Osteomalacia and osteitis fibrosa in a man ingesting aluminum hydroxide antacid. *Am J Med* 76:1137–1143, 1984
19. Maierhofer WJ, Gray RW, Cheung H, Lemann J Jr: Bone resorption stimulated by elevated serum 1,25(OH)2-vitamin D concentrations in healthy men. *Kidney Int* 24:555–560, 1983

59. Metabolic Bone Disease in Gastrointestinal, Hepatobiliary, and Pancreatic Disorders

D. Sudhaker Rao, M.B.B.S., F.A.C.P. and *Mahalakshmi Honasoge, M.B.B.S., F.A.C.P.

*Department of Medicine, University of Michigan, and *Bone and Mineral Division, Henry Ford Health System, Detroit, Michigan*

Increasing life expectancy, inadequate intake of vitamin D and calcium, and decreasing efficiency of calcium absorption with advancing age may contribute to the development of metabolic bone disease (MBD) in otherwise healthy individuals. The impact of these abnormalities on bone is only amplified in patients with various gastrointestinal, hepatobiliary, and pancreatic disorders. In addition, the morbidity and mortality related to the MBD is far greater in such patients than in patients with postmenopausal osteoporosis.

In a number of gastrointestinal, hepatobiliary, and pancreatic diseases, there is impaired absorption (1–5) and/or increased catabolism of vitamin D and its metabolites (6) and malabsorption of calcium (7,8). In a few patients there may even be an increased urinary and/or fecal loss of calcium and calcidiol (25-hydroxyvitamin D). Symptoms related to the underlying malabsorption syndrome may not always be obvious. Occasionally, MBD may be the only presenting manifestation of an occult malabsorption syndrome (9,10). Careful and systematic evaluation is therefore needed to uncover such abnormalities.

The prevalence and the type of MBD in gastrointestinal diseases varies with the duration, type, and severity of malabsorption. MBD is uncommon, for instance, in patients with pancreatic insufficiency, but its prevalence may approach 50% to 70% in those with gluten enteropathy. Conversely, prior history of gastrectomy and celiac sprue are strong risk factors for osteoporosis (11–14). Because of the varied response of the skeleton to alterations in mineral and vitamin D nutrition, the spectrum of bone disease in gastrointestinal disorders may range from subjective impression of "decreased bone density" seen on routine skeletal roentgenograms, to severe osteomalacia with its classic clinical, biochemical, radiologic, and histologic findings. All gradations between these two extremes may be encountered. In addition, estrogen deficiency, smoking, excess alcohol consumption, and therapy with corticosteroids, sucralfate (which has a high aluminum content),

cholestyramine, and immunosuppressive agents may also modify the expression of bone disease.

Based on morphologic and kinetic characteristics (15,16), it is possible to identify three distinct types of bone lesions in patients with various gastrointestinal disorders. The salient histomorphometric features are summarized in Table 1, and the individual bone lesions are discussed below in detail.

SECONDARY HYPERPARATHYROIDISM WITH OR WITHOUT VITAMIN D DEFICIENCY

Secondary hyperparathyroidism with or without vitamin D deficiency is characterized by increased surface and volume, but not the thickness of osteoid (Table 1). In patients with vitamin D deficiency additional features of reduced adjusted mineral apposition rate (AjAR) and prolongation of mineralization lag time (Mlt; usually <100 days) will be present (hypovitaminosis D osteopathy; HVO-I). In both types there is accelerated loss of mainly cortical bone. Serum calcium (Ca), phosphate (P), and Ca × P product are normal but serum total alkaline phosphatase (AP), or bone-specific AP (BSAP) may be elevated in up to 80% of the patients. There is biochemical evidence of secondary hyperparathyroidism with increased levels of serum parathyroid hormone (PTH). Although 24-hour urine calcium is usually <100 mg/day, it varies with dietary intake. Clinically, patients are asymptomatic at this stage of the disease, bone density is reduced and most patients present mainly with skeletal fractures. Bone pain, muscle weakness, and pseudofractures are uncommon.

OSTEOMALACIA

Osteomalacia is characterized by osteoid thickness (O.Th) of >15 μm and an Mlt of >100 days. Both the surface

TABLE 1. *Morphologic and kinetic characteristics of bone diseases*

Measurement	Secondary HPT		Osteomalacia		
	D+	D-(HVO-I)	HVO-II	HVO-III	LTO
Osteoid surface (% BS)	↑	↑	↑↑	↑↑	N
Osteoid volume (% BV)	N	N/	↑↑	↑↑	N
Osteoid thickness (μm)	N	N/	↑↑	↑↑	N/↓
Mlt(days)	N	<100	>100	>100	<100
Osteoclast surface (% MdS)	↑	↑	↑↑	↑↑	N/↓
BFR (μm3/μm2/year)	↑	↑	↓	0	N/↓

BFR, bone formation rate; BS, bone surface; BV, bone volume; D+, no vitamin D depletion; D-, vitamin D depletion; HPT, hyperparathyroidism; HVO, hypovitaminosis D osteopathy (stages I, II, and III); LTO, low-turnover osteoporosis; MdS, mineralized surface; Mlt, mineralization lag time; N, normal; ↑, increased; ↓, decreased.

and volume, as well as the thickness, of osteoid are increased (Table 1). Within this group two further stages are identified: HVO-II, in which some mineralization of osteoid still occurs, and HVO-III where mineralization ceases to occur. Biochemical abnormalities are common in osteomalacia with reductions in serum levels of Ca, P, and Ca × P product, and elevations in AP, BSAP, and PTH. Patients are symptomatic with diffuse bone pain and muscle weakness at this stage of the disease, and may present with waddling gait that is typical of osteomalacia. Classic radiologic features of osteomalacia such as pseudofractures, biconcave vertebrae, triradiate pelvis, and protrusio acetabuli are seen only in this group.

Two additional types of osteomalacia (focal and atypical) that are not related to vitamin D depletion are recognized on careful analysis of bone histomorphometry. These two variants of osteomalacia that may be seen during therapy with sodium fluoride or etidronate are discussed in more detail in Chapter 65.

LOW-TURNOVER OSTEOPOROSIS

Low-turnover osteoporosis is probably the most common and least understood form of MBD in patients with gastrointestinal disorders. It is characterized by normal or reduced O.Th, decreased bone formation rate (Table 1), and slight reduction in AjAR resembling in some ways postmenopausal or age-related osteoporosis. Protein and other micronutrient deficiencies, and low serum levels of insulin-like growth factor-1 (IGF-1; Rao DS, *unpublished data*) might contribute to the development of this bone disease. Vertebral compression fractures are more common than in the other two types of bone lesions. Biochemical abnormalities are less frequent and secondary hyperparathyroidism is usually absent. Symptoms are usually related to the attendant skeletal fractures.

Two specific points deserve emphasis: (i) secondary hyperparathyroidism is a consistent feature in all patients with vitamin D depletion leading to an accelerated loss of mainly cortical bone; and (ii) both the age-related or postmenopausal osteoporosis that frequently accompany the vitamin D-related bone disease and the low turnover of osteoporosis described above do not respond to therapy with vitamin D or its metabolites. Currently, transiliac bone biopsy after tetracycline labeling (see Chapter 25) is the only definitive way of determining the exact nature of the underlying bone disease. In the future, the availability of biochemical markers of bone turnover may obviate the need for bone biopsy.

SPECIFIC ASPECTS OF METABOLIC BONE DISEASES IN GASTROINTESTINAL DISORDERS

Postgastrectomy Bone Disease (1–3,11,13,17,18)

Metabolic bone disease following gastrectomy or the more recent gastric stapling procedure is much more common than is generally appreciated. This is partly due to the incorrect notion that bone disease after gastric resection or exclusion surgery occurs infrequently because of the routine fortification of milk and other dairy products with vitamin D in this country. Indeed, gastrectomy alone accounts for half of all cases of osteomalacia seen in this country followed by intestinal malabsorption, primarily biliary cirrhosis and pancreatic insufficiency (19). Furthermore, gastrectomy is a known risk factor for postmenopausal osteoporosis (11,12). Several factors contribute to the development of bone disease following gastrectomy. These include poor dietary intake or self-imposed restriction of dairy products to avoid diarrhea and dumping syndrome; the anatomic changes in the gastrointestinal tract resulting in impaired absorption of vitamin D and its metabolites (Fig. 1) and of calcium; rapid transit of

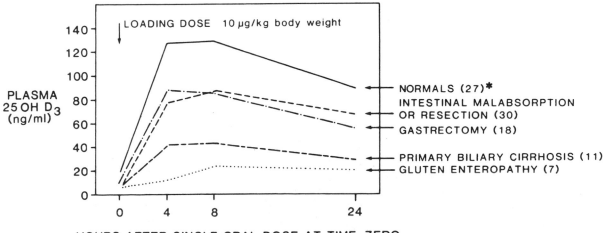

FIG. 1. Calcidiol absorption in normal subjects and in patients with various gastrointestinal disorders. Only the mean values were used to construct the curves for the sake of clarity. There is wide variation both in normal subjects and in patients. The scatter is much wider at 4 hours than at 8 hours, but the mean level at 4 and 8 hours for each group is significantly lower than in normal persons. Data were compiled from published reports as well as from personal experience. *Numbers in parentheses represent the total number of normal subjects and patients studied.

food; increased catabolism of vitamin D and its metabolites; and phosphate depletion due to excessive use of phosphate-binding antacids. It is important to note that sucralfate, a drug that contains excess aluminum, may cause aluminum-related osteomalacia (see Chapters 65–67) (20), especially in patients with impaired renal function. Patients with Billroth II or total gastrectomy appear to be more at risk of developing MBD than those who have had Billroth I operation.

Bone disease is seldom detected early, and most patients present 5 or more years after gastrectomy. The onset is insidious, and there is frequent association of osteoporosis. Many patients are asymptomatic in the early postoperative period, and the bone loss can be detected only by measurement of bone density (see Chapter 23). Routine skeletal surveys are neither sensitive nor specific to be useful for screening purposes. Hypocalcemia and hypophosphatemia are uncommon early in the course and tend to occur when the bone disease has advanced to HVO stage II or III. Elevated serum levels of AP or BSAP may suggest an underlying bone disease, and thus serves as a useful screening test to detect early vitamin D depletion and is available through commercial laboratories. When there is decreased bone density or low serum calcidiol level or both, bone histology is almost always abnormal. Approximately 20% to 30% of such patients will have osteomalacia as defined previously, and the remainder show evidence of secondary hyperparathyroidism or low-turnover osteoporosis.

As vitamin D depletion becomes more severe, usually a function of the time since gastrectomy, patients develop diffuse bone pain, muscle weakness, and a typical waddling gait. When bone disease is far advanced, pseudofractures, the classic radiologic sign of osteomalacia are present. Bone histology shows either HVO-II or HVO-III and the clinical syndrome resembles more closely the traditional descriptions of osteomalacia. Hypocalcemia, hypophosphatemia, and elevated serum levels of AP or BSAP are uniform findings at this stage of the disease. Although treatment will greatly improve the clinical status of the patient, recovery of the cortical bone mineral deficit is negligible and patients are at risk of fractures for the rest of their lives. It is therefore important to diagnose the bone disease at the earliest possible time to prevent long-term morbidity. This policy is no different from that of iron, folate, or vitamin B_{12} deficiency.

Despite similar risk factor(s) it is unclear why some patients develop HVO and others low-turnover osteoporosis after gastrectomy. General malnutrition, protein and other "micronutrient" deficiencies, and low serum levels of IGF-1 may contribute to the pathogenesis of the latter. As might be expected, low-turnover osteoporosis does not respond to vitamin D therapy. Therapeutic strategies similar to those employed in the management of osteoporosis might offer promise.

Intestinal Disorders (9,10,14,21–27)

In patients with intestinal disease, resection, or bypass, there is impaired absorption of both vitamin D (Fig. 1) and calcium; in some patients there may even be an increased endogenous fecal loss of calcium and vitamin D. The degree of malabsorption of vitamin D and calcium is quite variable and, in general, depends on the severity of intestinal malabsorption. In Crohn's disease, for instance, vitamin D depletion is uncommon in the absence of intestinal resection or concomitant cholestyramine therapy. In gluten enteropathy, on the other hand, vitamin D depletion is common because of the more severe malabsorption (Fig. 1). Osteomalacia may occur in 50% to 70% of such patients and occasionally may be the only presenting manifestation of gluten enteropathy (9,10). Low-turnover bone disease is probably more common, and osteomalacia is less common in patients with inflammatory bowel disease (IBD) than in patients who have had previous gastrectomy. Furthermore, the clinical expression of bone disease is modified by other factors such as sun exposure, general malnutrition (and consequently low IGF-1 levels?), frequent use of corticosteroids, bile acid sequestrants, total parenteral nutrition (see Chapter 66), and the menopausal status. Impaired skeletal growth and decreased bone density have been reported in children and adolescents with IBD, especially in patients receiving corticosteroids. Both low-turnover osteoporosis and osteomalacia are seen in adults with IBD (24). Rate of bone loss is greater in men treated with corticosteroids (25) and in perimenopausal women in whom bone loss can be prevented by estrogen therapy (26).

In patients with intestinal bypass surgery for morbid obesity, bone disease may develop even when prophylactic vitamin D therapy is instituted soon after surgery. This suggests that other nutritional deficiencies (protein, albumin, or other micronutrients) may contribute to osteoblast dysfunction and to the pathogenesis of MBD (22). Both osteopenia and osteoporosis are more common and severe than in patients with gastrectomy. Gastric stapling, which has replaced intestinal bypass procedure, has also been reported to produce osteomalacia (19).

No systematic studies of bone disease are available in patients with celiac sprue to determine the exact nature and magnitude of the problem. However, it has been estimated that MBD is two- to threefold more common in such patients compared to the general population (14). Conversely, the prevalence of undiagnosed celiac sprue is higher among patients with osteoporosis (14). Calcidiol absorption is severely impaired, and in the authors' experience the absorption test is both diagnostic and therapeutic (Fig. 1). In a few patients, the abnormal calcidiol absorption test has led to the diagnosis of celiac disease in the absence of overt symptoms of malabsorption (Rao DS, *unpublished data*). Measurement of serum antigliadin antibodies may be useful in detecting occult celiac disease in patients presenting with MBD, but the false-positive rate is unacceptably high. Occasionally, patients may even develop autonomous hypercalcemic secondary hyperparathyroidism requiring parathyroidectomy (28). Even though a gluten-free diet plus vitamin D and calcium supplementation results in dramatic clinical improvement, increased risk of fractures persists due to irreversible loss of mainly cortical bone.

Hepatobiliary Diseases (29–38)

Because of the large functional reserve, abnormalities of bone and mineral metabolism are relatively uncommon in the usual types of parenchymal liver diseases. Bone disease in chronic alcoholism is probably related to the direct effect of alcohol on bone rather than to the associated liver disease. In obstructive liver diseases, such as primary biliary cirrhosis or biliary atresia in children, abnormalities of bone and mineral metabolism are commonplace. Factors that contribute to MBD include inadequate intake of dairy products because of anorexia; impaired absorption of dietary vitamin D and calcidiol (Fig. 1); urinary and fecal loss of vitamin D and its metabolites; binding of vitamin D or its metabolites by bile acid-sequestering agents; and impaired 25-hydroxylation of vitamin D in the liver. Other factors, such as corticosteroid and immunosuppressive therapy, malnutrition, decreased sun exposure, and possibly "hepatotoxins," may also influence the nature and the severity of MBD.

Biochemical abnormalities are more common and pronounced than in patients with gastrectomy or malabsortion syndrome. Hypocalcemia, when present, is usually due to the associated hypoalbuminemia or hypoproteinemia. Because serum levels of AP are uniformly elevated in various liver diseases, its significance in detecting an underlying bone disease is negated unless serum levels of BSAP are measured. Low calcidiol levels may be related to the reduced vitamin D-binding proteins. Secondary hyperparathyroidism is less common than in patients with gastrectomy or intestinal malabsorption.

Osteopenia and low-turnover osteoporosis are more common than osteomalacia. Indeed, osteomalacia as defined by rigorous criteria has occurred only in two cases (19). Both the lack of clinically significant bone disease and the infrequency of osteomalacia are probably related to the fact that skeletal manifestations become less clinically relevant due to the serious nature of the liver disease. However, in a small number of patients bone disease may contribute to the morbidity of already ill patients. With improvement in long-term survival, MBD may dominate the clinical course of their illness, just as renal osteodystrophy has become a major problem in patients receiving maintenance hemodialysis.

Bone pain, when present, is often related to multiple long bone and rib fractures as a result of severe cortical bone loss rather than to osteomalacia. Even in asymptomatic patients vertebral compression fractures may occur. Muscle weakness is also unrelated to vitamin D depletion in the majority of patients.

Treatment of hepatic osteodystrophy is unsatisfactory at present, except in those with unequivocal osteomalacia. Bone histology after tetracycline labeling is mandatory in planning therapeutic options in these patients. Because of severe impairment of liver function either calcidiol or calcitriol (1,25-dihydroxyvitamin D) is preferred to vitamin D in patients with vitamin D depletion.

Bone disease following liver transplantation confers significant morbidity and is being recognized with greater frequency (39–41). Unlike renal osteodystrophy, which frequently improves after kidney transplantation, hepatic osteodystrophy deteriorates following liver transplantation. The incidence of vertebral fractures is increased in patients with liver transplantation, especially during the first year after surgery (40). In some patients, the onset of skeletal fractures is quite rapid over a period of a few months. One of us (D. S. Rao) has seen a 16-year-old patient develop seven spontaneous vertebral fractures in 6 months! The nature of the bone disease prior to the liver transplantation, immobilization, direct toxic effects of immunosuppressive agents, and possibly the deficiency of IGF-1 may all contribute to this serious problem. At present, treatment of post transplant bone disease is unsatisfactory. Calcitonin and vitamin D metabolites have been used with variable results. A therapeutic trial with IGF-1 and/or growth hormone may be worth pursuing.

Pancreatic Insufficiency (42–45)

Because intestinal mucosal integrity is preserved in patients with pancreatic insufficiency, MBD is uncommon in most such patients. Malabsorption of calcium and/or vitamin D due to profound steatorrhea, poor nutrition, and frequent history of alcoholism (46) may all predispose such patients to the development of MBD. Hypocalcemia is more common in patients with acute than with chronic pancreatic disease. Other biochemical abnormalities are less common than in patients with celiac sprue with a comparable degree of steatorrhea. Low serum levels of calcidiol, when present, are usually a reflection of poor dietary intake.

In cystic fibrosis, the most severe form of exocrine pancreatic insufficiency, MBD may be more common than is currently appreciated. Osteomalacia, however, is distinctly rare. With improvement in life expectancy, MBD may become a major clinical problem in patients with cystic fibrosis. Reduced bone density and increased bone fractures and bone deformities (kyphosis) have been found with greater frequency in patients with cystic fibrosis compared to the general population (43,45). Gonadal dysfunction, a common feature in such patients, may contribute to the development of MBD. An occasional patient may even develop autonomous hypercalcemic secondary hyperparathyroidism (the so-called tertiary) requiring parathyroidectomy (19), analogous to that seen in patients with longstanding untreated celiac sprue (28). Systematic studies of bone histomorphometry in patients with chronic pancreatic insufficiency or cystic fibrosis are not available and therefore the spectrum of bone disease in such patients remains unknown. In men with cystic fibrosis treatment consists of vitamin D and calcium supplementation to assure adequate daily intake and correction of hypogonadism. However, hormone replacement therapy may aggravate pulmonary dysfunction in women with cystic fibrosis. Follow-up of patients with cystic fibrosis should include routine yearly measurement of at least bone density as well as serum levels of Ca, BSAP, and calcidiol.

PREVENTION AND MANAGEMENT OF MBD IN PATIENTS WITH VARIOUS GASTROINTESTINAL DISORDERS

Prevention of MBD depends on the awareness of its existence in an appropriate clinical setting and the ability to screen the population at risk. Since the evolution of MBD in these patients is often asymptomatic, the prevention program must begin before significant irreversible cortical bone loss has occurred. Yearly screening of patients at risk with serum levels of AP or BSAP and calcidiol appears reasonable. Whether this is cost-effective is unknown, but considering the morbidity that an undiagnosed HVO confers, the cost appears justifiable. Bone density, serum PTH, and biochemical markers of bone turnover are indicated when serum BSAP is elevated or calcidiol is reduced or both.

Calcidiol Absorption Test (1–5,47)

Availability of sensitive assays for measurement of serum calcidiol concentration has made it possible to test for the presence of calcidiol malabsorption directly in various gastrointestinal disorders (Fig. 1). The test also provides an additional advantage of rapid repletion of body stores in patients with significant vitamin D depletion. The test is performed by administering 10 μg/kg of body weight of calcidiol as a single oral dose in the fasting state. Serum levels of calcidiol are measured at 4-hour intervals for 24 hours. A modified short test measuring only preabsorptive and 4- and 8-hour postabsorptive levels also provides adequate information. Although the test does not replace other specific tests for malabsorption syndrome, it has reasonable diagnostic and a definite therapeutic utility. Figure 1 shows typical absorption curves of calcidiol in various gastrointestinal diseases (47).

With the availability of calcidiol for therapeutic use and the ability to monitor its serum concentrations, it is prudent to use this preparation. Doses should be adjusted to maintain a serum calcidiol level of 30–50 ng/ml. Although oral vitamin D is effective in many patients, variable bioavailability, chemical deterioration, and problems in monitoring the dose make these preparations unsuitable for long-term management. Calcidiol, on the other hand, is available in gelatin-coated capsules, is less subject to chemical deterioration, has a shorter half-life (which reduces potential for toxicity), can easily be monitored by serum levels, and its conversion to calcitriol remains under homeostatic control. In conditions such as primary biliary cirrhosis, calcidiol may be the drug of choice because of defective 25-hydroxylation of vitamin D. In most patients with HVO as a result of gastrointestinal disorders, renal function is normal; therefore, there is little justification for the use of calcitriol. Oral calcium intake of 1–2 g/day should be insured. Serial measurements of serum levels of PTH, bone density, and biochemical markers of bone turnover should be performed to assess the efficacy of treatment.

Because many patients require lifelong therapy, periodic monitoring of serum levels of Ca and AP as well as renal function is necessary. Hypercalcemia, although rare, may occur at any time and should be treated promptly as discussed in Chapter 27. Education of patients about the nature of their bone disease, necessity for lifelong therapy and follow-up, and the potential for future risk of fractures even after resolution of HVO is essential both for compliance and to avoid complications related to calcidiol toxicity. It is equally important to identify other risk factors for MBD, such as smoking, excess alcohol consumption, estrogen deficiency, poor sunlight exposure, and physical inactivity, and take appropriate steps to modify these risk factors. It is worth reemphasizing that HVO in its early stages is asymptomatic but causes significant irreversible cortical bone loss and increased fracture risk. Therapy only repletes body stores and alleviates symptoms but rarely reverses bone loss. It is therefore necessary to keep all patients with gastrointestinal disorders under lifelong surveillance to avoid preventable morbidity.

REFERENCES

1. Stamp TCB: Intestinal absorption of 25-hydroxycholecalciferol. *Lancet* 2:121–123, 1974
2. Gertner JM, Lilburn M, Domenech M: 25-Hydroxycholecalciferol absorption in steatorrhoea and postgastrectomy osteomalacia. *BMJ* 1:1310–1312, 1977
3. Krawitt EL, Chastenay BF: 25-hydroxy vitamin D absorption test in patients with gastrointestinal disorders. *Calcif Tissue Int* 32:183–187, 1980
4. Compston JE, Creamer B: Plasma levels and intestinal absorption of 25-hydroxyvitamin D in patients with small bowel resection. *Gut* 18:171–175, 1977
5. Compston JE, Thompson RPH: Intestinal absorption of 25-hydroxyvitamin D and osteomalacia in primary biliary cirrhosis. *Lancet* 1:721–724, 1977
6. Clements MR, Davies M, Hayes ME, et al: The role of 1,25-dihydroxyvitamin D in the mechanism of acquired vitamin D deficiency. *Clin Endocrinol* 37:17–27, 1992
7. Sjoberg HE, Nilsson LH: Retention of oral ^{47}Ca in patients with intestinal malabsorption: regional enteritis and pancreatic-insufficiency. *Scand J Gastroenterol* 5:265–273, 1970
8. Harris OD, Philips HM, Cooke WT: ^{47}Ca studies in adult coeliac disease and other gastrointestinal conditions with particular reference to osteomalacia. *Scand J Gastroenterol* 5:169–175, 1970
9. Hajjar ET, Vincenti F, Salti CS: Gluten-induced enteropathy; osteomalacia as a principal manifestation. *Arch Intern Med* 134:565–567, 1974
10. De-Boer WA, Tytgat GN: A patient with osteomalacia as single presenting symptom of gluten-sensitive enteropathy. *J Intern Med* 232:81–85, 1992
11. Rao DS, Kleerekoper M, Rogers M, Frame B, Parfitt AM: Is gastrectomy a risk factor for osteoporosis? In: Christiansen C et al. (ed) *Osteoporosis*. Denmark, pp 775–777, 1984
12. Mellstrom D, Johansson C, Johnell O, et al: Osteoporosis, metabolic aberrations, and increased risk for vertebral fractures after partial gastrectomy. *Calcif Tissue Int* 53:370–377, 1995
13. Kobayashi S, Takahashi C, Kuroda T, Sugenoya A, Lida F, Katoh K: Calcium regulating hormones and bone mineral content in patients after subtotal gastrectomy. *Surg Today* 24:295–298, 1994
14. Walters JRF: Bone mineral density in coeliac disease. *Gut* 35:150–151, 1994
15. Rao DS, Villanueva AR, Mathews M, et al: Histologic evolution of vitamin D depletion in patients with intestinal malabsorption or dietary deficiency. In: Frame B, Potts JT Jr (eds) *Clinical Disorders of Bone and Mineral Metabolism*. Amsterdam, Excerpta Medica, pp 224–226, 1983
16. Parfitt AM, Drezner MK, Glorieux FH, et al: Bone histomorphometry: standardization of nomenclature, symbols, and units. Report of the ASBMR histomorphometry nomenclature committee. *J Bone Min Res* 2:595–610, 1987
17. Bisballe S, Eriksen EF, Melsen F, Mosekilde L, Sorensen OH, Hessov I: Osteopenia and osteomalacia after gastrectomy: interrelations between biochemical markers of bone remodeling, vitamin D metabolites and bone histomorphometry. *Gut* 32:1303–1307, 1991
18. Imawari M, Kozawa K, Akanuma Y, Koizumi S, Itakura H, Kosaka K: Serum 25-hydroxyvitamin D and vitamin D binding protein levels and mineral metabolism after partial and total gastrectomy. *Gastroenterology* 79:255–258, 1980
19. Honasoge M, Rao DS: Metabolic bone disease in gastrointestinal,

hepatobiliary, and pancreatic disorders and total parenteral nutrition. *Curr Op Rheumatol* 7:249–254, 1995

20. Chines A, Pacifici R: Antacid and sucralfate-induced hypophosphatemic osteomalacia: a case report and review of literature. *Calcif Tissue Int* 47:291–295, 1990

21. Compston JE, Ayers AB, Horton LWL, Tighe JR, Creamer B: Osteomalacia after small-intestinal resection. *Lancet* 1:9–12, 1978

22. Parfitt AM, Miller MJ, Frame B, et al: Metabolic bone disease after intestinal bypass for treatment of obesity. *Ann Intern Med* 89:193–199, 1978

23. Genant HD, Mall JC, Wagonfeld JB, van der Horst J, Lanzl LH: Skeletal demineralization and growth retardation in inflammatory bowel disease. *Invest Radiol* 11:541–549, 1976

24. Hessov I, Mosekilde L, Melsen F, et al: Osteopenia with normal vitamin D metabolites after small bowel resection for Crohn's disease. *Scand J Gastroenterol* 19:691–696, 1984

25. Motley RJ, Clements D, Evans WD, et al: A four-year longitudinal study of bone loss in patients with inflammatory bowel disease. *Bone Min* 23:95–104, 1993

26. Clements D, Compston JE, Evans WD, Rhodes J: Hormone replacement therapy prevents bone loss in patients with inflammatory bowel disease. *Gut* 34:1543–1546, 1993

27. Lupattelli G, Fuscaldo G, Castellucci B, Ciuffetti G, Pelli MA, Mannarino E: Severe osteomalacia due to gluten-sensitive enteropathy. *Ann Ital Med Int* 9:40–43, 1994

28. Bolla G, Disdler P, Harle JR, et al: Hyperparathyroidie tertiaire revelatrice d'une maladie coeliaque de l'adulte. *Presse Med* 23:346–348, 1994

29. Dibble JB, Sheridan P, Hampshire R, Hardy GJ, Losowsky MS: Evidence for secondary hyperparathyroidism in the osteomalacia associated with chronic liver disease. *Clin Endocrinol* 15:373–383, 1981

30. Reed JS, Meredith SC, Nemchansky BA, Rosenberg IH, Bover JL: Bone disease in primary biliary cirrhosis: reversal of osteomalacia with oral 25-hydroxyvitamin D. *Gastroenterology* 79:512–517, 1980

31. Matloff DS, Kaplan MM, Neer RM, Goldberg MJ, Bitman W, Wolfe HI. Osteoporosis in primary biliary cirrhosis: effects of 25-hydroxyvitamin D treatment. *Gastroenterology* 83:97–102, 1982

32. Herlong FH, Recker RR, Maddrey WC: Bone disease in primary biliary cirrhosis: histologic features and response to 25-hydroxyvitamin D. *Gastroenterology* 83:103–108, 1982

33. Lindor KD: Management of osteopenia of liver disease with special emphasis on primary biliary cirrhosis. *Semin Liver Dis* 13:367–372, 1993

34. Soriano H, Shulman RJ, Levy M, et al: Hepatic osteodystrophy in chronic cholestasis: evidence for multifactorial etiology. *J Pediatr Gastroenterol Nutr* 19:345, 1994

35. Hodgson SF, Dickson ER, Eastell R, Eriksen EF, Bryant SC: Rates of cancellous bone remodeling and turnover in osteopenia associated with primary biliary cirrhosis. *Bone* 14:819–827, 1993

36. Stellon AJ, Webb A, Compston JE, Williams R: Low bone turnover state in primary biliary cirrhosis. *Hepatology* 7:137–142, 1987

37. Crippin JS, Jorgenson RA, Dickson ER, Lindor KD: Hepatic osteodystrophy in primary biliary cirrhosis: effects of medical treatment. *Am J Gastroenterol* 89:47–50, 1994

38. Bonkovsky HL, Hawkins M, Steinberg K, et al: Prevalence and prediction of osteopenia in chronic liver disease. *Hepatology* 12:273–280, 1990

39. Katz IA, Epstein S: Perspective in post-transplantation bone disease. *J Bone Min Res* 7:123–126, 1992

40. Navasa M, Monegal A, Guanabens N, et al: Bone fractures in liver transplant patients. *Br J Rheumatol* 33:52–55, 1994

41. Hawkins FG, Leon M, Lopez MB, et al: Bone loss and turnover in patients with transplantation. *Hepatogastroenterology* 41:158–161, 1994

42. Hahn TJ, Squires AE, Halstead LR, Stonninger DB: Reduced serum 25-hydroxyvitamin D concentration and disordered mineral metabolism in patients with cystic fibrosis. *J Pediatr* 94:38–42, 1979

43. Henderson RC, Specter BB: Kyphosis and fractures in children and young adults with cystic fibrosis. *J Pediatr* 125:208–212, 1994

44. Bachrach LK, Loutit CW, Moss RB. Osteopenia in adults with cystic fibrosis. *Am J Med* 96:27–34, 1994

45. De Schepper J, Smitz J, Dab I, Piepsz A, Jonckheer M, Bergmann P: Low serum bone gamma-carboxyglutamic acid protein concentrations in patients with cystic fibrosis: correlation with hormonal parameters and bone mineral density. *Horm Res* 39:197–201, 1993

46. Diez A, Puig J, Serrano S, et al: Alcohol induced bone disease in the absence of severe chronic liver damage. *J Bone Miner Res* 9:825–831, 1994

47. Rao DS: Bone and mineral metabolism. In: Haubrick WS, Schaftner F, Berk JE (eds) *Bockus Gastroenterology*. 5th ed. Philadelphia, WB Saunders, pp 3464–3471, 1995

60. Vitamin D-Dependent Rickets

Uri A. Liberman, M.D., Ph.D. and *Stephen J. Marx, M.D.

*Division of Endocrinology and Metabolic Diseases, Rabin Medical Center—Beilinson Campus, and Sackler School of Medicine, Tel Aviv University, Petch-Tikva, Israel; and *Genetics and Endocrinology Section, National Institute of Diabetes and Digestive and Kidney Diseases, National Institutes of Health, Bethesda, Maryland*

Pseudovitamin D deficiency or vitamin D-dependent rickets (VDDR) type I and II are rare inborn errors of vitamin D metabolism, characterized by all of the classical clinical, radiologic, biochemical, and histologic features of vitamin D deficiency (Chapter 58) despite adequate vitamin D intake and without a therapeutic response to an accepted vitamin D replacement therapy. The two syndromes differ (Table 1) in the circulating concentration of 1,25-dihydroxyvitamin D [1,25(OH)$_2$D], the therapeutic response to 1α-hydroxylated active vitamin D metabolites, and obviously in the primary defect in vitamin D metabolism.

VITAMIN D-DEPENDENT RICKETS TYPE I (VDDR-I)

Prader et al. (1) in 1961 were the first to report two young children with VDDR-I and to coin the phrase "pseudovitamin D deficiency" to describe this syndrome. The disease manifests itself before 2 years of age and often during the first 6 months of life. Complete remission could be obtained but was dependent on continuous therapy with high doses of vitamin D. Family studies revealed this to be a genetic disorder with a pattern suggestive of autosomal recessive inheri-

TABLE 1. *Vitamin D-dependent rickets (VDDR)*

| | Serum concentrations | | | | |
	Calcium	25(OH)D	1,25(OH)$_2$D	iPTH	Presumed defect
VDDR I	↓	N–↑	↓↓	↑	renal 25OHD 1-hydroxylase
VDDR II	↓	N–↑	N–↑	↑	intracellular 1,25(OH)$_2$D receptor

tance (2) and linkage analysis assigned the gene responsible for the disease to chromosome 12q14. It was shown very recently that decidua cells isolated from term placenta of two patients with VDDR-I were unable to synthesize calcitriol in contrast to control decidual cells (2A). This may imply that there is a defect in the renal tubular 25-hydroxyvitamin D 1α-hydroxylase as well. Several indirect measurements support this notion. First, serum concentrations of 25-hydroxyvitamin D (25(OH)D) were normal or markedly elevated in patients treated with high doses of vitamin D or 25(OH)D$_3$. Second, blood levels of 1,25(OH)$_2$D were very low in several studies of children with VDDR-I. Finally, while massive doses of vitamin D and 25(OH)D$_3$ (1000–3000 μg/day and 200 to 900 μg/day, respectively, 100–300 times the recommended daily dose) are required to maintain remission of rickets in VDDR-I, 0.25–1.0 μg/day of 1,25(OH)$_2$D$_3$ (a normal physiologic dose) are sufficient to achieve the same effect. Taken together, these observations support the thesis that many if not all patients with VDDR-I have a hereditary defect in the renal tubular 25(OH)D-1-hydroxylase. The beneficial therapeutic effect of high circulating levels of 25(OH)D in patients with VDDR-I treated with vitamin D or 25(OH)D$_3$ where 1,25(OH)$_2$D concentrations remain low has several possible explanations. First, 25(OH)D at high concentrations may activate the specific intracellular receptor for 1,25(OH)$_2$D whose affinity of 25(OH)D is about two orders of magnitude lower than for the active hormone (Chapter 13). Second, high concentrations of the substrate 25(OH)D may drive the local production of 1,25(OH)$_2$D in some tissues in a paracrine or autocrine manner. Finally, a metabolite of 25(OH)D may act directly on target tissues.

A similar syndrome has been studied in a mutant strain of pigs (3) in which the mode of inheritance as well as the clinical, radiologic, and biochemical pictures are similar to that of the human disease. In a recent study (4) of piglets affected by this disease, circulating levels of 25(OH)D were elevated, 1,25(OH)$_2$D were low or undetectable, concentrations of specific [^{3}H]1,25(OH)$_2$D$_3$ binding sites were normal, and no 25(OH)D-1-hydroxylase activity could be measured in renal cortical homogenates. Thus, there is strong evidence that the disease state in the pig is caused solely by an inherited defect in the renal 25(OH)D-1-hydroxylase system. It is likely that a similar defect occurs in human VDDR-I.

VITAMIN D-DEPENDENT RICKETS TYPE II (VDDR-II)

In 1978, Brooks et al. (5) described a patient with hypocalcemia, osteomalacia, and elevated circulating levels of 1,25(OH)$_2$D. Treatment with vitamin D$_3$ resulted in a further increase in serum 1,25(OH)$_2$D levels and corrected the hypocalcemia of the patient. The term "vitamin D-dependent rickets type II" was suggested to describe this disorder. Based on additional case reports, in which about half of the patients with this disorder did not respond to any form of vitamin D therapy and therefore were not dependent on the vitamin, and some *in vivo* and *in vitro* studies to be discussed, the term VDDR-II seems to be a misnomer. We therefore suggest the term "hereditary resistance to 1,25(OH)$_2$D" as more appropriate to describe this syndrome. However, due to convention and convenience the term VDDR-II will be retained in this chapter.

Clinical Manifestations

The clinical, radiologic, histologic, and biochemical characteristics common to all patients with VDDR-II are rickets and/or osteomalacia of varying severity; no history or biochemical evidence of vitamin D or calcium deficiency; hypocalcemia and/or secondary hyperparathyroidism; no remission with physiologic doses of vitamin D or its active metabolites; and increased serum levels of 1,25(OH)$_2$D before or during treatment with calciferol preparations (6).

Patients with VDDR-II show the highest serum levels of 1,25(OH)$_2$D found in any living system. These levels could represent the end result of synergistic action of three potential stimulators of the 25(OH)D-1-hydroxylase, namely, hypocalcemia, secondary hyperparathyroidism, and hypophosphatemia; or they might also reflect an additional defect in regulation of the renal hydroxylase.

There are fewer than 50 known kindreds with this syndrome (a partial list in references 6–22 and personal communications). Contrary to the homogeneity of the clinical and biochemical presentation of VDDR-I, a marked heterogeneity exists in VDDR-II.

Affected children appear normal at birth, and the metabolic bone disease presents early, usually before 2 years of age. However, late onset of the disease was reported in several sporadic cases, presenting in some patients in their teens (5); in one patient the onset of osteomalacia was at 45 years of age (10). All cases with late presentation have been normocalcemic, and they represent the mildest form of the disease.

A peculiar feature of the syndrome that appears in about two thirds of the kindreds is alopecia that varies from sparse hair to total alopecia without eyelashes (Fig. 1). In some patients, additional ectodermal anomalies, such as multiple milia, epidermal cysts (Fig. 1), and oligodontia, appear as well (9). The alopecia may be obvious at birth but usually develops during the first months of life. Alopecia seems to be a marker of a more severe form of the disease as judged by the earlier age of the presentation of the disease, the marked clin-

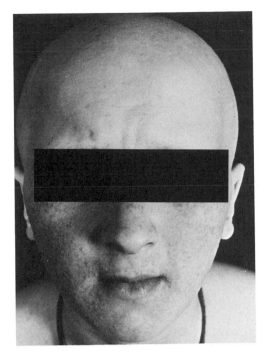

FIG. 1. A patient with VDDR-II: total alopecia, multiple milia, and epidermal cysts.

ical aberrations, the number of patients who did not respond to treatment with high doses of vitamin D and metabolites (in contrast to the complete remission achieved in almost all patients with normal hair), and the high levels of serum 1,25(OH)$_2$D recorded during successful and unsuccessful therapy (6,23). Though some patients with alopecia have a satisfactory calcemic response to high doses of vitamin D and metabolites, none have shown improvement of hair growth.

The notion that total alopecia is probably a direct consequence of resistance to 1,25(OH)$_2$D is supported by the following observations: (i) Alopecia is present in kindreds with different biochemical and molecular defects in the 1,25 (OH)$_2$D receptor-effector system; (ii) high-affinity uptake of [^{3}H]1,25(OH)$_2$D$_3$ occurred in the nucleus of the outer root sheath cells of the hair follicle of rodents; and (iii) the epidermis and hair follicles contain a calcium-binding protein that is at least partially vitamin D-dependent. Alopecia has been observed only with end-organ resistance to 1,25(OH)$_2$D and has not been noted with hereditary or acquired states associated with low-circulating levels of 1,25(OH)$_2$D. Thus, either the deficiency in vitamin D action is more severe in VDDR-II or, alternatively, 1,25(OH)$_2$D may have an effect on differentiation of the hair follicle in the fetus that is unrelated to mineral homeostasis.

Parental consanguinity and multiple siblings with the same defect occur in about half of the reported kindreds with VDDR-II, suggesting an autosomal recessive mode of inheritance in these and perhaps all kindreds. Parents of patients appear phenotypically normal. However, *in vitro* studies of cultured cells (see the following discussion) from parents of two kindreds with VDDR-II revealed heterogeneity of their 1,25(OH)$_2$D$_3$ receptor (VDR), i.e., expression of both a normal and an abnormal VDR allele. The affected children expressed only the abnormal allele (24,25). There is a striking clustering of patients close to the Mediterranean, and most of the patients reported from Europe and North America are descendants of families originating from around the Mediterranean as well. Notable exceptions are several kindreds reported from Japan (10,11,22).

Classification by Cellular Defect

Studies on the nature of the intracellular defect in the 1,25(OH)$_2$D receptor-effector system of patients with VDDR-II became possible with demonstration that cells originating from tissues easily accessible for biopsy contain receptors for the hormone that are similar if not identical to those of classical target tissues. The cells used are mainly dermal fibroblasts, but keratinocytes, cells derived from bone, and, recently, peripheral blood mononuclear (PBM) cells [mitogen-stimulated T-lymphocytes and Epstein–Barr (EB) virus–transformed lymphocytes] have been used as well (6,12–16,25–28). These cells are used to assess most of the steps in 1,25(OH)$_2$D action from cellular uptake to bioresponse and to elucidate the molecular aberrations in the hormone receptor protein and the nuclear DNA that encodes for it (24,25). The latter became feasible with the recent cloning and sequencing of the human VDR chromosomal gene.

Several methods have been used to characterize the hormone–receptor interaction, including binding capacity and affinity of [^{3}H]1,25(OH)$_2$D$_3$ to intact cells, nuclei, or high-salt-soluble extract (cytosol) (6,12,13,16); measurements of receptor content by monoclonal antibodies (24,29,29A); and characterization of the hormone–receptor complex on continuous sucrose gradient and heterologous DNA-cellulose columns (6,13,19,30). For studies on the molecular defects, isolation, amplification, and sequencing of genomic VDR DNA, as well as cloning and sequencing of VDR cDNA and recreation of the mutant VDR *in vitro,* have been utilized. *In vitro* bioeffects of 1,25(OH)$_2$D on the various cells have been assayed by induction of the 25(OH)D-24-hydroxylase in skin- and bone-derived cells (17,31–33), osteocalcin synthesis in cells derived from bone (33), inhibition of cell proliferation in PBM cells (27,28) and dermal fibroblasts (15,34), a mitogenic effect on dermal fibroblasts (34), and stimulation of cyclic cGMP production in cultured skin fibroblasts (35).

Heterogeneity of the cellular and molecular defects of vitamin D receptor-effector system had been revealed in studies of different kindreds with VDDR-II. However, based on the hormone–receptor–nuclear interaction three different classes of intracellular defects have been identified.

1. Hormone binding defects. These include:
   a. Markedly decreased capacity (number of binding sites was about 10% of controls) in one patient, who did not respond to prolonged treatment with high doses of active calciferol metabolites (14).
   b. Decreased hormone binding affinity. [^{3}H]1,25(OH)$_2$D$_3$ binding affinity is reduced 20- to 30-fold with normal binding capacity of soluble (cytosolic) dermal fibroblasts extract. A complete remission of the disease in these patients could be achieved by high doses of vitamin D or its active metabolites (21).

c. No hormone binding. Unmeasurable specific binding of $[^3H]1,25(OH)_2D_3$ to either high-salt-soluble cell extract and/or intact cells or nuclei. This is the most common abnormality observed. In the majority of these patients, high concentrations of $1,25(OH)_2D$ in serum or culture medium did not evoke a biological or biochemical response in vivo or in vitro. Recently, different point mutations in the DNA region transcribing the hormone binding domain of VDR were described (29,29A,36). In five affected kindreds the nucleotide substitution resulted in a stop codon in the coding sequence (which was different for each kindred), thus causing a truncated receptor having no or only a nonfunctional part of the hormone binding site of the VDR. In an additional patient a missense mutation resulted in the substitution of arginine by leucine (36). It is of interest that in a cotransfection assay normal transcription could be induced in the presence of 1000-fold higher levels of the hormone than were needed for the wild-type VDR. This may indicate that the mutation caused an extreme decrease in the affinity of the receptor to $1,25(OH)_2D_3$.

2. Deficient nuclear localization. Normal or near-normal binding affinity and capacity of $[^3H]1,25(OH)_2D_3$ binding to soluble cell extract. Normal binding to heterologous DNA but unmeasurable localization of $[^3H]1,25(OH)_2D_3$ to nuclei in intact cells (12,16,37). An identical defect was demonstrated with cells cultured from a bone biopsy of one patient (12) and in mitogen-stimulated PBM cells from several kindreds (22). These patients were treated successfully with high doses of vitamin D and its active metabolites (7,12,22,37). No mutation was found on sequencing VDR cDNA of some of these patients (37, and personal communication).

3. Normal or near-normal $[^3H]1,25(OH)_2D_3$ binding to soluble cell extract and to nuclei of intact cells, but decreased affinity of the hormone–receptor complex to heterologous DNA (19,25,30). No biological response to high doses of vitamin D or its active metabolites either in vivo or in vitro was documented in almost all patients with this type of defect (9,19,30). Recently, a single nucleotide missense mutation within exon 2 or 3 encoding the DNA binding domain of the VDR was demonstrated in genomic DNA isolated from fibroblasts and/or EB virus-transformed lymphocytes from members from eight unrelated kindreds with this defect (25,25A,38–40). Different single-nucleotide mutations were found with the exception of two unrelated patients that share the same defect. All mutations caused a single amino acid substitution localized to the region of the two zinc fingers of the vitamin D receptor protein. This region is essential for DNA binding of the hormone–receptor complex. It is worthwhile mentioning that the DNA binding domain of the VDR is evolutionarily highly conserved throughout all members of the v-ERB-A-related proteins that include the receptors for steroid hormones, thyroid hormones, and retinoic acid.

Measurements of an in vitro bioresponse of cells to $1,25(OH)_2D_3$ were carried out in less than half of the kindreds with VDDR-II. Induction of 25(OH)D-24-hydroxylase by $1,25(OH)_2D_3$ in cultured dermal fibroblasts showed an invariable correlation to the therapeutic response to vitamin D and metabolites in vivo (17,31,32,37,40).

Treatment

If the predictive therapeutic value of the in vitro bioresponse to $1,25(OH)_2D_3$ could be substantiated, it may eliminate the need for expensive and time-consuming therapy trials with vitamin D and metabolites. In the meantime, it is mandatory to treat every patient with VDDR-II, regardless of the type of receptor defect. An adequate therapeutic trial must include (i) vitamin D alone for the mildest cases, though in more severe typical cases therapy should be initiated with high doses of vitamin D analogs that will ensure maintenance of high serum concentrations of $1,25(OH)_2D$ (this can be accomplished by treatment with $1,25(OH)_2D_3$ or $1\alpha(OH)D_3$ at daily doses in the range of up to 6 µg per kilogram body weight or a total of 30–60 µg); (ii) supplemental calcium of up to 3 g elementary calcium per day; and (iii) a duration of therapy (about 3–5 months) sufficient to mineralize depleted bones and thus allow recovery from the hypocalcemia of "hungry bones." Close follow-up is essential and consists of clinical signs and symptoms; bone x-rays; serum levels of calcium, phosphorus, alkaline phosphatase, and creatinine; urinary excretion of calcium, phosphorus, and creatinine; parameters of parathyroid function; and serum $1,25(OH)_2D$ levels. Failure of therapy may be considered if no change in any of these parameters occurs during the treatment period while $1,25(OH)_2D$ serum levels are maintained above 100 times the mean normal range. It was reported recently that remarkable clinical and biochemical remission including catch-up growth and histologic healing of defective osteoid mineralization was achieved by long-term therapy with high-dose oral calcium in one patient (41) or long-term intracaval infusion of calcium in several unusual patients with VDDR-II who did not respond to adequate trial with active vitamin D metabolites (33,42,43). These important studies imply that clinical remission could be achieved by calcium administration even in the most resistant patients with VDDR-II.

CONCLUSION

In summary, two inborn errors in vitamin D metabolism are presented and discussed. The important message is not just the description of a rare curiosity of nature but rather the finding that rare aberrations of natural metabolic processes are important to unveil basic physiologic, biochemical, and molecular mechanisms in general and in human beings in particular.

REFERENCES

1. Prader A, Illig R, Heierli E: Eline besondere Form der primaren vitamin D-resistenten Rachitis mit Hypocalcemie und autosomal-dominanten Erbgang: Die hereditare Pseudo-Mangelrachitis. Helv Paediatr Acta 16:452–468, 1961
2. Scriver CR, Fraser D, Kooh SW: Hereditary rickets. In: Heath

D, Marx SJ (eds) *Calcium Disorders*. Butterworth, London, 1982

2A. Glorieux FH, Azabian A, Delvin EE: Pseudo-vitamin D deficiency: Absence of 25-hydroxyvitamin D 1α-hydroxylase activity in human placenta decidual cells. *J Clin Endocrinol Metab* 80: 2255–2258, 1995

3. Harmeyer JV, Grabe C, Winkley I: Pseudovitamin D deficiency rickets in pigs. An animal model for the study of familial vitamin D dependency. *Exp Biol Med* 7:117–125, 1982

4. Fox J, Maunder EMW, Ranall VA, Care AD: Vitamin D dependent rickets type I in pigs. *Clin Sci* 69:541–548, 1985

5. Brooks MH, Bell NH, Love L, Stern PH, Ordei E, Queener SJ, Hamstra AJ, DeLuca HF: Vitamin D dependent rickets type II, resistance of target organs to 1,25-dihydroxyvitamin D. *N Engl J Med* 293:996–999, 1978

6. Marx SJ, Liberman UA, Eil C, Gamblin GT, DeGrange DA, Balsan S: Hereditary resistance to 1,25-dihydroxyvitamin D. Recent Prog *Hormone Res* 40:589–620, 1984

7. Marx SJ, Spiegel AM, Brown EM, Gardner DG, Downs RW Jr, Attie M, Hamstra AJ, DeLuca HF: A familial syndrome of decrease in sensitivity of 1,25-dihydroxyvitamin D. *J Clin Endocrinol Metab* 47:1303–1310, 1978

8. Rosen JF, Fleischman AR, Finberg L, Hamstra A, DeLuca HF: Rickets with alopecia: an inborn error of vitamin D metabolism. *J Pediatrics* 94:729–735, 1979

9. Liberman UA, Samuel R, Halabe A, Kauli R, Edelstein S, Weisman Y, Papapoulos SE, Clemens TL, Fraher LJ, O'Riordan JLH: End-organ resistance to 1,25-dihydroxy cholecalciferol. *Lancet* 1: 504–506, 1980

10. Fujita T, Nomura M, Okajima S, Suzuya H: Adult-onset vitamin D-resistant osteomalacia with unresponsiveness to parathyroid hormone. *J Clin Endocrinol Metab* 50:927–931, 1980

11. Tsuchiya Y, Matsuo N, Cho H, Kumagai M, Yasaka A, Suda T, Orimo H, Shiraki M: An unusual form of vitamin D-dependent rickets in a child: alopecia and marked end-organ hyposensitivity to biological active vitamin D. *J Clin Endocrinol Metab* 51:685–690, 1980

12. Eil C, Liberman UA, Rosen JF, Marx SJ; A cellular defect in hereditary vitamin D-dependent rickets type II: defective nuclear uptake of 1,25-dihydroxyvitamin D in cultured skin fibroblasts. *N Engl J Med* 304:1588–1591, 1981

13. Feldman D, Chen T, Cone C, Hirst M, Shari S, Benderli A, Hochberg Z: Vitamin D resistant rickets with alopecia: cultured skin fibroblasts exhibit defective cytoplasmic receptors and unresponsiveness to 1,25(OH)$_2$D$_3$. *J Clin Endocrinol Metab* 55: 1020–1025, 1982

14. Balsan A, Garabedian M, Liberman UA, Eil C, Bourdeau A, Guillozo H, Grimberg R, DeDeunff MJ, Lieberherr M, Guimbaud P, Broyer M, Marx SJ: Rickets and alopecia with resistance to 1,25-dihydroxyvitamin D: two different clinical courses with two different cellular defects. *J Clin Endocrinol Metab* 57:803–811, 1983

15. Clemems TL, Adams JC, Horiuchi N, Gilchrist BA, Cho H, Ysuchiya Y, Matsuo N, Suda T, Holick MF: Interaction of 1,25-dihydroxyvitamin D3 with keratinocytes and fibroblasts from skin of a subject with vitamin D-dependent rickets type II: a model for the study of action of 1,25-dihydroxyvitamin D$_3$. *J Clin Endocrinol Metab* 56:824–830, 1983

16. Liberman UA, Eil C, Marx SJ: Resistance of 1,25-dihydroxyvitamin D: Association with heterogeneous defects in cultured skin fibroblasts. *J Clin Invest* 71:192–200, 1983

17. Chen TL, Hirst MA, Cone CM, Hochberg Z, Tietze HU, Feldman D: 1,25-dihydroxyvitamin D resistance, rickets and alopecia: analysis of receptors and bioresponse in cultured skin fibroblasts from patients and parents. *J Clin Endocrinol Metab* 59:383–388, 1984

18. Hochberg Z, Benderli Z, Levy J, Weisman Y, Chen T, Feldman D: 1,25-dihydroxyvitamin D resistance, rickets, and alopecia. *Am J Med* 77:805–811, 1984

19. Hirst MA, Hochman HI, Feldman D: Vitamin D resistance and alopecia: a kindred with normal 1,25-dihydroxyvitamin D3 binding, but decreased receptor affinity for deoxyribonucleic acid. *J Clin Endocrinol Metab* 60:490–495, 1985

20. Fraher LJ, Karmali R, Hinde FRJ, Hendy GN, Jani H, Nicholson L, Grant D, O'Riordan JLH: Vitamin D-dependent rickets type II:

extreme end organ resistance to 1,25-dihydroxyvitamin D$_3$ in a patient without alopecia. Eur J Pediatr 145:389–395, 1986

21. Castells S, Greig F, Fusi MA, Finberg L, Yasumura S, Liberman UA, Eil C, Marx SJ: Severely deficient binding of 1,25-dihydroxyvitamin D to its receptor in a patient responsive to high doses of this hormone. *J Clin Endocrinol Metab* 63:252–256, 1986

22. Tajkeda E, Kuroda Y, Saijo T, Naito E, Kobashi H, Yokota I, Miyao M; 1α-hydroxyvitamin D$_3$ treatment of three patients with 1,25-dihydroxyvitamin D-receptor-defect rickets and alopecia. *Pediatrics* 80:97–101, 1987

23. Marx SJ, Bliziotes MM, Nanes M: Analysis of the relation between alopecia and resistance to 1,25-dihydroxyvitamin D. *Clin Endocrinol* 25:373–381, 1986

24. Malloy PJ, Hochberg Z, Pike JW, Feldman D: Abnormal binding of vitamin D receptors to deoxyribonucleic acid in a kindred with vitamin D dependent rickets, type II. *J Clin Endocrinol Metab* 68: 263–269, 1989

25. Hughes MR, Malloy PJ, Kieback DG, Kesterson RA, Pike JW, Feldman D, O'Malley BW: Point mutations in the human vitamin D receptor gene associated with hypocalcemia rickets. *Science* 242:1702–1705, 1988

25a. Sone T, Marx SJ, Liberman UA, Pike JW: A unique point mutation in the human vitamin D receptor chromosomal gene confers hereditary resistance to 1,25-dihydroxyvitamin D$_3$. *Mol Cell Endocrinol* 4:623–631, 1990

26. Liberman UA, Eil C, Holst P, Rosen JF, Marx JS: Hereditary resistance to 1,25-dihydroxyvitamin D: defective function of receptors for 1,25-dihydroxyvitamin D in cells cultured from bone. *J Clin Endocrinol Metab* 57:958–962, 1983

27. Koren R, Ravid A, Liberman UA, Hochberg Z, Weisman J, Novogrodsky A: Defective binding and function of 1,25-dihydroxyvitamin D$_3$ receptors in peripheral mononuclear cells of patients with end-organ resistance to 1,25-dihydroxyvitamin D. *J Clin Invest* 76:2012–2015, 1985

28. Takeda E, Kuzoda Y, Saijo T, Toshima K, Naito E, Kobashi H, Iwakuni Y, Miyao M: Rapid diagnosis of vitamin D-dependent rickets type II by use of phytohemagglutinin-stimulated lymphocytes. *Clin Chim Acta* 155:245–250, 1986

29. Malloy PJ, Hochberg Z, Tiosano D, Pike JW, Hughes MR, Feldman D: The molecular basis of hereditary 1,25-dihydroxyvitamin D$_3$ resistant rickets in seven related families. *J Clin Invest* 86: 2017–2079, 1990

29a. Weise RJ, Goto H, Prahl JM, Marx SJ, Thomas M, Al-Aqeel A, DeLuca HF: Vitamin D-dependency rickets type II: truncated vitamin D receptor in three kindreds. *Mol Cell Endocrinol* 90:197–201, 1993

30. Liberman UA, Eil C, Marx SJ: Receptor positive hereditary resistance to 1,25-dihydroxyvitamin D: chromatography of hormone-receptor complexes on DNA-cellulose shows two classes of mutation. *J Clin Endocrinol Metab* 62:122–126, 1986

31. Griffin JE, Zerwekh JE: Impaired stimulation of 25-hydroxyvitamin D-24-hydroxylase in fibroblasts from a patient with vitamin D-dependent rickets, type II. *J Clin Invest* 72:1190 -1199, 1983

32. Gamblin GT, Liberman UA, Eil C, Downs RW Jr, DeGrange DA, Marx SJ: Vitamin D-dependent rickets type II, defective induction of 25-hydroxyvitamin D$_3$-24-hydroxylase by 1,25-dihydroxyvitamin D$_3$ in cultured skin fibroblasts. *J Clin Invest* 75:954–960, 1985

33. Balsan S, Garabedian M, Larchet M, Gorski AM, Cournot G, Tau C, Bourdeau A, Silve C, Ricour C: Long-term nocturnal calcium infusions can cure rickets and promote normal mineralization in hereditary resistance to 1,25-dihydroxyvitamin D. *J Clin Invest* 77:1661–1667, 1986

34. Barsony J, McKoy W, DeGrange DA, Liberman UA, Marx SJ: Selective expression of a normal action of 1,25-dihydroxyvitamin D$_3$ receptor in human skin fibroblasts with hereditary severe defects in multiple action of this receptor. *J Clin Invest* 83:2093–2101, 1989

35. Barsony J, Marx SJ: Receptor-mediated rapid action of 1α-25-dihydroxy-cholecalciferol: increase of intracellular cGMP in human skin fibroblasts. *Proc Natl Acad Sci USA* 85:1223–1226, 1988

36. Kristjansson K, Rut AR, Hewison M, O'Riordan JLF, Hughes MR: Two mutations in the hormone binding domain of the vita-

min D receptor cause tissue resistance to 1,25 dihydroxyvitamin D3. *J Clin Invest* 92:12–16, 1993

37. Hewison M, Rut AR, Kristjansson K, Walker RE, Dillon MJ, Hughes MR, O'Riordan JLH: Tissue resistance to 1,25-dihydroxyvitamin D without a mutation in the vitamin D receptor gene. *Clin Endocrinol* 39:663–670, 1993

38. Yagi H, Ozono K, Miyake H, Nagashima K, Kuraum T, Pike JW: A new point mutation in the doxyribonucleic acid-binding domain of the vitamin D receptor in a kindred with hereditary 1,25-dihydroxyvitamin D resistant rickets. *J Clin Endocrinol Metab* 76:509–512, 1993

39. Saijjo T, Ito M, Takeda E, Mahbubul Huq AHM, Naito E, Yokota I, Sine T, Pike JW, Kuroda Y: A unique mutation in the vitamin D receptor gene in three Japanese patients with vitamin D-dependent rickets type II: utility of single-strand conformation polymorphism analysis for heterozygous carrier detection. *Am J Hum Genet* 49:668–673, 1991

40. Rut AR, Hewison K, Kristjansson K, Luisi B, Hughes MR, O'Riordan JLH: Two mutations causing vitamin D resistant rickets: modelling on the basis of steroid hormone receptor DNA-binding domain crystal structures. *Clin Endocrinol* 41:581–590, 1994

41. Sakati N, Woodhouse NTY, Niles N, Harji H, DeGrange DA, Marx SJ: Hereditary resistance to 1,25-dihydroxyvitamin D: clinical and radiological improvement during high-dose oral calcium therapy. *Hormone Res* 24:280–287, 1986

42. Weisman Y, Bab I, Gazit D, Spirer Z, Jaffe M, Hochberg Z: Long-term intracaval calcium infusion therapy in end-organ resistance to 1,25-dihydroxyvitamin D. *Am J Med* 83:984–990, 1987

43. Bliziotes M, Yergey AL, Nanes MS, Muenzer J, Begley MG, Vieira NE, Kher KK, Brandi ML, Marx SJ: Absent intestinal response to calciferols in hereditary resistance to 1,25-dihydroxyvitamin D: documentation and effective therapy with high dose intravenous calcium infusions. *J Clin Endocrinol Metab* 66:294–300, 1988

61. Hypophosphatemic Vitamin D-Resistant Rickets

Francis H. Glorieux, M.D, Ph.D.

Departments of Surgery, Pediatrics, and Human Genetics, McGill University, and Genetics Unit, Shriners Hospital, Montreal, Quebec, Canada

Bone growth and mineralization require adequate availability of calcium and phosphate, the two major constituents of hydroxyapatite, which is the crystalline part of bone tissue. Defective supply of either calcium or phosphate will result in impaired mineralization, which will cause rickets at the growth plate level and osteomalacia at the corticoendosteal level. Thus in growing individuals, both lesions will be present, whereas by definition only osteomalacia can possibly develop in adults.

Deficiency in calcium, as a consequence of either insufficient intake (1) or vitamin D simple deficiency or abnormal metabolism (2), will induce hypocalcemia, rickets, and osteomalacia. The latter will be characterized by osteopenia, as a consequence of the increased resorption induced by hyperparathyroidism secondary to hypocalcemia.

In chronic hypophosphatemia, although clinical and radiologic manifestations of rickets are similar to those seen in calcium deficiency, osteomalacia is characterized by an accumulation of unmineralized osteoid along the trabeculae. Because calcemia is normal, there is no secondary hyperparathyroidism and therefore no increased osteoclast activity or excessive resorption. Consequently, bone mass is not decreased. It is, in fact, often measured above normal values for age.

CLASSIFICATION OF HYPOPHOSPHATEMIC SYNDROMES

There are acquired and congenital forms of hypophosphatemia. In most instances, the acquired forms can be controlled by acting on the underlying causes (insufficient phosphate intake, increased renal loss secondary to a mesenchymal tumor or an altered tubular function). However, the inherited syndromes present a challenge sometimes for

diagnosis and always for management. The most frequent of the hypophosphatemic syndromes was described more than 50 years ago by Albright (3) who coined the term "hypophosphatemic vitamin D-resistant rickets." It is inherited as an X-linked dominant trait (4) with the mutant gene being located in the distal part of the short arm of the X chromosome (5); hence it is now referred to as X-linked hypophosphatemia (HYP). In 1976, a homologous mutation was discovered in the mouse (Hyp) (6). The high degree of conservatism of the mammalian X chromosome and comparative mapping of the man and mouse gonosomes (7) support the contention of a close analogy between the HYP and Hyp mutations. Active studies have thus been pursued in parallel in the two species to better understand the phenotypic expression of the abnormal genes.

CLINICAL EXPRESSION

The classic triad, fully expressed in hemizygous male patients, is made of (i) hypophosphatemia, (ii) lower limb deformities, and (iii) stunted growth rate. Although low serum phosphate (P) is evident early after birth, it is only at time of weight bearing that leg deformities and progressive departure from normal growth rate become sufficiently striking to attract attention and make parents seek medical opinion. An often overlooked clinical sign is the appearance of the teeth. There is no enamel hypoplasia in HYP, as opposed to what is seen in hypocalcemic rickets. Hypophosphatemic rickets rather presents with dentin defects not apparent on examination but that may cause dental abscesses and early decay in the young adult. In several families, isolated hypophosphatemia can be found in some heterozygous females. Thus this trait is considered as the marker for the mutation (4). These healthy trait carriers provide evidence that hypophosphatemia and renal P waste cannot solely explain the abnormal phenotype.

BASIC DEFECT

Several recent studies based on genetic linkage and multi-locus analysis have allowed fine mapping of the HYP gene to the Xp22.1-22.2 region of the X chromosome between markers DXS41 and DXS43. There is, however, accumulating evidence for possible locus heterogeneity in X-linked hypophosphatemic rickets (8). The question will be resolved by the identification of the mutant gene(s) by positional cloning. A major step in that direction has been made by the isolation of a candidate gene in the HYP region (9). This gene, called *PEX*, codes for a membrane-bound endopeptidase. Further characterization of its full sequence and tissue expression will be needed to dissect out its role in phosphate homeostasis. Once this is completed it will allow for comparisons among affected families and between species (mouse and man).

The most intriguing question regarding HYP concerns the primary lesion causing the disease. It has long been accepted that hypophosphatemia is the consequence of a primary inborn error of phosphate transport probably located in the proximal nephron. It is noteworthy that the defect is less severe in female heterozygotes than it is in male hemizygotes (10). This gene–dose effect indicates that the observed defect is close to the abnormal gene product. The abnormality in the Hyp mouse has been localized to the brush border of the proximal tubular cells (11). The possibility that it would be secondary to the presence of a humoral hypophosphatemic factor (12) has received experimental support from kidney cross-transplantation studies in the mouse model (13). However, these findings would not explain the gene–dose effect present in humans but not readily evident in the murine model.

Because of the close link between the phosphate repletion status and 1,25-dihydroxyvitamin D (1,25D) synthesis, the metabolism of this hormone has been extensively studied in mutant individuals. It is important to point out that there is no simple 1,25D deficiency (as seen in vitamin D pseudodeficiency) and that there is no close correlation between extracellular P concentration and 1,25D synthesis. Rather, the reported inappropriate response of 1,25D synthesis to a low phosphate challenge (14), although there is no abnormality in the response to a low calcium challenge (15), points to the vitamin D metabolism abnormality being secondary to the primary P transport defect and its consequences on intracellular P economy.

Studies both in man and mouse indicate that defective bone formation in X-linked hypophosphatemia is linked to an intrinsic osteoblast defect. The hypomineralized periosteocytic lesions (HPLs), which are a hallmark of HYP, never completely disappear even after active mineralization has been restored at the endosteal surfaces. After more than 2 years of efficient therapy, HPLs are still present around 20% of the osteocytes in the newly formed osteons (16). As HPLs are never present in other chronic hypophosphatemic states, this observation gives substance to the early proposal that there may be an osteoblast primary metabolic defect in HYP (17). The lesions are also present in the Hyp mouse (18) where an abnormal osteoblast response to 1,25D has been demonstrated (19). Studies recently conducted with osteoblasts isolated from mouse calvaria have provided morphologic evidence that Hyp osteoblasts, even when transplanted in a normal environment are unable to produce adequate amounts of mineralized matrix (20). Although more work will be needed to precisely characterize the osteoblast defect, it is tempting to speculate that the osteoblast shares, with the renal tubular cell, a gene product which would specifically affect phosphate transport and, in an ancillary fashion, 1,25D synthesis.

RESPONSE TO TREATMENT

Based on the established renal P waste, therapy has centered on often aggressive P replacement (1–3 g elemental P/day in 4–5 doses). To offset the hypocalcemic effect of P supplementation, which has sometimes caused severe secondary hyperparathyroidism, large (20–75,000 IU/day) amounts of vitamin D were added to the regimen. With adequate compliance to such a combined treatment, growth rate improved markedly and there was radiologic evidence of healed rickets (21,22). The early observation that heterozygous girls responded better to treatment than hemizygous boys (21) has been recently substantiated supporting the concept of a gene–dose effect in this X-linked dominant disorder (23). However, histologic studies of iliac crest bone biopsies showed that the osteomalacic component of the bone disease was hardly improved (24). It was only by substituting 1,25D to vitamin D at the dose of 30–70 ng/kg/day that improvement and sometimes healing of the mineralization defect was observed on the trabecular surfaces (25–28).

LONG-TERM EFFECTS OF TREATMENT

Except for occasional osmotic diarrhea, P supplementation has not caused any harmful effects. Coated tablets should be preferred to liquid forms, as they provide a slower rate of absorption. Tablets are also made of a mixture of sodium and potassium salts, avoiding the high sodium load so frequent with the solutions.

Before 1978, large amounts of vitamin D were administered to offset the hypocalcemic effect of P supplementation and the ensuing iatrogenic hyperparathyroidism. This was often difficult to control and several cases of autonomous hyperparathyroidism were encountered that could only be treated surgically (21). The substitution of 1,25D for vitamin D has now allowed a more precise control of parathyroid (PTH) secretion throughout the treatment period. It thus appears that 1,25D, through its direct effect on PTH release, is able to maintain PTH levels within acceptable limits together with ensuring adequate bone modeling and remodeling (27–29). Interestingly, this may also be the case for $24,25(OH)_2D_3$. A placebo-controlled trial based on the addition of the metabolite (10 µg/day) to the standard protocol (1,25D and phosphate) has shown that better control of the therapy-induced hyperparathyroidism was achieved over a 2-year period (30). A detailed report is forthcoming.

One major concern with long-term administration of 1,25D is a possible deterioration of renal function through interstitial nephrocalcinosis. Indeed frequent ultrasound observations of echodense renal pyramids have been reported (31). Histologic studies have confirmed that they correspond to mineral deposits exclusively made of calcium phosphate (32). Whether the induction of such deposits is primarily related to the phosphate load or to the long-term use of 1,25D is not clear at present. Such findings are, however, not directly related to evidence of decreased renal function. Our experience with 18 patients treated for an average of 8 years indicates that two thirds of them present with profiles of increased echogenicity of the renal pyramids (too quickly labeled nephrocalcinosis), but no alteration of renal function (unpublished data). Thus long-term use of 1,25D associated with supplemental P and with frequent monitoring of urinary calcium excretion to avoid episodes of hypercalciuria should be considered a safe and efficient way to control the clinical expression of the HYP mutation. When hypercalciuria develops, adjustment of the 1,25D dosage is necessary.

Because stunted growth is a major consequence of the HYP phenotype, the use of recombinant human growth hormone (rhGH), as a third therapeutic component, was also advocated (33,34). The hormone increased serum P levels, and over a 24-week period, appeared to positively affect growth rate, in 11 HYP children. These results have recently been substantiated by a long-term (3 years) study showing that adding rhGH (0.6 IU/kg/week) to phosphate and 1,25D had a significant positive effect on growth in young HYP patients (34). Other such studies will be needed before concluding that the basic treatment protocol should be uniformly modified.

TREATMENT OF ADULT PATIENTS

With early initiation of therapy and good compliance throughout the growing period, clinical results are usually satisfactory in terms of stature achieved and prevention of lower limb deformities. An important question is whether one should maintain the demanding treatment schedule combining 1,25D and phosphate, after fusion of the epiphyseal plates. Because growth has ceased and bone turnover is reduced, the appropriateness of maintaining a high phosphate intake can rightly be questioned. The demonstration that in 18 symptomatic HYP adult patients, who received P +1,25D for 4 years, the treatment resulted in significant clinical and histomorphometric improvement (35) suggests that such an approach is worthwhile. Its optimal duration remains, however, unresolved. Because strict compliance to P supplements on a 5 dose per day schedule is difficult, one may envisage that continuing 1,25D alone, through its stimulation of bone turnover and intestinal phosphate absorption, would maintain the good results obtained with the combined therapy. Preliminary observations in 6 HYP patients indicate that 1,25D alone (at a dose of 1–2 μg/day) has positively influenced the parameters of bone mineralization over an 11- to 17-month period (unpublished data). This study, still in progress, should allow us to better define our long-term strategy of metabolic and clinical control of adult HYP patients.

CONCLUSION

Despite the persistent questions about the pathogenesis of HYP, medical control of its clinical expression has greatly improved over the past 15 years. The combination of large amounts of phosphate salts and supraphysiologic doses of 1,25D has allowed normal growth and adequate bone matrix mineralization. With close and careful follow-up the regimen is safe, and no deleterious effects on renal function are to be expected. Uncertainty continues with regard to the treatment of asymptomatic adult subjects.

ACKNOWLEDGMENTS

This work was supported by the Shriners of North America.

REFERENCES

1. Marie PJ, Pettifor JM, Ross FP, Glorieux FH: Histologic osteomalacia due to dietary calcium deficiency in children. N Engl J Med 307:584, 1982
2. Glorieux FH, Pettifor JM: Metabolic bone disease. In: Kelly VC (ed) Practice of Pediatrics. vol 7. New York, Harper and Row, p 34, 1984
3. Albright F, Butler AM, Bloomberg E: Rickets resistant to vitamin D therapy. Am J Dis Child 54:529, 1937
4. Winters RW, Graham JB, Williams TF, McFalls VW, Burnett CH: A genetic study of familial hypophosphatemia and vitamin D-resistant rickets with a review of the literature. Medicine 37:97, 1958
5. Thakker RV, Read AP, Davies KE, Whyte WP, Weksberg R, Glorieux FH, Davies M, Mountford RC, King A, Kim GS, Harris R, O'Riordan JLH: Bridging markers defining the map position of X-linked hypophosphatemic rickets. J Med Genet 24:756, 1987
6. Eicher EM, Southard JL, Scriver CR, Glorieux FH: Hypophosphatemia: mouse model for human familial hypophosphatemic (vitamin D-resistant) rickets. Proc Natl Acad Sci USA 73:4667, 1976
7. Davisson MT: X-linked genetic homologies between mouse and man. Genomics 1:213, 1987
8. Rowe PSN: Molecular biology of hypophosphatemic rickets and oncogenic osteomalacia. Hum Genet 94:457, 1994
9. Francis F, Henning S, Korn B, et al: A gene (PEX) with homologies to endopeptidases is mutated in patients with X-linked hypophosphatemic rickets. Nat Genet 11:150, 1995
10. Glorieux F, Scriver CR: Loss of a PTH sensitive component of phosphate transport in X-linked hypophosphatemia. Science 175:997, 1972
11. Tenenhouse HS, Scriver CR, McInnes RR, Glorieux FH: Renal handling of phosphate in vivo and in vitro by the X-linked hypophosphatemic male mouse (Hyp/Y). Evidence for a defect in the brush border membrane. Kidney Int 14:236, 1978
12. Bonjour J-P, Caverzasio J, Muhlbauer R, Trechsel U, Troehler U: Are 1,25(OH)$_2$D$_3$ production and tubular phosphate transport regulated by one common mechanism which would be defective in X-linked hypophosphatemic rickets? In: Norman AW, Schaefer K, Herrath D, Grigoleit H-G (eds) Vitamin D: Chemical, Biochemical and Clinical Endocrinology of Calcium Metabolism. New York, Walter de Gruyter, pp 427–433, 1982
13. Nesbitt T, Coffman TM, Griffiths R, Drezner MK: Cross-transplantation of kidneys in normal and Hyp mice. Evidence that the Hyp mouse phenotype is unrelated to an intrinsic renal defect. J Clin Invest 89:1453, 1992
14. Lobaugh B, Drezner MK: Abnormal regulation of renal 25-dihydroxyvitamin D-1α-hydroxylase activity in the X-linked hypophosphatemic mouse. J Clin Invest 71:400, 1983
15. Meyer RA Jr, Gray RW, Roos BA, Kiebzak GM: Increased

plasma 1,25-dihydroxyvitamin D after low calcium challenge in X-linked hypophosphatemic mice. *Endocrinology* 111:174, 1982

16. Marie PJ, Glorieux FH: Relation between hypomineralized periosteocytic lesions and bone mineralization in vitamin D-resistant rickets. *Calcif Tissue Int* 35:443, 1983
17. Frost HM: Some observations on bone mineral in a case of vitamin D resistant rickets. *Henry Ford Hosp Med Bull* 6:300, 1958
18. Glorieux FH, Ecarot-Charrier B: X-linked vitamin D-resistant rickets: Is osteoblast activity defective? In: Cohn DV, Martin TJ, Meunier PJ (eds) *Calcium Regulation and Bone Metabolism.* vol 9. Amsterdam, Excerpta Medica, pp 227–231, 1987
19. Yamamoto T, Ecarot B, Glorieux FH: Abnormal response of osteoblasts from Hyp mice to 1,25-dihydroxyvitamin D_3. *Bone* 13:209, 1992
20. Ecarot-Charrier E, Glorieux FH, Travers R, Desbarats M, Bouchard F, Hinek A: Defective bone formation by transplanted Hyp mouse bone cells into normal mice. *Endocrinology* 123:768, 1988
21. Glorieux FH, Scriver CR, Reade TM, Goldman H, Roseborough A: The use of phosphate and vitamin D to prevent dwarfism and rickets in X-linked hypophosphatemia. *N Engl J Med* 281:481, 1972
22. Verge CF, Lam A, Simpson JM, Cowell CR, Howard NJ, Silink M: Effects of therapy in X-linked hypophosphatemic rickets. *N Engl J Med* 325:1843, 1991
23. Petersen DJ, Boniface AM, Schranck FW, Rupich RC, Whyte MP: X-linked hypophosphatemic rickets: a study (with literature review) of linear growth response to calcitriol and phosphate therapy. *J Bone Min Res* 7:583, 1992
24. Glorieux FH, Bordier PJ, Marie P, Delvin EE, Travers R: Inadequate bone response to phosphate and vitamin D in familial hypophosphatemic rickets. In: Massry S, Ritz E, Rapada A (eds) *Homeostasis of Phosphate and Other Minerals.* New York, Plenum Press, pp 227–232, 1980
25. Glorieux FH, Marie PJ, Pettifor JM, Delvin EE: Bone response to phosphate salts, ergocalciferol and calcitriol in hypophosphatemic vitamin-D resistant rickets. *N Engl J Med* 303:1023, 1980

26. Costa T, Marie PJ, Scriver CR, Cole DEC, Reade TM, Nogrady B, Glorieux FH, Delvin EE: X-linked hypophosphatemia. Effect of calcitriol on renal handling of phosphate, serum phosphate, and bone mineralization. *J Clin Endocrinol Metab* 52:463, 1981
27. Drezner MK, Lyles KW, Haussler MR, Harrelson JM: Evaluation of a role for 1,25-dihydroxyvitamin D in the pathogenesis and treatment of X-linked hypophosphatemic rickets and osteomalacia. *J Clin Invest* 66:1020, 1980
28. Harrell RM, Lyles KW, Harrelson JM, Friedman NE, Drezner MK: Healing of bone disease in X-linked hypophosphatemic rickets/osteomalacia. Induction and maintenance with phosphorus and calcitriol. *J Clin Invest* 75:1858, 1985
29. Bettinelli A, Bianchi ML, Mazazucchi E, Gandolini G, Appliani AC: Acute effects of calcitriol and phosphate salts on mineral metabolism in children with hypophosphatemic rickets. *J Pediatrics* 118:373, 1991
30. Carpenter T, Insogna K, Glorieux FH, Travers R, Carey D, Horst R, Comite F, Keller M: 24,25(OH)2D3 ameliorates hyperparathyroidism and improves skeletal findings in X-linked hypophosphatemic rickets. *J Bone Min Res* 10:S300, 1995
31. Goodyer PR, Kronick JB, Jequier S, Reade TM, Scriver CR: Nephrocalcinosis and its relationship to treatment of hereditary rickets. *J Pediatrics* 111:700, 1987
32. Alon U, Donaldson DL, Hellerstein S, Warady BA, Harris DJ: Metabolic and histologic investigation of the nature of nephrocalcinosis in children with hypophosphatemic rickets and in the Hyp mouse. *J Pediatrics* 120:899, 1992
33. Wilson DM, Lee PDK, Morris AH, Reiter EO, Gertner JM, Marcus R, Quarmby VE, Rosenfeld RG: Growth hormone therapy in hypophosphatemic rickets. *Am J Dis Child* 145:1165, 1991
34. Saggese G, Baroncelli GI, Bertelloni S, Perri G: Long-term growth hormone treatment in children with renal hypophosphatemic rickets: effects on growth, mineral metabolism, and bone density. *J Pediatrics* 127:395, 1995
35. Sullivan W, Carpenter T, Glorieux FH, Travers R, Insogna K: A prospective trial of phosphate and 1,25-dihydroxyvitamin D_3 therapy in symptomatic adults with X-linked hypophosphatemic rickets. *J Clin Endocrinol Metab* 75:879, 1992

62. Tumor-Induced Rickets and Osteomalacia

Marc K. Drezner, M.D.

*Departments of Medicine and Cell Biology, and Sarah W. Stedman Center for Nutritional Studies,
Duke University Medical Center, Durham, North Carolina*

Although McCance (1) described the first case of oncogenic osteomalacia-rickets in 1947, Prader et al. (2) first recognized the causal role of a tumor in this syndrome in 1959. Since that time there have been reports of approximately 102 patients (1–83) in whom rickets and/or osteomalacia has been induced with various types of tumors (Table 1). With time the name of the syndrome has varied and included oncogenous osteomalacia and tumor-induced osteomalacia. In at least 54 cases a tumor has been clearly documented as causing the osteomalacia-rickets, since the metabolic disturbances improved or completely disappeared on removal of the tumor. In the remainder of cases, patients had inoperable lesions and investigators could not determine the effects of tumor removal on the syndrome or surgery did not result in complete resolution of the syndrome during the period of observation. In any case, with greater awareness of the disease, physician-scientists have recognized >40% of known affected subjects within the past decade. The syndrome is characterized, in general, by remission of the unexplained bone disease after resection of

the coexisting tumor. Patients usually present with bone and muscle pain, muscle weakness, and, occasionally, recurrent fractures of long bones. Additional symptoms common to younger patients are fatigue, gait disturbances, slow growth, and skeletal abnormalities, including bowing of the lower extremities. The duration of symptoms before diagnosis ranges from 2.5 months to 19 years with an average of >2.5 years. The age at diagnosis is generally the sixth decade with a range of 7–74 years. Approximately 18% of the patients are younger than 20 years at presentation.

The biochemical findings characterizing this disorder prior to tumor removal include hypophosphatemia and an abnormally low renal tubular maximum for the reabsorption of phosphorus per liter of glomerular filtrate (TmP/GFR), indicative of renal phosphate wasting. The serum phosphorus values average from 0.7 to 2.4 mg/dl. After removal of the tumor the level returns to normal. Additional abnormalities include gastrointestinal malabsorption of phosphorus, which coupled with renal phos-

TABLE 1. *Tumor-induced osteomalacia*

Reference	Age/Sex	Symptom Duration (yrs.)	Serum phosphorus Pre-op (mg/dl)	Serum phosphorus Post-op (mg/dl)	Tumor type
McCance (1)	15/F	9.0	2.1	4.7	Degenerated osteoid
Prader et al. (2)	11/F	1.0	1.9	4.1	Giant cell granuloma
Hauge (3)	55/M		2.1	4.7	Malignant neuroma
Yoshikawa et al. (4)	54/F	6.0	0.9	5.4	Cavernous hemangioma
Krane (5)	56/M	3.0	1.4	3.2	Giant cell tumor
Salassa et al. (6)	38/M	4.0	1.4	4.6	Sclerosing hemangioma
	30/M	3.0	1.2	3.3	Sclerosing hemangioma
Evans and Azzopardi (7)	47/F	1.5	1.7	3.6	Primary bone tumor (type ?)
Olefsky et al. (8)	40/M	10.0	1.1	3.5	Ossifying mesenchymal tumor
Pollack et al. (9)	9/F	1.5	1.7	4.8	Nonossifying fibroma
Moser and Fessel (10)	54/M	1.0	1.7		Nonossifying fibroma
Willhoite (11)	11/F	3.5	1.7	4.4	Ossifying mesenchymal tumor
Linovitz et al. (12)	36/M	9.0	1.4	4.0	Hemangiopericytoma
	51/M	4.0	0.9	1.6	Hemangioma
Renton and Shaw (13)	53/F	5.0	1.2		Hemangiopericytoma
	58/M	14.0	1.6		Hemangiopericytoma
	43/F	2.0	1.5	1.8	Hemangiopericytoma
Morita (14)	30/M	5.0	0.7	3.5	Fibrous xanthoma
Aschinberg et al. (15)	12/M	7.0	1.0	3.9	Fibroangioma
Drezner and Feinglos (16)	42/F	8.0	1.3	3.2	Giant cell tumor of bone
Yoshikawa et al. (17)	18/M	5.0	1.5	4.0	Benign osteoblastoma
	18/F	5.0	1.2	5.0	Benign osteoblastoma
Wyman et al. (18)	44/M	5.0	1.2	3.5	Sarcoma
Leite et al. (19)	50/M				Hemangiofibroma
Lau et al.(20)			2.0	4.1	Sclerosing hemangioma
Werner et al. (21)			1.9		Atypical chondroma
Turner and Dalinka (22)	56/F	8.0			Cavernous hemangioma
Nortman et al. (23)	49/F	4.0	1.5	1.5	Mesenchymoma
Daniels and Weisenfeld (24)	34/M	0.8	1.8		Hemangioma
Fukumoto et al. (25)	27/F		1.5	3.1	Osteoblastoma
Lejeune et al. (26)	62/F	2.5	1.8	3.6	Benign connective tissue
Crouzet et al. (27)	37/M	6.0	1.7	3.4	Hemangiopericytoma
Camus et al. (28)	37/F	1.0	2.2	3.2	Hemangioma
	37/M	9.0	1.6	3.4	Hemangiopericytoma
	72/M	0.5	1.8	3.4	Neuroma
Sweet et al. (29)	25/F	1.0	1.5	2.7	Hemangiopericytoma
Lyles et al. (30)	61/M	0.5	1.4		Prostatic carcinoma
	74/M	4.0	1.7		Prostatic carcinoma
Nitzan et al. (31)	26/M	2.0	1.5	3.1	Brown tumor
Asnes et al. (32)	14/F	1.0	1.7	3.8	Nonossifying fibroma
Parker et al. (33)	15/M	1.0	2.1	4.2	Nonossifying fibroma
Chacko and Joseph (34)	56/F	5.0	1.7	1.2	Hemangiopericytoma
Hioco et al. (35)	65/F				Cavernous hemangioma
Barcelo et al. (36)	44/F	3.0	1.3		Fibroangioma
Nomura et al. (37)	29/M	2.0	1.3	3.6	Osteosarcoma
Ryan and Reiss (38)	64/M	4.0	1.8	2.1	Primary bone tumor (type ?)
	66/F	2.5	1.3		Type ?
Firth et al. (39)	44/M	1.0	1.2	2.4	Malignant chondroblastoma
Taylor et al. (40)	57/M	0.3	1.5		Oat cell carcinoma
Leehey et al. (41)	20/M	1.0	1.6	3.5	Nonossifying fibroma
Seshadri et al. (42)	73/M		1.7		Giant cell tumor
	40/F		1.1		Hemangiopericytoma
	14/M		2.2		Odontogenic fibroma
Cotton and Van Puffelen (43)	44/M	1.0	1.2	2.4	Malignant chondroblastoma
Murphy et al. (44)	4 Patients		2.0		Prostatic carcinoma
Gitelis et al. (45)	44/F	0.3	1.4	2.6	Hemangiopericytoma
	48/F	3.0	1.2	3.8	Mesenchymal tumor (type ?)
Rico et al. (46)	31/M	9.0	0.9	4.7	Histocytoma
Carey et al. (47)	7/M	5.0	2.6		Epidermal nevi
	23/F	14.0	1.2		Epidermal nevi
Siris et al. (48)	44/M	2.0	2.1	3.5	Vascular mesenchymoma

TABLE 1. *Continued.*

Reference	Age/Sex	Symptom Duration (yrs.)	Serum phosphorus		Tumor type
			Pre-op (mg/dl)	Post-op (mg/dl)	
Reid et al. (49)	57/F	16.0	1.1	2.7	Mixed mesenchymal tumor
Prowse and Brooks (50)	73/M	1.0	1.6	3.4	Diffuse giant cell tumor
Sparagana (51)	19/M	0.5	1.6	3.9	Ossifying fibroma
	50/M	3.0	1.8	3.7	Low-grade fibrosarcoma
Rao et al. (52)	69/F		2.4	3.1	Myelomatosis
	70/F		2.4	3.0	Chronic lymphoeytic leukemia
McClure and Smith (53)	60/F	2.0	1.2		Hemangiopericytoma
Miyauchi et al. (54)	54/M	7.0	1.0	3.9	Hemangiopericytoma
Konishi et al. (55)	40/F	10.0	1.0		Neurofibromatosis
Nitzan et al. (56)	53/M	19.0	2.0	6.0	Fibrosarcoma
McGuire et al. (57)	34/F	1.0	1.3	4.1	Mesenchymal tumor
Schultze et al. (58)	51/M	6.0	2.1	3.8	Hemangiopericytoma
Leicht et al. (59)	34/F	2.0	1.2	4.0	Synovial sarcoma
Uchida et al. (60)	53/F	17.0	1.5	6.0	Tumor of bone
Papotti et al. (61)	62/M	2.0	1.6		Hemangiopericytoma
	24/F	1.8	1.6		Chondroid, giant cell tumor
	38/F	2.0	1.2		Hemangiopericytoma
Dent and Gartner (63)	52/M		2.1		Polyostotic fibrous dysplasia
	8/F		2.1		Polyostotic fibrous dysplasia
Saville et al. (64)	55/M	0.6	2.2		Neurofibromatosis
Boriani and Campanacci (66)	18/M	0.3			Osteoblastoma
Castleman and McNeely (67)	53/M	6.0	1.4		Giant cell tumor
Robertson (68)	60/F	3.0			Hemangiopericytoma
Kabdi (69)	70/M	0.3	1.8		Prostatic carcinoma
Moncrieff et al. (70)	10/M	2.5	1.6	4.4	Nonossifying fibroma
Cramer et al. (71)	69/M	1.0	1.9	2.7	Transitional cell carcinoma
Ioakimidis et al. (72)	57/M	7.0	1.2	2.5	Mesenchymal tumor
Lee et al. (73)	66/F	3.0	1.8		Giant cell granuloma
Harvey et al. (74)	32/F	12.0	1.8		Mesechymal chondrosarcoma
Cehreli et al. (75)	46/M	3.0	1.1	Normal	Osteochondroblastoma
Schapira et al. (76)	24/M	4.0	1.3	4.2	Mesenchymal tumor
Shaker et al. (77)	46/M		1.2-1.9		Small cell carcinoma
Yu et al. (78)	58/F				Mesenchymal spindle cell tumor
Linsey et al. (79)	54/F	0.5	1.8		Angiofibroma
Nuovo et al. (80)	13/F	0.2	1.7	4.1	Nonossifying fibroma
	9/M	0.5	1.9	3.2	Hemangiopericytoma
	56/F				Hemangioendothelioma
Hernberg and Edgren (81)	39/F	7.0	2.3		Neurofibromatosis
Hosking et al. (82)	66/M	0.5	1.4		Prostatic carcinoma
Weidner et al. (83)	37/F	1.5	1.6	4.8	Primitive mesenchymal tumor
	34/M	1.0	1.6	4.2	Giant cell chondroma
Cai et al. (84)	47/F	7.0	1.4	4.4	Sclerosing hemangioma

phorus wasting, results in a negative phosphorus balance. Serum 25(OH)D is normal (in 15 of 19 patients) and serum 1,25(OH)$_2$D overtly low (in 19 of 23 patients) or inappropriately normal relative to the hypophosphatemia. Aminoaciduria, most frequently glycinuria, and glucosuria is occasionally present. Radiographic abnormalities include generalized osteopenia, pseudofractures, and coarsened trabeculae, as well as widened epiphyseal plates in children.

TUMORS

The tumors present in patients with tumor-induced osteomalacia have been of mesenchymal origin in the large majority of patients (Table 1). However, the frequent occur-

rence of Looser zones in the radiographs of moribund patients with carcinomas of epidermal and endodermal derivation (62) indicates that the disease may be secondary to a variety of tumor types. Indeed the recent observation of tumor-induced osteomalacia concurrent with breast carcinoma (63), prostate carcinoma (30,44,82), oat cell carcinoma (41), small cell carcinoma (77), multiple myeloma and chronic lymphocytic leukemia (53) supports this conclusion. The occurrence of osteomalacia in patients with widespread fibrous dysplasia of bone (63,64), neurofibromatosis (55,65), and linear nevus sebaceous syndrome (47) could also be tumor- induced. Proof of a causal relationship has been precluded by the multiplicity of lesions and the consequent inability to effect surgical care. However, in one case of fibrous dysplasia, removal of virtually all of the abnormal bone did result in appropriate biochemical and radiographic improvement (64).

The mesenchymal tumors induced with this osteomalacia syndrome have been variably described as sclerosing angioma, benign angiofibroma, hemangiopericytoma, chondrosarcoma, primitive mesenchymal tumor, soft parts chondroma-like tumor, and giant cell tumor of bone. The diversity of these diagnostic labels underscores the morphologic complexity of these tumors. However, Weidner and Cruz (65) recently established that the histologically polymorphous mesenchymal tumors can be subdivided into four distinct morphologic patterns: (i) primitive-appearing, mixed connective tissue tumors; (ii) osteoblastoma-like tumors; (iii) nonossifying fibroma-like tumors; and (iv) ossifying fibroma-like tumors. The most common of these, the mixed connective tissue variant, occurred in soft tissue, behaved in a benign fashion, and is characterized by variable numbers of primitive-appearing stromal cells growing in poorly defined sheets and punctuated by clusters of osteoclast-like giant cells. Vascularity is also often prominent but in less vascular areas poorly developed cartilage or foci of osteoid or bone is commonly present. The cartilage-like areas sometimes exhibit considerable dystrophic calcification. Likely the primitive stromal cells are the source of the hormonal factor(s) that causes the syndrome. However, immunohistochemical studies have shown no evidence of epithelial, neural, vascular, or neuroendocrine differentiation in these cells. Indeed, these cells are organelle-poor and do not have neurosecretory granules. This, of course, does not preclude them from secreting hormonally active substances (probably protein in nature). Whether similar mesenchymal elements exist in the epidermal and endodermal tumors associated with the syndrome remains unknown. However, fibrous mesenchymal components are present in many neural tumors and metastatic carcinoma of the prostate is frequently an osteoblastic lesion induced with varying degrees of fibrous tissue proliferation. Thus, it is possible that the expression of tumor-induced osteomalacia, concurrent with the presence of epidermal or endodermal tumors, depends on the presence and activity of such mesenchymal elements in many cases.

Regardless of the cell type responsible for the syndrome, the tumors at fault are often small, difficult to locate, and present in obscure areas. In this regard, many of the reported lesions have been located in a relatively inaccessible area within bone, such as within the femur or tibia, the nasopharynx, or a sinus. Alternatively, small lesions have been found in the popliteal region, the groin, and the suprapatellar area. In any case, a careful and thorough examination is necessary to document or exclude the presence of such a tumor.

PATHOPHYSIOLOGY

The pathophysiologic basis underlying tumor-induced osteomalacia remains unknown. Such incomplete understanding of the disorder undoubtedly relates to its infrequent occurrence and, consequently, the few physiologic studies of the disease. Nevertheless, most investigators agree that tumor production of a humoral factor(s) that may affect multiple functions of the proximal renal tubule, particularly phosphate reabsorption (resulting in hypophosphatemia), is the probable pathogenesis of the syndrome. This possibility has been supported by (i) the presence of phosphaturic activity in tumor extracts from three of four patients with tumor-induced osteomalacia (15,17,20), (ii) the absence of parathyroid hormone and calcitonin from these extracts and the apparent cyclic AMP-independent action of the extracts; (iii) the occurrence of hypophosphatemia and increased urinary phosphate excretion in heterotransplanted tumor-bearing athymic nude mice (54), (iv) the demonstration that extracts of the heterotransplanted tumor inhibited renal 25-hydroxyvitamin D-1α-hydroxylase activity in cultured kidney cells (54), and (v) the coincidence of aminoaciduria and glycosuria with renal phosphate wasting in some affected subjects, indicative of complex alterations in proximal renal tubular function (16). Indeed, partial purification of "phosphatonin" from a cell culture derived from a sclerosing hemangioma causing tumor-induced osteomalacia has reaffirmed this possibility (84). These studies reveal that the putative phosphatonin is a peptide with molecular weight of 8–25 kd that does not alter glucose or alanine transport but inhibits sodium-dependent phosphate transport in a cyclic AMP-independent fashion. Moreover, the activity of the phosphatonin is not blocked by a parathyroid hormone receptor antagonist. However, recent studies that document the presence in various disease states of additional phosphate transport inhibitors (85) indicate that the tumor-induced osteomalacia syndrome is heterogeneous and "phosphatonin" may be a family of hormones. In fact, the complexity of the syndrome may reach greater proportions because additional recent observations indicate that some mesenchymal tumors from affected subjects do not secrete phosphaturic factors into culture medium (56). Thus, the pathogenesis of the disorder may be more complicated than is currently appreciated.

In any case, abnormal vitamin D metabolism is an additional factor that likely contributes to the pathogenesis of the tumor-induced osteomalacia. Several observations support this possibility including (i) the decreased circulating 1,25(OH)₂D level observed in virtually all patients who manifest the characteristic syndrome; (ii) rapid normalization of the serum 1,25(OH)₂D concentration after surgical removal of the coincident tumor and in association with resolution of the biochemical abnormalities of the syndrome; and (iii) diminished renal 25(OH)D-1α-hydroxylase activity in heterotransplanted tumor-bearing athymic nude mice (66) and in kidney cell cultures exposed to tumor extracts (54).

The interrelationship between the abnormal renal phosphate transport and the defect in vitamin D metabolism evident in affected subjects remains unknown. An innate heterogeneity in the pathogenesis of the syndrome cannot be excluded. However, an interplay between these abnormalities likely contributes to the phenotypic expression of the disorder in the majority of patients.

In contrast to these observations, patients with tumor-induced osteomalacia secondary to hematogenous malignancy manifest abnormalities of the syndrome due to a distinctly different mechanism. In these subjects the nephropathy induced with light chain proteinuria results in the decreased renal tubular reabsorption of phosphate characteristic of the disease. To date at least 15 patients have been reported who potentially manifest this form of the disorder (53). In many instances, however, the diagnosis of tumor-induced osteomalacia was not considered. Nevertheless, at least in some cases of this syndrome, renal tubular damage may be mediated by tissue deposition of light chains or of some other immunoglobulin derivative with similar toxic effects on the kidney. Thus, light chain nephropathy must be considered one possible mechanism for the tumor-induced osteomalacic syndrome.

DIFFERENTIAL DIAGNOSIS

The tumor-induced osteomalacia syndrome has all of the classic biochemical and radiologic criteria of the hypophosphatemic osteomalacias. Diagnosis is therefore dependent on a diligent search for tumors in all patients with hypophosphatemic vitamin D-resistant rachitic/osteomalacic disease. Tumors may range from small to large and from benign to malignant. Moreover, the tumor may be present for many years before the clinical appearance of bone disease. Thus, regardless of the temporal association between the onset of the osteomalacia and the clinical awareness of tumor, tumor-induced osteomalacia should be considered. Indeed, where possible resection of any associated tumor should be attempted to both confirm the diagnosis and possibly to induce resolution of the syndrome.

When the tumor cannot be totally resected, diagnosis remains inferential. However, several observations can support the diagnosis: (i) a normal serum 25(OH)D level; (ii) a selective deficiency of 1,25(OH)$_2$D, manifested by a decreased serum concentration; (iii) presence of light chain proteinuria; (iv) demonstration of phosphaturic activity in tumor extracts; and/or (v) induction of the tumor-induced osteomalacia syndrome in athymic nude mice upon heterotransplantation of tumor tissue from affected subjects.

In the absence of tumor and/or family history of disease, and after exclusion of common causes of osteomalacia, the possibility of adult onset hypophosphatemic osteomalacia with or without Fanconi's syndrome must be considered. This syndrome may result from acquired or genetic causes and age of onset is extremely variable. Biochemical abnormalities are indistinguishable from those in patients with tumor-induced osteomalacia. Thus, in the absence of genetic transmission of the disorder, careful long-term follow-up for tumor occurrence must be maintained in all patients with hypophosphatemic osteomalacia.

TREATMENT

The first and foremost treatment of tumor-induced osteomalacia is complete resection of the associated tumor. However, recurrence of mesenchymal tumors, such as giant cell tumors of bone, or inability to resect completely certain malignancies, such as prostatic carcinoma, has resulted in the need to develop effective therapeutic intervention for the tumor-induced osteomalacia syndrome. Historically, pharmacologic doses of vitamin D have been used in an effort to heal the bone disease. For the most part, the trials have been short and the results have not been assessed in detail. Nevertheless, it appears certain that this treatment does not cure

the rachitic or osteomalacic components of the syndrome. Moreover, no resolution of the abnormal biochemistries ensues.

More recently, administration of 1,25(OH)$_2$D alone or in combination with phosphorus supplementation has served as effective therapy for the tumor-induced osteomalacia. In this regard, Drezner and Feinglos (16) and Lobaugh et al. (86) have noted striking improvement of the biochemical and bone abnormalities of the syndrome in response to calcitriol (2.0–3.0 µg/day). In two such patients the serum phosphorus level increased from pretreatment levels of 1.5 ± 0.7 and 2.2 ± 0.1 mg/dl to normal values of 3.7 ± 0.03 and 2.8 ± 0.08 mg/dl, respectively. Similarly, the renal TmP/GFR rose from an abnormally low level, 0.8 ± 0.03 and 1.9 ± 0.03 mg/dl, to normal 3.0 ± 0.01 and 2.8 ± 0.09 mg/dl. Commensurately, evidence of bone healing was present in bone biopsies from these subjects.

In contrast, several investigators have observed only modest symptomatic, biochemical, and histologic improvement in response to calcitriol. However, in general such patients responded well to combination therapy with pharmacologic amounts of 1,25(OH)$_2$D and phosphorus (59). Phosphorus supplementation (2–4 g/day) directly replaces the ongoing renal loss of inorganic phosphorus, whereas calcitriol (1.5–3 µg/day) serves to replace insufficient renal production of the sterol and to enhance renal phosphate reabsorption. Such therapy normalizes the biochemical abnormalities of the syndrome and results in healing of the osteomalacia. These data indicate that patients with tumor-induced osteomalacia may benefit from a combination drug regimen.

COMPLICATIONS OF THERAPY

Little information is available regarding the long-term consequences of therapy in patients with tumor-induced osteomalacia. The doses of medicines used, however, raise the possibility that nephrolithiasis, nephrocalcinosis, and hypercalcemia may frequently complicate the therapeutic course. Indeed, hypercalcemia secondary to parathyroid hyperfunction has been documented in five affected subjects, representing approximately 5% of the reported cases. All of these patients had received phosphorus (as part of a combination regimen with vitamin D$_2$ or 1,25(OH)$_2$D), which may have stimulated parathyroid hormone secretion and ultimately led to parathyroid autonomy. Thus, careful assessment of parathyroid function, serum and urinary calcium, and renal function are essential to ensure safe and efficacious therapy.

REFERENCES

1. McCance RA: Osteomalacia with looser's nodes (milkman's syndrome) due to a raised resistance to vitamin D acquired about the age of 15 years. *Q J Med* 16:33–46, 1947
2. Prader AV, Illig R, Uehilinger E, Stalder G: Rachitis infolge knochentumors. *Helv Paediatr Acta* 14:554–565, 1959
3. Hauge BM: Vitamin D-resistant osteomalacia. *Acta Med Scand* 153:271–282, 1956
4. Yoshikawa S, Kawabata M, Hatsuyama Y, Hosokawa 0, Fujita T: Atypical vitamin D-resistant osteomalacia. Report of a Case. *J Bone Joint Surg* 45-A:998–1007, 1964

5. Krane SM: Case records of the Massachusetts General Hospital. *N Engl J Med* 273:1330, 1965
6. Salassa RM, Jowsey J, Arnaud CD: Hypophosphatemic osteomalacia induced with "nonendocrine" tumors. *N Engl J Med* 1970; 283:65–70.
7. Evans DJ, Azzopardi JG: Distinctive tumours of bone and soft tissue causing acquired vitamin-D-resistant osteomalacia. *Lancet* 11:353–354, 1972
8. Olefsky J, Kempson R, Jones H, Reaven G: "Tertiary" hyperparathyroidism and apparent "cure" of vitamin D-resistant rickets after removal of an ossifying mesenchymal tumor of the pharynx. *N Engl J Med* 286:740–745, 1972
9. Pollack JA, Schiller AL, Crawford JD: Rickets and myopathy cured by removal of a nonossifying fibroma of bone. *Pediatrics* 52:364–371, 1973
10. Moser CR Fessel WJ: Rheumatic manifestations of hypophosphatemia. *Arch Intern Med* 134:674–678, 1974
11. Willhoite DR: Acquired rickets and solitary bone tumor. The question of a causal relationship (abstract). *Clin Orthop* 109:210–211, 1975
12. Linovitz RJ, Resnick D, Keissling P, Kondon JJ, Sehler B, Nejdl RJ, Rowe JH, Deftos LJ: Tumor-induced osteomalacia and rickets: a surgically curable syndrome. Report of two cases. *J Bone Joint Surg* 58–A:419–423, 1976
13. Renton P, Shaw DG: Hypophosphatemic osteomalacia secondary to vascular tumors of bone and soft tissue. *Skel Radiol* 1:21–24, 1975
14. Morita M: [A case of adult onset vitamin D-resistant osteomalacia induced with soft tissue tumor.] *Kotsu Taisha [Bone Metabolism]* 9:286–291, 1976
15. Aschinberg LC, Soloman LM, Zeis PM, Justice P, Rosenthal IM: Vitamin D-resistant rickets induced with epidermal nevus syndrome: demonstration of a phosphaturic substance in the dermal lesions. *J Pediatrics* 91:56–60, 1977
16. Drezner MK, Feinglos MN: Osteomalacia due to 1,25-dihydroxycholecalciferol deficiency. Association with a giant cell tumor of bone. *J Clin Invest* 60:1046–1053, 1977
17. Yoshikawa S, Nakamura T, Takagi M, Imamura T, Okano K, Sasaki S: Benign osteoblastoma as a cause of osteomalacia. A report of two cases. *J Bone Joint Surg* 59-B(3):279–289, 1977
18. Wyman AL, Paradinas FJ, Daly JR: Hypophosphataemic osteomalacia induced with a malignant tumour of the tibia: report of a case. *J Clin Pathol* 30:328–335, 1977
19. Leite MOR, Borelli A, de Ulhoa Cintra AB: Osteomalacia hipofosfatemica associada a hemangio-fibroma. Consideracoes etiopaogenicas. *Rev Hosp Clin Fac Med San Paulo* 33:65–67, 1978
20. Lau K, Strom MC, Goldberg M, Goldfarb S, Gray RW, Lemann R Jr, Agus ZS: Evidence for a humoral phosphaturic factor in oncogenic hypophosphatemic osteomalacia (abstract). *Clin Res* 27:421A, 1979
21. Werner M, Cohen L, Bar RS, Strottmann MP, DeLuca H: Regulation of phosphate and calcium metabolism by vitamin D metabolites: studies in a patient with oncogenic osteomalacia [abstract]. *Arthritis Rheum* 22:672–673, 1979
22. Turner ML, Dalinka MK: Osteomalacia: uncommon causes. *AJR* 133:539–540, 1979
23. Nortman DF, Coburn JW, Brautbar N, Sherrard DJ, Haussler MR, Singer FR, Brickman AS, Barton RT: Treatment of mesenchymal tumor induced osteomalacia (MTAO) with 1,25(OH)₂D₃. Report of a case. In: Norman AW (ed) *Vitamin D: Basic Research and Its Clinical Application. Proceedings of the Fourth Workshop on Vitamin D.* Berlin, De Gruyter, pp 1167–1168, 1979
24. Daniels RA, Weisenfeld I: Tumorous phosphaturic osteomalacia. Report of a case induced with multiple hemangiomas of bone. *Am J Med* 67:155–159, 1979
25. Fukumoto Y, Tarui S, Tsukiyama K, Ichihara K, Moriwaki K, Nonaka K, Mizushima T, Kobayashi Y, Dokoh S, Fukunaga M, Morita R: Tumor-induced vitamin D-resistant hypophosphatemic osteomalacia induced with proximal renal tubular dysfunction and 1,25-dihydroxyvitamin D deficiency. *J Clin Endocrinol Metab* 49:873–878, 1979
26. Lejeune E, Bouvier M, Meunier P, Vauzelle JL, Deplante JP, David L, Llorca G, Andre-Fouet E: L'osteomalacie des tumeurs mesenchymateuses. A propos d'une noouvelle observation. *Rev Rhumat* 46:187–193, 1979
27. Crouzet J, Camus JP, Gatti JM, Descamps H, Beraneck L: Osteomalacie hypophosphoremique et hemangiopericytome de la voute du crane. *Rev Rhum Mal Osteoartic* 47:523–528, 1980
28. Camus JP, Courzet J, Prier A, Guillemant S, Ulmann A, Koeger AC. Osteomalacies hypophosphoremiques gueries par l'ablation de tumeurs benignes du tissu conjonctif: etude de trois observations avec dosages pre-et post-operatoires des metabolites de la vitamine D. *Ann Med Interne* 131:422–426, 1980
29. Sweet RA, Males JL, Hamstra AJ, Deluca HF: Vitamin D metabolite levels in oncogenic osteomalacia. *Ann Intern Med* 93: 279–280, 1980
30. Lyles KW, Berry WR, Haussler M, Harrelson JM, Drezner MK: Hypophosphatemic osteomalacia: association with prostatic carcinoma. *Ann Intern Med* 93:275–278, 1980
31. Nitzan DW, Marmary Y, Azaz B: Mandibular tumor-induced muscular weakness and osteomalacia. *Oral Surg Oral Med Oral Pathol* 52:253–256, 1981
32. Asnes RS, Berdon WE, Bassett CA: Hypophosphatemic rickets in an adolescent cured by excision of a nonossifying fibroma. *Clin Pediatrics* 20:646–648, 1981
33. Parker MS, Klein I, Haussler MR, Mintz DH: Tumor-induced osteomalacia. Evidence of a surgically correctable alteration in vitamin D metabolism. *JAMA* 245:492–493, 1981
34. Chacko V, Joseph B: Osteomalacia induced with hemangiopericytoma. *J Indian Med Assoc* 76:173–175, 1981
35. Hioco J, Chanzy MO, Hioco F, Voisin MC, Villiaumey J: Osteomalacia with mesenchymal tumors—two new cases (abstract). *Rev Rhumat Special* 890, 1981
36. Barcelo P Jr, Asensi E, Paso M, Obach J, Barcelo P Sr: Osteomalacia hipofosforemica secundaria as histiocitoma fibroso vascular [abstract]. *Rev Rhumat Special* 1352, 1981
37. Nomura G, Koshino Y, Morimoto H, Kida H, Noura S, Tamai K: Vitamin D resistant hypophosphatemic osteomalacia induced with osteosarcoma of the mandible. Report of a case. *Jpn J Med* 21:35–39, 1982
38. Ryan EA, Reiss E: Oncogenous osteomalacia. Review of the world literature and report of two new cases. *Am J Med* 77:501–512, 1984
39. Firth RG, Grant CS, Riggs BL: Development of hypercalcemic hyperparathyroidism after long-term phosphate supplementation in hypophosphatemic osteomalacia. Report of two cases. *Am J Med* 78:669–673, 1985
40. Taylor HC, Fallon MD, Velasco ME: Oncogenic osteomalacia and inappropriate antidiuretic hormone secretion due to oat-cell carcinoma. *Ann Intern Med* 101:786–788, 1984
41. Leehey DJ, Ing TS, Daugirdas JT: Fanconi syndrome induced-with a non–ossifying fibroma of bone. *Am J Med* 78:708–710, 1985
42. Seshadri MS, Cornish CJ, Mason RS, Posen S: Parathyroid hormone-like bioactivity in tumours from patients with oncogenic osteomalacia. *Clin Endocrinol* 23:689–697, 1985
43. Cotton GE, Van Puffelen P: Hypophosphatemic osteomalacia secondary to neoplasia. *J Bone Joint Surg* 68A:129–133, 1986
44. Murphy P, Wright G, Rai GS: Hypophosphatemic osteomalacia induced with prostatic carcinoma. *Br Med J* 290:1945, 1985
45. Gitelis S, Ryan WG, Rosenberg AG, Templeton AC: Adult-onset hypophosphatemic osteomalacia secondary to neoplasm: a case report and review of the pathophysiology. *J Bone Joint Surg* 68A: 134–138, 1986
46. Rico H, Fernandez-Miranda E, Sanz J, Gomez-Castresana F, Escriba A, Hernandez ER, Krsnik I: Oncogenous osteomalacia: a new case secondary to a malignant tumor. *Bone* 7:325–329, 1986
47. Carey DE, Drezner MK, Hamdan JA, Mange M, Ashmad MS, Mubarak S, Nyhan WL: Hypophosphatemic rickets/osteomalacia in linear sebaceous nevus syndrome: a variant of tumor-induced osteomalacia. *J Pediatrics* 109:994–1000, 1986
48. Siris ES, Clemens TL, Dempster DW, Shane E, Segre GV, Lindsay R, Bilezekian JP: Tumor-induced osteomalacia: kinetics of calcium phosphorus and vitamin D metabolism and characteristics of bone histomorphometry. *Am J Med* 82:307–312, 1987

49. Reid IR, Teitelbaum SL, Dusso A, Whyte MP: Hypercalcemic hyperparathyroidism complicating oncogenic osteomalacia: effect of successful tumor resection on mineral homeostasis. *Am J Med* 83:350–354, 1987

50. Prowse M, Brooks PM: Oncogenic hypophosphatemic osteomalacia induced with a giant cell tumour of a tendon sheath. *Aust NZ J Med* 17:330–332, 1987

51. Sparagana M: Tumor-induced osteomalacia: long-term follow-up of two patients cured by removal of their tumors. *J Surg Oncol* 36:198–205, 1987

52. Rao DS, Parfitt AM, Villanueva AR, Dorman PJ, Kleerekoper M: Hypophosphatemic osteomalacia and adult Fanconi syndrome due to light-chain nephropathy: another form of oncogenous osteomalacia. *Am J Med* 82:333–338, 1987

53. McClure J, Smith PS: Oncogenic osteomalacia. *J Clin Pathol* 40: 446–453, 1987

54. Miyauchi A, Fukase M, Tsutsumi M, Fujita T: Hemangiopericytoma-induced osteomalacia: tumor transplantation in nude mice causes hypophosphatemia and tumor extracts inhibit renal 25-hydroxyvitamin D-1-hydroxylase activity. *J Clin Endocrinol Metab* 67:46–53, 1988

55. Konishi K, Nakamura M, Yamakawa H, Suzuki H, Saruta T, Hanaoka H, Davatchi T: Case report: hypophosphatemic osteomalacia in von Recklinghausen neurofibromatosis. *Am J Med Sci* 301:322–328, 1991

56. Nitzan DW, Horowitz AT, Darmon D, Friedlaender MM, Rubinger D, Stein P, Bab I, Popovtzer MM, Silver J: Oncogenous osteomalacia: a case study. *Bone Mineral* 6:191–197, 1989

57. McGuire MH, Merenda JT, Etzkorn JR, Sundaram M: Oncogenic osteomalacia: a case report. *Clin Orthop Rel Res* 244:305–308, 1989

58. Schultze G, Delling G, Faensen M, Haubold R, Loy V, Molzahn M, Pommer W, Semier J, Trempenau B. Onkogene hypophosphatamische Osteomalazie. *Kurze Originalien and Falberichte* 114:1073–1078, 1989

59. Leicht E, Biro G, Langer H.-J: Tumor-induced osteomalacia: pre- and postoperative biochemical findings. *Horm Metab Res* 22: 640–643, 1990

60. Uchida H, Yokoyama S, Kashima K, Nakayama I, Shimizu K, Masumi S: Oncogenic vitamin D resistant hypophosphatemic osteomalacia (benign ossifying mesenchymal tumor of bone): case report. *Jpn J Clin Oncol* 21:218–226, 1991

61. Papotti M, Foschini MP, Isia G, Rizzi G, Betts C, Eusebi V: Hypophosphatemic oncogenic osteomalacia: report of three new cases. *Tumori* 74:599–607, 1988

62. Dent CE, Stamp TCB: Vitamin D rickets and osteomalacia. In: Avioli LV, Krane S (eds) *Metabolic Bone Disease.* vol 1. New York, Academic Press, p 237, 1978

63. Dent CE, Gertner JM: Hypophosphatemic osteomalacia in fibrous dysplasia. *Q J Med* 45:411–420, 1976

64. Saville PD, Nassim JR, Stevenson FH: Osteomalacia in von Recklinghausen's neurofibromatosis: metabolic study of a case. *Br Med J* 1:1311–1313, 1955

65. Weidner N, Cruz DS: Phosphaturic mesenchymal tumors: a polymorphous group causing osteomalacia or rickets. *Cancer* 59: 1442–1454, 1987

66. Boriani S, Campanacci: Osteoblastoma associated with osteomalacia (presentation of a case and review of the literature). *Ital J Orthop Traumatol* 4:379–382, 1978

67. Castleman B, McNeely BU. Case records of the Massachusetts General Hospital: case 38—1965. *N Engl J Med* 273:494–504, 1965

68. Robertson A: Case of the winter season. *Semin Roentgenol* 18:5–6, 1983

69. Kabadi UM: Osteomalacia associated with prostatic cancer and osteoblastic metastases. *Urology* 21:65–67, 1983

70. Moncrieff MW, Brenton DP, Arthur LJH: Case of tumour rickets. *Arch Dis Child* 53:740–745, 1978

71. Cramer SF, Aikawa M, Cebelin M: Neurosecretory granules in small cell invasive carcinoma of the urinary bladder. *Cancer* 47: 724–730, 1981

72. Ioakimidis DE, Dendrinos GK, Frangia KB, Babiolakis DN, Chilas GI, Lyberopoulos KL, Kontomerkos TK. Tumor induced osteomalacia. *J Rheumatol* 21:1162–1164, 1994

73. Lee HK, Sung WW, Dolodnik P, Shimshi M: Bone scan in tumor-induced osteomalacia. *J Nucl Med* 36:247–249, 1995

74. Harvey JN, Gray C, Belchetz PE: Oncogenous osteomalacia and malignancy. *Clin Endocrinol* 37:379–384, 1992

75. Cehreli C, Alakavuklar MN, Cavdar C, Basdemir G, Undar B, Akkoc N, Payzin B, Oztop F: Oncogenous osteomalacia—report of a case. *Acta Oncologica* 33:975–980, 1994

76. Schapira D, Izhak OB, Nachtigal A, Burstein A, Shalom RB, Shagrawi I, Best LA: Tumor-induced osteomalaica. *Semin Arthitis Rheum* 25:35–46, 1995

77. Shaker JL, Brickner RC, Divgi AB, Raff H, Findling JW: Case report: renal phosphate wasting, syndrome of inappropriate antidiuretic hormone and ectopic corticotropin production in small cell carcinoma. *Am J Med Sci* 310:38–41, 1995

78. Yu GH, Katz RL, Raymond AK, Gagel RF, Allison A, McCutcheion I: Oncogenous osteomalacia: fine needle aspiration of a neoplasm with a unique endocrinologic presentation. *Acta Cytol* 39:831–832, 1995

79. Linsey M, Smith W, Yamauchi H, Bernstein L: Nasopharyngeal angiofibroma presenting as adult osteomalacia: case report and review of the literature. *Laryngoscope* 93:1328–1331, 1982

80. Nuovo MA, Dorfman HD, Sun C-CJ, Chalew S: Tumor-induced osteomalacia and rickets. *Am J Surg Pathol* 13:588–589, 1989

81. Hernberg CA, Edgren W: Looser-Milkman's syndrome with neurofibromatosis Recklinghause and general decalcification of the skeleton. *Acta Medica Scand* 136:26–33, 1949

82. Hosking DJ, Chamberlain MJ, Whortland-Webb WR: Osteomalacia and carcinoma of prostate with major redistribution of skeletal calcium. *Br J Radiol* 48:451–456, 1975

83. Weidner N, Bar RS, Weiss D, Strottmann MP: Neoplastic pathology of oncogenic osteomalacia/rickets. *Cancer* 55:1691–1705, 1985

84. Cai Q, Hodgson SF, Kao PC, Lennon VA, Klee GG, Zinsmiester AR, Kumar R: Brief report: inhibition of renal phosphate transport by a tumor product in a patient with oncogenic osteomalacia. *N Engl J Med* 330:1645–1649, 1994

85. Kumar R, Haugen JD, Wieben ED, Londowski JM, Cai Q: Inhibitors of renal epithelial phosphate transport in tumor induced osteomalacia and uremia. *Proc Am Assoc Physicians* 107:296–305, 1995

86. Lobaugh B, Burch WM Jr, Drezner MK: Abnormalities of vitamin D metabolism and action in the vitamin D-resistant rachitic and osteomalacic diseases. In: Kumar R (ed) *Vitamin D.* Boston, Martinus Nijhoff, pp 665–720, 1984

63. Hypophosphatasia

Michael P. Whyte, M.D.

Division of Bone and Mineral Diseases, Washington University School of Medicine; and Metabolic Research Unit, Shriners Hospital for Crippled Children, St. Louis, Missouri

Hypophosphatasia is a rare heritable type of rickets or osteomalacia (1,2). Approximately 300 cases have been reported. The disorder occurs in all races with an incidence of about 1 per 100,000 live births for the severe forms. This inborn error of metabolism is characterized by a reduction of activity of the tissue-nonspecific (liver/bone/kidney) isoenzyme of alkaline phosphatase (TNSALP). Activity of the tissue-specific intestinal, placental, and germ cell ALP isoenzymes is not reduced (3).

Although there is overlap between the various clinical forms of hypophosphatasia, four principal types are reported depending on the age at which skeletal lesions are discovered: perinatal, infantile, childhood, and adult. When dental manifestations alone are present, the condition is called odontohypophosphatasia. In general, the earlier the presentation of skeletal problems, the more severe the clinical course (1,2).

CLINICAL PRESENTATION

Although some TNSALP is present in all tissues, hypophosphatasia affects predominantly the skeleton and dentition. The severity of clinical expression is, however, remarkably variable, e.g., death may occur *in utero* or symptoms may never appear (1,2).

Perinatal hypophosphatasia manifests during gestation. The pregnancy may be complicated by polyhydramnios. Typically, extreme skeletal hypomineralization (causing short and deformed limbs and caput membranaceum) is present at birth. Rarely, unusual bony spurs appear on long bones. Some newborns survive briefly but suffer increasing respiratory compromise, unexplained fever, anemia (perhaps from encroachment on the marrow space by excessive osteoid), failure to gain weight, irritability, periodic apnea with cyanosis and bradycardia, intracranial hemorrhage, and seizures. This is a lethal condition (1,2).

Infantile hypophosphatasia becomes clinically apparent before 6 months of age. Development often seems normal until poor feeding, inadequate weight gain, hypotonia, and wide fontanels are noted. Progressive rachitic deformities then manifest. Hypercalcemia and hypercalciuria can cause recurrent vomiting, nephrocalcinosis, and occasionally significant renal compromise. Despite widely "open" fontanels (actually hypomineralized areas of calvarium), functional craniosynostosis is common. Raised intracranial pressure can cause bulging of the anterior fontanel, proptosis, and papilledema. Mild hypertelorism and brachycephaly can be present. A flail chest predisposes to pneumonia. Infantile hypophosphatasia may show progressive deterioration during the months after diagnosis and is fatal in about 50% of patients. The prognosis seems to improve with survival beyond infancy (1,2).

Childhood hypophosphatasia varies greatly in clinical severity. Premature loss of deciduous teeth (<age 5)) from hypoplasia or aplasia of dental cementum is a clinical hallmark. Odontohypophosphatasia is present when radiographs show no evidence of skeletal disease. The incisors are typically lost first, but in severe cases the entire dentition can be affected. There is only minimal tooth root resorption. Dental radiographs often show enlarged pulp chambers and root canals that characterize "shell teeth." When rickets is present, delayed walking with a waddling gait, short stature, and a dolichocephalic skull with frontal bossing are often present. Childhood hypophosphatasia may improve spontaneously, but recurrence of skeletal disease during adulthood is likely (1,2).

Adult hypophosphatasia usually presents during middle age, often with painful and poorly healing recurrent metatarsal stress fractures. Pain in the thighs or hips may be due to femoral pseudofractures. About 50% of affected adults will have a history of rickets and/or premature loss of deciduous teeth during childhood. Loss or extraction of adult teeth is also common. Chondrocalcinosis occurs frequently and calcium pyrophosphate dihydrate crystal deposition disease and calcific periarthritis affect some patients (see below) (4). Recurrent stress fractures heal slowly; persistent femoral pseudofractures will mend following intramedullary rodding (5).

LABORATORY FINDINGS

Hypophosphatasia is diagnosed from a consistent clinical history and physical findings, radiologic evidence of rickets or osteomalacia, and the presence of low serum ALP activity (hypophosphatasemia) (1). One must recognize that there are changes in the normal range for serum ALP activity with age and that rarely other conditions and treatments can cause hypophosphatasemia (6).

The rickets/osteomalacia of hypophosphatasia is unusual in that serum levels of calcium and inorganic phosphate (Pi) are not reduced. In fact, hypercalciuria and hypercalcemia occur frequently in perinatal and infantile hypophosphatasia apparently from dyssynergy between gut absorption of calcium and defective skeletal growth and mineralization (some severely affected patients also show progressive skeletal demineralization). Children and adults with hypophosphatasia actually have serum Pi levels that are above mean levels for controls, and about 50% of patients are frankly hyperphosphatemic. Enhanced renal reclamation of Pi (increased TmP/GFR) accounts for this finding. In serum, vitamin D and parathyroid hormone levels are usually normal (1).

Three phosphocompounds accumulate endogenously in hypophosphatasia (1): phosphoethanolamine (PEA), inorganic pyrophosphate (PPi), and pyridoxal 5′-phosphate (PLP). Demonstration of phosphoethanolaminuria supports the diagnosis but is not specific. Urinary PEA levels can be modestly increased in a variety of other disorders, and normal levels can occur in mild cases of hypophosphatasia. Assay of PPi in plasma and urine remains a research technique. An elevated plasma level of PLP is a sensitive and specific marker for hypophosphatasia (subjects should not be taking vitamin B_6 supplements when tested). In general, the greater the plasma PLP level, the more severe the clinical manifestations (1,3).

RADIOLOGIC FINDINGS

Perinatal hypophosphatasia has pathognomonic findings (7). Marked skeletal undermineralization occurs with severe rachitic changes. In extreme cases, the skeleton may be so poorly mineralized that only the base of the skull is visualized. In less remarkable cases, the calvarium may be ossified at central portions of the membranous bones and thereby give the illusion that the sutures are open and widely separated. Fractures are common.

Infantile hypophosphatasia causes characteristic but less severe changes. Abrupt transition from relatively normal appearing diaphyses to hypomineralized metaphyses may suggest a sudden metabolic deterioration. Progressive skeletal demineralization can occur. Skeletal scintigraphy may help to show premature closure of cranial sutures that appear "widened" on radiographs.

Childhood hypophosphatasia often causes "tongues" of radiolucency to project from rachitic growth plates into metaphyses (Fig. 1). True premature fusion of cranial sutures can cause a "beaten-copper" appearance of the skull.

Adult hypophosphatasia is associated with osteopenia, recurrent poorly healing stress fractures, chondrocalcinosis, and proximal femoral pseudofractures.

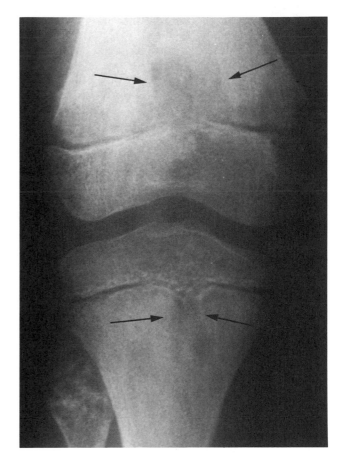

FIG. 1. The metaphysis of the proximal tibia of this 10-year-old boy with mild childhood hypophosphatasia shows a subtle but characteristic "tongue" of radiolucency *(arrows)*. Note, however, that his rickets does not manifest with widening of the growth plate.

HISTOPATHOLOGIC FINDINGS

Nondecalcified sections of bone reveal typical histologic features of rickets or osteomalacia in all clinical forms of hypophosphatasia except odontohypophosphatasia. However, biochemical or histochemical measurement of ALP activity in bone would distinguish hypophosphatasia from other disorders.

Open cranial "sutures" are actually uncalcified osteoid. Dental histopathology shows aplasia or hypoplasia of cementum. Enlarged pulp chambers ("shell teeth") indicate impaired dentinogenesis. These changes do vary from tooth to tooth.

INHERITANCE

Perinatal and infantile hypophosphatasia are inherited as autosomal recessive disorders. Parents of severely affected patients may have low or low normal serum ALP activity, mildly elevated plasma PLP levels, and modest phosphoethanolaminuria. Challenge with vitamin B_6 (pyridoxine)

orally is followed by a distinctly abnormal increase in plasma PLP levels in carriers and especially in patients (3).

The mode of inheritance for the milder forms of hypophosphatasia is less clear. Some cases of odontohypophosphatasia and adult-onset disease may reflect clinical expression in heterozygotes for whom the disorder was transmitted as an autosomal dominant trait (see below) (1,2).

BIOCHEMICAL/GENETIC DEFECT

In keeping with an inborn error of metabolism that selectively affects the TNSALP isoenzyme, autopsy studies of perinatal and infantile hypophosphatasia patients demonstrate profound deficiency of ALP activity in liver, bone, and kidney, but not in the intestine or placenta. Missense mutations in the TNSALP gene have been discovered in severe forms of hypophosphatasia (8). Some patients, however, may have a regulatory defect involving TNSALP (1). Childhood and adult hypophosphatasia can be due to compound heterozygosity for TNSALP missense mutations (8).

PATHOGENESIS

Studies of vitamin B_6 metabolism in hypophosphatasia indicate that TNSALP acts to regulate the extracellular concentration of a variety of phosphocompounds (3). Accumulation of PPi, an inhibitor of hydroxyapatite crystal growth, may account for the impaired skeletal mineralization (3). Recent development of a "knockout" mouse model for hypophosphatasia should help to further clarify the role of TNSALP (9).

TREATMENT

There is no established medical therapy. It is important to avoid traditional treatments for rickets or osteomalacia (e.g., vitamin D sterols and mineral supplementation) because serum levels of calcium, Pi, 25(OH)D, and 1,25(OH)$_2$D are not reduced (1). Furthermore, vitamin D may exacerbate any predisposition to hypercalcemia and hypercalciuria.

The hypercalcemia of perinatal or infantile hypophosphatasia will respond to restriction of dietary calcium and/or to glucocorticoid therapy. Fractures in children and adults do mend, however, this process may be slow, and delayed healing after osteotomy with casting has been observed. Placement of load-sharing intramedullary rods, rather than load-sparing plates, is best for the acute or prophylactic treatment of fractures and pseudofractures in adults (5). Dentures may be necessary for some affected children.

PRENATAL DIAGNOSIS

Perinatal hypophosphatasia can be detected prenatally. Combined use of serial ultrasonography (with attention to the limbs as well as skull), assay of ALP activity in amniotic fluid cells by an experienced laboratory, and radiologic study of the fetus have been used successfully for prenatal diagnosis of this form of hypophosphatasia in the second trimester

(10). First-trimester diagnosis using chorionic villus samples and a monoclonal antibody-based TNSALP assay has been achieved (11). Recently, DNA-based techniques have also proven helpful for assessment of the infantile form (10).

REFERENCES

1. Whyte MP: Hypophosphatasia. In: Scriver CR, Beaudet AL, Sly WS, Valle D (eds) *The Metabolic and Molecular Bases of Inherited Disease.* 7th ed. New York, McGraw-Hill, pp 4095–4112, 1995
2. Caswell AM, Whyte MP, Russell RGG: Hypophosphatasia and the extracellular metabolism of inorganic pyrophosphate: clinical and laboratory aspects. *Crit Rev Clin Lab Sci* 28:175–232, 1992
3. Whyte MP: Hypophosphatasia and the role of alkaline phosphatase in skeletal mineralization. *Endocr Rev* 15:439–461, 1994
4. Chuck AJ, Pattrick MG, Hamilton E, Wilson R, Doherty M: Crystal deposition in hypophosphatasia: a reappraisal. *Ann Rheum Dis* 48:571–576, 1989
5. Coe JD, Murphy WA, Whyte MP: Management of femoral fractures and pseudofractures in adult hypophosphatasia. *J Bone Joint Surg* 68A:981–990, 1986
6. Weinstein RS, Whyte MP: Heterogeneity of adult hypophosphatasia: report of severe and mild cases. *Arch Intern Med* 141:727–731, 1981
7. Shohat M, Rimoin DL, Gerber HE, Lachman RS: Perinatal hypophosphatasia: clinical, radiologic, and morphologic findings. *Pediatr Radiol* 21:421–427, 1991
8. Henthorn PS, Raducha M, Fedde KN, Lafferty MA, Whyte MP: Different missense mutations at the tissue-nonspecific alkaline phosphatase gene locus in autosomal recessively inherited forms of mild and severe hypophosphatasia. *Proc Natl Acad Sci USA* 89:9924–9928, 1992
9. Waymire KG, Mahuren JD, Jaje JM, Guilarte TR, Coburn SP, MacGregor GR: Mice lacking tissue non-specific alkaline phosphatase die from seizures due to defective metabolism of vitamin B-6. *Nature Genet* 11:45–51, 1995
10. Henthorn PS, Whyte MP: Infantile hypophosphatasia: successful prenatal assessment by testing for tissue-nonspecific alkaline phosphatase gene mutations. *Prenat Diagn* 15:1001–1006, 1995
11. Brock DJH, Barron L: First-trimester prenatal diagnosis of hypophosphatasia: experience with 16 cases. *Prenat Diagn* 11:387, 1991

64. Fanconi Syndrome and Renal Tubular Acidosis

Russell W. Chesney, M.D.

Department of Pediatrics, University of Tennessee; and LeBonheur Children's Medical Center, Memphis, Tennessee

Osteomalacia with or without rickets is a common feature of Fanconi syndrome and certain forms of renal tubular acidosis. The renal Fanconi syndrome is characterized by a generalized defect in renal proximal tubule transport capacity including impaired reabsorption of glucose, phosphate, amino acids, bicarbonate, uric acid, citrate and other organic acids, and low-molecular-weight proteins (less than 50,000 kd). Calcium, magnesium, sodium, potassium, and water are also excreted in excess (1). This syndrome is often the ultimate expression of toxic and/or metabolic injury to the proximal tubule; hence, the syndrome has many associated disorders that play a role in its pathogenesis (Tables 1 and

2). Familial and hereditary disorders associated with the syndrome are listed in Table 1 and acquired conditions in Table 2. Because the syndrome represents a global tubulopathy and has a large number of associated disorders, the most likely pathogenic sequence involves deranged intracellular metabolic regulation rather than a defect in individual solute or ion transport sites. The occurrence of the syndrome in patients with disorders of mitochondrial respiration and myopathy stress the importance of intact energy production in proximal tubular function (1). Abnormal intracellular metabolism could result either in a reduction in high-energy phosphate compounds necessary for active transport

TABLE 1. *Familial and hereditary disorders associated with Fanconi syndrome*

Primary or idiopathic disorders (no identifiable associated disorder)
1. Familial
2. Sporadic hereditary disorders
   1. Cystinosis (Lignac–Fanconi disease)
   2. Lowe syndrome
   3. Hereditary fructose intolerance
   4. Tyrosinemia, type I (tyrosinosis)
   5. Galactosemia
   6. Glycogen storage disease
   7. Wilson's disease
   8. Others
      A. Hereditary mitochondrial myopathy with lactic acidemia
      B. Metachromatic leukodystrophy
      C. Subacute necrotizing encephalomyelopathy (Leigh syndrome)
      D. Hereditary nephritis (Alport syndrome)
      E. Medullary cystic disease

TABLE 2. *Acquired disorders associated with Fanconi syndrome*

1. Disorders of protein metabolism/excretion
   a. Multiple myeloma
   b. Benign monoclonal gammopathy
   c. Light chain nephropathy
   d. Amyloidosis
   e. Sjögren syndrome
   f. Nephrotic syndrome
2. Immunologic disorders
   a. Interstitial nephritis with anti-TBM antibody
   b. Renal transplantation
   c. Malignancy
3. Other renal disorders
   a. Balkan nephropathy
   b. Paroxysmal nocturnal hemoglobinuria
   c. Renal vein thrombosis in newborn infant
4. Vitamin D disorders with secondary hyperparathyroidism
   a. Vitamin D deficiency
   b. Vitamin D-dependent rickets
5. Disorders linked with drug, heavy metal, or other toxin exposure
A. Drug-related courses
   a. Outdated, degraded tetracycline
   b. Methyl-3-chromone
   c. 6-Mercaptopurine
   d. Gentamicin and aminoglycoside antibiotics
   e. Valproic acid
   f. Streptozotocin
   g. Isophthalanilide
   h. Ifosfamide
B. Heavy metal exposure
   a. Cadmium
   b. Lead
   c. Mercury
   d. Uranium
   e. *cis*-Platinum
C. Other toxin exposure
   a. Paraquat poisoning
   b. Lysol burn
   c. Toluene inhalation (glue sniffing)

processes, or in defective membrane biosynthesis or epithelial integrity (2). The syndrome has also been seen in association with vitamin D deficiency (3), although autosomal recessive cystine storage disease (cystinosis) and light chain myeloma are the most common causes in children and adults, respectively (4). Some cases of Fanconi syndrome are not linked to any of the known associations, and these idiopathic cases can be seen in both children and adults by a sporadic, recessive, dominant, or sex-linked hereditary pattern (4).

Renal tubular acidosis (RTA) is a disorder in which the kidney is incapable of conserving bicarbonate; thus, patients develop a decline in plasma bicarbonate concentrations and systemic metabolic acidosis (5). The underlying renal defect consists of a reduction in tubular bicarbonate reabsorption, the inability to secrete protons (H^+) so that a pH gradient between blood and the lumen cannot be formed, or the back-diffusion of previously secreted hydrogen ions across a cell membrane that cannot sustain a pH gradient (5). The causes and associations with RTA are given in Table 3. A current classification of the types of RTA considers a distal tubular hydrogen ion gradient limited form (type I), a proximal tubular bicarbonate wasting form (type II), and a hyperkalemic form (type IV). The term type III is no longer used and is thought to have represented a hybrid of types I and II. The magnitude of bicarbonate wasting into the urine is greatest in type II and least in type IV (2). Some patients with RTA will have a limited gradient defect and demonstrate renal bicarbonate wasting and a low plasma bicarbonate concentration but no systemic metabolic acidosis; this type is difficult to classify.

McSherry (6) has divided type IV RTA into several subtypes: Subtype 1 is related to aldosterone deficiency in the absence of overt intrinsic renal insufficiency, and subtype 2 arises from hyporeninemic hypoaldosteronism. Another subtype is associated with partial or total end-organ resistance to aldosterone. If these patients have total lack of responsiveness to the hormone, with high circulating values of aldosterone, this disorder is termed "pseudohypoaldosteronism."

Metabolic bone disease is a feature of both Fanconi syndrome and RTA (1–6); each will be discussed individually. Both rickets and osteomalacia are common in many forms of Fanconi syndrome (Table 4). Ascribed mechanisms for this metabolic bone disorder include hypophosphatemia due to phosphaturia, increased urinary calcium excretion, abnormal vitamin D metabolism, and renal insufficiency (7). Since 85% to 90% of filtered phosphate is reabsorbed by the S1 and S2 segments of the proximal tubule, the global defect in proximal tubule transport capacity limits phosphate reclamation. Despite any other alterations in mineral or hormone regulation in Fanconi syndrome, this persistent phosphaturia is a major factor in the development and maintenance of rickets and/or osteomalacia because phosphate levels in the extracellular fluid are diminished. This hypophosphatemic osteomalacia can result in osteonecrosis as a result of microfractures (8) and may be a late feature of lifelong Fanconi syndrome (9). Hypercalci-

TABLE 3. *Classification of RTA*

Site	Hereditary	Acquired
Proximal tubule	**RTA type II** Familial transient (infants)	**RTA type II** Drugs Acetazolamide Mafenide acetate Sulfanilamide Chronic active hepatitis Associated with tetralogy of Fallot
	Fanconi syndrome Familial Sporadic Cystinosis Wilson's disease Galactosemia Hereditary fructose intolerance Lowe syndrome Tyrosinemia Pyruvate carboxylase deficiency	**Fanconi syndrome** Drugs Outdated tetracycline Methyl-5-chrome 6-Mercaptopurine Cephalothin Gentamicin Heavy metals: Pb, Cd, Hg, U Secondary hyperparathyroidism Immunologic disorders Multiple myeloma Monoclonal gammopathy Systemic lupus Sjögren syndrome Renal transplantation Amyloidosis Burkitt's lymphoma Interstitial nephritis Balkan nephropathy Nephrotic syndrome Osteopetrosis Paroxysmal nocturnal hemoglobinuria
Distal tubule	**RTA type I** Primary Secondary Hereditary fructose intolerance Ehlers–Danlos syndrome Fabry's disease Hereditary elliptocytosis Medullary sponge kidney Hypercalciuria Polycystic kidney disease Associated with nerve deafness	**RTA type I** Sporadic Metabolic disorders Hyperthyroidism with nephrocalcinosis Hypothyroidism Primary hyperparathyroidism with nephrocalcinosis Galactorrhea with hyperprolactinemia Idiopathic hypercalciuria Hypomagnesemia Hypergammaglobulinemic states Idiopathic Hyperglobulinemic purpura Cryoglobulinemia Sjogren syndrome Systemic lupus erythematosus Sarcoidosis Hodgkin's disease Tuberculosis Takayusu's arteritis Chronic active hepatitis Thyroiditis Starvation and malnutrition Hepatic cirrhosis Primary biliary cirrhosis Acute tubular necrosis Pyelonephritis Renal transplantation Obstructive uropathy Drugs Lithium Amphotericin B Toluene Analgesics

TABLE 3. *Continued.*

Site	Hereditary	Acquired

	RTA type IV
	Combined aldosterone, glucocorticoid
	    deficiency
	21-Hydroxylase deficiency
	Aldosterone deficiency (isolated)
	Corticosterone methyl oxidase deficiency
		RTA type IV
		Combined aldosterone, glucocorticoid
		    deficiency
		Addison's disease
		Bilateral adrenalectomy
		Aldosterone deficiency (isolated)
		    Primary, idiopathic
		    Secondary, deficient renin secretion
		    Chronic renal parenchymal disease
		    Diabetic nephropathy
		    Interstitial nephritis
		    Obstructive uropathy
		    Renal transplantation
		Drugs
		    Nonsteroidal anti-inflammatory
		Secondary (without hyporeninemia)
		Drugs
		    Heparin
		    Converting enzyme inhibitors
		    Adrenal insensitivity to AII

	Pseudohypoaldosteronism of infancy, type 1
	21-Hydroxylase deficiency
		Pseudohypoaldosteronism
		    Secondary
		        Interstitial nephritis
		Drugs
		    Spironolactone
		    Amiloride
		    Triamterene

	Aldosterone deficiency plus resistance 21-Hydroxylase deficiency Pseudohypoaldosteronism, type II	Aldosterone deficiency plus resistance Secondary Chronic renal parenchymal disease Obstructive uropathy Renal transplantation Lupus nephritis

	RTA combined types I and IV
	SS hemoglobinopathy
	SC hemoglobinopathy
		RTA combined types I and IV
		Secondary
		    Chronic renal parenchymal disease
		    Obstructive uropathy
		Drugs
		    Amiloride
		    Triamterene

uria and nephrocalcinosis are especially common in Wilson's disease, in which both a proximal and a distal RTA are present; hence the finding of calcium deposition in the renal interstitium. Nevertheless, the serum calcium concentration is not reduced, and hypocalcemia probably does not cause metabolic bone disease.

Abnormalities of vitamin D metabolism have been described in Fanconi syndrome. As indicated, vitamin D deficiency can result in a proximal tubulopathy resembling Fanconi syndrome that is reversed by vitamin D treatment (3). Galactosemia, Wilson's disease, tyrosinemia, Fanconi–Bickel syndrome, and fructose intolerance could result in sufficient hepatic damage and cirrhosis to impair the 25-hydroxylation of vitamin D (10). The circulating values of $1,25(OH)_2D$ are either low or normal but are not elevated, as would be anticipated in the face of hypophosphatemia and secondary hyperparathyroidism (11). Whenever $1,25(OH)_2D$ values are reduced, bone demineralization appears to be greater (12). This reduction in $1,25(OH)_2D$ circulating values

may be related to impaired proximal tubule cell metabolism or to structural changes in this tissue, since the $25(OH)D-1\alpha$-hydroxylase is localized to proximal tubule cell mitochondria (2). Other researchers, however, have shown reduced production of $1,25(OH)_2D$ only when renal insufficiency is demonstrable (13), especially in cystinosis, a disorder associated with progressive renal insufficiency (7).

Light chain nephropathy may result in bone disease due to defective vitamin D metabolism (reflected in low serum $1,25(OH)_2D$ values) and hypophosphatemic osteomalacia (14).

Osteomalacia has also been reported as being related to the presence of a tumor that possibly elaborated a tubulopathic substance, now termed phosphotonin, resulting in the features of Fanconi syndrome (15). As in oncogenous rickets, removal of the bone tumor reverses all signs of Fanconi syndrome, including metabolic bone disease.

Wilson's disease has been associated with hypoparathyroidism, which could also contribute to the development of

TABLE 4. *Factors contributing to osteomalacia and rickets in Fanconi syndrome*

1. Hypophosphatemia due to a renal tubular phosphate hyperexcretion
2. Hypercalciuria—probably a minor component
3. Vitamin D deficiency
   A. Malabsorption
   B. Failure of 25-hydroxylation in disorders associated with Fanconi syndrome and cirrhosis
4. Reduced 1α-hydroxylation of 25(OH)D
   A. Not responsive to hypophosphatemic stimulus
   B. Result of proximal tubule damage, which also leads to global proximal tubulopathy
   C. Renal insufficiency, especially in nephropathic cystinosis and chronic idiopathic Fanconi syndrome with renal insufficiency
   D. Kappa light chain deposition in the proximal tubule in myeloma or leukemia
5. Mesenchymal tumor-elaborating substance, which results in the complex tubulopathy and osteomalacia
6. Hypoparathyroidism in Wilson's disease, presumably due to copper deposition in the parathyroid glands
7. Chronic renal transplant rejection resulting in a global tubulopathy with phosphaturia and steroid-induced osteopenia

TABLE 5. *Causes of osteomalacia/rickets in renal tubular acidosis*

1. Bone resorption and hypercalciuria in association with type I RTA
2. Osteomalacia and/or rickets with type II RTA as part of Fanconi syndrome (see Table 4); predominately related to hypophosphatemia
3. Vitamin D deficiency
4. Defect in the conversion of 25(OH)D to 1,25(OH)$_2$D
   A) Animal model
   B) Possible presence in humans
5. Type IV RTA associated with renal insufficiency and renal osteodystrophy
6. Association between osteopetrosis and RTA with carbonic anhydrase

osteomalacia. This association is presumably related to copper deposition in the parathyroid glands (16).

Bone disease may occur in association with Fanconi syndrome found in patients with chronic rejection of a renal transplant (17). Presumably the bone disease is due to phosphaturic hypophosphatemia and steroid-induced osteopenia related to the use of glucocorticoids as part of antirejection therapy.

Many patients with cystinosis have been stated to demonstrate osteoporosis (4). These patients have not undergone bone biopsies using modern histomorphometric analysis and double tetracycline labeling. Many of these patients are malnourished and have bone roentgenograms that display a severe degree of osteopenia that has been termed osteomalacia and/or osteoporosis.

The therapy of osteomalacia/rickets in Fanconi syndrome is predicated on the cause of the bone disease. In general, oral phosphate supplements, either in the form of neutral phosphate or Joulie's solution, are provided at doses between 1 and 4 g daily given in 4–6 daily divided doses (4). In patients with vitamin D deficiency, treatment with appropriate doses may reverse the bone disease (3,7). Many patients with Fanconi syndrome and osteomalacia will benefit from therapy with the 1α-hydroxylated vitamin D analogs or dihydrotachysterol (DHT) in appropriate doses (4,9–13). In patients with myeloma, therapy of the underlying monoclonal gammopathy is often curative, but oral phosphate and vitamin D may also be required. Finally, in patients with the unexpected occurrence of osteomalacia and Fanconi syndrome, a bone scan may be indicated to seek a nonossifying fibroma that hopefully can then be fully extirpated.

Osteomalacia and/or rickets in RTA also has several causes (Table 5). Rickets is rare in children with RTA type I, as is osteomalacia in adults with the same condition (2,18). Nevertheless, these patients have erosion of bone as a result

of systemic metabolic acidosis and release of calcium from bone as calcium carbonate is used as a buffer (2). This additional calcium is excreted into the urine, and many of these patients are hypercalciuric by any criteria used, with a urine calcium level greater than 4 mg/kg/day or a urine calcium/creatinine ratio greater than 0.2. Calcium excretion decreases with correction of metabolic acidosis (19). Hence, oral NaHCO$_3$ or Shohl's solution will reverse this bone demineralization. As noted by numerous groups, nephrocalcinosis may persist long after correction of systemic metabolic acidosis (2).

Rickets and osteomalacia are common features of RTA type II, particularly if the proximal tubular bicarbonaturia is a component of a more global tubulopathy. The mechanisms and therapy for metabolic bone disease in RTA type II are covered in the previous section on the Fanconi syndrome. Nephrocalcinosis and hypercalciuria are not as common, since the final urine pH in proximal RTA is often acidic and thus the deposition of calcium phosphate complexes is not favored (5).

In type II RTA, which is isolated, systemic metabolic acidosis presumably results in demineralization; however, this has not been systematically evaluated.

Certain patients with vitamin D deficiency on a nutritional basis show evidence of bicarbonate wasting, although this is not usually an isolated event (2). In view of experimental studies in animals, an impaired conversion of 25(OH)D to 1,25(OH)$_2$D may be a consequence of systemic metabolic acidosis (20). A somewhat similar study in normal men who were made acidotic by an ammonium chloride challenge indicated impaired conversion of vitamin D to its active metabolite (21). However, this effect was seen only acutely. Chronic acidosis did not impair conversion of 25(OH)D to 1,25(OH)$_2$D in a study in children with RTA types I and II. Several had never been treated with bicarbonate therapy and had normal values of 1,25(OH)$_2$D in serum (22). Hence, there is little evidence for the role of impaired metabolic conversion in bone demineralization.

Whenever type IV RTA is associated with renal insufficiency, renal osteodystrophy may be expected to occur as renal failure progresses (2).

A rare form of RTA is associated with *osteopetrosis* (2). This is discussed elsewhere but clearly does not result in bone demineralization.

The therapy of RTA includes correction of systemic metabolic acidemia by oral $NaHCO_3$ therapy; the doses vary according to the nephron segment affected. Type I RTA is generally treated with 1–2 mEq/kg/24 hr of oral $NaHCO_3$, but higher doses may be needed in young children (19). Type II RTA requires 10–15 mEq/kg/24 hr or slightly lower doses if thiazides are used in addition (2). Thiazides reduce plasma volume and thereby enhance tubule bicarbonate reabsorption. Patients with type IV disease may also require fluorinated glucocorticoids in supraphysiologic doses that augment potassium secretion (2). Hypercalciuria and bone resorption are reversed by $NaHCO_3$ therapy.

REFERENCES

1. Chesney RW, Jones DP: Renal tubular syndromes. In: Gonick HC (ed) *Current Nephrology*. vol 19. Chicago, Mosby Yearbook, 1995
2. Baum M: The cellular basis of Fanconi syndrome. *Hosp Pract* 137–148, Nov 15, 1994
3. Chesney RW, Harrison HE: Fanconi syndrome following bowel surgery and hepatitis reversed by 25-hydroxycholecalciferol. *J Pediatrics* 86:857–861, 1975
4. Brewer ED: The Fanconi syndrome: clinical disorders. In: Gonick HC, Buckalew VM (eds) *Renal Tubular Disorders*. New York, Marcel Dekker, pp 475–544, 1985
5. Battle DC, Kurtzman NA: The defect in distal tubular acidosis. In: Gonick HC, Buckalew VM (eds) *Renal Tubular Disorders*, New York, Marcel Dekker, pp 281–306, 1985
6. McSherry E: Renal tubular acidosis in childhood. *Kidney Int* 20: 799–809, 1982
7. Friedman AL, Chesney RW: Isolated renal tubular defects. In: Schrier R, Gottschalk C (eds) *Diseases of the Kidney*. 6th ed. Boston, Little Brown, pp 611–634, 1993
8. Gaucher A, Thomas JL, Netter P, Faure G: Osteomalacia, pseudosacroiliitis and necrosis of the femoral heads in Fanconi syndrome in an adult. *J Rheumatol* 8:512–515, 1981
9. Brenton DP, Isenberg DA, Ainsworth DC, Garrod P, Krywawych S, Stamp TC: The adult presenting idiopathic Fanconi syndrome. *J Inherit Metab Dis* 4:211–215, 1981
10. Kitagawa T, Akatsuka A, Owada M, Mano T: Biologic and therapeutic effects of 1-alpha-hydroxycholecalciferol in different types of Fanconi syndrome. *Contrib Nephrol* 22:107–119, 1980
11. Baran DT, March TW: Evidence for a defect in vitamin D metabolism in a patient with incomplete Fanconi syndrome. *J Clin Endocrinol Metab* 59:998–1001, 1984
12. Colussi G, DeFerrari ME, Surean M, Malberti F, Rombola G, Ponlomero G, Galvanini G, Minetti L: Vitamin D metabolites and osteomalacia in the human Fanconi syndrome. *Proc Eur Dial Transplant Assoc* 21:756–760, 1985
13. Steinberg R, Chesney RW, Schulman J, DeLuca HF, Phelps M: Circulating vitamin D metabolites in nephropathic cystinosis. *J Pediatrics* 120:592–594, 1983
14. Rao DS, Parfitt AM, Villanueva AR, Dorman PJ, Kleerekoper M: Hypophosphatemic osteomalacia and adult Fanconi syndrome due to light chain nephropathy. Another form of oncogenous osteomalacia. *Am J Med* 82:333–338, 1987
15. Cai Q, Hodgson SF, Kao PC: Inhibition of renal phosphate transport by a tumor product in a patient with oncogenic osteomalacia. *N Engl J Med* 330:1645-1647, 1994.
16. Carpenter TO, Carnes DL, Anast CS: Hypoparathyroidism in Wilson's disease. *N Engl J Med* 309:873–877, 1983
17. Friedman AL, Chesney RW: Fanconi syndrome in renal transplantation. *Am J Nephrol* 1:45–47, 1981
18. Brenner RJ, Spring DB, Sebastian A: Incidence of radiographically evident bone disease, nephrocalcinosis and nephrolithiasis in various types of renal tubular acidosis. *N Engl J Med* 307:217–221, 1982
19. Rodriguez-Soriano J, Vallo A, Vastillo G: Natural history of primary distal renal tubular acidosis treated since infancy. *J Pediatrics* 101:669–676, 1982
20. Lee SW, Russell J, Avioli LV: 25-hydroxycholecalciferol to 1,25-dihydroxycholecalciferol: conversion impaired by systemic metabolic acidosis. *Science* 195:994, 1977
21. Kraut JF, Gordon EM, Ranson JC: Effect of chronic metabolic acidosis on vitamin D metabolism in humans. *Kidney Int* 24:644–648, 1983
22. Chesney RW, Kaplan BS, Phelps M, De Luca HG: Renal tubular acidosis does not alter circulating values of calcitriol. *J Pediatrics* 104:51–55, 1984

65. Drug-Induced Osteomalacia

Daniel D. Bikle, M.D., Ph.D.

Department of Medicine, University of California, San Francisco; and Veterans Affairs Medical Center, San Francisco, California

Bone formation requires calcium and phosphate. Vitamin D through its active metabolites provides for adequate amounts of calcium and phosphate in addition to regulating the differentiation and function of the bone cells involved. Osteomalacia results from the reduction in mineralization of the matrix, demonstrated histomorphometrically as increased osteoid thickness and osteoid surface area coupled with decreased mineral apposition rate and active mineralizing surface area. Drugs that result in deficiencies in calcium, phosphate, and the active vitamin D metabolites or that interfere with their deposition in or action on bone could lead to osteomalacia. Drugs affecting the vitamin D endocrine system include blockers of vitamin D production (sun screens could play this role in an otherwise marginally deficient individual), inhibitors of vitamin D absorption (e.g., cholestyramine), modifiers of vitamin D metabolism (anticonvulsants such as phenytoin, antituberculous agents such as rifampicin, proximal renal tubule toxins such as cadmium), or antagonists of vitamin D action at the target tissue (e.g., glucocorticoids). Phosphate deficiency can be induced by ingestion of aluminum-containing antacids that prevent its absorption from the intestine or by proximal renal tubule toxins that result in renal phosphate wasting. Calcium deficiency as a cause of osteomalacia has only been demonstrated conclusively in children ingesting a very low calcium diet, although theoretically drugs that interfere with intestinal calcium absorption or accelerate its excretion by the kidney could lead to osteomalacia. Even in the presence of adequate levels of vitamin D, calcium, and phosphate, direct inhibitors of bone mineralization such as bisphospho-

TABLE 1. *Drugs causing osteomalacia*

A. Disruption of vitamin D endocrine system
  1. Block vitamin D production
    ? Sun screens
  2. Inhibit vitamin D absorption
    Cholestyramine
  3. Interfere with vitamin D metabolism
    a. 25(OH)D production
      Phenytoin
      Phenobarbital
      Rifampicin
    b. 1,25(OH)$_2$D production
      Cadmium
  4. Antagonize vitamin D action
    Glucocorticoids
B. Disruption of phosphate homeostasis
  1. Inhibit phosphate absorption
    Aluminum-containing antacid
  2. Induce renal phosphate wasting
    Cadmium
    Lead
C. Disruption of bone mineralization
  Aluminum
  Fluoride
  Bisphosphonates

nates, aluminum, and fluoride can lead to osteomalacia. Thus, drugs can cause osteomalacia by several mechanisms, and any one drug may do so by several mechanisms as summarized in Table 1. This chapter will focus on those drugs for which clinical evidence linking them to the development of osteomalacia is reasonably secure.

BLOCKERS OF VITAMIN D PRODUCTION

Lack of sunlight is a well-appreciated risk factor for the development of osteomalacia in adults and rickets in children. The association of sunlight exposure with the development of skin cancer has led some authorities to claim that all sunlight exposure is harmful and that sun screens should be used to protect against the harmful rays. The degree to which this recent campaign to eliminate solar exposure will increase the incidence of vitamin D deficiency and osteomalacia remains for future investigation.

INHIBITORS OF VITAMIN D ABSORPTION

Vitamin D like other fat-soluble vitamins is absorbed in the jejunum and ileum by a process facilitated by bile acids. Bile acid-binding resins such as cholestyramine and colestipol have the potential to interfere with vitamin D absorption. The development of osteomalacia has been described in a patient with Crohn's disease following ileal resection who was treated with cholestyramine (1). This patient was successfully treated with 25 hydroxyvitamin D [25(OH)D] (calcifediol). The relative contribution of cholestyramine to the onset of osteomalacia in this patient predisposed to vitamin D deficiency on the basis of the underlying disease is difficult to assess, but this case report indicates that in the marginally vitamin D-deficient patient bile acid binding resins may suffice

to precipitate osteomalacia, and their impact on vitamin D absorption should be monitored with serum 25(OH)D levels.

INTERFERENCE WITH VITAMIN D METABOLISM

Vitamin D must be metabolized first in the liver to 25(OH)D, then in the kidney to 1,25(OH)$_2$D and other metabolites to be active. Drugs that induce the drug-metabolizing enzymes in the liver can accelerate the catabolism of vitamin D and its metabolites. Anticonvulsants are the best studied of these drugs with respect to their ability to induce osteomalacia or rickets. Rifampicin may also accelerate vitamin D metabolite catabolism, but the link between rifampicin and osteomalacia is less well established (2).

Early reports suggested that 20% to 65% of epileptics receiving anticonvulsants developed signs of rickets or osteomalacia especially if institutionalized (3–8). Such patients are at increased risk of fractures during their epileptic fits, and the low serum calcium may aggravate the seizure disorder. Outpatient populations appear to be at much lower risk of developing clinically significant bone disease (9–16), although biochemical abnormalities (reduced serum and urine calcium and serum 25(OH)D, elevated serum parathyroid hormone (PTH) and alkaline phosphatase), reduced bone density, and increased osteoid on bone biopsy are observed in 10% to 40% of patients on long-term anticonvulsant therapy (11–19). In ambulatory subjects definitive histomorphometric evidence of osteomalacia is seldom found.

The high rate of bone disease in institutionalized patients, regardless of anticonvulsant therapy, emphasizes the importance of nutrition and sunlight, which can be lacking in this setting. However, anticonvulsant therapy clearly compounds this problem. Two of the most frequently used anticonvulsants, phenobarbital and phenytoin, induce liver drug-metabolizing enzymes and increase the metabolism and clearance of vitamin D (20,21). Anticonvulsants such as sodium valproate, which do not induce the hepatic drug-metabolizing enzymes, have little or no impact on serum calcium and 25(OH)D levels (22,23). *In vitro* studies suggest that phenobarbital and phenytoin have direct inhibitory effects on parathyroid hormone (PTH)–stimulated bone resorption (24) and intestinal calcium absorption (25), but the relevance of these studies to the *in vivo* situation is unclear.

Numerous studies point out that the well-nourished patient exposed to adequate amounts of sunlight will seldom develop clinically significant bone disease as a result of anticonvulsant therapy. However, patients on anticonvulsants require higher intakes of vitamin D to achieve positive calcium balance (26), with doses up to 4000 units (100 μg) per day sometimes being required to normalize 25(OH)D levels (27).

ANTAGONISTS OF VITAMIN D ACTION

Glucocorticoids interfere with intestinal calcium absorption by a little-understood mechanism. As such, they provide one means of treating vitamin D toxicity. However, as discussed elsewhere, glucocorticoids cause osteoporosis not osteomalacia, and are not direct antagonists of vitamin D at the receptor level. At present, there are no known drugs in clinical use that directly interfere with the actions of $1,25(OH)_2D$ at the target tissue level.

INHIBITORS OF PHOSPHATE ABSORPTION

Hypophosphatemia is a central feature of a number of diseases presenting as osteomalacia or rickets including X-linked hypophosphatemic rickets, oncogenic hypophosphatemic osteomalacia, and various forms of Fanconi syndrome. These feature renal phosphate wasting and reduced $1,25(OH)_2D$ production. In contrast, the major drug-induced form of hypophosphatemic osteomalacia is caused by excessive ingestion of aluminum-containing antacids, which inhibit intestinal phosphate absorption. Such patients present with little or no urine phosphate excretion and increased $1,25(OH)_2D$ levels (28–30). Serum and urine calcium levels tend to be high. This syndrome is uncommon and needs to be distinguished from that in patients with renal failure given aluminum-containing antacids to normalize serum phosphate who develop osteomalacia because of the aluminum-induced inhibition of bone mineralization (see below). The absence of aluminum in the bone biopsy sample helps identify those patients who develop osteomalacia on the basis of the antacid-induced hypophosphatemia rather than aluminum-induced inhibition of mineralization (31). Treatment consists of discontinuing the aluminum-containing antacid, and healing of the bone lesions may be expedited with supplemental vitamin D and phosphate.

INHIBITORS OF BONE MINERALIZATION

Aluminum

The two principal situations in which aluminum-induced osteomalacia is found are hemodialysis and total parenteral nutrition (32). The sources of aluminum include antacids used to control serum phosphate levels in renal failure patients, nondeionized water used during dialysis, and aluminum contamination of various components used during total parenteral nutrition. Unlike patients with antacid-induced hypophosphatemia, patients with aluminum-induced osteomalacia generally have normal or even high serum phosphate levels and low $1,25(OH)_2D$ levels. Patients with renal failure have a lower than expected PTH level and often become hypercalcemic at low doses of $1,25(OH)_2D$ which generally fail to treat the osteomalacia. Awareness of this complication of aluminum and reduction of the aluminum exposure of the patients has reduced if not totally eliminated the incidence of aluminum-induced osteomalacia. Deferoxamine is currently being used with success to reduce the body load of aluminum and reverse the osteomalacia (33). This form of drug-induced osteomalacia is covered in greater depth in the chapters concerned with renal osteodystrophy and total parenteral nutrition.

Bisphosphonates

Etidronate is the first bisphosphonate approved for clinical use, initially for the treatment of Paget's disease and more recently for the treatment of hypercalcemia of malignancy. The bisphosphonates are nonhydrolyzable analogs of pyrophosphate, an inhibitor of mineralization, and the original experimental applications of the bisphosphonates were to prevent ectopic calcification. Therefore, it was no surprise when the early studies with etidronate as therapy for Paget's disease resulted in a patchy, hypocellular form of osteomalacia (34). This effect appeared to be direct in that no changes in serum calcium and vitamin D metabolite levels were observed, and phosphate levels tended to be increased at least early in treatment (34,35). These early studies utilized 20 mg/kg doses. Subsequent studies with lower doses indicated that most of the reduction in alkaline phosphatase and urinary hydroxyproline levels observed at 20 mg/kg doses could be achieved with 6 months of treatment using a 5 mg/kg dose (the current recommended therapy for Paget's disease) without increasing the risk of nontraumatic fractures or mineralization defects on bone biopsy (36). However, even this lower dose (effectively 400 mg/day because the tablets each contain 200 mg) proved capable of inducing a patchy form of osteomalacia in some subjects (37). Fractures, when they occur, tend to involve lytic lesions of Paget's disease so that the presence of such lesions are a relative contraindication to the use of etidronate.

Etidronate is the first-generation bisphosphonate. Pamidronate, a second-generation bisphosphonate, has been approved for treatment of hypercalcemia of malignancy. However, it is also effective therapy for Paget's disease. Pamidronate is given intravenously because of its poor oral absorption and gastric side effects. Pamidronate appears to have a less inhibitory effect on bone mineralization than etidronate (38,39). However, one recent study of 20 patients with Paget's disease treated with pamidronate showed a patchy form of osteomalacia (focal areas of increased osteoid) in several of the subjects treated with 180- to 360-mg doses over a 6- to 9-week period (40). Alendronate is the first of the third-generation bisphosphonates to be approved for clinical use, and it is expected to be widely used for treatment of osteoporosis. At this point, no reports of osteomalacia caused by alendronate have been published, but this potential complication warrants close scrutiny.

FLUORIDE

Fluoride has attracted attention as a therapeutic agent for osteoporosis because it is an effective stimulator of new bone growth (41). How fluoride stimulates new bone formation is not clear. Fluoride is rapidly and extensively accumulated into bone and teeth where x-ray crystallographic data show stabilization by fluoride of the hydroxyapatite crystal (42). Numerous clinical studies have demonstrated increased bone mineral density in subjects treated with fluoride, especially in bones with a high cancellous bone component, yet decreased fracture risk has been hard to document in carefully performed, double-blind, placebo-controlled trials (43,44). At least part of the problem is that the new bone stimulated by fluoride often shows evidence of abnormal mineralization (45–47). This mineralization defect is aggravated by conditions of low calcium intake but is not completely prevented by the coadministration of adequate amounts of calcium and vitamin D (48). Conceivably, the painful lower extremity syndrome seen in some subjects treated with fluoride is the consequence of the imbalance between matrix production and mineralization leading to microfractures (49). More controversial is the possibility that fluoride treatment increases the risk of hip fracture, again hypothesized to involve the imbalance between matrix formation and mineralization (50,51). Regardless of whether or not fluoride increases the risk of fracture, its ability to disrupt the normal mineralization of bone matrix, the production of which it so potently stimulates, limits the usefulness of this unique stimulator of bone formation.

REFERENCES

1. Compston JE, Horton LW: Oral 25-hydroxyvitain D3 in treatment of osteomalacia associated with ileal resection and cholestyramine therapy. *Gastroenterology* 74:900–902, 1978
2. Perry W, Erooga MA, Brown J, Stamp TC: Calcium metabolism during rifampicin and isoniazid therapy for tuberculosis. *J R Soc Med* 75:533–536, 1982
3. Dent CE, Richens A, Rowe DJ, Stamp TC: Osteomalacia with long-term anticonvulsant therapy in epilepsy. *Br Med J* 4:69–72, 1970
4. Richens A, Rowe DJ: Disturbance of calcium metabolism by anticonvulsant drugs. *Br Med J* 4:73–76, 1970
5. Hunter J, Maxwell JD, Stewart DA, Parsons V, Williams R: Altered calcium metabolism in epileptic children on anticonvulsants. *Br Med J* 4:202–204, 1971
6. Tolman KG, Jubiz W, Sannella JJ, Madsen JA, Belsey RE, Goldsmith RS, Freston JW: Osteomalacia associated with anticonvulsant drug therapy in mentally retarded children. *Pediatrics* 56:45–50, 1975
7. Hunt PA, Wu-Chen ML, Handal NJ, Chang CT, Gomez M, Howell TR, Hartenberg MA, Chan JC: Bone disease induced by anticonvulsant therapy and treatment with calcitriol(1,25-dihydroxyvitamin D3). *Am J Dis Child* 140:715–718, 1986
8. Offermann G, Pinto V, Kruse R: Antiepileptic drugs and vitamin D supplementation. *Epilepsia* 20:3–15, 1979
9. Livingston S, Berman W, Pauli LL: Anticonvulsant drugs and vitamin D metabolism. *JAMA* 224:1634–1635, 1973
10. Fogelman I, Gray JM, Gardner MD, Beastall GH, McIntosh WB, Allam BF, Boyce BF, Boyle IT, Lawson DH: Do anticonvulsant drugs commonly induce osteomalacia? *Scott Med J* 27:136–142, 1982
11. Pylypchuk G, Oreopoulos DG, Wilson DR, Harrison JE, McNeill KG, Meema HE, Ogilvie R, Sturtridge WC, Murray TM. Calcium metabolism in adult outpatients with epilepsy receiving long-term anticonvulsant therapy. *Can Med Assoc J* 118:635–638, 1978
12. Keck E, Gollnick B, Reinhardt D, Karch D, Peerenboom H, Kruskemper HL: Calcium metabolism and vitamin D metabolite levels in children receiving anticonvulsant drugs. *Eur J Pediatr* 139:52–55, 1982
13. Ashworth B, Horn DB: Evidence of osteomalacia in an outpatient group of adult epileptics. *Epilepsia* 18:37–43, 1977
14. Hoikka V, Savolainen K, Alhava EM, Sivenius J, Karjalainen P, Parvianinen M: Anticonvulsant osteomalacia in epileptic outpatients. *Ann Clin Res* 14:129–132, 1982
15. Bogliun G, Beghi E, Crespi V, Delodovici L, d'Amico P: Anticonvulsant drugs and bone metabolism. *Acta Neurol Scand* 74:284–288, 1986
16. Weinstein RS, Bryce GF, Sappington LJ, King DW, Gallagher BB: Decreased serum ionized calcium and normal vitamin D metabolite levels with anticonvulsant drug treatment. *J Clin Endocrinol Metab* 58:1003–1009, 1984
17. Hahn TJ, Hendin BA, Scharp CR, Haddad JGJ: Effect of chronic anticonvulsant therapy on serum 25-hydroxycalciferol levels in adults. *N Engl J Med* 287:900–904, 1972
18. Hahn TJ, Hendin BA, Scharp CR, Boisscau VC, Haddad JG,Jr:. Serum 25-hydroxycalciferol levels and bone mass in children on chronic anticonvulsant therapy. *N Engl J Med* 292:550–554, 1975
19. Christiansen C, Rodbro P: Treatment of anticonvulsant osteomalacia with vitamin D. *Calcif Tissue Res* 21 Suppl:252–259, 1976
20. Matheson RT, Herbst JJ, Jubiz W, Freston JW, Tolman KG: Absorption and biotransfomation of cholecalciferol in drug-induced osteomalacia. *J Clin Pharmacol* 16:426–432, 1976
21. Hahn TJ, Birge SJ, Scharp CR, Avioli LV: Phenobarbital-induced alterations in vitamin D metabolism. *J Clin Invest* 51: 741–748, 1972
22. Gough H, Goggin T, Bissessar A, Baker M, Crowley M, Callaghan N: A comparative study of the relative influence of different anticonvulsant drugs, UV exposure and diet on vitamin D and calcium metabolism in out-patients with epilepsy. *Q J Med* 59:569–577, 1986
23. Davie MW, Emberson CE, Lawson DE, Roberts GE, Barnes JL, Barnes ND, Heeley AF: Low plasma 25-hydroxyvitamin D and serum calcium levels in institutionalized epileptic subjects: associated risk factors, consequences and response to treatment with vitamin D. *Q J Med* 52:79–91, 1983
24. Hahn TJ, Scharp CR, Richardson CA, Halstead LR, Kahn AJ, Teitelbaum SL: Interaction of diphenylhydantoin (phenytoin) and phenobarbital with hormonal mediation of fetal rat bone resorption in vitro. *J Clin Invest* 62:406–414, 1978
25. Corradino RA: Diphenylhydantoin: direct inhibition of the vitamin D3-mediated calcium absorptive mechanism in organ–cultured duodenum. *Biochem Pharmacol* 25:863–864, 1976
26. Peterson P, Gray P, Tolman KG: Calcium balance in drug-induced osteomalacia: response to vitamin D. *Clin Pharmacol Ther* 19:63–67, 1976
27. Collins N, Maher J, Cole M, Baker M, Callaghan N: A prospective study to evaluate the dose of vitamin D required to correct low 25-hydroxyvitamin D levels, calcium, and alkaline phosphatase in patients at risk of developing antiepileptic drug-induced osteomalacia. *Q J Med* 78:113–122, 1991
28. Godsall JW, Baron R, Insogna KL: Vitamin D metabolism and bone histomorphometry in a patient with antacid-induced osteomalacia. *Am J Med* 77:747–750, 1984
29. Carmichael KA, Fallon MD, Dalinka M, Kaplan FS, Axel L, Haddad JG: Osteomalacia and osteitis fibrosa in a man ingesting aluminum hydroxide antacid. *Am J Med* 76:1137–1143, 1984
30. Pivnick EK, Kerr NC, Kaufman RA, Jones DP, Chesney RW: Rickets secondary to phosphate depletion. A sequela of antacid use in infancy. *Clin Pediatr* 34:73–78, 1995
31. Kassem M, Eriksen EF, Melsen F, Mosekilde L: Antacid-induced osteomalacia: a case report with a histomorphometric analysis. *J Intern Med* 229:275–279, 1991
32. Nebeker HG, Coburn JW: Aluminum and renal osteodystrophy. *Annu Rev Med* 37:79–95, 1986
33. Felsenfeld AJ, Rodriguez M, Coleman M, Ross D, Llach F: Desferrioxamine therapy in hemodialysis patients with aluminum-associated bone disease. *Kidney Int* 35:1371–1378, 1989
34. Smith R, Russell RG, Bishop MC, Woods CG, Bishop M: Paget's disease of bone. Experience with a diphosphonate (disodium etidronate) in treatment. *Q J Med* 42:235–256, 1973
35. Gibbs CJ, Aaron JE, Peacock M: Osteomalacia in Paget's disease treated with short term, high dose sodium etidronate. *Br Med J* 292:1227–1229, 1986
36. Khairi MR, Altman RD, DeRosa GP, Zimmermann J, Schenk RK, Johnston CC: Sodium etidronate in the treatment of Paget's disease of bone. A study of long-term results. *Ann Intern Med* 87:656–663, 1977
37. Boyce BF, Smith L, Fogelman I, Johnston E, Ralston S, Boyle IT: Focal osteomalacia due to low-dose diphosphonate therapy in Paget's disease. *Lancet* 1:821–824, 1984
38. Fenton AJ, Gutteridge DH, Kent GN, Price RI, Retallack RW, Bhagat CI, Worth GK, Thompson RI, Watson IG, Barry-Walsh C: Intravenous aminobisphosphonate in Paget's disease: clinical,

biochemical, histomorphometric and radiological responses. *Clin Endocrinol* 34:197–204, 1991

39. Harinck HI, Bijvoet OL, Blanksma HJ, Dahlinghaus-Nienhuys PJ: Efficacious management with aminobisphosphonate (APD) in Paget's disease of bone. *Clin Orthop* 79–98, 1987
40. Adamson BB, Gallacher SJ, Byars J, Ralston SH, Boyle IT, Boyce BF: Mineralisation defects with pamidronate therapy for Paget's disease. *Lancet* 342:1459–1460, 1993
41. Farley JR, Wergedal JE, Baylink DJ: Fluoride directly stimulates proliferation and alkaline phosphatase activity of bone-forming cells. *Science* 222:330–332, 1983
42. Eanes ED, Reddi AH: The effect of fluoride on bone mineral apatite. *Metab Bone Dis Rel Res* 2:3–10, 1979
43. Riggs BL, Hodgson SF, O'Fallon WM, Chao EY, Wahner HW, Muhs JM, Cedel SL, Melton LJ: Effect of fluoride treatment on the fracture rate in postmenopausal women with osteoporosis. *N Engl J Med* 322:802–809, 1990
44. Kleerekoper M, Mendlovic DB: Sodium fluoride therapy of postmenopausal osteoporosis. *Endocr Rev* 14:312–323, 1993
45. Jowsey J, Riggs BL, Kelly PJ, Hoffmann DL: Effect of com-
bined therapy with sodium fluoride, vitamin D and calcium in osteoporosis. *Am J Med* 53:43–49, 1972
46. Briancon D, Meunier PJ: Treatment of osteoporosis with fluoride, calcium, and vitamin D. *Orthop Clin North Am* 12:629–648, 1981
47. Baylink DJ, Bernstein DS: The effects of fluoride therapy on metabolic bone disease. A histologic study. *Clin Orthop* 55:51–85, 1967
48. Compston JE, Chadha S, Merrett AL: Osteomalacia developing during treatment of osteoporosis with sodium fluoride and vitamin D. *Br Med J* 281:910–911, 1980
49. Schnitzler CM, Solomon L: Histomorphometric analysis of a calcaneal stress fracture: a possible complication of fluoride therapy for osteoporosis. *Bone* 7:193–198, 1986
50. Gutteridge DH, Price RI, Kent GN, Prince RL, Michell PA: Spontaneous hip fractures in fluoride-treated patients: potential causative factors. *J Bone Min Res* 5 Suppl 1:S205–S215, 1990
51. Bayley TA, Harrison JE, Murray TM, Josse RG, Sturtridge W, Pritzker KP, Strauss A, Vieth R, Goodwin S: Fluoride-induced fractures: relation to osteogenic effect. *J Bone Min Res* 5 Suppl 1:S217–S222, 1990

66. Metabolic Bone Disease of Total Parenteral Nutrition

Gordon L. Klein, M.D., M.P.H.

Department of Pediatrics, University of Texas Medical Branch, Galveston, Texas

Total parenteral nutrition (TPN) is a therapeutic regimen designed to provide for the administration of all nutritional requirements in a concentrated solution infused into either a central or a peripheral vein. This method of treatment is generally used in patients with gastrointestinal disease severe enough to prevent adequate oral or enteral nutrition. Because parenteral requirements for various nutrients are unknown and because the purity of individual intravenous solutions is variable, TPN therapy may be subject to the inadequate provision of certain nutrients as well as to the inadvertent contamination of solutions with toxic substances. Bone disease may be a manifestation of the various deficiencies or toxicities.

Bone disease resulting from inadequate provision of calcium or phosphate in the TPN solution has been discussed in Chapter 58. This chapter deals with bone disease brought about by aluminum toxicity in adults. It also covers the role of aluminum in the metabolic bone disease in infants and children receiving long-term TPN therapy.

BONE DISEASE IN ADULTS

Clinical Presentation

The initial and, in many cases, only clinical presentation of bone disease in a group of patients studied in Los Angeles and Seattle was periarticular bone pain, especially in weight-bearing bones, lower back, or ribs. The pain presented from 2 to 36 months after initiation of TPN therapy, increased in intensity, and did not respond to narcotic analgesics. In some instances movement was so painful that patients confined themselves to bed. Improvement occurred only when TPN treatment was discontinued (1, Fig. 1). However, only about 20% of the patients evaluated prospectively were symptomatic.

Roentgenographic Findings

Approximately 80% of patients evaluated had diffuse osteopenia (1). Photon absorptiometry of the radius in one patient revealed decreased bone mineral content. Neutron activation studies in a similar series of patients in Toronto revealed that bone mass decreased to the level seen in osteoporosis in 60% of the subjects, whereas 40% had intermediate values between normal and osteoporotic (2).

Histologic Evaluation

Within 4 months of initiating TPN treatment, hyperkinetic, rapidly turning over bone (increased formation and resorption) was described, which changed to low-turnover osteomalacia after at least 1 year of therapy (3). Patchy osteomalacia was found in patients from Los Angeles and Seattle who had bone biopsies performed after at least 1 year of TPN. Increased unmineralized osteoid and decreased bone formation were seen (Fig. 2).

Biochemical Features

In both the Canadian and American reports, serum calcium and phosphorus levels were normal or mildly elevated.

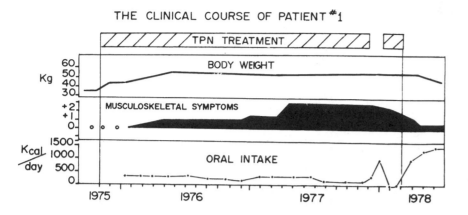

THE CLINICAL COURSE OF PATIENT #1

FIG. 1. Changes in bone pain in relation to TPN therapy in the index case with TPN bone disease. (Modified from ref. 1.)

Serum levels of alkaline phosphatase were often elevated, but the cholestatic complications of TPN treatment interfered with interpretation. A striking hypercalciuria, often with negative calcium balance, was found in most TPN patients. Because the hypercalciuria resolved when TPN was stopped, and because the urinary calcium excretion was not related to serum levels of immunoreactive parathyroid hormone (iPTH), the hypercalciuria was thought to be due to increased filtered load of calcium from the exogenously administered calcium and possibly the protein load in the TPN solutions (1,4).

Serum levels of immunoreactive PTH were in the low normal range, whereas serum levels of 1,25-dihydroxyvitamin D [1,25(OH)$_2$D[were very low, giving rise to the possibility of TPN-induced hypoparathyroidism. However, when calcium was removed from the TPN solution in two patients, serum PTH levels rose without any detectable rise in serum levels of 1,25(OH)$_2$D. Serum levels of 25-hydroxyvitamin D 25(OH)D and 24,25-dihydroxyvitamin D were normal (5). Cessation of TPN treatment in one patient with low serum levels of 1,25(OH)$_2$D resulted in a rise in serum levels to normal within 6 weeks after discontinuing TPN treatment (5), thus raising the possibility that a component of the TPN solution was acting as a toxin.

Aluminum

Because osteomalacia with decreased bone formation had been observed in patients with renal failure undergo-

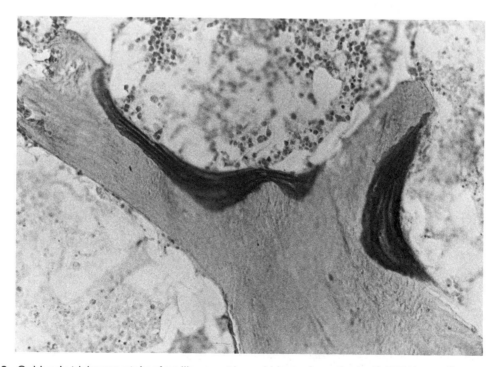

FIG. 2. Goldner's trichrome stain of an iliac crest bone biopsy of a patient with TPN bone disease, magnification ×160. Mineralized bone is shown in gray; unmineralized osteoid is shown in black. This patient has patchy areas of excessive unmineralized osteoid, one of the diagnostic features of osteomalacia. (Photo courtesy of Dr. DJ Sherrard, VA Medical Center, Seattle, WA.)

ing hemodialysis and because aluminum accumulation in bone had been previously observed (6), bone biopsies were obtained from TPN patients. Aluminum content in biopsy specimens was elevated, up to 30 times normal, and elevated aluminum levels were also found in plasma and urine (7). Analysis of the TPN solutions revealed that casein hydrolysate was found to contain large quantities of aluminum, up to 1 mg/L, which provided a parenteral aluminum intake of 2000–3000 μg/day (7). Substitution for casein hydrolysate of a synthetic amino acid mixture containing only about 2% of the aluminum in casein resulted in an acute decline in plasma aluminum concentration and urinary aluminum excretion. However, aluminum retention by tissues such as bone persisted for up to 3 years after discontinuation of casein (4,8).

The primary route of aluminum excretion is urinary. However, patients receiving TPN have relatively normal renal function (7). One possibility for the accumulation of aluminum in patients with normal renal function is the fact that plasma ultrafilterable aluminum is only about 5% of total plasma aluminum (8). Therefore, most circulating aluminum is protein-bound and not filtered. We have suggested that there are at least two pools of aluminum in the body: a rapidly exchangeable pool that is quickly depleted on reduction or cessation of aluminum loading and a slowly exchangeable pool, which may represent a tissue pool in equilibrium with plasma.

Proposed Pathogenesis of the Adult Form of TPN Bone Disease

Aluminum has been localized by aurin tricarboxylic acid stain to the mineralization front of bone, both in patients with TPN bone disease and in those with dialysis osteomalacia (Chapters 25,67). Under conditions of chronic aluminum loading, the extent of surface-stainable aluminum in bone correlates very closely with quantitative bone aluminum determined by flameless atomic absorption spectroscopy. However, surface-stainable bone aluminum was inversely correlated with rate of bone formation (6, Fig. 3). It remains unknown as to whether aluminum impairs bone formation directly by affecting bone, indirectly by accumulating in the parathyroid glands and interfering with PTH secretion (6), or by altering vitamin D metabolism (6), or by a combination of these mechanisms.

Role of Vitamin D

Removal of vitamin D from the TPN solutions resulted in low serum levels of 25(OH)D but no clinical or histologic manifestations of bone disease (3). In another study patients receiving chronic parenteral nutrition failed to develop osteomalacia even though they received amounts of vitamin D comparable to the quantities postulated to produce osteomalacia in aluminum-loaded patients (9). Although vitamin D is in standard multivitamin mixes for parenteral use, the role of vitamin D in the pathogenesis of TPN bone disease remains open to question.

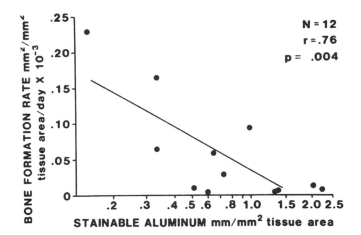

FIG. 3. Correlation between bone formation rate and stainable aluminum in patients receiving total parenteral nutrition who had received casein hydrolysate. The values for bone aluminum are plotted on a logarithmic scale. (From ref. 6, with permission.)

Treatment and Prevention

Replacement of casein hydrolysate, the chief source of aluminum from the TPN solutions, with a synthetic amino acid solution resulted in reduction of bone pain and hypercalciuria, improvement in bone formation rate, and return of serum levels of 1,25(OH)$_2$D to normal (4). Whether aluminum reduction was the only factor resulting in improvement is not certain because the amounts of protein and vitamin D$_2$ in the TPN solution were also reduced (4). The reduction in protein content may have corrected the hypercalciuria, though it was probably not responsible for the increase in bone formation rate (4). It is also unlikely that the reduction in vitamin D content played a major role in the increased bone formation rate.

A recent report showed that bone histology in TPN patients is heterogeneous in the absence of stainable bone aluminum (10). Bone formation rate was not lower than in normal subjects but was higher than that in aluminum-toxic TPN patients (10). Another study describes low-turnover TPN bone disease in the absence of stainable bone aluminum but with elevated serum aluminum levels (11).

Bone biopsies in aluminum-loaded patients who had casein hydrolysate removed from their TPN solutions showed inverse relationships between bone formation rate and surface-stainable aluminum and between bone formation rate and plasma aluminum (4). This latter relationship suggests that plasma aluminum, even before it accumulates in bone, reduces bone formation. It would appear that TPN bone disease can be reduced or eliminated if care is taken to avoid contamination of the solution with calcium-containing additives. Because the current aluminum content of TPN solutions is highly variable, measurements of aluminum in blood, urine, and TPN solution is advisable in patients who develop bone disease while receiving TPN therapy.

Two concerns remain. First, the attribution of metabolic bone disease to TPN therapy may be mistaken if preexisting bone disease is not excluded. Malabsorption of vitamin D, calcium, or phosphorus, for example, could result in osteomalacia secondary to gastrointestinal disease. Elderly women requiring TPN treatment may have postmenopausal osteoporosis. Therefore, evaluation of bone density, histology, and biochemistry early in the course of TPN therapy can help to determine the presence of preexisting metabolic bone disease.

Second, the recent report of long-term persistence of low bone density in TPN patients (12) suggests that either TPN treatment fails to improve osteopenia produced by a preexisting condition or TPN treatment itself contributes to the persistence of this problem in a still unspecified way.

BONE DISEASE IN INFANTS

Long-term treatment with TPN has been associated with rickets or osteopenia in premature infants (13). Although insufficient provision of calcium or phosphate may be primarily responsible for the rickets, aluminum loading may be a complicating factor. Evidence supporting this is as follows:

Significant quantities of aluminum may still be found in TPN solutions, mainly in calcium and phosphate salts, heparin, and albumin (13). These sources can result in aluminum concentrations of some TPN solutions from 30 to 306 μg/L (14,15) (see Table 1).

This concentration of aluminum can result in aluminum administration to premature infants of 15–30 μg/kg/day (15). Adult patients receiving TPN with normal renal function who were loaded with aluminum to the point of bone toxicity received 60 μg/kg/day, whereas others receiving long-term TPN therapy with crystalline amino acids instead of casein hydrolysate received only 1 μg/kg/day. The latter groups had no evidence of elevated serum, urine, or bone content of aluminum (15). Thus, premature infants receive aluminum in TPN solutions intermediate between known safe and known toxic amounts.

Because renal function in premature infants is developmentally reduced, the risk of aluminum retention is increased. Older term infants receiving chronic TPN treatment retain approximately 75% of the intravenous aluminum load (13).

In premature infants aluminum has been observed to accumulate in bone, blood, and urine, occasionally to high levels (13,14). Autopsy specimens of vertebrae from two infants who died while receiving TPN revealed a positive aurin tricarboxylic acid stain for aluminum at the level of the mineralization front (14). Thus, premature infants receiving TPN therapy may accumulate aluminum in bone at the mineralization front in a manner similar to that of adults.

Although accumulation of aluminum at the mineralization front in premature infants is not by itself evidence of aluminum toxicity, aluminum accumulation in bone has been associated with decreased bone formation and osteomalacia in adults (6).

In addition, long-term TPN therapy in three infants led to rickets despite the provision of 1000 IU (25 μg) daily vitamin D2 in the TPN solution. The rickets finally resolved after high-dose vitamin D2 (ergocalciferol in oil) was given (12). The reason for vitamin D-dependent rickets with long-term TPN therapy is unclear. However, all three patients were subsequently found to have accumulated large quantities of aluminum.

Treatment and Prevention

Every attempt should be made to provide, especially to premature infants, as much calcium and phosphate as permitted by the TPN solution. Until manufacturers reduce the aluminum content of these products, periodic monitoring of infants receiving TPN for roentgenographic evidence of bone disease is recommended. Periodic determinations of serum levels of calcium, phosphorus, PTH, 25(OH)D, and 1,25(OH)$_2$D can identify associated hyperparathyroidism and vitamin D deficiency (low 25(OH)D). If bone disease persists despite maximal calcium and phosphate supplementation, and if 24-hour urine excretion of calcium and phosphorus does not exceed intake, then aluminum in plasma, urine, and the TPN solution should be obtained. Specimens must be collected in plastic containers and sent to a specialized laboratory for analysis.

Plasma aluminum concentration exceeding 100 μg/L and/or urine aluminum/creatinine (μg/mg) greater than 0.3 (normal <0.05) require analysis of the components of the TPN solution for aluminum content: Inform the hospital pharmacy of the source(s) of the high levels of aluminum so that they may inform the manufacturer and possibly stop or reduce TPN. Although deferoxamine therapy has been useful in chelating aluminum from the bones of adults with dialysis osteomalacia, there has been insufficient experience with this drug in infants to recommend its general use. Moreover, use of deferoxamine in one infant was reported to be associated with sustained hypocalcemia (16), raising concerns about its safety in this age group.

TABLE 1. *Sources of aluminum in common intravenously administered products*[a]

Solution	Number of lots tested	Aluminum content, μg/L	Ref.
Potassium phosphate	3	16,598±1801	13
Sodium phosphate	1	5977	13
10% Calcium	5	5056±335	13
Heparin (1000±gm/ml)	3	684±761	13
25% Normal serum albumin	4	1822±2503	13
Trace metal solution	7	972±108	11

[a]Values are given as mean ± SD.

REFERENCES

1. Klein GL, Targoff CM, Ament ME, Sherrard DJ, Bluestone R, Young JH, Norman AW, Coburn JW: Bone disease associated with total parenteral nutrition. *Lancet* 2:1041–1044, 1980
2. Harrison JE, Jeejeebhoy KN, Track NS: The effect of total parenteral nutrition (TPN) on bone mass. In: Coburn JW, Klein GL (eds) *Metabolic Bone Disease in Total Parenteral Nutrition.* Baltimore, Urban and Schwarzenberg, pp 53–61, 1985
3. Jeejeebhoy KN, Shike M, Sturtridge WC, Tam CS, Jones G, Murray TM, Harrison JE: TPN bone disease at Toronto. In: Coburn JW, Klein GL (eds) *Metabolic Bone Disease in Total Parenteral Nutrition.* Baltimore, Urban and Schwarzenberg, pp 17–29, 1985
4. Vargas JH, Klein GL, Ament ME, Ott SM, Sherrard DJ, Horst RL, Berquist WE, Alfrey AC, Slatopolsky E, Coburn JW: Metabolic bone disease of total parenteral nutrition: course after changing from casein to amino acids in parenteral solutions with reduced aluminum content. *Am J Clin Nutr* 48:1070–1078, 1988
5. Klein GL, Horst RL, Norman AW, Ament ME, Slatopolsky E, Coburn JW: Reduced serum levels of 1α,25-dihydroxyvitamin D during long term parenteral nutrition. *Ann Intern Med* 94:638–643, 1981
6. Ott SM, Maloney NA, Klein GL, Alfrey AC, Ament ME, Coburn JW, Sherrard DJ: Aluminum is associated with low bone formation in patients receiving chronic parenteral nutrition. *Ann Intern Med* 98:910–914, 1983
7. Klein GL, Alfrey AC, Miller NL, Sherrard DJ, Hazlet TK, Ament ME, Coburn JW: Aluminum loading during total parenteral nutrition. *Am J Clin Nutr* 35:1425–1429, 1982
8. Klein GL, Ott SM, Alfrey AC, Sherrard DJ, Hazlet TK, Miller NL, Maloney NA, Berquist WE, Ament ME, Coburn JW: Aluminum as a factor in the bone disease of long-term parenteral nutrition. *Trans Assoc Am Phys* 95:155–164, 1982
9. Shike M, Shils ME, Heller A, Alcock N, Vigorita V, Brockman R, Holick MF, Lane J, Flombaum C: Bone disease in prolonged parenteral nutrition: osteopenia without mineralization defect. *Am J Clin Nutr* 44:89–98, 1986
10. Lipkin EW, Ott SM, Klein GL: Heterogeneity of bone histology in parenteral nutrition patients. *Am J Clin Nutr* 46:673–680, 1987
11. DeVernejoul MC, Messing B, Modrowski D, Bielakoff J, Buisine A, Miravet L: Multifactorial low remodeling bone disease during cyclic total parenteral nutrition. *J Clin Endocrinol Metab* 60:109–113, 1985
12. Saitta JC, Ott SM, Sherrard DJ et al: Metabolic bone disease in adults in long-term parenteral nutrition: Longitudinal study with regional densitometry and bone biopsy. *J Parenter Enter Nutr* 17:214–219, 1993
13. Sedman AB, Klein GL, Merritt RJ, Miller NL, Weber KO, Gill WL, Anand H, Alfrey AC: Evidence of aluminum loading in infants receiving intravenous therapy. *N Engl J Med* 312:1337–1343, 1985
14. Koo WWK, Kaplan LA, Bendon R, Succop P, Tsang RC, Horn J, Steichen JJ: Response to aluminum in parenteral nutrition during infancy. *J Pediatrics* 109:877–883, 1986
15. Klein GL: Unusual sources of aluminum. In: DeBroe ME, Coburn JW (eds) *Aluminum and Renal Failure.* Boston, Kluwer Academic, pp 203–211, 1990
16. Klein GL, Snodgrass WR, Griffin MP, Miller NL, Alfrey AC: Hypocalcemia complicating deferoxamine therapy in an infant with parenteral nutrition-associated aluminum overload: evidence for a role of aluminum in the bone disease of infants. *J Pediatr Gastroenterol Nutr* 9:400–403, 1989

67. Renal Osteodystrophy in Adults and Children

William G. Goodman, *Jack W. Coburn, †Eduardo Slatopolsky, and ‡Isidro B. Salusky

*Departments of Radiological Sciences, *Medicine, and ‡Pediatrics and Nephrology, University of California, Los Angeles School of Medicine, Los Angeles, California; and *West Los Angeles Veterans Affairs Medical Center; and †Department of Medicine, Barnes-Jewish Hospital, St. Louis, Missouri*

The physiologic control of mineral metabolism is a closely integrated process that involves the kidneys, intestine, parathyroid glands, and bone. With the onset of renal disease, mineral homeostasis becomes substantially altered, and the development of renal failure has widespread consequences for bone and various soft tissues. In its broadest sense, the term renal osteodystrophy encompasses the full range of disorders of mineral metabolism that affect the skeleton and other organs in patients with chronic renal disease.

The kidneys regulate the external balances of calcium, phosphorus, magnesium, and other minerals by modulating their excretion in the urine, and they serve not only as target organs for the actions of parathyroid hormone (PTH) but as a site for the degradation of PTH. In addition, cells of the proximal nephron are the primary site of production of 1,25-dihydroxyvitamin D, or calcitriol, a hormone with diverse actions in a variety of tissues. Calcitriol is a major regulator of intestinal calcium absorption, a key determinant of parathyroid hormone (PTH) synthesis, and an important modifier of cell proliferation and differentiated function both in bone and in cartilage. Renal excretion also provides the major route of removal for certain exogenous and endogenous substances, such as aluminum and β_2-microglobulin, that can lead to specific bone and joint disorders if retained in the body of patients with end-stage renal disease (1,2). Because even modest reductions in renal function substantially alter the kidney's excretory and metabolic capacities, mineral homeostasis becomes increasingly compromised in patients with progressive renal failure (3).

Disturbances in the control of PTH secretion, hyperplasia of the parathyroid glands, and alterations in the metabolism of vitamin D are key elements in the pathogenesis of renal osteodystrophy. Other factors such as aluminum can also affect PTH secretion and bone metabolism either directly or indirectly (4–6), and complex interactions among these pathogenic considerations ultimately determine the type of skeletal disorder that develops in patients with renal failure. Generally, the renal bone diseases are classified as either high-turnover lesions, which are due to persistently elevated serum PTH levels, or low-turnover lesions, which are related either to excess bone aluminum deposition or to normal or reduced serum PTH levels (7). Each group of disorders is considered separately below, but it should be noted that the skeletal manifestations in individual patients can reflect the combined response to more than one pathogenic process (8,9). The histopathologic lesions of renal bone disease probably represent portions of a continuum that encompasses both the low-turnover and high-turnover skeletal disorders.

HIGH-TURNOVER BONE DISEASE (SECONDARY HYPERPARATHYROIDISM)

Several factors contribute to sustained increases in PTH secretion and, ultimately, to parathyroid gland hyperplasia and high-turnover lesions of bone in patients with chronic renal failure. Among these are hyperphosphatemia due to diminished renal phosphorus excretion, hypocalcemia, impaired renal calcitriol production, alterations in the control of PTH gene transcription secretion, and skeletal resistance to the calcemic actions of PTH (3).

Phosphorus retention and hyperphosphatemia have been recognized for many years as important factors in the pathogenesis of secondary hyperparathyroidism. Secondary hyperparathyroidism can be prevented in experimental animals with chronic renal failure when dietary phosphorus intake is lowered in proportion to glomerular filtration rate (10), and phosphate restriction can reduce serum PTH levels in patients with moderate renal failure (11,12). Phosphorus retention promotes the secretion of PTH in several ways. First, hyperphosphatemia can lower serum ionized calcium levels directly, thereby stimulating PTH release. Second, phosphorus impairs renal 1α-hydroxylase activity, which diminishes the conversion of 25-hydroxyvitamin D to 1,25-dihydroxyvitamin D; high rates of transepithelial phosphate transport in the proximal tubule may be responsible for this change when glomerular filtration is reduced (12). Third, phosphorus retention may directly enhance PTH synthesis without associated changes in serum ionized calcium or calcitriol levels.

Impaired renal calcitriol production and low serum levels of 1,25-dihydroxyvitamin D account, at least in part, for intestinal calcium malabsorption and for low serum calcium levels in many patients with progressive renal failure (13). A decrease in vitamin D receptor expression in parathyroid tissue in chronic renal failure may also interfere with the normal feedback inhibition of PTH gene transcription by 1,25-dihydroxyvitamin D, leading to excess PTH secretion (14). Although calcitriol up-regulates its own receptor in normal parathyroid tissues (15), it is not known as to whether the reduction in vitamin D receptor expression in chronic renal failure is due to low circulating levels of the hormone, to the hyperplastic state of the parathyroids, or to differences in cell function that are a consequence of the uremic environment.

Controversy persists about several key factors that regulate PTH secretion in chronic renal failure. *In vitro* studies of dispersed parathyroid cells in tissue culture suggest that the regulation of PTH release by calcium is abnormal in parathyroid cells obtained from patients with chronic renal failure and that higher calcium levels are required to achieve similar reductions in PTH release in hyperplastic parathyroid tissues compared with normal glands (16). Such findings underlie the concept that the set point for calcium-regulated PTH release is greater than normal in secondary hyperparathyroidism (17); moreover, some reports have suggested that calcitriol corrects this abnormality and lowers the set point for calcium-regulated PTH release in patients with renal failure and secondary hyperparathyroidism (18,19).

However, the results of several recent clinical studies indicate that the regulation of PTH secretion by calcium does not differ from normal in patients with secondary hyperparathyroidism (20–23). Set point estimates were no greater in patients with advanced secondary hyperparathyroidism than in normal subjects, and values did not differ in patients with osteitis fibrosa or adynamic lesions of renal osteodystrophy (20,22,23). Treatment with calcitriol did not alter values for the set point despite marked histologic improvement in the skeletal changes of secondary hyperparathyroidism (21). Such findings suggest that differences in functional parathyroid gland size, rather than disturbances in the regulation of PTH release by calcium, account for the wide variation in serum PTH levels in patients with chronic renal failure (Fig. 1).

Because of the potent inhibitory effects of 1,25-dihydroxyvitamin D on parathyroid cell growth, disturbances in the metabolism of vitamin D may be particularly important in determining the degree of parathyroid hyperplasia and the extent of parathyroid gland enlargement in chronic renal failure (24). Fukuda et al. reported that vitamin D receptor expression was lower in parathyroid tissues exhibiting a nodular rather than a diffuse histologic pattern of parathyroid gland hyperplasia (25). Interestingly, the extent of glandular enlargement is frequently greater in the nodular form of parathyroid hyperplasia (26). Clonal expansion of subpopulations of parathyroid cells and selected chromosomal deletions are additional factors that may influence the degree of parathyroid gland hyperplasia in end-stage renal disease (27).

Skeletal resistance to the calcemic action of PTH may further contribute to the development of hypocalcemia and secondary hyperparathyroidism in chronic renal failure. The calcemic response to infusions of parathyroid extract is subnormal in patients with moderate to advanced renal failure, and the correction of hypocalcemia during PTH infusions is less rapid than in normal individuals (28). Abnormalities in vitamin D metabolism are largely responsible for these changes.

Because PTH increases both osteoblastic and osteoclastic activity in bone, sustained elevations in serum PTH levels promote bone formation and turnover. Serum PTH values generally correspond to the extent of bone resorption surface, to the number of osteoclasts, and to the rate of bone formation as measured in iliac crest bone biopsy specimens. If the biochemical severity of secondary hyperparathyroidism becomes advanced, radiographic and histologic features of osteitis fibrosa cystica develop. The skeletal changes in patients with secondary hyperparathyroidism due to chronic renal failure are usually more pronounced than in primary hyperparathyroidism, probably due to the higher serum levels of PTH. Serum PTH values are often 5–10 times above the upper limit of normal in patients with secondary hyper-

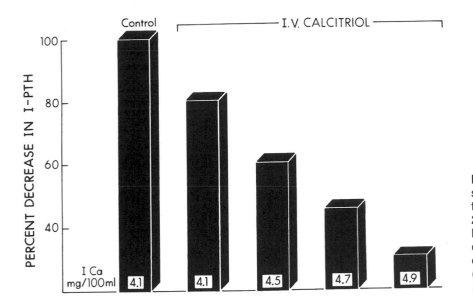

FIG. 1. Effect of intravenous calcitriol on serum ionized calcium and immunoreactive parathyroid hormone (iPTH) levels in 20 patients undergoing maintenance hemodialysis. Serum iPTH values decrease before changes in ionized calcium levels can be demonstrated. (Adapted from Slatopolsky E, et al: *J Clin Invest* 74:21, 1984, with permission.)

parathyroidism due to end-stage renal disease, and they may reach levels that are 20–40 times normal.

LOW-TURNOVER BONE DISEASE (ADYNAMIC LESIONS OF BONE AND OSTEOMALACIA)

In the past, secondary hyperparathyroidism was an almost invariable consequence of chronic renal failure and the most common skeletal lesion of renal osteodystrophy. Recent evidence indicates, however, that many patients do not have markedly elevated serum PTH levels at the time that regular dialysis is begun; values may be only minimally elevated or fall within the normal range. Moreover, approximately 40% of patients undergoing regular hemodialysis and more than half of adult patients receiving peritoneal dialysis have serum PTH levels that are typically associated with normal or reduced rates of bone formation and turnover (29).

The adynamic lesion currently accounts for most cases of low-turnover bone disease in patients with chronic renal failure, whereas osteomalacia is less frequently encountered. Bone formation and turnover are reduced in both disorders, but osteomalacia is characterized by an additional defect in the mineralization of newly formed bone; thus, unmineralized bone collagen, or osteoid, accumulates in osteomalacia, whereas the amount of osteoid is normal or reduced in the adynamic lesion.

In the 1970s and 1980s, aluminum intoxication was largely responsible for the development of these two skeletal lesions in patients with chronic renal failure. Evidence of bone aluminum deposition was a prominent finding both in patients with adynamic lesions and in those with osteomalacia, and bone histology improved markedly when aluminum overload was effectively treated.

Aluminum adversely affects bone and mineral metabolism in several ways (9). Both the proliferation of osteoblasts and the differentiation of precursor cells into mature osteoblasts are impaired by aluminum, and decreases in osteoblastic number are a characteristic finding in aluminum-related bone disease. Aluminum also diminishes basal and hormone-stimulated osteoblastic activity *in vitro,* and it impairs the release of PTH from parathyroid cells (4). Together, these changes contribute to marked reductions in collagen synthesis and mineralized bone formation during aluminum loading *in vivo,* and they are sufficient to account for the development of adynamic lesions in some patients (9).

In addition, deposits of aluminum in bone are often found within the mineralization front, which is located at the junction between surface osteoid seams and adjacent mineralized bone (9). The calcification of newly formed bone collagen is initiated at this site, and several studies indicate that aluminum disrupts the mineralization process directly, at least in part, by slowing the rate of formation and growth of hydroxyapatite crystals (6).

The relative severity of the reductions in collagen synthesis and skeletal mineralization ultimately determines whether overt histologic osteomalacia or adynamic bone develops after aluminum loading. Collagen synthesis is diminished in both lesions, but the defect in skeletal mineralization is more severe in patients with osteomalacia; thus, mineralization lags behind collagen synthesis, leading to osteoid accumulation and thickened osteoid seams. In contrast, the rates of mineralization and collagen synthesis are reduced to a similar degree in patients with adynamic lesions, and osteoid volume and osteoid seam thickness remain normal or low.

Several factors increase the risk of aluminum-related bone disease in patients with chronic renal failure, including previous parathyroidectomy, a history of renal transplantation and graft failure, bilateral nephrectomy, and diabetes mellitus. Also, citrate forms soluble complexes of aluminum in aqueous solutions, and it markedly enhances intestinal aluminum absorption. The administration of citrate together with aluminum-containing medications can lead to acute aluminum intoxication (30,31).

Persistently high serum PTH levels appear to partially offset the adverse effects of aluminum on bone; thus, aluminum-related bone disease may not be seen despite evidence of skeletal aluminum deposition in patients with established secondary hyperparathyroidism. This may account for the greater risk of aluminum-related bone disease in patients who have undergone parathyroidectomy or in those with diabetes because the serum levels of PTH are generally low in these two conditions. Marked increases in bone aluminum content and overt aluminum-related osteomalacia may develop after parathyroidectomy in patients undergoing regular dialysis if there is ongoing exposure to aluminum (32,33).

Adequate water purification methods for the preparation of dialysis solutions and the avoidance of aluminum-containing, phosphate-binding agents have markedly reduced the incidence of aluminum-related bone disease in the contemporary dialysis population. As such, other causes of adynamic renal osteodystrophy are now more frequently encountered. Diabetes, corticosteroid therapy, and increasing age account for the finding of adynamic skeletal changes in some patients; however, the widespread use of active vitamin D sterols and the administration of large doses of oral calcium carbonate for the management of phosphate retention in patients with end-stage renal disease are likely contributors to the increasing prevalence of this disorder in the general dialysis population (29). High levels of calcium in dialysis solutions may also play a role. As noted previously, both calcium and vitamin D reduce PTH secretion. Because PTH is a major determinant of the rate of bone remodeling in chronic renal failure, oversuppression of parathyroid gland function may lead to the development of adynamic renal osteodystrophy. The long-term consequences of this disorder in the absence of aluminum toxicity remain to be determined.

In cases of aluminum toxicity, low serum PTH levels are generally attributed to frequent episodes of hypercalcemia and the direct inhibitory effects of aluminum on PTH secretion (29); however, serum calcium levels are also higher in patients with adynamic bone without evidence of bone aluminum deposition than in subjects with secondary hyperparathyroidism (34). This finding probably reflects diminished calcium uptake by the skeleton due to low rates of bone remodeling; as such, persistently high serum calcium levels may further suppress parathyroid gland function.

Although low serum PTH levels contribute to the diminished rates of bone formation and turnover that characterize the adynamic lesion, they do not explain the mineralization defect of osteomalacia; thus, additional pathogenic factors must be considered in patients with this disorder. Evidence of vitamin D deficiency, as judged by low serum levels of 25-hydroxyvitamin D, was noted in some dialysis patients with osteomalacia in England (35), but this is an uncommon finding in the United States. It is likely that differences in sunlight exposure and in the amount of vitamin D in fortified foods and nutritional supplements account for this disparity. Long-term therapy with phenytoin and/or phenobarbital has been associated osteomalacia in nonuremic patients, and a higher incidence of symptomatic bone disease was reported in dialysis patients receiving these drugs (36). Persistent hypocalcemia and/or hypophosphatemia can lead to osteomalacia in some patients with chronic renal failure. Overall Improvements in nutritional management

and the decreased use of aluminum-containing medications has diminished the prevalence of the osteomalacic form of renal osteodystrophy.

HISTOLOGIC FEATURES OF RENAL OSTEODYSTROPHY

The use of bone biopsy has contributed substantially to our understanding of renal bone disease. Quantitative histomorphometry of bone provides information about the relative amounts of mineralized and unmineralized bone, the length and thickness of osteoid seams, the extent of resorption surfaces, the numbers of osteoblasts and osteoclasts, and the presence or absence of marrow fibrosis. Measurements of bone formation can also be obtained using the technique of double tetracycline labeling. The tetracyclines are deposited in bone at sites of active mineralization, and their presence can be demonstrated in thin sections of tissue examined by fluorescence microscopy. Where new bone has been formed, double bands of tetracycline fluorescence can be seen, and the amount of mineralized tissue deposited during the labeling interval is circumscribed by the two labels; as such, bone formation can be measured directly. This information is often essential for the correct diagnostic interpretation of biopsy material from patients with renal osteodystrophy.

Methods for achieving double tetracycline labeling of bone differ among laboratories, but the following approach is suitable for patients with chronic renal failure. Patients are given either demeclocycline, 300 mg orally twice a day, or tetracycline HCl, 500 mg orally 4 times a day, for 2 or 3 days followed by a 10- to 20-day interval during which no tetracycline is given. A second course of oral tetracycline HCl, 500 mg twice a day, is then given for another 2 or 3 days. Bone biopsy should be obtained 3–7 days after finishing of the second course of oral tetracycline. For pediatric patients, 2-day courses of tetracycline are recommended for each label, and doses should not exceed 10 mg/kg/day.

In addition to standard histologic assessments, special staining procedures can be used to demonstrate deposits of aluminum, iron, and amyloid in bone, and the bone aluminum content can be measured by atomic absorption spectroscopy in small samples obtained at the time of biopsy. Iliac crest bone biopsy can be done safely in the outpatient setting with little morbidity both in adults and in children.

High-Turnover Bone Disease

Osteitis fibrosa is the most common of high-turnover lesions of renal osteodystrophy both in adults and in children (7,8). Overall, the disorder represents the response of bone to persistently high serum levels of PTH. There is histologic evidence of active bone resorption with increases in the number and size of osteoclasts and an increase in the number of resorption bays, or Howship's lacunae, within cancellous bone. Fibrous tissue may be found immediately adjacent to bony trabeculae, or it may accumulate more extensively within the marrow space (Fig. 2A); partial or complete fibrous replacement of individual bony trabeculae occurs in advanced cases.

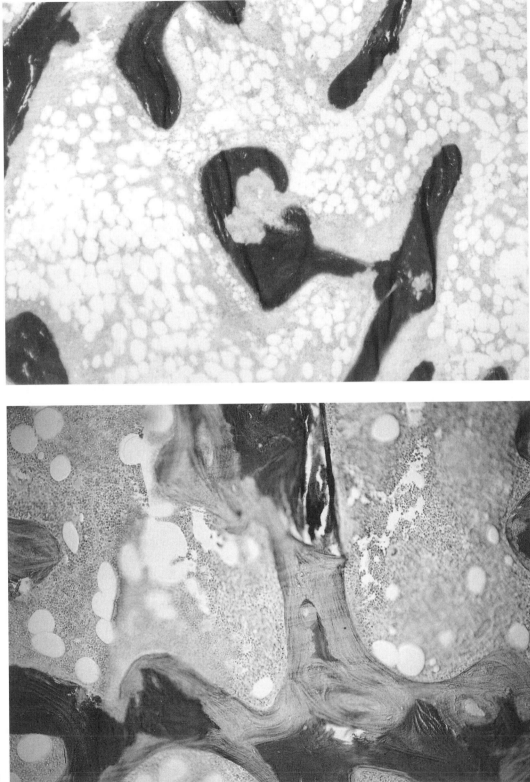

FIG. 2. A: Goldner stained section of undecalcified bone from a hemodialysis patient with osteitis fibrosa; magnification 50×. Mineralized bone stains green *(light)* and osteoid appears red *(dark)*. Fibrous tissue has accumulated within the marrow space immediately adjacent to bone, and the serrated margins along the bone surface represent sites of osteoclastic bone resorption. **B:** Goldner-stained section of undecalcified bone from a hemodialysis patient with osteomalacia; magnification 50×. Mineralized bone stains green *(light)* and osteoid appears red *(dark)*. The total amount of osteoid is markedly increased; osteoid seams are wide and have a multilaminant appearance.

Osteoblastic activity is also increased in patients with osteitis fibrosa (7,8), and the combined increase in osteoblastic and osteoclastic activity accounts for the high rate of bone remodeling and turnover in secondary hyperparathyroidism. Bone formation is increased, and values are often 3–4 times greater than the upper limit of normal. The number of osteoblasts is substantially increased, and a greater proportion of the surface of cancellous bone is covered with newly formed osteoid. Overall, the amount of osteoid is moderately elevated, but many osteoid seams have a woven appearance similar to that of a straw basket; this finding is characteristic of skeletal disorders in which collagen synthesis and bone formation are markedly increased, and it reflects the disordered arrangement of collagen fibrils within osteoid seams.

Patients with modest increases in osteoclastic activity and bone formation and in whom there is little or no evidence of peritrabecular fibrosis are classified as having mild lesions of renal osteodystrophy. This disorder is a less severe manifestation of hyperparathyroid bone disease (7,8). Serum PTH levels are elevated, but values are substantially lower than in patients with overt osteitis fibrosa (34,37); other biochemical and roentgenographic manifestations of secondary hyperparathyroidism are also present. Because the histologic features are much less striking than in overt osteitis fibrosa, tetracycline-based measurements of bone formation are useful for distinguishing this subgroup of patients from those with normal bone or adynamic lesions (7,8).

Low-Turnover Bone Disease

Osteomalacia is the most striking histologic manifestation of low-turnover bone disease. Excess osteoid, or unmineralized bone collagen, accumulates in bone due to a primary defect in mineralization. Osteoid seams are wide, and they often have a multi-lamellar appearance (Fig. 2B); the extent of bone surfaces covered with osteoid is also increased. In contrast, osteoblastic activity is markedly reduced, and bone formation often cannot be measured because of the lack of tetracycline uptake into bone. In patients with aluminum-related osteomalacia the bone aluminum content is elevated. Deposits of aluminum can be seen along trabecular bone surfaces using histochemical staining methods (7,8,38), and the histologic severity of osteomalacia generally corresponds to the amount of surface-stainable aluminum (39).

Bone biopsies from patients with the adynamic lesion of renal osteodystrophy exhibit normal or reduced amounts of osteoid, no tissue fibrosis, diminished numbers of osteoblasts and osteoclasts, and low or unmeasurable rates of bone formation (7,8,40). This disorder was originally described in patients with evidence of aluminum toxicity, and aluminum deposition along trabecular bone surfaces was a prominent finding (40). *In vivo* experimental studies suggest that this disorder may be the forerunner of overt histologic osteomalacia when bone aluminum is the underlying cause (41); thus, bone aluminum levels are not as high in this subgroup of patients compared to those with aluminum-related osteomalacia.

Currently, the majority of adult and pediatric dialysis patients with adynamic lesions of renal osteodystrophy do not have evidence of bone aluminum deposition, and the overall prevalence of this disorder in patients undergoing both hemodialysis and peritoneal dialysis has risen substantially (8,42). Adynamic bone is now the most common histologic manifestation of renal osteodystrophy in adults undergoing peritoneal dialysis (37). Apart from aluminum, other factors that contribute to the development of adynamic bone include the use of large doses of calcium-containing, phosphate-binding antacids and the administration of active vitamin D sterols early in the clinical management of secondary hyperparathyroidism. Diabetes, corticosteroid therapy, and increasing age are additional causative factors (43).

Occasionally patients demonstrate histologic features of both osteitis fibrosa and osteomalacia. This combination of findings is termed the mixed lesion of renal osteodystrophy (44). Patients usually have biochemical evidence of secondary hyperparathyroidism together with findings that are more characteristic of those with impaired bone formation and mineralization. Persistent hypocalcemia is present in some patients, and this can contribute to defective skeletal mineralization (44). Mixed lesions of renal osteodystrophy may be seen in patients with osteitis fibrosa who are in the process of developing aluminum-related bone disease or in patients with aluminum-related osteomalacia who are undergoing treatment with deferoxamine (45); thus, mixed renal osteodystrophy can represent a transitional state between the high-turnover lesions of secondary hyperparathyroidism and the low-turnover disorders of osteomalacia or adynamic bone (9).

CLINICAL MANIFESTATIONS

The signs and symptoms of renal osteodystrophy are rather nonspecific, and various laboratory and roentgenographic abnormalities often fail to correspond with the severity of the clinical manifestations (3). Common clinical features include bone pain, muscle weakness, skeletal deformities, and extraskeletal calcifications. In children, growth retardation is a prominent feature.

Bone Pain

Bone pain is very common in patients with renal osteodystrophy; its onset is usually insidious, and symptoms progress gradually over many months. The pain is frequently diffuse and nonspecific, but it is often aggravated by weight bearing or by changes in posture. When localized, the lower back, hips, and legs are most often affected. The appendicular skeleton can also be involved, and pain in the heel or ankles may be a presenting complaint (3). Occasionally, the initial manifestation is that of a acute arthritis or periarthritis that is not relieved by massage or by application of local heat. Severe bone pain is more common in patients with aluminum-related bone disease than in those with osteitis fibrosa, and it is a prominent clinical feature of this disorder (46). There is marked variation among patients, however, and some with advanced secondary hyperparathyroidism are severely incapacitated. The physical examination is generally unremarkable unless fractures or skeletal deformities are present.

Muscle Weakness

Proximal myopathy develops in some patients with advanced renal failure. Symptoms appear very slowly, and weakness and aching are the most common manifestations both in adults and in children (3). The physiologic basis of this disorder is not understood, and several factors may contribute. Favorable clinical responses have been noted in some patients after treatment with calcitriol or 25-hydroxyvitamin D, following parathyroidectomy, after successful renal transplantation or during the treatment of aluminum-related bone disease with deferoxamine (3). The role of abnormal vitamin D metabolism in the pathogenesis of uremic myopathy remains uncertain, but a careful evaluation must be done to exclude severe secondary hyperparathyroidism or aluminum toxicity. In those with prominent symptoms of muscle pain and weakness, an empiric therapeutic trial of calcitriol or 25-hydroxyvitamin D is warranted.

Skeletal Deformities

Bone deformities are a major manifestation of renal osteodystrophy, particularly in children with longstanding renal failure. The frequency of skeletal deformity in pediatric patients is probably related to the high rates of bone growth and skeletal modeling that characterize the immature skeleton. Bone deformities may affect either the axial or appendicular skeleton.

The pattern of deformity varies with age in children with chronic renal failure. In patients <3–4 years old, the changes of secondary hyperparathyroidism most often resemble those of vitamin D-deficiency rickets; characteristic features include rachitic rosary, Harrison grooves, and enlargement of the wrists and ankles due to a widening of the metaphysis beneath the growth plate in long bones. Craniotabes and frontal bossing of the skull occur in children who develop renal failure in the first 2 years of life (47).

The onset of overt renal failure before the age of 10 years is often associated with deformities of long bones; bowing is the most frequent change. Genu valgum is a common manifestation at any age, and ulnar deviation of hands, pes varus, "swelling" of the wrists, ankles, or medial ends of clavicles due to metaphyseal widening and pseudoclubbing are frequently observed. Despite regular treatment with vitamin D sterols, 20% to 25% of pediatric patients undergoing long-term dialysis may require corrective orthopedic procedures for skeletal deformities (48).

Slipped epiphyses are another common complication of renal bone disease in pediatric patients. The disorder usually occurs in association with severe secondary hyperparathyroidism (47), and the femoral epiphysis is most often affected. Dental abnormalities, including enamel defects and malformations of the teeth, are typical in children with congenital renal disease because of disturbances in mineral metabolism that develop early in life (47).

In adults with aluminum-related bone disease, skeletal deformities are confined predominantly to the axial skeleton; changes include lumbar scoliosis, kyphosis, and distortion of the thoracic cage. Adult patients with severe osteitis fibrosa may develop rib deformities and pseudoclubbing.

Growth Retardation

Children with chronic renal failure almost invariably exhibit growth retardation; among the factors that contribute are chronic acidosis, malnutrition, renal bone disease, and abnormal somatomedin metabolism (49). Treatment with calcitriol may improve linear growth in some children (50), but consistent increases in growth rate have not been observed in most children undergoing maintenance dialysis during treatment with vitamin D, 1α-hydroxyvitamin D, or calcitriol.

Extraskeletal Manifestations

Several types of soft tissue calcification can be detected by radiographic examination. Among the most frequent are tumoral or peri-articular calcifications; these are occasionally associated with acute periarticular inflammation, and the clinical presentation may suggest an episode of acute arthritis. Soft tissue calcifications are common when serum phosphorus levels are greater than 8–9 mg/dl or when the calcium-phosphorus ion product exceeds 75. Soft tissue calcifications can regress substantially if sustained reductions in serum phosphorus levels can be achieved. Although extraskeletal calcifications are more common with advancing age, they can occur in children with end-stage renal disease.

The most frequent form of vascular calcification in patients with renal failure is localized to the medial layer of small and medium-sized arteries (Mockerberg's sclerosis); this type of calcification is diffuse and continuous along the vessel wall (Fig. 3). Involvement is most common in diabetic patients, and the roentgenographic appearance differs from the irregular pattern of calcified intimal plaques. Medial calcifications are usually asymptomatic, but palpation of the peripheral pulses and blood pressure measurements may be rendered difficult in affected limbs. Vascular calcifications are best detected by lateral views of the ankle or anteroposterior views of the hands or feet using magnification techniques with macroradioscopy (51). The importance of a high serum calcium-phosphorus ion product in the development of vascular calcifications has been questioned, but a concerted effort should be made to avoid values above 65–70 (52).

In extreme cases, there may be ischemic necrosis of the skin, muscle, and/or subcutaneous tissues; this syndrome is known as "calciphylaxis" but its pathogenesis is not understood. Some patients have advanced secondary hyperparathyroidism, and parathyroidectomy may provide significant clinical improvement. Calciphylaxis can be seen in patients with advanced renal failure, in those receiving regular dialysis, and in patients with functioning renal allografts (53).

Visceral calcifications are somewhat infrequent, and they may differ in chemical composition from vascular calcifications; the lungs, heart, kidneys, skeletal muscle and stomach are mainly involved. Pulmonary calcifications can cause restrictive lung disease that may be severe and progressive, and the disorder often persists even after successful kidney transplantation or parathyroidectomy.

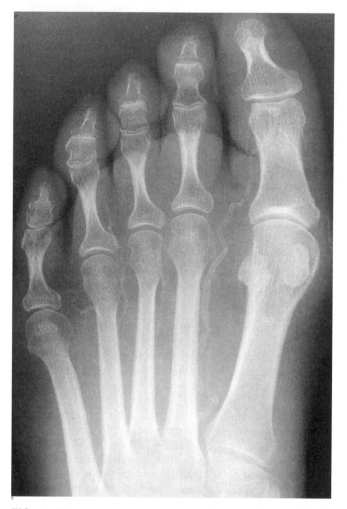

FIG. 3. Radiography of the foot of a long-term dialysis patient demonstrating extensive medial calcification of the arteries.

Amyloidosis in Patients with Chronic Renal Failure

Most adult patients with end-stage renal disease who are treated with dialysis for more than 7–10 years develop amyloid deposits with a unique amyloid fibril protein that is derived from β₂-microglobulin (β₂M), a normal plasma constituent. These patients present with multiple bone cysts, pathologic fractures, carpal tunnel syndrome, scapulohumeral arthritis, and spondyloarthropathy (2,54–56); the predilection for this syndrome to affect the musculoskeletal system with skeletal and articular symptoms can lead to difficulty in separating it from other forms of renal osteodystrophy.

β₂-Microglobulin is a low-molecular-weight protein of approximately 12,000 daltons that is produced by many cells, particularly lymphoid cells and other cells with high rates of turnover. In cells of this type, β₂M stabilizes the structure of the MHC class I antigen on the cell surface, but β₂M is released when the complexes are shed from the cell membrane. Approximately 180-250 mg of β₂M is normally generated each day. Almost all available β₂M is filtered at the glomerulus, and it is then catabolized by cells of the renal tubules (55,57). With advanced renal failure, β₂M accumulates in the plasma, and levels increase to values 50 times greater than normal in anuric dialysis patients (58).

Histologically, β₂M amyloid fibrils are similar in appearance to amyloid AA; however, β₂M amyloid deposits are predominantly osteoarticular, leading to musculoskeletal manifestations (55,57). The slow rate of appearance and the predilection for bone and articular structures both suggest that elevated serum β₂M levels do not fully account for the clinical syndrome observed in patients with chronic renal failure. Increased age-related glycosylation products (59), certain specific proteases (60), and inhibitors of other proteases (61) have each been suggested as factors that lead to the deposition of β₂M amyloid in bony structures and in synovial tissues. In rare cases, systemic deposits occur, and these may be fatal (62).

The clinical features of amyloid deposition rarely appear before 5 years of dialysis therapy, and the disorder is more common in patients who start regular dialysis after the age of 50 years (63). Carpal tunnel syndrome is the most frequent clinical feature, but shoulder pain, other arthritic complaints, and bone lesions are common. Deposits of β₂M are found in periarticular structures, joints, bone (Fig. 4), and tendon sheaths. Far less commonly, the liver, spleen, rectal mucosa, or blood vessels are involved.

Skeletal manifestations include generalized arthritis, erosive arthritis, and joint effusions. Scapulohumeral involvement with shoulder pain is a common clinical presentation. Generalized arthritis can lead to pain and stiffness, decreased joint mobility, joint effusions and deformities. Characteristically, pain is worse at night or when the patient must sit quietly for a few hours during dialysis sessions; joint motion or activity can provide temporary relief. Erosive arthritis can involve the metacarpophalangeal joints, the interphalangeal joints, the shoulders, wrists, and knees; effusions sometimes occur at these sites. The cervical spine is the most common site of destructive spondyloarthropathy (64).

Roentgenographically, bone cysts are most common at the ends of long bones, particularly the femoral head and proximal humerus, and they may also be found in the metacarpal and carpal bones. Multiple cystic lesions are common, and serial radiographs often demonstrate cyst enlargement with time. Cystic deposits of β₂M may resemble brown tumors of osteitis fibrosa; however, their location and the presence of multiple rather than solitary cysts suggest that amyloid deposition is responsible. Cystic changes most commonly occur at sites of tendinous insertions, and pathologically these may represent "amyloidomas" that have replaced trabecular bone (Fig. 4). Fractures sometimes occur at these sites, and hip fractures in dialysis patients commonly arise at sites of β₂M deposition (65)). Ultrasound examinations of the shoulder are a simple noninvasive method to assess progressive tendinous involvement with β₂M amyloid deposits (66)).

The fraction of patients afflicted with amyloidosis increases progressively with the duration of dialysis therapy; thus, 70% to 80% of adult patients treated with hemodialysis for 10 or more years will have clinical features of β₂M amyloidosis (56,57)). The distinction between this disorder and either severe secondary hyperparathyroidism or aluminum-related bone disease can be difficult, and thorough clinical,

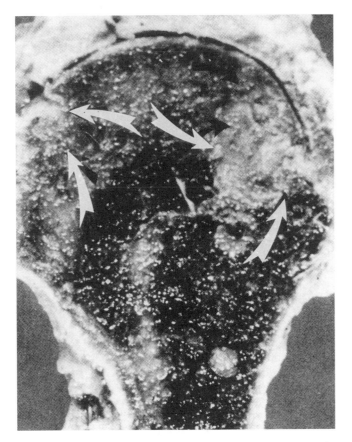

FIG. 4. Postmortem photograph showing extensive deposits of amyloid within the femoral head *(white arrows)*: such areas appear as cystic lesions on roentgenographs. (From van den Broucke JM, et al: *Kidney Int* 33:S-35, 1988, with permission.)

biochemical, and radiographic evaluations are required; $\beta_2 M$ amyloidosis can coexist with either high-turnover or low-turnover lesions of renal osteodystrophy (65).

The overall clinical management of amyloidosis in patients with end-stage renal disease has thus far proven unsatisfactory. The carpal tunnel syndrome may respond to surgical correction but it often recurs. The use of highly permeable dialysis membranes can achieve slightly lower serum levels of $\beta_2 M$, but there is no evidence that this intervention alters the progression of established disease (55,57). There is some evidence that patients treated from the onset of long-term dialysis with polyacrylonitrile (PAN) membranes have a delayed appearance of certain clinical features of dialysis amyloidosis compared with those treated with conventional cellulosic dialyzers (63). Successful renal transplantation is followed by symptomatic relief in most patients, but there is no evidence that bony or soft tissue lesions actually regress after renal transplantation (67).

BIOCHEMICAL FEATURES OF RENAL OSTEODYSTROPHY

When the glomerular filtration rate falls below 30% of normal, hyperphosphatemia is common, and phosphate-binding agents and dietary phosphorus restriction are often needed to correct and/or prevent this disorder. Although hemodialysis and continuous ambulatory peritoneal dialysis (CAPD) remove substantial amounts of phosphorus, additional efforts to control hyperphosphatemia are required in most patients undergoing regular dialysis.

Serum calcium levels are often subnormal in patients with advanced renal failure. With the initiation of hemodialysis, calcium levels usually increase, and they may return to normal. The magnitude of the rise in serum calcium values is partly related to the calcium concentration in dialysate. In patients treated with CAPD who are not receiving vitamin D supplements, serum calcium levels often remain at the lower limit of normal.

The development of hypercalcemia in patients undergoing regular dialysis warrants an immediate and thorough investigation. Conditions associated with hypercalcemia include marked hyperplasia of the parathyroid glands due to severe secondary hyperparathyroidism, aluminum-related bone disease, therapy with calcitriol or other vitamin D sterols, administration of calcium carbonate or other calcium-containing compounds, immobilization, malignancy, and granulomatous disorders such as sarcoidosis or tuberculosis with extrarenal production of 1,25-dihydroxyvitamin D (3). Patients with adynamic bone, even in the absence of aluminum toxicity, have higher basal serum calcium levels than subjects with other skeletal lesions of renal osteodystrophy, and episodes of hypercalcemia are common (34). Because skeletal calcium uptake is limited in the adynamic lesion, calcium entering the extracellular fluid from dialysate or after absorption from the intestine cannot be adequately buffered, and serum calcium levels rise. Reducing the dose of calcium-containing, phosphate-binding agents and lowering dialysate calcium concentrations can usually correct hypercalcemia in patients with adynamic renal osteodystrophy.

In advanced renal failure, serum magnesium levels often rise due to reduced renal magnesium excretion, but they remain within the upper range of normal or slightly elevated when the concentration of magnesium in dialysate is maintained between 0.5 and 0.8 mEq/L (68). The use of magnesium-containing laxatives or antacids can abruptly raise serum magnesium levels in patients with renal failure (69), and such agents should be avoided in patients with diminished renal function. Serum magnesium levels must be measured frequently and regularly if magnesium-containing medications are used.

Serum alkaline phosphatase values are fair markers of the severity of secondary hyperparathyroidism in patients with renal failure. Osteoblasts normally express large amounts of the bone isoenzyme of alkaline phosphatase, and serum levels are usually elevated when osteoblastic activity and bone formation are increased. High levels generally reflect the extent of histologic change in patients with high-turnover lesions of renal osteodystrophy, and values frequently correlate with serum PTH levels (70). Alkaline phosphatase measurements are also useful for monitoring the skeletal response to treatment with vitamin D sterols in patients with osteitis fibrosa; values that decrease over weeks or months usually indicate histologic improvement. Serum alkaline phosphatase levels may increase early in the course of treatment with the chelating agent deferoxamine in patients with aluminum-related bone disease.

Serum alkaline phosphatase levels are less useful for distinguishing between high-turnover and low-turnover lesions of bone. Although values are generally elevated in patients with secondary hyperparathyroidism, they can also be high in patients with aluminum-related osteomalacia (71). Normal serum alkaline phosphatase levels are more common, however, in patients with severe aluminum toxicity arising from aluminum-contaminated dialysis fluids. In pediatric patients undergoing peritoneal dialysis, alkaline phosphatase levels have been a poor predictor of bone histology, and values can be elevated in patients with either osteitis fibrosa or osteomalacia (8).

Increases in isoenzymes of alkaline phosphatase that originate in nonskeletal tissues, particularly liver, can account for high plasma levels in patients with renal failure; consequently, confirmation of a skeletal source of alkaline phosphatase activity should be obtained. This can be achieved by measuring the heat-labile fraction of the enzyme if reliable techniques are available. In clinical practice, measuring other liver enzymes that reflect biliary tract dysfunction, such as γ-glutamyltranspeptidase or 5'-nucleotidase, is useful for excluding hepatic sources of alkaline phosphatase.

Serum osteocalcin levels, or bone Gla-protein, can also be used as an index of osteoblastic activity in patients with chronic renal failure (72). Values are generally elevated in chronic renal failure, but measurements can be useful in separating patients with high-turnover lesions of secondary hyperparathyroidism from those with low-turnover lesions such as osteomalacia and adynamic bone (72,73).

Serum PTH levels vary widely in patients with advanced renal failure, but currently available assays are useful for the assessment of patients with renal osteodystrophy. In the past, most radioimmunoassays for PTH utilized antisera directed against epitopes located in the carboxy terminal or midportions of the PTH molecule. Results obtained by these methods were difficult to interpret because biologically inactive peptide fragments that cross-reacted with carboxy- and midregion antisera were retained in the plasma of patients with chronic renal failure (74). Because the initial 34 amino acid sequence of the PTH molecule determines its receptor binding, more reliable assays for PTH utilize antisera directed at the amino terminal portion of the molecule or double-antibody methods to measure the intact hormone (75,76). Although a number of PTH assays are available commercially, the relationship between the histologic findings in bone and the serum levels of immunoreactive PTH in patients with renal disease has been validated in relatively few of them; therefore. proper interpretation of the results of PTH assays must be made with knowledge about their value as an indicator of bone histology.

For patients with chronic renal failure, amino terminal assays, or assays that use double-antibody methods to measure the intact PTH molecule are highly recommended. Amino terminal measurements provide good discrimination between patients with osteitis fibrosa and those with either osteomalacia or mild lesions of secondary hyperparathyroidism, and serum levels correspond with the degree of marrow fibrosis (77). Amino terminal PTH values are also lower in patients with aluminum-related bone disease than

in patients with other histologic subtypes of renal osteodystrophy, but values remain elevated in some patients with evidence of bone aluminum toxicity (77). Thus, although patients with aluminum-related bone disease generally have lower serum PTH levels than those with osteitis fibrosa (Fig. 5), bone aluminum deposition must be documented by bone biopsy, and high serum PTH values do not exclude this diagnostic possibility.

Several recent reports confirm the utility of intact PTH measurements using an immunoradiometric assay in the assessment of patients with renal osteodystrophy (34,78,79). Cohen-Solal et al. found that intact PTH measurements were superior to other assays for separating patients with secondary hyperparathyroidism from those with adynamic lesions of bone (78). Most patients with bone biopsy-proven secondary hyperparathyroidism have serum intact PTH levels above 250–300 pg/ml, or 25–30 pM. In contrast, values in patients with adynamic lesions are usually below 150 pg/ml, or 15 pM, and levels frequently fall below 100 pg/ml, or 10 pM. Both in children and in adults with chronic renal failure, intact serum PTH levels that are 2–3 times the upper limit of normal for subjects with normal renal function correspond to normal rates of bone formation as documented by bone biopsy (78,79).

Plasma aluminum levels are elevated in patients with chronic renal failure and in those treated with maintenance

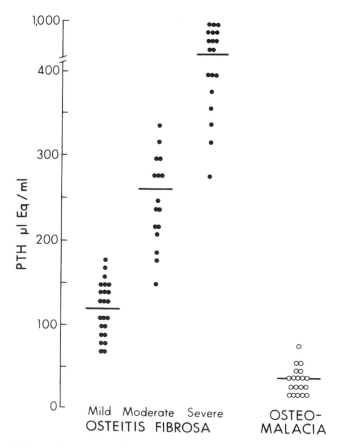

FIG. 5. Serum parathyroid hormone levels in adult dialyzed patients with mild, moderate, and severe osteitis fibrosa. Patients with osteomalacia have low values for iPTH.

dialysis if there is ongoing exposure to aluminum-containing medications or to inadequately purified dialysate water (80–82). The reported range of normal for plasma aluminum in humans varies considerably among laboratories, in part due to differences in methodology. Electrothermal atomic absorption spectrometry is an accurate and reproducible method for measuring aluminum in tissues and plasma, and values from reliable reference laboratories in normal subjects are usually less than 10 µg/L. Levels of 15–40 µg/L are common in patients undergoing regular dialysis who have previously ingested aluminum-containing medications (83,84), whereas values above 50 µg/L suggest some degree of aluminum loading. Aluminum levels in plasma reflect recent exposure to aluminum via either contaminated dialysate or aluminum-containing medications. Accordingly, plasma aluminum levels should be monitored at regular intervals in patients undergoing maintenance dialysis, particularly in those who continue to use aluminum-containing, phosphate-binding antacids.

Although plasma aluminum levels may correspond to the amount of aluminum ingested orally (Fig. 6), they do not accurately reflect the tissue stores of aluminum (85). Bone and liver represent major sites of aluminum deposition within the body, but tissue aluminum levels do not correspond to plasma values. Serum aluminum levels may fall substantially after aluminum-containing medications have been withdrawn despite evidence of substantial tissue stores of aluminum.

Deferoxamine (DFO) is a chelating agent that binds to aluminum, and infusions of DFO can mobilize aluminum from various tissues and markedly increase plasma aluminum levels in patients with aluminum-related bone disease. Deferoxamine has been used to treat patients with aluminum intoxication, often with dramatic clinical results

(86,87). Infusion of DFO can be used as a diagnostic test for the noninvasive assessment of aluminum loading in patients with chronic renal failure (83).

The DFO infusion test is completed as follows: patients are given a standardized intravenous dose of deferoxamine, 40 mg/kg in 100 ml of 5% dextrose solution, over 2 hours immediately after a hemodialysis procedure; plasma aluminum levels are measured before and 24–48 hours after the infusion. An increase in plasma aluminum greater than 300 µg/L above preinfusion levels is often a better predictor of bone aluminum deposition in symptomatic patients than measurements of basal plasma aluminum (83).

Unfortunately, the magnitude of the rise in plasma aluminum after DFO infusions is not highly specific when applied to the broader dialysis population (88). Hodsman et al. reported that dialysis patients with secondary hyperparathyroidism can exhibit substantial increases in plasma aluminum following infusions of DFO despite little evidence of stainable aluminum in bone biopsy specimens (84). Thus, some patients with osteitis fibrosa have high tissue levels of aluminum and a positive DFO infusion test but no histologic evidence of bone aluminum toxicity. Such patients may be at risk, however, of developing aluminum-related bone disease after parathyroidectomy or with prolonged treatment with maintenance dialysis.

ROENTGENOGRAPHIC FEATURES OF RENAL OSTEODYSTROPHY

Osteitis Fibrosa

Subperiosteal erosions are one of the most consistent radiographic findings in patients with secondary hyperparathyroidism, and the extent of this change often corresponds to the serum levels of PTH and alkaline phosphatase (89). Patchy osteosclerosis is also common, and this accounts for the classic "rugger jersey" appearance of the spine on lateral views of the thoracic vertebrae and the "salt-and-pepper" appearance of the skull. Skeletal roentgenographs may be normal, however, in patients with mild to moderate osteitis fibrosa. In contrast, subperiosteal erosions may be found in patients with aluminum-related bone disease and osteomalacia (90), emphasizing the need for independent biochemical or histologic confirmation of the diagnosis of secondary hyperparathyroidism.

Subperiosteal erosions can be detected at the surfaces of the digital phalanges (Fig. 7), at the distal ends of the clavicles, beneath the surfaces of the ischium and pubis, at the sacroiliac joints, and at the junction of the metaphysis and diaphysis of long bones. Fine-grain films and a hand lens of 6–7× magnification can help to detect erosions in radiographs of the hands (91). In pediatric patients, metaphyseal changes, i.e., growth zone lesions, are common, and these have been described as "rickets-like lesions." Mehls et al. demonstrated that this radiographic finding of secondary hyperparathyroidism differs from that of true vitamin D deficiency (47). Both subperiosteal erosions of the digits and growth zone lesions are best demonstrated by examining x-ray films of the hands; the presence of growth zone changes is a reliable indicator of the severity of secondary

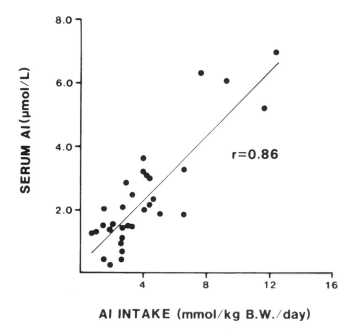

FIG. 6. Relationship between oral aluminum intake from aluminum hydroxide and serum aluminum levels in pediatric patients undergoing continuous ambulatory peritoneal dialysis. (From Salusky IB, et al: *J Pediatrics* 105:717, 1984, with permission.)

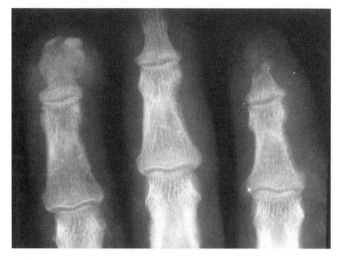

FIG. 7. Radiograph of the left hand showing abundant subperiosteal erosions of the phalanges in a patient with severe secondary hyperparathyroidism. The abnormalities are most pronounced on the radial surfaces.

hyperparathyroidism in children as judged by the serum levels of PTH and alkaline phosphatase (89).

Slipped epiphyses are among the most striking clinical and radiographic manifestations of renal osteodystrophy in children, and they are usually a consequence of advanced osteitis fibrosa in uremic children (47). The age of the patient often determines the site affected. In preschool children, epiphyseal slippage occurs in either the upper or lower femoral region or in the distal tibial epiphysis but not in the distal radius or distal ulna. In contrast, the upper femoral epiphysis and the distal epiphyses of the forearm are affected most often in older children. Severe epiphyseal slippage can lead to gross deformities of the skeleton with ulnar deviation of the hands and abnormalities in gait.

Osteomalacia

The roentgenographic features of osteomalacia are less specific than those of secondary hyperparathyroidism. Indeed, pseudofractures are the only pathognomonic finding in adult patients. These are straight, wide radiolucent bands in the cortex oriented perpendicular to the longitudinal axis of the bone. Fractures of the ribs and hips and compression fractures of the vertebral bodies are more common in dialysis patients with osteomalacia than in those with osteitis fibrosa (46).

Rickets-like lesions have also been described in pediatric patients with aluminum-related bone disease and osteomalacia, and these changes may resolve after treatment with deferoxamine (92). Rachitic lesions in pediatric patients are not specific, however, for any particular histologic lesion, and bone biopsy is usually required to determine the type of bone disease in pediatric patients with end-stage renal failure.

Amyloidosis

Cystic changes in bone, particularly if they are large, suggest amyloid deposition in bone. Cysts most commonly involve the metacarpals and regions immediately adjacent to large joints near the site of tendon insertions; the hip, wrist, proximal humerus, pubic ramus, and proximal tibia are affected most often, but the carpal and tarsal bones may also be involved (Fig. 8). X-rays may reveal fractures at the site of cyst formation. Multiple bone cysts suggest the presence of amyloidosis, whereas brown tumors more often occur as isolated cystic lesion, usually in the ribs or jaw.

Bone Scan

The compounds used most frequently for skeletal scintigraphy are technetium-labeled bisphosphonates, mainly ^{99}Tc-methylene diphosphonate. Bone scans can be useful for evaluating the severity of skeletal disease in patients with advanced renal failure, and they can help in assessing the response to therapy. Bone scintigraphy may reveal pseudofractures or extraskeletal calcifications, and local increases in the uptake of tracer can occur in areas of amyloid deposition. Patients with osteitis fibrosa often exhibit symmetric increases in isotope activity in the skull, mandible, sternum, shoulders, vertebral bodies, and distal portions of the femur and tibia; these findings have been termed the "superscan." In contrast, the skeletal uptake of isotopic tracers is less in patients with aluminum-related osteomalacia than in those with osteitis fibrosa (93). Despite these general trends, the findings on bone scan often do not agree closely with data obtained by histologic assessment (94); as such, bone scans

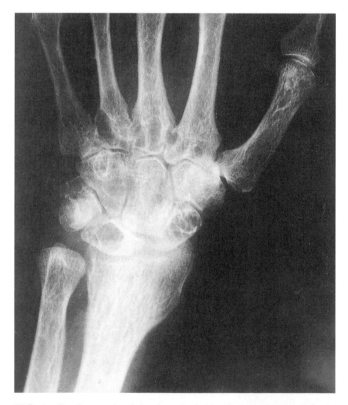

FIG. 8. Radiograph of the hand of a long-term hemodialysis patient showing cystic lesions due to β_2-microglobulin amyloidosis. (From Grateau G, et al: *Am J Kidney Dis* 11:231, 1988, with permission.)

provide supportive information, but they are of limited diagnostic value in the assessment of patients with renal bone disease.

TREATMENT OF RENAL OSTEODYSTROPHY

The successful clinical management of patients with renal osteodystrophy include interventions designed to correct or to counteract several major pathogenic factors. Important objectives include: (i) the maintenance of normal serum calcium and phosphorus levels; (ii) the prevention of extraskeletal calcifications; (iii) the avoidance of exposure to toxic agents such as aluminum and excess iron; (iv) the judicious use of vitamin D sterols; and (v) the appropriate use of chelating agents such as deferoxamine to treat aluminum intoxication.

Dietary Adjustments

Adequate control of serum phosphorus levels is important for the prevention of soft tissue calcifications and for the management of secondary hyperparathyroidism in patients with advanced renal failure. Dietary phosphorus restriction also may lower serum PTH levels in some patients with moderate renal failure (12). The dietary intake of phosphorus normally ranges from 1.0 to 1.8 g/day in adults, but it must be lowered to 400–800 mg/day to prevent hyperphosphatemia in patients with renal failure. Such diets are generally unpalatable, and long-term compliance is difficult to achieve (95). Consequently, phosphate-binding antacids are usually required to adequately control hyperphosphatemia when the glomerular filtration rate decreases to 25% to 30% of normal.

Phosphate-Binding Agents

Phosphate-binding antacids diminish intestinal phosphate absorption by forming poorly soluble complexes with phosphorus in the intestinal lumen. In the past, aluminum-containing, phosphate-binding gels were widely used, but aluminum loading and aluminum toxicity may develop because only limited amounts of aluminum are removed by dialysis and renal excretion is impaired (85). Both the duration of treatment and the daily dose of aluminum ingested influence the extent of aluminum retention in tissues (96–98). Generally, these compounds should be avoided in patients with end-stage renal disease. If aluminum-containing agents are used, the duration of treatment should be limited, doses must be kept as low as possible, and the concurrent administration of citrate-containing compounds must be carefully avoided. Aluminum levels in plasma should also be monitored at regular intervals.

A variety of calcium-containing compounds have been employed to lower intestinal phosphorus absorption, but calcium carbonate is currently the most widely utilized agent. Calcium carbonate can adequately control serum phosphorus levels in patients undergoing maintenance dialysis (Fig. 9) although hypercalcemia remains the major side effect (99,100). The regular use of dialysate containing 2.5

mEq/L rather than 3.5 mEq/L of calcium can reduce the frequency of hypercalcemic episodes in patients ingesting calcium carbonate (101,102).

When used as a phosphate-binding agent, calcium carbonate should be ingested with meals to increase the efficiency of phosphate binding and to minimize intestinal calcium absorption. Doses in individual patients range from 4 to 15 g/day. Some patients require combined therapy with aluminum hydroxide and calcium carbonate to achieve adequate control of serum phosphorus levels. Fournier et al. reported that only 50% of adult patients undergoing long-term dialysis achieved adequate control of serum phosphorus levels when calcium carbonate was given as the only phosphate-binding agent (103). The adverse effects associated with the use of very large doses of oral calcium in patients with renal failure remain to be determined. Of greatest concern is the development of soft tissue and vascular calcifications, but no increase in the prevalence of vascular calcification was found in adult patients treated for 3 years (104).

Calcium acetate has also been used to control hyperphosphatemia in patients with chronic renal failure (105,106). *In vitro* studies and short-term *in vivo* assessments indicate that calcium acetate binds more phosphorus than equivalent doses of either calcium carbonate or aluminum hydroxide. The frequency of hypercalcemic episodes was no less, however, in patients given calcium acetate than in those receiving calcium carbonate (107).

Calcium citrate is an effective phosphate-binding agent, but the role of citrate in enhancing intestinal aluminum absorption is a major concern for patients who may be given other medications that contain aluminum (30,108). Generally, calcium citrate should be avoided in patients with chronic renal failure. Magnesium oxide was reported to be ineffective or poorly tolerated in two studies (109), whereas magnesium carbonate was effective when used in conjunction with magnesium-free dialysate in patients undergoing regular hemodialysis (110).

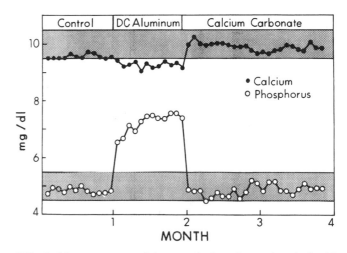

FIG. 9. Mean serum calcium and phosphorus levels in 20 adult dialyzed patients during the three phases of the 4-month study. (From Slatopolsky E, et al: *N Engl J Med* 315:157, 1986, with permission.)

Vitamin D Sterols

Despite dietary phosphate restriction, maintenance of an adequate dietary calcium intake, the use of appropriate levels of calcium in dialysate, and the regular use of phosphate-binding agents, a substantial proportion of patients receiving regular dialysis develop secondary hyperparathyroidism. Consequently, the administration of active vitamin D sterols is required in many patients. Although calcifediol, or 25-hydroxyvitamin D, 1α-hydroxyvitamin D, and dihydrotachysterol have all proven to be effective in the management of secondary hyperparathyroidism, calcitriol is by far the most widely used agent in the United States.

The efficacy of daily oral doses of calcitriol in the treatment of patients with symptomatic renal osteodystrophy has been documented in several clinical trials (111,112). Bone pain diminishes, muscle strength and gait posture improve, and osteitis fibrosa frequently resolves either partially or completely (113). When measured using reliable assays, serum PTH levels decrease in patients who respond favorably to treatment. Growth velocity has been reported to increase during calcitriol therapy in some children with chronic renal failure (50).

Similar findings have been reported in patients treated with daily doses of oral 1α-hydroxyvitamin D, which undergoes 25-hydroxylation in the liver to form calcitriol (114,115); this agent is widely used in Europe and Japan. Overall, calcitriol and 1α-hydroxyvitamin D are similarly effective for the treatment of secondary hyperparathyroidism in patients with chronic renal failure. Doses of oral calcitriol in most clinical trials have ranged from 0.25 to 1.5 μg/day. Hypercalcemia is the most common side effect, but most adult patients tolerate daily doses of 0.25–0.50 μg without marked increases in serum calcium levels; children may require somewhat larger daily oral doses of calcitriol.

Treatment is started using small doses, and these are periodically adjusted to maintain serum calcium levels between 10.5 and 11.0 mg/dl; such an approach lowers serum PTH levels in many patients (89). Because the biological half-life of calcitriol is relatively short, episodes of hypercalcemia resolve within several days after treatment is withheld.

The development of hypercalcemia during calcitriol therapy may predict the underlying type of skeletal lesion. When hypercalcemia occurs after many weeks or months of treatment and previously elevated serum PTH and alkaline phosphatase levels have returned toward normal, it is likely that osteitis fibrosa has substantially resolved. In contrast, hypercalcemia that occurs within the first several weeks of treatment suggests the presence of aluminum-related bone disease or severe secondary hyperparathyroidism (113). If there is evidence of autonomous hyperparathyroidism, parathyroidectomy may be required.

Large intermittent doses of oral calcitriol have also been used to treat secondary hyperparathyroidism in patients undergoing regular dialysis (116,117). When given two or three times per week, the cumulative weekly dose of calcitriol that can be delivered is greater, and higher peak serum levels of 1,25-dihydroxyvitamin D are achieved after each dose. As such, intermittent large oral doses of calcitriol may be more effective than smaller daily doses in reducing PTH gene transcription and lowering serum PTH levels in patients with secondary hyperparathyroidism. Dosage regimens have ranged from 0.5–1.0 μg to 3.5–4.0 μg thrice weekly or 2.0–5.0 μg twice weekly; low doses should be used initially, and adjustments must be based on frequent measurements of serum calcium and phosphorus levels.

Slatopolsky et al. initially demonstrated that the intravenous administration of calcitriol thrice weekly markedly lowered serum PTH levels in adult hemodialysis patients (118). A portion of this response appears to be independent of changes in serum ionized calcium, findings which suggest that calcitriol may have direct *in vivo* effects to reduce PTH synthesis and/or release (118). Intravenous calcitriol is now the most widely used approach for the treatment of secondary hyperparathyroidism in patients undergoing regular hemodialysis. Advantages of intravenous calcitriol include assured patient compliance, convenience of therapy because doses are given during regularly scheduled hemodialysis treatments, and the ability to achieve very high serum levels of 1,25-dihydroxyvitamin D after bolus intravenous injections (119). As with intermittent oral calcitriol therapy, the calcemic response to thrice weekly doses of intravenous calcitriol is less than with daily oral calcitriol; thus, larger weekly doses of 1,25-dihydroxyvitamin D can be given that may enhance the delivery of calcitriol to the parathyroid glands and promote its suppressive effect on PTH secretion (119).

Unfortunately, intravenous calcitriol therapy is not feasible for patients undergoing peritoneal dialysis. Intraperitoneal calcitriol administration can lower serum PTH levels in patients with secondary hyperparathyroidism (120), but concern about increasing the risk of peritonitis by using the intraperitoneal route of drug administration makes this therapeutic alternative less appealing than intermittent oral calcitriol for those receiving peritoneal dialysis.

An intermittent, rather than a daily, schedule of calcitriol administration may improve therapeutic efficacy in patients with established secondary hyperparathyroidism. Bone formation and turnover may fall dramatically, however, during both intermittent oral and intermittent intravenous calcitriol therapy. As such, adynamic lesions of bone develop in some patients. Serum PTH levels should be monitored during intermittent calcitriol therapy, and the dose of calcitriol should be reduced substantially or discontinued when values fall to levels that are 3–4 times the upper limit of normal.

Parathyroidectomy

Certain events indicate the need to consider parathyroid surgery in patients with advanced secondary hyperparathyroidism. In all instances, the diagnosis of aluminum-related bone disease must be considered and excluded prior to parathyroidectomy, and evidence of severe secondary hyperparathyroidism should be adequately documented by biochemical, radiographic, and, if necessary, bone histologic criteria (3). Specific indications for parathyroidectomy include (i) persistent hypercalcemia with serum calcium levels above 11.5–12.0 mg/dl; (ii) intractable pruritus that does not respond to intensive dialysis or to other medical interventions; (iii) progressive extraskeletal calcifications and/or persistent hyperphosphatemia despite the continued and appropriate use of dietary phosphorus restriction and phosphate-binding agents; (iv) severe bone pain or fractures; and (v) development of calciphylaxis (121). Other causes of hypercalcemia such as sarcoidosis, malignancy, and excessive calcium or vitamin D intake must also be considered and excluded. Because the risk of aluminum toxicity is greater after parathyroidectomy, aluminum hydroxide should be avoided, and calcium carbonate should be used as the sole phosphate-binding agent after parathyroid surgery.

There is ongoing disagreement about the use of subtotal vs. total parathyroidectomy in patients with chronic renal failure. The substantial incidence of recurrent secondary hyperparathyroidism in patients undergoing subtotal parathyroidectomy is a legitimate concern, and the availability of calcitriol and other active vitamin D sterols greatly facilitates the management of hypocalcemia after total parathyroidectomy. For patients who may subsequently undergo renal transplantation, the preservation of some parathyroid tissue with subtotal parathyroidectomy may help to maintain calcium homeostasis when renal function is restored. The implantation of parathyroid tissue removed at surgery into the forearm or other sites is not recommended. Such grafts occasionally spread locally into surrounding tissues leading to recurrent hyperparathyroidism, and adequate surgical resection may be difficult.

Management of Aluminum Intoxication

The clinical manifestations and histologic features of aluminum-related bone disease have been shown to improve during deferoxamine (DFO) therapy in patients undergoing regular dialysis (86,88). Aluminum removal during both hemodialysis and peritoneal dialysis increases substantially after intravenous or subcutaneous doses of DFO (122,123). After 4–10 months of therapy, clinical improvement has been observed in a large proportion of patients with severe bone disease (86,124). Analgesic use decreased and patients who were confined to bed or a wheelchair were able to resume walking without assistance.

Typical biochemical changes after DFO treatment include reductions in serum calcium and increases in serum alkaline phosphatase levels, findings consistent with an improvement in skeletal mineralization. Serum PTH levels rise modestly in most patients, but it is not known as to whether this change is due to aluminum removal from the parathyroid glands or to a fall in serum calcium levels. Serial bone biopsies generally show an increase in bone formation and improvements in mineralization; indeed, some patients with low-turnover lesions of bone may develop osteitis fibrosa (86). The amount of surface stainable aluminum in bone decreases in most patients who improve with treatment, but patients who have undergone previous parathyroidectomy may respond less well or not at all (86). As such, adequate parathyroid gland function may be important for skeletal recovery in patients with aluminum intoxication.

Unfortunately, serious and often lethal infections with *Rhizopus* and *Yersinia* species have been documented in dialysis patients given DFO (125–129). In one series, 6 of 131 patients treated with DFO over a 3-year period were affected (125). The chelation of iron by DFO enhances iron delivery to certain organisms, increasing their pathogenic potential (130–132). These observations raise serious concerns about appropriate use of DFO for the treatment of aluminum intoxication in patients undergoing regular dialysis.

Deferoxamine should be given only to patients with symptomatic aluminum intoxication, and evidence of tissue toxicity should be fully documented before therapy is begun. Doses of DFO should not exceed 0.5–1.0 g/week, and plasma aluminum levels should be measured regularly. In asymptomatic patients with aluminum deposition in bone, bone histology and bone formation can improve without the use of DFO after completely withdrawing aluminum-containing medications and using calcium carbonate as the sole phosphate-binding agent (133).

BONE AND MINERAL METABOLISM IN RENAL TRANSPLANT RECIPIENTS

Although the restoration of kidney function after successful renal transplantation corrects many of the disturbances that lead to renal osteodystrophy, disorders of bone and mineral metabolism remain a major clinical problem in renal transplant recipients. Indeed, as many as 80% to 90% of patients have histologic evidence of bone disease 5 years after transplantation (134,135). In these patients, alterations in bone and mineral homeostasis can be a manifestation of preexisting renal osteodystrophy or the result of changes peculiar to the posttransplant setting.

Hypercalcemia is not uncommon after renal transplantation; its frequency corresponds to the duration of previous dialysis treatment and probably to the degree of parathyroid gland hyperplasia at the time of transplantation (136). Several other factors also contribute. The presence of a functioning renal allograft rapidly corrects the deficit in renal 1,25-dihydroxyvitamin D production that is characteristic of chronic renal failure, and calcitriol synthesis is further enhanced by the resolution of hyperphosphatemia. Since the reversal of parathyroid gland hyperplasia may take many months or years, most patients exhibit persistently high serum PTH levels in the immediate posttransplant period, and this change also promotes renal calcitriol production. Overall, these factors lead to increased intestinal calcium absorption, enhanced calcium mobilization from bone, and increased renal tubular calcium reabsorption, each of which can contribute to the development of hypercalcemia.

Hypercalcemia during the first several months after renal transplantation can be quite severe, and serum calcium levels may reach 15 mg/dl. Hypercalcemia can lead to allograft dysfunction, and peripheral ischemia may develop on rare occasion due to extensive vascular calcification, i.e., calciphylaxis (53). Those with advanced secondary hyperparathyroidism prior to transplantation are at greatest risk. More often, the degree of hypercalcemia after renal transplantation is less severe. Serum calcium levels usually range from 10.5 to 12.0 mg/dl in such cases, and episodes of hypercalcemia are intermittent and of short duration; the disorder usually resolves within 12 months (137). In 4% to 10% of patients, mild to moderate hypercalcemia can persist for more than a year and as long as 5 years. Serum calcium levels between 10.5 and 12.0 mg/dl are usually well tolerated without adverse effects on renal allograft function (138), but elective parathyroidectomy should be considered when serum calcium levels persistently exceed 12.5 mg/dl more than 1 year following renal transplantation (139).

Hypophosphatemia is common in the early postoperative period after renal transplantation. Persistent secondary hyperparathyroidism is the major contributor, leading to reduced renal tubular phosphate reabsorption and increased renal phosphate excretion. Primary defects in the tubular reabsorption of phosphorus occasionally occur, however, and some patients excrete large amounts of phosphorus in the urine despite normal levels of PTH in serum. Pharmacologic doses of glucocorticoids also increase renal phosphorus excretion, and this may further aggravate renal phosphate wasting (140).

The clinical manifestations of hypophosphatemia are variable; some patients complain of malaise, fatigue, and proximal muscle weakness (141). Although hypophosphatemia can persist for many months, osteomalacia rarely develops (142). Symptomatic patients with serum phosphorus levels below 1.0 mg/dl should be given oral phosphorus supplements, and the serum phosphorus level should be monitored regularly. In those who require supplemental phosphorus, potassium rather than sodium salts should be used to avoid extracellular volume expansion which increases renal phosphate excretion by lowering phosphate reabsorption in the proximal nephron.

Osteopenia is common following renal transplantation, and evidence of reduced bone mass is found in nearly all patients within 5 years (134,135,143). Substantial decreases in bone mass have been documented within the first 6–18 months after renal transplantation; these changes are associated with histologic evidence of diminished bone formation and turnover, findings consistent with the known effects of glucocorticoids on bone (144). The development of osteopenia is not confined, however, to renal transplant recipients, and reductions in bone mass have been demonstrated in patients undergoing cardiac and hepatic transplantation (145).

The use of large, immunosuppressive doses of corticosteroids is generally considered to be a major contributor to the development of osteopenia in transplant recipients. Glucocorticoids directly inhibit osteoblastic activity and collagen synthesis, and they impede the differentiation of progenitor cells into fully mature osteoblasts. Glucocorticoids also accelerate bone resorption by lowering intestinal calcium absorption, thereby inducing a mild state of secondary hyperparathyroidism.

The effects of cyclosporine on human bone have not been well characterized. Movsowitz et al. demonstrated increases in bone remodeling with reductions in cancellous bone volume, but there was no change in the serum levels of calcium, magnesium, 1,25-dihydroxyvitamin D, or PTH in rats given cyclosporine (146). Stewart and coworkers reported that cyclosporine inhibited *in vitro* bone resorption in a dose-dependent manner during incubations with PTH, 1,25-dihydroxyvitamin D, and interleukin-1 (147). Although preliminary data in humans suggest that cyclosporine may decrease the incidence of osteonecrosis in renal transplant recipients by lowering the dose of prednisone required for adequate immunosuppression (148), the effects of this immunosuppressive agent on bone and mineral metabolism require further investigation.

Measures that are effective for the prevention of bone loss in transplant recipients have yet to be identified, but few studies have been done. Newer synthetic derivatives of prednisolone, such as deflazacort, are effective immunosuppressive agents, and they appear to have fewer adverse effects on bone and mineral metabolism. Such agents may be of benefit for the management of transplant recipients in the future but await fuller clinical evaluation.

Osteonecrosis, or avascular necrosis, is by far the most debilitating skeletal complication associated with transplantation surgery. Approximately 15% of patients will develop osteonecrosis within 3 years of renal transplantation (149,150). The occurrence of osteonecrosis in patients undergoing cardiac, hepatic, and bone marrow transplantation as well as in those with systemic lupus erythematosus given high doses of corticosteroids strongly suggests that glucocorticoids play a critical pathogenic role (151,152).

The mechanism by which corticosteroids contribute to the development of osteonecrosis has not been established. These agents may promote the accumulation of fat cells within the marrow space, thereby increasing intraosseous hydrostatic pressure and altering blood flow within bone (153). Alternatively, corticosteroids may interfere with the process of microfracture repair, leading to a loss of the structural integrity of bone.

Osteonecrosis usually begins in weight-bearing areas; the femoral head and femoral neck are the sites most commonly affected in adults, but the distal femur, proximal tibia, and humeral head can also be affected (154). Osteonecrosis can occur at several sites in an individual patient. Thus, Ibels et al. found two sites of involvement in 85% of renal transplant recipients whereas three or more areas were affected in 27% of patients (155). Risk factors for osteonecrosis include the cumulative dose of corticosteroids, advanced age, and duration of dialysis prior to transplantation.

ACKNOWLEDGMENTS

Supported in part by USPHS grants RR-00865 and DK-35423.

REFERENCES

1. Goodman WG: Aluminum metabolism and the uremic patient. In: Simpson DJ (ed) *Nutrition and Bone Development.* New York, Oxford University Press, pp 269–294, 1990
2. Kleinman KS, Coburn JW: Amyloid syndromes associated with hemodialysis. *Kidney Int* 35:567–575, 1989
3. Coburn JW, Slatopolsky E: Vitamin D, parathyroid hormone, and the renal osteodystrophies. In: Brenner B, Rector F (eds) *The Kidney.* 4th ed. Philadelphia, WB Saunders, p 2076, 1990
4. Morrissey J, Rothstein M, Mayor G: Suppression of parathyroid hormone secretion by aluminum. *Kidney Int* 23:699–704, 1983
5. Sedman AB, Alfrey AC, Miller NL, Goodman WG: Tissue and cellular basis for impaired bone formation in aluminum-related osteomalacia in the pig. *J Clin Invest* 79:86–92, 1987
6. Blumenthal NC, Posner AS: In vitro model of aluminum-induced osteomalacia: inhibition of hydroxyapatite formation and growth. *Calcif Tissue Int* 36:439–441, 1984
7. Sherrard DJ, Ott SM, Maloney NA, Andress DL, Coburn JW: Uremic osteodystrophy: Classification, cause and treatment. In:

Frame B, Potts J (eds) *Clinical Disorders of Bone and Mineral Metabolism*. Amsterdam, Excerpta Medica, pp 254–259, 1983

8. Salusky IB, Coburn JW, Brill J, et al: Bone disease in pediatric patients undergoing dialysis with CAPD or CCPD. *Kidney Int* 33: 975–982, 1988

9. Goodman WG, Leite Duarte ME: Aluminum: effects on bone and role in the pathogenesis of renal osteodystrophy. *Min Electrolyte Metab* 17:221–232, 1991

10. Slatopolsky E, Caglar S, Pennell JP, et al: On the pathogenesis of hyperparathyroidism in chronic experimental renal insufficiency in the dog. *J Clin Invest* 50:492–499, 1971

11. Llach F, Massry SG: On the mechanism of secondary hyperparathyroidism in moderate renal insufficiency. *J Clin Endocrinol Metab* 61:601–606, 1985

12. Portale AA, Booth BE, Halloran BP, Morris RC Jr: Effect of dietary phosphorus on circulating concentrations of 1,25-dihydroxyvitamin D and immunoreactive parathyroid hormone in children with moderate renal insufficiency. *J Clin Invest* 73: 1580–1589, 1984

13. Coburn JW, Kopple JD, Brickman AS: Study of intestinal absorption of calcium in patients with renal failure. *Kidney Int* 3: 264–272, 1973

14. Korkor AB: Reduced binding of 3H-1,25-dihydroxyvitamin D in the parathyroid glands of patients with renal failure. *N Engl J Med* 316:1573–1577, 1987

15. Strom M, Sandgren ME, Brown TA, DeLuca HF: 1,25-Dihydroxyvitamin D_3 up-regulates the 1,25-dihydroxyvitamin D_3 receptor in vivo. *Proc Natl Acad Sci USA* 86:9770–9773, 1989

16. Brown EM, Wilson RE, Eastman RC, Pallotta J, Marynick S: Abnormal regulation of parathyroid hormone release by calcium in secondary hyperparathyroidism due to chronic renal failure. *J Clin Endocrinol Metab* 54:172–179, 1982

17. Felsenfeld AJ, Llach F: Parathyroid gland function in chronic renal failure. *Kidney Int* 43:771–789, 1993

18. Delmez JA, Tindira C, Grooms P, Dusso A, Windus DW, Slatopolsky E. PTH suppression by intravenous 1,25-dihydroxyvitamin D. A role for increased sensitivity to calcium. *J Clin Invest* 83:1349–1355, 1989

19. Dunlay R, Rodriguez M, Felsenfeld AJ, Llach F. Direct inhibitory effect of calcitriol on parathyroid function (sigmoidal curve) in dialysis. *Kidney Int* 36:1093–1098, 1989

20. Ramirez JA, Goodman WG, Gornbein J, et al: Direct in vivo comparison of calcium-regulated PTH secretion in normal volunteers and patients with secondary hyperparathyroidism. *J Clin Endocrinol Metab* 76:1489–1494, 1993

21. Ramirez JA, Goodman WG, Belin T, Gales B, Segre GV, Salusky IB: Calcitriol therapy and calcium-regulated PTH secretion in patients with secondary hyperparathyroidism. *Am J Physiol (Endocrinol Metab)* 267:E961–967, 1994

22. Goodman WG, Belin T, Gales B, Jüppner H, Segre GV, Salusky IB: Calcium-regulated parathyroid hormone release in patients with mild or advanced secondary hyperparathyroidism. *Kidney Int* 148:1553–1558, 1995

23. Sanchez CP, Goodman WG, Ramirez JA, Gales B, Belin TR, Segre GV, Salusky IB: Calcium-regulated parathyroid hormone secretion in adynamic renal osteodystrophy. *Kidney Int* 48:838–843, 1995

24. Szabo A, Merke J, Beier E, Mall G, Ritz E: 1,25(OH)2 vitamin D_3 inhibits parathyroid cell proliferation in experimental uremia. *Kidney Int* 35:1049–1056, 1989

25. Fukuda N, Tanaka H, Tominaga Y, Fukagawa M, Kurokawa K, Seino Y. Decreased 1,25-dihydroxyvitamin D_3 receptor density is associated with a more severe form of parathyroid hyperplasia in chronic uremic patients. *J Clin Invest* 92:1436–1443, 1993

26. DeFrancisco AM, Ellis HA, Owen JP, et al: Parathyroidectomy in chronic renal failure. *Q J Med (New Series)* 55:289–315, 1985

27. Arnold A, Brown MF, Ureña P, Gaz RD, Sarfati E, Drüeke TB: Monoclonality of parathyroid tumors in chronic renal failure and in primary parathyroid hyperplasia. *J Clin Invest* 95:2047–2053, 1995

28. Massry SG, Coburn JW, Lee DBN, Jowsey J, Kleeman CR: Skeletal resistance to parathyroid hormone in renal failure. *Ann Intern Med* 78:357–364, 1973

29. Pei Y, Hercz G, Greenwood C, et al: Non-invasive prediction of

aluminum bone disease in hemo- and peritoneal dialysis patients. *Kidney Int* 41:1374–1382, 1992

30. Molitoris BA, Froment DH, Mackenzie TA, Huffer WH, Alfrey AC: Citrate: a major factor in the toxicity of orally administered aluminum compounds. *Kidney Int* 36:949–953, 1989

31. Froment DP, Molitoris BA, Buddington B, Miller N, Alfrey AC: Site and mechanism of enhanced gastrointestinal absorption of aluminum by citrate. *Kidney Int* 36:978–984, 1989

32. de Vernejoul MC, Marchais S, London G, Morieux C, Bielakoff J, Miravet L: Increased bone aluminum deposition after subtotal parathyroidectomy in dialyzed patients. *Kidney Int* 27:785–791, 1985

33. Felsenfeld AJ, Harrelson JM, Gutman RA, Wells SA, Drezner MK: Osteomalacia after parathyroidectomy in patients with uremia. *Ann Intern Med* 960:34–39, 1982

34. Salusky IB, Ramirez JA, Oppenheim WL, Gales B, Segre GV, Goodman WG: Biochemical markers of renal osteodystrophy in pediatric patients undergoing CAPD/CCPD. *Kidney Int* 45:253–258, 1994

35. Eastwood JB, Harris E, Stamp TCB, de Wardener HE: Vitamin D deficiency in the osteomalacia of chronic renal failure. *Lancet* 2: 1209–1211, 1976

36. Pierides AM, Ellis HA, Ward M, et al: Barbiturate and anticonvulsant treatment in relation to osteomalacia with haemodialysis and renal transplantation. *Br Med J* 1:190–193, 1976

37. Sherrard DJ, Hercz G, Pei Y, et al: The spectrum of bone disease in end-stage renal failure—an evolving disorder. *Kidney Int* 43: 436–442, 1993

38. Llach F, Felsenfeld AJ, Coleman MD, Pederson JA: Prevalence of various types of bone disease in dialysis patients. In: Robinson RR (ed) *Nephrology, Proceedings of the Ninth International Congress of Nephrology*. vol II. New York, Springer-Verlag, pp 1375–1382, 1984

39. Hodsman AB, Sherrard DJ, Alfrey AC, et al: Bone aluminum and histomorphometric features of renal osteodystrophy. *J Clin Endocrinol Metab* 54:539–546, 1982

40. Andress DL, Maloney NA, Endres DB, Sherrard DJ: Aluminum-associated bone disease in chronic renal failure: high prevalence in a long-term dialysis population. *J Bone Min Res* 1:391–398, 1986

41. Goodman WG: Short-term aluminum administration in the rat: reductions in bone formation without osteomalacia. *J Lab Clin Med* 103:749–57, 1984

42. Parisien M, Charhon SA, Arlot M, et al: Evidence for a toxic effect of aluminum on osteoblasts: a histomorphometric study in hemodialysis patients with aplastic bone disease. *J Bone Min Res* 3:259–267, 1988

43. Pei Y, Hercz G, Greenwood C, et al: Risk factors for renal osteodystrophy: A multivariant analysis. *J Bone Min Res* 10:149–156, 1995

44. Sherrard DJ, Baylink DJ, Wergedal JE, Maloney NA: Quantitative histological studies on the pathogenesis of uremic bone disease. *J Clin Endocrinol Metab* 39:119–135, 1974

45. Sherrard DJ: Renal osteodystrophy. *Semin Nephrol* 6:56–67, 1986

46. Llach F, Felsenfeld AJ, Coleman MD, Keveney JJ Jr, Pederson JA, Medlock TR: The natural course of dialysis osteomalacia. *Kidney Int* 29:S74–79, 1986

47. Mehls O. Renal osteodystrophy in children: etiology and clinical aspects. In: Fine RN, Gruskin AB (eds) *Endstage Renal Disease in Children*. Philadelphia, WB Saunders, pp 227–250, 1984

48. Salusky IB, Brill J, Oppenheim W, Goodman WG: Features of renal osteodystrophy in pediatric patients receiving regular peritoneal dialysis. *Semin Nephrol* 9:37–42, 1989

49. Stickler GB, Bergen BJ: A review: short stature in renal disease. *Pediatr Res* 7:978–982, 1973

50. Chesney RW, Moorthy AV, Eisman JA, Tax DK, Mazess RB, De Luca HF: Increased growth after long-term oral 1,25–vitamin D_3 in childhood renal osteodystrophy. *N Engl J Med* 298:238–242, 1978

51. Meema HE, Oreopoulos DG, Rapoport A: Serum magnesium and arterial calcification in end-stage renal disease. *Kidney Int* 32: 388–394, 1987

52. Ibels LS, Alfrey AC, Huffer WE, Craswell PW, Anderson JT,

Weil R III: Arterial calcification and pathology in uremic patients undergoing dialysis. *Am J Med* 66:790–796, 1979

53. Gipstein RM, Coburn JW, Adams JA, et al: Calciphylaxis in man: A syndrome of tissue necrosis and vascular calcification in 11 patients with chronic renal failure. *Arch Intern Med* 136:1273–1280, 1976

54. Bardin T, Kuntz D, Zingraff J, Voisin MC, Zelmar A, Lansaman J: Synovial amyloidosis in patients undergoing long-term hemodialysis. *Arthritis Rheum* 28:1052–1058, 1985

55. Koch KM: Dialysis-related amyloidosis. *Kidney Int* 41:1416–1429, 1992

56. Bazzi C, Arrigo G, Luciani L, et al: Clinical features of 24 patients on regular hemodialysis treatment (RDT) for 16-23 years in a single unit. *Clin Nephrol* 44:96–107, 1995

57. Zingraff J, Drüeke T: Can the nephrologist prevent dialysis-related amyloidosis? *Am J Kidney Dis* 18:1–11, 1991

58. Gejyo F, Homma N, Suzuki M, Arakawa KM: Serum levels of β-2-microglobulin as a new form of amyloid protein in patients undergoing long-term hemodialysis. *N Engl J Med* 314:585–586, 1986

59. Miyata T, Inagi R, Iida Y, et al: Involvement of β2-microglobulin modified with advanced glycation end products in the pathogenesis of hemodialysis-associated amyloidosis. Induction of human monoctye chemotaxis and macrophage secretion of tumor necrosis factor-a and interleukin-1. *J Clin Invest* 93:521–528, 1994

60. Linke RP, Hampl H, Lobeck H, et al: Lysine-specific cleavage of β2-microglobulin in amyloid deposits associated with hemodialysis. *Kidney Int* 36:675–681, 1989

61. Campistol JM, Shirahama T, Abraham CR, et al: Demonstration of plasma proteinase inhibitors in β2-microglobulin amyloid deposits. *Kidney Int* 42:915–923, 1992

62. Campistol JM, Cases A, Torras A, et al: Visceral involvement of dialysis amyloidosis. *Am J Nephrol* 7:390–393, 1987

63. van Ypersele de Strihou C, Jadoul M, Malghem J, Maldague B, Jamart J: The Working Party on Dialysis Amyloidosis. Effect of dialysis membrane and patient's age on signs of dialysis-related amyloidosis. *Kidney Int* 39:1012–1019, 1991

64. Ohashi K, Hara M, Kawai R, et al: Cervical discs are most susceptible to beta2-microglobulin amyloid deposition in the vertebral column. *Kidney Int* 41:1646–1654, 1992

65. Onishi S, Andress DL, Maloney NA, Coburn JW, Sherrard DJ: Bone deposition of beta-2-microglobulin in hemodialysis patients. *Kidney Int* 39:990–995, 1991

66. McMahon LP, Radford J, Dawborn JK: Shoulder ultrasound in dialysis-related amyloidosis. *Clin Nephrol* 35:227–232, 1991

67. Jadoul M, Malgehm J, Pirson Y, Maldague B, van Ypersele de Strihou CA: Effect of renal transplantation on the radiological signs of dialysis amyloid osteoarthropathy. *Clin Nephrol* 32:194–197, 1989

68. Stewart WK, Fleming LW: The effects of dialysate magnesium on plasma and erythocyte magnesium and potassium concentrations during maintenance haemodialysis. *Nephron* 10:221–231, 1973

69. Guillot AP, Hood VL, Runge CF, Gennari FJ: The use of magnesium-containing phosphate binders in patients with end-stage renal disease on maintenance hemodialysis. *Nephron* 30:114–117, 1982

70. Hruska KA, Teitelbaum SL, Kopelman R, et al: The predictability of the histological features if uremic bone disease by non-invasive techniques. *Metab Bone Dis Relat Res* 1:39–44, 1978

71. Coburn JW, Norris KC: Diagnosis of aluminum-related bone disease and treatment of aluminum toxicity with deferoxamine. *Semin Nephrol* 6 (Suppl 1):12–21, 1986

72. Charhon SA, Delmas PD, Malaval L, et al: Serum bone Gla-protein in renal osteodystrophy: comparison with bone histomorphometry. *J Clin Endocrinol Metab* 63:892–897, 1986

73. Epstein S, Traberg H, Raja R, et al: Serum and dialysate osteocalcin levels in hemodialysis and peritoneal dialysis patients and after renal transplantation. *J Clin Endocrinol Metab* 60:1253–1256, 1985

74. Freitag J, Martin KJ, Hruska KA, et al: Impaired parathyroid hormone metabolism in patients with chronic renal failure. *N Engl J Med* 298:29–32, 1978

75. Segre GV: Amino-terminal radioimmunoassays for parathyroid hormone. In: Frame B, Potts JT Jr (eds) *Clinical Disorders of Bone and Mineral Metabolism.* Amsterdam, Excerpta Medica, pp 14–17, 1983

76. Nussbaum SR, Zahradnik RJ, Lavigne JR, et al: Highly sensitive two-site immunoradiometric assay of parathyrin, and its clinical utility in evaluating patients with hypercalcemia. *Clin Chem* 33:1364–1367, 1987

77. Andress DL, Endres DB, Ott SM, Sherrard DJ: Parathyroid hormone in aluminum bone disease: a comparison of parathyroid hormone assays. *Kidney Int* 29 (Suppl 18):S87–90, 1986

78. Cohen-Solal ME, Sebert JL, Boudailliez B, et al: Comparison of intact, midregion, and carboxy-terminal assays of parathyroid hormone for the diagnosis of bone disease in hemodialyzed patients. *J Clin Endocrinol Metab* 73:516–524, 1991.

79. Quarles LD, Lobaugh B, Murphy G: Intact parathyroid hormone overestimates the presence and severity of parathyroid-mediated osseous abnormalities in uremia. *J Clin Endocrinol Metab* 75:145–150, 1992

80. Pierides AM, Edwards WG Jr, Cullu US Jr, McCall JT, Ellis HA: Hemodialysis encephalopathy with osteomalacic fractures and muscle weakness. *Kidney Int* 18:115–124, 1980

81. Felsenfeld AJ, Gutman RA, Llach F, Harrelson JM: Osteomalacia in chronic renal failure: a syndrome previously reported only with maintenance dialysis. *Am J Nephrol* 2:147–154, 1982

82. Coburn JW, Nebeker HG, Hercz G, et al: Role of aluminum accumulation in the pathogenesis of renal osteodystrophy. In: Robinson RR (ed) *Nephrology.* vol. 2. New York, Springer-Verlag, pp 1383–1395, 1984

83. Milliner DS, Nebeker HG, Ott SM, et al: Use of the deferoxamine infusion test in the diagnosis of aluminum-related osteodystrophy. *Ann Intern Med* 101:775–779, 1984

84. Hodsman AB, Hood SA, Brown P, Cordy PE: Do serum aluminum levels reflect underlying skeletal aluminum accumulation and bone histology before or after chelation by deferoxamine. *J Lab Clin Med* 106:674–681, 1985

85. Alfrey AC: Aluminum metabolism. *Kidney Int* 29 (Suppl 18):S8–S11, 1986

86. Ott SM, Andress DL, Nebeker HG, et al: Changes in bone histology after treatment with desferrioxamine. *Kidney Int* 29 (Suppl 18):S108–113, 1986

87. Ackrill P, Ralston AJ, Day JP, Hodge KC: Successful removal of aluminum from a patient with dialysis encephalopathy. *Lancet* 2:692–693, 1980

88. Malluche HH, Smith AJ, Abreo K, Faugere MC: The use of deferoxamine in the management of aluminium accumulation in bone in patients with renal failure. *N Engl J Med* 311:140–144, 1984

89. Salusky IB, Fine RN, Kangarloo H, et al: "High-dose" calcitriol for control of renal osteodystrophy in children on CAPD. *Kidney Int* 32:89–95, 1987

90. Shimada H, Nakamura M, Marumo F: Influence of aluminium on the effect of 1-alpha-(OH)D3 on renal osteodystrophy. *Nephron* 35:163–170, 1983

91. Meema HE, Schatz DL: Simple radiologic demonstration of cortical bone loss in thyrotoxicosis. *Radiology* 97:9–15, 1970

92. Andreoli SP, Smith JA, Bergstein JM: Aluminum bone disease in children: radiographic features from diagnosis to resolution. *Radiology* 156:663–667, 1985

93. Karsenty G, Vigneron N, Jorgetti V, et al: Value of the 99-mTc-methylene diphosphonate bone scan in renal osteodystrophy. *Kidney Int* 29:1058–1065, 1986

94. Hodson EM, Howman-Gilles RB, Evans RB, et al: The diagnosis of renal osteodystrophy: A comparison of technitium99 pyrophosphate bone scintography with other techniques. *Clin Nephrol* 16:24–28, 1981

95. Barsotti G, Guiducci A, Ceardella G, Giovannetti S: Effects on renal function of a low-nitrogen diet supplemented with essential amino acids and ketoanalogues and of hemodialysis and free protein supply in patients with chronic renal failure. *Nephron.* 27:113–117, 1981

96. Sedman AB, Miller NL, Warady BA, Lum GM, Alfrey AC: Aluminum loading in children with chronic renal failure. *Kidney Int* 26:201–204, 1984

97. Winney RJ, Cowie JF, Robson JS: The role of plasma aluminum in the detection and prevention of aluminum toxicity. *Kidney Int* 29 (Suppl 18):S91–95, 1986

98. Salusky IB, Foley J, Nelson P, Goodman WG: Aluminum accumulation during treatment with aluminum hydroxide and dialysis in children and young adults with chronic renal disease. *N Engl J Med* 324:527–531, 1991

99. Salusky IB, Coburn JW, Foley J, Nelson P, Fine RN: Effects of oral calcium carbonate on control of serum phosphorus and changes in plasma aluminum levels after discontinuation of aluminum-containing gels in children receiving dialysis. *J Pediatrics* 108:767–770, 1986

100. Slatopolsky E, Weerts C, Lopez-Hilker S, et al: Calcium carbonate is an effective phosphate binder in patients with chronic renal failure undergoing dialysis. *N Engl J Med* 315:157–161, 1986

101. Mactier RA, Van Stone J, Cox A, Van Stone M, Twardowski Z: Calcium carbonate is an effective phosphate binder when dialysate calcium concentration is adjusted to control hypercalcemia. *Clin Nephrol* 28:222–226, 1987

102. Slatopolsky E, Weerts C, Norwood K, et al: Long-term effects of calcium carbonate and 2.5 mEq/liter calcium dialysate on mineral metabolism. *Kidney Int* 36:897–903, 1989

103. Fournier A, Moriniere PH, Sebert JL, et al: Calcium carbonate, an aluminum-free agent for control of hyperphosphatemia, hypocalcemia and hyperparathyroidism in uremia. *Kidney Int* 29:S115–119, 1986

104. Renaud H, Atik A, Herve M, et al: Evaluation of vascular calcinosis risk factors in patients on chronic hemodialysis: lack of influence of calcium carbonate. *Nephron* 48:28–32, 1988

105. Schiller LR, Santa Ana CA, Sheikh MS, Emmett M, Fordtran JS: Effect of the time of administration of calcium acetate on phosphorus binding. *N Engl J Med* 320:1110–1113, 1989

106. Mai ML, Emmett M, Sheikh MS, Santa Ana CA, Schiller L, Fordtran JS: Calcium acetate, an effective phosphorus binder in patients with renal failure. *Kidney Int* 36:690–695, 1989

107. Schaefer K, Scheer J, Asmus G, Umlauf E, Hagemann J, von Herrath D: The treatment uraemic hyperphosphataemia with calcium acetate and calcium carbonate: A comparative study. *Nephrol Dial Transplant* 6:171–175, 1991

108. Bakir AA, Hryhorczuk DO, Berman E, Dunea G: Acute fatal hyperaluminemic encephalopathy in undialyzed and recently dialyzed uremic patients. *Trans Am Soc Artif Intern Organs* 32:171–176, 1986

109. Oe PL, Lips P, van der Muelen J, et al: Long-term use of magnesium hydroxide as a phosphate binder in patients on hemodialysis. *Clin Nephrol* 28:180–185, 1987

110. O'Donovan R, Baldwin D, Hammer M, et al: Substitution of aluminum salts by magnesium salts in control of dialysis hyperphosphatemia. *Lancet* 1:880–882, 1986

111. Baker LR, Muir JW, Sharman VL, et al: Controlled trial of calcitriol in hemodialysis patients. *Clin Nephrol* 26:185–191, 1986

112. Berl T, Berns AS, Huffer WE, et al: 1,25-Dihydroxycholecalciferol effects in chronic dialysis. A double-blind controlled study. *Ann Intern Med* 88:774–780, 1978

113. Ott SM, Maloney NA, Coburn JW, Alfrey AC, Sherrard DJ: The prevalence of bone aluminum deposition in renal osteodystrophy and its relation to the response to calcitriol therapy. *N Engl J Med* 307:709–713, 1982

114. Pierides AM, Simpson W, Ward MK, Ellis HA, Dewar JH, Kerr DNS: Variable response to long-term 1a-hydroxycholecalciferol in hemodialysis osteodystrophy. *Lancet* 1:1092–1095, 1976

115. Kanis JA, Henderson RG, Heynen G, et al: Renal osteodystrophy in nondialysed adolescents: long-term treatment with 1α-hydroxycholecalciferol. *Arch Dis Child* 52:473–481, 1977

116. Fukagawa M, Kitaoka M, Kaname S, et al: Suppression of parathyroid gland hyperplasia by 1,25(OH)2D3 pulse therapy. *N Engl J Med* 315:421–422, 1990

117. Martin KJ, Bullal HS, Domoto DT, Blalock S, Weindel M. Pulse oral calcitriol for the treatment of hyperparathyroidism in patients on continuous ambulatory peritoneal dialysis: preliminary observations. *Am J Kidney Dis* 19:540–545, 1992

118. Slatopolsky E, Weerts C, Thielan J, Horst RL, Harter H, Martin KJ: Marked suppression of secondary hyperparathyroidism by intravenous administration of 1,25-dihydroxycholecalciferol in uremic patients. *J Clin Invest* 74:2136–2143, 1984

119. Salusky IB, Goodman WG, Horst R, et al: Pharmakokinetics of calcitriol in CAPD/CCPD patients. *Am J Kidney Dis* 16:126–132, 1990

120. Delmez JA, Dougan CS, Gearing BK, et al: The effects of intraperitoneal calcitriol on calcium and parathyroid hormone. *Kidney Int* 31:795–799, 1987

121. Llach F. Parathyroidectomy in chronic renal failure: indications, surgical approach, and the use of calcitriol. *Kidney Int* 38 Suppl 29:S29, 1990

122. Hercz G, Salusky IB, Norris KC, Fine RN, Coburn JW: Aluminum removal by peritoneal dialysis: intravenous vs. intraperitoneal deferioxamine. *Kidney Int* 30:944–948, 1986

123. Milliner DS, Hercz G, Miller JH, Shinaberger JH, Nissenson AR, Coburn JW: Clearance of aluminum by hemodialysis: Effect of deferoxamine. *Kidney Int* 29 (Suppl 18):S100–103, 1986

124. Coburn JW, Norris KC, Nebeker HG: Osteomalacia and bone disease arising from aluminum. *Semin Nephrol* 6:68–89, 1986

125. Windus DW, Stokes TJ, Julian BA, Fenves AZ: Fatal Rhizopus infections in hemodialysis patients receiving deferoxamine. *Ann Intern Med* 107:678–680, 1987

126. Boelaert JR, Valcke, Vanderbroucke DH: Yersinia enterocolitica bacteraemia in hemodialysis. *Proc EDTA* 22:283, 1985

127. Gallant T, Freedman MH, Vellend H, Francombe WH: Yersinia sepsis in patients with iron overload treated with deferoxamine. *N Engl J Med* 314:1643, 1986

128. Hoen B, Renoult E, Jonon B, Kessler M: Septicemia due to Yersinia enterocolitica in a long-term hemodialysis patient after a single desferrioxamine administration. *Nephron* 50:378–379, 1988

129. Segal R, Zoller KA, Sherrard DJ, Coburn JW: Mucormycosis: a life-threatening complication of deferoxamine therapy in long-term dialysis patients. *Kidney Int* 33:238(Abstract), 1988

130. Abe F, Inaba H, Katoh T, Hotchi M: Effects of iron and desferrioxamine of Rhizopus infection. *Mycopathologica* 110:81–91, 1990

131. Van Cutsem J, Boelaert JR: Effects of deferoxamine, feroxamine and iron on experimental mucormycosis (zygomycosis). *Kidney Int* 36:1061–1068, 1989

132. Robins-Browne RM, Prpic JK: Effects of iron and desferrioxamine on infections with Yersinia enterocolitica. *Infect Immun* 47:774–779, 1985

133. Hercz G, Andress DL, Nebeker HG, Shinaberger JH, Sherrard DJ, Coburn JW: Reversal of aluminum-related bone disease after substituting calcium carbonate for aluminum hydroxide. *Am J Kidney Dis* 11:70–75, 1988

134. Kober M, Schneider H, Reinold HM, et al: Development of renal osteodystrophy afer kidney transplantation. *Kidney Int* 28:378, 1985

135. Bonomini V, Felelli C, DiFelice A, Buscaroli A: Bone remodelling after renal transplantation. *Adv Exp Med Biol* 178:207–216, 1984

136. Conceicao SC, Wilkinson R, Feest TJ, et al: Hypercalcemia following renal transplantation: causes and consequences. *Clin Nephrol* 16:235–244, 1981

137. Diethelm AG, Edwards RP, Whelchel JD: The natural history and surgical treatment of hypercalcemia before and after renal transplantation. *Surg Gynecol Obstet* 154:481–490, 1982

138. Deierhoi MH, Diethelm AG: Management of hyperparathyroidism following renal transplantation. *Transplant Management* 2:3–10, 1991

139. D'Alessandro AM, Melzer JS, Pirsch JD, et al: Tertiary hyperparathyroidism after renal transplantation: operative indications. *Surgery* 106:1049–1056, 1989

140. Ingbar S, Kon E, Burnett C, et al: The effects of cortisone on the renal tubular transport of uric acid, phosphorus, and electrolytes in patients with normal renal and adrenal function. *J Lab Clin Med* 38:533–541, 1951

141. Goodman M, Solomons CC, Miller PD: Distinction between the common symptoms of the phosphate-depletion syndrome and glucocorticoid-induced disease. *Am J Med* 65:868–872, 1978

142. Felsenfeld AJ, Gutman RA, Drezner M, Llach F: Hypophosphatemia in long-term renal transplant recipients: effects on bone histology and 1,25-dihydroxycholecalciferol. *Min Electrolyte Metab* 12:333–341, 1986

143. Nielsen HE, Melsen F, Christensen MS: Aseptic necrosis of bone following renal transplantation. *Acta Med Scand* 202:27, 1977

144. Julian BA, Laskow DA, Dubovsky J, Dubovsky EV, Curtis JJ,

Quarles LD. Rapid loss of vertebral mineral density after renal transplantation. *N Engl J Med* 325:544–550, 1991

145. McDonald JA, Dunstan CR, Dilworth P, et al: Bone loss after liver transplantation. *Hepatology* 14:613–619, 1991

146. Movsowitz C, Epstein S, Fallon M, Ismail F, Thomas S: Cyclosporin-A in vivo produces severe osteopenia in the rat: effect of dose and duration of administration. *Endocrinology* 123: 2571–2577, 1988

147. Stewart PJ, Green OC, Stern PH: Cyclosporine A inhibits calcemic hormone-induced bone resorption in vitro. *J Bone Miner Res* 1:285–291, 1986

148. Landmenn J, Renner N, Gacher A, et al: Cyclosporin A and osteonecrosis of the femoral head. *J Bone Joint Surg* 69A:1226–1228, 1987

149. Slatopolsky E, Martin K: Glucocorticoids and renal transplant osteonecrosis. *Adv Exp Med Biol* 171:353–359, 1984

150. Parfrey PS, Farge D, Parfrey NA, et al: The decreased incidence of aseptic necrosis in renal transplant recipients: a case control study. *Transplantation* 41:182–187, 1986

151. Isono SS, Woolson ST, Schurman DJ: Total joint arthroplasty for steroid-induced osteonecrosis in cardiac patients. *Clin Orthop* 217:201–208, 1987

152. Enright H, Haake R, Weisorf D: Avascular necrosis of bone: a common serious complication of allogeneic bone marrow transplantation. *Am J Med* 89:733–738, 1990

153. Ficat RP: Idiopathic bone necrosis of the femoral head. Early diagnosis and treatment. *J Bone Joint Surg* 67B:3–9, 1985

154. Van Damme-Lombaerts R, Pirson Y, Squifflet JP, et al: The avascular necrosis of bone after renal transplantation in children. *Tranplant Proc* 17:184–186, 1985

155. Ibels LS, Alfrey AC, Huffer WE, et al: Aseptic necrosis of bone following renal transplantation: experience in 194 transplant recipients and review of the literature. *Medicine (Baltimore)* 57: 25–45, 1978

Genetic, Developmental, and Dysplastic Skeletal Disorders

VI. Introduction

Michael P. Whyte, M.D.

*Division of Bone and Mineral Diseases, Washington University School of Medicine; and Metabolic Research Unit,
Shriners Hospital for Crippled Children, St. Louis, Missouri*

Physicians are confronted with a great diversity of rare genetic, developmental, and dysplastic skeletal disorders (1–5). Some are simply radiologic curiosities; others are challenging clinical problems. Some cause focal bony abnormalities; others result in generalized disturbances of bone growth or modeling, or osteosclerosis or osteopenia. A few are associated with overt derangements in mineral homeostasis. Several are important because they are heritable and therefore offer clues concerning normal mechanisms of skeletal homeostasis and mineral metabolism. Cumulatively, the number of affected subjects is substantial (1–5).

This section provides a concise overview of a number of the more common or more revealing of the genetic, developmental, and dysplastic skeletal disorders, beginning with a description of some of the conditions that are traditionally grouped together as sclerosing bone dysplasias (1,2,4). A discussion of several additional important heritable or sporadic developmental and dysplastic skeletal disorders follows.

REFERENCES

1. Beighton P (ed): *McKusick's Heritable Disorders of Connective Tissue.* Mosby-Year Book, St. Louis, 1993
2. Royce PM, Steinmann B (eds): *Connective Tissue and Its Heritable Disorders.* Wiley-Liss, New York, 1993
3. Scriver CR, Beaudet AL, Sly WS, Valle D: *The Metabolic and Molecular Bases of Inherited Disease,* 7th ed. McGraw-Hill Books, New York, 1995
4. Frame B, Honasoge M, Kottamasu SR: *Osteosclerosis, Hyperostosis, and Related Disorders.* Elsevier, New York, 1987
5. Wynne-Davies R, Hall CM, Apley AG: *Atlas of Skeletal Dysplasias.* Churchill Livingstone, Edinburgh, 1985

68. Sclerosing Bone Dysplasias

Michael P. Whyte, M.D.

*Division of Bone and Mineral Diseases, Washington University School of Medicine; and
Metabolic Research Unit, Shriners Hospital for Crippled Children, St. Louis, Missouri*

Focal or generalized osteosclerosis is caused by many rare (primarily hereditary) dysplastic conditions, as well as by a variety of dietary, metabolic, endocrine, hematologic, infectious, and neoplastic diseases (Table 1). The following sections discuss the principal disorders among the sclerosing bone dysplasias.

OSTEOPETROSIS

Osteopetrosis (marble bone disease) was first described in 1904 by Albers-Schönberg (1). More than 300 cases have been reported. Two major clinical forms are well delineated—the autosomal dominant adult (benign) type that is associated with few or no symptoms (2) and the autosomal recessive infantile (malignant) type that, if untreated, is typically fatal during infancy or early childhood (3). A rarer autosomal recessive (intermediate) form presents during childhood with some of the signs and symptoms of malignant osteopetrosis, but its impact on life expectancy is not well characterized (4). A fourth clinical type, inherited as an autosomal recessive trait, was formerly called the syndrome of osteopetrosis with renal tubular acidosis and cerebral calcification, but it is now understood to be an inborn error of metabolism, carbonic anhydrase II deficiency (see later section). Neuronal storage disease with malignant osteopetrosis has been reported in several subjects and seems to reflect a distinct phenotype (5). There also appear to be especially rare forms of osteopetrosis, called lethal, transient infantile, and postinfectious (6).

Although the diversity of clinical and hereditary types makes it apparent that several different gene defects and biologic disturbances cause osteopetrosis in humans, the pathogenesis of all true forms is expressed through a failure of osteoclast-mediated resorption of the skeleton. Consequently, primary spongiosa (calcified cartilage deposited during endochondral bone formation) persists and causes characteristic histopathologic changes (see later) (7). For some other conditions, the term *osteopetrosis* has been incorrectly used to refer generically to a skeleton that, although it appears sclerotic on radiographic study, is without these histologic features. Accordingly, it is important to recognize that therapeutic approaches for true forms of osteopetrosis, for which the pathogenesis is partly elucidated, may be inappropriate for these other, generally enigmatic, disorders.

Clinical Presentation

Infantile osteopetrosis presents during infancy (3). Occurrence within sibships and an increased incidence of parental consanguinity indicate that this phenotype is transmitted as an autosomal recessive trait. Nasal stuffiness resulting from malformation of the mastoid and paranasal sinuses is often an early symptom. Cranial foramina do not widen fully, and this defect can gradually cause palsies of the optic, oculomotor, and facial nerves. There is failure to thrive. Eruption of the dentition is delayed. Bones may appear to be dense on radiologic study, but they are actually fragile and can fracture. Some patients develop hydrocephalus; sleep apnea may occur. Retinal degeneration is another cause of blindness. Recurrent infection with spontaneous bruising and bleeding are common problems and appear to be a consequence of myelophthisis, and hematopoietic failure due to many osteoclasts and abundant fibrous tissue crowd together in bone marrow spaces. Hypersplenism and hemolysis can worsen anemia. Physical examination shows short stature, frontal bossing, a large head, an "adenoid" appearance, nystagmus, hepatosplenomegaly, and genu valgum. Untreated children usually die during the first decade of life from hemorrhage, pneumonia, severe anemia, or sepsis (3).

Intermediate osteopetrosis causes short stature. Some patients develop cranial nerve deficits, macrocephaly, ankylosed teeth that predispose to osteomyelitis of the jaw, mild or occasionally moderately severe anemia, and recurrent fracture (4).

Adult osteopetrosis is a developmental condition in which radiologic abnormalities became apparent during childhood. In some kindreds, alternate generations are skipped, and carriers show no radiologic disturbances. Although most patients are asymptomatic (2), the long bones are brittle and fractures may occur. Facial palsy, deafness, osteomyelitis of the mandible, compromised vision or hearing, psychomotor delay, carpal tunnel syndrome, and osteoarthritis are additional clinical problems. Studies from Denmark propose that there are two types of adult osteopetrosis, distinguishable, in part, by their radiologic appearances, somewhat different clinical expressions, and biochemical findings (8).

Neuronal storage disease with osteopetrosis is associated with severe skeletal manifestations and the additional features of epilepsy and neurodegenerative disease (5). Lethal osteopetrosis results in stillbirth (6). Transient infantile osteopetrosis resolves during the first few years of life (6).

Radiologic Features

Generalized osteosclerosis is the principal radiologic finding in the osteopetrosis (9). There is a symmetrical increase in bone mass. In the severe forms, all three principal components of skeletal development are disturbed, causing diminished skeletal growth, modeling, and remodeling. The skeleton may be uniformly dense, but alternating sclerotic and lucent bands are commonly noted in the iliac wings and near the ends of the long bones, where diaphyses and metaphyses are typically broadened and may have an "Erlenmeyer flask"

TABLE 1. *Disorders that cause osteosclerosis*

Dysplasias
  Craniodiaphyseal dysplasia
  Craniometaphyseal dysplasia
  Dysosteosclerosis
  Endosteal hyperostosis
  van Buchem disease
  Sclerosteosis
  Frontometaphyseal dysplasia
  Infantile cortical hyperostosis (Caffey's disease)
  Melorheostosis
  Metaphyseal dysplasia (Pyle's disease)
  Mixed sclerosing bone dystrophy
  Oculodento-osseous dysplasia
  Osteodysplasia of Melnick and Needles
  Osteoectasia with hyperphosphatasia (hyperostosis
    corticalis)
  Osteopathia striata
  Osteopetrosis
  Osteopoikilosis
  Progressive diaphyseal dysplasia (Engelmann's disease)
  Pycnodysostosis
Metabolic
  Carbonic anhydrase II deficiency
  Fluorosis
  Heavy metal poisoning
  Hypervitaminosis A,D
  Hyper-, hypo-, and pseudohypoparathyroidism
  Hypophosphatemic osteomalacia
  Milk-alkali syndrome
  Renal osteodystrophy
Other
  Axial osteomalacia
  Fibrogenesis imperfecta osseum
  Intravenous drug abuse (hepatitis C-associated
    osteosclerosis)
  Ionizing radiation
  Lymphomas
  Mastocytosis
  Multiple myeloma
  Myelofibrosis
  Osteomyelitis
  Osteonecrosis
  Paget's disease
  Sarcoidosis
  Skeletal metastases
  Tuberous sclerosis

Updated and reproduced with permission, from: Whyte MP, Murphy WA. Osteopetrosis and other sclerosing bone disorders. In: Avioli LV, Krane SM (eds) *Metabolic Bone Disease*, 2nd ed. WB Saunders, Philadelphia, 1990.

deformity (Fig. 1). Rarely, the distal phalanges are eroded (a finding more characteristic of pycnodysostosis). Pathologic fracture of long bones is not uncommon. Rachitic changes in growth plates may occur (10). In the axial skeleton, the cranium is usually thickened and dense, especially at the base, and the paranasal and mastoid sinuses are underpneumatized (Fig. 2).Vertebrae may show, on lateral view, a "bone-in-bone" (endobone) configuration.

The two proposed types of adult osteopetrosis manifest progressive osteosclerosis from childhood, with either (i) marked thickening of the cranial vault and diffusely increased density of the spine without endobone formation (type I), or (ii) selective thickening of the base of the skull together with typical vertebral end-plate sclerosis that causes an endobone, or "rugger jersey," appearance of the spine (type II) (8). In both types, skeletal modeling defects are absent.

In the various forms of osteopetrosis, scintigrapic abnormalities of the skeleton include fractures and osteomyelitis (11). Magnetic resonance imaging (MRI) may help to monitor patients with severe disease who undergo bone marrow transplantation, because successful engraftment will enlarge marrow spaces (12) (see later). The cranial computed tomography (CT) and MRI findings of infants and children have been characterized (13).

Laboratory Findings

In infantile osteopetrosis, serum calcium levels generally reflect dietary intake (14). Hypocalcemia can occur and may be severe enough to cause rickets. Secondary hyperparathyroidism with elevated serum levels of calcitriol is commonly

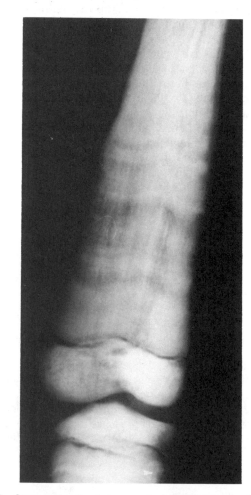

FIG. 1. Osteopetrosis. Anteroposterior radiograph of the distal femur of a 10-year-old boy shows a widened metadiaphyseal region with characteristic alternating dense and lucent bands. (From: Whyte MP, Murphy WA. Osteopetrosis and other sclerosing bone disorders. In: Avioli LV, Krane SM (eds) *Metabolic Bone Disease*, 2nd ed. WB Saunders, Philadelphia, 1990.)

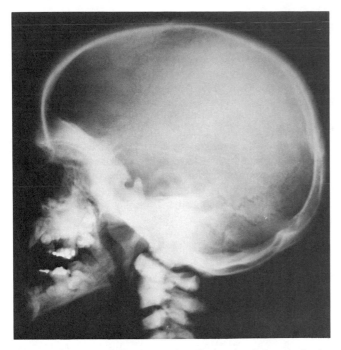

FIG. 2. Osteopetrosis. Lateral radiograph of the skull of a 13-year-old boy shows osteosclerosis, especially apparent at the base. (From: Whyte MP, Murphy WA. Osteopetrosis and other sclerosing bone disorders. In: Avioli LV, Krane SM (eds) *Metabolic Bone Disease*, 2nd ed. WB Saunders, Philadelphia, 1990.)

present (15). Acid phosphatase (ACP) activity is often increased in serum. Creatine kinase brain isoenzyme (BB-CK) is aberrantly present in serum in genuine forms of osteopetrosis (16). Both ACP and BB-CK appear to originate from the defective osteoclasts (16).

In adult osteopetrosis, standard biochemical indices of mineral homeostasis are usually described as unremarkable. However, more recent studies indicate that immunoreactive parathyroid hormone (PTH) levels and BB-CK activity in serum are often increased in patients with type II disease (8,16).

Histopathologic Findings

The radiologic features of the osteopetroses are usually diagnostic (9). Nevertheless, the failure of osteoclasts to resorb skeletal tissue provides a histologic finding that is pathognomonic (17): remnants of mineralized primary spongiosa persist as islands or bars of calcified cartilage within mature bone (Fig. 3). Absence of these structures in adult type I osteopetrosis on iliac crest biopsy (8,18) indicates that this disorder is not a genuine form of osteopetrosis (16).

In osteopetrosis, osteoclasts may be present in increased, normal, or decreased numbers. In the infantile form, these multinucleated cells are usually abundant and are found at bone surfaces, but their nuclei are especially numerous, and characteristic ruffled borders or clear zones are absent (19). Fibrous tissue often crowds the marrow spaces (19). Adult osteopetrosis may show increased amounts of osteoid, and osteoclasts can be few and lack ruffled borders or can be especially numerous and large (18). A common histologic finding is "woven" bone (17).

Etiology and Pathogenesis

Although most forms of human osteopetrosis appear to be transmitted as autosomal traits, the molecular defects or gene loci are unknown, except for carbonic anhydrase II deficiency (see next section) (6). The pathogenesis of all

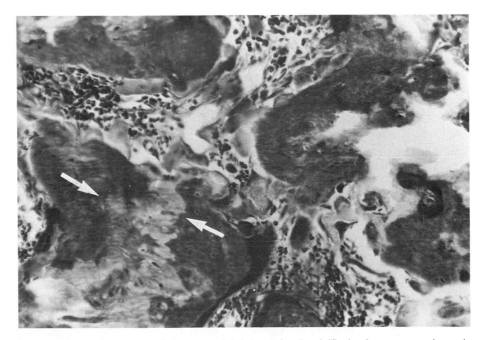

FIG. 3. Osteopetrosis. A characteristic area of lightly stained calcified primary spongiosa *(arrows)* is found within darkly stained mineralized bone (×150).

true forms, however, involves diminished osteoclast-mediated skeletal resorption (20,21). The potential causes of osteoclast failure are complex (21). Abnormalities in the osteoclast stem cell itself, or in its microenvironment, in the mature osteoclast, or in the bone matrix, could be at fault (6,7). The few cases of osteopetrosis with neuronal storage disease (characterized by accumulation of ceroid lipofuscin), may involve a primary lysosomal defect (5). Virus like inclusions have been found in some of the osteoclasts of a few sporadic cases of benign osteopetrosis, but their significance is uncertain (22). Synthesis of an abnormal PTH (23), or defective production of interleukin-2 (24) or superoxide (25)—factors necessary for bone resorption—may also be fundamental defects. Leukocyte function studies in the infantile form have revealed abnormalities in circulating monocytes and granulocytes (25,26). Ultimately, impaired bone resorption causes skeletal fragility because few collagen fibrils properly connect osteons, and there is defective remodeling of woven bone to compact bone (7).

Treatment

Because the etiology, precise pathogenesis, prognosis, and patterns of inheritance for the various forms of osteopetrosis differ, a correct diagnosis of the particular subtype is especially important before therapy is attempted. Intermediate osteopetrosis is relatively benign compared to the infantile type. Infants or young children with carbonic anhydrase II deficiency may have radiologic features consistent with malignant osteopetrosis, yet serial studies can show spontaneous gradual resolution of their bony sclerosis. Correct diagnosis from among the various forms of osteopetrosis may require investigation of the family and careful evaluation of the patient's disease progression.

Bone Marrow Transplantation

Bone marrow transplantation (BMT) has remarkably improved a few cases of infantile osteopetrosis (27). Transplanted osteoclasts, but not osteoblasts, were shown to be of donor origin in one affected infant (28), an observation that supported the hypothesis that osteopetrosis is caused by defective osteoclast-mediated bone resorption, and that the progenitor cell for the osteoclast is normally derived from marrow (28). Patients with severely crowded marrow spaces appear less likely to benefit from BMT. Accordingly, histomorphometric studies of bone may help to prognosticate the outcome of this procedure. Use of marrow from human leukocyte antigen (HLA)-nonidentical donors warrants continued study (29). It is understandable that BMT may not benefit all patients (6), because a variety of defects (not all of which are intrinsic to marrow, including osteoclast precursors) may cause osteopetrosis. Successful BMT can cause hypercalcemia as osteoclast function begins (30).

Hormonal and Dietary Treatments

Some success in the treatment of osteopetrosis was reported with a calcium-deficient diet alone. However, supplementation of dietary calcium may be necessary for symptomatic hypocalcemia and rickets in some severely affected infants or children (10).

Large oral doses of calcitriol, together with limited dietary calcium intake to prevent hypercalciuria/hypercalcemia, occasionally improves infantile osteopetrosis as dramatically as does successful BMT (31). Calcitriol appears to be helpful by stimulating dormant osteoclasts. Unfortunately, some patients appear to become resistant to this treatment (20,25). Long-term infusion of PTH was helpful for one infant (23), perhaps by stimulating calcitriol synthesis. The observation that leukocytes from severely affected cases have diminished production of superoxide has led to clinical, laboratory, and histopathologic evidence of successful response to recombinant human interferon gamma 1-b therapy (20,25).

High-dose glucocorticoid treatment stabilizes patients with pancytopenia and hepatomegaly from infantile osteopetrosis. Prednisone and a low-calcium/high-phosphate diet may be an alternative to BMT (32).

Supportive

Hyperbaric oxygenation can be an important adjunctive treatment for osteomyelitis of the jaw. Surgical decompression of the optic and facial nerves may benefit some patients.

Early prenatal diagnosis of osteopetrosis by ultrasound has generally been unsuccessful. Conventional radiographic studies occasionally diagnose malignant osteopetrosis late in pregnancy (33).

Carbonic Anhydrase II Deficiency

In 1983, the autosomal recessive syndrome of osteopetrosis with renal tubular acidosis (RTA) and cerebral calcification was discovered to be an inborn error of metabolism caused by deficiency of the carbonic anhydrase II (CA II) isoenzyme (34).

Clinical Presentation

Description of nearly 50 cases of CA II deficiency has revealed considerable clinical variability among affected families (35). The perinatal history is typically unremarkable, but then, in infancy or early childhood, patients may develop a fracture or show failure to thrive, developmental delay, or short stature. Mental subnormality is common but not invariable. Compression of the optic nerves and dental malocclusion are additional complications. RTA may explain the hypotonia, apathy, and muscle weakness that trouble some patients. Periodic hypokalemic paralysis has been described. Although fracture is unusual, recurrent breaks in long bones may cause significant morbidity (34). Life expectancy does not appear to be shortened, but to date the oldest subjects reported have been young adults (36,37).

Radiologic Features

Carbonic anhydrase II deficiency resembles other forms of osteopetrosis on radiologic study, except that cerebral calcification develops during childhood and the defects in skeletal modeling and the osteosclerosis may diminish spontaneously (rather than increase) over years (38). The changes on x-ray of the skeleton have been present at diagnosis in all cases, although one patient had only subtle findings at birth. Computed tomography has demonstrated that the cerebral calcification appears between 2 and 5 years of age, increases during childhood, affects gray matter of the cortex and basal ganglia, and is similar if not identical to that of idiopathic hypoparathyroidism or pseudohypoparathyroidism.

Laboratory Findings

Bone marrow examination is unremarkable. If anemia is present, it is generally mild and likely to be of nutritional origin. Metabolic acidosis occurs as early as the neonatal period. Both proximal and distal RTA have been described (39); however, occurrence of distal (type I) RTA seems to be better documented. Additional studies are required to clarify the pathogenesis of the abnormality in acid–base homeostasis (39). Aminoaciduria and glycosuria are absent (36).

Autopsy studies have not been reported (37). Histopathologic examination of bone from four individuals who represented two affected families revealed characteristic bars—areas of unresorbed calcified primary spongiosa (38).

Etiology and Pathogenesis

The CA isoenzymes accelerate the first step in the reaction $CO_2 + H_2O \rightarrow H_2CO_3 \rightarrow H^+ + HCO_3^-$. Accordingly, they function importantly in acid–base regulation.

Carbonic anhydrase II is present in many tissues, such as brain, kidney, erythrocytes, cartilage, lung, and gastric mucosa (40). The other CA isoenzymes have a more limited tissue distribution.

All of 21 patients from 12 unrelated kindreds of diverse ethnic and geographic origin were shown to have selective deficiency of CA II in erythrocytes (36). Autosomal recessive inheritance for CA II deficiency is supported by the observation that red cell CA II levels in carrier parents are approximately half the normal level (36,37).

Although deficiency of CA II remains to be shown in tissues other than erythrocytes, the presence of osteopetrosis, RTA, and cerebral calcification in patients with this disorder suggests that there is a global deficiency of CA II and that this isoenzyme has an important function in bone, kidney, and perhaps brain (36,37). Mutations in the CA II gene have been identified in several patients (40).

Treatment

Renal tubular acidosis in CA II deficiency has been treated by bicarbonate supplementation, but the long-term impact of this therapy is unknown. Transfusion of CA-II-replete erythrocytes to one affected woman did not correct her systemic acidosis (41).

PYCNODYSOSTOSIS

Pycnodysostosis is the skeletal dysplasia that is believed to have affected the French impressionist painter Henri de Toulouse-Lautrec (1864–1901) (42). More than 100 cases from 50 kindreds have been described since the condition was delineated in 1962 (43). The disorder is transmitted as an autosomal recessive trait; parental consanguinity has been reported for about 30% of patients. Most case descriptions have come from Europe or the United States, but the dysplasia has been found in Israelis, Indonesians, Asian Indians, and Africans. Pycnodysostosis appears to be especially common in Japanese (44).

Clinical Presentation

Pycnodysostosis is generally diagnosed during infancy or early childhood because of disproportionate short stature and dysmorphic features that include fronto-occipital prominence, relatively large cranium, obtuse mandibular angle, small facies and chin, high-arched palate, dental malocclusion with retained deciduous teeth, proptosis, bluish sclerae, and a beaked and pointed nose (45). The anterior fontanel and other cranial sutures are usually open. Fingers are short and clubbed from acro-osteolysis or aplasia of terminal phalanges, the fingernails are hypoplastic, and hands are small and square. The thorax is narrow and there may be pectus excavatum, kyphoscoliosis, and increased lumbar lordosis. Recurrent fractures typically involve the lower limbs and cause genu valgum deformity. Patients are, however, usually able to walk independently. Visceral manifestations and rickets have been described. Mental retardation affects about 10% of cases (45). Adult height ranges from 4 ft 3 in to 4 ft 11 in. Recurrent respiratory infections and right heart failure from chronic upper airway obstruction due to micrognathia occur in some patients.

Radiologic Features

Pycnodysostosis shares many radiologic features with osteopetrosis; for example, both disorders cause generalized osteosclerosis and are associated with recurrent fractures. The osteosclerosis is developmental and uniform, it first becomes apparent in childhood, and it increases with age. However, the marked modeling defects of the severe forms of osteopetrosis do not occur in pycnodysostosis, although long bones have thick cortices and narrow medullary canals. Additional findings that help to differentiate pycnodysostosis from osteopetrosis include delayed closure of cranial sutures and fontanels (prominently the anterior) (Fig. 4), obtuse mandibular angle, wormian bones, gracile clavicles that are hypoplastic at their lateral segments, hypoplasia or aplasia of the distal phalanges and ribs, and partial absence of the hyoid bone (46). Endobones and radiodense striations are also absent (9). The calvarium and base of the skull are sclerotic, and the orbital ridges are radiodense. Hypoplasia of facial bones, sinuses, and terminal phalanges are characteristic. Vertebrae are sclerotic, yet their transverse processes are uninvolved; anterior and posterior concavities occur. Lumbosacral spondylolisthesis is not uncommon, and lack of segmentation of the atlas and axis may be present. Madelung deformity can affect the forearms.

Laboratory Findings

Serum calcium and inorganic phosphate levels and alkaline phosphatase activity are usually unremarkable. Anemia

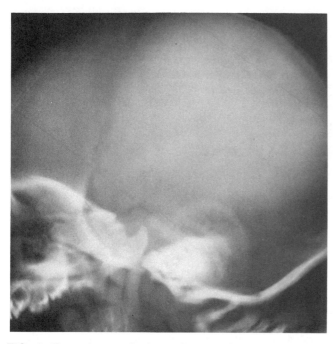

FIG. 4. Pycnodysostosis. Lateral radiograph of the skull of an infant shows that the cranial sutures are markedly widened. The base is sclerotic. (From Whyte MP, Murphy WA. Osteopetrosis and other sclerosing bone disorders. In: Avioli LV, Krane SM (eds) *Metabolic Bone Disease*, 2nd ed. WB Saunders, Philadelphia, 1990.)

is not a problem. Histopathologic study of bone shows cortical bone structure that appears to be normal despite the appearance of decreased osteoclastic and osteoblastic activity (47). Skeletal turnover may be decreased. Electron microscopy of bone from two patients suggested that degradation of collagen could be defective, perhaps from an abnormality in the bone matrix or in the osteoclast itself (48). In chondrocytes, abnormal inclusions have been described.

Etiology and Pathogenesis

The genetic basis for pycnodysostosis is unknown. Absorption of dietary calcium has been noted to be markedly increased. Both the rate of bone accretion and the size of the exchangeable calcium pool can be reduced (49). Accordingly, diminished rates of bone resorption may explain the osteosclerosis. Virus like inclusions were found in the osteoclasts of two affected brothers (50).

Treatment

There is no effective medical therapy for pycnodysostosis. Fractures of the long bones are typically transverse. They usually heal at a satisfactory rate, although delayed union and massive callus formation have been reported. Internal fixation of long bones is formidable because of their hardness. Extraction of teeth is similarly difficult; fracture of the jaw has occurred (45). Osteomyelitis of the mandible may require

treatment with a combined antibiotic and surgical approach. The orthopedic problems have recently been briefly reviewed (51).

PROGRESSIVE DIAPHYSEAL DYSPLASIA (CAMURATI-ENGELMANN'S DISEASE)

Progressive diaphyseal dysplasia was characterized by Cockayne in 1920 (52). Camurati reported that the condition was heritable. Engelmann described the severe typical form in 1929 (53). This developmental disorder is transmitted as an autosomal dominant trait. Descriptions of more than 100 cases show that the clinical and radiologic penetrance is quite variable (54). The characteristic feature is new bone formation that occurs gradually on both the periosteal and endosteal surfaces of long bones. All races appear to be affected. In severe cases, osteosclerosis is widespread and the skull and axial skeleton are also involved. Some carriers have no radiographic changes but bone scintigraphy is abnormal.

Clinical Presentation

Progressive diaphyseal dysplasia typically presents during childhood with limping or a broad-based and waddling gait, leg pain, muscle wasting, and decreased subcutaneous fat in the extremities. The condition may be mistaken for a form of muscular dystrophy (55). Severely affected patients have a characteristic body habitus that includes an enlarged head with prominent forehead, proptosis, and thin limbs with thickened bones but with little muscle mass. Cranial nerve palsies may develop when the skull is affected. Puberty is sometimes delayed. Raised intracranial pressure can occur. Physical findings include palpable bony enlargement and skeletal tenderness. Some patients have hepatosplenomegaly, Raynaud's phenomenon, and other findings suggestive of vasculitis (56). Although radiologic studies typically show progressive disease, the clinical course is variable, and remission of symptoms seems to occur in some patients during adulthood (57).

Radiologic Features

The principal radiologic feature of progressive diaphyseal dysplasia is cortical hyperostosis of major long bone diaphyses from proliferation of new bone on both periosteal and endosteal surfaces (9). The sclerosis is fairly symmetrical and gradually spreads to involve metaphyses (epiphyses are spared) (Fig. 5). The tibiae and femora are most commonly involved; less frequently, the radii, ulnae, humeri, and occasionally the short tubular bones are affected. The scapulae, clavicles, and pelvis may also become thickened. Typically, the shafts of long bones gradually widen and develop irregular surfaces. The age of onset, rate of progression, and degree of osteosclerosis are very variable. With relatively mild disease, especially in adolescents or young adults, radiographic and scintigraphic abnormalities may be confined to the long bones of the lower limbs. Maturation of the new bone increases the osteosclerosis. In severely affected children, some areas of the skeleton can appear osteopenic.

Bone scanning generally reveals focally increased radionuclide accumulation in affected areas (58). Clinical, radiologic, and scintigraphic findings are generally concordant. In some affected subjects, however, bone scans can be unremarkable despite considerable radiologic abnormality. This association seems to reflect advanced but quiescent disease (58). Markedly increased radioisotope accumulation with minimal radiologic findings can reflect early and active skeletal disease (58). MR and CT findings for cranial involvement have recently been described (59).

Laboratory Findings

Routine biochemical parameters of bone and mineral metabolism are typically normal, although serum alkaline phosphatase activity, urinary hydroxyproline levels, and the erythrocyte sedimentation rate are elevated in some patients. Modest hypocalcemia and significant hypocalciuria occur in some affected subjects who have severe disease and appear to reflect their positive calcium balance (57). Mild anemia and leukopenia may also be present (56).

New bone formation along diaphyses is the characteristic feature of progressive diaphyseal dysplasia. Peripheral to the original bony cortex, disorganized newly formed woven bone undergoes centripetal maturation and then incorporation into the cortex (54). Electron microscopy of muscle has shown myopathic changes and vascular abnormalities (55).

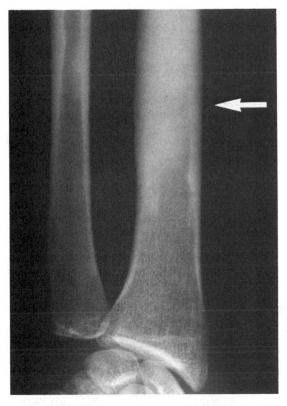

FIG. 5. Progressive diaphyseal dysplasia (Camurati-Engelmann's disease). The distal radius of this 20-year-old woman has a characteristic area of patchy thickening *(arrow)* of the periosteal and endosteal surfaces of the diaphysis.

Etiology and Pathogenesis

Progressive diaphyseal dysplasia is caused by an autosomal gene defect that remains to be mapped and characterized. Some especially mild cases were reported to be an autosomal recessive condition (i.e., Ribbing's disease) (60). However, sporadic cases do occur, and mild clinical forms can be transmitted as an autosomal dominant trait with variable penetrance.

The clinical and laboratory features of the disease when severe, together with its responsiveness to glucocorticoid treatment, have led some to suggest that progressive diaphyseal dysplasia is a systemic condition (i.e., an inflammatory connective tissue disease) (56).

Aberrant differentiation of monocytes/macrophages to fibroblasts, and hence to osteoblasts, has been discussed as a fundamental pathogenetic feature (61).

Treatment

Progressive diaphyseal dysplasia is a chronic and somewhat unpredictable disorder (62). Symptoms may remit during adolescence or adulthood. Since its initial use in 1967 for this disorder, glucocorticoid therapy (typically prednisone given in small doses on an alternate day schedule) has become a well-documented effective treatment that can not only relieve bone pain but also normalize histologic abnormalities in affected bone (63). Complete relief of localized pain has followed surgical removal of the affected area of diaphysis forming a "cortical window" (64).

ENDOSTEAL HYPEROSTOSIS

In 1955, van Buchem and colleagues first described the entity *hyperostosis corticalis generalisata* (65). This report subsequently led to characterization of the disorders that are considered endosteal hyperostoses.

van Buchem Disease

This is an autosomal recessive, clinically severe condition (65) that is differentiated from an autosomal dominant, more mild, benign form of endosteal hyperostosis (Worth type) (65,66). Nevertheless, van Buchem disease is considerably less common than the cumulative number of reports in the literature might suggest (67).

Clinical Presentation

van Buchem disease has been described in children and adults; sex distribution seems to be equal. Progressive asymmetrical enlargement of the jaw occurs during puberty. The mandibles of affected adults are markedly thickened with wide angles, but there is no prognathism, and dental malocclusion is uncommon. Affected subjects may be symptom free; however, recurrent facial nerve palsy, deafness, and optic atrophy from narrowing of cranial foramina are common and can begin as early as infancy. Long bones may become painful with applied pressure, but they are not fragile, and joint range of motion is generally normal. Sclerosteosis had, until recently (68), been differentiated from van Buchem disease because patients are excessively tall and have syndactyly (see later sections).

Radiologic Features

Endosteal cortical thickening that produces a dense and homogeneous diaphyseal cortex and narrows the medullary canal is the major radiologic feature of van Buchem disease. The hyperostosis is selectively endosteal; long bones are properly modeled. Generalized osteosclerosis also includes the base of the skull, facial bones, vertebrae, pelvis, and ribs. The mandible becomes enlarged (Fig. 6). Cranial CT findings have been reported (69).

Laboratory Findings

Alkaline phosphatase activity in serum is primarily of skeletal origin and may be increased; calcium and inorganic phosphate levels are unremarkable.

Van Buchem and colleagues suggested that the excessive bone was essentially of normal quality.

Etiology and Pathogenesis

Summarized evidence indicates that van Buchem disease and sclerosteosis reflect the same genetic defect, so their

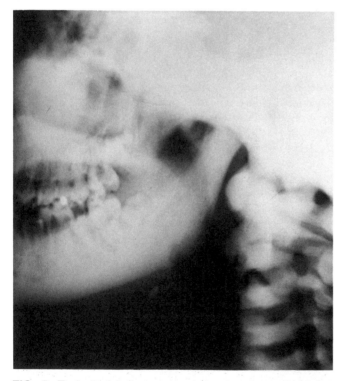

FIG. 6. Endosteal hyperostosis. Lateral radiograph of the mandible and facial bones of a 9-year-old boy with van Buchem disease shows dense sclerosis of all osseous structures. (From Whyte MP, Murphy WA. Osteopetrosis and other sclerosing bone disorders. In: Avioli LV, Krane SM (eds) *Metabolic Bone Disease*, 2nd ed. WB Saunders, Philadelphia, 1990.)

clinical/radiologic differences are explained by the epistatic effects of modifying genes (68).

Treatment

There is no specific medical therapy. Surgical decompression of narrowed foramina may help to alleviate cranial nerve palsies (70). Surgery has also been used to recontour the mandible (71).

Sclerosteosis

Sclerosteosis (cortical hyperostosis with syndactyly), like van Buchem disease (see the preceding section), is an autosomal recessive form of endosteal hyperostosis. It occurs primarily in the Afrikaners of South Africa. Patients who live elsewhere are also often of Dutch ancestry (68). Initially, sclerosteosis was distinguished from van Buchem disease by some radiographic differences and the presence of syndactyly, but more recent studies suggest that both disorders are caused by the same primary gene defect (68).

Clinical Presentation

At birth, only syndactyly may be noted (72). During early childhood, there is overgrowth and attendant sclerosis of the skeleton that involves especially the skull and causes facial disfigurement. Affected subjects are tall and heavy beginning in childhood. Understandably, the term *gigantism* has been used to refer to their appearance. Deafness and facial palsy due to nerve entrapment are also presenting problems. The mandible has a rather square configuration. Raised intracranial pressure and headache may be sequellae of a small cranial cavity. The brainstem can become compressed. Syndactyly from either cutaneous or bony fusion of the middle and index fingers is typical but of variable severity. The fingernails are dysplastic. Patients are not prone to fracture and their intelligence is normal. Life expectancy may be shortened (73).

Radiologic Features

Except when syndactyly is present, the skeleton of sclerosteosis is normal in early childhood. The principal radiologic feature is progressive bony thickening that causes widening of the skull and prognathism (74). In the long bones, modeling defects occur and the cortices are thickened. Syndactyly, most often involving the index and long finger, is common. The vertebral pedicles, ribs, pelvis, and tubular bones may also become somewhat dense. Computed tomography has shown fusion of the ossicles and narrowing of the internal auditory canals and cochlear aqueducts, which can explain the associated deafness (69).

Histopathologic Findings

In an American kindred with sclerosteosis, histomorphometric analysis of the calvarium of one patient following *in vivo* tetracycline labeling showed dense thickened trabeculae and osteoidosis where the rate of bone formation was increased; osteoclastic bone resorption appeared to be quiescent (74).

Etiology and Pathogenesis

Enhanced osteoblast activity with failure of osteoclasts to compensate for the increased bone formation appears to explain the osteosclerosis of sclerosteosis (75). No abnormality of calcium homeostasis or of pituitary gland function has been documented (76). The pathogenesis of the neurologic defects has been described in detail (75). Comparison of sclerosteosis and van Buchem disease suggests that both disorders are caused by abnormalities in the same gene and that the phenotypic variation results from epistatic effects of modifying genes (68).

Treatment

There is no specific medical treatment for sclerosteosis. Surgical correction of syndactyly is especially difficult if there is bony fusion. Correction of prognathism is complicated by dense mandibular bone. Management of associated neurologic dysfunction has been reviewed (75).

OSTEOPOIKILOSIS

Osteopoikilosis literally translated means spotted bones. This condition is a radiologic curiosity that is transmitted as an autosomal dominant trait with a high degree of penetrance (77). Patients in some kindreds may also have a form of connective tissue nevus called *dermatofibrosis lenticularis disseminata*; the disorder is then called the Buschke-Ollendorff syndrome (78). Although the bony lesions of osteopoikilosis are not symptomatic, incorrectly diagnosed patients may be subjected to rigorous and expensive studies for other important disorders, including metastatic disease to the skeleton (79).

Clinical Presentation

Osteopoikilosis is typically an incidental discovery that follows a radiologic study. Musculoskeletal pain is described in many cases but is probably coincidental. The nevi usually involve the lower trunk or extremities and present before puberty; occasionally they are congenital. This dermatosis characteristically appears as small asymptomatic papules; however, they are sometimes yellow or white discs or plaques, deep nodules, or streaks (78).

Radiologic Features

The characteristic radiologic finding is numerous small foci of bony sclerosis in cancellous bone that are of variable shape (usually round or oval) (9). Commonly affected areas are the ends of the short tubular bones, the metaepiphyseal regions of the long bones, and the tarsal, carpal, and pelvic bones (Fig. 7). The foci do not change in shape and size for

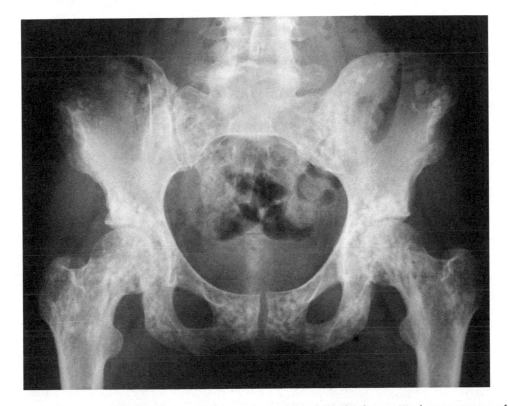

FIG. 7. Osteopoikilosis. Characteristic features shown here include the spotted appearance of the pelvis and metaepiphyseal regions of the femora. (From: Whyte MP. Rare disorders of skeletal formation and homeostasis. In: Becker KN (ed) *Principles and Practice of Endocrinology Bone Metabolism*, 2nd ed. Lippincott-Raven Publishers, Philadelphia, 1995.)

decades, but they may mimic metastatic lesions. Radionuclide accumulation is not increased on bone scintigraphy (79).

Histopathologic Studies

Dermatofibrosis lenticularis disseminata is characterized by excessive amounts of unusually broad, markedly branched, interlacing elastin fibers in the dermis; the epidermis is normal (79).

The foci of osteosclerosis are thickened trabeculae that merge with surrounding normal bone, or islands of cortical bone that include haversian systems. Mature lesions seem to be remodeling slowly (80).

Treatment

Osteopoikilosis does not require treatment. Nevertheless, family members at risk should be screened with a radiograph of the hand/wrist and knee after childhood and educated concerning the disorder.

OSTEOPATHIA STRIATA

Osteopathia striata is characterized by linear striations at the ends of long bones and in the ileum (9). Like osteopoikilosis, it is a radiographic curiosity when the skeletal findings occur alone. However, osteopathia striata is also a feature of a variety of clinically important syndromes, including osteopathia striata with cranial sclerosis (81) and osteopathia striata with focal dermal hypoplasia (82).

Clinical Presentation

When osteopathia striata occurs alone, it is benign. This form can be transmitted as an autosomal dominant trait. The musculoskeletal symptoms that may have led to the radiologic studies are probably unrelated. When there is cranial sclerosis, however, cranial nerve palsies are common (81). This clinical type is also inherited as an autosomal dominant trait.

Osteopathia striata with focal dermal hypoplasia (Goltz syndrome) is a serious X-linked recessive condition in which affected boys have widespread linear areas of dermal hypoplasia through which adipose tissue can herniate. They also have a variety of additional bony defects in their limbs (82).

Radiologic Features

Gracile linear striations in the cancellous regions of the skeleton, particularly in the metaepiphyseal portions of the long bones and in the periphery of the iliac bones, is the characteristic radiologic finding (Fig. 8) (9). The carpal, tarsal, and tubular bones of the hands and feet are less commonly and more subtly affected. The striations will remain unchanged in appearance for years. Radionuclide accumulation is not increased during bone scintigraphy (79).

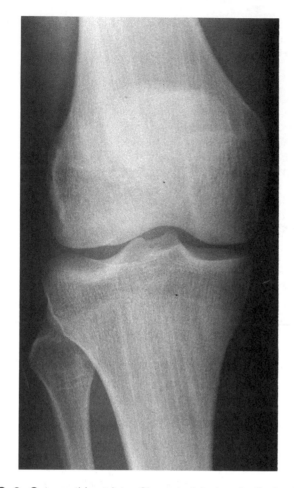

FIG. 8. Osteopathia striata. Characteristic longitudinal striations are present in the femur and tibia of this 17-year-old girl.

Histopathologic Findings

Histopathologic studies have not been described.

Treatment

Medical treatment for the osteopathia striata per se is not necessary. Although the characteristic skeletal findings are unlikely to be misdiagnosed, radiologic screening of individuals at risk would seem prudent after childhood.

In one family with osteopathia striata and cranial sclerosis, the diagnosis was reportedly made prenatally by ultrasound examination (83).

MELORHEOSTOSIS

Melorheostosis, from the Greek, refers to flowing hyperostosis of the limbs. The radiologic findings in the skeleton have been likened to the appearance of melted wax that has dripped down the side of a candle. Since its initial description in 1922 (84), about 200 cases have been reported (85,86). No Mendelian pattern of inheritance has been found; the disorder occurs sporadically.

Clinical Presentation

Melorheostosis typically manifests during childhood. Usually there is monomelic involvement; bilateral disease, when it occurs, is generally asymmetric. Cutaneous changes that overlie affected skeletal regions are not uncommon. Of 131 patients reported in one investigation, 17% had linear scleroderma-like areas and hypertrichosis. Fibromas, fibrolipomas, capillary hemangiomas, lymphangiectasis, and arterial aneurysms also occur (87,88). Soft-tissue abnormalities are often noted before the hyperostosis is discovered. Pain and stiffness are the major symptoms. Affected joints may become contracted and deformed. In affected children, leg length inequality occurs from soft tissue contractures and premature fusion of epiphyses. The skeletal changes appear to progress most rapidly during childhood. During the adult years, melorheostosis may gradually extend or fail to progress (89). Nevertheless, pain is a more frequent symptom in adults because of subperiosteal new bone formation.

Radiologic Features

Irregular, dense, eccentric hyperostosis that affects both the cortex and the adjacent medullary canal of a single bone, or several adjacent bones, is the characteristic radiologic finding in melorheostosis (Fig. 9) (9,86). Any anatomic region or bone may be affected, but the lower extremities

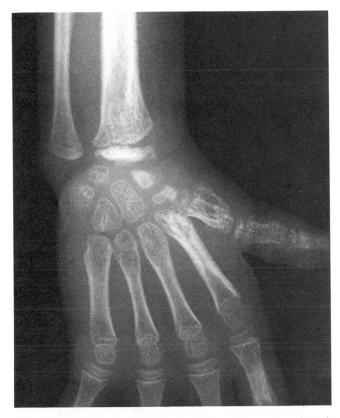

FIG. 9. Melorheostosis. Characteristic patchy osteosclerosis is most apparent in the radius and second metacarpal of this 8-year-old girl.

are most commonly involved. Bone tissue may also develop in soft tissues that are adjacent to affected skeletal areas, particularly near joints. Melorheostotic bone has increased blood flow and avidly accumulates radionuclide during bone scintigraphy (90).

Laboratory Findings

Routine laboratory studies (e.g., serum calcium and inorganic phosphate levels and alkaline phosphatase activity) are normal in melorheostosis.

Histologic Findings

The skeletal lesion in melorheostosis is characterized by endosteal thickening during infancy and childhood and then periosteal new bone formation during adulthood (86). Bony lesions are sclerotic with thickened irregular lamellae that may occlude haversian systems. Marrow fibrosis may also be present (86). Unlike in true scleroderma, the collagen of the sclerodermatous skin lesions of melorheostosis is normal appearing. Thus, this dermatosis has been called linear melorheostotic scleroderma (87,91).

Etiology and Pathogenesis

The distribution of melorheostosis and its associated soft-tissue lesions in sclerotomes, myotomes, and dermatomes suggests that a segmentary embryogenetic defect explains this sporadic condition (87,91). The linear scleroderma may reflect the primary abnormality that extends deep into the skeleton to cause the hyperostosis.

Treatment

Surgical correction of contractures has been difficult; recurrent deformity is common. Distraction techniques have been associated with promising results (92).

MIXED SCLEROSING BONE DYSTROPHY

Mixed sclerosing bone dystrophy is a rare skeletal dysplasia in which radiologic features of osteopoikilosis, osteopathia striata, melorheostosis, cranial sclerosis, and additional skeletal defects occur together in various combinations in one individual (93).

Clinical Presentation

Patients may experience the symptoms and complications that are typically associated with the individual patterns of osteosclerosis; for example, cranial sclerosis with skull enlargement may result in cranial nerve palsy, and melorheostosis can cause bone pain (93).

Radiologic Features

Two or more patterns of osteosclerosis (osteopoikilosis, osteopathia striata, melorheostosis, cranial sclerosis, generalized cortical hyperostosis, focal osteosclerosis, or progressive diaphyseal dysplasia) occur in one individual. Just a portion of the skeleton may be affected.

Bone scanning shows increased radionuclide uptake in the areas of greatest osteosclerosis (93,94).

Histopathologic Findings

Although the term *osteopetrosis* has been used to describe generalized osteosclerosis in some subjects, histopathologic study has failed to show remnants of calcified primary spongiosa (see the prededing section on osteopetrosis) (93,94).

Etiology and Pathogenesis

Delineation of mixed sclerosing bone dystrophy suggests a common pathogenesis for the individual component osteosclerotic patterns. However, osteopoikilosis and most forms of osteopathia striata are clearly heritable, whereas mixed sclerosing bone dystrophy in its most florid presentation, like melorheostosis, appears to be a sporadic disorder (93,94).

Treatment

There is no specific medical treatment. Contractures or neurovascular compression by osteosclerotic lesions may require surgical intervention.

AXIAL OSTEOMALACIA

Axial osteomalacia is characterized radiologically by coarsening of the trabecular pattern of the axial but not the appendicular skeleton (95). Fewer than 20 patients have been described. Most affected subjects appear to have been sporadic cases, but dominant transmission has been reported (96); thus, additional family studies are necessary.

Clinical Presentation

Most patients with axial osteomalacia have been middle-aged or elderly men; a few middle-aged women have been described. Radiologic manifestations, however, are likely to be detectable much earlier (96). The majority of cases have presented with dull, vague, and chronic axial skeletal pain (often in the cervical region) that prompts radiologic study. Family histories are usually negative for skeletal disease.

Radiologic Features

Abnormalities are limited essentially to the spine and pelvis, where trabeculae are coarsened and form a pattern like that in other types of osteomalacia (97). However, Looser's zones (a radiologic hallmark of osteomalacia) have not been reported. The cervical spine and ribs seem most severely affected; the lumbar spine is abnormal to a lesser degree. Two patients had features of ankylosing spondylitis (98). Radiologic survey of the appendicular skeleton is unremarkable.

Laboratory Studies

In four patients, serum inorganic phosphate levels tended to be low (98). In others, osteomalacia occurred despite normal serum levels of calcium, inorganic phosphate, 25-hydroxyvitamin D [25(OH)D], and 1,25-dihydroxyvitamin D [1,25(OH)$_2$D]. Serum alkaline phosphatase activity (bone isoenzyme) may be increased.

Histopathologic Findings

Iliac crest specimens have distinct corticomedullary junctions, but the cortices can be especially wide and porous. Trabeculae are of variable thickness; total bone volume may be increased. Collagen has a normal lamellar pattern on polarized-light microscopy. There is increased width and extent of osteoid seams on trabecular bone surfaces and in cortical spaces. Tetracycline labeling confirms the defective skeletal mineralization and results in fluorescent "labels" that are single, irregular, and wide (96). Osteoblasts are flat and inactive-appearing "lining" cells, with reduced Golgi zones and rough endoplasmic reticulum, and increased amounts of cytoplasmic glycogen, but they do stain intensely for alkaline phosphatase activity. Changes of secondary hyperparathyroidism are absent (96).

Etiology and Pathogenesis

Axial osteomalacia has been postulated to result from an osteoblast defect (99). Electron microscopic studies of iliac crest bone from one patient (96) revealed osteoblasts that had an inactive appearance but were able to form matrix vesicles within abundant osteoid.

Treatment

Effective medical therapy has not been reported. The natural history for axial osteomalacia, however, seems relatively benign. Methyltestosterone and stilbestrol have been tested unsuccessfully (99). Vitamin D$_2$ (as much as 20,000 U/day for 3 years) was similarly without beneficial effect (99). Slight improvement in skeletal histology, but not in symptoms, was reported for calcium and vitamin D$_2$ therapy in a study of four cases (98). Long-term follow-up of one patient showed that symptoms and radiologic findings did not change (99).

FIBROGENESIS IMPERFECTA OSSIUM

Fibrogenesis imperfecta ossium was first described in 1950 (100). Fewer than ten cases have been reported (101,102). Although radiologic studies suggest that there is generalized osteopenia, the coarse and dense appearance of trabecular bone explains why it is included among the osteosclerotic disorders. The clinical, biochemical, radiologic, and histopathologic features of fibrogenesis imperfecta ossium and axial osteomalacia have been carefully contrasted (100).

Clinical Presentation

Fibrogenesis imperfecta ossium typically presents during middle age or later. Both sexes are affected. Gradual onset of intractable skeletal pain that rapidly progresses is the characteristic symptom that precedes a debilitating course with progressive immobility. Spontaneous fractures are also a prominent clinical feature. Patients generally become bedridden. Physical examination typically shows marked bony tenderness.

Radiologic Features

Radiologic changes are noted throughout the skeleton, except in the skull. Initially, there may be only osteopenia and a slightly abnormal appearance of trabecular bone (102). Subsequently, the changes become more consistent with osteomalacia (i.e., further alterations of the trabecular bone pattern, heterogeneous bone density, and thinning of cortical bone). The corticomedullary junctions become indistinct as cortices are replaced by an abnormal pattern of trabecular bone. Areas of the skeleton may have a mixed lytic and sclerotic appearance (100–102). The generalized osteopenia causes the remaining trabeculae to appear coarse and dense in a fish-net pattern. Pseudofractures may develop. Deformities secondary to fractures can be present, although bony contours are typically normal. Some patients have a "rugger jersey" spine that should not be confused with a similar radiographic finding in osteopetrosis or in renal osteodystrophy. The shafts of long bones may show periosteal reaction. In fibrogenesis imperfecta ossium and axial osteomalacia, the distribution of the radiographic abnormalities (generalized versus axial) helps to distinguish the two conditions. However, the histopathologic features are also clearly different (100).

Laboratory Findings

Serum calcium and inorganic phosphate levels are normal, but alkaline phosphatase activity is increased. Acute agranulocytosis and macroglobulinemia have been reported. Hydroxyproline levels in urine may be normal or increased (102). Typically, there is no aminoaciduria or other evidence of renal tubular dysfunction.

Histopathologic Findings

The bony lesion is a form of osteomalacia, although the amount of affected bone varies considerably from area to area (102). Aberrant collagen is found in regions with abnormal mineralization patterns, but it is unremarkable in other tissues. Cortical bone in the shaft of the femora and tibiae may demonstrate the least abnormality. Osteoid seams are thick. Osteoblasts and osteoclasts can be abundant. Polarized-light microscopy shows that the abnormal bone collagen fibrils lack birefringence. Electron microscopy reveals that the collagen fibrils are thin and randomly organized in a "tangled" pattern. In some regions, peculiar circular matrix structures of 300 to 500 nm diameter have been noted (102). Unless bone specimens are viewed with polarized-light or electron microscopy, fibrogenesis imperfecta ossium can be mistaken for osteoporosis or other forms of osteomalacia (102).

Etiology and Pathogenesis

The etiology is unknown. Genetic factors have not been implicated, because this condition has been reported only sporadically. It seems to be an acquired disorder of collagen synthesis in lamellar bone. Subperiosteal bone formation and collagen synthesis in nonosseous tissues appears to be normal.

Treatment

There is no specific medical therapy. Temporary clinical improvement may occur (102). Treatment with vitamin D_2 (or an active metabolite) together with calcium supplementation has been tried without significant benefit. Indeed, ectopic calcification occurred with high-dose vitamin D_2 therapy in one patient. Synthetic salmon calcitonin, sodium fluoride, and $24,25(OH)_2D$ have also been tested, but without apparent benefit (102). Treatment with melphalan and prednisolone appeared to benefit one patient (103).

PACHYDERMOPERIOSTOSIS

Pachydermoperiostosis (hypertrophic osteoarthropathy: primary or idiopathic) causes clubbing of the digits; hyperhidrosis and thickening of the skin, especially of the face and forehead; and periosteal new bone formation that occurs prominently in the distal limbs. Autosomal dominant inheritance with variable expression is established (104), but autosomal recessive transmission also seems to occur (105).

Clinical Presentation

Men appear to be more severely affected than women, and blacks more commonly than whites. The age at presentation is variable, but symptoms typically first manifest during adolescence (104,105). All three principal features (pachydermia, cutis verticis gyrata, periostitis) are present in some affected individuals; others have just one or two of these findings. Clinical expression develops during the course of a decade, but the disorder then becomes quiescent (106). Progressive gradual enlargement of the hands and feet can result in a "pawlike" appearance. Some patients are described as acromegalic. Arthralgias of the ankles, knees, wrists, and elbows are common. Occasionally, the small joints are also painful. Acro-osteolysis has also been reported. Symptoms of pseudogout can occur. Chondrocalcinosis, with calcium pyrophosphate crystals in synovial fluid, has been found in one patient. Stiffness and limited mobility of both the appendicular and the axial skeleton can develop. Compression of cranial or spinal nerves has been described. Cutaneous changes include coarsening, thickening, furrowing, pitting, and oiliness of especially the scalp and face. Fatigue is not uncommon. Myelophthisic anemia with extramedullary hematopoiesis may occur. Life expectancy is normal (106).

Radiologic Features

Severe periostitis that thickens and scleroses the distal portions of the tubular bones—typically the tibia, fibula, radius, and ulna—is the principal radiologic abnormality (Fig. 10). The metacarpals, tarsals/metatarsals, clavicles, pelvis, base of the skull, and phalanges may also be affected. Clubbing is obvious, and acro-osteolysis can occur. The spine is rarely involved. Ankylosis of joints, especially in the hands and in the feet, may occur in older patients (9).

The principal consideration in the differential diagnosis for pachydermoperiostosis is secondary hypertrophic osteoarthropathy (pulmonary or otherwise). The radiologic features of this condition are, however, somewhat different. In secondary hypertrophic osteoarthropathy, the periosteal reaction typically has a smooth, undulating appearance (107). In pachydermoperiostosis, periosteal proliferation is more exuberant, has an irregular appearance, and often involves epiphyses. Bone scanning in either condition reveals symmetrical, diffuse, regular uptake along the cortical margins of long bones, especially in the legs. This feature results in a "double stripe" sign.

Laboratory Findings

Synovial fluid examination typically does not reveal evidence of inflammation.

Periosteal new bone formation roughens the surface of cortical bone (108). This newly formed osseous tissue undergoes cancellous compaction and can accordingly be difficult to distinguish from the original cortex (108). However, there may be osteopenia of trabecular bone from quiescent formation (9). Mild cellular hyperplasia and thickening of subsynovial blood vessels is found near synovial membranes (109). Electron microscopy demonstrates layered basement membranes.

Etiology and Pathogenesis

No gene defects have been identified. A controversial hypothesis suggests that some unknown circulating factor acts on the vasculature initially to cause hyperemia, and it thereby alters soft tissues, but later blood flow is reduced (105).

Treatment

There is no established medical treatment. Painful synovial effusions may respond to nonsteroidal anti-inflammatory drugs (110). Colchicine was reported to be an effective medication for arthralgias, clubbing, folliculitis, and pachy-

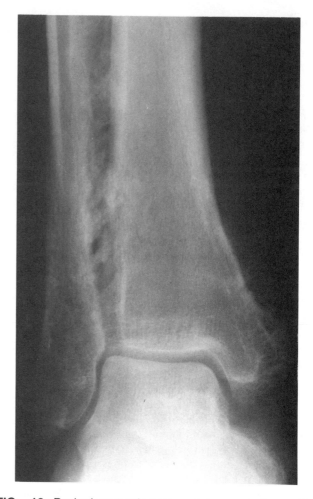

FIG. 10. Pachydermoperiostosis. Anteroposterior radiograph of the ankle shows ragged periosteal reaction along the interosseous membrane between the tibia and fibula (note also the proliferative bone formation along the medial malleolus). (From: Whyte MP. Rare disorders of skeletal formation and homeostasis. In: Becker KN (ed) *Principles and Practice of Endocrinology and Metabolism,* 2nd ed. Lippincott-Raven Publishers, Philadelphia, 1995.)

derma in one patient (111). Contractures or neurovascular compression by osteosclerotic lesions may require surgical intervention.

HEPATITIS C-ASSOCIATED OSTEOSCLEROSIS

In 1992, a new syndrome was characterized which features remarkably severe, developmental, generalized osteosclerosis in hepatitis C-positive former intravenous drug abusers (112).

Periosteal, endosteal, and trabecular bone thickening occurs throughout the skeleton except in the cranium (Fig. 11). The forearms and legs are painful. Densitometric studies show bone mass that may be 200% to 300% above mean values for age and sex. Skeletal remodeling can be abnormally rapid and respond to calcitonin therapy. Gradual spontaneous remission in pain and normalization of bone remodeling may occur. Tainted blood exposure is characteristic (113).

OTHER SCLEROSING BONE DYSPLASIAS

Table 1 lists the relatively large number of conditions that cause focal or generalized increases in skeletal mass (114). Of note, sarcoidosis characteristically causes cysts within coarsely reticulated bone; occasionally, however, sclerotic areas are found in the axial skeleton or in long tubular bones. These skeletal changes may occur well after the pulmonary disease is arrested. Although multiple myeloma typ-ically presents with generalized osteopenia or with discrete osteolytic lesions, widespread osteosclerosis can occur. Lymphoma, myelosclerosis, and mastocytosis are additional hematologic causes of increased bone mass. Metastatic car-cinoma, primarily prostatic, commonly causes osteosclero-sis. Diffuse osteosclerosis is also a relatively frequent radio-logic finding in secondary hyperparathyroidism (as with renal disease), but it can occur in primary hyperparathy-roidism as well. Intoxication with vitamin A or vitamin D, heavy metal poisoning, milk-alkali syndrome, ionizing radi-ation, osteomyelitis, and osteonecrosis are additional etiolo-gies for increased bone mass (114).

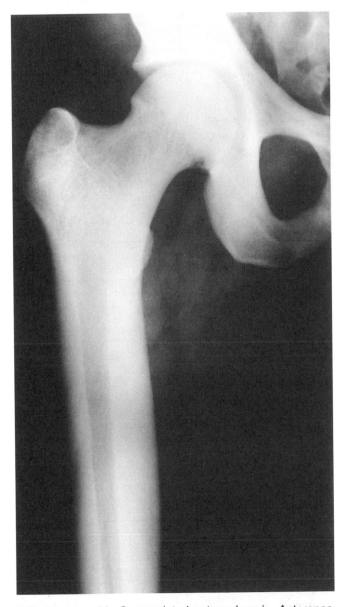

FIG. 11. Hepatitis C-associated osteosclerosis. Anteropos-terior view of the proximal right femur of this middle-aged, former intravenous drug abuser shows diffuse bony sclerosis with marked cortical thickening. The medullary cavity is nar-row and the periosteal margins of the cortex are mildly con-vex, suggesting endosteal and periosteal bone apposition, respectively. The cortices of the greater and lesser trochanters are relatively spared. The trabecular pattern in the femoral neck is especially prominent [From Whyte et al., *J Bone Miner Res* 11:554–558, 1996.]

REFERENCES

1. Albers-Schönberg H: Rontgenbilder einer seltenen, Knochen-erkrankung. *Meunch Med Wochenschr* 51:365, 1904
2. Johnston CC Jr, Lavy N, Lord T, et al.: Osteopetrosis: A clinical, genetic, metabolic, and morphologic study of the dominantly inherited, benign form. *Medicine* 47:149–167, 1968
3. Loria-Cortes R, Quesada-Calvo E, Cordero-Chaverri E: Osteope-trosis in children: A report of 26 cases. *J Pediatr* 91:43–47, 1977
4. Kahler SG, Burns JA, Aylsworth AS: A mild autosomal recessive form of osteopetrosis. *Am J Med Genet* 17:451–464, 1984
5. Jagadha V, Halliday WC, Becker LE, Hinton D: The association of infantile osteopetrosis and neuronal storage disease in two brothers. *Acta Neuropathol* 75:233–240, 1988
6. Whyte MP: Recent advances in osteopetrosis. In: Cohn DV, Gen-nari C, Tashian AH (eds) *Calcium-Regulating Hormones and Bone Metabolism.* Elsevier, Amsterdam, pp 420–430, 1992
7. Marks SC Jr: Osteopetrosis—Multiple pathways for the intercep-tion of osteoclast function. *Appl Pathol* 5:172–183, 1987
8. Bollerslev J: Autosomal dominant osteopetrosis: Bone metabo-lism and epidemiological, clinical and hormonal aspects. *Endocr Rev* 10:45–67, 1989
9. Resnick D, Niwayama G: *Diagnosis of Bone and Joint Disorders,* 3rd ed. WB Saunders, Philadelphia, 1995
10. Oliveira G, Boechat MI, Amaral SM, et al.: Osteopetrosis and rickets: An intriguing association. *Am J Dis Child* 140:377–378, 1986
11. Park H-M, Lambertus J: Skeletal and reticuloendothelial imaging in osteopetrosis: Case report. *J Nucl Med* 18:1091–1095, 1977
12. Rao VM, Dalinka MK, Mitchell DG, et al.: Osteopetrosis: MR characteristics at 1.5 T. *Radiology* 161:217–220, 1986
13. Elster AD, Theros EG, Key LL, Chen MYM: Cranial imaging in autosomal recessive osteopetrosis (parts I & II). *Radiology* 183:129–144, 1992
14. Key LL, Carnes D, Holtrop M, et al.: Treatment of congenital osteopetrosis with high dose calcitriol. *N Engl J Med* 310:409–415, 1984
15. Cournot G, Trubert-Thil CL, Petrovic M, Boyle A, Cormier C, Girault D, Fischer A, Garabedian M: Mineral metabolism in infants with malignant osteopetrosis: Heterogeneity in plasma 1,25-dihydroxyvitamin D levels and bone histology. *J Bone Miner Res* 7:1–10, 1992
16. Whyte MP, Chines A, Silva DP Jr, Landt Y, Ladenson JH: Crea-tine kinase brain isoenzyme (BB-CK) presence in serum distin-guishes osteopetrosis among the sclerosing bone disorders. *J Bone Miner Res* 1996 (in press)
17. Revell PA: *Pathology of Bone.* Springer-Verlag, Berlin, 1986
18. Bollerslev J, Steiniche T, Melsen F, Mosekilde L: Structural and histomorphometric studies of iliac crest trabecular and cortical bone in autosomal dominant osteopetrosis: A study of two radio-logical types. *Bone* 10:19–24, 1989
19. Helfrich MH, Aronson DC, Everts V, Mieremet RHP, Gerritsen EJA, Eckhardt PG, Groot CG, Scherft JP: Morphologic features of bone in human osteopetrosis. *Bone* 12:411–419, 1991
20. Whyte, MP: Chipping away at marble bone disease *(editorial). N Engl J Med* 332:1639–1640, 1995
21. Teitelbaum SL, Tondravi MM, Ross FP: Osteoclast biology. In:

Marcus R, Feldman D, Kelsey J (eds) *Osteoporosis.* Academic Press, San Diego, 61–94, 1996

22. Mills BG, Yabe H, Singer FR: Osteoclasts in human osteopetrosis contain viral-nucleocapsid-like nuclear inclusions. *J Bone Miner Res* 3:101–106, 1988

23. Glorieux FH, Pettifor JM, Marie PJ, et al.: Induction of bone resorption by parathyroid hormone in congenital malignant osteopetrosis. *Metab Bone Dis Rel Res* 3:143–150, 1981

24. Key LL, Ries WL, Schiff R: Osteopetrosis associated with interleukin-2 deficiency *(abstract). J Bone Miner Res* 2(suppl II):85, 1987

25. Key LL, Rodriguiz RN, Willi SM, Wright NM, Hatcher HC, Eyre DR, Cure JK, Griffin PP, Ries WL: Recombinant human interferon gamma therapy for osteopetrosis. *N Engl J Med* 332:1594–1599, 1995

26. Beard CJ, Key L, Newburger PE, et al.: Neutrophil defect associated with malignant infantile osteopetrosis. *J Lab Clin Med* 108:498–505, 1986

27. Kaplan FS, August CS, Fallon MD, et al.: Successful treatment of infantile malignant osteopetrosis by bone-marrow transplantation: A case report. *J Bone Joint Surg (Am)* 70:617–623, 1988

28. Coccia PF, Krivit W, Cervenka J, et al.: Successful bone-marrow transplantation for infantile malignant osteopetrosis. *N Engl J Med* 302:701–708, 1980

29. Orchard PJ, Dickerman JD, Mathews CHE, et al.: Haploidentical bone marrow transplantation for osteopetrosis. *Am J Pediatr Hematol Oncol* 9:335–340, 1987

30. Rawlinson PS, Green RH, Coggins AM, Boyle IT, Gibson BE: Malignant osteopetrosis: Hypercalcaemia after bone marrow transplantation. *Arch Dis Child* 66:638–639, 1991

31. Key LL Jr: Osteopetrosis: A genetic window into osteoclast function. In: *Cases Metab Bone Dis* 2(3), pp 1–12, 1987

32. Dorantes LM, Mejia AM, Dorantes S: Juvenile osteopetrosis: Effects of blood and bone of prednisone and low calcium, high phosphate diet. *Arch Dis Child* 61:666–670, 1986

33. Ogur G, Ogur E, Celasun B, Baser I, Imirzalioglu N, Ozturk T, Alemdaroglut A: Prenatal diagnosis of autosomal recessive osteopetrosis, infantile type, by X-ray evaluation. *Prenat Diagn* 15:477–481, 1995

34. Sly WS, Hewett-Emmett D, Whyte MP, et al.: Carbonic anhydrase II deficiency identified as the primary defect in the autosomal recessive syndrome of osteopetrosis with renal tubular acidosis and cerebral calcification. *Proc Natl Acad Sci USA* 80:2752–2756, 1983

35. Whyte MP: Carbonic anhydrase II deficiency. *Clin Orthop* 294:52–63, 1993

36. Sly WS, Whyte MP, Sundaram V, et al.: Carbonic anhydrase II deficiency in 12 families with the autosomal recessive syndrome of osteopetrosis with renal tubular acidosis and cerebral calcification. *N Engl J Med* 313:139–145, 1985

37. Sly WS, Hu PY: The carbonic anhydrase II deficiency syndrome: Osteopetrosis with renal tubular acidosis and cerebral calcification. In: Scriver CR, Beaudet AL, Sly WS, Valle D (eds) *The Metabolic and Molecular Bases of Inherited Disease,* 7th ed. McGraw-Hill, New York, 4113–4124, 1995

38. Whyte MP, Murphy WA, Fallon MD, et al.: Osteopetrosis, renal tubular acidosis and basal ganglia calcification in three sisters. *Am J Med* 69:64–74, 1980

39. Sly WS, Whyte MP, Krupin T, et al.: Positive renal response to acetazolamide in carbonic anhydrase II-deficient patients. *Pediatr Res* 19:1033–1036, 1985

40. Roth DE, Venta PJ, Tashian RE, Sly WS: Molecular basis of human carbonic anhydrase II deficiency. *Proc Natl Acad Sci USA* 89:1804–1808, 1992

41. Whyte MP, Hamm LL III, Sly WS: Transfusion of carbonic anhydrase-replete erythrocytes fails to correct the acidification defect in the syndrome of osteopetrosis, renal tubular acidosis, and cerebral calcification (carbonic anhydrase II deficiency). *J Bone Miner Res* 3:385–388, 1988

42. Maroteaux P, Lamy M: The malady of Toulouse-Lautrec. *JAMA* 191:715–717, 1965

43. Maroteaux P, Lamy M: La pycnodysostose. *Presse Med* 70:999–1002, 1962

44. Sugiura Y, Yamada Y, Koh J: Pycnodysostosis in Japan: Report of six cases and a review of Japanese literature. *Birth Defects* X(12):78–98, 1974

45. Elmore SM: Pycnodysostosis: A review. *J Bone Joint Surg* 49A:153–162, 1967

46. Wolpowitz A, Matisson A: A comparative study of pycnodysostosis, cleidocranial dysostosis, osteopetrosis and acro-osteolysis. *S Afr Med J* 48:1011–1118, 1974

47. Soto TJ, Mautalen CA, Hojman D, et al.: Pycnodysostosis, metabolic and histologic studies. In: *Birth Defects* V(4):109–115, 1969

48. Everts V, Aronson DC, Beertsen W: Phagocytosis of bone collagen by osteoclasts in two cases of pycnodysostosis. *Calcif Tissue Int* 37:25–31, 1985

49. Cabrejas ML, Fromm GA, Roca JF, et al.: Pycnodysostosis: Some aspects concerning kinetics of calcium metabolism and bone pathology. *Am J Med Sci* 271(2):215–220, 1976

50. Beneton MNC, Harris S, Kanis JA: Paramyxovirus-like inclusions in two cases of pycnodysostosis. *Bone* 8:211–217, 1987

51. Edelson JG, Obad S, Geiger R, On A, Artul HJ: Pycnodysostosis: Orthopedic aspects, with a description of 14 new cases. *Clin Orthop* 280:263–276, 1992

52. Cockayne EA: A case for diagnosis. *Proc R Soc Med* 13:132–136, 1920

53. Engelmann G: Ein fall von osteopathia hyperostotica (sclerotisans) multiplex infantilis. *Fortschr Geb Roentgen* 39:1101–1106, 1929

54. Hundley JD, Wilson FC: Progressive diaphyseal dysplasia: Review of the literature and report of seven cases in one family. *J Bone Joint Surg* 55(A):461–474, 1973

55. Naveh Y, Ludatshcer R, Alon U, et al.: Muscle involvement in progressive diaphyseal dysplasia. *Pediatrics* 76:944–949, 1985

56. Crisp AJ, Brenton DP: Engelmann's disease of bone—A systemic disorder? *Ann Rheum Dis* 41:183–188, 1982

57. Smith R, Walton RJ, Corner BD, et al.: Clinical and biochemical studies in Engelmann's disease (progressive diaphyseal dysplasia). *Q J Med* 46:273–294, 1977

58. Kumar B, Murphy WA, Whyte MP: Progressive diaphyseal dysplasia (Engelmann's disease): Scintigraphic-radiologic-clinical correlations. *Radiology* 140:87–92, 1981

59. Applegate LJ, Applegate GR, Kemp SS: MR of multiple cranial neuropathies in a patient with Camurati-Engelmann disease: Case report. *Am Soc Neuroradiol* 12:557–559, 1991

60. Shier CK, Krasicky GA, Ellis BI, Kottamasu SR: Ribbing's disease: Radiographic-scintigraphic correlation and comparative analysis with Engelmann's disease. *J Nucl Med* 28:244–248, 1987

61. Labat ML, Bringuier AF, Seebold C, Moricard Y, Meyer-Mula C, Laporte P, Talmage RV, Grubb SA, Simmons DJ, Milhaud G: Monocytic origin of fibroblasts: Spontaneous transformation of blood monocytes into neo-fibroblastic structures in osteomyelosclerosis and Engelmann's disease. *Biomed Pharmacother* 45:289–299, 1991

62. Kaftori JK, Kleinhaus U, Neveh Y: Progressive diaphyseal dysplasia (Camurati-Engelmann): Radiographic follow-up and CT findings. *Radiology* 164:777–782, 1987

63. Naveh Y, Alon U, Kaftori JK, et al.: Progressive diaphyseal dysplasia: Evaluation of corticosteroid therapy. *Pediatrics* 75:321–323, 1985

64. Fallon MD, Whyte MP, Murphy WA: Progressive diaphyseal dysplasia (Engelmann's disease): Report of a sporadic case of the mild form. *J Bone Joint Surg* 62(A):465–472, 1980

65. van Buchem FSP, Prick JJG, Jaspar HHJ: *Hyperostosis Corticalis Generalisata Familiaris (Van Buchem's Disease).* Excerpta, Amsterdam, 1976

66. Perez-Vicente Jr, Rodriguez de Castro E, Lafuente J, et al.: Autosomal dominant endosteal hyperostosis. Report of a Spanish family with neurological involvement. *Clin Genet* 31:161–169, 1987

67. Eastman JR, Bixler D: Generalized cortical hyperostosis (van Buchem disease): Nosologic considerations. *Radiology* 125:297–304, 1977

68. Beighton P, Barnard A, Hamersma H, et al.: The syndromic status of sclerosteosis and van Buchem disease. *Clin Genet* 25:175–181, 1984

69. Hill SC, Stein SA, Dwyer A, Altman J, Dorwart R, Doppman J:

Cranial CT findings in sclerosteosis. *Am J Neuroradiol* 7:505–511, 1986

70. Ruckert EW, Caudill RJ, McCready PJ: Surgical treatment of van Buchem disease. *J Oral Maxillofac Surg* 43:801–805, 1985

71. Schendel SA: van Buchem disease: Surgical treatment of the mandible. *Ann Plast Surg* 20:462–467, 1988

72. Beighton P, Durr L, Hamersma H: The clinical features of sclerosteosis: A review of the manifestations in twenty-five affected individuals. *Ann Intern Med* 84:393–397, 1976

73. Barnard AH, Hamersma H, Kretzmar JH, et al.: Sclerosteosis in old age. *S Afr Med J* 58:401–403, 1980

74. Beighton P, Cremin BJ, Hamersma H: The radiology of sclerosteosis. *Br J Radiol* 49:934–939, 1976

75. Stein SA, Witkop C, Hill S, et al.: Sclerosteosis, neurogenetic and pathophysiologic analysis of an American kinship. *Neurology* 33:267–277, 1983

76. Epstein S, Hamersma H, Beighton P: Endocrine function in sclerosteosis. *S Afr Med J* 55:1105–1110, 1979

77. Berlin R, Hedensio B, Lilja B, et al.: Osteopoikilosis—A clinical and genetic study. *Acta Med Scand* 18:305–314, 1967

78. Uitto J, Starcher BC, Santa-Cruz DJ, et al.: Biochemical and ultrastructural demonstration of elastin accumulation in the skin of the Buschke-Ollendorff syndrome. *J Invest Derm* 76:284–287, 1981

79. Whyte MP, Murphy WA, Seigel BA: 99m Tc-pyrophosphate bone imaging in osteopoikilosis, osteopathia striata, and melorheostosis. *Radiology* 127:439–443, 1978

80. Lagier R, Mbakop A, Bigler A: Osteopoikilosis: A radiological and pathological study. *Skeletal Radiol* 11:161–168, 1984

81. Rabinow M, Unger F: Syndrome of osteopathia striata, macrocephaly, and cranial sclerosis. *Am J Dis Child* 138:821–823, 1984

82. Happle R, Lenz W: Striation of bones in focal dermal hypoplasia: Manifestation of functional mosaicism? *Br J Dermatol* 96:133–138, 1977

83. Kornreich L, Grunebaum M, Ziv N, Shuper A, Mimouni M: Osteopathia striata, cranial sclerosis with cleft palate and facial nerve palsy. *Eur J Pediatr* 147:101–103, 1988

84. Léri A, Joanny J: Une affection non decrite des os. Hyperostose "en coulée" sur toute la longueur d'un membre ou "melorheostose." *Bull Mem Soc Med Hop Paris* 46:1141–1145, 1922

85. Murray RO, McCredie J: Melorheostosis and sclerotomes: A radiological correlation. *Skeletal Radiol* 4:57–71, 1979

86. Campbell CJ, Papademetriou T, Bonfiglio M: Melorheostosis: A report of the clinical, roentgenographic, and pathological findings in fourteen cases. *J Bone Joint Surg* 50(A):1281–1304, 1968

87. Miyachi Y, Horio T, Yamada A, et al.: Linear melorheostotic scleroderma with hypertrichosis. *Arch Dermatol* 115:1233–1234, 1979

88. Applebaum RE, Caniano DA, Sun C-C, et al.: Synchronous left subclavian and axillary artery aneurysms associated with melorheostosis. *Surgery* 99:249–253, 1986

89. Colavita N, Nicolais S, Orazi C, Falappa PG: Melorheostosis: Presentation of a case followed up for 24 years. *Arch Orthop Trauma Surg* 106:123–125, 1987

90. Davis DC, Syklawer R, Cole RL: Melorheostosis on three-phase bone scintigraphy: Case report. *Clin Nucl Med* 17:561–564, 1992

91. Wagers LT, Young AW Jr, Ryan SF: Linear melorheostotic scleroderma. *Br J Dermatol* 86:297–301, 1972

92. Atar D, Lehman WB, Grant AD, Strongwater AM: The Ilizarov apparatus for treatment of melorheostosis: Case report and review of the literature. *Clin Orthop* 281:163–167, 1992

93. Whyte MP, Murphy WA, Fallon MD, et al.: Mixed-sclerosing-bone-dystrophy: Report of a case and review of the literature. *Skeletal Radiol* 6:95–102, 1981

94. Pacifici R, Murphy WA, Teitelbaum SL, Whyte MP: Mixed-sclerosing-bone-dystrophy: 42-year follow-up of a case reported as osteopetrosis. *Calcif Tissue Int* 38:175–185, 1986

95. Frame B, Frost HM, Ormond RS, et al.: Atypical axial osteomalacia involving the axial skeleton. *Ann Int Med* 55:632–639, 1961

96. Whyte MP, Fallon MD, Murphy WA, et al.: Axial osteomalacia: clinical, laboratory and genetic investigation of an affected mother and son. *Am J Med* 71:1041–1049, 1981

97. Christman D, Wenger JJ, Dosch JC, et al.: L'osteomalacie axiale: Analyse compare avec la fibrogenese imparfaite. *J Radiol* 62:37–41, 1981

98. Nelson AM, Riggs BL, Jowsey JO: Atypical axial osteomalacia: Report of four cases with two having features of ankylosing spondylitis. *Arthritis Rheum* 21:715–722, 1978

99. Condon JR, Nassim JR: Axial osteomalacia. *Postgrad Med* 47:817–820, 1971

100. Christman D, Wenger JJ, Dosch JC, et al.: L'osteomalacie axiale analyse compare avec la fibrogenese imparfaite. *J Radiol* 62:37–41, 1981

101. Swan CHJ, Shah K, Brewer DB, et al.: Fibrogenesis imperfecta ossium. *Q J Med* 45:233–253, 1976

102. Lang R, Vignery AM, Jenson PS: Fibrogenesis imperfecta ossium with early onset: Observations after 20 years of illness. *Bone* 7:237–246, 1986

103. Ralphs JR, Stamp TCB, Dopping-Hepenstal PJC, Ali SY: Ultrastructural features of the osteoid of patients with fibrogenesis imperfecta ossium. *Bone* 10:243–249, 1989

104. Rimoin DL: Pachydermoperiostosis (idiopathic clubbing and periostosis). Genetic and physiologic considerations. *N Engl J Med* 272:923–931, 1965

105. Matucci-Cerinic M, Lott T, Jajic IVO, Pignone A, Bussani C, Cagnoni M: The clinical spectrum of pachydermoperiostosis (primary hypertrophic osteoarthropathy). *Medicine* 79:208–214, 1991

106. Herman MA, Massaro D, Katz S: Pachydermoperiostosis—Clinical spectrum. *Arch Intern Med* 116:919–923, 1965

107. Ali A, Tetalman M, Fordham EW: Distribution of hypertrophic pulmonary osteoarthropathy. *Am J Roentgenol* 134:771–780, 1980

108. Vogl A, Goldfischer S: Pachydermoperiostosis: Primary or idiopathic hypertrophic osteoarthropathy. *Am J Med* 33:166–187, 1962

109. Lauter SA, Vasey FB, Huttner I, Osterland CK: Pachydermoperiostosis: Studies on the synovium. *J Rheumatol* 5:85–95, 1978

110. Cooper RG, Freemont AJ, Riley M, Holt PJL, Anderson DC, Jayson MIV: Bone abnormalities and severe arthritis in pachydermoperiostosis. *Ann Rheum Dis* 51:416–419, 1992

111. Matucci-Cerinic M, Fattorini L, Gerini G, Lombardi A, Pignone A, Petrini N, Lotti T: Cochicine treatment in a case of pachydermoperiostosis with acroosteolysis. *Rheumatol Int* 8:185–188, 1988

112. Whyte MP, Teitelbaum SL, Reinus WR: Doubling skeletal mass during adult life: The syndrome of diffuse osteosclerosis after intravenous drug abuse. *J Bone Miner Res* 11:554–558, 1996

113. Whyte MP, Reasner CA: Hepatitis C-associated osteosclerosis after blood transfusion. *(submitted)*

114. Frame B, Honasoge M, Kottamasu SR: *Osteosclerosis, Hyperostosis, and Related Disorders*. Elsevier, New York, 1987

69. Fibrous Dysplasia

Michael P. Whyte, M.D.

Division of Bone and Mineral Diseases, Washington University School of Medicine; and Metabolic Research Unit, Shriners Hospital for Crippled Children, St. Louis, Missouri

Fibrous dysplasia is a sporadic developmental disorder characterized by a unifocal or multifocal expanding fibrous lesion of bone-forming mesenchyme that often results in fracture and/or deformity. The condition affects both sexes.

McCune-Albright syndrome refers to patients with fibrous dysplasia (generally polyostotic) and patches of skin pigmentation, called café-au-lait spots, who also have hyperfunction of one or more endocrine glands.

Somatic mosaicism for "activating" mutations in the Gsα subunit of the receptor/adenylate cyclase-coupling G protein (which stimulates cAMP production) cause all types of fibrous dysplasia (see the following).

CLINICAL PRESENTATION

Mono-ostotic fibrous dysplasia characteristically develops during the second or third decade of life; polyostotic disease generally manifests before 10 years of age (1). The mono-ostotic form is most common. Typically, an expansile bony lesion causes fracture or deformity and may occasionally entrap nerves. The skull and long bones are affected most often. Sarcomatous degeneration of involved skeletal sites occurs with somewhat increased frequency (incidence <1%), especially when the facial bones or femora are involved (2). Pregnancy may reactivate previously quiescent lesions (3).

In the McCune-Albright syndrome, café-au-lait spots are hyperpigmented macules with rough borders (Fig. 1) compared to the smooth borders of these lesions in neurofibromatosis (i.e., "Coast-of-Maine" versus "Coast-of-California," respectively) (4). Typically, the endocrinopathy is pseudoprecocious puberty in girls due to early ovarian activity. Less commonly, there is thyrotoxicosis, Cushing syndrome, acromegaly, hyperprolactinemia, hyperparathyroidism, or pseudoprecocious puberty in boys (5–8). In some patients with widespread skeletal lesions, renal phosphate wasting causes hypophosphatemic bone disease. This situation resembles an oncogenic form of rickets or osteomalacia (see Chapter 62) (9).

RADIOLOGIC FEATURES

Femora, tibiae, ribs, and facial bones are involved most frequently, but any skeletal site can be affected (10). Small bones show radiographic features in about 50% of patients with polyostotic disease. In the long bones, the lesions may be found either in the metaphysis or in the diaphysis. Typically, they are well defined and are characterized by thin cortices and a ground glass appearance (Fig. 2). Occasionally, the lesions are lobulated with trabeculated areas of radiolucency.

LABORATORY FINDINGS

Although serum alkaline phosphatase activity may be elevated, calcium and inorganic phosphate levels are usually normal.

Both mono-ostotic and polyostotic bone lesions have a similar histologic appearance. They are anatomically well defined but are not encapsulated. Characteristically, spindle-shaped fibroblasts form "swirls" within marrow spaces. Haphazardly arranged trabeculae are composed of woven bone. Cartilage is found within these lesions more often when there is polyostotic involvement. Cystic regions, which are lined by multinucleated giant cells, may be present. These findings resemble the histopathology of hyperparathyroidism (osteitis fibrosa cystica), but an important distinction is that osteoblasts are absent in fibrous dysplasia rather than plentiful in hyperparathyroid bone disease (1).

ETIOLOGY AND PATHOGENESIS

Recently, mono-ostotic and polyostotic fibrous dysplasia were associated with the same activating mutation in the Gsα protein discovered in 1991 in the McCune-Albright

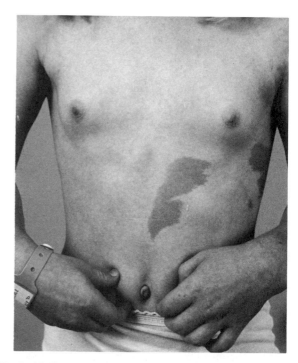

FIG. 1. McCune-Albright syndrome. Characteristic café-au-lait spots (rough border) are present on the left abdomen and chest of this $3^{10}/_{12}$-year-old girl who also has precocious breast development.

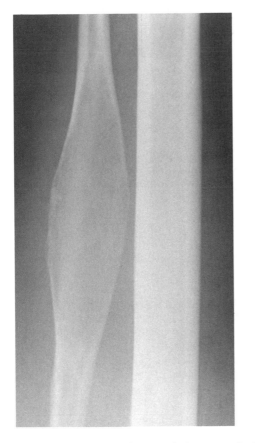

FIG. 2. Fibrous dysplasia. A characteristic expansile lesion with ground glass appearance has caused thinning of the cortex in the mid-diaphyseal region of the right fibula of this young man.

syndrome (11–14). The skeletal lesion appears to result from the formation of imperfect bone, because mesenchymal cells do not fully differentiate to osteoblasts. Endocrine hyperfunction in the McCune-Albright syndrome is generally due to end-organ hyperactivity (5,15). Recent studies of growth hormone and prolactin hypersecretion in this syndrome suggest that some patients have defective hypothalamic regulation of the pituitary and/or an embryologic abnormality in pituitary cell differentiation and function (15).

TREATMENT

There is no specific medical treatment for the skeletal disease of fibrous dysplasia. Spontaneous healing of the bone lesions does not occur. In most patients with mild disease, the radiologic appearance of bone defects does not change. In more severe cases, individual lesions may progress, and new ones can appear (10). Fractures generally mend well. Nevertheless, stress or fissure fractures can be difficult to detect and treat. When the skull is involved, neurologic assessment and careful follow-up are necessary, because nerve compression may require surgical intervention. Preliminary reports describe some relief from bone pain and radiologic improvement following pamidronate therapy (16).

In the McCune-Albright syndrome, an aromatase inhibitor, testolactone, can control the precocious puberty of affected girls (17), although some may escape from control after several years of treatment (18). Calcitriol and inorganic phosphate supplementation have not been extensively evaluated for associated hypophosphatemic bone disease, but they have reversed radiographic features of rickets in some of our patients *(personal observation)*.

REFERENCES

1. Harris WH, Dudley HR Jr, Barry RJ: The natural history of fibrous dysplasia: An orthopedic, pathological and roentgenographic study. *J Bone Joint Surg* 44(A):207–233, 1962
2. Johnson CB, Gilbert EF, Gottlieb LI: Malignant transformation of polyostotic fibrous dysplasia. *South Med J* 72:353–356, 1979
3. Kaplan FS, Fallon MD, Boden SD, Schmidt R, Senior M, Haddad JG: Estrogen receptors in bone in a patient with polyostotic fibrous dysplasia (McCune-Albright Syndrome). *N Engl J Med* 319:241–245, 1988
4. Schwindinger WF, Levine MA: McCune-Albright syndrome. *Trends Endocrinol Metab* 4:238–242, 1993
5. Harris RI; Polyostotic fibrous dysplasia with acromegaly. *Am J Med* 78:538–542, 1985
6. Feuillan PP, Jones J, Ross JL: Growth hormone hypersecretion in a girl with McCune-Albright syndrome: Comparison with controls and response to a dose of long-acting somatostatin analog. *J Endocrinol Metab* 80:1357–1360, 1995
7. Cavanah SF, Dons RF: McCune-Albright syndrome: How many endocrinopathies can one patient have? *South Med J* 86:364–367, 1993
8. Shenker A, Weinstein LS, Moran A, Pescovitz OH, Charest NJ, Boney CM, Van Wyk JJ, Merino MJ, Feuillan PP, Spiegel AM: Severe endocrine and nonendocrine manifestations of the McCune-Albright syndrome associated with activating mutations of stimulatory G protein Gs. *J Peds* 123:509–518, 1993
9. Lever EG, Pettingale KW: Albright's syndrome associated with a soft-tissue myxoma and hypophosphatemic osteomalacia. Report of a case and review of the literature. *J Bone Joint Surg* 65(B): 621–626, 1983
10. Resnick D, Niwayama G: *Diagnosis of Bone and Joint Disorders,* 3rd ed. WB Saunders, Philadelphia, 1995
11. Weinstein LS, Shenker A, Gejman PV, Merino MJ, Friedman E, Spiegel AM: Activating mutations of the stimulatory G protein in the McCune-Albright syndrome. *N Engl J Med* 325:1688–1695, 1991
12. Schwindinger WF, Francomano CA, Levine MA: Identification of a mutation in the gene encoding the α subunit of the stimulatory G protein of adenylyl cyclase in McCune-Albright syndrome. *Proc Natl Acad Sci (USA)* 89:5152–5156, 1992
13. Shenker A, Weinstein LS, Sweet DE, Spiegel AM: An activating Gs alpha mutation is present in fibrous dysplasia of bone in the McCune-Albright syndrome. *J Endocrinol Metab* 79:750–755, 1994
14. Shenker A, Chanson P, Weinstein LS, Chi P, Spiegel AM, Lomri A, Marie PJ: Osteoblastic cells derived from isolated lesions of fibrous dysplasia contain activating somatic mutations of the Gsa gene. *Hum Molec Genet* 4:1675–1676, 1995
15. Cuttler L, Jackson JA, Saeed uz-Zafar M, Levitsky LL, Mellinger RC, Frohman LA: Hypersecretion of growth hormone and prolactin in McCune-Albright syndrome. *J Clin Endocrinol Metab* 68:1148–1154, 1989
16. Liens D, Delmas PD, Meunier PJ: Long-term effects of intravenous pamidronate in fibrous dysplasia of bone. *Lancet* 343: 953–954, 1994
17. Feuillan PP, Foster CM, Pescovitz OH, Hench KD, Shawker T, Dwyer A, Malley JD, Barnes K, Loriaux DL, Cutler GB Jr: Treatment of precocious puberty in the McCune-Albright syndrome with the aromatase inhibitor testolactone. *N Engl J Med* 315:1115–1119, 1986
18. Feuillan PP, Jones J, Cutler GB Jr: Long-term testolactone therapy for precocious puberty in girls with the McCune-Albright syndrome. *J Endrocrinol Metab* 77:647–651, 1993

70. Osteogenesis Imperfecta

Michael P. Whyte, M.D.

Division of Bone and Mineral Diseases, Washington University School of Medicine; and
Metabolic Research Unit, Shriners Hospital for Crippled Children, St. Louis, Missouri

Osteogenesis imperfecta (OI), also called brittle bone disease, is a heritable disorder of connective tissue. The pathogenesis of nearly all clinical types (Table 1) centers on a qualitative or quantitative abnormality of the most abundant protein in bone, type I collagen (1–3). The hallmark of OI is osteopenia associated with recurrent fracture and skeletal deformity (4). However, type I collagen is also present in teeth, ligaments, skin, sclerae, and elsewhere, and many patients with OI have tooth disease caused by defective formation of dentin (dentinogenesis imperfecta) as well as abnormalities of other tissues that contain this fibrous protein (1–4).

Severity of clinical expression of OI is extremely variable and ranges from stillbirth to perhaps lifelong absence of symptoms. The classification system devised by Sillence (5) according to clinical/hereditary features has been useful in providing a framework for prognostication and a foundation for further biochemical/molecular studies. However, this classification system has limitations, and molecular findings have provided important new interpretations for the modes of inheritance, especially those of the severe forms (1,6). The clinical heterogeneity of OI is now better understood because of the identification of a great variety of molecular defects within the genes that encode the two large protein strands (the pro-α_1 and pro-α_2 chains) of the type I collagen heterotrimer (1,7).

CLINICAL PRESENTATION

The differential diagnosis for OI in infants and children includes idiopathic juvenile osteoporosis, Cushing's disease, homocystinuria, congenital indifference to pain, and child abuse (see Chapter 51). However, the disturbances in type I collagen biosynthesis that result in OI usually engender signs and symptoms that enable a correct diagnosis to be made easily from the patient's medical history, physical findings, and radiographic features. A positive family history is especially helpful, but many patients represent new mutations. Patients can manifest ligamentous laxity with joint hypermobility, diaphoresis, susceptibility to bruises, fragile and discolored teeth, and hearing loss (which occurs in about 50% of patients younger than age 30 and nearly all patients who are older) (8). Deafness is typically from conductive or mixed pathogenesis, but it sometimes results from sensorineural problems (8). Scleral discoloration ranges from a blue or gray tint that may be startling or subtle. With severe OI, other signs and symptoms include a high-pitched voice, short stature, scoliosis, hernia, disproportionately large head compared to body size, triangular face, and thoracic deformity. The thoracic deformity predisposes to pneumonia which can be life threatening. Mitral valve clicks are not uncommon, but cardiac disease is unusual. Patients with even the most deformed skeletons are generally of normal intelligence. Variable severity of OI can occur even among affected individuals in a single family or kindred (4).

CLINICAL TYPES

The classification scheme devised by Sillence (Table 1) is based on the clinical manifestations and apparent mode of inheritance of OI (5). This classification scheme remains useful but has been greatly clarified by revelations of the heterogeneous biochemical/molecular defects and their modes of genetic transmission, especially for the more severe types of OI (1–3).

Type I OI features sclerae with bluish discoloration (especially apparent during childhood), relatively mild osteopenia with infrequent fractures (deformity is uncommon or mild), and deafness (30% incidence) that first manifests during early adulthood. Typically, height is normal. Elderly women with this most mild form of OI can be mistaken as having osteoporosis if they present with fracture during middle age, because radiologic findings generally do not distinguish between the two disorders. More cortical osteocytes may be detected by iliac crest biopsy in these patients than in patients with osteoporosis (9,10). Type I OI has been subclassified into I-A and I-B disease depending on the absence or (more rarely) the presence, respectively, of dentinogenesis imperfecta. Type I OI is transmitted as an autosomal dominant trait. However, approximately one third of cases reflect new mutations.

Type II OI is often fatal within the first few days or weeks of life from respiratory complications. Affected newborns are often premature and small for gestational age and have short, bowed limbs, numerous fractures, markedly soft skulls, and small thoraces.

Type III OI is characterized by progressive skeletal deformity from recurrent fracture, and short stature that results in part from fragmentation of growth plates (5). Dental manifestations of OI are common.

Type IV OI is transmitted as an autosomal dominant trait and, until recently, was considered rare. Now, more frequently this type of OI explains multigeneration disease (1). The sclerae have normal color, but skeletal deformity, dental disease, and hearing loss are typical features.

RADIOLOGIC FEATURES

Characteristic findings are manifested in severely affected patients (11). The cardinal observations are generalized osteopenia, modeling defects of long bones, and deformity from recurrent fractures. Modeling (shaping) defects are caused by diminished periosteal bone formation that retards

TABLE 1. *Clinical heterogeneity and biochemical defects in osteogenesis imperfecta (OI)*

OI type	Clinical features	Inheritance	Biochemical defects
I	Normal stature, little or no deformity, blue sclerae, hearing loss in about 50% of individuals. Dentinogenesis imperfecta is rare and may distinguish a subset.	AD	Decreased production of type I procollagen. Substitution for residue other than glycine in triple helix of α1(I).
II	Lethal in the perinatal period, minimal calvarial mineralization, beaded ribs, compressed femurs, marked long bone deformity, platyspondyly.	AD (new mutation) AR (rare)	Rearrangements in the COL1A1 and COL1A2 genes. Substitutions for glycyl residues in the triple-helical domain of the α1(I) α2(I) chain. Small deletion in α2(I) on the background of a null allele.
III	Progressively deforming bones, usually with moderate deformity at birth. Sclerae variable in hue, often lighten with age. Dentinogenesis imperfecta is common, hearing loss is common. Stature very short.	AD AR	Frameshift mutation that prevents incorporation of pro α2(I) into molecules. (Noncollagenous defects.) Point mutations in the α1(I) or α2(I) chain.
IV	Normal sclerae, mild to moderate bone deformity, and variable short stature. Dentinogenesis imperfecta is common, and hearing loss occurs in some.	AD	Point mutations in the α2(I) chain. Rarely, point mutations in the α1(I) chain. Small deletions in the α2(I) chain.

AD, autosomal dominant; AR, autosomal recessive.
(From: Byers PH. Disorders of collagen biosynthesis and structure. In: Scriver CR, Beaudet AL, Sly WS, Valle D (eds) *The Metabolic and Molecular Bases of Inherited Disease,* 7th ed. McGraw Hill, New York, 4029–4077, 1995.)

circumferential widening of bones. Cortices appear thin. Multiple and recurrent fractures deform vertebrae as well as long bones (Fig. 1). In some severely affected infants, micromelia occurs with major long bones that are short but "thick" in their external diameter. Wormian bones (Fig. 2) of significant number and size in the skull are a common but not pathognomonic feature of OI (12). Platybasia, which can progress to basilar impression, and excessive pneumatization of the frontal and mastoid sinuses are common in severely affected patients (12). The pelvis can have a triradiate-

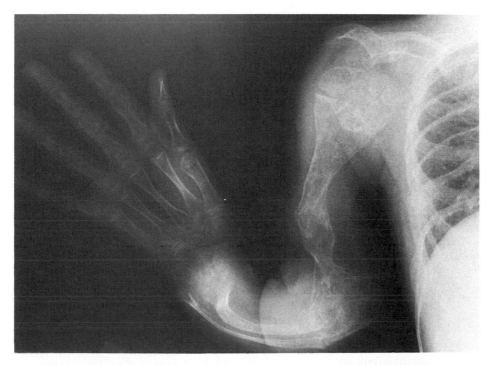

FIG. 1. Osteogenesis imperfecta. Severe changes of OI are present in the upper limb of this 14-year-old boy, including marked osteopenia with characteristic thinning of bony cortices, evidence of old fractures, gracile ribs, and limb deformities. (From: Whyte MP. Hereditary disorders of bone and mineral metabolism. In: Monolagas SC, Olefsky JM (eds) *Metabolic Bone and Mineral Disorders.* Churchill Livingston, New York, 1988.)

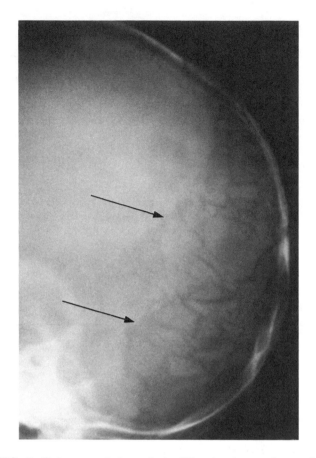

FIG. 2. Osteogenesis imperfecta. Wormian bones *(arrows),* although not pathognomonic of OI, may be found near the lambdoidal suture of the posterior occiput. (From: Whyte MP. Rare disorders of skeletal formation and homeostasis. In: Becker KN (ed) *Principles and Practice of Endocrinology and Metabolism,* 2nd ed. Lippincott-Raven Publishers, Philadelphia, 1995.)

shaped appearance. Osteoarthritis is a frequent problem for ambulatory adults with skeletal deformity.

Radiologic abnormalities may increase markedly during growth—a feature that helps to define progressively deforming, type III OI. "Popcorn" calcifications are unusual developmental defects in the regions of the epiphyses and metaphyses of major long bones (predominantly near the ankles and knees) that occur most often in type III OI patients (13). This finding is believed to result from traumatic fragmentation and then disordered maturation of growth plate cartilage. The complication may severely limit long bone growth and thereby contribute importantly to short stature. This problem is encountered during childhood, but it then "resolves" during puberty when the growth plates fuse as the cartilage becomes fully mineralized.

When fractures occur in OI, they are often transverse but heal at normal rates. Occasionally, there is exuberant callus formation that has been mistaken for skeletal malignancy.

LABORATORY FINDINGS

Routine biochemical studies of bone and mineral metabolism are typically unremarkable; however, elevations in serum alkaline phosphatase activity and urinary levels of hydroxyproline occur in some patients. Recently, hypercalciuria has been found to be a common finding, especially in severely affected children, but their renal function does not appear to be compromised (14).

Bone histology often reflects the abnormal skeletal matrix, especially in severely affected patients. Polarized-light microscopy can reveal an abundance of disorganized (woven) bone or abnormally thin collagen bundles in areas of lamellar osseous tissue. Numerous osteocytes are found in the cortical bone of some patients. This finding appears to reflect a decreased amount of bone production by individual osteoblasts, yet many cells are active at one time. Subsequently, the overall rate of skeletal turnover can be rapid, as shown by *in vivo* tetracycline labeling (15).

ETIOLOGY AND PATHOGENESIS

Table 1 summarizes the types of biochemical/molecular defects that have been identified in the various clinical types of OI (1). They include low levels of type I collagen synthesized by skin fibroblasts, and various mutations within the pro-α_1 and pro-α_2 type I collagen genes. The large and complex nature of type I collagen is such that nearly all affected families with OI have "private" mutations in one of these two genes. The interested reader is referred elsewhere for detailed discussion (1,7).

TREATMENT

Although there has been considerable progress in the elucidation of the biochemical/molecular defects that cause OI, there is no established medical therapy. Bisphosphonate treatment seems promising but requires further study, especially in growing children (16). Mouse models for OI provide a new way to test potential therapeutic approaches (17,18). Treatment is supportive and may require expert orthopedic, rehabilitative, and dental intervention to care for recurrent fractures, limb deformities, kyphoscoliosis, dental sequellae, etc. Rodding of long bones and bracing of the lower limbs has enabled some affected children to walk. Stapes surgery has been used for hearing loss (19). The current management of OI has been recently reviewed (20).

National support groups (e.g., Osteogenesis Imperfecta Foundation, Inc., U.S.A.) are important sources of comfort and lay-language information for patients and their families.

Genetic counseling should be periodically updated when appropriate, as progress in this area has been considerable. In fact, we now know that although rare patients with type II OI represent homozygosity for an autosomal recessive trait, most cases result from new dominant mutations or reflect germline mosaicism for such mutations. Hence, the recurrence risk of this most severe OI phenotype is now estimated to be 5% to 10% (1).

Prenatal diagnosis of severe OI by a variety of techniques, particularly ultrasound examination at 14 to 18 weeks gestation, has been quite successful (21).

REFERENCES

1. Byers PH: Disorders of collagen biosynthesis and structure. In: Scriver CR, Beaudet AL, Sly WS, Valle D, (eds) *The Metabolic and Molecular Bases of Inherited Disease,* 7th ed. McGraw-Hill, New York, pp 4029–4077, 1995
2. Tsipouras P: Osteogenesis imperfecta. In: *McKusick's Heritable Disorders of Connective Tissue,* 5th ed. St. Louis, Mosby pp 281–314, 1993
3. Byers P: Osteogenesis imperfecta. In: Royce PM, Steinmann B (eds) *Connective Tissue and Its Heritable Disorders.* Wiley-Liss, New York, pp 317–350, 1993
4. Albright JA, Millar EA: Osteogenesis imperfecta (symposium). *Clin Orthop* 159:1–156, 1981
5. Sillence D: Osteogenesis imperfecta: An expanding panorama of variants. *Clin Orthop* 159:11–25, 1981
6. Byers PH, Tsipouras P, Bonadio JF, Starman BJ, Schwartz RC: Perinatal lethal osteogenesis imperfecta (OI type II): A biochemically heterogeneous disorder usually due to new mutations in the genes for type I collagen. *Am J Hum Genet* 42:237–248, 1988
7. Byers PH, Wallis GA, Willing MC: Osteogenesis imperfecta: Translation of mutation to phenotype. *Med Genet* 28:433–442, 1991
8. Pedersen U: Hearing loss in patients with osteogenesis imperfecta. *Scand Audiol* 13:67–74, 1984
9. Revell PA: *Pathology of Bone.* Springer-Verlag, Berlin, 1986
10. Falvo KA, Bullough PG: Osteogenesis imperfecta: A histometric analysis. *J Bone Joint Surg (Am)* 55:275–286, 1973
11. Resnick D, Niwayama G: *Diagnosis of Bone and Joint Disorders,* 3rd ed. WB Saunders, Philadelphia, 1995
12. Cremin B, Goodman H, Prax M, Spranger J, Beighton P: Wormian bones in osteogenesis imperfecta and other disorders. *Skeletal Radiol* 8:35–38, 1982
13. Goldman AB, Davidson D, Pavlor H, Bullough PG: "Popcorn" calcifications: A prognostic sign in osteogenesis imperfecta. *Radiology* 136:351–358, 1980
14. Chines A, Boniface A, McAlister W, Whyte M: Hypercalciuria in osteogenesis imperfecta: A follow-up study to assess renal effects. *Bone* 16:333–339, 1995
15. Baron R, Gertner JM, Lang R, Vighery A: Increased bone turnover with decreased bone formation by osteoblasts in children with osteogenesis imperfecta tarda. *Pediatr Res* 17:204–207, 1983
16. Devogelaer JP, Malghem J, Maldague B, Nagant de Deuxchaisnes C: Radiological manifestations of bisphosphonate treatment with ADP in a child suffering from osteogenesis imperfecta. *Skeletal Radiol* 16:360–363, 1987
17. Cassella JP, Pereira R, Khillan JS, Prockop LJ, Garrington N, Sli SY: An ultra-structural, microanalytical, and spectroscopic study of bone from a transgenic mouse with a COL1.A1 pro-alpha-1 mutation. *Bone* 15:611–619, 1994
18. Prockop DJ, Colige A, Helminen H, Khillan JS, Pereira R, Vandenberg P: Mutations in type 1 procollagen that cause osteogenesis imperfecta: Effects of the mutations on the assembly of collagen into fibrils, the basis of phenotypic variations, and potential antisense therapies. *J Bone Miner Res* 6(suppl 2):S489–492, 1993
19. Garretsen TJ, Cremers CW: Stapes surgery in osteogenesis imperfecta: Analysis of postoperative hearing loss. *Ann Otol Rhinol Laryngol* 100:120–130, 1991
20. Binder H, Conway A, Hason S, Gerber LH, Marini J, Weintrob J: Comprehensive rehabilitation of the child with osteogenesis imperfecta. *Am J Med Genet* 45:265–269, 1993
21. Thompson EM: Non-invasive prenatal diagnosis of osteogenesis imperfecta. *Am J Med Genet* 45:201–206, 1993

71. Chondrodystrophies and Mucopolysaccharidoses

Michael P. Whyte, M.D.

Division of Bone and Mineral Diseases, Washington University School of Medicine; and Metabolic Research Unit, Shriners Hospital for Crippled Children, St. Louis, Missouri

Beginning in the 1960s, concerted efforts to classify the skeletal dysplasias led to recognition of more than 80 such entities (1). Most appeared to be heritable. The resulting classification, however, was essentially descriptive because the biochemical basis was unknown for nearly all of these conditions, and the molecular/genetic defects were largely unapproachable. Hence, the nomenclature for the bone dysplasias has been based on the parts of the skeleton that are most involved, according to radiologic study (1–4).

OSTEOCHONDRODYSPLASIAS

The term *osteochondrodysplasia* comprises a group of conditions among the skeletal dysplasias (5,6). Each disorder is characterized by abnormal growth or development of cartilage and/or bone (see refs. 1,5,6 for review of clinical nomenclature).

Osteochondrodysplasias are, in turn, subdivided into several groups, some of which feature defects in the growth of tubular bones and/or the spine. These conditions are frequently referred to as chondrodysplasias (1). The region of the long bones that is most affected (epiphysis, metaphysis,

or diaphysis) is the basis for the subclassifications of epiphyseal, metaphyseal, or diaphyseal dysplasia (1–3). When the vertebrae are also deformed, these disorders are grouped as spondyloepiphyseal dysplasia, and so on (Fig. 1).

Chondrodysplasias that feature primarily metaphyseal defects (metaphyseal dysplasia and spondylometaphyseal dysplasia) may be confused, from their radiographic appearance, with forms of rickets (Fig. 2). However, biochemical parameters of bone and mineral metabolism are typically not abnormal in metaphyseal dysplasias and the skeleton is generally well mineralized. Indeed, the configuration of the metaphyseal defects can lead to an accurate diagnosis by the experienced radiologist. When abnormalities of the spine are present (Fig. 3), the correct diagnosis should be especially apparent.

Recently, progress with recombinant DNA technology has led to impressive success at mapping the genes that cause skeletal dysplasias and to understanding some of them at the molecular/biochemical level (7,8). Defects in a variety of genes in these disorders reveal that the encoded proteins are essential for normal skeletal development. Abnormalities in the type I, II, IX, and X collagen genes are now

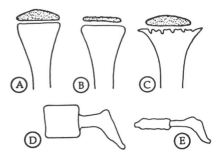

Involvement	Disease Category
A+D	Normal
B+D	Epiphyseal dysplasia
C+D	Metaphyseal dysplasia
B+E	Spondyloepiphyseal dysplasia
C+E	Spondylometaphyseal dysplasia
B+C+E	Spondyloepimetaphyseal dysplasia

FIG. 1. Chondrodysplasias. Classification based on radiologic involvement of long bones and vertebrae (1). (From: Rimoin DL, Lachman RS. The chondrodysplasias. In: Emery AEH, Rimoin DL (eds) *Principles and Practice of Medical Genetics.* Churchill Livingstone, London, 1983.)

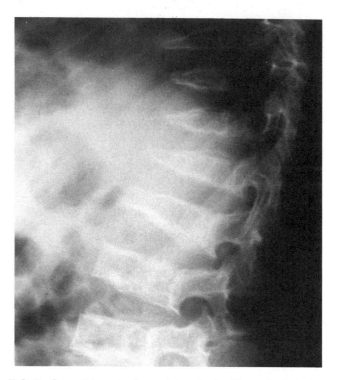

FIG. 3. Spondylometaphyseal dysplasia. Characteristic dysplastic changes at 11 years of age are present in the vertebrae of the patient shown in Fig. 2 and establish a spondylometaphyseal rather than a metaphyseal dysplasia.

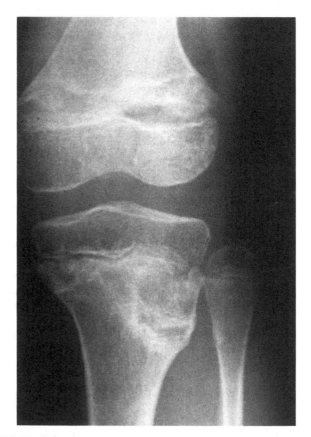

FIG. 2. Spondylometaphyseal dysplasia. The irregularity of the metaphyses in the knees of this 8⁹/₁₂-year-old girl are sometimes mistaken for rickets.

known to cause osteogenesis imperfecta, spondyloepiphyseal dysplasia, multiple epiphyseal dysplasia, and metaphyseal dysplasia (Schmid type), respectively. Cartilage-oligomeric-matrix-protein gene mutations can be the basis for multiple epiphyseal dysplasia and pseudoachondroplasia. Fibroblast growth factor receptor-3 gene defects cause achondroplasia. The elastin and fibrillin genes are involved in Williams and Marfan syndromes, respectively. Hence, a number of skeletal dysplasias can now be regarded as types of "metabolic bone disease," and the number of such conditions will continue to grow (7,8).

MUCOPOLYSACCHARIDOSES

The mucopolysaccharidoses are a group of inborn errors of metabolism that result from diminished activity of the lysosomal enzymes that degrade glycosaminoglycans (acid mucopolysaccharides) (9,10). Accumulation of these complex carbohydrates within marrow cells leads to skeletal change that is generally referred to as dysostosis multiplex. However, the degree of severity and precise bony manifestations vary according to the specific disorder (1–4). (See refs. 9,10 for recent, detailed descriptions.)

Dysostosis multiplex is characterized by the following general radiographic features: osteoporosis with coarsened trabeculae, macrocephaly, dyscephaly, a J-shaped sella turcica, oar-shaped ribs, widened clavicles, oval or hook-shaped vertebral bodies, dysplasia of the capital femoral epiphyses, coxa valga, epiphyseal and metaphyseal dysplasia, proximal tapering of the 2nd and 5th metacarpals, and dysplasia of long tubular bones (3,4).

REFERENCES

1. Rimoin DL, Lachman RS: The chondrodysplasias. In: Emery AEH, Rimoin DL (eds) *Principles and Practice of Medical Genetics.* Churchill Livingstone, London, 1983
2. Wynne-Davies R, Hall CM, Apley AG: *Atlas of Skeletal Dysplasias,* Churchill Livingstone, Edinburgh, 1985
3. Resnick D, Niwayama G: *Diagnosis of Bone and Joint Disorders,* 3rd ed. WB Saunders, Philadelphia, 1995
4. Taybi H, Lachman RS: *Radiology of Syndromes, Metabolic Disorders, and Skeletal Dysplasias,* 4th ed. Mosby, St. Louis, 1996
5. Rimoin DL, Lachman RS: Genetic disorders of the osseous skeleton. In: *McKusick's Heritable Disorders of Connective Tissue,* 5th ed, pp 557–689, 1993
6. Horton WA, Hecht JT: The chondrodysplasias. In: Royce PM, Steinmann B (eds) *Connective Tissue and Its Heritable Disorders.* Wiley-Liss, New York, pp 641–675, 1993
7. Whyte MP: Recent progress in metabolic bone disease: Clinical and basic aspects with special emphasis on hypophosphatasia, osteogenesis imperfecta, and vitamin D resistant rickets. *Jpn J Inherit Metab Dis* 11:1–10, 1995
8. Horton WA: Molecular genetics of the human chondrodysplasias—1995. *Eur J Hum Genet* 3:357–373, 1995
9. Leroy JG, Wiesmann U: Disorders of lysosomal enzymes. In: Royce PM, Steinmann B (eds) *Connective Tissue and Its Heritable Disorders.* Wiley-Liss, New York, pp 613–639, 1993
10. Neufeld EF, Muenzer J: The mucopolysaccharidoses. In: Scriver CR, Beaudet AL, Sly WS, Valle D (eds) *The Metabolic and Molecular Bases of Inherited Disease,* 7th ed. McGraw-Hill, New York, 2465–2494, 1995

Acquired Disorders of Cartilage and Bone

VII. Introduction

Michael P. Whyte, M.D.

Division of Bone and Metabolic Diseases, Washington University School of Medicine; and Metabolic Research Unit,
Shriners Hospital for Crippled Children, St. Louis, Missouri

Physicians who specialize in the care of patients with metabolic bone diseases encounter a considerable number and variety of acquired disorders of cartilage and bone. Among these conditions are skeletal neoplasms, problems that result from disruption of the vascular supply to the skeleton, and diseases that are characterized by proliferation or infiltration of the marrow spaces by specific types of cells. In certain "metabolic" bone diseases and some skeletal dysplasias, there is predisposition to neoplastic transformation (e.g., Paget's disease, fibrous dysplasia), metabolic disturbances can cause skeletal ischemia (e.g., Cushing syndrome, storage diseases), and infiltrative marrow disorders may be associated with aberrant mineral homeostasis (e.g., sarcoidosis). This section provides an overview of some of the principal acquired disturbances of cartilage and bone.

72. Skeletal Neoplasms

Michael P. Whyte, M.D.

*Division of Bone and Mineral Diseases, Washington University School of Medicine; and Metabolic Research Unit,
Shriners Hospital for Crippled Children, St. Louis, Missouri*

GENERAL CONSIDERATIONS

Among the acquired disorders of cartilage and bone are a variety of neoplasms. Some are malignant and cause considerable morbidity; some metastasize and result in death. Others are benign and can even heal spontaneously. Rarely, some of these tumors behave as though they are transitional, with both benign and malignant characteristics. Diagnosis and treatment of bone tumors is a complex discipline. Only a brief overview is provided here. The reader may wish to refer to several reviews of this topic (1–5).

Histopathologic classification of skeletal neoplasms is based on the cell or tissue type from which they appear to have originated (Table 1). The source of the tumor is usually revealed by the kind of tissue that the neoplastic cells make, such as osteoid or cartilage. However, in a few instances (e.g., giant cell tumor of bone), the cell or tissue of origin is unknown (1–5).

Biologic behavior of bone tumors also importantly influences their classification (see later). Within the two major categories, benign and malignant, there are skeletal neoplasms with different degrees of aggressivity. Biologic behavior reflects the capacity of the tumor to exceed its natural barriers. Such barriers may include a tumor capsule (the shell of fibrous tissue or bone around the neoplasm), a reactive zone (composed in part of either fibrous tissue or bone that forms between the capsule and normal tissue), and any adjacent articular cartilage, cortical bone, or periosteum (1–6).

Skeletal neoplasms will be properly managed only if there is a thorough understanding of their clinical presentation and natural history, as well as use of current staging procedures, which often require histopathologic examination (6). Proper choice of therapy may include medical and/or surgical approaches (1–8). Optimum patient management requires multidisciplinary expertise (2). Improved radiologic imaging studies, histopathologic methods, cytogenetic and molecular testing (9), surgical techniques, and chemotherapeutic regimens have all led to better survival and function of patients with skeletal sarcomas. Chemotherapy has improved the treatment of early metastatic deposits (2,10–12). Consequently, aggressive limb-salvaging procedures are now possible with survival rates that were previously achieved only by radical amputation (1,4,7,11,13–17).

Benign Bone Tumors

Benign skeletal tumors, with only rare exception, do not metastasize. Nevertheless, as a group, their biologic behavior can still be rather variable and may range from completely inactive to quite aggressive. Fortunately, the behavior can often be predicted by noting the clinical presentation and examining the radiologic features of the specific neoplasm (18,19); sometimes histopathologic inspection is essential as well (1,3–5). As discussed later, benign tumors can be classified generally as inactive, active, or aggressive (1).

Inactive benign bone tumors are also sometimes called latent or static. They are encapsulated by mature fibrous tissue or by cortical bone like material, and they do not expand or deform surrounding skeletal tissue. Each neoplasm will have only a minimal (if any) reactive zone, and their histopathologic appearance is that of a benign tumor, with a low cell-to-matrix ratio, a well-differentiated matrix, and no cellular hyperchromasia, anaplasia, or pleomorphism. Inactive benign tumors are usually asymptomatic (1–5).

Active benign bone tumors can deform or destroy adjacent cortical bone or joint cartilage as they grow, but they do not metastasize. They are encapsulated within fibrous tissue, although a thin reactive zone can develop. These lesions generally cause mild symptoms but may lead to pathologic fracture (1–5).

Aggressive benign bone tumors are not uncommon in children. They demonstrate invasive properties like those of low-grade malignancies. Their reactive zone forms a capsule or pseudocapsule that prevents the neoplasm itself from extending directly into normal tissue, but the tumor can resorb and destroy adjacent bone and spread to nearby skeletal compartments. Despite their aggressive behavior, the cytologic features are benign—including a well-differentiated matrix. These tumors cause symptoms and can result in pathologic fracture (1–5).

Malignant Bone Tumors

Malignant skeletal tumors can metastasize. Nevertheless, as a group, their biologic behavior also varies considerably (1–5). Some grow slowly with a low probability of spreading, so that there is typically a long interval between the discovery of the primary neoplasm and the development and recognition of metastases. Others are biologically very aggressive and not only cause rapid and extensive local tissue destruction, but also have a high incidence of metastases so that primary and metastatic lesions are frequently recognized together. The biologic behavior of malignant skeletal tumors can usually be predicted by their clinical, radiologic (18,19), and histopathologic features (1,4,5). Assessment of the histopathologic type and grade is the best predictor of biologic activity and is of paramount importance for successful treatment and accurate prognostication (see later) (1–6).

Low-grade sarcomas invade local tissues but grow slowly and have a low risk of metastasizing. They are usually

TABLE 1. *Common skeletal neoplasms*

Tissue origin	Benign	Malignant
Osseous		Classic osteosarcoma
		Parosteal osteosarcoma
		Periosteal osteosarcoma
Cartilaginous	Enchondroma	Primary chondrosarcoma
	Exostosis	Secondary chondrosarcoma
Fibrous	Nonossifying fibroma	Fibrosarcoma
		Malignant fibrous histiocytoma
Reticuloendothelial		Ewing's sarcoma
		Multiple myeloma
Unknown	Giant cell tumor in bone	

From: refs. 1–5.

asymptomatic and manifest as gradually growing masses. Nevertheless, the histopathologic features of malignancy are present, such as anaplasia, pleomorphism, and hyperchromasia, together with a few mitotic cells. The tumor capsule can be disrupted in many areas, and there may be an extensive reactive zone that forms a pseudocapsule and contains satellite tumor nodules that slowly erode the various natural barriers. Over time and after repeatedly unsuccessful surgical excision with tumor recurrence, there is a risk of transformation to a high-grade sarcoma (1–5).

High-grade sarcomas readily extend beyond their reactive zone. They seem to have minimal pseudoencapsulation. Their margins are poorly demarcated. Metastases may appear in seemingly uninvolved areas of the same bone and often in the medullary canal. Extension to nearby tissues destroys cortical bone, joint capsules, and articular cartilage. These tumors show all of the histopathologic features that typify malignancy and produce a poorly differentiated (immature) matrix (1–5).

Diagnosis of Bone Tumors

A thorough history and complete physical examination are the foundation for successful diagnosis and management of skeletal neoplasms (20). The patient's age, the presence or absence of predisposing conditions (e.g., Paget's bone disease), and the anatomic site of the lesion provide important clues to the precise diagnosis (see later).

Radiologic studies should be selected both to help establish the tumor type and to provide staging information that will be critical for choosing treatment and for understanding the patient's prognosis (1–6,21). The tumor stage reflects the neoplasm's location and extent, as well as its biologic activity or grade, and is based in part on the presence or absence of metastases (6). Radiographs establish the tumor location, often suggest the underlying histopathologic type (18,19), help to evaluate its extent, and guide the selection of additional staging studies. Clinical and radiologic examination is completed prior to biopsy or other surgical procedures (6,20).

Bone scanning helps to determine if multiple areas of neoplasm are present and if the extent of skeletal involvement exceeds that indicated by conventional radiographs. Avidity for radionuclide uptake generally reflects the tumor's biologic activity (18,19,22,23).

Computed tomography is very useful for precisely defining the anatomic extent of the primary lesion, detecting destruction of spongy or cortical bone, assessing compartmental changes, and locating neurovascular structures that may be impinged upon by tumor or are located near planned surgery (24,25). This technique also supplements conventional radiography for detecting pulmonary metastases.

Magnetic resonance imaging is especially helpful for defining tumor soft-tissue extension and for showing any disruption of the marrow spaces (23,25–28).

Angiography can help plan limb-salvage operations, because this procedure may show involvement of major neurovascular bundles (1,2).

Arthrography helps to demonstrate joint involvement and thus is useful for determining whether a cartilaginous tumor is of intra-articular or extra-articular origin (1,4).

Biopsy and histopathologic study are essential for successful staging and treatment of many skeletal neoplasms (1–6,29). Open (incisional) biopsy is typically the technique of choice if a malignant lesion is suspected, because it secures sufficient tissue for study (1). However, this technique carries a greater risk of tumor contamination of uninvolved tissues (e.g., by dissecting hematoma) than closed biopsy. Accordingly, open biopsy can potentially compromise a limb-salvage procedure because of added risk of local recurrence. Therefore, careful attention must be paid to where the incision for biopsy is made and to the surgical technique (1–6). Accessible benign tumors may be removed by incisional biopsy as they are intracapsular, or with *en bloc* marginal incision (2,4,7).

INDIVIDUAL TYPES OF SKELETAL NEOPLASIA

Benign and Transitional Bone Tumors

Benign skeletal neoplasms occasionally originate from marrow elements, but most often they are derived from cartilage or bone (30). Typically, these tumors develop before skeletal maturation is complete or during the early adult years, and they are most common in areas of rapid bone growth and cellular metabolism (i.e., the epiphyses and metaphyses of the major long bones) (1–4,31). In some patients or families with particular heritable disorders, benign skeletal tumors (e.g., enchondromas and exostoses) are multiple and have a significantly increased risk of malignant transformation. Most benign skeletal tumors, however, are solitary lesions and are associated with a good prognosis (1–5,31). The following paragraphs describe the principal types.

Nonossifying fibroma is the most common bone tumor (32,33). This lesion is often called a fibrous cortical defect. It is the outcome of a focal developmental abnormality in periosteal bone formation that results in an area of failed ossification. Nonossifying fibromas most commonly occur in the metaphyses of the distal femur or distal tibia and are located eccentrically, in or near the bony cortex (18,19). They are somewhat more common in boys than in girls, develop during childhood or adolescence, and are active lesions that enlarge throughout childhood yet typically do not cause symptoms. However, when more than 50% of the diameter of a long bone is involved, pathologic fracture can occur (32,33). Radiologic study may show a well-demarcated radiolucent zone with apparent trabecularization that results in a multilocular or even in a septated appearance (Fig. 1). Some cortical bone erosion may be present. The radiologic pattern can be considered diagnostic, and further staging is typically unnecessary (18,19). After puberty with skeletal maturation, nonossifying fibromas become inactive or latent and ultimately ossify. Surgical intervention is usually unnecessary unless pathologic fracture is a significant

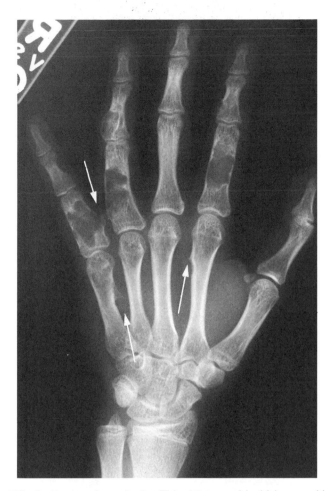

FIG. 2. Enchondromatosis. This 13-year-old girl has multiple, lucent, benign-appearing lesions of the phalanges. Each has produced expansion of the bone as well as cortical scalloping and thinning. Several periosteum-based chondromas are present that show reactive bone formation at their margins *(arrows)*.

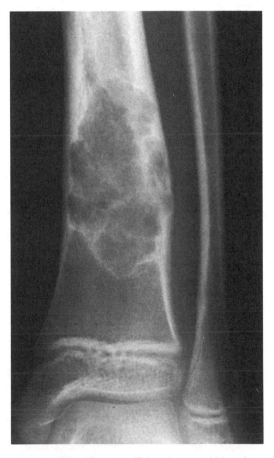

FIG. 1. Nonossifying fibroma. This 11-year-old boy has a typical benign-appearing lesion of his distal left tibia. It is an ovoid, radiolucent fibrous tumor located at the metadiaphyseal junction that is slightly expansile and has a multiloculated appearance with regions of cortical scalloping and thinning.

risk. Intracapsular curettage is effective, but bone grafting or other stabilizing techniques for fracture prevention or treatment may be required (1–4,32,33). Rarely, nonossifying fibromas cause oncogenic rickets (see Chapter 62).

Enchondroma is a benign and typically asymptomatic tumor of cartilage caused by focal disruption of endochondral bone formation. It can be considered a dysplasia of the central growth plate (34). Enchondromas appear as though they arise in the metaphysis, and they may eventually become incorporated into the diaphysis. Solitary lesions are noted, typically in adolescence or during early adulthood. They most commonly involve small tubular bones of the hands or feet or the proximal humerus, but they can occur in any bone. Several distinct disorders feature multiple enchondromas (enchondromatosis, Ollier's disease, and Maffucci syndrome). Fewer than 1% of asymptomatic solitary tumors undergo malignant transformation. However, with enchondromatosis, the risk of malignant degeneration has been estimated to be 10% (1–4,31,34).

Radiographs show a medullary radiolucent lesion with a well-defined but only slightly thickened bony margin (Fig. 2)

(18,19). This defect may enlarge slowly during its active phase in adolescence, but, when the tumor becomes latent during the adult years, it calcifies to produce a diffusely punctate or stippled appearance (Fig. 3). In time, enchondromas become surrounded by dense reactive osseous tissue. Skeletal scintigraphy typically reflects the tumor's biologic activity and shows increased radioisotope uptake in the reactive zone (greatly increased uptake suggests malignant transformation). Accordingly, it is prudent to secure for young adults with multiple enchondromas a baseline bone scan and radiographs.

Biopsy is often not necessary, because the lesion's identity is revealed by typical radiography (18,19). Histopathologic examination may be required, however, to distinguish benign from low-grade malignant enchondromas. Here, the patient's age is an especially important consideration (34).

Solitary asymptomatic enchondromas are generally benign and require no treatment, although periodic follow-up is indicated. If they become symptomatic and begin to enlarge, careful surveillance is necessary (34). Imaging techniques may be helpful to search for evidence of malignancy (23,24). Surgical treatment would then be indicated.

Osteocartilaginous exostosis (osteochondroma) is a common developmental dysplasia of cartilage involving the peripheral region of a growth plate (31,34). It can arise in

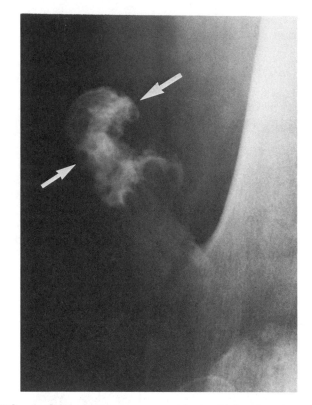

FIG. 4. Osteocartilagenous exostosis (osteochondroma). This 51-year-old woman has a typical pedunculated exostosis of her distal femur. The cortex and trabecular components of the exostosis are continuous with the host bone. Note how the exostosis slants away from the knee joint. The osteocartilagenous cap *(arrows)* is densely mineralized.

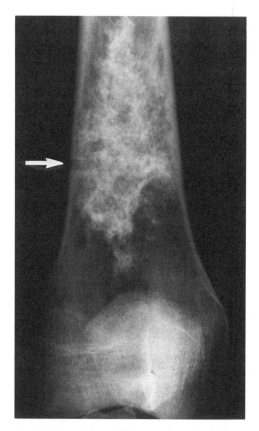

FIG. 3. Enchondroma. This 43-year-old woman has an extensively calcified lesion of the metadiaphyseal region of her distal femur. The calcification is amorphous and dense with little radiolucent component *(arrow* indicates a biopsy needle track). This lesion is differentiated from a bone infarction, which typically has a dense, linearly marginated periphery.

any bone that derives from cartilage, but it usually involves a long bone. Typically, either end of a femur, the proximal humerus or tibia, the pelvis, or the scapula is affected. Exostoses present as hard painful masses that are fixed to bone. They enlarge during childhood but become latent in adulthood. These lesions can irritate overlying soft tissues and may form a fluid-filled bursa. Generally they are solitary, but multiple hereditary exostoses are well-characterized entities that can cause significant angular deformity of the lower limbs, clubbing of the radius, and short stature (35). A painful and enlarging exostosis in an adult, especially in the pelvis or shoulder girdle, should suggest malignant transformation to a chondrosarcoma (31,34,35).

Radiologic study may show either a flat, sessile, or pedunculated metaphyseal bony lesion of variable density that is typically well defined and covered by a radiolucent cartilaginous cap (Fig. 4). A characteristic feature of an exostosis is continuity of the tumor bone with metaphyseal bone (18,19). The diagnosis is rarely difficult. Following malignant transformation, there may be a soft tissue mass on computed tomography or magnetic resonance imaging, and skeletal scintigraphy will demonstrate suddenly or considerably increased tracer uptake.

The cartilaginous cap of an exostosis appears histopathologically like a poorly organized growth plate. The trabeculae are not remodeled and thus contain cartilage cores (primary spongiosa)—the histopathologic hallmark of osteopetrosis (see Chapter 68).

Excisional treatment of an active exostosis should include the cartilaginous cap and overlying perichondrium to minimize the risk of recurrence (1,3,4,34). There is about a 5% recurrence rate following marginal excision of a solitary lesion. Malignant degeneration occurs in fewer than 1% of solitary lesions, but the risk is almost 10% for multiple hereditary exostoses (34).

Giant cell tumor of bone (osteoclastoma) is a common benign bone neoplasm. The cellular origin, however, is unknown (1–4,36). Men are more frequently affected than women, typically at 20 to 40 years of age. These tumors cause chronic and deep pain that mimics an arthropathy. Pathologic fracture or effusion into the knee is a typical presentation. The epiphysis of a distal femur or proximal tibia is frequently affected. However, the distal radius, proximal humerus, distal tibia, and sacrum are also commonly involved. Often, giant cell tumors enlarge to occupy most of the epiphysis and portions of the adjacent metaphysis, and they can penetrate into subchondral bone and may even invade articular cartilage. In contrast to other benign skeletal neoplasms, they occasionally metastasize. Accordingly, giant cell tumors of bone are sometimes referred to as transitional neoplasms (3).

Radiologic studies show a relatively large lucent abnormality that is surrounded by an obvious reactive zone (18,19). The cortex can appear eroded from the endosteal surface (Fig. 5). A trabecular bone pattern may fill in the tumor cavity. Bone scanning can demonstrate decreased tracer uptake at the center of the lesion (the "doughnut"

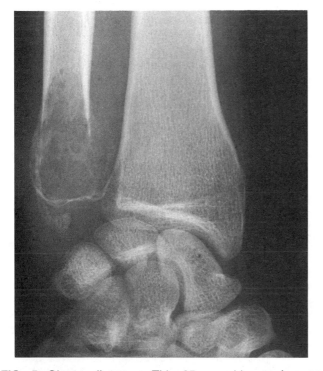

FIG. 5. Giant cell tumor. This 25-year-old man has an expansile, destructive, lucent lesion of the distal ulna. The lesion extends to the end of the bone.

sign). Histopathologic examination shows numerous, scattered, multinucleated giant cells in a proliferative stroma; mitoses are occasionally present (5).

Curettage with bone grafting or use of cement is the treatment of less advanced lesions. Recurrent or advanced tumors are removed with *en bloc* wide excision and reconstructive surgery (1–5,7).

Malignant Bone Tumors

Myeloma, the most common cancer of the skeleton, is a tumor of bone marrow origin. Nevertheless, a considerable variety of malignant tumors commonly arise from bone, cartilage, fibrous tissue, histiocytes, and perhaps endothelial tissue in the skeleton (1–5,31–34). Malignant bone tumors typically cause skeletal pain that is especially prominent at night. Accordingly, this symptom, particularly in adolescents or young adults, is reason for evaluation. The treatment of these neoplasms is complex and is primarily based on the tumor grade and staging (1–6). Only general comments are provided in this subsection, in which the principal types among these entities are discussed.

Multiple myeloma typically develops during middle age and affects multiple skeletal sites. Constitutional symptoms can include bone pain, fever, malaise, fatigue, and weight loss. There is often anemia, thrombocytopenia, and renal failure (37). Hypercalcemia, resulting from the elaboration of osteoclast-activating factors, occurs at some time in the disease course of about 20% to 40% of patients (38). The diagnosis is made by examination of the bone marrow for plasmacytosis and demonstration of paraproteinemia by serum and urine immunoelectrophoresis (37).

Radiologic findings may include classic discrete osteolytic lesions, but generalized osteopenia is actually a more common presentation. Bone scintigraphy can seem unusual because there may be little tracer uptake in foci of osteolysis (18,19).

Myeloma is radiation sensitive and treatable by chemotherapy. Reossification of tumor sites can occur within several months of therapy. Prevention of pathologic fractures may require surgical stabilization (37).

Osteosarcoma (osteogenic sarcoma) is the most common primary malignancy of the skeleton (1–4,39–44). There are about 1,100 to 1,500 new cases in the United States yearly. Typically, this bone cancer develops before age 30, and male patients somewhat outnumber female patients. Although most are the classic variety, there are variants of osteosarcoma that include parosteal, periosteal, and telangiectatic types that have somewhat different presentations and prognoses (see later) (39–44).

Classic osteosarcoma characteristically arises in the metaphysis of a long bone where there is the most rapid growth. It primarily affects teenagers. In about 50% of cases, these tumors develop near the knee in the distal femur or proximal tibia. Other commonly involved sites are the humerus, proximal femur, and pelvis, but they can arise *de novo* anywhere in the skeleton. They also derive from malignant transformation of Paget's bone disease (Chapter 75) (45).

Typically, an osteosarcoma presents as a tender bony mass. Pain is severe and unremitting. Pathologic fracture can occur. Osteosarcomas are aggressive neoplasms that readily penetrate metaphyseal cortical bone, and the majority have already infiltrated surrounding soft tissues at diagnosis. At presentation, about 50% of affected adolescents show penetration of their growth plates with epiphyseal involvement, about 20% have metastases elsewhere in the cancerous bone, and, in approximately 10% of these patients, tumor has spread to lymph nodes or lung (39–44).

Radiologic study shows a destructive lesion that is composed of amorphous osseous tissue with poorly defined margins (18,19,44). Some osteosarcomas are predominately osteoblastic and radiologically dense; others are predominately osteolytic and radiolucent. Some have a mixed pattern (18,19). Cortical bone destruction is often apparent (Fig. 6). A characteristic "sunburst" configuration results from spicules of amorphous neoplastic osseous tissue that forms perpendicular to the affected bone's long axis. This is in contrast to the parallel or "onion skin" appearance of reactive periosteal new bone. Codman's triangle results from periosteal reaction and elevation that demarcates a triangular area of cortical bone (see Fig. 8 for illustration). Bone scintigraphy shows intense uptake of tracer and may disclose more widespread disease than is indicated by conventional radiographs. Computed tomography, magnetic resonance imaging, and angiography are helpful, as discussed previously. Microscopic examination typically

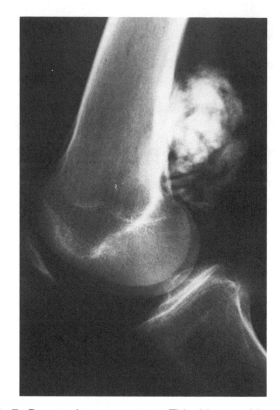

FIG. 7. Parosteal osteosarcoma. This 30-year-old woman has a very densely mineralized mass arising from the periosteal surface of the distal femoral metaphysis posteriorly. This tumor has lobular calcification and is attached to the femur by a broad pedicle.

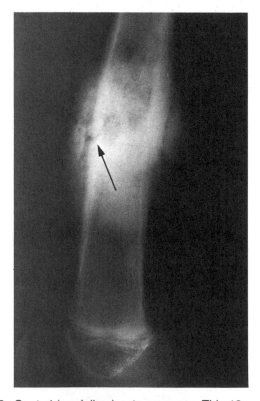

FIG. 6. Central (medullary) osteosarcoma. This 12-year-old boy has a sclerotic diaphyseal lesion that arose in the medullary cavity. It has penetrated the cortex and produced a densely mineralized mass surrounding the femur. Portions of the cortex appear to have been destroyed (arrow), whereas other regions are thickened.

shows a very malignant stroma that produces an amorphous and immature osteoid in a trabecular pattern (1–5).

Use of chemotherapy preoperatively (4,10–12,39,40) has significantly improved the prognosis for this malignancy and has enabled many osteosarcoma patients to be managed by limb-salvage procedures instead of radical amputation (7,15,17).

Parosteal osteosarcomas are juxtacortical (i.e., they develop between the bony cortex and the soft tissue as a surface neoplasm). Adolescents and young adults are most commonly affected by these slowly growing, low-grade tumors that typically occur as a fixed and painless mass posteriorly on the distal femur or medially on the proximal humerus. They are less aggressive than classic osteosarcomas and can be separated for a considerable length of time from the parent bone by a narrow radiolucent region of soft tissue. Eventually, they may involve the underlying skeleton and degenerate into a high-grade osteosarcoma (1–5,39).

Radiologic study typically reveals a densely ossified, broad-based, fusiform mass that seems to encircle the metaphyseal region of a long bone (Fig. 7) (18,19). Reactive tissue initially separates the neoplasm from the underlying bone that is destroyed once the tumor penetrates the normal cortex and the medullary canal becomes involved. Parosteal osteosarcomas have mature trabeculae with cement lines similar to those seen in Paget's disease; however, a low-grade malignant stroma is present. This tumor is often misdiagnosed as benign. Limb-salvage with wide marginal excision is the usual treatment for less advanced disease. The prognosis is good. Chemotherapy is typically not used unless there has been dedifferentiation (1–5,39).

Periosteal osteosarcoma often presents as a painless growing mass that extends from the surface of a bone into soft tissue (1–5,39). This is an uncommon variant of classic osteosarcoma that principally affects young adults. Radiologic study shows a poorly mineralized mass found primarily on a bone surface in an area of cortical erosion. The crater like lesion has irregular margins and is associated with periosteal reaction (18,19). Penetration by this neoplasm through cortical bone into the medullary canal is more rapid than for parosteal osteosarcoma. If this complication has occurred, the frequency of pulmonary metastasis is greater—a feature that contributes to its poorer prognosis. Bone scintigraphy shows avid tracer uptake. Computed tomography reveals a mass that fills a shallow cortical bone defect but contains minimal calcification. Malignant mesenchymal stroma with neoplastic osteoid occurs in and around areas of mature cartilage (1,2,4,5).

Periosteal osteosarcoma is often treated by excision with a wide margin (1,2,7,12,17,39). Adjuvant chemotherapy is used when the tumor has regions of high-grade malignancy (1–5,10,12).

Chondrosarcoma occurs most often between 40 and 60 years of age, when this neoplasm presents as a primary tumor (1–5,34,46). In about 25% of patients, malignant transformation has occurred in a preexisting enchondroma or osteocartilaginous exostosis. Thus, chondrosarcomas usually involve the pelvis, proximal femur, or shoulder girdle. Patients experience persistent dull ache that can mimic arthritis as the initial symptom. Variants of the classic form of chondrosarcoma include a high-grade dedifferentiated tumor, an intermediate-grade clear cell type, and a low-grade juxtacortical tumor. The particular designation depends on the histopathologic pattern and anatomic location (1,4,5,34,46).

Radiographs show a subtle radiolucent lesion that contains hazy or speckled calcification in a diffuse "salt and pepper" or "popcorn" pattern (18,19). Primary chondrosarcomas can develop either within the medullary canal or on the surface of a bone where they can destroy the cortex and form a mass. On histopathologic examination, it can be difficult to demonstrate that high-grade tumors are cartilaginous in origin or that low-grade tumors are actually malignant (5,34,46).

Treatment of chondrosarcomas depends on the tumor stage. Limb amputation may be necessary for higher grade tumors. Adjuvant chemotherapy or radiation therapy has been disappointing (1–5,34).

Ewing sarcoma is a highly malignant neoplasm that arises from nonmesenchymal cells in the bone marrow (2,3,47–52). This cancer harbors a t(11:12) (q24;q12) translocation (50–52). It typically presents in 10- to 15-year-old children and is more common in boys than in girls (50–52). Initial manifestations are an enlarging and tender soft tissue swelling together with weight loss, malaise, fever, and lethargy. The erythrocyte sedimentation rate may be elevated, and there can be leukocytosis and anemia. The diaphysis of the femur is most commonly involved; alternatively,

an ilium, tibia, fibula, or rib is affected. When this cancer occurs in the pelvis, it is usually found late and therefore has an especially poor prognosis (47–52).

Radiologic study typically reveals a diaphyseal lesion of patchy density that destroys cortical bone and frequently causes an "onion skin" appearance of reactive periosteum (Fig. 8) (18,19). Bone scanning may show intense tracer uptake that extends considerably beyond the radiographic abnormality.

Chemotherapy can be followed by wide excision or radiation therapy, depending on, among other factors, the anatomic site. Newer therapeutic approaches have reduced the incidence of pulmonary metastases and have markedly improved survival (1–5,34,49–52).

Malignant fibrous histiocytoma occurs more frequently in soft tissues than in the skeleton and is less common than benign fibrous tumors (1–5,33). This cancer affects adults and often originates in Paget's bone disease or at the site of a skeletal infarct. Typically, this is an aggressive sarcoma that readily spreads in the lymphatics. Bone is infiltrated early on, and pathologic fracture is a common presenting sign.

Radiologic study reveals a poorly defined radiolucent lesion that causes cortical bone erosion (18,19). The

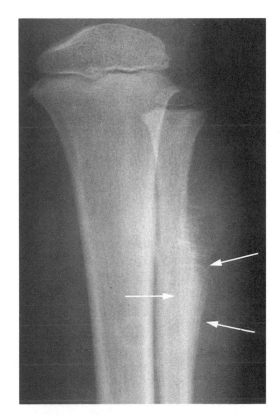

FIG. 8. Ewing sarcoma. This 5-year-old boy has a subtle permeative lesion of the proximal diaphysis of his fibula. The tumor is characterized by layered (onion skin) periosteal reaction forming a Codman's triangle *(arrows)* and by "sunburst" new bone formation more proximally, which is characteristically oriented perpendicularly to the long axis of the bone. A large soft tissue mass is associated with the skeletal defects.

histopathologic pattern is variable from area to area; extremely large and bizarre histiocytic cells are found in some sections, and undifferentiated cells that resemble histiocytic lymphoma are noted in others. Areas that contain fibrous tissue may suggest that the tumor is a fibrosarcoma. Special stains and electron microscopy can be required to establish the correct diagnosis (1,4,5). Staging studies direct the therapy, which may require radical resection or amputation and perhaps chemotherapy (1,2). The prognosis is guarded (33).

Fibrosarcoma is a painful neoplasm that typically arises in a major long bone of an adolescent or young adult (1–5,33). Radiologic study reveals a poorly defined and destructive lucent lesion in a metaphysis (18,19). Low-grade and high-grade fibrosarcomas have similar radiologic and histopathologic appearances. Accordingly, electron microscopy may be necessary to reveal the collagenous composition of the matrix of a high-grade tumor (1,2,4,33). Therapy depends on the staging results (6,33).

Metastatic bone tumors are considerably more common than primary skeletal malignancies (with a ratio of about 25 to 1) (1–5). Prostate, breast, thyroid, lung, and kidney cancers are the primary neoplasms that commonly metastasize to bone. There is a predilection for deposition of malignant cells within blood-forming marrow spaces in the spine, ribs, skull, pelvis, and metaphyses of long bones (particularly the femur and humerus). In children, metastases within the skeleton usually reflect a neuroblastoma, leukemia, or Ewing sarcoma. In teenagers or young adults, lymphomas are the predominant source. After age 30, an adenocarcinoma is the likely primary. Osteoblastic metastases most commonly derive from carcinoma of the prostate or breast. Osteolytic metastases may come from the lung, thyroid, kidney, or gastrointestinal tract (18,19). In a significant number of patients, a primary neoplasm is not evident and staging studies with biopsy are performed to explore the possibility of a primary skeletal sarcoma (1–6).

REFERENCES

1. Adler C-P, Kozlowski K (eds): *Primary Bone Tumors and Tumorous Conditions in Children: Pathologic and Radiologic Diagnosis.* Springer-Verlag, London, 1993
2. Lewis MM (ed): *Musculoskeletal Oncology: A Multidisciplinary Approach.* WB Saunders, Philadelphia, 1992
3. Moser RP Jr (ed): *Cartilaginous Tumors of the Skeleton.* Hanley and Belfus, Philadelphia, 1990
4. Mirra JM, Picci P, Gold RH: *Bone Tumors: Clinical, Radiologic, and Pathologic Correlations.* Lea & Febiger, Philadelphia, 1989
5. Unni KK: *Bone Tumors.* Churchill Livingstone, New York, 1988
6. Heare TC, Enneking WF, Heare MM: Staging techniques and biopsy of bone tumors. *Orthop Clin North Am* 20:273–285, 1989
7. Lewis MM: *Bone Tumor Surgery: Limb-Sparing Techniques.* Lippincott, Philadelphia; Gower Medical Publishers, New York, 1988
8. Mankin HJ, Springfield DS, Gebhardt MC, Tomford WW: Current status of allografting for bone tumors. *Orthopedics* 15:1147–1154, 1992
9. Bridge JA: Cytogenetic and molecular cytogenetic techniques in orthopaedic surgery. *J Bone Joint Surg Am* 75:606–614, 1993
10. Jaffe N: Chemotherapy for malignant bone tumors. *Orthop Clin North Am* 20:487–503, 1989
11. Sweetnam R: Malignant bone tumor management: 30 years of achievement. *Clin Orthop* 247:67–73, 1989
12. Eilber FR, Rosen G: Adjuvant chemotherapy for osteosarcoma. *Semin Oncol* 16:312–323, 1989
13. Nichter LS, Menendez LR: Reconstructive considerations for limb salvage surgery. *Orthop Clin North Am* 24:511–521, 1993
14. McDonald DJ: Limb-salvage surgery for treatment of sarcomas of the extremities. *Am J Roentgenol* 163:509–513, 1994
15. Langlais F, Tomeno B (eds): *Limb Salvage: Major Reconstruction in Oncologic and Nontumoral Conditions.* Springer-Verlag, Berlin, 1991
16. Springfield DS, Schmidt R, Graham-Pole J, Marcus RB Jr, Spanier S, Enneking WF: Surgical treatment of osteosarcoma. *J Bone Joint Surg* 70A:1124–1130, 1988
17. Simon MA: Limb salvage for osteosarcoma. *J Bone Joint Surg* 70A:307–310, 1988
18. Edeiken J, Dalinka M, Karasick D: *Edeiken's Roentgen Diagnosis of Diseases of Bone,* 4th ed. Williams and Wilkins, Baltimore, 1990
19. Resnick D, Niwayama G: *Diagnosis of Bone and Joint Disorders,* 2nd ed. WB Saunders, Philadelphia, 1988
20. Simon MA, Finn HA: Diagnostic strategy for bone and soft-tissue tumors. *J Bone Joint Surg Am* 75:622–631, 1993
21. Moser RP Jr, Madewell JE: An approach to primary bone tumors. *Radiol Clin North Am* 25:1049–1093, 1987
22. Brown ML: Bone scintigraphy in benign and malignant tumors. *Radiol Clin North Am* 31:731–738, 1993
23. Murphy WA Jr: Imaging bone tumors in the 1990s. *Cancer* 67:1169–1176, 1991
24. Magid, D: Two-dimensional and three-dimensional computed tomographic imaging in musculoskeletal tumors. *Radiol Clin North Am* 31:426–447, 1993
25. Sundaram M, McGuire MH: Computed tomography or magnetic resonance for evaluating the solitary tumor or tumor-like lesion of bone? *Skeletal Radiol* 17:393–401, 1988
26. Berquist TM: Magnetic resonance imaging of primary skeletal neoplasms. *Radiol Clin North Am* 31:411–424, 1993
27. Redmond OM, Stack JP, Dervan PA, Hurson BJ, Carney DN, Ennis JT: Osteosarcoma: Use of MR imaging and MR spectroscopy in clinical decision making. *Radiology* 172:811–815, 1989
28. DeSchepper AMA, Degryse HRM: *Magnetic Resonance Imaging of Bone and Soft Tissue Tumors and Their Mimics: A Clinical Atlas.* Kluwer Academic Publishers, Boston, 1989
29. Simon MA, Biermann JS: Biopsy of bone and soft-tissue lesions. *J Bone Joint Surg Am* 75:616–621, 1993
30. Giudici MA, Moser RP Jr, Kransdorf MJ: Cartilaginous bone tumors. *Radiol Clin North Am* 31:237–259, 1993
31. Schubiner JM, Simon MA: Primary bone tumors in children. *Orthop Clin North Am* 18:577–595, 1987
32. Hudson TM, Stiles RG, Monson DK: Fibrous lesions of bone. *Radiol Clin North Am* 31:279–297, 1993
33. Marks KE, Bauer TW: Fibrous tumors of bone. *Orthop Clin North Am* 20:377–393, 1989
34. Greenspan A: Tumors of cartilage origin. *Orthop Clin North Am* 20:347–366, 1989
35. Merchan EC, Sanchez-Herrera S, Gonzalez JM: Secondary chondrosarcoma. Four cases and review of the literature. *Acta Orthopaed Belg* 59:76–80, 1993
36. Manaster BJ, Doyle AJ: Giant cell tumors of bone. *Radiol Clin North Am* 31:299–323, 1993
37. Osserman EF, Merlini G, Butler VP Jr: Multiple myeloma and related plasma cell dyscrasias. *JAMA* 258:2930–2937, 1987
38. Mundy GR: *Calcium Homeostasis: Hypercalcemia and Hypocalcemia.* Martin Dunitz, London, 1989
39. Meyers PA: Malignant bone tumors in children: Osteosarcoma. *Hematol Oncol Clin North Am* 1:655–665, 1987
40. Taylor WF, Ivins JC, Unni KK, Beabout JW, Golenzer HJ, Black LE: Prognostic variables in osteosarcoma: Multi-institutional study. *J Natl Cancer Inst* 81:21–30, 1989
41. Dahlin D, Coventry MB: Osteogenic sarcoma: A study of six hundred cases. *J Bone Joint Surg* 49A:101–110, 1967
42. Klein MJ, Kenan S, Lewis M: Osteosarcoma: Clinical and pathological considerations. *Orthop Clin North Am* 20:327–345, 1989
43. Eckardt JJ (ed): Newest knowledge of osteosarcoma (symposium). *Clin Orthop* 270, 1991
44. Edeiken-Monroe B, Edeiken J, Jacobson HG: Osteosarcoma. *Semin Roentgenol* 24:153–173, 1989

45. Hadjipavlou A, Lander P, Srolovitz H, Enker IP: Malignant transformation in Paget disease of bone. *Cancer* 70:2802–2808, 1992
46. Welkerling H, Dreyer T, Delling G: Morphological typing of chondrosarcoma: A study of 92 cases. *Virchows Arch A Pathol Anat Histopathol* 418:419–425, 1991
47. Horowitz ME, Tsokos MG, DeLaney TF: Ewing's sarcoma. *CA Cancer J Clin* 42:300–320, 1992
48. Eggli KD, Quiogue T, Moser RP Jr: Ewing's sarcoma. *Radiol Clin North Am* 31:325–337, 1993
49. Meyers PA: Malignant bone tumors in children: Ewing's sarcoma. *Hematol Oncol Clin North Am* 1:667–673, 1987
50. Womer RB: The cellular biology of bone tumors. *Clin Orthop* 262:12–21, 1991
51. Selleri L, Hermanson GG, Eubanks JH, Lewis KA, Evans GA: Molecular localization of the t(11;22) (q24;q12) translocation of Ewing sarcoma by chromosomal in situ suppression hybridization. *Proc Natl Acad Sci USA* 88:887–891, 1991
52. O'Connor MI, Pritchard DJ: Ewing's sarcoma. *Clin Orthop* 262:78–87, 1991

73. Ischemic Bone Disease

Michael P. Whyte, M.D.

Division of Bone and Mineral Diseases, Washington University School of Medicine; and Metabolic Research Unit, Shriners Hospital for Crippled Children, St. Louis, Missouri

Regional interruption of blood flow to the skeleton causes this important acquired disorder of cartilage and bone (1–3). Ischemia, if sufficiently severe and prolonged, will kill osteoblasts and chrondrocytes. Clinical problems may arise because subsequent resorption of necrotic areas of bone and cartilage during skeletal repair compromises bone strength and predisposes to fracture (4).

A change in skeletal density is the principal radiologic feature of ischemic bone disease (2,3). However, radiographic changes may take several months to appear. Characteristic radiologic signs include crescent-shaped subchondral radiolucencies, patchy areas of sclerosis and lucency, bony collapse, and diaphyseal periostitis, although joint space is initially preserved despite the affected epiphyseal region.

A variety of conditions cause ischemic bone disease (Table 1) and a great number of clinical presentations occur based primarily on the affected skeletal region. Legg-Calvé-Perthes disease is discussed in some detail first, because it represents an archetypal form of ischemic bone disease. A few additional important clinical presentations are reviewed subsequently.

LEGG-CALVÉ-PERTHES DISEASE

Legg-Calvé-Perthes disease (LCPD) can be defined as idiopathic ischemic necrosis (osteonecrosis) of the capital femoral epiphysis in children (5–7). It is a common, complex, and controversial pediatric problem that affects boys more frequently than girls (4:1 to 5:1). Typically, LCPD presents between 2 and 12 years of age; the mean age at diagnosis is 7 years. When it first manifests later in life, the term "adolescent ischemic necrosis" is used to indicate the poorer prognosis that occurs when adults suffer ischemic bone disease (see later). Usually, one hip is involved, but bilateral disease troubles about 20% of patients. Familial incidence varies from 1% to 20% (5–7).

Although the etiology of LCPD is as yet unknown, the pathogenesis seems to be fairly well understood. Interruption of blood flow to the capital femoral epiphysis is the fundamental skeletal insult. Ischemia at this site in children may occur from raised intracapsular pressure that results from congenital or developmental abnormalities, episodes of synovitis, venous thrombosis, or perhaps increased blood viscosity (5–7). Most, if not all, of the capital femoral epiphysis is rendered ischemic. Consequently, marrow cells, osteoblasts, and osteocytes may die. Endochondral ossification ceases temporarily because blood flow to chondrocytes in the growth plate is impaired. Articular cartilage, however, remains intact initially because it depends on synovial fluid for nourishment. Revascularization then follows and proceeds from the periphery to the center of the capital femoral epiphysis. New bone is deposited on the surface of dead, subchondral cortical or central trabecular bone. Subsequently, the critical process of removal of necrotic bone begins, during which time the rate of bone resorption exceeds the rate of reparative new bone formation. As a result, the subchondral bone is weakened.

If there is no fracture in the area of reparative bone resorption, the child may remain asymptomatic with eventual healing. However, if fracture does occur, there will be symptoms. Furthermore, trabecular bone collapse can cause a second episode of ischemia (5–7). Longitudinal growth of the proximal femur can be stunted, because the disrupted blood flow disturbs the physis and metaphysis. Premature closure of the growth plate may occur. As reossification of the capital femoral epiphysis takes place, the femoral head will remodel and remold its shape according to mechanical forces acting on it (2,3,5–7).

Children with LCPD typically limp, complain of pain in a knee or anterior thigh, and have limited mobility of the hip (especially with abduction or internal rotation). The Trendelenburg sign may be positive. If treatment is not successful, adduction and flexion contractures of the hip can develop, and thigh muscles can atrophy.

TABLE 1. *Causes of ischemic necrosis of cartilage and bone*

Endocrine/metabolic
  Glucocorticoid therapy
  Cushing syndrome
  Alcohol abuse
  Gout
  Osteomalacia
Storage diseases (e.g., Gaucher's disease)
Hemoglobinopathies (e.g., sickle cell disease)
Trauma (e.g., dislocation, fracture)
Dysbaric conditions
Collagen vascular disorders
Irradiation
Pancreatitis
Renal transplantation
Idiopathic, familial

From: Edeiken J, Dalinka M, Karasick D. *Edeiken's Roentgen Diagnosis of Diseases of Bone,* 4th ed. Williams and Wilkins, Baltimore, 1990; and Resnick D, Niwayama G. *Diagnosis of Bone and Joint Disorders,* 3rd ed. WB Saunders, Philadelphia, 1995.

Laboratory investigation may show a slightly elevated erythrocyte sedimentation rate. Radiologic examination, which should include anteroposterior and "frog" lateral views for diagnosis and follow-up, often reveals a bone age that is 1 to 3 years delayed (2,3). Sequential studies typically demonstrate cessation of growth of the capital femoral epiphysis, resorption of necrotic bone, subchondral fracture, reossification, and, finally, healing (Fig. 1). Magnetic reso-

nance imaging (MRI) is a helpful technique because signal intensity patterns change with circulatory compromise, soft tissues as well as bone are visualized, and containment of the femoral head can be assessed (8).

The short-term prognosis for LCPD depends on the severity of femoral head deformity at the completion of the healing phase. The long-term outcome is conditioned by how much secondary degenerative osteoarthritis develops. In general, the more extensive the involvement of the capital femoral epiphysis, the worse the prognosis. Girls appear to have poorer outcomes than boys, because they tend to have greater involvement of the capital femoral epiphysis and mature earlier. Earlier sexual maturation means less time for femoral head modeling before closure of the growth plates. Onset at 2 to 6 years of age is associated with the least femoral head deformity; onset after 10 years of age has a poor outcome (5–9).

Treatment for LCPD is directed principally by the orthopedic surgeon (10). Prevention of femoral head deformity is a major goal. Significant deformity, not mild, predisposes to osteoarthritis. Osteoarthritis seems to be greatest for children who have "loss of containment" of the femoral head by the acetabulum. Hip subluxation, and loss of motion from muscle spasm and contractures, disproportionately increase mechanical stresses on some regions of the femoral head. The objective of treatment is to improve the coverage of the femoral head by the acetabulum, thus allowing it to act as a mold during reparative reossification. Prevention of subluxation of the femoral head with elimination of irritability and restoration and maintenance of the range of motion of the hip are primary concerns of therapy (5–7). Appropriate

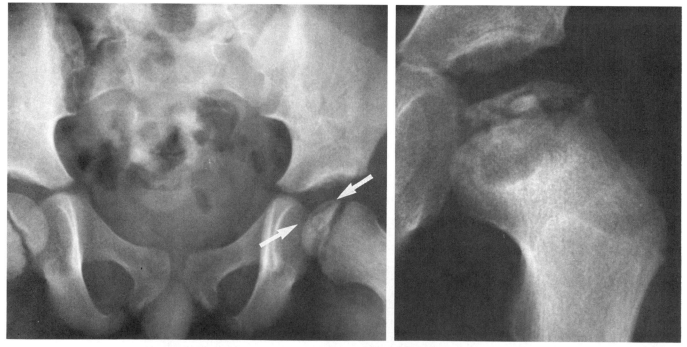

A   B

FIG. 1. Legg-Calvé-Perthes disease. **A:** The affected left capital femoral epiphysis of this 4-year-old boy is denser and smaller than the contralateral normal side. It shows a radiolucent area that forms the "crescent sign" *(arrows)* indicative of subchondral bone collapse. **B:** Seven months later, there is flattening of the capital femoral epiphysis with widening and irregularity of the femoral neck.

management may be observation alone, intermittent treatment of symptoms with periodic bed rest, stretching exercises to maintain hip range of motion, and early or late surgical prevention or correction of deformity (10,11). Bed rest does not appear to substantially decrease compressive forces that may stimulate healing and bone modeling if properly distributed (6). Casts, orthoses, or a "stirrup" crutch may achieve containment. Operative approaches may include osteotomy. Surgical procedures for deformities used later in the course of treatment include muscle release and abduction casting, osteotomy, and partial excision of the femoral head (5–7,10,11). Periodic radiographic follow-up is essential, and arthrography, bone scintigraphy, and especially MRI can also be useful (6,8).

The long-term results of these treatments remain controversial. Whether containment is useful, and which method of achieving containment is best, are clinical questions that are being actively studied (5–7,10,11).

OTHER CLINICAL PRESENTATIONS

Numerous other clinical presentations for ischemic bone disease occur in children and adults (Table 2) (1–3). Symptoms result primarily from skeletal disintegration. The specific diagnosis depends on the patient's age, the anatomic site, and the size of the area of bone where blood flow has been interrupted. Legg-Calvé-Perthes disease is an excellent illustration that disruption of the microvasculature of the

TABLE 2. *Common sites of osteochondrosis and ischemic necrosis of bone*

Adult skeleton
  Osteochondritis dissecans (König)
  Osteochondrosis of lunate (Kienböck)
  Fractured head of femur (Axhausen, Phemister)
  Proximal fragment of fractured carpal scaphoid
  Fractured head of humerus
  Fractured talus
  Osteonecrosis of the knee (spontaneous or idiopathic
    ischemic necrosis)
  Idiopathic ischemic necrosis of the femoral head
Developing skeleton
  Osteochondrosis of femoral head (Legg-Calvé-Perthes)
  Slipped femoral epiphysis
  Vertebral epiphysitis affecting secondary ossification
    centers (Scheuermann)
  Vertebral osteochondrosis of primary ossification centers
    (Calvé)
  Osteochondrosis of tibial tuberosity (Osgood-Schlatter)
  Osteochondrosis of tarsal scaphoid (Köhler)
  Osteochondrosis of medial tibial condyle (Blount)
  Osteochondrosis of primary ossification center of patella
    (Köhler) and of secondary ossification center (Sinding
    Larsen)
  Osteochondrosis of os calcis (Sever)
  Osteochondrosis of head of second metatarsal (Freiberg)
    and of other metatarsals and metacarpals
  Osteochondrosis of the humeral capitellum (Panner)

From: Edeiken J, Dalinka M, Karasic D (eds). *Edeiken's Roentgen Diagnosis of Diseases of Bone,* 4th ed. Williams & Wilkins, Baltimore, 937, 1990.

skeleton predisposes especially subchondral bone to infarction. However, several general mechanisms for vascular insufficiency may lead to ischemic bone disease, such as traumatic rupture, internal obstruction, and external pressure compromising blood flow. Arteries, veins, or sinusoids may be directly affected. The resulting ischemic bone disease has been referred to as avascular, aseptic, ischemic, or idiopathic necrosis (1–3). A considerable variety of conditions can cause ischemic bone disease (Table 1).

The pathogenesis of disrupted blood flow in ischemic bone disease is incompletely understood (1–3). For many types of nontraumatic ischemic necrosis, the predisposed sites of the skeleton seem to recapitulate the conversion of red marrow to fatty marrow with aging (2). This process occurs from distal to proximal in the appendicular skeleton. As the transition occurs, there is a decrease in marrow blood flow. Accordingly, disorders that increase the size and/or number of fat cells within critical areas of medullary space (e.g., alcohol abuse, Cushing syndrome) may ultimately compress sinusoids and infarct bone. However, fat embolization, hemorrhage, and abnormalities in the quality of susceptible bone tissue may also be pathogenetic factors in some types of traumatic or nontraumatic ischemic bone disease (2).

Radiologic features of ischemic bone disease depend on the amount of skeletal revascularization, reossification, and resorption of infarcted bone (2,3). Revascularization occurs within 6 to 8 weeks of the ischemic event and may cause trabecular bone resorption (radiolucent bands near necrotic areas). New bone formation then occurs on dead bone surfaces. Over months or years, dead bone may, or may not, be slowly resorbed. Osteosclerosis will occur if new bone encases dead bone and/or if there is bony collapse.

Histopathologic study is consistent with the pathogenesis that is suggested radiographically. It demonstrates that these various processes of skeletal death and repair are focal and may be occurring simultaneously (Fig. 2) (4).

Following infarction, necrotic bone does not change density for at least 10 days (2). Currently, MRI is the most sensitive way to detect ischemic necrosis of the skeleton and therefore is particularly useful early on, although occasionally false negatives do occur (8,12,13). Bone scintigraphy with 99m-technetium diphosphonate, although not specific, can also detect osteonecrosis before radiographic changes are apparent (14,15). Prior to the process of revascularization, the infarcted area shows decreased radioisotope uptake. Later, increased tracer accumulation will occur. Computed tomography is especially helpful for detecting ischemic necrosis of the femoral head, because the bony anatomy there normally assumes an asterisk shape at the center that is distorted by new bone formation (16).

The various clinical presentations of ischemic bone disease (Table 2) are sometimes divided into two major anatomic categories: diaphysometaphyseal and epiphysometaphyseal (2).

Diaphysometaphyseal ischemia can be caused by dysbaric disorders, hemoglobinopathies, collagen vascular diseases, thromboembolic conditions, gout, storage disorders (e.g., Gaucher's disease), acute or chronic pancreatitis, pheochromocytoma, and other conditions. Typically, this category involves large bones (especially the distal femur or proximal

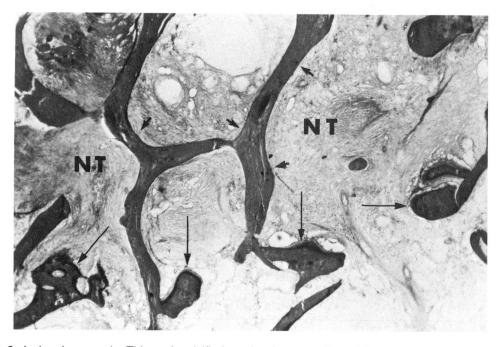

FIG. 2. Ischemic necrosis. This undecalcified section from an affected femoral head shows a typical area of dead bone *(arrows)* with a smooth acellular surface. A band of necrotic tissue (NT) is visible. Reparative bone formation is occurring in adjacent areas where darkly stained, newly synthesized osteoid is covered by osteoblasts *(arrowheads)* (Goldner stain; ×160).

tibia) where radiologic changes extend into the metaphysis. Such lesions are often symmetrical; however, the size of the involved areas can vary considerably. Small bones, however, may be affected, for example in the hands and feet of infants with sickle cell anemia. New bone deposition delineates infarcted bone especially well on radiographic study.

Epiphysometaphyseal infarcts can result from dysbaric conditions, sickle cell disease, Cushing syndrome, gout, trauma, storage problems, and other disorders. When the lesions are small, they are typically found in children or young adults and occur without a history of injury, though occult trauma may actually be important in their pathogenesis. Thrombosis, disease of arterial walls, or abnormalities within adjacent bone such as those occurring in Gaucher's disease or histiocytosis-X (see Chapter 74) may cause this category of ischemic bone disease.

Osteochondrosis refers to a traumatic ischemic necrosis that typically affects a skeletal growth or ossification center (2). *Osteochondritis dissecans* describes a small epiphysometaphyseal infarct that can cause fracture immediately adjacent to a joint space. This lesion appears as a small, dense, button like area of osseous tissue that is separated from the bone by a radiolucent band. This bone fragment can become loose and enter the joint, but it may also heal. Larger infarcts are often also idiopathic, occur frequently in adults, and typically involve the hip and the femoral condyles. Large areas of ischemic bone can collapse, thus flattening joint surfaces and destroying articular cartilage. Ultimately, this complication will lead to osteoarthritis (Fig. 3). Very extensive epiphysometaphyseal infarction results from trauma or sys-

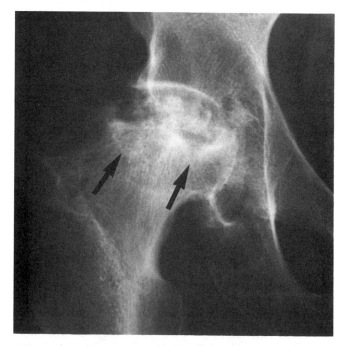

FIG. 3. Ischemic (avascular) necrosis. This 50-year-old man has advanced avascular necrosis of the femoral head. Note that much of the femoral head has been resorbed, with resultant collapse of the articular surface. The necrotic area is fragmented. A sclerotic zone of reparative tissue *(arrows)* indicates the interface between viable and necrotic tissues. The acetabular cartilage is focally thin. This finding indicates that he is developing secondary osteoarthritis.

temic disease and frequently involves the femoral head; an example of this is LCPD (2).

Eponyms for specific presentations of osteochondrosis or ischemic necrosis of the skeleton are numerous (e.g., Blount's disease, Scheuermann's disease) and are widely used. However, classification according to the involved anatomic site is more understandable. Table 2 matches the eponym with the affected skeletal region and helps to illustrate that the patient's age is an important factor for determining which areas of the skeleton are at risk (2).

Treatment of ischemic bone disease varies according to the site and size of the lesion, and the patient's age. Conservative or surgical approaches may be appropriate (1,17,18).

REFERENCES

1. Mankin HJ. Nontraumatic necrosis of bone (osteonecrosis). *N Engl J Med* 326:1473–1479, 1992
2. Edeiken J, Dalinka M, Karasick D: *Edeiken's Roentgen Diagnosis of Diseases of Bone,* 4th ed. Williams and Wilkins, Baltimore, 1990
3. Resnick D, Niwayama G: *Diagnosis of Bone and Joint Disorders,* 3rd ed. WB Saunders, Philadelphia, 1995
4. Chang CC, Greenspan A, Gershwin ME: Osteonecrosis: Current perspectives on pathogenesis and treatment. *Semin Arthritis Rheum* 23:47–69, 1992
5. Katz JE: *Legg-Calvé-Perthes Disease.* Praeger, New York, 1984
6. Conway JJ: A scintigraphic classification of Legg-Calvé-Perthes disease. *Semin Nucl Med* 23:274–295, 1993
7. Wenger DR, Ward WT, Herring JA: Current concepts review: Legg-Calvé-Perthes disease. *J Bone Joint Surg* 73(A):778–788, 1991
8. Lang P, Genant HK, Jergesen HE, Murray WR: Imaging of the hip joint. Computed tomography versus magnetic resonance imaging. *Clin Orthop* 274:135–153, 1992
9. Mukherjee A, Fabry G: Evaluation of the prognostic indices in Legg-Calvé-Perthes disease: Statistical analysis of 116 hips. *J Pediatr Orthop* 10:153–158, 1990
10. Herring JA: The treatment of Legg-Calvé-Perthes disease. A critical review of the literature. *J Bone Joint Surg* 76(A):448–458, 1994
11. Paterson DC, Leitch JM, Foster BK: Results of innominate osteotomy in the treatment of Legg-Calvé-Perthes disease. *Clin Orthop* 266:96–103, 1991
12. Mitchell MD, Kundel HL, Steinberg ME, Kressel HY, Alavi A, Axel L: Avascular necrosis of the hip: Comparison of MR, CT, and scintigraphy. *Am J Roentgenol* 147:67–71, 1986
13. Mitchell DG, Rao VM, Dalinka MK, et al.: Femoral head avascular necrosis: Correlation of MR imaging, and clinical findings. *Radiology* 162:709–715, 1987
14. Bonnarens F, Hernandez A, D'Ambrosia RD: Bone scintigraphic changes in osteonecrosis of the femoral head. *Orthop Clin North Am* 16:697–703, 1985
15. Spencer JD, Maisey M: A prospective scintigraphic study of avascular necrosis of bone in renal transplant patients. *Clin Orthop* 194:125–135, 1985
16. Dihlmann W: CT analysis of the upper end of the femur: The asterisk sign and ischemic bone necrosis of the femoral head. *Skeletal Radiol* 8:251–258, 1982
17. Crenshaw AH: *Campbell's Operative Orthopaedics,* 8th ed. CV Mosby, St. Louis, 1992
18. Smith SW, Fehring TK, Griffin WL, Beaver WB: Core decompression of the osteonecrotic femoral head. *J Bone Joint Surg* 77(A):674–680, 1995

74. Infiltrative Disorders of Bone

Michael P. Whyte, M.D.

Division of Bone and Mineral Diseases, Washington University School of Medicine; and Metabolic Research Unit, Shriners Hospital for Crippled Children, St. Louis, Missouri

Several important and interesting skeletal disorders are associated with abnormal proliferation or infiltration of specific cell types within the marrow spaces. Reviewed briefly here are systemic mastocytosis and histiocytosis-X.

SYSTEMIC MASTOCYTOSIS

Systemic mastocytosis is characterized by increased numbers of mast cells in the viscera—principally the liver, spleen, gastrointestinal tract, and lymph nodes. However, the skin can contain numerous hyperpigmented macules that reflect dermal mast cell accumulation, a problem called *urticaria pigmentosa* (Fig. 1). Bone marrow is also typically involved, causing the skeletal pathology. The etiology of systemic mastocytosis is unknown (1–3). Persistence of mast cell disease following successful bone marrow transplantation for an additional condition suggests that a defective myeloid precursor cell is not involved in the pathogenesis (4,5).

Symptoms of systemic mastocytosis are largely a result of the release of mediator substances from the mast cells and include generalized pruritus, urticaria, flushing, episodic hypotension, diarrhea, weight loss, peptic ulcer, and syncope. With cutaneous involvement, histamine release occurs from stroking the skin causing urtication (Darier's sign). Skeletal symptoms occur relatively infrequently; they include bone pain or tenderness from deformity resulting from fracture (1–3,6–9). Patients often succumb to a granulocytic neoplasm (10).

Radiologic abnormalities of the skeleton are common in systemic mastocytosis (about 70% of patients). The features have been thoroughly characterized (11,12). Radiographs typically show diffuse, poorly demarcated, sclerotic, and lucent areas where red marrow is present (i.e., the axial skeleton) (Fig. 2). However, circumscribed lesions can occur, especially in the skull and in the extremities. These focal findings can be mistaken for metastatic disease. Lytic areas are often small and have a surrounding rim of osteosclerosis.

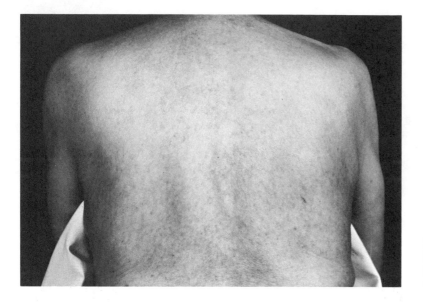

FIG. 1. Systemic mastocytosis. Numerous characteristic hyperpigmented macules (urticaria pigmentosa) are present on the back of this 61-year-old woman.

Progression of the radiologic changes can occur as regional involvement becomes generalized (11,12). Focal bony changes may be absent despite extensive accumulation of mast cells in the skeleton. Generalized osteopenia (without focal bony abnormalities) can also be a common presen-

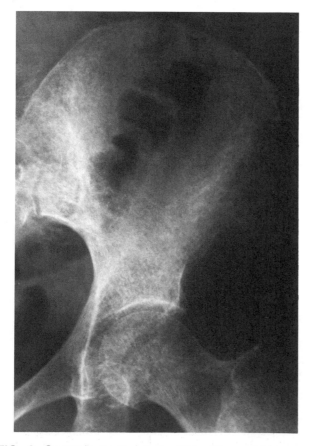

FIG. 2. Systemic mastocytosis. This 81-year-old woman has characteristic diffuse punctuate radiolucencies of her pelvis and hip that indicate a permeative process in the bone marrow.

tation (6,7,9), but this has a relatively benign prognosis (13). Bone scintigraphy is not only an effective way to detect involved skeletal areas (14) but can provide information regarding disease activity and prognosis (15).

Histopathologic correlates of systemic mastocytosis in the skeleton are also well characterized (6,16,17). In fact, examination of undecalcified sections of bone can be a particularly effective way to establish the diagnosis. Iliac crest biopsy may be superior for this purpose to bone marrow aspiration or biopsy (6,16,17). Undecalcified sections of iliac crest show multiple nodules of 150 to 450 micron in diameter that resemble granulomas. Within the granulomas are characteristic oval or spindle-shaped cells, eosinophils, lymphocytes, and plasma cells. The spindle-shaped cells resemble histiocytes or fibroblasts, but they contain granules that stain metachromatically and are actually a type of mast cell (Fig. 3). In addition, the marrow contains increased numbers of these mast cells individually or in small aggregates (6,16,17). Studies with tetracycline show that skeletal remodeling is rapid (16,17).

The treatment of systemic mastocytosis is discussed in a number of reviews (1–3,18–21). Recently, severe bone pain from advanced bone disease has been found to respond to radiotherapy (22).

HISTIOCYTOSIS-X

Histiocytosis-X was the term first used in 1953 to unify what had been regarded as three distinct entities: Letterer-Siwe disease, Hand-Schüller-Christian disease, and eosinophilic granuloma (23–25). The Langerhans cell was recognized as the pathognomonic feature that appeared to link these three disorders. Histiocytosis-X seems to result from some poorly understood dysfunction of the immune system. Nevertheless, it is an extremely heterogeneous condition. The tripartite distinction for histiocytosis-X continues to be used because of the generally different clinical courses and prognoses for each of the three subtypes (23–25).

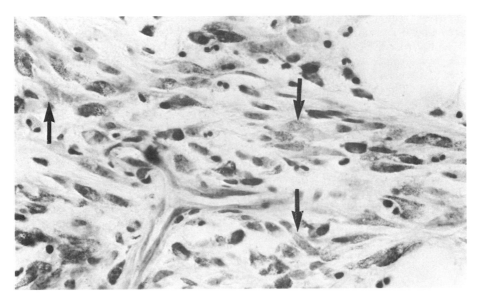

FIG. 3. Mast cell granuloma. A nondecalcified specimen of iliac crest shows a characteristic mast cell granuloma that contains numerous spindle-shaped mast cells *(arrows)*. (Toluidine blue stain, ×220.)

About 1200 cases of histiocytosis-X are diagnosed yearly in the United States. Sex incidence is equal. Northern Europeans are affected more commonly than Hispanics, and the condition is rare in blacks. Many tissues and organs can be diseased, including brain, lung, oropharynx, gastrointestinal tract, skin, and bone marrow. Diabetes insipidus is common in affected children and adults because of pituitary infiltration. Prognosis is age related: infants and the elderly have poor outcomes.

The signs and symptoms of the three principal clinical forms are described briefly.

Letterer-Siwe disease presents between the ages of several weeks and 2 years, with hepatosplenomegaly, lymphadenopathy, anemia, a tendency to hemorrhage, fever, failure to grow, and skeletal lesions. It may end fatally after just several weeks (23–25).

Hand-Schüller-Christian disease is a chronic disorder that begins in early childhood, although symptoms may not manifest until the third decade (23–25). The classic triad consists of exophthalmos, diabetes insipidus, and bony lesions. However, this presentation occurs in only 10% of cases. The most common skeletal manifestation is osteolytic lesions in the skull, with overlying soft tissue nodules (Fig. 4) (26,27). Proptosis is associated with destruction of orbital bones. There may by spontaneous remissions and exacerbations. Soft tissue nodules may remit without treatment.

Eosinophilic granuloma occurs most frequently in children between 3 and 10 years of age, and it is rare past the age of 15 years (23–25). A solitary and painful lesion in a flat bone is the most common finding (26,27). There may be a soft tissue mass. The calvarium is usually affected, although any bone can be involved. The prognosis is excellent, with monostotic lesions responding well to x-ray therapy or healing spontaneously.

The radiologic findings in the skeleton are similar in the three disorders (11,12,26,27). Single bony foci are most common. Nevertheless, multiple-affected areas can occur and show progressive enlargement. Individual lesions are well defined, punched-out appearing, osteolytic, and destructive with scalloped edges. They vary from a few millimeters to several centimeters in diameter. Fewer than half of these radiolucencies show marginal reactive osteosclerosis. Membranous bone as well as long bones can be affected. In the long bones, these defects occur in the medullary canal where there is erosion of the endosteal cortex (commonly in

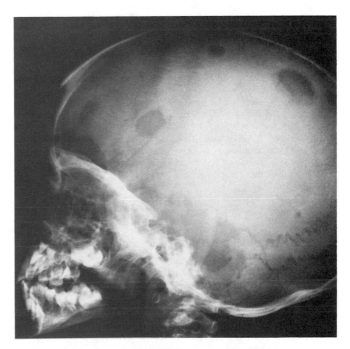

FIG. 4. Hand-Schüller-Christian disease. This 2⁴/₁₂-year-old boy has multiple, well-defined, beveled-edge, lucent lesions of the skull. Note the extensive destruction of the paranasal sinuses and at the base of the skull.

the metaphyseal or epiphyseal regions). Periosteal reaction is frequent and produces a solid layer of new bone. In the skull, the bony tables can be eroded. Destruction of orbital bones may or may not be associated with exophthalmos. Vertebra plana (i.e., flattened vertebrae) can result from spinal involvement in young children. Radionuclide accumulation is poor during bone scanning (11,12). Biochemical parameters of mineral homeostasis are usually normal.

Histiocytosis-X tends to be benign and self-limiting when there is no systemic involvement. Treatment modalities for severe disease include chemotherapy, radiation therapy, and immunotherapy (28). Methylprednisolone injected into lesions is an effective procedure (27). Central nervous system involvement is often treated by radiation therapy. Allogeneic bone marrow transplantation was reported to have been successful in a severe case with poor prognosis (29).

REFERENCES

1. Travis WD, Li CY, Bergstrahl EJ, Yam LI, Swee RG: Systemic mast cell disease: Analysis of 58 cases and literature review. *Medicine* 67:345–368, 1988
2. Friedman BS, Metcalfe DD: Mastocytosis. *Prog Clin Biol Res* 297:163–173, 1989
3. Gruchalla RS: *Mast cells and mastocytosis: Developments over the last decade.* University of Texas Health Science Center at Dallas, Dallas, 1993
4. Ronnov-Jessen D, Nielsen PL, Horn T: Persistence of systemic mastocytosis after allogeneic bone marrow transplantation in spite of complete remission of the associated myelodysplastic syndrome. *Bone Marrow Transplant* 8:413–415, 1991
5. Van Hoof A, Criel A, Louwagie A, Vanvuchelen J: Cutaneous mastocytosis after autologous bone marrow transplantation. *Bone Marrow Transplant* 8:151–153, 1991
6. Fallon MD, Whyte MP, Teitelbaum SL: Systemic mastocytosis associated with generalized osteopenia: Histopathological characterization of the skeletal lesion using undecalcified bone from two patients. *Hum Pathol* 12:813–820, 1981
7. Harvey JA, Anderson HC, Borek D, Morris D, Lukert BP: Osteoporosis associated with mastocytosis confined to bone: Report of two cases. *Bone* 10:237–241, 1989
8. Cook JV, Chandy J: Systemic mastocytosis affecting the skeletal system. *J Bone Joint Surg* 71B:536, 1989
9. Lidor C, Frisch B, Gazit D, Gepstein R, Hallel T, Mekori YA: Osteoporosis as the sole presentation of bone marrow mastocytosis. *J Bone Miner Res* 5:871–876, 1990
10. Lawrence JB, Friedman BS, Travis WD, Chinchilli VM, Metcalfe DD, Gralnick HR: Hematologic manifestations of systemic mast cell disease: A prospective study of laboratory and morphologic features and their relation to prognosis. *Am J Med* 91:612–624, 1991
11. Edeiken J, Dalinka M, Karasick D: *Edeiken's Roentgen Diagnosis of Diseases of Bone,* 4th ed. Williams and Wilkins, Baltimore, 1990
12. Resnick D, Niwayama G: *Diagnosis of Bone and Joint Disorders,* 3rd ed. WB Saunders, Philadelphia, 1995
13. Andrew SM, Freemont AJ: Skeletal mastocytosis. *J Clin Pathol* 46:1033–1035, 1993
14. Arrington ER, Eisenberg B, Hartshorne MF, Vela S, Dorin RI: Nuclear medicine imaging of systemic mastocytosis. *J Nucl Med* 30:2046–2048, 1989
15. Chen CC, Andrich MP, Mican JM, Metcalfe DD: A retrospective analysis of bone scan abnormalities in mastocytosis: Correlation with disease category and prognosis. *J Nucl Med* 35:1471–1475, 1994
16. de Gennes C, Kuntz D, de Vernejoul MC: Bone mastocytosis: A report of nine cases with a bone histomorphometric study. *Clin Orthop* 279:281–291, 1992
17. Chines A, Pacifici R, Avioli LV, Teitelbaum SL, Korenblat PE: Systemic mastocytosis presenting as osteoporosis: A clinical and histomorphometric study. *J Clin Endocrinol Metab* 72:140–144, 1991
18. Gasior-Chrzan B, Falk ES: Systemic mastocytosis treated with histamine H1 and H2 receptor antagonists. *Dermatology* 184:149–152, 1992
19. Metcalfe DD: The treatment of mastocytosis: An overview. *J Invest Dermatol* 96:55S–59S, 1991
20. Póvoa P, Ducla-Soares J, Fernandes A, Palma-Carlos AG: A case of systemic mastocytosis: Therapeutic efficacy of ketotifen. *J Intern Med* 229:475–477, 1991
21. Kluin-Nelemans HC, Jansen JH, Breukelman H, Wolthers BG, Kluin PM, Kroon HM, Willemze R: Response to interferon alfa-2b in a patient with systemic mastocytosis. *N Engl J Med* 326:619–623, 1992
22. Johnstone PA, Mican JM, Metcalfe DD, DeLaney TF: Radiotherapy of refractory bone pain due to systemic mast cell disease. *Am J Clin Oncol* 17:328–330, 1994
23. Osband ME, Pochedley C: Histiocytosis X. *Hematol Oncol Clin North Am* 1:1–165, 1987
24. Raney RB Jr, D'Angio GJ: Langerhans' cell histiocytes (histiocytosis X): Experience at the Children's Hospital of Philadelphia, 1970–1984. *Med Pediatr Oncol* 17:20–28, 1989
25. Osband ME: Histiocytosis X: Langerhans' cell histiocytosis. *Hematol Oncol Clin North Am* 1:737–751, 1987
26. Alexander JE, Seibert JJ, Berry DH, Glasier CM, Williamson SL, Murphy J: Prognostic factors for healing of bone lesions in histiocytosis X. *Pediatr Radiol* 18:326–332, 1988
27. Bollini G, Jouve JL, Gentet JC, Jacquemier M, Bouyala JM: Bone lesions in histiocytosis X. *J Pediatr Orthop* 11:469–477, 1991
28. Greenberger JS, Crocker AC, Vawter G, Jaffe N, Cassady JR: Results of treatment of 127 patients with systemic histiocytosis (Letterer-Siwe syndrome, Schüller-Christian syndrome and multifocal eosinophilic granuloma). *Medicine* 60:311–388, 1981
29. Ringdén O, Aohström L, Lönnqvist B, Boaryd I, Svedmyr E, Gahrton G: Allogeneic bone marrow transplantation in a patient with chemotherapy-resistant progressive histiocytosis X. *N Engl J Med* 316:733–735, 1987

SECTION VIII

Paget's Disease

75. Paget's Disease of Bone

Ethel S. Siris, M.D.

Department of Medicine, Columbia University, College of Physicians and Surgeons, New York, New York

Paget's disease of bone is a localized disorder of bone remodeling. The process is initiated by increases in osteoclast-mediated bone resorption, with subsequent compensatory increases in new bone formation, resulting in a disorganized mosaic of woven and lamellar bone at affected skeletal sites. This structural change produces bone that is expanded in size, less compact, more vascular, and more susceptible to deformity or fracture than normal bone (1). Clinical signs and symptoms will vary from one patient to the next depending on the number and location of affected skeletal sites, as well as on the rapidity of the abnormal bone turnover. It is believed that most patients are asymptomatic, but a substantial minority may experience a variety of symptoms, including bone pain, secondary arthritic problems, bone deformity, excessive warmth over bone from hypervascularity, and a variety of neurologic complications caused in most instances by compression of neural tissues adjacent to pagetic bone.

ETIOLOGY

The etiology of Paget's disease remains unknown. However, existing data from several different areas of investigation have provided some useful working hypotheses. First, Paget's disease appears to have a significant genetic component. Fifteen percent to 30% of patients with Paget's disease from several clinical series have positive family histories of the disorder (2). Genetic analyses of multiple affected kindreds support an autosomal dominant pattern of inheritance (3). There are data indicating that Paget's disease may be linked to human leukocyte antigen (HLA), and one report describes an increased frequency of HLA-DQw 1 antigen in pagetic subjects with either positive or negative family histories of the disease (4). Familial aggregation studies in a United States population (5) suggest that the risk of a first-degree relative of a pagetic subject developing the condition is 7 times greater than is the risk for someone who does not have an affected relative. Moreover, the risk increases if the first-degree relative has more severe disease and an early age at diagnosis. The data suggest that the predicted cumulative incidence to age 90 is about 2% in people without affected first-degree relatives and over 9% in people with one or more affected first-degree relatives.

Ethnic and geographic clustering of Paget's disease has also been described, with the intriguing observation that the disorder is quite common in some parts of the world but relatively rare in others. Clinical observations indicate that the disease is most common in Europe, North America, Australia, and New Zealand. Studies surveying radiologists have computed prevalence rates in hospitalized patients over age 55 in several European cities and have found the highest percentages in England (4.6%) and France (2.4%),

with other Western European countries reporting slightly lower prevalences (e.g., 0.7% to 1.7% in Ireland, 1.3% in Spain and West Germany, and 0.5% in Italy and Greece) (6). There is a remarkable focus of Paget's disease in Lancashire, England, where 6.3% to 8.3% of people over age 55 in several Lancashire towns had x-rays revealing Paget's disease (7).

Prevalence rates appear to decrease when moving north to south in Europe, except for the finding that Norway and Sweden have a particularly low rate (0.3%) (6). Few data are available from Eastern Europe, but Russian colleagues indicate that Paget's disease is not uncommon in that country. The disorder is seen in Australia and in New Zealand at rates of 3% to 4% (8). Paget's disease is distinctly rare in Asia, particularly in China, India, and Malaysia, although occasional cases of Indians living in the United States have been documented. Similar radiographic studies have described 0.01% to 0.02% prevalences in several areas of sub-Saharan Africa (8). A recent study has described the characteristics of 278 cases in Israel, of which all patients were Jewish and none Arabs (9). In another recent observation, a relatively high frequency of Paget's disease in Argentina was recognized to be restricted to an area surrounding Buenos Aires and predominantly occurring in patients descended from European immigrants (10).

It is estimated—based on very few studies—that up to 3% of people over the age of 55 living in the United States have Paget's disease, making it second only to osteoporosis in terms of numbers of people with the disorder. It is believed that most Americans with Paget's disease are Caucasian, of Anglo-Saxon or European descent. The disorder is described in African Americans, and most clinical series from hospitals in major American cities report having black patients (2,11).

There are also data that support a viral etiology for Paget's disease. It has been proposed that the changes in bone remodeling occur as a result of a viral infection of osteoclasts in pagetic bone. Inclusions that resemble viral nucleocapsids have been described in the nuclei and cytoplasm of osteoclasts at pagetic sites, but not in nonpagetic osteoclasts from the same patients or from normal subjects (12,13). The viruslike particles resemble members of the paramyxovirus family, but debate has continued for over a decade as to whether the putative virus is respiratory syncytial, measles, canine distemper, some mutation of one or more of these, or some other paramyxovirus. *In situ* hybridization studies have reported the detection of measles virus or canine distemper virus transcripts in pagetic osteoclasts (14,15). Studies of osteoclast precursors from Paget's disease patients show evidence of measles virus messenger ribonucleic acid (mRNA), including mutations of a specific region of the viral nucleocapsid gene (16). There have also been studies suggesting that interleukin-6 may play a role in regulating the behavior of the osteoclast line in Paget's disease (17). A current "unifying" hypothesis suggests that the large, functionally hyperactive osteoclasts in pagetic bone are a product of a virus-mediated increase in cell fusion between osteoclasts and osteoclast progenitor cells that migrate to pagetic sites. Despite the lack of definitive proof of a viral etiology, many investigators believe that a common viral infection, perhaps early in life, in a genetically susceptible host predisposes to an osteoclast lesion that is manifested in adulthood (typically in the fifth or sixth decade) as the abnormality that produces Paget's disease.

PATHOLOGY

Histopathologic Findings in Paget's Disease

The initiating lesion in Paget's disease is an increase in bone resorption. This occurs in association with an abnormality in the osteoclasts found at affected sites, as previously described. Pagetic osteoclasts are more numerous than normal and contain substantially more nuclei than do normal osteoclasts, with up to 100 nuclei per cell noted by some investigators.

In response to the increase in bone resorption, numerous osteoblasts are recruited to pagetic sites where active and rapid new bone formation occurs. Although some ultrastructural variation in morphology of these osteoblasts is occasionally seen, no inclusion bodies are found, and it is believed by many investigators that the osteoblasts are inherently normal (18).

In the earliest phases of Paget's disease, increased osteoclastic bone resorption dominates, a picture appreciated radiographically by an advancing lytic wedge or "blade of grass" lesion in a long bone or by osteoporosis circumscripta as seen in the skull. At the level of the bone biopsy, the structurally abnormal osteoclasts are abundant. After this, there is a combination of increased resorption and relatively tightly coupled new bone formation, produced by the large numbers of osteoblasts present at these sites. During this phase, and presumably because of the accelerated nature of the process, the new bone that is made is abnormal. Newly deposited collagen fibers are laid down in a haphazard rather than a linear fashion, creating more primitive woven bone. The woven bone pattern is not specific for Paget's disease, but it does reflect a high rate of bone turnover. The endproduct is the so-called mosaic pattern of woven bone plus irregular sections of lamellar bone linked in a disorganized way by numerous cement lines representing the extent of previous areas of bone resorption. The bone marrow becomes infiltrated by excessive fibrous connective tissue and by an increased number of blood vessels, explaining the hypervascular state of the bone.

Bone matrix at pagetic sites is usually normally mineralized, and tetracycline labeling shows increased calcification rates. It is not unusual, however, to find areas of pagetic biopsies in which widened osteoid seams are apparent, perhaps reflecting inadequate calcium-phosphorus products in localized areas where rapid bone turnover heightens mineral demands.

In time, the hypercellularity at a locus of affected bone may diminish, leaving the endproduct of a sclerotic, pagetic mosaic without evidence of active bone turnover. This is so-called burned-out Paget's disease. Typically, all phases of the pagetic process can be seen at the same time at different sites in a particular subject.

Scanning electron microscopy affords an excellent view of the chaotic architectural changes that occur in pagetic bone and provides the visual imagery that makes the loss of structural integrity comprehensible. Figure 1 compares the appearances of normal and of pagetic bone utilizing this technique. Similarly, a view of the mosaic bone pattern of Paget's disease contrasted with an apparent early restoration toward normal after treatment can be seen in Fig. 2.

Biochemical Parameters of Paget's Disease

Increases in the urinary excretion of biomarkers of bone resorption [classically, total hydroxyproline has been measured, but more recently newer markers such as collagen cross-links are used (19)] reflect the primary lesion in Paget's disease, the increase in bone resorption. Increases in osteoblastic activity are associated with elevated levels of serum alkaline phosphatase. In untreated patients, the values of these two markers rise in proportion to each other, offering a reflection of the preserved coupling between resorption and formation. From the clinical perspective, the degree of elevation of these indices offers an approximation of the extent or severity of the abnormal bone turnover, with higher levels reflecting a more active, ongoing localized metabolic process. Interestingly, the patients with the highest alkaline phosphatase elevation (e.g., 10 times the upper limit of normal or greater) typically have involvement of the skull as at least one site of the disorder. Active monostotic disease (other than skull) may have lower biochemical values than polyostotic disease. Lower values (e.g., less than 3 times the upper limit of normal) may reflect a lesser extent of involvement (i.e., fewer sites on bone scans or radiographs) or a burned-out form of Paget's disease, especially in a very elderly person known to have had extensive polyostotic disease in the past. However, minimal elevations in a patient with highly localized disease (e.g., the proximal tibia) may be associated with symptoms and clear progression of disease at the affected site over time.

In addition to offering some estimate of the degree of abnormal bone turnover, the hydroxyproline and alkaline phosphatase measurements are useful in observing the disorder over time and especially for monitoring the effects of treatment. Currently approved therapies generally reduce these parameters by about 50% in up to two thirds of patients, and these measurements provide the physician with an indication of the efficacy of a particular regimen. As newer treatments become available (see the following sections), urinary markers such as hydroxyproline, pyridinium cross-links, or the N-telopeptide measurements may serve as rapid predictors of eventual pharmacologic response, as dramatic decreases in bone resorption may quickly occur with some of the potent new bisphosphonates. The serum alkaline phosphatase may decrease into the normal range

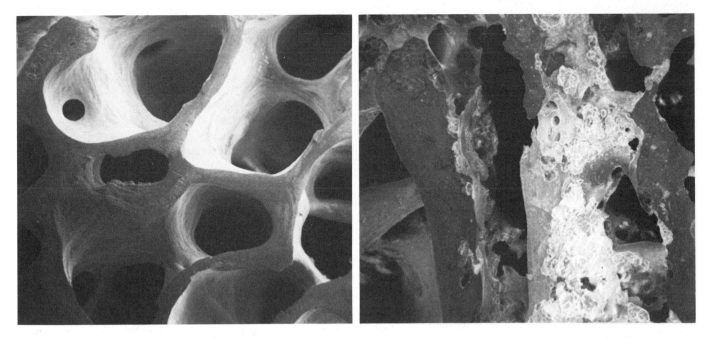

FIG. 1. Scanning electron microscope sections of normal bone *(left)* and pagetic bone *(right)*. Both samples were taken from the iliac crest. The normal bone shows the plates and marrow spaces to be well preserved, whereas the pagetic bone has totally lost this architectural appearance. Extensive pitting of the pagetic bone is apparent, due to dramatically increased osteoclastic bone resorption. (Photographs courtesy of Dr. David Dempster; reproduced, with permission, from: Siris ES, Canfield RE. Paget's disease of bone. In: Becker KL (ed) *Principles and Practice of Endocrinology and Metabolism,* 2nd ed. JB Lippincott, Philadelphia, 1995.)

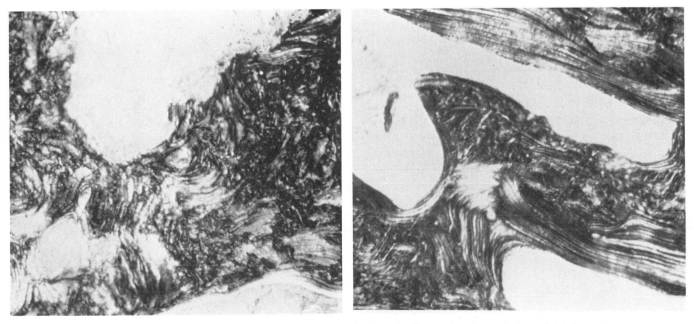

FIG. 2. This figure demonstrates iliac crest bone with Paget's disease under polarized light. The view at the *left* shows typical woven bone; the one on the *right* is a section from the same area 6 months after treatment with etidronate, showing a more lamellar pattern after treatment. (Courtesy of Dr. Pierre Meunier.)

after a period of several weeks to 2 to 3 months or more, as an indication of true "remission" with some of these agents.

Several investigators have examined the usefulness of serum osteocalcin measurements in Paget's disease. This test appears to be substantially less sensitive than serum alkaline phosphatase in this disorder and has not yet shown utility in the monitoring of these patients. As improved assays of serum bone-specific alkaline phosphatase emerge, they may prove to have considerable value in this condition.

Serum calcium levels are typically normal in Paget's disease. Clinical experience indicates that the serum calcium may occasionally become elevated in two types of situations. First, if a patient with active, usually extensive Paget's disease is immobilized, the loss of the weight-bearing stimulus to new bone formation may transiently uncouple resorption and accretion, so that increasing hypercalciuria and hypercalcemia may occur. Alternatively, when a raised serum calcium is discovered in an otherwise healthy, ambulatory patient with Paget's disease, coexistent primary hyperparathyroidism may be the cause. Inasmuch as increased levels of parathyroid hormone (PTH) can drive the intrinsic pagetic remodeling abnormality to even higher levels of activity, correction of primary hyperparathyrodism in such cases is indicated. It is currently believed that the coexistence of these two common disorders is a clinical coincidence.

Several investigators have commented on the 15% to 20% prevalence of secondary hyperparathyroidism (associated with normal levels of serum calcium) in Paget's disease, typically seen in patients with very high levels of serum alkaline phosphatase (20,21). The increase in PTH is believed to reflect the need to increase calcium availability to bone during phases of very active pagetic bone formation, particularly in subjects in whom dietary intake of calcium is inadequate. Secondary hyperparathyroidism and transient decreases in serum calcium may be found in some patients being treated with potent new bisphosphonates, reflecting an effective and rapid suppression of bone resorption in the setting of ongoing new bone formation (22). Later, as restoration of coupling occurs with time, PTH levels fall. In these cases of secondarily increased PTH, it is desirable to be certain that the patient's intake of calcium is at least 1 g/day.

Elevations in serum uric acid and serum citrate have been described in Paget's disease and are of unclear clinical significance (1). Gout has been noted in this disorder, but it is uncertain whether it is more common in pagetic patients than in nonpagetic subjects. Hypercalciuria may occur in some patients with Paget's disease, presumably because of the increased bone resorption, and kidney stones are occasionally found as a consequence of this abnormality (1).

CLINICAL FEATURES

Paget's disease affects both men and women, with most series describing a slight male predominance. It is rarely observed to occur below the age of 25, it is thought to develop after the age of 40 in most instances, and it is most commonly diagnosed in people in their 50s. In a survey of over 800 selected patients, 600 of whom had symptoms, the

average age at diagnosis was 58 (23). It seems likely that many patients have the disorder for a period of time before any diagnosis is made, especially since it is often an incidental finding.

It is important to emphasize the localized nature of Paget's disease. It may be monostotic, affecting only a single bone or portion of a bone (Fig. 3), or may be polyostotic, involving two or more bones. Sites of disease are often asymmetrical. A patient might have a pagetic right femur with a normal left, involvement of only half the pelvis, or involvement of several noncontiguous vertebral bodies. Clinical observation suggests that in most instances, sites affected with Paget's disease when the diagnosis is made are

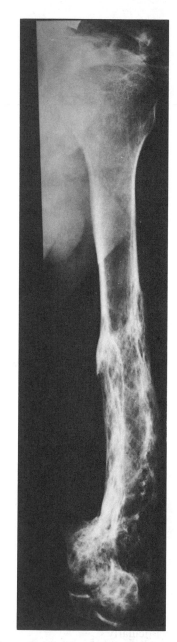

FIG. 3. Radiograph of a humerus showing typical pagetic change in the distal half, with cortical thickening, expansion, and mixed areas of lucency and sclerosis, contrasted with normal bone in the proximal half.

the only ones that will show pagetic change over time. Although progression of disease within a given bone may occur, the sudden appearance of new sites of involvement years after the initial diagnosis is uncommon. This information can be very reassuring for patients who often worry about extension of the disorder to new areas of the skeleton as they age.

The most common sites of involvement include the pelvis, femur, spine, skull, and tibia. The bones of the upper extremity, as well as the clavicles, scapulae, ribs, and facial bones, are less commonly involved, and the hands and feet are only rarely affected. It is generally believed that most patients with Paget's disease are asymptomatic and that the disorder is most often diagnosed when an elevated serum alkaline phosphatase is noted on routine screening or when a radiograph taken for an unrelated problem reveals typical skeletal changes. The development of symptoms or complications of Paget's disease is influenced by the particular areas of involvement, the interrelationships between affected bone and adjacent structures, and the extent of metabolic activity.

Signs and Symptoms

Bone pain from a site of pagetic involvement, experienced either at rest or with motion, is probably the most common symptom. The direct cause of the pain may be difficult to characterize and requires careful evaluation. Pagetic bone has an increased vascularity, leading to a warmth of the bone that some patients perceive as an unpleasant sensation. Small transverse lucencies along the expanded cortices of involved weight-bearing bones or advancing, lytic, blade of grass lesions may occasionally cause pain. It is postulated that microfractures frequently occur in pagetic bone and can cause discomfort for a period of days to weeks.

A bowing deformity of the femur or tibia (Fig. 4) can lead to pain for several possible reasons. A bowed limb is typically shortened, resulting in specific gait abnormalities that can lead to abnormal mechanical stresses. Clinically severe secondary arthritis can occur at joints adjacent to pagetic bone, (e.g., the hip, knee, or ankle). The secondary gait problems may also lead to arthritic changes on the contralateral nonpagetic side, particularly at the hip.

Back pain in pagetic patients is another difficult symptom to assess. Nonspecific aches and pains may emanate from enlarged pagetic vertebrae in some instances; vertebral compression fractures may also be seen. In the lumbar area, spinal stenosis with neural impingement may arise, producing radicular pain and possibly motor impairment. Degenerative changes in the spine may accompany pagetic changes, and it is useful for the clinician to determine which symptoms arise as a consequence of the pagetic process and which result from degenerative disease of nonpagetic vertebrae. Kyphosis may occur, or there may be a forward tilt of the upper back, particularly when a compression fracture or spinal stenosis is present. Treatment options will differ, depending on the basis of the symptoms. When Paget's disease affects the thoracic spine, there may rarely be syndromes of direct spinal cord compression with motor and

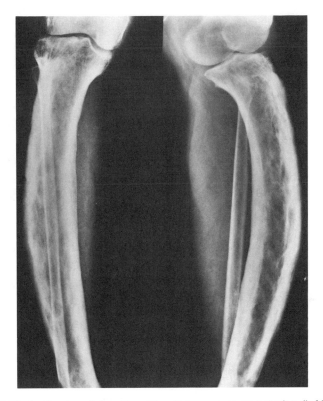

FIG. 4. Bowing deformity of the tibia on anteroposterior *(left)* and lateral views. The deformity leads to poor alignment at the knee and ankle and to a shortened limb.

sensory changes. Several cases of apparent direct cord compression with loss of neural function have now been documented to have resulted from a vascular steal syndrome, whereby hypervascular pagetic bone "steals" blood from the neural tissue (24).

Paget's disease of the skull, demonstrated radiographically in Fig. 5, may be asymptomatic, but common complaints in up to one third of patients with skull involvement may include an increase in head size with or without frontal bossing or deformity, or headache, sometimes described as a bandlike tightening around the head. Hearing loss may occur as a result of isolated or combined conductive or neurosensory abnormalities. Other cranial nerve palsies (such as II, VI, and VII) are described less often. With extensive skull involvement, a softening of the base of the skull may produce platybasia, or flattening, with the development of basilar invagination, so that the odontoid process begins to extend upward as the skull sinks downward upon it. This feature can be appreciated by various radiographic measures including skull x-rays and computed tomography or magnetic resonance imaging scans. Although many patients with severe skull changes may have radiographic evidence of basilar invagination, a relatively small number develop a very serious complication, such as direct brain stem compression or an obstructive hydrocephalus and increased intracranial pressure caused by blockage of cerebrospinal fluid (CSF) flow. Pagetic involvement of the facial bones may cause facial deformity, dental problems, and, rarely, narrowing of the airway. Mechanical changes of these types may lead to a nasal intonation when the patient is speaking.

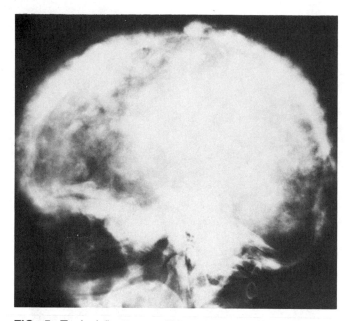

FIG. 5. Typical "cotton-wool" appearance of an enlarged pagetic skull with marked osteoblastic change. The patient had an increase in head size, and deafness.

Fracture through pagetic bone is an occasional and serious complication. These fractures may be either traumatic or pathologic, particularly involving long bones with active areas of advancing lytic disease; the most common involve the femoral shaft or subtrochanteric area (25). The increased vascularity of actively remodeling pagetic bone (i.e., with a moderately increased serum alkaline phosphatase) may lead to substantial blood loss in the presence of fractures due to trauma. Fractures may also occur in the presence of areas of malignant degeneration, a rare complication of Paget's disease. Far more common are the small fissure fractures along the convex surfaces of bowed lower extremities, which may be asymptomatic, stable, and persistent for years, but sometimes a more extensive transverse lucent area extends medially from the cortex and may lead to a clinical fracture with time. As described in following sections, there are data indicating that blade of grass lytic areas as well as these larger transverse fractures may respond to treatment with calcitonin and heal. These types of lesions warrant radiographic follow-up over time. Conversely, the smaller fissure fractures typically do not change with treatment and, in the absence of new pain, rarely require extensive radiographic monitoring. In most cases, fracture through pagetic bone heals normally, although some groups have reported as high as a 10% rate of nonunion.

Neoplastic degeneration of pagetic bone is a relatively rare event, occurring with an incidence of less than 1%. This abnormality has a grave prognosis, typically manifesting itself as new pain at a pagetic site. The most common site of sarcomatous change appears to be the pelvis, with the femur and humerus next in frequency (26). Typically, these lesions are osteolytic. The majority of the tumors are classified as osteogenic sarcomas, although both fibrosarcomas and chondrosarcomas are also seen. Current treatment regimens emphasize maximal resection of tumor mass and chemotherapy (or sometimes radiotherapy), but death from massive local extension of disease or from pulmonary metastases occurs in the majority of cases in 1 to 3 years.

Benign giant cell tumors may also occur in bone affected by Paget's disease. These lesions may present as localized masses at the affected site. Radiographic evaluation may disclose lytic changes. Biopsy reveals clusters of large osteoclasts, which some authors believe represent reparative granulomas (27). These tumors may show a remarkable sensitivity to glucocorticoids, so in many instances the mass will disappear after treatment with prednisone or dexamethasone (28).

DIAGNOSIS

When Paget's disease is suspected, the diagnostic evaluation should include a careful medical history and physical examination. Gout, pseudogout, and arthritis are all possible complications of Paget's disease. Rarely, patients with underlying intrinsic heart disease may develop congestive heart failure in the presence of severe Paget's disease. There are also reports suggesting that patients may have an increased incidence of calcific aortic disease (29). Angioid streaks are seen on funduscopic examination of the eye in some patients with polyostotic Paget's disease. The possibility of a positive family history and a symptom history should be ascertained. The physical exam should also note the presence or absence of warmth, tenderness, or bone deformity in the skull, spine, pelvis, and extremities, as well as evidence of loss of range of motion at major joints or leg length discrepancy.

Laboratory tests include measurement of serum alkaline phosphatase and 24-hour urinary hydroxyproline or perhaps a newer marker of bone resorption, as described earlier. Many investigators prefer to express the urinary hydroxyproline as a ratio to creatinine (mg/g) in order to have a more accurate and precise value. Radiographic studies (bone scans and conventional radiographs) complete the initial evaluation. Bone biopsy is not usually indicated, as the characteristic radiographic and laboratory findings are diagnostic in most instances.

Bone scans are the most sensitive means of identifying pagetic sites and are most useful for this purpose. Scans are nonspecific, however, and can also be positive in nonpagetic areas that have degenerative changes or, more ominously, may reflect metastatic disease. Plain radiographs of bones noted to be positive on the bone scan provide the most specific information, because the changes noted on the radiograph are usually characteristic to the point of being pathognomonic. Examples of these are shown in Figs. 3, 4, and 5. Enlargement or expansion of bone, cortical thickening, coarsening of trabecular markings, and typical lytic and sclerotic changes may be found. Radiographs also provide data on the status of the joints adjacent to involved sites, identify fissure fractures, indicate the degree to which lytic or sclerotic lesions predominate, and demonstrate the presence or absence of deformity or fracture.

Repeat scans or radiographs are usually unnecessary in observing patients over time, unless new symptoms develop or current symptoms become significantly worse. The possibility of an impending fracture or, rarely, of sarcomatous change should be borne in mind in these situations.

The characteristic radiographic and clinical features of Paget's disease usually eliminate problems with differential diagnosis. However, an older patient may occasionally present with severe bone pain, elevations of the serum alkaline phosphatase and urinary hydroxyproline, a positive bone scan, and less-than-characteristic radiographic areas of lytic or blastic change. Here, the possibility of metastatic disease to bone or some other form of metabolic bone disease (e.g., osteomalacia with secondary hyperparathyroidism) must be considered. Old radiographs and laboratory tests are very helpful in this setting, as normal studies a year earlier would make a diagnosis of Paget's disease less likely. A similar dilemma occurs when someone with known and established Paget's disease develops multiple painful new sites; here, too, the likelihood of metastatic disease must be carefully considered, and bone biopsy for a tissue diagnosis may be indicated.

TREATMENT

Antipagetic Therapy

Specific antipagetic therapy consists of those agents capable of suppressing the activity of pagetic osteoclasts. Currently approved agents available by prescription in the United States include salmon and human calcitonin, both given by subcutaneous injection, and three bisphosphonate compounds: orally administered etidronate and alendronate, and intravenously administered pamidronate. Plicamycin, a cytotoxic anticancer agent previously called mithramycin, although not specifically approved for Paget's disease by the Food and Drug Administration (FDA) (it is approved for the management of hypercalcemia), has been used in the past for refractory cases but has largely been replaced by pamidronate. Several investigational bisphosphonates, such as risedronate, tiludronate, and zoledronate, are currently in clinical trials in the United States. Clodronate, neridronate, dimethyl pamidronate, and ibandronate are being studied and used clinically in other parts of the world. The newer bisphosphonates are progressively more potent than the earlier ones, offering the potential for greater disease suppression and frank remission (i.e., normalization of pagetic indices) for prolonged periods of time. Gallium nitrate, approved in the United States for the treatment of cancer hypercalcemia, is also being studied for efficacy in Paget's disease, and preliminary reports suggest that its use can lower pagetic indices in many patients (30). Other symptomatic treatment for Paget's disease, including analgesics, anti-inflammatory drugs, and selected orthopedic and neurosurgical interventions, also have roles in management.

Indications for treatment and choices of therapeutic agents continue to be issues of debate among clinicians who treat Paget's disease. The potential benefits of antipagetic agents as a group should be understood as a preface to discussion of the advantages and disadvantages of each specific antipagetic medication currently available in the United States. Two logical indications for treatment of Paget's disease are to relieve symptoms and to prevent future complications. It has been clearly demonstrated that suppression of the pagetic process by any of the available classes of agents can effectively ameliorate certain symptoms in the majority of patients. Symptoms such as bone aches or pain (probably the most common complaints of Paget's disease), excessive warmth over bone, headache due to skull involvement, low back pain secondary to pagetic vertebral changes, and some syndromes of neural compression (e.g., radiculopathy and some examples of slowly progressive brainstem or spinal cord compression) are the most likely to be relieved. Pain due to a secondary arthritis from pagetic bone involving the spine, hip, knee, ankle, or shoulder may or may not respond to antipagetic treatment. Filling in of osteolytic blade of grass lesions in weight-bearing bones has been reported in some treated cases. On the other hand, a bowed extremity or other bone deformity will not change after treatment, and deafness is unlikely to improve, although limited studies suggest progression of hearing loss may be slowed (31).

In the absence of potentially responsive symptoms, the indications for treatment are less clear. It has not been proved that a reduction in substantially elevated pagetic indices will prevent future complications. However, as shown in Fig. 2, there is a restoration toward a more normal, lamellar pattern of bone in biopsy specimens after suppression of pagetic activity. It is also known that active, untreated disease may continue to undergo a persistent degree of abnormal bone turnover for many years. Thus, in the view of many investigators, the presence of moderately active asymptomatic disease (i.e., a serum alkaline phosphatase 3 to 4 times the upper limit of normal or more) at sites where the potential for later problems or complications exists (weight-bearing bones, areas near major joints, vertebral bodies, extensively involved skull) is an indication for treatment. Patients with monostotic disease of a tibia or femur with a minimal elevation of alkaline phosphatase (e.g., 1.5 to 2 times the upper limit of normal) are also treatment candidates, as progression of disease in such bones is likely over time. The need for treatment is particularly valid in patients who are young, for whom many years of coexistence with the disorder are likely. Although controlled studies are not available to prove efficaciousness, the use of antipagetic therapy prior to elective surgery on pagetic bone is recommended. The goal here is to reduce the hypervascularity associated with moderately active disease (e.g., a threefold or more elevation in serum alkaline phosphatase) to reduce the amount of blood loss at operation.

Calcitonin

The polypeptide hormones, salmon and human calcitonin, are both available therapeutically as synthetic formulations for parenteral administration. These agents have been widely studied over the past 20 years (32,33). At present, the forms approved for use in Paget's disease in the United States must be injected subcutaneously or intramuscularly. A nasal spray formulation of salmon calcitonin was recently approved for use in postmenopausal osteoporosis and will thus be available (though not yet specifically FDA approved) for use in Paget's disease.

Salmon calcitonin preparations for Paget's disease include Calcimar (Rhone-Poulenc-Rorer, Collegeville,

Pennsylvania) or Miacalcin (Sandoz, East Hanover, New Jersey) in a 400-U vial (2 cc). The usual starting dose is 100 U (0.5 cc), generally self-injected subcutaneously, initially on a daily basis. Symptomatic benefit may be apparent in a few weeks, and the biochemical benefit is usually seen after 3 to 6 months of treatment. After this period, many clinicians reduce the dose to 50 to 100 U every other day or three times weekly. Often, maintenance with 50 U three times weekly after the first few months of therapy is quite satisfactory. Patients with moderate to severe disease may require indefinite treatment to maintain a 50% reduction in the biochemical indices and symptomatic relief, but milder or monostotic disease may allow discontinuation of treatment for prolonged periods of time.

Escape from the efficacy of salmon calcitonin may sometimes occur after a variable period of benefit. In some cases this may be due to a postulated down-regulation of receptors, but in other instances it may be a consequence of the development of neutralizing antibodies to the salmon polypeptide (34). Partly for this reason, human calcitonin, an agent somewhat less potent on a mass basis, was eventually developed and is an FDA-approved therapy for Paget's disease. The human calcitonin preparation, Cibacalcin (Ciba, Summit, New Jersey), is provided in a prefilled syringe containing 0.5 mg, a dose probably equivalent to 150 to 200 U of Calcimar or Miacalcin. Cibacalcin is not available in pharmacies at the time of this writing, but physicians can obtain it directly from Ciba for those patients requiring it.

These agents are fairly similar in effectiveness, although for individual patients one or the other may be preferred. Each may cause a slight decrease in serum calcium after the injection, usually of no clinical significance, during the early months of treatment. More troublesome in a small minority of patients is the development of nausea or queasiness, with or without flushing of the skin of the face and ears. These annoying side effects may last from a few minutes to several hours after each injection, although many patients can avoid them by experimenting with taking the agent at bedtime, with food, without food, and so on. Some clinicians find that full doses of Cibacalcin are more likely to cause side effects, a problem significantly reduced by decreasing the daily dose. Although these side effects are unpleasant, they do not appear to be serious or harmful, and most patients develop tolerance to them. Despite the requirement for parenteral administration, many patients who experience benefit from these agents gladly tolerate the need for injection.

Intranasal calcitonin (Miacalcin Nasal Spray, Sandoz, East Hanover, New Jersey) appears to have a lower incidence of the side effects described above. The dose in Paget's disease with the present formulation is not clear at this time, but it will probably be in the range of 200 to 400 U per day. It is anticipated that many patients will be quite accepting of an intranasal form as compared with injections, and this agent may play a significant role in treatment of patients for whom calcitonin is a preferred treatment.

Etidronate

Etidronate is the first bisphosphonate to have been used clinically in the United States for Paget's disease (35,36). It is commercially available as Didronel (Procter and Gamble, Cincinnati, Ohio) in a 200- or 400-mg tablet. Although only a small percentage of the administered dose is absorbed, 5 mg/kg/day will provide a 50% lowering of biochemical indices and a reduction in symptoms in perhaps two thirds of patients, much as is observed with the calcitonins and over similar time frames.

The dose of etidronate is limited by the fact that this agent, like other bisphosphonates, inhibits not only bone resorption but also the mineralization of newly forming bone when high doses are administered for prolonged periods of time. For this reason, the recommended regimen for the agent is 5 mg/kg/day (i.e., 400 mg in most patients) for a 6-month period, followed by at least 6 months of no treatment. Over several years of repeated 6-months-on, 6-or-more-months-off cycles, long-term benefit with maintenance of lower levels of pagetic biochemical activity is possible in a majority of patients. A failure to adhere to a cyclic regimen can induce bone pain and, occasionally, fracture due to focal osteomalacia secondary to excessive etidronate effect. However, careful cyclic management is extremely well tolerated by the great majority of patients. Occasionally, mild transient diarrhea may occur with etidronate, but this does not usually require more than a day or two of withholding the agent, after which it may be taken again. Rarely, patients have some aches and pains, which are usually mild and transient as well. More severe new pain in patients taking etidronate warrants stopping the drug and evaluating the patient before continuing therapy, to be certain that lytic disease or impending fracture—particularly in a weight-bearing extremity—has not been exacerbated.

Pamidronate

With the relatively recent approval of pamidronate more than 15 years after the approval of etidronate and salmon calcitonin, a new philosophy of and approach to management have become available to the clinician. The newer bisphosphonates, such as pamidronate and those still under clinical investigation, offer great promise for several reasons. First, they are substantially more potent than earlier bisphosphonates and may permit normalization of pagetic indices rather than only partial suppression. Second, the effects may be longer lasting, so a limited course of treatment may provide many months of suppression. Third, all of the newer bisphosphonates have a much more favorable ratio of inhibition of bone resorption to inhibition of mineralization, so the threat of focal osteomalacia should be markedly reduced if not eliminated.

At the time of this writing, an optimal regimen for pamidronate remains controversial, and the literature is replete with numerous approaches, as has recently been discussed (37), all of which seem to be effective. The package insert for pamidronate, available as Aredia (Ciba, Summit, New Jersey), recommends three daily infusions of 30 mg each, over 4 hours each time, in 500 cc of saline or dextrose solution. In my own experience, I find that patients with relatively mild disease may experience a substantial reduction of alkaline phosphatase to normal or near normal with a single 60-mg infusion given over 3 to 4 h in 500 cc of 5%

dextrose in water. Patients with more moderate to severe disease may require multiple infusions of 60 mg infused as described and given on a once weekly or biweekly basis, primarily based on physician and patient convenience. Total doses of 240 to 480 mg may be required in some cases, given over a number of weeks. Suppression of urinary markers can often be noted at once, but the serum alkaline phosphatase may take up to 3 months to reach its nadir. Giving three to four doses and then reassessing at 3 months with the possibility of more treatment is a reasonable approach until more is learned about the use of the agent. A successful course of therapy may result in up to 1 year of continued disease suppression. Side effects may include a low-grade fever the day after the first dose, flulike symptoms in the first 24 hours after an infusion (decreasing in likelihood with repeated dosing), and the possibility of mild and transient hypocalcemia, hypophosphatemia, and lymphopenia. Venous irritation may arise, especially if insufficient volume of fluid is used. It is desirable to provide oral calcium supplements at a dose of 500 mg two or three times daily to prevent or ameliorate the reduction in serum calcium and concomitant rise in PTH.

Overall, pamidronate offers the new opportunity to titrate the dosage required to the individual patient, with the possibility of normalization or near normalization of biochemical indices and the potential for substantial and prolonged reduction in disease progression in many patients. In my view, it is most useful in patients with mild disease, in whom a single infusion may afford long-term benefit in a very cost-effective manner, and in severe and refractory cases, in whom neither oral etidronate nor a calcitonin may offer optimal benefit. The need for outpatient intravenous administration of multiple doses may be expensive and inconvenient in some cases. However, the rapid onset of symptomatic improvement and overall potency of the agent make it the drug of choice for cases with neurologic compression syndromes, for severe and painful lytic disease with or without impending fracture, and as a pretreatment of active Paget's disease prior to elective surgery to shrink the hypervascularity of the pagetic bone and decrease the amount of bleeding at operation. There has been one report of asymptomatic mineralization abnormalities with dosing in the usual clinical range (38), but this is not the general experience.

Alendronate

Approved by the FDA for the treatment of Paget's disease in the fall of 1995, alendronate (sold as Fosamax, from Merck, West Point, Pennsylvania) is an orally administered aminobisphosphonate that is much more potent than etidronate and that is not associated with mineralization problems at therapeutically effective doses. In a study of 89 patients with moderate to severe disease who received 6 months of either alendronate 40 mg daily or etidronate 400 mg per day, alendronate led to a normalized serum alkaline phosphatase in over 63% of subjects, compared with 17% for etidronate; overall, alendronate led to a mean fall in alkaline phosphatase of 79% compared with 44% with etidronate (39). Alendronate appeared to be as well tolerated

as etidronate in this study, although symptoms of upper gastrointestinal discomfort or nausea, or the less common but more serious complication of esophageal ulceration, should be watched for at the 40 mg dose. The recommended dose is 40 mg daily for 6 months to be taken on arising in the morning with 8 oz of tap water. The patient is instructed not to take anything else by mouth (except more water) and not to lie down for at least 30 minutes after the dose. It is important with alendronate, as with pamidronate, that patients be replete in vitamin D and have a daily calcium intake of 1000 mg to avoid hypocalcemia early in the treatment course. Retreatment guidelines are incomplete until follow-up data on study patients become available, but several investigators have given a second 6-month course to previously treated patients once suppressed alkaline phosphatase values began to rise again, typically many months to a year or more after the end of the initial treatment.

Other Emerging Bisphosphonates

Tiludronate is another orally administered bisphosphonate that is not associated with mineralization problems at clinically effective doses. Clinical trials with this agent are concluding and it may become available if approved within the next 2 years. A recent publication reported that in 128 patients in an open study, there was a 60% reduction in serum alkaline phosphatase and excellent patient tolerance when 400 mg was provided daily for 6 months (40). Preliminary reports with risedronate, a very potent bisphosphonate also in clinical trials, indicate that a dose of 30 mg for 84 days followed by a 112-day-off drug period reduced the excess alkaline phosphatase by 77% at the 112-day point (41). Finally, both zoledronate (in the United States) and ibandronate (being studied in Europe) appear to have antibone-resorbing activity with microgram amounts given as a 1-hour infusion or as an intravenous bolus, indicating the tremendous potencies that may be available with these newest agents.

Plicamycin

Previously called mithramycin, this agent is a potent and somewhat toxic treatment for Paget's disease that is generally reserved by most investigators for severely affected or refractory patients or for individuals with syndromes of neural compression in whom rapid therapy is desirable (42). It is anticipated that pamidronate and emerging bisphosphonates will replace plicamycin in most cases, but the drug still remains a potentially useful therapy in selected situations as noted. At doses of 15 to 25 µg/kg per 6 to 8 h infusion, this agent can quickly lower pagetic indices over a few days. Regimens consisting of an infusion every second to third day for up to 5 to 10 infusions have been successfully utilized to reverse spinal cord compression. Even when full resolution of a serious neurologic problem is not achieved, pretreatment with plicamycin (often together with dexamethasone) substantially reduces the hypervascularity associated with active pagetic bone turnover. If surgical decompression is then undertaken, there may be much less bleeding.

Plicamycin typically causes nausea and vomiting during the course of treatment, and elevations of hepatocellular enzymes and sometimes of blood urea nitrogen (BUN) are seen as toxic side effects. At the doses used in Paget's disease, marrow toxicity, particularly directed against platelets, is uncommon, but platelet counts should be monitored. Plicamycin also typically induces hypocalcemia after each infusion, with restoration toward normal in 24 to 36 hours, and adequacy of calcium and vitamin D intake are required.

Choice of Agents

Each of the approved therapies described above has a valuable role in the treatment of Paget's disease. Etidronate has been in use for nearly 20 years, is an oral formulation that has very few side effects at the 5-mg/kg/day dose, and has been well accepted by patients. For many patients with moderate disease, it remains an appropriate choice. It should be avoided in patients with extensive osteolytic disease in weight-bearing bones.

Pamidronate is a more potent bisphosphonate; its dose can be titrated for the individual patient's particular characteristics. Individualizing the regimen may lead to more frequent monitoring, and the use of multiple 60-mg infusions can become quite expensive. Some patients prefer an oral agent to the intravenous therapy. However, for patients with mild disease for whom one infusion per year will suffice, or with severe disease or very symptomatic disease, it is a very effective therapy.

Alendronate is another very potent bisphosphonate that normalized alkaline phosphatase in over 60% of patients in the clinical trial described above. It appears to have greater efficacy than etidronate, but the mode of administration and the need for caution in patients with active upper gastrointestinal disease must be borne in mind by prescribing clinicians.

The calcitonins, like etidronate, have been in use for more that 20 years, offering very good and often rapid symptomatic benefit and great safety for many patients. Annoying side effects in a significant minority, as well as the need for parenteral administration and high cost compared with etidronate when given at full doses daily, do influence patient acceptance. The nasal spray will probably enhance compliance, but it is unclear if equivalent doses will enter the circulation with the intranasal route.

Other Therapies

Analgesics and nonsteroidal anti-inflammatory agents (NSAIDs) may be tried empirically with or without antipagetic therapy to relieve pain. Pagetic arthritis (i.e., osteoarthritis caused by deformed pagetic bone at a joint space) may cause periods of pain that are often helped by the NSAIDs.

Surgery on pagetic bone may be necessary in the setting of established or impending fracture. Elective joint replacement, although more complex with Paget's disease than with osteoarthritis, is often very successful in relieving refractory pain. Rarely, osteotomy is performed to alter bowing deformity. Neurosurgical intervention is sometimes required in cases of spinal cord compression, spinal stenosis, or basilar invagination with neural compromise. Although medical management may be beneficial and adequate in some instances, all cases of serious neurologic compromise require immediate neurologic and neurosurgical consultation to allow the appropriate plan of management to be developed. As improved therapies emerge, long-term suppression of pagetic activity may have a preventive role in Paget's disease and may obviate the need for surgical management in many cases.

REFERENCES

1. Singer FR: *Paget's Disease of Bone.* Plenum, New York, 1977
2. Siris ES, Canfield RE, Jacobs TP: Paget's disease of bone. *Bull NY Acad Med* 56:285–304, 1980
3. Mc Kusick VA: *Heritable Disorders of Connective Tissue.* CV Mosby, St. Louis, pp 718–723, 1972
4. Singer FR, Mills BG, Park MS, et al.: Increased HLA-DQw-1 antigen frequency in Paget's disease of bone. *Proc 7th annual meeting American Society for Bone and Mineral Research.* Washington, DC, p 128, 1985
5. Siris ES, Ottman R, Flaster E, Kelsey JL: Familial aggregation of Paget's disease of bone. *J Bone Miner Res* 6:495–500, 1991
6. Barker DJ: The epidemiology of Paget's disease of bone. *Br Med Bull* 40:396–400, 1984
7. Barker DJP, Chamberlain AT, Guyer PB, Gardner MJ: Paget's disease of bone: The Lancashire focus. *Br Med J* 280:1105–1107, 1980
8. Barry HC: *Paget's Disease of Bone.* Edinburgh: E&S Livingstone, 1969
9. Dolev E, Samuel R, Foldes J, Brickman M, Assia A, Liberman U: Some epidemiological aspects of Paget's disease in Israel. *Semin Arthritis Rheum* 23:228, 1994
10. Mautalen C, Pumarino H, Blanco MC, Gonzalez D, Ghiringhelli G, Fromm G: Paget's disease: The South American experience. *Semin Arth Rheum* 23:226–227, 1994
11. Guyer PB, Chamberlain AT: Paget's disease of bone in two American cities. *Br Med J* 280:985, 1980
12. Rebel A, Bregeon C, Basle M, Malkani K, Patezour A, Filmon R: Osteoclastic inclusions in Paget's disease of bone. *Rev Rhum Mal Osteoartic* 42:637–641, 1975
13. Mills BG, Singer FR: Nuclear inclusions in Paget's disease of bone. *Science* 194:201–202, 1976
14. Gordon MT, Mee AP, Anderson DC, Sharpe PT: Canine distemper virus transcripts sequenced from pagetic bone. *J Bone Miner Res* 19:159–174, 1992
15. Cartwright EJ, Gordon MT, Freemont AJ, Anderson DC, Sharpe PT: Paramyxovirus and Paget's disease. *J Med Virol* 40:133–141, 1993
16. Reddy SV, Singer FR, Roodman GD: Bone marrow mononuclear cells from patients with Paget's disease contain measles virus nucleocapsid messenger ribonucleic acid that has mutations in a specific region of the sequence. *J Clin Endocrinol Metab* 80:2108–2111, 1995
17. Roodman GD, Kurihara N, Ohsaki Y, et al.: Interleukin-6: A potential autocrine/paracrine factor in Paget's disease of bone. *J Clin Invest* 89:46–52, 1992
18. Rebel A, Basle M, Pouplard A, et al.: Bone tisssue in Paget's disease of bone: Ultrastructure and immunocytology. *Arthritis Rheum* 23:1104–1114, 1980
19. Uebelhart D, Ginetys E, Chapuy MC, Delmas PD: Urinary excretion of pyridinium crosslinks. A new marker of bone resorption in metabolic bone disease. *Bone Miner* 8:87–96, 1990
20. Meunier PJ, Coindre JM, Edouard CM, Arlot ME: Bone histomorphometry in Paget's disease: Quantitative and dynamic analysis of pagetic and non-pagetic bone tissue. *Arthritis Rheum* 23:1095–1103, 1980
21. Siris ES, Clemens TP, McMahon D, et al.: Parathyroid function in Paget's disease of bone. *J Bone Miner Res* 4:75–79, 1989

22. Siris ES, Canfield RE: The parathyroids and Paget's disease of bone. In: Bilezikian J, Levine M, Marcus R (eds) *The Parathyroids.* Raven Press, New York, pp 823–828, 1994

23. Siris ES: Indications for medical treatment of Paget's disease of bone. In: Singer FR, Wallach S (eds) *Paget's disease of bone. Clinical assessment, present and future therapy.* Elsevier, New York, pp 44–56, 1991

24. Herzberg L, Bayliss E: Spinal cord syndrome due to non-compressive Paget's disease of bone: A spinal artery steal phenomenon reversible with calcitonin. *Lancet* 2:13–15, 1980

25. Barry HC: Orthopedic aspects of Paget's disase of bone. *Arthritis Rheum* 23:1128–1130, 1980

26. Wick MR, Siegal GP, Unni KK, McLeod RA, Greditzer HB: Sarcomas of bone complicating osteitis deformans (Paget's disease.) *Am J Surg Pathol* 5:47 – 59, 1981

27. Upchurch KS, Simon LS, Schiller AL, et al.: Giant cell reparative granulomas of Paget's disease of bone: A unique clinical entity. *Ann Intern Med* 98:35–40, 1983

28. Jacobs, TP, Michelsen J, Polay J, et al.: Giant cell tumor in Paget's disease of bone. Familial and geographic clustering. *Cancer* 44:742–747, 1979

29. Strickenberger SA, Schulman SP, Hutchins GM: Association of Paget's disease of bone with calcific aortic valve disease. *Am J Med* 82:953–956, 1987

30. Bockman RS, Wilhelm F, Siris E, et al.: A multicenter, prospective trial of gallium nitrate in patients with advanced Paget's disease of bone. *J Clin Endocrinol Metab* 80:595–602, 1995

31. El-Sammaa M, Linthicum FH, House HP, House JW: Calcitonin as treatment for hearing loss in Paget's disease. *Am J Otol* 7:241–243, 1986

32. Woodhouse NJY, Bordier Ph, Fisher M, et al.: Human calcitonin in the treatment of Paget's bone disease. *Lancet* 1:1139–1143, 1971

33. DeRose J, Singer F, Avramides A, et al.: Response of Paget's disease to porcine and salmon calcitonins. Effects of long term treatment. *Am J Med* 47:9–15, 1974

34. Singer FR, Ginger K: Resistance to calcitonin. In: Singer FR, Wallach S (eds) *Paget's disease of bone. Clinical assessment, present and future therapy.* Elsevier, New York, 75–85, 1991

35. Altman RD, Johnston CC, Khairi MRA, Wellman H, Serafini AN, Sankey RR: Influence of disodium etidrorate on clinical and laboratory manifestations of Paget's disease of bone (osteitis deformans). *N Engl J Med* 379–1384, 1973

36. Canfield R, Rosner W, Skinner J, et al.: Diphosphonate therapy of Paget's disease of bone. *J Clin Endocrinol Metab* 44:96–106, 1977

37. Siris ES: Perspectives: A practical guide to the use of pamidronate in the treatment of Paget's disease. *J Bone Miner Res* 9:303–304, 1994

38. Adamson BB, Gallacher SJ, Byars J, et al.: Mineralisation defects with pamidronate therapy for Paget's disease. *Lancet* 342:1459–1460, 1993

39. Siris E, Weinstein RS, Altman R, et al.: Comparative study of alendronate vs. etidronate for the treatment of Paget's disease of bone. *J Clin Endocrinol Metab* 81:961–967, 1996

40. Reginster JY, Treves R, Renier JC: Efficacy and tolerability of a new formulation of oral tiludronate (tablet) in the treatment of Paget's disease of bone. *J Bone Miner Res* 9:615–619, 1994

41. Brown J, Kylstra JW, Bekker P, et al.: Risedronate in Paget's disease: Preliminary results of a multicenter study. *Semin Arthritis Rheum* 23:272, 1994

42. Ryan WG, Schwartz TB, Perlia CP: Effects of mithramycin on Paget's disease of bone. *Ann Intern Med* 70:549–557, 1969

Extraskeletal (Ectopic) Calcification and Ossification

IX. Introduction

Michael P. Whyte, M.D.

Division of Bone and Mineral Diseases, Washington University School of Medicine; and
Metabolic Research Unit, Shriners Hospital for Crippled Children, St. Louis, Missouri

A significant number and variety of disorders cause extraskeletal deposition of calcium and phosphate (Table 1). In some, mineral is precipitated as amorphous calcium phosphate or as hydroxyapatite crystals; in others, bone tissue is formed. The pathogenesis of the ectopic mineralization in these conditions is generally ascribed to one of three mechanisms (Table 1). First, a supranormal calcium-phosphate solubility product in extracellular fluid can cause metastatic calcification. Alternatively, mineral may be deposited as dystrophic calcification into metabolically impaired or dead tissue, despite normal serum levels of calcium and phosphate. Third, ectopic ossification, or true bone formation, occurs in a few disorders for which the pathogenesis is poorly understood.

Discussed briefly in this section are these three mechanisms for extracellular calcification or ossification. Afterwards, descriptions of three principal disorders illustrate each pathogenesis.

MECHANISMS FOR EXTRACELLULAR CALCIFICATION AND OSSIFICATION

Calcium and inorganic phosphate are normally present in serum or extracellular fluid at concentrations that form a

TABLE 1. *Disorders associated with extraskeletal calcification or ossification*

Metastatic calcification
Hypercalcemia
Milk-alkali syndrome
Hypervitaminosis D
Sarcoidosis
Hyperparathyroidism
Renal failure
Hyperphosphatemia
Tumoral calcinosis
Hyperparathyroidism
Pseudohypoparathyroidism
Cell lysis following chemotherapy for leukemia
Renal failure
Dystrophic calcification
Calcinosis (universalis or circumscripta)
Childhood dermatomyositis
Scleroderma
Systemic lupus erythematosis
Posttraumatic
Ectopic ossification
Myositis ossificans (posttraumatic)
Burns
Surgery
Neurologic injury
Fibrodysplasia (myositis) ossificans progressiva

metastable solution: i.e., their levels are too low for spontaneous precipitation but high enough to cause hydroxyapatite $[3Ca_3(PO_4)_2 \cdot Ca(OH)_2]$ formation once crystal nucleation has begun (1). Normally, the presence of a variety of inhibitors of mineralization, such as inorganic pyrophosphate, helps to prevent ectopic calcification from occurring in healthy tissues (2). The pathogenesis of metastatic and dystrophic calcification is partially understood at the cell level. The process typically involves mineral accumulation within matrix vesicles and sometimes within mitochondria (2). The pathogenesis of ectopic ossification is largely an enigma.

Metastatic calcification is a risk of significant hypercalcemia or hyperphosphatemia (especially both), regardless of the cause (Table 1). In fact, therapy with phosphate supplements during mild hypercalcemia, or treatment with vitamin D or calcium during mild hyperphosphatemia, may trigger this problem (3).

Direct precipitation of mineral occurs when the calcium-phosphate solubility product in extracellular fluid is exceeded. A value of 75 for this parameter (mg/dl × mg/dl) is commonly taken as the level that, if surpassed, is associated with mineral precipitation. However, the critical value at which renal calcification might occur is not precisely defined and may vary with age (3). In adults, some consider 70 to be the maximal safe value for the kidney. It is possible that children can tolerate a somewhat higher level, because they normally have higher serum phosphate levels than adults, but this is not well established (3). Mineral deposition can occur ectopically from hyperphosphatemia despite concomitant hypocalcemia.

The mineral that is deposited in metastatic calcification may be amorphous calcium phosphate initially, but hydroxyapatite is formed soon after (2). The pattern of deposition varies somewhat between hypercalcemia and hyperphosphatemia, but deposition occurs irrespective of the specific underlying condition or mechanism for the disturbed mineral homeostasis. There is a predilection for precipitation into certain tissues.

Hypercalcemia is typically associated with mineral deposits in the kidneys, lungs, and fundus of the stomach. In these acid-secreting organs or tissues, a local alkaline milieu may account for the calcium deposition. In addition, the media of large arteries, elastic tissue of the endocardium (especially the left atrium), conjunctiva, and periarticular soft tissues are often affected. However, the predisposition for these sites is not well understood. In the kidney, hypercalciuria may cause calcium phosphate casts to form within the tubule lumen, or calculi to develop in the calyces or pelvis. Furthermore, calcium phosphate may precipitate in peritubular tissues. In the lung, calcification affects the alveolar walls and the pulmonary venous system. Well-established causes of metastatic calcification mediated by hyper-

calcemia include the milk-alkali syndrome, hypervitaminosis D, sarcoidosis, and hyperparathyroidism (Table 1).

Hyperphosphatemia of sufficient severity to cause
metastatic calcification occurs with idiopathic hypoparathyroidism or pseudohypoparathyroidism, and with the massive
cell lysis (release of cellular phosphate) that can follow
chemotherapy for leukemia (Table 1). Renal insufficiency is
commonly associated with metastatic calcification—the
mechanism may involve hyperphosphatemia, hypercalcemia, or both. Of interest, but unexplained, is the fact that
ectopic calcification is more common in pseudohypoparathyroidism (type I) than in idiopathic hypoparathyroidism despite comparable elevations in serum phosphate
levels. Furthermore, the location of ectopic calcification in
pseudohypoparathyroidism and hypoparathyroidism (e.g.,
cerebral basal ganglion) is different from that which occurs
from hypercalcemia. With hyperphosphatemia, calcification
of periarticular subcutaneous tissues is characteristic and
may be related to tissue trauma from the movement of
joints.

Dystrophic calcification occurs despite a normal serum
calcium-phosphate solubility product. Injured tissue of any
kind is predisposed to this type of extraskeletal calcification. Apparently, such tissue can release material that has
nucleating properties. One example of this phenomenon is
the caseous lesion of tuberculosis. What local factor predisposes to the precipitation of calcium salts is unknown.
Indeed, several mechanisms seem likely. It is clear that
mineral precipitation into injured tissue is even more striking and more severe when either the calcium or the phosphate level in extracellular fluid is increased. The
deposited mineral, as for metastatic calcification, may be
either amorphous calcium phosphate or crystalline hydroxyapatite.

The term *calcinosis* refers to an important type of dystrophic calcification that commonly occurs in (or under) the
skin with connective tissue disorders—particularly dermatomyositis (discussed in this section), scleroderma, and systemic lupus erythematosus. Other etiologies for calcinosis
include metastases, and trauma that produces necrotic tissue. As the symptoms of the acute connective tissue disease
and the inflammatory process in the subcutaneous tissues

subside, painful masses of calcium phosphate appear under
the skin. Calcinosis may involve a relatively localized area
with small deposits in the skin and subcutaneous tissues,
especially over the extensor aspects of the joints and the fingertips (calcinosis circumscripta); or it may be widespread
and not only in the skin and subcutaneous tissues, but deeper
in periarticular regions and areas of trauma as well (calcinosis universalis). The lesions of calcinosis are small- or
medium-sized, hard nodules that can cause muscle atrophy
and contractures.

Ectopic ossification is associated with two principal etiologies. It is called myositis ossificans when it occurs with
the fasciitis that follows neurologic injury, surgery, a burn,
or trauma. It also occurs as a principal feature of a separate,
heritable entity—fibrodysplasia (myositis) ossificans progressiva—a condition in which the pathogenesis is especially unclear and controversial. Some consider the primary
reason for the ectopic bone formation in this latter condition
to be a muscle abnormality (myositis ossificans progressiva), whereas others think a connective tissue defect is
more likely (fibrodysplasia ossificans progressiva). In these
various conditions, "true" bone tissue is formed. The bone is
lamellar, is actively remodeled by osteoblasts and osteoclasts, has haversian systems, and sometimes contains marrow. Apparently, the injured or diseased tissue contains the
necessary precursor cells and inductive signals to form
osseous tissue.

Described in the following chapters are three conditions—tumoral calcinosis, dermatomyositis, and fibrodysplasia ossificans progressiva—that are principal examples
of each type of ectopic mineralization.

REFERENCES

1. Fawthrop FW, Russell RGG: Ectopic calcification and ossification. In: Nordin BEC, Need AG, Morris HA (eds) *Metabolic
Bone and Stone Disease,* 3rd ed. Churchill Livingstone, Edinburgh, pp 325–338, 1993
2. Anderson HC: Calcific diseases: A concept. *Arch Pathol Lab
Med* 107:341–348, 1983
3. Harrison HE, Harrison HC: *Disorders of Calcium and Phosphate
Metabolism in Childhood and Adolescence.* WB Saunders,
Philadelphia, 291–304, 1979

76. Tumoral Calcinosis

Michael P. Whyte, M.D.

Division of Bone and Mineral Diseases, Washington University School of Medicine; and
Metabolic Research Unit, Shriners Hospital for Crippled Children, St. Louis, Missouri

Tumoral calcinosis, first described in 1899, is a heritable disorder that is characterized clinically by periarticular metastatic calcification (1). More than 2000 cases have been described. Mineral deposition develops as soft tissue masses around the major joints. Typically, the shoulder and hip regions are affected, although areas adjacent to additional joints may become involved (2). Visceral calcification does not occur, but segments of vasculature may contain mineral deposits. Hyperphosphatemia is a pathogenetic factor in many patients (3,4). The differential diagnosis includes periarticular metastatic calcification from hypercalcemia associated with renal failure, milk-alkali syndrome, sarcoidosis, and vitamin D intoxication.

CLINICAL PRESENTATION

Most patients in North America are black. About one third of cases are familial. Autosomal recessive inheritance is usually described, although autosomal dominant transmission has also been reported (1,2). There is no gender preference. Tumoral calcinosis often presents in childhood, but characteristic masses have been noted first in infancy or in old age. Hyperphosphatemic patients are usually black, have a positive family history for tumoral calcinosis, manifest the disease before age 20 years, and have multiple lesions (4). This is a lifelong disorder.

The soft tissue tumors of ectopic calcification are typically painless and grow at variable rates. After 1 or 2 years, they may be the size of an orange or grapefruit and weigh 1 kg or more. Often they are hard, lobulated, and firmly attached to deep fascia. Occasionally, the masses infiltrate into muscles and tendons (4). Because the deposits are extracapsular, joint range of motion is not impaired unless the tumors are particularly large. There can, however, be compression of adjacent neural structures. The lesions can also ulcerate the skin and form a sinus tract that drains a chalky fluid; this complication may lead to infection. Other potential problems from tumoral calcinosis include anemia, low-grade fever, regional lymphadenopathy, splenomegaly, and amyloidosis. Some patients have features of pseudoxanthoma elasticum (i.e., skin and vascular calcifications and angioid streaks in the retina). A dental abnormality featuring short bulbous roots and calcific deposits that often obliterate pulp chambers is characteristic of tumoral calcinosis (2,5).

RADIOLOGIC EXAMINATION

The tumors typically appear as large aggregations of irregular, densely calcified lobules that are confined to soft tissues (Fig. 1). The early lesion may involve hemorrhage and histiocyte accumulation (6). Radiolucent fibrous septae account for the lobular appearance. Occasionally, fluid layers are seen within the lobules. The joints per se are unaffected. Bone texture and density are also unremarkable. Periarticular masses that are radiologically indistinguishable from those of tumoral calcinosis also occur in chronic renal failure when mineral homeostasis is poorly controlled.

A "diaphysitis" has been recognized using radiographs, computerized tomography (CT), or magnetic resonance imaging (MRI) in some cases of tumoral calcinosis. This finding may be confused with osteomyelitis or neoplasm (7). New bone formation occurs along the endosteal surface of the diaphysis, perhaps from calcific myelitis. When only calcific myelitis is present, CT and MRI are excellent tools for diagnosis (7). Bone scanning, however, is the best method to detect and localize the calcified masses.

LABORATORY FINDINGS

Serum calcium levels and alkaline phosphatase activity are usually normal. Hyperphosphatemia and increased serum calcitriol levels occur in some patients (4,8).

The TmP/GFR (phosphate transport maximum/glomerular filtration rate) may be supranormal, but renal function is otherwise unremarkable. Patients are in positive calcium/phosphate balance. Renal studies reflect both the ongoing calcium and phosphate retention, and some patients are frankly hypocalciuric. The chalky fluid found in lesions is predominantly hydroxyapatite (9,10).

HISTOPATHOLOGY

The masses of tumoral calcinosis are essentially foreign body granuloma reactions that form multilocular, cystic structures. The cysts have tough connective tissue capsules and their fibrous walls contain numerous foreign body giant cells. They are filled with calcareous material in a viscous milky fluid. Occasionally, spicules of spongy bone and cartilage are found as well.

ETIOLOGY AND PATHOGENESIS

The genetic basis for tumoral calcinosis is unknown (1). The precise pathogenesis is poorly understood but may lie within the renal tubule cell. Increased renal reclamation of filtered phosphate appears to be an important pathogenetic factor. In hyperphosphatemic patients, enhanced renal tubular reabsorption of phosphate occurs independently of suppressed serum parathyroid hormone (PTH) levels (4,8). Deranged regulation of renal 25-hydroxyvitamin D, 1α-hydroxylase causes increased calcitriol synthesis. Consequently, there is enhanced absorption of dietary calcium and suppression of serum PTH levels (4,8).

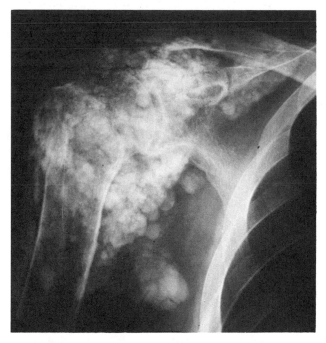

FIG. 1. Tumoral calcinosis. Typical lobular periarticular calcifications are present in the region of the right shoulder of this middle-aged man.

The masses may begin as calcific bursitis but then grow into adjacent fascial planes. Tissue damage with fat necrosis can be a pathogenetic factor (10). The major clinical complications of tumoral calcinosis are related to the metastatic calcifications that occur around joints and in skin, marrow, teeth, and blood vessels.

TREATMENT

Surgical removal of subcutaneous calcified masses may be helpful if they are painful, interfere with function, or are cosmetically unacceptable. When excision of a tumor is complete, recurrence appears to be unlikely (11).

Radiation therapy and cortisone treatment have not been effective. Phosphate-binding antacids (together with dietary phosphate and calcium deprivation) have been helpful (3,12,13). Although it might appear that if large apatite crystals were already in place administration of phosphate-binding antacids might not be effective, dissolution of calcific tumors after aluminum hydroxide therapy has been reported

(3,12,13). Furthermore, reduction of phosphate levels in extracellular fluid could help to prevent re-formation of mineral deposits (3). Preliminary studies indicate that calcitonin therapy may also be efficacious by enhancing renal clearance of phosphate (14). Phosphaturia caused by acetazolamide was helpful in one patient (15).

REFERENCES

1. McKusick VA: *Mendelian Inheritance in Man: Catalogs of Autosomal Dominant, Autosomal Recessive, and X-Linked Phenotypes,* 10th ed. The Johns Hopkins University Press, Baltimore, 1992
2. Lyles KW, Burkes EJ, Ellis GJ, et al.: Genetic transmission of tumoral calcinosis: Autosomal dominant with variable clinical expressivity. *J Clin Endocrinol Metab* 60:1093–1096, 1985
3. Mozaffarian G, Lafferty FW, Pearson OH: Treatment of tumoral calcinosis with phosphorus deprivation. *Ann Intern Med* 77:741–745, 1972
4. Prince MJ, Schaefer PC, Goldsmith RS, Chausmer AB: Hyperphosphatemic tumoral calcinosis: Association with elevation of serum 1,25-dihydroxy-cholecalciferol concentrations. *Ann Intern Med* 96:586–591, 1982
5. Burkes EJ Jr, Lyles KW, Dolan EA, Giammara B, Hanker J: Dental lesions in tumoral calcinosis. *Oral Pathol Med* 20:222–227, 1991
6. Slavin RE, Wen J, Kumar WJ, Evans EB: Familial tumoral calcinosis. A clinical, histopathologic, and ultrastructural study with an analysis of its calcifying process and pathogenesis. *Am J Surg Pathol* 17:788–802, 1993
7. Martinez S, Vogler JB, Harrelson JM, Lyles KW: Imaging of tumoral calcinosis: New observations. *Radiology* 174:215–222, 1990
8. Lyles KW, Halsey DL, Friedman NE, Lobaugh B: Correlations of serum concentrations of 1,25-dihydroxyvitamin D, phosphorus, and parathyroid hormone in tumoral calcinosis. *J Clin Endocrinol Metab* 67:88–92, 1988
9. Boskey AL, Vigorita VJ, Sencer O, Stuchin SA, Lane JM: Chemical, microscopic and ultrastructural characterization of mineral deposits in tumoral calcinosis. *Clin Orthop* 178:258–270, 1983
10. Kindbolm L-G, Gunterberg B: Tumoral calcinosis: An ultrastructural analysis and consideration of pathogenesis. *APMIS* 96:368–376, 1988
11. Noyez JF, Murphree SM, Chen K: Tumoral calcinosis, a clinical report of eleven cases. *Acta Orthop Belg* 59:249–254, 1993
12. Davies M, Clements MR, Mawer EB, Freemont AJ: Tumoral calcinosis: Clinical and metabolic response to phosphorus deprivation. *Q J Med* 242:493–503, 1987
13. Gregosiewicz A, Warda E: Tumoral calcinosis: Successful medical treatment. *J Bone Joint Surg* 71A:1244–1249, 1989
14. Salvi A, Cerudelli B, Cimino A, Zuccato F, Giustina G: Phosphaturic action of calcitonin in pseudotumoral calcinosis *(letter).* *Horm Metab Res* 15:260, 1983
15. Yamaguchi T, Sugimoto T, Imai Y, Fukase M, Fujita T, Chihara K: Successful treatment of hyperphosphatemic tumoral calcinosis with long-term acetazolamide. *Bone* 16:247S–250S, 1995

77. Dermatomyositis

Michael P. Whyte, M.D.

*Division of Bone and Mineral Diseases, Washington University School of Medicine; and
Metabolic Research Unit, Shriners Hospital for Crippled Children, St. Louis, Missouri*

Dermatomyositis is a multisystem connective tissue disorder, caused by small vessel vasculitis, that is characterized by nonsuppurative inflammation of especially skin and striated muscle (1–5). Dystrophic calcification often follows episodes of inflammation.

CLINICAL PRESENTATION

There are more female than male patients. One sees two peak ages of incidence: childhood (5 to 15 years) and adulthood (50 to 60 years). When dermatomyositis manifests before age 16, it is called the juvenile or the childhood form (1–5). The adult form is associated with malignancy.

In childhood dermatomyositis, the patient's sex and the age of onset of symptoms do not appear to influence the severity of calcinosis. Calcification is generally noted 1 to 3 years after the disease onset and usually subsequent to the acute phase. Mineral deposits develop for 1 to 3 years. Although the dystrophic calcification then typically remains stable, some regression may occur, and spontaneous resolution of calcinosis has been reported (1–5).

In calcinosis universalis, mineral deposition occurs throughout the subcutaneous tissues, but primarily in periarticular regions or in areas that are subject to trauma (Fig. 1). In calcinosis circumscripta, the deposits are more localized and typically occur around joints. The ectopic calcification can cause pain, ulcerate the skin, limit mobility, and predispose to abscess formation.

LABORATORY FINDINGS

Hypercalcemia with hypercalciuria and hyperphosphaturia may occur. Elevated levels of gamma-carboxyglutamic acid have been found in the urine of children with dermatomyositis—especially if there is calcinosis (6).

RADIOLOGIC FINDINGS

In childhood dermatomyositis, four types of dystrophic calcification occur (7):

1. Superficial masses (small circumscribed nodules or plaques) within the skin
2. Deep discrete subcutaneous nodular masses (see Fig. 1) near joints that can impair movement (calcinosis circumscripta)
3. Deep, linear, sheet-like deposits within intramuscular fascial planes (calcinosis universalis)
4. Lacy reticular subcutaneous deposits that encase the torso to form a generalized "exoskeleton"

Children with severe disease that is refractory to medical therapy seem to be especially prone to developing exoskeleton-like calcifications. The exoskeleton is in turn associated with severe calcinosis and poor physical function.

ETIOLOGY AND PATHOGENESIS

Childhood dermatomyositis appears to be a form of complement-mediated microangiopathy (8). The precise cause of the dystrophic calcification, however, is unknown. Immune deficiencies may predispose the patient to this complication (9). Calcinosis seems to occur in the majority of long-term survivors and may reflect a scarring process. This hypothesis is supported by the observation that mineral deposition seems to occur primarily in the muscles that were most severely affected during the acute phase of the disease. Electron microscopy shows that the calcification consists of hydroxyapatite crystals.

A variety of mechanisms have been considered for the dystrophic calcification, including release of alkaline phosphatase or discharge of free fatty acids from diseased muscle that, in turn, directly precipitate calcium or first bind acid mucopolysaccharides. Increased urinary levels of gamma-carboxylated peptides suggest that calcium-binding proteins may be responsible for the mineral deposition.

TREATMENT

High-dose prednisone therapy soon after the onset of symptoms seems to be important for minimizing the risk of calcinosis and for ensuring good functional recovery (1,2,10). If the response is only incomplete, consideration is given to additional immunosuppressive agents (2,4). Accumulating evidence indicates that phosphate-binding antacid therapy may reverse the mineral deposition (11). In a small clinical trial, warfarin sodium treatment to decrease gamma-carboxylation was not associated with changes in calcium or phosphorus excretion or in a reduction of calcinosis (12). Troublesome calcium deposits can be removed surgically.

PROGNOSIS

The clinical course of dermatomyositis in children is variable. Some have long-term relapsing or persistent disease, whereas others recover. When recovery is incomplete, there may be severe residual weakness, joint contractures, and calcinosis. The calcinosis may be the principal cause of long-term disability.

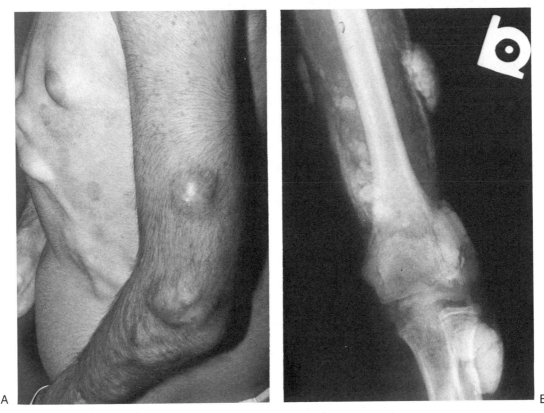

FIG. 1. *Calcinosis universalis* in childhood dermatomyositis. **A:** Characteristic subcutaneous nodules are apparent in the left arm and anterior chest wall of this 15-year-old boy. **B:** The nodules in this boy's arm are composed of dense lobular calcifications. In addition, the muscles of the upper arm are encased in a characteristic calcified sheath.

REFERENCES

1. Pachman LM: Juvenile dermatomyositis: Pathophysiology and disease expression. *Pediatr Clin North Am* 42:1071–1098, 1995
2. Kaye SA, Isenberg DA: Treatment of polymyositis and dermatomyositis. *Br J Hosp Med* 52:463–468, 1994
3. Pachman LM: Juvenile dermatomyositis: New clues to diagnosis and pathogenesis. *Clin Exp Rheumatol* 12(suppl 10):S69–73, 1994
4. Ansell BM: Juvenile dermatomyositis. *J Rheumatol Suppl* 33:60–62, 1992
5. Olson JC: Juvenile dermatomyositis. *Dermatologica* 11:57–64, 1992
6. Lian JB, Pachman LM, Gundberg CM, Partridge REH, Maryjowski MC: Gamma-carboxyglutamate excretion and calcinosis in juvenile dermatomyositis. *Arthritis Rheum* 25:1094–1100, 1982
7. Blane CE, White SJ, Braunstein EM, Bowyer SL, Sullivan DB: Patterns of calcification in childhood dermatomyositis. *Am J Roentgenol* 142:397–400, 1984
8. Kissel JT, Mendell JR, Rammohan KW: Microvascular deposition of complement membrane attack complex in dermatomyositis. *N Engl J Med* 314:329–334, 1986
9. Moore EC, Cohen F, Douglas SD, Gutta V: Staphylococcal infections in childhood dermatomyositis—association with the development of calcinosis, raised IgE concentrations and granulocyte chemotactic defect. *Ann Rheum Dis* 51(3):378–383, 1992
10. Bowyer SL, Blane CE, Sullivan DB, Cassidy JT: Childhood dermatomyositis: Factors predicting functional outcome and development of dystrophic calcification. *J Pediatr* 103:882–888, 1983
11. Wang W-J, Lo W-L, Wong CK: Calcinosis cutis—juvenile dermatomyositis: Remarkable response to aluminum hydroxide therapy *(letter)*. *Arch Dermatol* 124:1721–1722, 1988
12. Moore SE, Jump AA, Smiley JD: Effect of warfarin sodium therapy on excretion of 4-carboxy-L-glutamic acid in scleroderma, dermatomyositis, and myositis ossificans progressiva. *Arthritis Rheum* 29:344–351, 1986

78. Fibrodysplasia (Myositis) Ossificans Progressiva

Michael P. Whyte, M.D., *Frederick S. Kaplan, M.D., and †Eileen Shore, Ph.D.

Division of Bone and Mineral Diseases, Washington University School of Medicine; and Metabolic Research Unit,
*Shriners Hospital for Crippled Children, St. Louis, Missouri; and *Division of Metabolic Bone Disease,*
**†Departments of Orthopaedic Surgery and Medicine, The University of Pennsylvania School of Medicine, Philadelphia, Pennsylvania*

Fibrodysplasia ossificans progressiva (myositis ossificans progressiva) is a rare heritable disorder of connective tissue characterized by two principal features: first, congenital skeletal malformations of the great toes; second, recurrent episodes of painful soft-tissue swelling that lead to progressive heterotopic ossification in characteristic anatomic patterns (1,2).

Posttraumatic myositis ossificans, a different condition, is characterized by bone and cartilage in soft tissue (typically muscle, but also in tendons, ligaments, joint capsules, and fascia). Early on, an injured mass may be painful, warm, and of doughy consistency. About 4 to 6 weeks after the trauma, mineralization is apparent on routine radiographs. A biopsy specimen may be mistaken for an osteosarcoma because of mitotic figures and cellular pleomorphism. However, true malignancy rarely occurs. The heterotopic ossification that follows hip replacement and spinal cord injury is also true bone.

Fibrodysplasia ossificans progressiva (FOP) was first described in 1692; more than 600 cases have been reported (1,2). The disorder is among the rarest of human afflictions, with an estimated incidence of one per two million live births in Great Britain (1). Currently, we know of fewer than 200 individuals with FOP worldwide. Although Caucasian patients have been described most often, the disorder has been reported in all ethnic groups (1,2). Autosomal dominant transmission with variable expressivity is established (3–5). However, reproductive fitness is low, and the majority of cases develop sporadically. Gonadal mosaicism appears to explain the disorder when isolated in sibships.

CLINICAL PRESENTATION

Fibrodysplasia ossificans progressiva can be suspected at birth, before soft-tissue lesions occur, if the typical congenital skeletal malformations are recognized (1,2). The most characteristic is shortening of big toes, with malformations in the cartilaginous anlage of the first metatarsal and proximal phalanx (1,2,7,8). Although the toe may appear to be deformed (hallux valgus), it is actually malformed (Fig. 1). In some cases, the thumbs may also be strikingly short. Synostosis and hypoplasia of the phalanges are typical (8). Nevertheless, the digital anomalies are not pathognomonic. Usually, FOP is diagnosed only when soft-tissue swellings and radiologic evidence of heterotopic ossification are noted.

The severity of FOP differs from patient to patient (9), although most affected individuals become completely immobilized and confined to a wheelchair by the third decade (1,2,10). Typically, episodes of soft-tissue swelling begin during the first decade of life (11). Occasionally, the onset is as late as early adulthood, yet there are also reports of *in utero* involvement. Painful, tender, and rubbery soft-tissue lesions appear spontaneously, or they may appear to be precipitated by minor trauma including intramuscular childhood immunizations (12). Swellings develop rapidly during the course of several days. Fever may occur during periods of induration and can mistakenly suggest an infectious process (1,2). Typically, lesions occur in paraspinal muscles in the back or in the limb girdles and may last for several weeks (11). Aponeuroses, fascia, tendons, ligaments, and connective tissue of voluntary muscles may be affected. Although some swellings may regress spontaneously, most mature through an endochondral pathway to contain true heterotopic bone (13). The episodes of induration recur at unpredictable frequencies. Some patients will seem to enter periods of disease quiescence. However, once ossification appears, it is permanent.

Gradually, the bony masses immobilize joints and cause muscle contractures and deformity, particularly in the neck and shoulders. Ossification around the hips, typically present by the third decade of life, commonly prevents ambulation (10). Involvement of the muscles of mastication (injured by injection of local anesthetic or over-stretching of the jaw during dental procedures) can severely limit movement of the jaw and ultimately impair nutrition (14). Ankylosis of the spine and rib cage further restrict mobility and may imperil cardiopulmonary function (1,2,8). Scoliosis is a common finding and is associated with asymmetric bars of heterotopic bone connecting the rib cage to the pelvis (Figs. 1,2) (15). Hypokyphosis results from early ossification of the paravertebral musculature. Restrictive lung disease and predisposition to pneumonia may follow. The diaphragm, extraocular muscles, heart, and smooth muscles are characteristically spared (1,2,8). Although secondary amenorrhea may develop, successful reproduction has been reported (1,2). Hearing impairment (beginning in late childhood or adolescence) and alopecia also occur with increased frequency (8).

RADIOLOGIC FEATURES

Skeletal anomalies and soft-tissue ossification are the characteristic radiologic features of FOP (16). The principal malformations involve the great toe, although other digital anomalies of the feet and hands may occur. Exostoses are frequent (1,2). A remarkable feature of FOP is developmental fusion of cervical vertebrae that may be confused with Klippel-Feil syndrome or Still's disease (1,2,16). The femoral necks may be broad and short. The remainder of the skeleton does not have anomalies (16).

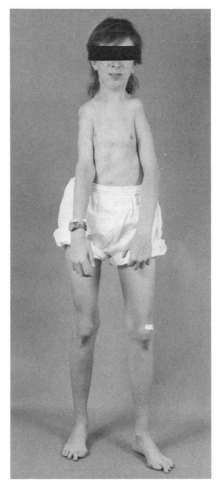

FIG. 1. Fibrodysplasia (myositis) ossificans progressiva. Severe underdevelopment of the chest has occurred from ectopic bone formation in the thorax of this 16-year-old boy. Note also the feet with characteristic malformations of the great toes.

Ectopic ossification occurs and progresses in several regular patterns or gradients: proximally before distally, axially before appendicularly, cranially before caudally, and dorsally before ventrally (11). The paraspinal muscles are involved early in life, with subsequent progression to the shoulders and hips. The ankles, wrists, and jaw may be affected, but later.

Of interest, there is radiographic evidence of normal modeling and remodeling of the heterotopic skeleton (17). Modeling changes include: (i) tubular and flat bones with mature cortical and trabecular organization; (ii) well-defined cortical–endosteal borders enclosing medullary canals; and (iii) metaphyseal funnelization in isolated ossicles or at sites of synostoses (17). Remodeling changes include: (i) osteosclerosis from use (weightbearing) and osteopenia from disuse, and (ii) absence of pathologic fractures or stress fractures from fatigue failure. Bone scans suggest that remodeling of mature heterotopic bone is normal (17). Fractures respond similarly in the heterotopic and normotopic skeleton (18).

Bone scans are abnormal before ossification can be demonstrated by conventional radiographs (19). Computer-ized tomography and magnetic resonance imaging of early lesions has been described (20,21).

LABORATORY FINDINGS

Routine biochemical studies of mineral metabolism are usually normal, although alkaline phosphatase activity in serum may be increased, especially during flare-ups (1,2,22).

HISTOPATHOLOGY

The soft-tissue masses are initially composed of one or more edematous skeletal muscles. Ligaments, tendons, and joint capsules may also be affected. Edema of fascial planes is one of the earliest findings (13). Subsequently, a dense fibroproliferative lesion is formed, and it is indistinguishable from aggressive juvenile fibromatosis (13,23). Misdiagnosis is common but can be avoided by correctly examining the *toes* (13,23). Immunostaining with a monoclonal antibody against bone morphogenetic protein (BMP) 2/4 is intense in the fibroproliferative cells of FOP lesions, but not in the fibroproliferative cells of aggressive fibromatosis (23). Endochondral ossification is the major pathway for heterotopic bone formation (13). Mature osseous lesions have haversian systems. Cancellous bone containing hematopoietic tissue will eventually form.

ETIOLOGY AND PATHOGENESIS

The autosomal gene defect that causes FOP has not been mapped within the human genome (3). The genes that

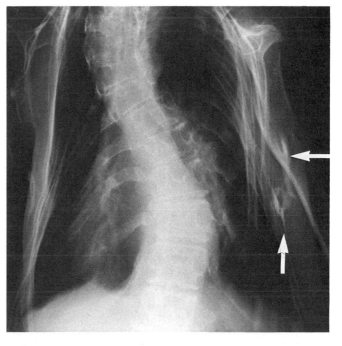

FIG. 2. The thorax of the boy shown in Fig. 1 was markedly narrowed by the ectopic bone within the chest wall (arrows) at 15 years of age. Scoliosis was also present and contributed to the restrictive lung disease that soon after proved lethal.

encode BMPs have been proposed as candidates for FOP (24). Disregulation of BMP4 gene expression has been reported recently (25). Similarities between FOP and the decapentaplegic mutation of *Drosophila* may represent clues to the etiology and pathogenesis (24).

TREATMENT

There is no established medical treatment for FOP (1,2). The rarity of the disorder, its variable severity, and the fluctuating clinical course pose substantial difficulties for evaluating potential therapies. Adrenocorticotrophic hormone, corticosteroids, binders of dietary calcium, intravenous infusion of ethylenediaminetetraacetic acid (EDTA), nonsteroidal anti-inflammatory agents, radiotherapy, disodium etidronate, and warfarin (to inhibit gamma-carboxylation of osteocalcin) are ineffective (1,2,8,26–28). Accordingly, medical intervention is currently supportive.

Physical therapy to maintain joint mobility may be harmful if too aggressive and may provoke or exacerbate lesions (8). Surgical release of joint contractures is generally unsuccessful and risks new, trauma-induced heterotopic ossification (8). Removal of lesions is often followed by their recurrence. Osteotomy of ectopic bone to mobilize a joint is usually counterproductive because of robust heterotopic ossification at the operative site. Spinal bracing is ineffective and surgical intervention is associated with numerous complications (15). Dental therapy should preclude routine injection of local anesthetics and stretching of the jaw (1,2,14). Newer dental techniques for focused administration of anesthetic are available. All intramuscular injections should be avoided (12). Guidelines for general anesthesia have been reported (29). Measures against recurrent pulmonary infections and onset of cardiopulmonary complications of restrictive lung disease are important.

PROGNOSIS

Despite widespread heterotopic ossification and severe disability, some subjects live productive lives into the seventh decade. Most, however, die earlier from pulmonary complications secondary to restricted ventilation and pneumonia from chest wall involvement (1,2,8).

REFERENCES

1. Connor JM: Fibrodysplasia ossificans progressiva. In: Royce PM, Steinmann B (eds) *Connective Tissue and Its Heritable Disorders.* Wiley-Liss, New York, pp 603–611, 1993
2. Beighton P: Fibrodysplasia ossificans progressiva. In: Beighton P (ed) *Heritable Disorders of Connective Tissue.* Mosby, St. Louis, pp 501–518, 1993
3. McKusick VA: *Mendelian Inheritance in Man: Catalogs of Autosomal Dominant, Autosomal Recessive, and X-Linked Phenotypes,* 11th ed. The Johns Hopkins University Press, Baltimore, 1994
4. Connor JM, Skirton H, Lunt PW: A three generation family with fibrodysplasia ossificans progressiva. *J Med Genet* 30:687–689, 1993
5. Kaplan FS, McCluskey W, Hahn GV, Tabas JA, Muenke M, Zasloff MA: Genetic transmission of fibrodysplasia ossificans progressiva: Report of a family. *J Bone Joint Surg* 75A:1214–1220, 1993
6. Janoff HB, Muenke M, Johnson LO, et al.: Fibrodysplasia ossificans progressiva in two half-sisters. Evidence for maternal mosaicism. *Am J Med Genet* 61:320–324, 1996
7. Rogers JG, Geho WB: Fibrodysplasia ossificans progressiva: A survey of forty-two cases. *J Bone Joint Surg* 61A:909–914, 1979
8. Connor JM, Evans DAP: Fibrodysplasia ossificans progressiva: The clinical features and natural history of 34 patients. *J Bone Joint Surg* 64B:76–83, 1982
9. Janoff HB, Tabas JA, Shore EM, et al.: Mild expression of fibrodysplasia ossificans progressiva: A report of 3 cases. *J Rheumatol* 22:976–978, 1995
10. Rocke DM, Zasloff M, Peeper J, Cohen RB, Kaplan FS: Age and joint-specific risk of initial heterotopic ossification in patients who have fibrodysplasia ossificans progressiva. *Clin Orthop* 301:243–248, 1994
11. Cohen RB, Hahn GV, Tabas JA, et al.: The natural history of heterotopic ossification in patients who have fibrodysplasia ossificans progressiva. A study of 44 patients. *J Bone Joint Surg* 75A:215–219, 1993
12. Lanchoney TF, Cohen RB, Rocke DM, Zasloff MA, Kaplan FS: Permanent heterotopic ossification at the injection site after diphtheria-tetanus-pertussis immunizations in children who have fibrodysplasia ossificans progressiva. *J Pediatr* 126:762–764, 1995
13. Kaplan FS, Tabas JA, Gannon FH, Finkel G, Hahn GV, Zasloff MA: The histopathology of fibrodysplasia ossificans progressiva: An endochondral process. *J Bone Joint Surg* 75A:220–230, 1993
14. Janoff HB, Cohen R, Shafritz A, Shore EM, Zasloff M, Kaplan FS: Submandibular swelling in patients who have fibrodysplasia ossificans progressiva. *J Bone Miner Res* 9(Suppl 1):S428, 1994
15. Shah PB, Zasloff MA, Drummond D, Kaplan FS: Spinal deformity in patients who have fibrodysplasia ossificans progressiva. *J Bone Joint Surg* 76A:1442–1450, 1994
16. Cremin B, Connor JM, Beighton P: The radiological spectrum of fibrodysplasia ossificans progressiva. *Clin Radiol* 33:499–508, 1982
17. Kaplan FS, Strear CM, Zasloff MA: Radiographic and scintigraphic features of modeling and remodeling in the heterotopic skeleton of patients who have fibrodysplasia ossificans progressiva. *Clin Orthop* 304:238–247, 1994
18. Einhorn TA, Kaplan FS: Traumatic fractures of heterotopic bone in patients who have fibrodysplasia ossificans progressiva. *Clin Orthop* 308:173–177, 1994
19. Fang MA, Reinig JW, Hill SC, et al.: Technetium-99m MDP demonstration of heterotopic ossification in fibrodysplasia ossificans progressiva. *Clin Nucl Med* 11:8–9, 1986
20. Reinig JW, Hill SC, Fang M, et al.: Fibrodysplasia ossificans progressiva: CT appearance. *Radiology* 159:153–157, 1986
21. Shirkhoda A, Armin A-R, Bis KG, Makris J, Irwin RB, Shetty AN: MR imaging of myositis ossificans: Variable patterns at different stages. *J Magne Reson Imaging* 5:287–292, 1995
22. Lutwak L: Myositis ossificans progressiva. Mineral, metabolic, and radioactive calcium studies of the effects of hormones. *Am J Med* 37:269–293, 1964
23. Gannon F, Kaplan FS, Olmsted E, Finkel G, Zasloff M, Shore E: Differential immunostaining with bone morphogenetic protein (BMP) 2/4 in early fibromatous lesions of fibrodysplasia ossificans progressiva and aggressive juvenile fibromatosis. *J Bone Miner Res* 10(suppl 1), S–508, 1995
24. Kaplan F, Tabas JA, Zasloff MA: Fibrodysplasia ossificans progressiva: A clue from the fly? *Calcif Tissue Int* 47:117–125, 1990
25. Shafritz A, Gannon F, Mitchell H, et al.: Disregulation of bone morphogenetic protein 4 (BMP4) gene expression in fibrodysplasia ossificans progressiva. *J Bone Miner Res* 10(suppl 1), S–191, 1995
26. Smith R, Russell RGG, Wood CG: Myositis ossificans progressiva. Clinical features of eight patients and their response to treatment. *J Bone Joint Surg* 58B:48–57, 1976
27. Moore SE, Jump AA, Smiley JD: Effect of warfarin sodium therapy on excretion of 4-carboxy-L-glutamic acid in myositis ossificans progressiva. *Arthritis Rheum* 29:344–351, 1986
28. Bar Oz B, Boneh A: Myositis ossificans progressiva: A 10-year follow-up on a patient treated with etidronate disodium. *Acta Paediatr* 83:1332–1334, 1994
29. Lininger TE, Brown EM, Brown M: General anesthesia and fibrodysplasia ossificans progressiva. *Anesth Analg* 68:175–176, 1989

SECTION X

Nephrolithiasis

X. Introduction

Murray J. Favus, M.D.

Bone Program, General Clinical Research Center, and Department of Medicine, The University of Chicago Medical Center, Chicago, Illinois

The first chapter in this section describes the clinical presentation, complications, natural history, pathogenesis, and medical treatment of common and rare forms of nephrolithiasis. The message is that stone recurrence rates are high and can largely be prevented by appropriate treatment. However, selection of therapy requires a knowledge of the metabolic disturbance that created the chemical milieu of the urine that favors crystal formation, growth, and aggregation. The second chapter addresses the problem of existing stones in the upper and lower urinary tract and how to remove them with lithotripsy. The location, size, and composition of stones susceptible to dissolution with lithotripsy are clearly stated. The recurrent stone former who has undergone successful lithotripsy is faced with the prospect of new stone formation if the metabolic abnormalities are not reversed. Therefore, the successful prevention of recurrent stones depends on careful evaluation and treatment, as described in the first chapter.

79. Nephrolithiasis

Fredric L. Coe, M.D., and Joan H. Parks, M.B.A.

Kidney Stone Program, Nephrology Section, Department of Medicine, University of Chicago Hospital, Chicago, Illinois

All kidney stones are aggregates of crystals mixed with a protein matrix, and all cause disease because of obstruction of urine flow in the renal collecting system, ureters, or urethra; bleeding; or local erosion into the kidney tissue. The common stone is calcium oxalate; this stone is small, recurrent, a cause of pain from passage and obstruction, and caused by metabolic disorders that mostly are treatable. Uric acid stones are uncommon (about 5% of all stones) and radiolucent but otherwise like calcium oxalate stones. Struvite stones, from infection, fill renal collecting systems, erode into the renal tissue, and cause obvious renal functional impairment. Cystine stones have only one cause, hereditary cystinuria. They grow large enough to fill the renal collecting system, begin in childhood, and can cause renal failure.

All stones need crystallographic analysis, by simple polarization microscopy, or x-ray diffraction when needed. Even if the first few stones are shown to contain uric acid, for example, the next may contain calcium oxalate or struvite. Radiographs are not helpful for identification except in the case of uric acid stones, which are lucent; the rest are similar, although some generalizations can be made: calcium oxalate stones resemble stars in the night sky, cystine stones are like eggs or staghorns and seem sculpted of a soft stone or wax, and struvite stones are mostly rugged, ringed staghorns that look like tree roots. We use flat plates to count stones; tomograms without prior radiocontrast injection are ideal but expensive.

Laboratory evaluation is to detect causes, so measure 24-hour urine calcium, oxalate, uric acid, citrate, pH, volume, and creatinine to estimate completeness of collection. How many urine samples is best? One is certainly minimal; we favor three for better surety, and, if we found stones, we would measure four. Blood tests are for hypercalcemia; the rest is vague and unsure. Hormone measurements are never proper for initial evaluation; a parathyroid hormone (PTH) measurement is obtained for patients who are hypercalcemic.

CALCIUM STONES

Just as bone mineral forms when a supersaturated extracellular fluid contacts an appropriate nucleation site, kidney stones form when urine or, more probably, tubule fluid becomes highly supersaturated with a calcium salt such as calcium oxalate or a calcium phosphate phase. What distinguish the two processes are the greater levels of supersaturation in urine compared to plasma, the presence in urine and tubule fluid of powerful inhibitors of the crystallization process, and the fact that calcium oxalate, not calcium phosphate, is the main constituent of stones.

The causes of calcium stones can have other effects. They increase urine calcium or oxalate concentration; lower urine volume, so concentrations of all solutes increase; lower urine citrate, which normally forms a soluble salt with calcium and prevents crystallization; raise levels of molecules (uric acid in particular) that can promote calcium oxalate nucleation; or cause abnormally high urine pH, which promotes calcium phosphate crystallization, or low urine pH, which promotes uric acid crystallization.

Hypercalciuric States

Idiopathic hypercalciuria (IH) (1), the most common hypercalciuric state, occurs in families, affects both sexes equally, and has a pattern of horizontal and vertical transmission like that of a mendelian dominant trait. About 50% of patients with calcium oxalate stones have IH and are detected by a daily urine calcium excretion rate above the usual normal limits of 300 mg (for men) and 250 mg (for women); by normal serum calcium level; and by the absence of other hypercalciuric conditions such as sarcoidosis, vitamin D intoxication, immobilization, hyperthyroidism, glucocorticoid excess, rapidly progressive osteoporosis, Paget's disease, and Cushing's disease (2). Hypercalciuria raises urine calcium oxalate supersaturation (3), especially after eating.

The mechanism of the hypercalciuria is surely intestinal calcium absorption at an abnormally high rate (4), and what controversy exists concerns the cause of the high absorption rate. The most satisfactory view is that 1,25-dihydroxyvitamin D or calcitriol levels in the serum are high as a primary defect; in eight studies, hypercalciuric patients had higher levels than normals (5–12). The high calcitriol levels can raise calcium absorption and suppress PTH secretion, leading to reduced renal tubule calcium reabsorption. After eating, calcium will enter the blood at a more rapid rate than normal, and tubule reabsorption will be low, so serum calcium levels can remain near normal despite high absorption rates, and the calcium can be excreted rapidly into the urine. Alternative theories include a primary renal tubule leak of calcium and a primary increase in intestinal calcium absorption. Neither would explain the common pattern of low PTH (9) and high calcitriol levels, but they could account for hypercalciuria in some selected patients with high PTH levels or normal calcitriol levels.

In addition to hyperabsorption of calcium, hypercalciuric patients conserve calcium less well than normal people when given a low calcium intake in the range of 200 to 500 mg daily. In balance studies, when total calcium absorption can be measured, their urine calcium clearly exceeds net calcium absorption on such diets, meaning that bone mineral is being mobilized into the urine. The reason for their labile bone mineral stores may partly be an excessive action of calcitriol. When given to normal men, this hormone promotes the same behavior as seen among infectious hepatitis patients, a loss of bone mineral during low-calcium diet (11,12). High levels of serum calcitriol are by no means universal among the patients, despite almost universal calcium hyperabsorption, suggesting that not only high serum levels but possibly also high levels of the calcitriol receptor could mediate excessive calcitriol effects. In rats bred for hypercalciuria, increased calcitriol receptor number is an established cause of increased calcitriol action (13).

Given the lability of bone mineral and the natural tendency of doctors to use low-calcium diets for treatment of hypercalciuria, one might expect reduced bone mineral density among IH patients, and to date five studies document just this (14). In particular, the patients whose hypercalciuria persists during low-calcium diet show decisively low bone mineral densities, whereas those with normal or near normal calcium retention during low-calcium diet (a minority) have normal bone mineral density. A clinical corollary of this finding must be caution concerning low-calcium diet as a treatment except among patients clearly able to respond to it with normal calcium conservation. Among patients otherwise prone to osteoporosis, low-calcium diet has an additional and obvious disadvantage. For these reasons, we favor its use in only very restricted circumstances.

Thiazide diuretic agents lower urine calcium excretion, calcium oxalate supersaturation (15), and the rate of stone production (16). Thiazide affects the connecting segment of the nephron (17), increasing calcium reabsorption rate, and presumably lowers calcium excretion in patients by a direct renal action. The drugs lower intestinal calcium absorption in patients who have severe hypercalciuria (18), but less than they lower urine calcium excretion, so calcium balance becomes more positive. Alternative treatments include low-calcium diet, sodium cellulose phosphate, and orthophosphate, all of which lower intestinal calcium absorption. The long-term effects of reduced calcium absorption, especially from low-calcium diet, may include reduced bone mineral stores, because hypercalciuric patients do not lower their urine calcium excretion rates to values as low as in normal people when both are given a very low calcium intake (9). Men who are given calcitriol in excess but at a dose that does not raise serum calcium above normal (11,12) also fail to lower urine calcium normally while eating a low-calcium diet.

Primary hyperparathyroidism causes hypercalciuria in about 5% of calcium stone formers (19); 85% have single enlarged glands, so-called adenoma; the rest have at least two enlarged glands, so-called hyperplasia (see Chapter 28). Serum calcium level is always increased, although the increase commonly is so mild that many values are needed to be sure hypercalcemia is present. Upper limits for our normal subjects are serum calcium levels of 10 mg/dl in women, and 10.1 mg/dl in men. Serum levels of at least half of our patients who have had curative surgery were all below 10.5 mg/dl (19). Urine calcium excretion is very high, despite the modest hypercalcemia, so a casual analysis can be misleading; extreme hypercalciuria and serum calcium levels of, for example, 10.1 mg/dl to 10.3 mg/dl can lead one to think of idiopathic hypercalciuria, and probably accounts for misleading accounts of "normocalcemic" primary hyperparathyroidism (20–22), each of which, in retrospect, was almost certainly an instance of mild hypercalcemia.

Among patients who have had curative surgery, serum PTH levels have been elevated between 80% and 100% using a carboxyl terminal assay, and between 60% and 80% with amino terminal or mild molecule assays (19), so PTH assay is more confirmatory than a structural basis of diagnosis. The best course is to establish if hypercalcemia is present, then to exclude other causes such as malignant tumors, sarcoidosis and other granulomatous diseases, vitamin D intoxication, thiazide use, lithium use, and the uncommon or rare disorders (19) (see Section IV). Familial hypocalciuric hypercalcemia is a mendelian dominant disorder, not a cause of stones, best diagnosed by family studies (19) (see Chapter 30). Low PTH levels are especially valuable to detect states of primary calcitriol excess (19). Serum calcitriol is increased in most patients (23–25) as a consequence of high PTH and low serum phosphorus level, and the calcitriol stimulates intestinal calcium absorption, causing most of the hypercalciuria. Bone mineral loss into the urine also occurs.

Treatment is surgical in patients with stone disease. Stone formation is greatly reduced, as urine calcium excretion falls promptly. We follow our patients to be sure that residual hypercalciuria is not present and that serum calcium levels remain normal.

Renal tubular acidosis (RTA) is ostensibly a cause of hypercalciuria (26), but we suspect it is as often a consequence as a cause (see Chapter 64). The defect associated with stones is reduced ability to lower urine pH; urine citrate excretion is very low, as a rule, and urine calcium is high. It is true that metabolic acidosis is a consequence of severe reductions of tubule ability to lower pH, because a pH lower than that of blood is needed to titrate urine buffers with protons and to trap ammonia as ammonium ion, for excretion. Metabolic acidosis lowers urine citrate excretion and raises urine calcium, so one is tempted to consider the high pH, high urine calcium, and low urine pH as an expected clustering based on known physiology.

However, we (27) have found that alkali treatment, which should lower urine calcium excretion, usually does not, although it may raise urine citrate excretion. Metabolic acidosis is not discernible in most patients. Early reports of RTA (28) included, as a majority, patients such as we have encountered, and labeled them as having "incomplete RTA." In families, idiopathic hypercalciuria and RTA both appear (29), and the hypercalciuria of our patients usually responds to thiazide. We are inclined to believe that the hypercalciuria comes first and that nephrocalcinosis, perhaps hypercalciuria itself, damages collecting ducts and causes the incomplete RTA.

The patients form stones composed mainly of calcium phosphate salts. High urine pH raises urine levels of dissociated phosphate, which forms brushite—calcium monohydrogen phosphate—and apatite. The stones are larger than calcium oxalate stones, and they grow faster, too.

Apart from sporadic and familial incomplete RTA, rare patients have complete RTA, usually inherited as an autosomal dominant trait. They have metabolic acidosis; their urine calcium excretions fall with alkali treatment. Diamox (acetazolamide) reduces bicarbonate reabsorption by the proximal tubule and causes alkaline urine and stones. The urine is alkaline because the drug is given in multiple doses, so bicarbonate levels fall, rise between doses, and fall again as the bicarbonate is excreted. Inherited or acquired proximal RTA is a steady defect and causes neither stones nor alkaline urine. Hyperkalemic "type 4" RTA—resulting from obstruction, low renin or aldosterone secretion rates, or renal disease (30)—causes an acid urine pH and not stones.

Hyperoxaluric States

Primary hyperoxaluria always comes from one of two hereditary enzyme defects that raise oxalate production (31). Oxalate is an endproduct, excreted only by the kidneys, which filter and secrete it (32). Urine oxalate excretion is above the usual normal limit of 40 mg daily (33), in the range of 80 to 120 mg. The oxalate crystallizes with calcium, causing stones that begin in childhood, and tubulointerstitial nephropathy, which leads to chronic renal failure. Renal tubular acidosis may be an early sign of nephropathy, causing an anion gap metabolic acidosis that raises the serum chloride level and lowers the bicarbonate level. Renal transplantation requires extensive dialytic preparation so that stored oxalate does not flood the graft and destroy it. Overproduction occurs from pyridoxine deficiency (in animals) and methoxyflurane anesthetic and occurs if one is so foolish or mistaken as to drink ethylene glycol (antifreeze) as a beverage. Treatment is with fluids, citrate (to reduce calcium ion levels), and pyridoxine, which may be helpful in low doses of 20 to 40 mg daily in some people. Others respond only to 300 to 400 mg daily, and some do not respond at all.

Enteric hyperoxaluria means that the colon absorbs oxalate excessively because small bowel malabsorption permits undigested fatty acids and bile acids to reach the colon epithelium and increase its permeability (34). Small bowel resection, intestinal bypass for obesity, and small bowel diseases such as Crohn's disease are common causes (35). Colectomy or ileostomy prevents the oxaluria. Urine oxalate is above normal, in the range of 75 to 150 mg daily. Urine citrate is low because of the alkali loss from the small bowel, and urine pH is low. Urine calcium usually is low, not high. Low-oxalate diet and low-fat diet reduce oxaluria; low fat reduces delivery of fatty acids to colon. Oral calcium, 1 to 4 g as calcium carbonate, taken with meals, crystallizes with oxalate in the gut lumen. Cholestyramine, 1 to 4 g with meals, adsorbs oxalate and also bile salts. The four treatments are synergistic and should be used together. Cholestyramine has important side effects of vitamin K depletion and reduced absorption of drugs.

In a way, dietary oxalate excess is an enteric oxaluria. Usual food culprits are nuts, pepper, chocolate, rhubarb, and spinach for a few devotees, and for the rest, mixtures of dark green vegetables and of fruits. Vitamin C in large doses may raise urine oxalate, and ascorbic acid itself may, in urine, break down to oxalic acid, giving a wrong impression of hyperoxaluria. Treatments are simply dietary.

Hyperuricosuric States

About 25% of calcium stone formers excrete more than 800 mg daily of uric acid (750 mg in women) and have no other apparent causes of their stones (36). Their urine pH is lower than the normal of 6.0, averaging 5.6 (37), so the uric acid can crystallize (38). Uric acid crystals can promote calcium oxalate crystallization (39) because they share structural features. Treatment with allopurinol reduced stone recurrence in a prospective, controlled trial (40), and neither allopurinol nor its metabolites affect calcium oxalate crystallization. The hyperuricosuria results from high purine intake (41) from meats, and dietary treatment should be effective, although it has not been tested. We recommend reducing diet purine intake and reserving allopurinol for those who produce more stones, unless stone disease has been so severe that maximal certainty of treatment is desired despite the risk of drug side effects.

Low Urine Citrate

Women with stones excrete only 550 mg of citrate daily, compared with 750 mg daily for normal women (42). This decisive abnormality ought to raise the risk of stones because citrate forms a soluble calcium salt, and what calcium is in the salt is not free to combine with oxalic acid. Normal men excrete no more citrate than women with stones, and men who form stones excrete about the same amount of citrate, so low urine citrate in men is not so much an abnormality as it is a trait that explains why men are four out of every five people with stones. Any oral alkali can raise urine citrate. We prefer citrate to sodium bicarbonate for its longer duration of action, and we use 25 to 50 mEq two or three times daily. Citrate treatment has not been tested by prospective controlled trials.

URIC ACID STONES

Mixed

About 12% of all calcium stones contain some uric acid (43), and patients who form the mixed stones from urine that is supersaturated with uric acid because its pH is below the normal level of 6.0. Hyperuricosuria is also common. The urine of mixed stone formers is like that of patients with hyperuricosuric calcium oxalate stones, and what distinguishes the two groups is simply that in one, uric acid is inferred as a promoter of calcium oxalate stones, and in the other, the uric acid crystals are seen in the stones themselves. Probably, if all of the stones of the former group were studied, uric acid would be found in some; the distinction is not so intrinsic as it is based on accident of how patients are studied and the relative proportions of uric acid to calcium oxalate in their stones.

Treatment includes reduced diet purine for hyperuricosuria, oral alkali to raise urine pH to 6 or 6.5, and thiazide for hypercalciuria, which may occur in some patients. The hyperuricosuric calcium oxalate stone formers are defined by absence of hypercalciuria or other cause of stones, so thiazide is not usually needed or appropriate.

Pure

Only about 5% of stone formers produce pure uric acid stones. Their urine is very acid, with pH values below 5.3, which is the pK of uric acid, and frequently below 5.0. Uric acid solubility in urine is just below 100 mg/L, whereas the salts of monohydrogen urate are relatively much more soluble, so urine pH values near the pK raise uric acid supersaturation drastically by raising the fraction of the total urate that is fully protonated. For example, average normal men excrete 650 mg of uric acid in 1.2 L of urine (37), a concentration of 540 mg/L; at pK 6.0, less than 10% is undissociated, whereas at pH 5.3 50% (270 mg/L) is undissociated (2.7 times above the solubility). Uric acid stones occur in people with gout and in others with familial uric acid stones. All have low urine pH, and the reason is unclear. Patients with ileostomy or who work in hot and dry places form scanty and acid urine, and uric acid stones. Treatment is always alkali to raise urine pH to 6, and reduced purine intake or allopurinol for hyperuricosuria.

STRUVITE STONES

Only microorganisms that have urease enzyme can produce struvite stones, by hydrolyzing urine urea to carbon dioxide and ammonia, so urinary infection is the only clinical cause of these "infection" stones. Struvite forms as the ammonia raises local pH to above 9; phosphate is fully dissociated and combines with urine magnesium and ammonium ion. Carbonate apatite is also formed from the carbonate and calcium because of high pH, so "pure" struvite stones always contain both crystals. Mixed stones also contain calcium oxalate, which is not particularly favored to form under the same circumstances as struvite and denotes the combination of metabolic and infection stone in the same patient.

Mixed

We find that about one third of struvite stones are mixed; patients begin their stone career with passage, and their prognosis for renal function and nephrectomy is excellent. Men are nearly one half of this group, and almost all men with struvite stones form mixed stones. Urine calcium excretion is above normal for the group in both sexes. Mean serum creatinine is normal. A few patients do have reduced creatinine clearance, which is rare among calcium stone formers (44).

Pure

Over half of this group are women. Stones are frequently staghorns that fill the renal collecting systems. Infection, bleeding, or flank pain, rather than stone passage, calls attention to the stones. Serum creatinine levels are above normal on average, creatinine clearance is low, and hypercalciuria is not usual. Thus, struvite stones seem to be a primary problem, not a complication of metabolic stones.

Treatment

Mixed or pure, these infected stones are treated by removal. Current practice is percutaneous nephrolithotomy, if the stones are over 2 cm in diameter, followed by extra-corporeal shock wave lithotripsy (ESWL) to fragment what is left, then a second look with percutaneous nephrolithotomy to remove all debris. If stones are less than 2 cm in diameter, ESWL is an adequate monotherapy. Antibiotic agents are best used before and after removal to sterilize the urinary tract.

CYSTINE STONES

Cystine, lysine, ornithine, and citrulline share a common set of transporters in gut and kidney that can be deficient by heredity, as one of at least three autosomal recessive diseases (45). Only cystine causes disease, and only because it is insoluble enough to crystallize into stones. The stones begin in childhood, may be staghorns, and recur throughout life unless treated well.

The solubility of cystine in urine is about 1 mM/L and varies about twofold from person to person. Excretion rates in normal people and also in heterozygotes are micromolar, so neither form cystine stones. In homozygous cystinuric people, excretion rates range from 1 to 15 mM daily, usual values being about 3 to 6 mM, so high fluid intake, of 3 to 6 liters daily, is adequate for most people. Nocturia is mandatory because cystine is excreted constantly. Alkaline pH increases cystine solubility, but only above pH 7.4, and to raise urine pH above serum pH requires a high dose of alkali, enough to overbalance total daily acid production. Calcium phosphate stones could be fostered. Even so, alkali is generally recommended.

If water and alkali fail to prevent stones, add a drug that forms a soluble disulfide with cysteine, such as d-penicillamine (45). Cystine is itself the cysteine disulfide and is in equilibrium with cysteine; the drug forms its own cysteine disulfide and lowers free cysteine concentration, and cystine dissociates into cysteine. All available drugs cause allergic side effects such as skin rash and serum sickness reactions and reduce smell and taste; the latter symptoms respond to zinc repletion. Thiola, long in European use, is now also available in the United States.

REFERENCES

1. Coe FL, Parks JH, Moore EM: Familial idiopathic hypercalciuria. *N Engl J Med* 300:337–340, 1979
2. Coe FL, Parks JH: Familial (idiopathic) hypercalciuria. In: Coe FL, Parks JH (eds) *Nephrolithiasis: Pathogenesis and Treatment,* 2nd ed. Yearbook Medical, Chicago, 108–138, 1988
3. Weber DV, Coe FL, Parks JH, et al.: Urinary saturation measurements in calcium nephrolithiasis. *Ann Intern Med* 90:180–184, 1979
4. Coe FL, Bushinsky DA: Pathophysiology of hypercalciuria. *Am J Physiol* 247:F1–F13, 1984
5. Haussler MR, Baylink J, Hughes MR, et al.: The assay of 1,25-dihydroxy vitamin D3: Physiologic and pathologic modulation of circulating hormone levels. *Clin Endocrinol* 5:151S–165S, 1976
6. Kaplan RA, Haussler MR, Deftos LJ, et al.: The role of 1-alpha,25-dihyroxyvitamin D in the mediation of intestinal hyperabsorption of calcium in primary hyperparathyroidism and absorptive hypercalciuria. *J Clin Invest* 59:756–760, 1977
7. Gray RW, Wilz DR, Caldas AE, et al.: The importance of phosphate in regulating plasma 1,25 (OH)2-vitamin D levels in humans: Studies in healthy subjects, in calcium stone formers, and in patients with primary hyperparathyroidism. *J Clin Endocrinol Metab* 45:299–306, 1977

8. Shen FH, Baylink DJ, Neilsen RL: Increased serum 1,25-dihydroxyvitamin D in idiopathic hypercalciuria. *J Lab Clin Med* 90: 955–962, 1977

9. Coe FL, Favus MJ, Crockett T, et al.: Effects of low calcium diet on urine calcium excretion, parathyroid function and serum 1,25(OH)2D3 levels in patients with idiopathic hypercalciuria and in normal subjects. *Am J Med* 72:25–31, 1982

10. Broadus AE, Insogna KL, Lang R, et al.: Evidence for disordered control of 1,25-dihyroxyvitamin D production in absorptive hypercalciuria. *N Engl J Med* 311:73–80, 1984

11. Adams ND, Gray RW, Lemann J Jr: The effects of oral CaCO3 loading and dietary calcium deprivation on plasma 1,25-dihydroxyvitamin D concentrations in healthy adults. *J Clin Endocrinol Metab* 48:1008–1016, 1979

12. Maierhofer WJ, Lemann J Jr, Gray RW, et al.: Dietary calcium and serum 1,25-(OH)2-vitamin D concentrations as determinants of calcium balance in healthy men. *Kidney Int* 26:752–759, 1984

13. Coe L, Parks JH, Asplin JR: The pathogenesis and treatment of kidney stones, medical progress. *N Engl J Med* 327:1141–1152, 1992

14. Li XQ, Tembe V, Horwitz GM, Bushinsky DA, Favus MJ: Increased intestinal vitamin D receptor in genetic hypercalciuric rats: A cause of intestinal calcium reabsorption. *J Clin Invest* 91: 661–667, 1993

15. Weber DV, Coe FL, Parks JH, et al.: Urinary saturation measurements in calcium nephrolithiasis. *Ann Intern Med* 90:180–184, 1979

16. Coe FL: Treated and untreated recurrent calcium nephrolithiasis in patients with idiopathic hypercalciuria, hyperuricosuria, or no metabolic disorder. *Ann Intern Med* 87:404–410, 1977

17. Costanzo LS: Localization of diuretic action in microperfused rat distal tubules: Ca and Na transport. *Am J Physiol* 248:F527–535, 1985

18. Coe FL, Parks JH, Bushinsky DA, Langman CV, Favus MJ: Chlorthalidone promotes mineral retention in patients with idiopathic hypercalciuria. *Kidney Int* 33:1140–1146, 1988

19. Coe FL, Parks JH: Primary hyperparathyroidism. In: Coe FL, Parks JH (eds) *Nephrolithiasis: Pathogenesis and Treatment,* 2nd ed. Yearbook Medical, Chicago, 59–107, 1988

20. Johnson RD, Conn JW: Hyperparathyroidism with a prolonged period of normocalcemia. *JAMA* 210:2063–2066, 1969

21. Yendt ER, Gagne RJA: Detection of primary hyperparathyroidism, with special reference to its occurrence in hypercalciuric females with "normal" or borderline serum calcium. *Can Med Assoc J* 98:331–336, 1968

22. Wills MR, Pak CYC, Hammond WG, et al.: Normocalcemic primary hyperparathyroidism. *Am J Med* 47:384–391, 1979

23. Broadus AE, Horst RL, Lang R, et al.: The importance of circulating 1,25-dihydroxyvitamin D in the pathogenesis of hypercalciuria and renal-stone formation in primary hyperparathyroidism. *N Engl J Med* 302:421–426, 1980

24. Pak CYC, Nicar MJ, Peterson R, et al.: A lack of unique pathophysiologic background for nephrolithiasis of primary hyperparathyroidism. *J Clin Endocrinol Metab* 55:536–542, 1981

25. LoCascio V, Adami S, Galvanini G, et al.: Substrate-product relation of 1-hydroxylase activity in primary hyperparathyroidism. *N Engl J Med* 313:1123–1130, 1985

26. Transbol I, Gill JR, Lifschitz M, et al.: Intestinal absorption and renal excretion of calcium in metabolic acidosis and alkalosis. *Acta Endocrinol* 155(suppl):217, 1971

27. Coe FL, Parks JH: Stone disease in distal renal tubular acidosis. *Ann Intern Med* 93:60–61, 1980

28. Albright F, Burnett CH, Parson W, et al.: Osteomalacia and late rickets: The various etiologies met in the United States with emphasis on that resulting from a specific form of renal acidosis, the therapeutic indications for each sub-group, and the relationship between osteomalacia and Milkman's syndrome. *Medicine (Baltimore)* 25:399–479, 1946

29. Buckalew VM Jr, Purvis ML, Shulman MG, et al.: Hereditary renal tubular acidosis. *Medicine (Baltimore)* 53:229–254, 1974

30. Wrong O, Davies HEF: The excretion of acid in renal disease. *Q J Med* 28:259–311, 1959

31. Williams HE, Smith LH Jr: Disorders of oxalate metabolism. *Am J Med* 45:715, 1968

32. Hagler L, Herman RH: Oxalate metabolism. *Am J Clin Nutr* (5 parts) 26:758,882,1006,1073,1242, 1973

33. Hodgkinson A, Wilkinson R: Plasma oxalate concentration and renal excretion of oxalate in man. *Clin Sci* 46:61, 1974

34. Kathpalia SC, Favus MJ, Coe FL: Evidence for size and change permselectivity of rat ascending colon: Effects of ricinoleate and bile salts on oxalic acid and neutral sugar transport. *J Clin Invest* 74:805–811, 1984

35. Smith LH, Fromm H, Hoffman AF: Acquired hyperoxaluria, nephrolithiasis and intestinal disease. *N Engl J Med* 286:1371, 1972

36. Coe FL, Kavalich AG: Hypercalciuria and hyperuricosuria in patients with calcium nephrolithiasis. *N Engl J Med* 291:1344, 1974

37. Coe FL, Strauss AL, Tembe V, et al.: Uric acid saturation in calcium nephrolithiasis. *Kidney Int* 17:662–668, 1980

38. Coe FL: Uric acid and calcium oxalate nephrolithiasis. *Kidney Int* 24:392–403, 1983

39. Deganello S, Coe FL: Epitaxy between uric acid and whewellite: Experimental verification. *Am J Physiol* 6:270–276, 1983

40. Ettinger B, Tang A, Citron JT, et al.: Randomized trial of allopurinol in the prevention of calcium oxalate calculi. *N Engl J Med* 315:1386–1389, 1986

41. Kavalich AG, Moran E, Coe FL: Dietary purine consumption by hyperuricosuric calcium oxalate kidney stone formers and normal subjects. *J Chronic Dis* 29:745, 1976

42. Parks JH, Coe FL: A urinary calcium-citrate index for the evaluation of nephrolithiasis. *Kidney Int* 30:85–90, 1986

43. Herring LC: Observations on the analysis of ten thousand urinary calculi. *J Urol* 88:545–562, 1962

44. Kristensen C, Parks JH, Lindheimer M, Coe FL: Reduced glomerular filtration rate, hypercalciuria and clinical morbidity in primary struvite nephrolithiasis. *Kidney Int* 32:749–753, 1987

45. Segal S, Thier SO: Cystinuria. In: Stanbury JB, Wyngaarden JB, Fredrickson DS, et al. (eds) *The Metabolic Basis of Inherited Disease,* 5th ed. McGraw-Hill, New York, 1774–1791, 1983

80. Urologic Aspects of Nephrolithiasis Management

James E. Lingeman, M.D.

Methodist Hospital Institute for Kidney Stone Disease, Indianapolis, Indiana

Over the last decade, extracorporeal shock wave lithotripsy (ESWL), percutaneous nephrolithotomy (PCNL), and ureteroscopy (URS) have largely supplanted surgical lithotomy for the management of nonpassable, symptomatic, upper urinary tract calculi (1–4). As experience and data have been published regarding these important new techniques, their advantages and disadvantages relative to one another have come into clearer focus. This brief overview will provide a perspective regarding the current roles and indications for ESWL, PCNL, and URS.

From the urologic perspective, classification of urolithiasis patients is a necessary prerequisite to a rational approach in choosing optimal therapy (Table 1). A basic assumption in choosing the most appropriate initial approach to a given urolithiasis problem is that it is important to achieve as complete removal of the offending stone material as possible.

NONSTAGHORN RENAL CALCULI

Most renal calculi requiring therapy fall into this category. Although most patients with nonstaghorn renal calculi are best approached initially with ESWL, a consensus has developed that the results achieved, no matter what lithotripter was utilized, will be inversely proportional to the amount of stone material (i.e., the stone burden) requiring treatment. As stone size (Fig. 1) and number (Fig. 2) increase, stone-free rates decrease. The critical role of stone burden in the outcome expected with ESWL has been confirmed by numerous investigators (3,5,6). Percutaneous nephrolithotomy, although more invasive than ESWL, does produce significantly higher stone-free rates than ESWL (2,3). Based on the preceding observations, a National Institutes of Health (NIH) Consensus Conference in 1988 concluded that renal stones smaller than 2 cm (which represent the vast majority of cases) are generally effectively managed with ESWL, but that stones larger than 2 cm should be approached initially with PCNL (7).

STAGHORN RENAL CALCULI

Staghorn renal calculi are stones that fill a substantial portion of the renal collecting system (Fig. 3). Typically, such stones will occupy the renal pelvis, and branches of the stone will extend into one or more of the calices. There is no widely accepted way to express the size of a staghorn calculus, and, as a result, stones of widely differing volumes are all referred to as staghorns. Our group has attempted to clarify this problem by promoting the use of stone surface area (8,9). Staghorn calculi most commonly represent the products of ureolysis (struvite and carbonate apatite), but stones made of cystine, uric acid, and calcium oxalate can also form staghorn stones. The American Urologic Association (AUA) has recently published clinical guidelines for the

TABLE 1. *Classification scheme for urolithiasis patients*

Nonstaghorn stones
Staghorn stones
Special considerations
UPJ obstruction
Horseshoe kidneys
Calyceal diverticula
Ureteral stones

UPJ, ureteropelvic junction.

management of staghorn calculi which will be briefly summarized in Table 2.

An untreated staghorn renal calculus is associated with a significant risk of renal loss and indeed mortality (10,11). In most instances, infected staghorn stones harbor urea-splitting organisms deep within the interstices of the stone material, rendering sterilization of the urine impossible. Elimination of future risk of ureolysis requires that all the offending calculous material be removed whenever possible. Given the large amount of stone burden represented by most staghorn stones, PCNL and/or open surgery are preferred to ESWL in most instances.

SPECIAL CONSIDERATIONS

A variety of congenital anomalies may affect the upper urinary tract; they increase the risk of urolithiasis because they result in obstruction and/or stasis [horseshoe kidney, ureteropelvic junction (UPJ) obstruction, calyceal diverticulum]. The occurrence of renal calculi in 8.5% to 31.4% of patients with horseshoe kidneys is at least in part a result of the impeded drainage presented by these often elongated and bizarre renal collecting systems (12,13). Although ESWL may be used to treat horseshoe kidneys, the results of treatment are considerably more sensitive to the location and stone burden than when treating normal renal units (Fig. 4). These results reflect the increased difficulty in fragmenting calculi within horseshoe kidneys with ESWL and also the difficulty of eliminating gravel from these unusual collecting systems. If the patient has a solitary stone larger than 2 cm in diameter, or if multiple stones are present, then PCNL is preferred because it provides significantly better results.

Obstruction remains a contraindication to ESWL and therefore patients with UPJ obstructions and renal calculi should be managed either with stone removal at the time of open surgical pyeloplasty or with PCNL at the time of endopyelotomy, a new endoscopic surgical alternative to open surgical pyeloplasty. Endopyelotomy is successful in 80% to 90% of instances and is easily combined with PCNL (14,15).

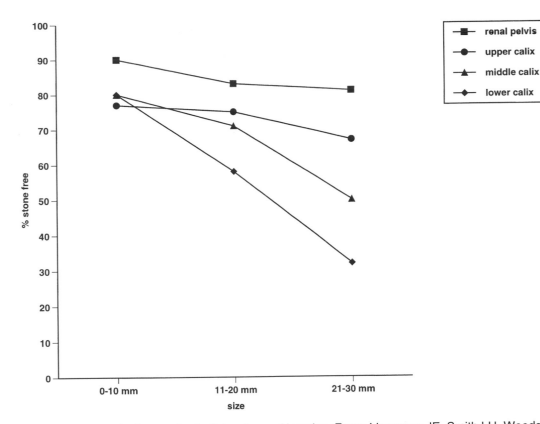

FIG. 1. ESWL results for renal calculi, by size and location. From: Lingeman JE, Smith LH, Woods JR, Newman DM. Bioeffects and long-term results of ESWL. In: Lingeman JE, Smith LH, Woods JR, Newman DM, eds. *Urinary Calculi: ESWL, Endourology, and Medical Therapy.* Lea & Febiger, Philadelphia, p 285, 1989.

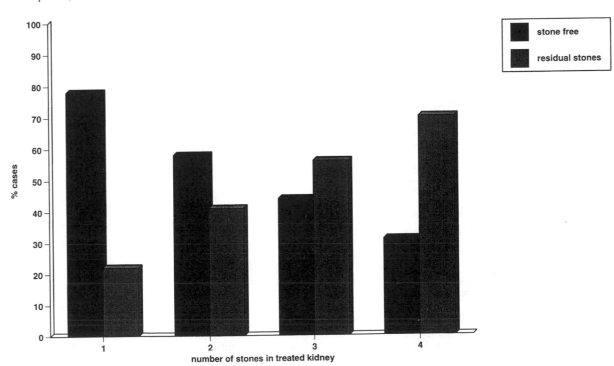

FIG. 2. Stone-free status after ESWL, as related to the number of stones treated. From: Lingeman JE, Smith LH, Woods JR, Newman DM. Bioeffects and long-term results of ESWL. In: Lingeman JE, Smith LH, Woods JR, Newman DM, eds. *Urinary Calculi: ESWL, Endourology, and Medical Therapy.* Lea & Febiger, Philadelphia, p 283, 1989.

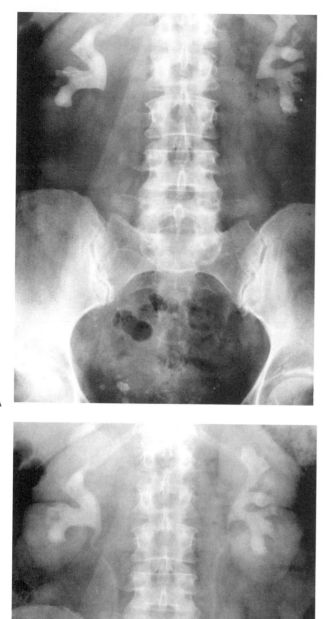

A

B

FIG. 3. KUB **(A)** and IVP **(B)** of a 56-year-old woman with bilateral staghorn calculi. She had a recurrent *Proteus mirabilis* urinary tract infection, and stone analysis revealed struvite and carbonate apatite. KUB, kidneys, ureters, and bladder; IVP, intravenous pyelogram.

TABLE 2. *American Urological Association clinical guidelines for staghorn calculi*

Standards
  A newly diagnosed struvite staghorn calculus represents an indication for active treatment intervention, as a policy of watchful waiting and observation is not in the best interest of the otherwise healthy patient with struvite staghorn calculi.
Guidelines
  Percutaneous stone removal, followed by ESWL and/or repeat percutaneous procedures as warranted, should be utilized for most patients with struvite staghorn calculi, with percutaneous lithotripsy being the first part of the combination therapy.
  ESWL monotherapy should not be used for most patients with struvite staghorn calculi as a first-line treatment choice.
  Open surgery (nephrolithotomy by any method) should not be used for most patients as a first-line treatment choice.
Options
  ESWL monotherapy and percutaneous lithotripsy monotherapy are equally effective treatment choices for small (<500 mm^2) struvite staghorn calculi in collecting systems that are of normal or near normal anatomy.
  Open surgery is an appropriate treatment alternative in unusual situations where a staghorn calculus is not expected to be removable by a reasonable number of percutaneous lithotripsy and/or ESWL procedures.
  For a patient with a poorly functioning, stone-bearing kidney, nephrectomy is a reasonable treatment alternative.

Recommendations for treatment are made with three levels of flexibility, based primarily on the strength of the scientific evidence for estimating outcomes of interventions. A standard is defined as the least flexible of the three; a guideline is more flexible, and an option is the most flexible.(From: ref. 23.)

When calyceal diverticula, although rare, are present, they are commonly complicated by the occurrence of renal calculi, presumably as a result of the stasis present within these nonsecretory cavities (Fig. 5). Typically, the ostium connecting a calyceal diverticulum to the rest of the renal collecting system is tiny, and this observation combined with their lack of urine production explains why few, if any, stone-containing calyceal diverticula can be successfully managed with ESWL (16,17). These uncommon cases are better managed via an endourologic approach (PCNL or URS) with or without concomitant fulguration of the diverticulum (16,18).

URETERAL CALCULI

Most ureteral calculi are small (<5 mm) and have a reasonable chance of spontaneous passage. However, when ureteral stones are larger or symptoms intractable, most ureteral calculi can be managed with ureteroscopy or ESWL. A recent trend in the management of ureteral calculi has been the increasing utilization of ESWL *in situ,* a technique that usually does not entail ureteral stenting or other instrumentation and that can often be accomplished with minimal anes-

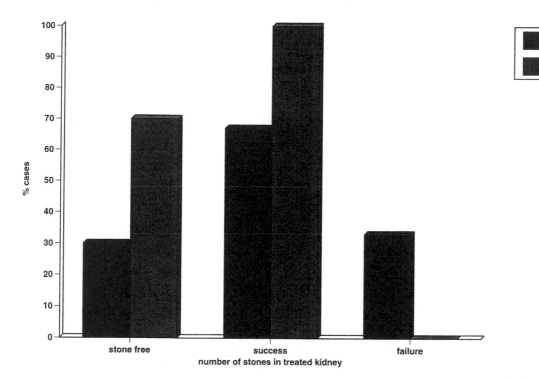

FIG. 4. Results of treatment of horseshoe kidney (nonstaghorn calculi), comparing ESWL and PCNL. (*Success* includes stone-free results and clinically insignificant residual fragments.) From: Lingeman JE, Smith LH, Woods JR, Newman DM. Bioeffects and long-term results of ESWL. In: Lingeman JE, Smith LH, Woods JR, Newman DM, eds. *Urinary Calculi: ESWL, Endourology, and Medical Therapy.* Lea & Febiger, Philadelphia, p 216, 1989.

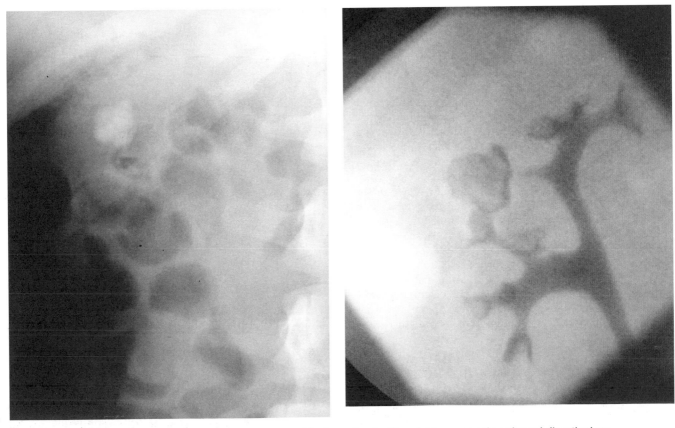

FIG. 5. KUB **(A)** and retrograde pyelogram **(B)** of a patient with a right upper pole calyceal diverticulum. This stone was calcium oxalate monohydrate.

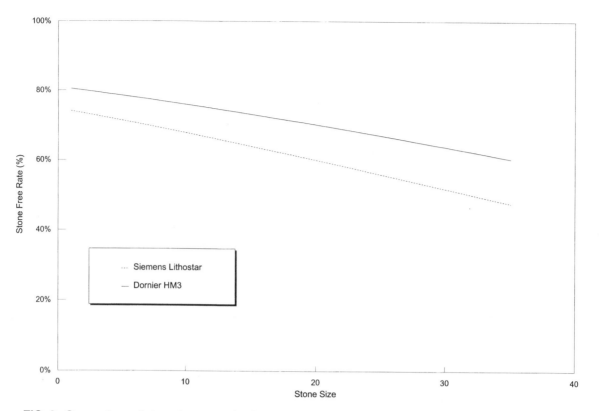

FIG. 6. Comparison of stone-free rates for Siemens Lithostar and unmodified Dornier HM3 lithotripters. From: Lingeman JE, Zafar FS. Lithotripsy systems. In: Smith AD, Lingeman JE, Preminger GM, et al. (eds) *Smith's Textbook of Endourology.* Quality Medical Publishers, St. Louis, p 581, 1996.

thetic requirements. However, as ureteral calculi are more difficult to fragment than renal calculi of comparable size, retreatment or other ancillary procedures are necessary in about one third of cases managed with ESWL *in situ.* Ultimately, approximately 80% to 85% of patients with ureteral calculi will become stone free with ESWL *in situ,* no matter where the stone is located in the ureter. Ureteroscopy, while more invasive, achieves better stone clearance in the lower ureter and is still commonly performed in this situation (19,20). For calculi in the mid- or upper ureter, ureteroscopy with rigid instruments is less successful than ESWL *in situ* or another commonly used ESWL technique (retrograde stone manipulation followed by ESWL to the kidney). In recent years, the advent of small (7.5 to 10 Fr.) flexible uretero-scopes combined with laser lithotripsy has increased the effectiveness of URS for upper ureteral calculi. In summary, at the present time, several effective and minimally invasive approaches for the management of ureteral calculi are available. The choice of treatment depends to a large extent on patient preferences and local circumstances (i.e., the availability of a lithotripter).

FUTURE TRENDS: NEW LITHOTRIPTERS

There are currently 29 ESWL devices marketed by 15 manufacturers (21). Interestingly, there is no evidence to date to suggest that newer lithotripters are more effective or safer than the original ESWL device, the Dornier HM3.

Newer lithotripters in general do have lessened anesthesia requirements than the original HM3, but this potential benefit appears to be counterbalanced by their lower efficacy (Fig. 6) (22). Because of its unsurpassed efficacy, the Dornier HM3 lithotripter remains in widespread use today.

SUMMARY

While 80% to 85% of symptomatic renal calculi are best managed initially with ESWL, it should be apparent that PCNL and URS retain significant roles in the current urologic management of the nephrolithiasis patient. Patients with substantial stone burden or anatomic abnormalities are usually preferentially managed initially with PCNL. ESWL *in situ* for the management of ureteral calculi is increasing in popularity. Ureteroscopy, particularly in the lower ureter, remains an attractive, widely available, cost-effective alternative.

REFERENCES

1. Lingeman JE, Woods JR, Toth PD, Evan AP, McAteer JA: The role of lithotripsy and its side effects. *J Urol* 141:793–797, 1989
2. Segura JW, Patterson DE, LeRoy AJ, Williams HJ, Barrett DM, Benson RC, May CR, Bender GE: Percutaneous removal of kidney stones: Review of 1,000 cases. *J Urol* 134:1077, 1985
3. Lingeman JE, Coury TA, Newman DM, Kahnoski RJ, Mertz JHO, Mosbaugh PG, Steele RE, Woods JR: Comparison of results and morbidity of percutaneous nephrostolithotomy and extracorporeal shock wave lithotripsy. *J Urol* 138:485, 1987

4. Lyon ES, Huffman JL, Bagley DH: Ureteroscopy and ureteral pyeloscopy. *Urology* 23:29, 1984
5. Politis G, Griffith DP: ESWL: Stone-free efficacy based on stone size and location. *World J Urol* 5:255, 1987
6. Psihrmas KE, Jewett MAS, Bombardier C, et al.: Lithostar extracorporeal shock wave lithotripsy: The first 1,000 patients. *J Urol* 147:1006, 1992
7. NIH Consensus Conference. Prevention and Treatment of Kidney Stones. *JAMA* 260:978, 1988
8. Lam HS, Lingeman JE, Russo R, Chua GT: Stone surface area determination techniques: A unifying concept of staghorn stone burden assessment. *J Urol* 148:1026–1029, 1992
9. Lam HS, Lingeman JE, Barron M, Newman DM, et al.: Staghorn calculi: Analysis of treatment results between initial percutaneous nephrostolithotomy and extracorporeal shock wave lithotripsy monotherapy with reference to surface area. *J Urol* 147:1219–1225, 1992
10. Rous SM, Turner WR: Retrospective study of 95 patients with staghorn calculus disease. *J Urol* 118:902, 1977
11. Blandy JP, Singh M: The case for a more aggressive approach to staghorn stones. *J Urol* 115:505, 1976
12. Evans WP, Resnick MI: Horseshoe kidney and urolithiasis. *J Urol* 125:620, 1981
13. Pitts WR, Muecke EC: Horseshoe kidneys: A 40-year experience. *J Urol* 113:743, 1975
14. Van Cangh PJ, Jorion JL, Wese FX, Opsomer RJ: Endoureteral pyelotomy: Percutaneous treatment of ureteral pelvic junction obstruction. *J Urol* 141:1317, 1989
15. Motola JA, Badlani GH, Smith AD: Results of 212 consecutive endopyelotomies: An eight-year follow up. *J Urol* 149:453, 1993
16. Jones JA, Lingeman JE, Steidle CP: The roles of extracorporeal shock wave lithotripsy and percutaneous nephrostolithotomy in the management of pyelocaliceal diverticula. *J Urol* 146:724–727, 1991
17. Mobley TB, Meyers DA, Grine WB, et al.: Low energy lithotripsy with Lithostar: Treatment results with 19,962 renal and ureteral calculi. *J Urol* 149:1419, 1993
18. Fuchs GJ, David RD: Flexible ureterorenoscopy, dilatation of narrow calyceal neck, and ESWL: A new, minimally invasive approach to stones in calyceal diverticula. *J Urol* 143:255, 1989
19. Lingeman JE, Sonda LP, Kahnoski RJ, Coury TA, Newman DM, Mosbaugh PG, Mertz JHO, Steele RE, Frank B: Ureteral stone management: Emerging concepts. *J Urol* 135:1172, 1986
20. Lyon ES: Ureteral calculi: Treatment in transition *(editorial)*. *J Urol* 139:1286, 1988
21. Lingeman JE: Update on ESWL. *AUA Update Series,* lesson 28, vol XIV, 1995
22. Lingeman JE, Zafar FS: Lithotripsy systems. In: Smith AD, Lingeman JE, Preminger GM, et al. (eds) *Smith's Textbook of Endourology.* Quality Medical Publishers, St. Louis, 553–589, 1996
23. Segura JW, Preminger GM, Assimos DG, Dretler SP, Kahn RI, Lingeman JE, Macaluso JN Jr., McCullough DL: Nephrolithiasis Clinical Guidelines Panel summary report on the management of staghorn calculi. *J Urol* 151:1648–1651, 1994

SECTION XI

Appendix

i. Growth Charts for Males and Females

Reg. No.

Surname

Forename

Date of Birth   /   /   .
                 Decimal Yr.

Notes/Treatment _____

_____

_____

_____

_____

_____

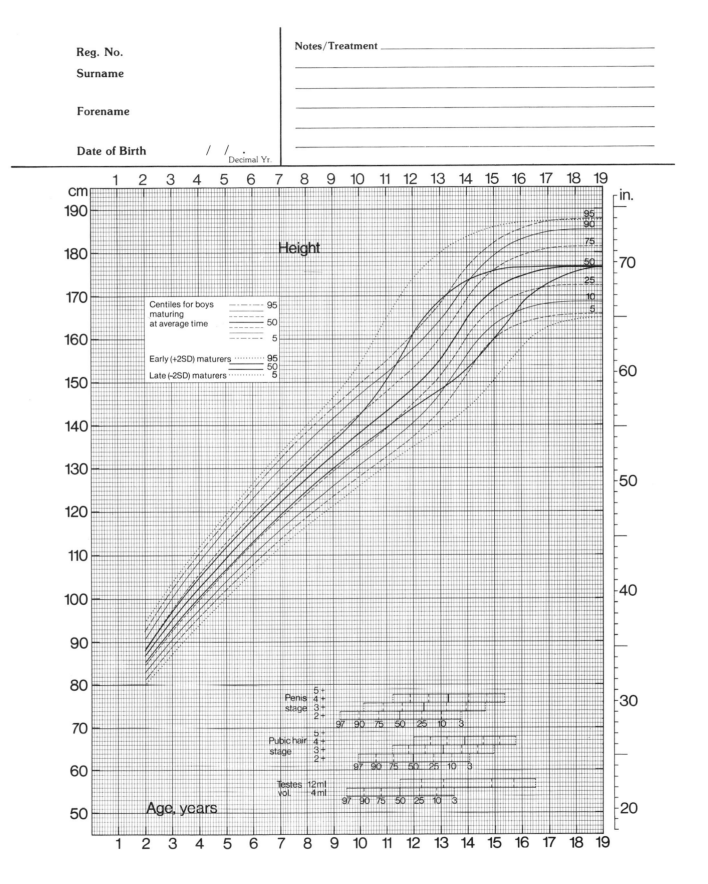

447

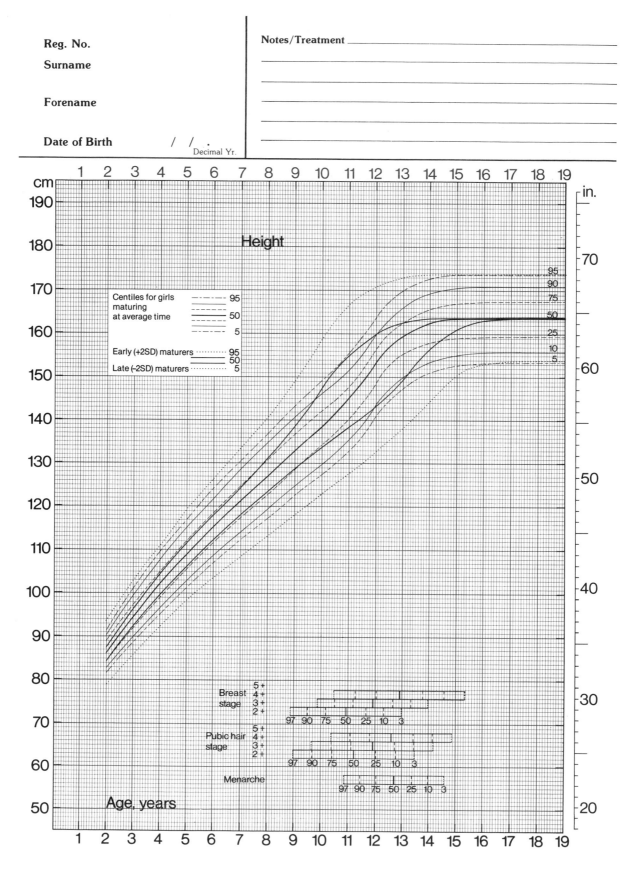

Reg. No.

Surname

Forename

Date of Birth   / / .
Decimal Yr.

Notes/Treatment _____

cm

190

180

Height

170

Centiles for girls
maturing
at average time

95
50
5

Early (+2SD) maturers
Late (−2SD) maturers

95
50
5

95
90
75
50
25
10
5

160

150

140

130

120

110

100

90

80

Breast
stage

5 +
4 +
3 +
2 +

97 90 75 50 25 10 3

70

Pubic hair
stage

5 +
4 +
3 +
2 +

97 90 75 50 25 10 3

60

Menarche

97 90 75 50 25 10 3

50

Age, years

in.

70

60

50

40

30

20

ii. Ossification Centers

Age-at-appearance percentiles for major postnatal ossification centers

| | Percentiles | | | | | |
| | Boys | | | Girls | | |
Ossification center	5th	50th	95th	5th	50th	95th
Head of humerus	37g	2w	4m	37g	2w	3m3
Proximal epiphysis of tibia	34g	2w	5w	34g	1w	2w
Coracoid process of scapula	37g	2w	4m2	37g	2w	5m
Cuboid of tarsus	37g	3w	3m3	37g	3w	2m
Capitate of carpus	—	3m	7m	—	2m	7m
Hamate of carpus	2w	3m3	10m	2w	2m1	7m
Capitulum of humerus	3w	4m	13m	3w	3m	9m1
Head of femur	3w	4m1	7m3	2w	4m	7m2
Third cuneiform of tarsus	3w	5m2	19m	—	2m3	14m3
Greater tubercle of humerus	3m	10m	2y4	2m2	6m1	13m3
Primary center, middle segment of 5th toe	—	12m2	3y10	—	9m	2y1
Distal epiphysis of radius	6m2	12m1	2y4	4m3	10m	20m2
Epiphysis, distal segment of 1st toe	8m2	12m3	2y1	4m3	9m2	20m1
Epiphysis, middle segment of 4th toe	5m	14m3	2y11	5m	11m	3y
Epiphysis, proximal segment of 3rd finger	9m1	16m2	2y5	5m	10m1	19m2
Epiphysis, middle segment of 3rd toe	5m	17m	4y3	2m3	12m1	2y6
Epiphysis, proximal segment of 2nd finger	9m2	17m	2y2	5m	10m2	19m3
Epiphysis, proximal segment of 4th finger	9m3	18m	2y5	5m	11m	20m
Epiphysis, distal segment of 1st finger	9m	17m1	2y8	5m	12m	20m3
Epiphysis, proximal segment of 3rd toe	11m	19m	2y6	6m1	12m3	22m3
Epiphysis of 2nd metacarpal	11m1	19m2	2y10	7m3	13m	20m1
Epiphysis, proximal segment of 4th toe	11m2	19m3	2y8	7m2	15m	2y1
Epiphysis, proximal segment of 2nd toe	11m3	21m	2y8	7m3	14m2	2y1
Epiphysis of 3rd metacarpal	11m2	21m2	3y	8m	13m2	23m1
Epiphysis, proximal segment of 5th finger	12m	22m1	2y10	8m	14m2	2y1
Epiphysis, middle segment of 3rd finger	12m1	2y	3y4	7m3	15m2	2y4
Epiphysis of 4th metacarpal	13m	2y	3y7	9m	15m2	2y2
Epiphysis, middle segment of 2nd toe	10m3	2y1	4y1	6m	14m1	2y3
Epiphysis, middle segment of 4th finger	12m	2y1	3y3	7m3	15m	2y5
Epiphysis of 5th metacarpal	15m1	2y2	3y10	10m2	16m2	2y4
First cuneiform of tarsus	10m3	2y2	3y9	6m	17m1	2y10
Epiphysis of 1st metatarsal	16m3	2y2	3y1	11m3	19m	2y3
Epiphysis, middle segment of 2nd finger	15m3	2y2	3y4	8m	17m2	2y7
Epiphysis, proximal segment of 1st toe	17m2	2y4	3y4	10m3	18m3	2y5
Epiphysis, distal segment of 3rd finger	15m3	2y5	3y9	8m3	17m3	2y8
Triquetrium of carpus	6m	2y5	5y6	3m2	20m2	3y9
Epiphysis, distal segment of 4th finger	16m2	2y5	3y9	8m3	18m1	2y10
Epiphysis, proximal segment of 5th toe	18m2	2y6	3y8	11m3	20m3	2y8
Epiphysis of 1st metacarpal	17m2	2y7	4y4	11m	19m1	2y8
Second cuneiform of tarsus	14m2	2y8	4y3	9m3	21m3	3y
Epiphysis of 2nd metatarsal	23m1	2y10	4y4	14m3	2y2	3y5
Greater trochanter of femur	23m	3y	4y4	11m2	22m1	3y
Epiphysis, proximal segment of 1st finger	22m1	3y	4y7	11m1	20m2	2y10
Navicular of tarsus	13m2	3y	5y5	9m1	23m1	3y7
Epiphysis, distal segment of 2nd finger	21m3	3y2	5y	12m3	2y6	3y4
Epiphysis, distal segment of 5th finger	2y1	3y4	5y	12m	23m2	3y6
Epiphysis, middle segment of 5th finger	23m1	3y5	5y10	10m3	23m3	3y7
Proximal epiphysis of fibula	22m2	3y6	5y3	16m	2y7	3y11
Epiphysis of 3rd metatarsal	2y4	3y6	5y	17m1	2y6	3y8
Epiphysis, distal segment of 5th toe	2y4	3y11	6y4	14m1	2y4	4y1
Patella of knee	2y6	4y	6y	17m3	2y6	4y
Epiphysis of 4th metatarsal	2y11	4y	5y9	21m1	2y10	4y1
Lunate of carpus	18m2	4y1	6y9	13m	2y8	5y8
Epiphysis, distal segment of 3rd toe	3y	4y4	6y2	16m2	2y9	4y1
Epiphysis of 5th metatarsal	3y1	4y5	6y4	2y1	3y3	4y11

449

Age-at-appearance percentiles for major postnatal ossification centers Continued.

	Percentiles					
	Boys			Girls		
Ossification center	5th	50th	95th	5th	50th	95th
Epiphysis, distal segment of 4th toe	2y11	4y5	6y5	16m2	2y7	4y1
Epiphysis, distal segment of 2nd toe	3y3	4y8	6y9	18m	2y11	4y6
Capitulum of radius	3y	5y3	8y	2y3	3y11	6y3
Scaphoid of carpus	3y7	5y8	7y10	2y4	4y1	6y
Greater multangular of carpus	3y7	5y11	9y	23m1	4y1	6y4
Lesser multangular of carpus	3y1	6y3	8y6	2y5	4y2	6y
Medial epicondyle of humerus	4y3	6y3	8y5	2y1	3y5	5y1
Distal epiphysis of ulna	5y3	7y1	9y1	3y4	5y5	7y8
Epiphysis of calcaneus	5y2	7y7	9y7	3y7	5y5	7y4
Olecranon of ulna	7y9	9y8	11y11	5y8	8y	9y11
Lateral epicondyle of humerus	9y3	11y3	13y8	7y2	9y3	11y3
Tubercle of tibia	9y11	11y10	13y5	7y11	10y3	11y10
Adductor sesamoid of 1st finger	11y	12y9	14y8	8y8	10y9	12y8
Acetabulum	11y11	13y7	15y4	9y7	11y6	13y5
Acromion	12y2	13y9	15y6	10y4	11y11	13y10
Epiphysis, iliac crest of hip	12y	14y	15y11	10y10	12y10	15y4
Accessory epiphysis, coracoid process of scapula	12y9	14y4	16y4	10y5	12y3	14y5
Ischial tuberosity	13y7	15y3	17y1	11y9	13y11	16y

From: Garn SM, et al. *Med Radiogr Photogr* 43:45–66, 1967.

g, gestational week; w, week; m, month; y, year. The number following m or y refers to the next smaller time unit (e.g., 9y4 = 9 years 4 months).

iii. Laboratory Values of Importance for Calcium Metabolism and Metabolic Bone Disease

Laboratory values of importance for calcium metabolism and metabolic bone disease[a]

Test	Source of specimen	Reference range		Reference range (SI units)
			mg/dl	mmol/L
Calcium, ionized	Serum or plasma	Cord:	5.5 ± 0.3	1.37 ± 0.07
		Newborn		
		3–24 h:	4.3–5.1	1.07–1.27
		24–48 h:	4.0–4.7	1.00–1.17
		Adult:	4.48–4.92	1.12–1.23
		>60 yr		1.13–1.30
			mg/dl	mmol/L
Calcium, total	Serum[b]	Child:	8.8–10.8	2.2–2.7
		Adult:	8.4–10.2	2.1–2.55
	Urine	Ca^{2+} in diet	mg/dl	mmol/d
		Free Ca^{2+}:	5–40	0.13–1.0
		Low to average:	50–150	1.25–3.8
		Average (20 mmol/d):	100–300	2.5–7.5
	Feces	Average: 0.64 g/d		16 mmol/d
Magnesium	Serum	1.3–2.1 mEq/L (higher in females during menses)		0.65–1.05 mmol/L
	Urine, 24-h	6.0–100 mEq/d		3.0–5.0 mmol/d
Phosphatase, acid	Serum	<3.0 ng/ml		<3.0 µg/L
Prostatic (RIA)		0.11–0.60 U/L		0.11–0.60 U/L
Roy, Brower, and				
Hayden, 37 C				
Phosphatase, alkaline	Serum			U/L
p-nitrophenyl phosphate,		Infant:		50–165
carbonate buffer, 30 C		Child:		20–150
		Adult:		20–70
		>60 yr:		30–75
Bowers and McComb, 30 C				25–90
IFFC, 30 C		Male:		30–90
		Female:		20–80
Phosphorus, inorganic	Serum		mg/dl	nmol/L
		Cord:	3.7–8.1	1.2–2.6
		Child:	4.5–5.5	1.45–1.78
		Thereafter	2.7–4.5	0.87–1.45
		>60 yr		
		Male:	2.3–3.7	0.74–1.2
		Female:	2.8–4.1	0.9–1.3
	Urine	Adult on diet containing 0.9–1.5 g P and 10 mg Ca/kg: <1.0 g/d		On diet containing 29–48 mmol P and 0.25 mmol Ca/kg: <32 mmol/d
		Unrestricted diet: 0.4–1.3 g/d		Unrestricted diet: 13–42 mmol/d
Tubular reabsorption of phosphate	Urine, 4 h (0800–1200 h), and serum	82%–95%		Fraction reabsorbed: 0.82–0.95
Vitamin A	Serum	30–65 µg/dl		1.05–2.27 mmol/L
Vitamin D_3, 25 hydroxy	Plasma	Summer: 15–80 ng/ml		37–200 nmol/L
		Winter: 14–42 ng/ml		35–105 nmol/L
Vitamin D_3, 1,25 dihydroxy	Serum	25–45 pg/ml		12–46 µmol/L

Laboratory values of importance for calcium metabolism and metabolic bone disease[a] Continued.

Test	Source of specimen	Reference range		Reference range (SI units)
Calcitonin[d]	Serum (Nichols RIA)	Basal	pg/ml	
		Male	<36	
		Female	<17	
		Pentagastrin		
		Male	<106	
		Female	<29	
	Serum (CIS 2-site IRMA)	Basal	pg/ml	
		Male	<10	
		Female	<10	
		Pentagastrin		
		Male	<30	
		Female	<30	
	Serum (Mayo Medical Lab)	Basal		
		Male	<19	
		Female	<14	
		Pentagastrin		
		Male	<110	
		Female	<30	
Parathyroid hormone[d]	Serum (intact, Mayo Lab)	Basal	1.0–5.0 pmol/L	
	Serum (intact, Nichols Institute)	Basal	10–65 pg/ml	
	Serum (mid-molecule, Nichols Institute)	Basal	50–330 pg/ml	
	Serum (N-terminal, Nichols Institute)	Basal	8–24 pg/ml	
Osteocalcin[d]	Serum (Nichols Institute)	Basal	1.6–9.2 ng/ml	
PTHrP[d]	Serum (intact, Nichols Institute)	Basal	<0.5 pmol/L	
Procollagen (PICP)	Plasma (Osteometer A/S)	Basal		
		Male	128 ng/ml	
		Female	115 ng/ml	
Pyridinium (PYD) crosslinks	Urine (Metra Biosystems)	Basal		
		Male	8–24 nM PYD/mM creatinine	
		Female	10–28 nM PYD/mM creatinine	
Type 1 collagen peptides	Urine (Osteometer A/S)	Basal		
		Female		
		(Premenopausal)	0.293 ± 0.155 µg/µmol creatinine (mean ± SD)	
		(Postmenopausal)	0.532 ± 0.229 µg/µmol creatinine	

[a]Laboratory values in this table were extracted from: Tietz NW. Reference ranges and laboratory values of clinical importance. In: Wyngaarden JB, Smith LH Jr (eds): *Cecil Textbook of Medicine*, 17th ed. Philadelphia: Saunders, 1985. This reference provides more detailed discussion of source material and units used in this table.

[b]Divide by 2 to get mEq/L.

[c]The total serum calcium can be corrected for alterations in the serum protein concentration by the following formula: Corrected total serum calcium (mg/dl) = observed total serum calcium + [(the normal mean albumin concentration - the observed albumin concentration) $\times$ 0.8]. In most situations, the normal mean albumin concentration equals 4 g/dl.

[d]The normal values listed include commercial assays. These are listed not to provide an endorsement for these assays, but because they are representative of values available for daily clinical use. It is likely that normal values in other research or commercial assays will vary to some extent.

iv. Mineral and Vitamin D RDAs for Infants, Children, and Adults

Recommended dietary allowances[a]   *Continues—*

	Age (yr)	Weight (kg/lb)	Height (cm/in)	Protein (g)	Vitamin A (µg RE)[b]	Vitamin D (µg)[c]	Vitamin E (mg Å-TE)[d]	Vitamin C (mg)
					Fat-soluble vitamins			
Infants	0–0.5	6/13	60/24	kg × 2.2	420	10	3	35
	0.5–1	9/20	71/28	kg × 2.2	400	10	4	35
Children	1–3	13/29	90/35	23	400	10	5	45
	4–6	20/44	112/44	30	500	10	6	45
	7–10	28/62	132/52	34	700	10	7	45
Males	11–14	45/99	157/62	45	1000	10	8	50
	15–18	66/145	176/69	56	1000	10	10	60
	19–22	70/154	177/70	56	1000	7.5	10	60
	23–50	70/154	178/70	56	1000	5	10	60
	51+	70/154	178/70	56	1000	5	10	60
Females	11–14	46/101	157/62	46	800	10	8	50
	15–18	55/120	163/64	44	800	10	8	60
	19–22	55/120	163/64	44	800	7.5	8	60
	23–50	55/120	163/64	44	800	5	8	60
	51+	55/120	163/64	44	800	5	8	60
Pregnant				+30	+200	+5	+2	+20
Lactating				+20	+400	+5	+3	+40

—Continues

	Thiamin (mg)	Riboflavin (mg)	Niacin (mg NE)[e]	Vitamin B$_6$ (mg)	Folacin (µg)[f]	Vitamin B$_{12}$ (µg)	Calcium (mg)	Phosphorus (mg)	Magnesium (mg)
	Water-soluble vitamins						Minerals		
Infants	0.3	0.4	6	0.3	30	0.5[g]	360	240	50
	0.5	0.6	8	0.6	45	1.5	540	360	70
Children	0.7	0.8	9	0.9	100	2.0	800	800	150
	0.9	1.0	11	1.3	200	2.5	800	800	200
	1.2	1.4	16	1.6	300	3.0	800	800	250
Males	1.4	1.6	18	1.8	400	3.0	1200	1200	350
	1.4	1.7	18	2.0	400	3.0	1200	1200	400
	1.5	1.7	19	2.2	400	3.0	800	800	350
	1.4	1.6	18	2.2	400	3.0	800	800	350
	1.2	1.4	16	2.2	400	3.0	800	800	350
Females	1.1	1.3	15	1.8	400	3.0	1200	1200	300
	1.1	1.3	14	2.0	400	3.0	1200	1200	300
	1.1	1.3	14	2.0	400	3.0	800[h]	800	300
	1.0	1.2	13	2.0	400	3.0	800	800	300
	1.0	1.2	13	2.0	400	3.0	800	800	300
Pregnant	+0.4	+0.3	+2	+0.6	+400	+1.0	+400	+400	+150
Lactating	+0.5	+0.5	+5	+0.5	+100	+1.0	+400	+400	+150

[a]Food and Nutrition Board, National Academy of Sciences/National Research Council (Revised 1980).

[b]Retinol equivalents. 1 retinol equivalent = 1 µg retinol or 6 µg; β carotene.

[c]As cholecalciferol, 10 µg cholecalciferol = 400 IU vitamin D.

[d]Å-Tocopherol equivalents. 1 mg *d*-Å-tocopherol = 1 Å-TE.

[e]One NE (niacin equivalent) is equal to 1 mg of niacin or 60 mg of dietary tryptophan.

[f]The folacin allowances refer to dietary sources as determined by *Lactobacillus casei* assay.

[g]The RDA for vitamin B$_{12}$ in infants is based on the average concentration of the vitamin in human milk, and other considerations such as intestinal absorption.

[h]As a result of the NIH Consensus Conference in Osteoporosis (1983), recommendations for calcium intake have been increased to 1000 mg/day and 1500 mg/day for pre- (after the age of 19) and post-menopausal women, respectively.

v. Formulary of Drugs Commonly Used in Treatment of Mineral Disorders

Formulary of drugs commonly used in treatment of mineral disorders[a]

Drug	Application in treatment of bone and mineral disorders	Dosage (adult)[b]	Rx Cat[c]	Notes[d]
Hormones and analogs				
1. Calcitonin				
Human (Cibacalcin) im or sc (0.5 mg vials)	Paget's disease	0.25–0.5 mg im or sc; q24h	Rx	
Salmon (Calcimar, Miacalcin) im or sc (100, 200 IU/ml) (sc preferred)	Paget's disease, osteoporosis, hypercalcemia	50–100 IU, im or sc; qod or qd for Paget's or osteoporosis; 4–6 IU/kg im or sc; qid for hypercalcemia	Rx	Modestly effective and short-lived in treatment of hypercalcemia
Nasal spray (200 IU/spray)		200 IU nasal qd for osteoporosis	Rx	
2. Estrogens				
Estinyl estradiol (Estinyl, Seminone), po (0.02, 0.05, 0.5 mg)	Postmenopausal osteoporosis	0.02–0.05 mg; qd 3/4 weeks	Rx	To reduce risk of . endometrial cancer, estrogens can be cycled with a progesterone during last 7–10 days or given concurrently with a progestin throughout the cycle (less break-through bleeding)
17B estradiol (Estrace), po (1, 2 mg)		1–2 mg; qd 3/4 weeks	Rx	
Transderm patch (Estraderm)		0.05–0.1 mg 2x/wk	Rx	
Conjugated equine estrogens (Premarin), po (0.3, 0.625, 0.9, 1.25, 2.5 mg)		0.625–1.25 mg qd 3/4 weeks	Rx	0.3 mg conjugated equine estrogens (CEE) with calcium may also be effective.
3. Glucocorticoids				
Prednisone (Deltasone), po (2.5, 5, 10, 20, 50 mg)	Hypercalcemia due to sarcoidosis, vitamin D intoxication, and certain malignancies such as multiple myeloma and related lymphoproliferative disorders	10–60 mg; qd	Rx	Long-term use results in osteoporosis and adrenal suppression. Other glucocorticoids with minimal mineralcorticoid activity can be used.
4. Parathyroid hormone				
Human 1–34 (Parathor), iv (200 U/vial)	Diagnosis of pseudo-hypoparathyroidism	200 U; over 10 min infusion	Rx	The use of PTH to treat osteoporosis is being evaluated.
5. Progesterone				
Medroxyprogesterone (Provera), po (2.5, 5, 10 mg)	Osteoporosis in conjunction with estrogens	10 mg; qd for final 7 to 10 days of cycle	Rx	The concurrent use of progesterone does not appear to reduce the protective cardiovascular effects of estrogen or diminish the potential risk for breast cancer.
Norethindrone (Micronor, Nor-QD, Norlutin), po (5 mg)		5 mg; qd for final 7 to 10 days of cycle 2.5 mg continuously with estrogen	Rx	

Formulary of drugs commonly used in treatment of mineral disorders[a] Continued.

Drug	Application in treatment of bone and mineral disorders	Dosage (adult)[b]	Rx Cat[c]	Notes[d]
6. Vitamin D preparations				
Cholecalciferol or D_3, po (125, 250, 400 U, often in combination with calcium)	Nutritional vitamin D deficiency, osteoporosis, malabsorption, hypoparathyroidism, refractory rickets	400–1000 U; as dietary supplement	OTC	
Ergocalciferol or D_2 (Calciferol), po (8000 U/ml drops; 25,000, 50,000 U tabs)		25,000–100,000 U; 3×/wk to qd	Rx, OTC	D_2 (or D_3) has been shown to reduce fractures and increase BMD in elderly women at 400–1000 U doses.
Calcifediol or 25(OH)D_3 (Calderol), (20, 50 mg)	Malabsorption, renal osteodystrophy	20–50 μg; 3×/wk to qd	Rx	25(OH)D_3 may be useful in treatment for steroid-induced osteoporosis.
Calcitriol or 1,25(OH)$_2D_3$ (Rocaltrol), po (0.25, 0.5 μg); (Calcijex), iv (1 or 2 μg/ml)	Renal osteodystrophy, hypoparathyroidism, refractory rickets	0.25–1.0 μg; qd to bid	Rx	Role of calcitriol in treatment of osteoporosis, psoriasis, and certain malignancies is being evaluated, primarily with new analogs.
Dihydrotachysterol (DHT), po (0.125, 0.2, 0.4 mg)	Renal osteodystrophy, hypoparathyroidism	0.2–1.0 mg; qd	Rx	
Bisphosphonates				
1. **Etidronate** (Didronel), po (200, 400 mg); iv (300 mg/6 ml vial)	Paget's disease, heterotopic ossification, hypercalcemia of malignancy	po: 5 mg/kg, qd for 6/12 mo for Paget's disease; 20 mg/kg, qd 1 mo before to 3 mo after total hip replacement; 10–20 mg/kg, qd for 3 mo after spinal cord injury for heterotopic ossification. iv: 7.5 mg/kg, qd for 3 d, given in 250–500 ml normal saline for hypercalcemia of malignancy.	Rx	Etidronate is the first-generation bisphosphonate. High doses may cause a mineralization disorder not seen with newer bisphosphonates.
2. **Alendronate** (Fosamax), po (10 mg)	Osteoporosis, Paget's disease	10 mg qd for osteoporosis; 40 mg qd for Paget's disease	Rx	
3. **Pamidronate** (Aredia), iv (30–90 mg/10 ml)	Hypercalcemia of malignancy, Paget's disease	60–90 mg given as a single intravenous infusion over 24 h for hypercalcemia of malignancy; 4-h infusions also effective for 30- or 60-mg doses. 30-mg doses over 4 h on 3 consecutive days for a total of 90 mg for Paget's disease	Rx	
Minerals				
1. **Bicarbonate, sodium**, po (325, 527, 650 mg)	Chronic metabolic acidosis leading to bone disease	Must be titrated for each patient	Rx, OTC	

Formulary of drugs commonly used in treatment of mineral disorders[a] Continued.

Drug	Application in treatment of bone and mineral disorders	Dosage (adult)[b]	Rx Cat[c]	Notes[d]
2. Calcium preparations				
Calcium carbonate (40% Ca), po (500, 650 mg)	Hypocalcemia (if symptomatic should be treated iv), osteoporosis, rickets, osteomalacia, chronic renal failure, hypoparathyroidism, malabsorption, enteric oxaluria	po: 400–2000 mg elemental Ca in divided doses; qd	OTC	Calcium carbonate is the preferred form because it has the highest percentage of calcium and is the least expensive, although calcium citrate may be somewhat better absorbed. In normal subjects, the solubility of the calcium salt has not been shown to affect its absorption from the intestine. In achlorhydric subjects, $CaCO_3$ should be given with meals.
Calcium citrate (Citracal) (21% Ca), po (950–1500 mg)				
Calcium chloride (36% Ca), iv (100% solution)				
Calcium bionate (6.5% Ca) (Neo-glucon), po (1.8 g in 5 ml)				
Calcium gluconate (9% Ca), po (500, 600, 1000 mg), iv (10% solution, 0.465 mEq/ml)		iv, 2–20 ml 10% calcium gluconate over several hours	Rx	Calcium gluconate is the preferred iv form because, unlike calcium chloride, it does not burn.
Calcium lactate (13% Ca), po (325, 650 mg)				
Calcium phosphate, dibasic (23% Ca), po (486 mg)				
Tricalcium phosphate (39% Ca) po (300, 600 mg)				
3. Fluoride preparations				
Fluoride, sodium (Luride, Fluoritab), po (2.25 mg/ml drops; 0.25, 0.5, 1.0 mg F tabs)	Dental prophylaxis in regions with non-fluoridated water	0.25–1 mg F, depending on age of child and fluoride content of water supply	Rx	Currently being investigated for treatment of osteoporosis at much higher doses. Also available combined with vitamins and other minerals or for topical application to teeth.
Florical (8.3 mg sodium fluoride and 364 mg calcium carbonate)	Osteoporosis	3–6 tablets/day		Fluoride is not FDA approved for treatment of osteoporosis
4. Magnesium preparations				
Magnesium oxide (Mag-Ox, Uro-Mag), po (84.5, 241.3 mg Mg)	Hypomagnesemia	240–480 mg elemental Mg; qd	OTC	Low magnesium often coexists with low calcium in alcoholics and malabsorbers. Also found in many antacids and vitamin formulations.
5. Phosphate preparations				
Neutra-Phos, po (250 mg P, 278 mg K, 164 mg Na)	Hypophosphatemia, vitamin-D-resistant rickets, hypercalcemia, hypercalciuria	po: 1–3 g in divided doses; qd	Rx, OTC	
Neutra-Phos-K, po (250 mg P, 556 mg K)				

Formulary of drugs commonly used in treatment of mineral disorders[a] Continued.

Drug	Application in treatment of bone and mineral disorders	Dosage (adult)[b]	Rx Cat[c]	Notes[d]
Fleet Phospha-Soda, po (815 mg P, 760 mg Na in 5 ml) In-Phos, iv (1 g P in 40 ml)		iv: 1.5 g over 6–8 h		iv phosphorus is seldom necessary and can be toxic if infusion is too rapid.
Hyper-Phos-K, iv (1 g P in 15 ml)				
Diuretics				
1. Thiazides				
Hydrochlorothiazide (Esidrix, Hydro-Diuril), po (25, 50, 100 mg)	Hypercalciuria, nephrolithiasis	25–50 mg; qd or bid	Rx	Other thiazides may also be effective but are less commonly used for this purpose. These uses are not FDA approved.
Chlorthalidone, po (25, 50 mg)				
2. Loop diuretics				
Furosemide (Lasix), po (20, 40, 80 mg), iv (10 mg/ml)	Hypercalcemia; if symptomatic, use iv	po: 20–80 mg, q6h as necessary; iv: 20–80 mg over several minutes, repeat as necessary	Rx	Ethacrynic acid may also be effective but is less commonly used for this purpose. These uses are not FDA approved.
Miscellaneous				
1. Mitramycin or plicamycin (Mithracin), iv (2.5 mg/vial)	Hypercalcemia of malignancy	25 μg/kg in 1 liter D5W or normal saline over 4–6 hr	Rx	Has been used in treatment of severe Paget's disease, but toxicity makes it treatment of last resort for this purpose and it has not been approved by the FDA for this purpose.
2. Gallium nitrate (Genite)	Hypercalcemia of malignancy	200 mg/m² qd in D5W for continuous infusion over 5 d	Rx	

[a]This table is not intended to be an official guideline.

[b]qd, every day; qod, every other day; bid, twice a day; tid, three times a day; qid, four times a day; sc, subcutaneously; im, intramuscularly; po, orally; iv, intravenously; IU, International Units.

[c]Rx Cat, prescription category: Rx, prescriptions required; OTC, over-the-counter preparations available.

[d]Where comments are not specifically aligned with preparations or their dosages, they apply to all preparations listed in that column.

vi. Structure of Naturally Occurring Vitamin D and Synthetic Analogs

Molecular weights, units, and mole equivalents for vitamin D, its metabolites, and important analogs[a]

Substance	Molecular weight	nmoles/ 1.00 μg	units/ 1.00 mg[b]	μg/unit[b]	nmoles/unit[b] 10 units	50 units	100 units
Cholecalciferol series							
D	384.3	2.60	40.0	25.0			
25(OH)D$_3$	400.3	2.49	38.4	26.0			
1,25(OH)$_2$D$_3$	416.3	2.40	36.9	27.1	0.65	3.25	6.50
24,25(OH)$_2$D$_3$	416.3	2.40	36.9	27.1			
25,26(OH)$_2$D$_3$	416.3	2.40	36.9	27.1			
1,24,25(OH)$_3$D$_3$	432.3	2.31	35.5	28.1			
Ergocalciferol series							
D$_2$	396.3	2.52	38.8	25.8			
25(OH)D$_2$	412.3	2.42	37.3	26.8			
1,25(OH)$_2$D$_2$	428.3	2.33	35.8	27.8	0.65	3.25	6.50
24,25(OH)$_2$D$_2$	428.3	2.33	35.8	27.8			
25,26(OH)$_2$D$_2$	428.3	2.33	35.8	27.8			
1,24,25(OH)$_3$D$_2$	444.3	2.25	34.6	28.9			
Analogs							
1(OH)D$_3$	400.3	2.49	38.4	26.0			
Dihydrotachysterol$_3$	385.3	2.59	39.9	25.0	0.65	3.25	6.50

[a]From: Norman AW. *Vitamin D: The Calcium Homeostatic Steroid Hormone.* Academic Press, New York, p 462, 1979.

[b]1.00 unit has been proposed by A. W. Norman (*J Nutr* 102:1243, 1972) to be 65.0 pmoles for all vitamin D compounds. For vitamin D$_3$, 1.0 IU is by definition (League of Nations, 1935) 0.025 μg, which is exactly equivalent to 65.0 pmoles.

CALCIUM ABSORPTION TEST

The calcium absorption test is useful for the evaluation and classification of hypercalciuric patients [1]. The test is performed by maintaining the patient on a 400-mg calcium diet for 1 wk or more prior to testing. The patient fasts for 10 to 12 h prior to the start of the test, except for access to distilled water. The test consists of three successive urine collections as shown in Fig. 1.

One hour before the start of the first urine collection and hourly thereafter, the patient is given 240 ml (8 oz) of distilled water. The oral calcium and milk may substitute for the distilled water at 120 min [2]. The serum and urine collections are analyzed as shown in the figure. Three pieces of information can be obtained from this study. First, the calcemic response (the magnitude of the increase of serum calcium after oral calcium) can be calculated. Second, the calciuric response (increase of urinary calcium excretion) is an index of the amount of calcium absorbed by the gastrointestinal tract. Third, measurement of nephrogenous cyclic AMP (cAMP) and its suppressibility by an oral calcium load is a sensitive dynamic parameter of parathyroid function. Specific calculations for each of these parameters is shown [2].

The *tubular reabsorption of phosphate* (TRP) is calculated from values obtained during the first urine collection using the following formula:

$$TRP = 1 - \frac{C_{Pi}}{C_{creat}} = 1 - \frac{S_{creat} \times U_{Pi}}{S_{Pi} \times U_{creat}} \text{ (all units in mg/dl)}$$

The TmP/GFR (tubular maximum of phosphate/glomerular filtration rate) is a relationship derived by Walton and Bijvoet [3] that utilizes both the serum phosphate concentration and the tubular reabsorption of phosphate to calculate an index of phosphate clearance. It can be calculated[a] from the nomogram shown in Fig. 2.

Calcemic Response

The calcemic response equals the serum calcium (mg/dl) during the third urine collection period minus the serum calcium during the first urine collection period.

Calciuric Response

The calciuric response equals the calcium excretion during period three minus the calcium excretion during period one. Calcium excretion is calculated from the following formula:

---

[a] A hypercard stack (MacIntosh computer) for computer calculation of the TmP/GF is available from LE Mallette, M.D., Ph.D., 2002 Holcombe Blvd. (111E), Houston, TX, 77030; it will be provided to anyone sending a blank disk and self-addressed, stamped envelope.

First urine
collection
$$= \frac{U_{calcium}}{U_{creat}} \times S_{creat} \text{ (all units in mg/dl)}$$

When the calculated value for period one is subtracted from the calculated value for period three, the result is the milligrams of calcium per 100 ml glomerular filtrate (GF).

The upper limit of normal for the calciuric response is 0.2 mg calcium/100 ml.

Suppression of Nephrogenous cAMP

Calculation of nephrogenous cAMP requires measurement of both plasma and urinary cAMP. The nephrogenous fraction is calculated by subtracting the fraction of the total cAMP that has been contributed by clearance of cAMP from the plasma. The first step required is calculation of the total urinary cAMP, in units of nmol/100 ml, by the following formula:

$$\frac{U_{cAMP} \text{ (nmol/100 ml)}}{U_{creat} \text{ (mg/dl)}} \times S_{creat} \text{ (mg/dl)}$$

The nephrogenous cAMP (in mmol/100 ml GF) is then calculated by subtracting the filtered load of cAMP (in nmol/100 ml of plasma) from the total urinary cAMP (in nmol/100 ml GF).

The Modified Ellsworth-Howard Test

The measurement of urinary cAMP and phosphate excretion after an intravenous injection of parathyroid hormone (PTH) is the preferred method for separation of hypoparathyroidism (secondary to parathyroid hormone deficiency) from pseudohypoparathyroidism [4]. There have been numerous modifications of the original test protocol over the years; the current protocol [5] utilizes synthetic human parathyroid hormone-(1–34) (PTH 1–34, recently approved by the Food and Drug Administration for this purpose.

Test Protocol

1. Have patient drink 200 ml of H_2O every 30 min from 0600 h to 1100 h.
2. Collect timed 30-min urine specimens from 0830 h to 1100 h for phosphate, creatinine, and cyclic AMP.
3. Draw serum samples at 0845 h, 1015 h, and 1045 h for creatinine and phosphate.
4. At approximately 0945 h, insert an indwelling catheter into a vein in the upper extremity.
5. From 1000 h to 1010 h, infuse teriparatide acetate (Rhone-Poulenc Rorer, Collegeville, Pennsylvania), 5 U per kg body weight (200 U maximum), intravenously at a steady rate.

459

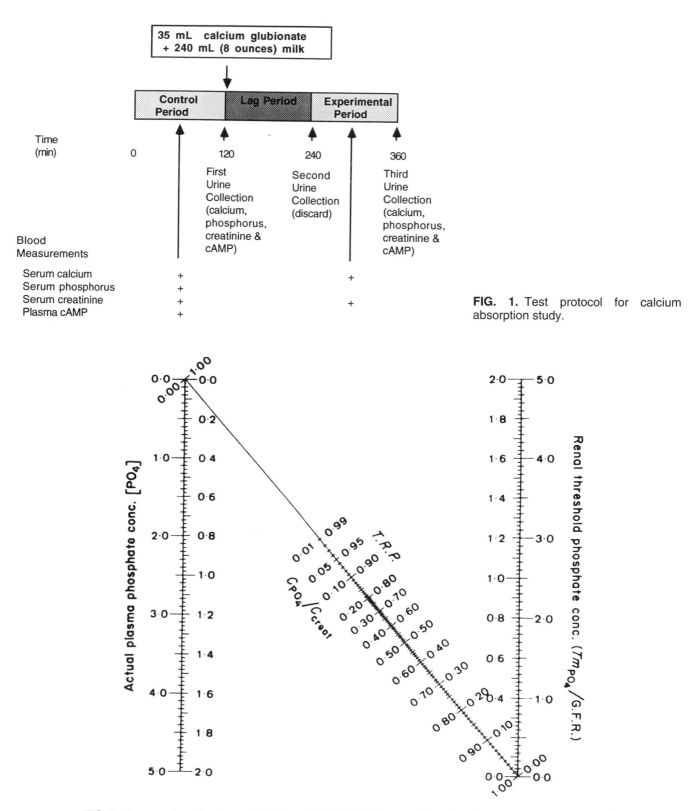

FIG. 1. Test protocol for calcium absorption study.

FIG. 2. A nomogram for the calculation of TmP/GFR. The renal threshold phosphate concentration or TmP/GFR is determined by passing a straight line through the observed serum or plasma phosphate concentration and the measured tubular reabsorption of phosphate (use equation in the text) and by reading the TmP/GFR from the rightmost axis. The data in this figure are presented as either mg/dl (left side of each axis) or mmol/L (right side of each axis). To use this nomogram all values must be expressed as a single type of unit. (From: Walton RJ, Bijvoet OLM. Nomogram for derivation of renal threshold phosphate concentration. *Lancet* 2:309, 1975, with permission.)

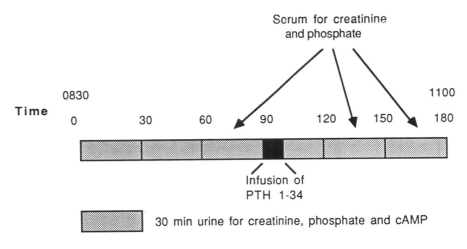

FIG. 3. Protocol for modified Ellsworth-Howard test.

6. Calculations for each parameter (Fig. 3) should be made for each collection. Posttreatment values are then compared with pretreatment values.

The formulas for calculation of response parameters are identical to those described for the calcium absorption test. Figure 4 provides an example of results utilizing this test in three patients to illustrate the differences in response in normal, pseudohypoparathyroid, and idiopathic hypoparathyroid patients.

The changes shown in Fig. 4 are illustrative of typical findings utilizing this technique, but they do not address the range of normal or abnormal values observed with these conditions. The reader is referred to a more complete discussion of the test for this purpose (4).

Suppression or Stimulation of Parathyroid Hormone Secretion

Suppression or stimulation of PTH secretion by increasing or decreasing the serum calcium concentration has been used in the past to diagnose several abnormalities of PTH secretion. The availability of sensitive and specific radioimmunoassays for intact and midregion PTH has eliminated the need for these studies in most clinical situations. Because induction of hypercalcemia or hypocalcemia may be associated with significant risk, these studies are not recommended outside of the research environment. References are provided for the interested reader (6,7).

STIMULATION OF CALCITONIN SECRETION

Measurement of the basal and stimulated serum calcitonin concentration is useful for diagnosis of C-cell hyperplasia and medullary thyroid carcinoma (8). Several different protocols are currently used.

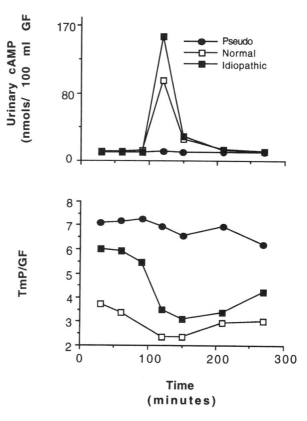

FIG. 4. Typical changes in the urinary cAMP and TmP/GF in a normal, a hypoparathyroid, and a pseudohypoparathyroid patient after an infusion of PTH 1–34 (200 U) performed by the protocol described in the text. In the normal and hypoparathyroid patients there is a prompt increase of the urinary cAMP; there is no increase in the pseudohypoparathyroid patient. The TmP/GFR is elevated in both the hypoparathyroid and pseudohypoparathyroid patients; in the hypoparathyroid patient there is a fall in the TmP/GFR after PTH 1–34 administration. (*Unpublished observations* of LE Mallette, JL Kirkland, RF Gagel, WM Law, H Heath III.)

Pentagastrin Test

The pentagastrin test (9) is performed as follows. After an overnight fast, a scalp vein needle with a three-way stopcock is placed in a large arm vein. A basal blood sample is taken, and then pentagastrin (0.5 μg/kg) is injected as a single bolus. [For a 70-kg patient, 35 μg of pentagastrin (Peptavlon, Ayerst Corporation, New York, New York, 0.14 ml of a 250-μg/ml solution) is diluted in 1 ml normal saline]. Blood samples for calcitonin are taken 2, 5, 10, and 15 min after the injection.

Combined Calcium and Pentagastrin Injection

Adding a short infusion of calcium prior to the pentagastrin injection has been reported to stimulate the release of calcitonin to a greater extent than either calcium or pentagastrin alone (10). Prior to the injection of pentagastrin, calcium gluconate (2 mg of elemental calcium/kg body weight) is infused over a 1-min period. The injection of pentagastrin follows immediately. The mean increase of the serum calcium concentration has been reported to be approximately 2.0 mg/dl.

Side Effects

Patients given pentagastrin almost always have side effects, which can include flushing, nausea, vomiting, urge to urinate, epigastric tightness, and tingling in the hands and feet. All of these symptoms subside within 2 to 3 min after the injection. The patient should be warned of these side effects prior to the injection. Although most patients consider the test to be unpleasant, family members at risk for hereditary medullary thyroid carcinoma return yearly for these studies. Pentagastrin injection has been used in children as young as 3 years of age for testing of hereditary medullary thyroid carcinoma, and it is well tolerated. There have been no reports of pentagastrin stimulation of catecholamine release, a point of some potential concern in multiple endocrine neoplasia, type II. There have been no reports that addition of calcium to the protocol results in additional side effects, although calcium may stimulate catecholamine secretion.

Normal Response

Pentagastrin stimulates a rapid release of calcitonin, with peak calcitonin values observed 2 to 5 min after injection, followed by a decline in the calcitonin concentration. Normal basal serum calcitonin values and the response to pentagastrin are generally greater in men than in women. Normal basal serum calcitonin values are generally less than 50 pg/ml (143 pmol/L), although there is considerable variation from assay to assay. After pentagastrin stimulation, there may be a twofold to fourfold increase in the serum calcitonin concentration, although the normal response range varies for each assay (see Appendix iii). The response after the combined calcium–pentagastrin test is usually greater. Abnormal test results are found most commonly in patients with abnormalities of the C-cell, including medullary thyroid carcinoma and C-cell hyperplasia, but other causes should also be considered, including chronic hypercalcemia, Hashimoto's thyroiditis, and ectopic production of calcitonin by other tumors.

GLUCOCORTICOID SUPPRESSION TEST

The glucocorticoid suppression test is performed by administration of hydrocortisone (100 mg per day orally for 10 days) in a hypercalcemic patient. The serum calcium and PTH concentrations are measured before and immediately after the completion of the course of hydrocortisone. There will frequently be a decrease of the serum calcium in patients with sarcoidosis, multiple myeloma, vitamin D intoxication, idiopathic hypercalcemia of infancy, and some malignant diseases with osseous metastases (11); if the decrease is great enough, there may be a concomitant increase of the serum parathyroid hormone concentration (12). The serum calcium in primary hyperparathyroidism is generally unchanged by glucocorticoid therapy (13).

REFERENCES

1. Broadus AE, Dominguez M, Bartter FC: Pathophysiological studies in idiopathic hypercalciuria: Use of an oral calcium tolerance test to characterize distinctive hypercalciuric subgroups. *J Clin Endocrinol Metab* 47:751–60, 1978
2. Felig P, Baxter JD, Broadus AE, Frohman LA (eds): *Endocrinology and Metabolism,* 2nd ed. McGraw-Hill, New York, p 1168, 1987
3. Walton RJ, Bijvoet OL: Nomogram for derivation of renal threshold phosphate concentration. *Lancet* 2:309, 1975
4. Mallette LE, Kirkland JL, Gagel RF, Law WM, Heath H III: Synthetic human parathyroid hormone-(1–34) for the study of pseudohypoparathyroidism. *J Clin Endocrinol Metab* 67:964–972, 1988
5. Mallette LE: Synthetic human parathyroid hormone 1–34 fragment for diagnostic testing. *Ann Intern Med* 109:800–804, 1988
6. Mallette LE, Tuma SN, Berger RE, Kirkland JL: Radioimmunoassay for the middle region of human parathyroid hormone using an homologous antiserum with a carboxy-terminal fragment of bovine parathyroid hormone as radioligand. *J Clin Endocrinol Metab* 54:1017–1024, 1982
7. Gidding SS, Minciotti AL, Langman CB: Unmasking of hypoparathyroidism in familial partial DiGeorge syndrome by challenge with disodium Edetate. *N Engl J Med* 319:1589–1591, 1988
8. Gagel RF, Tashjian AH Jr, Cummings T, Papathanasopoulos N, Kaplan MM, DeLellis RA, Wolfe HJ, Reichlin S: The clinical outcome of prospective screening for multiple endocrine neoplasia, type 2a—an 18 year experience. *N Engl J Med* 318:478–484, 1988
9. Hennessy JF, Wells SA Jr, Ontjes DA, et al.: A comparison of pentagastrin injection and calcium infusion as provocative agents for the detection of medullary carcinoma of the thyroid. *J Clin Endocrinol Metab* 39:487, 1974
10. Wells SA Jr, Baylin SB, Linehan WM, Farrell RE, Cox EB, Cooper CW: Provocative agents and the diagnosis of medullary carcinoma of the thyroid gland. *Ann Surg* 188:139–141, 1978
11. Dent CE, Watson L: Hyperparathyroidism and sarcordosis. *Br Med J* 1:646, 1966
12. Cushard WG Jr, Simon AB, Canterbury JM, Reiss E: Parathyroid function in sarcoidosis. *N Engl J Med* 286:395–398, 1972
13. Habener JF, Potts JT: Parathyroid physiology and primary hyperparathyroidism. In: Avioli LV, Krane SM (eds) *Metabolic Bone Disease,* vol II. Academic Press, New York, pp 96–97, 1978

viii. Bone Density Reference Data

The reference data displayed below were provided by the manufacturer for Hologic QDR Systems. All data, unless otherwise noted, were obtained from Caucasian sample populations. They are listed in 5-year age increments with mean ±2 standard deviations (95% confidence interval).

TABLE 1. *Normal bone mineral density (BMD) values of the AP Spine (L2 to L4) in females*

Age	BMD	DEV
20	1.051	0.110
25	1.072	0.110
30	1.079	0.110
35	1.073	0.110
40	1.056	0.110
45	1.030	0.110
50	0.997	0.110
55	0.960	0.110
60	0.920	0.110
65	0.878	0.110
70	0.840	0.110
75	0.805	0.110
80	0.775	0.110
85	0.754	0.110

TABLE 3. *Normal BMD values of the hip/femoral neck in females*

Age	BMD	DEV
20	0.895	0.100
25	0.894	0.100
30	0.886	0.100
35	0.871	0.100
40	0.850	0.100
45	0.826	0.100
50	0.797	0.100
55	0.766	0.100
60	0.733	0.100
65	0.700	0.100
70	0.667	0.100
75	0.636	0.100
80	0.607	0.100
85	0.581	0.100

TABLE 2. *Normal BMD values of the AP Spine (L2 to L4) in males*

Age	BMD	DEV
20	1.115	0.110
25	1.115	0.110
30	1.115	0.110
35	1.115	0.110
40	1.115	0.110
45	1.091	0.110
50	1.076	0.110
55	1.061	0.110
60	1.045	0.110
65	1.030	0.110
70	1.015	0.110
75	0.999	0.110
80	0.984	0.110
85	0.968	0.110

TABLE 4. *Normal BMD values of the hip/femoral neck in males*

Age	BMD	DEV
20	0.979	0.110
25	0.958	0.110
30	0.936	0.110
35	0.915	0.110
40	0.894	0.110
45	0.873	0.110
50	0.851	0.110
55	0.830	0.110
60	0.809	0.110
65	0.788	0.110
70	0.766	0.110
75	0.745	0.110
80	0.724	0.110
85	0.703	0.110

For additional information, please contact HOLOGIC, INC., 590 Lincoln Street, Waltham, MA 02154.

The following reference data were supplied by the manufacturer for HOLOGIC scanners. All data were based on ambulatory subjects free from chronic bone diseases and not currently taking medications that may affect bone.

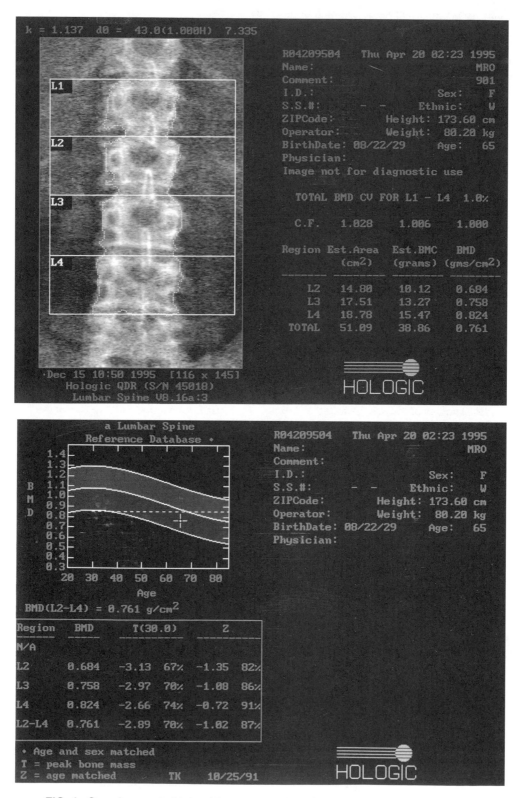

FIG. 1. Sample report obtained for lumbar spine of a 65-year-old female patient.

TABLE 5. *Mean BMD values for spine L2 to L4 (SD = 0.12 g/cm2) for reference US/Europe population*

Age	Female		Male	
	n	Mean	n	Mean
20–29	467	1.188	85	1.255
30–39	499	1.207	106	1.215
40–49	716	1.170	73	1.174
50–59	969	1.081	67	1.161
60–69	476	0.995	63	1.183
70–79	105	0.960	51	1.178

TABLE 6. *Mean female BMD values for femur regions (SD = 0.12 g/cm2)*

Age	n	Neck	Ward's	Trochanter
20–29	479	0.994	0.947	0.798
30–39	499	0.958	0.886	0.787
40–49	704	0.950	0.847	0.792
50–59	882	0.881	0.751	0.745
60–69	415	0.811	0.660	0.714
70–79	121	0.773	0.630	0.668

TABLE 7. *Mean male BMD values for femur regions (SD = 0.12 g/cm2)*

Age	n	Neck	Ward's	Trochanter
20–29	84	1.107	1.022	0.948
30–39	95	1.038	0.922	0.900
40–49	74	1.001	0.852	0.898
50–59	73	0.985	0.809	0.920
60–69	66	0.953	0.770	0.904
70–79	46	0.872	0.685	0.841

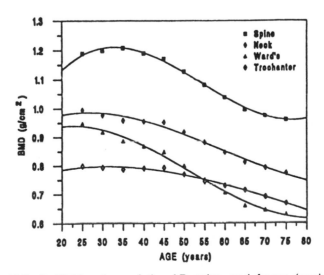

FIG. 2. BMD values of the AP spine and femur (neck, Ward's triangle, and trochanter) in Caucasian female reference subjects.

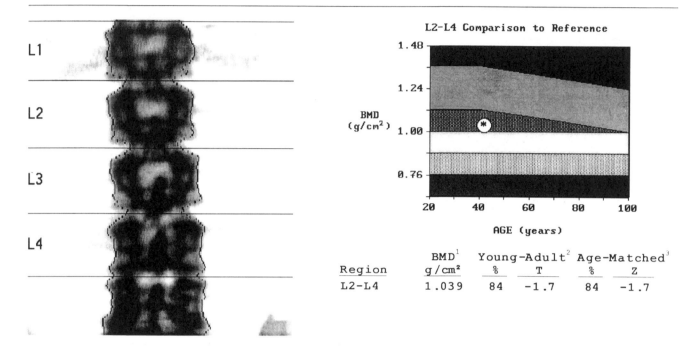

AP SPINE RESULTS
LUNAR CORPORATION
313 W. BELTLINE HWY., MADISON, WI 53713

Patient, Rkp   AP SPINE BONE DENSITY

Facility: Acquired: 09/15/95 (4.00)
42 years 12/01/52   Analyzed: 09/15/95 (4.00)
191.0cm 79.6kg White Male   Printed: 12/06/95 (4.00)
Physician: payner11.s01

L2-L4 Comparison to Reference

Region	BMD[1] g/cm²	Young-Adult[2] %	T	Age-Matched[3] %	Z
L2-L4	1.039	84	-1.7	84	-1.7

Image not for diagnosis
3.00:Medium DPX 0.6x1.2 1.68
813099:452773 1.385:5.0 263.79:195.56:142.67

FIG. 3. Sample report obtained for AP spine of a 42-year-old male patient.
[1]Statistically, 68% of repeat scans fall within 1 SD.
[2]USA AP spine reference population, ages 20–40.
[3]Matched for age, weight (males 25–100 kg; females 25–100 kg), ethnic background.

For additional information please contact LUNAR Corporation, 313 W. Beltline Highway, Madison, WI 53713.

Subject Index

Subject Index

Page numbers followed by f refer to figures and page numbers followed by t refer to tables.

ISBN 0-397-51763-7

9 780397 517633